Core Curriculum for

Neonatal Intensive Care Nursing

Core Curriculum for
Neonatal Intensive Care Nursing

Third Edition

Edited by

M. Terese Verklan, PhD, RNC, CCNS
Associate Professor, Neonatal Clinical Nurse Specialist
University of Texas Health Science Center at Houston
Director, Clinical Research
Memorial Hermann Healthcare System
Houston, Texas

Marlene Walden, PhD, RNC, NNP, CCNS
Assistant Professor, Baylor College of Medicine
Neonatal Nurse Practitioner and Nurse Scientist
Texas Children's Hospital
Houston, Texas

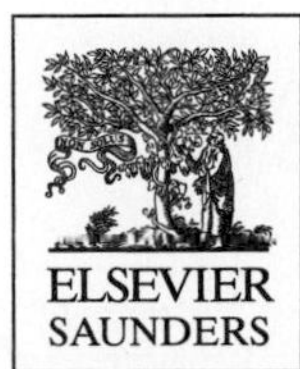

ELSEVIER
SAUNDERS

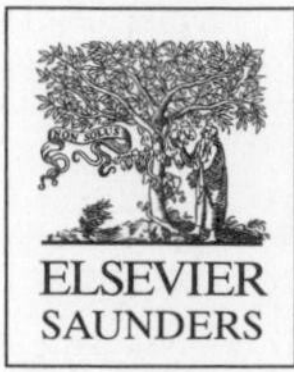

ELSEVIER
SAUNDERS

11830 Westline Industrial Drive
St. Louis, Missouri 63146

CORE CURRICULUM FOR NEONATAL INTENSIVE CARE NURSING

NOTICE

Nursing is an ever-changing field. Standard safety precautions must be followed, but as new research and clinical experience broaden our knowledge, changes in treatment and drug therapy may become necessary or appropriate. Readers are advised to check the most current product information provided by the manufacturer of each drug to be administered to verify the recommended dose, the method and duration of administration, and contraindications. It is the responsibility of the licensed prescriber, relying on experience and knowledge of the patient, to determine dosages and the best treatment for each individual patient. Neither the publisher nor the author assumes any liability for any injury and/or damage to persons or property arising from this publication.

Previous editions copyrighted 1999, 1993.
Library of Congress Cataloging-in-Publication Data

Core curriculum for neonatal intensive care nursing / edited by M. Terese Verklan, Marlene Walden.– 3rd ed.
p. ; cm.
Includes bibliographical references and index.
ISBN-13: 978-0-7216-0394-0 ISBN-10: 0-7216-0394-7
1. Neonatal intensive care–Outlines, syllabi, etc. I. Title: Neonatal intensive care nursing. II. Verklan, M. Terese. III. Walden, Marlene, 1956-
[DNLM: 1. Neonatal Nursing–methods–Outlines. 2. Intensive Care, Neonatal–methods–Outlines. WY 18.2 C7968 2004]
RJ253.5.C67 2004
618.92'01–dc22

2004046679

Executive Editor: Michael S. Ledbetter
Senior Developmental Editor: Laurie K. Gower
Publishing Services Manager: Catherine Jackson
Project Manager: Anne Gassett Konopka
Design Manager: Amy Buxton

ISBN-13: 978-0-7216-0394-0
ISBN-10: 0-7216-0394-7

Printed in the United States of America

Last digit is the print number: 9 8 7 6

To Mom and Dad, Cindy, Paul, and Theresa George—Thank you for showing me I have no boundaries.

MTV

To my loving parents, Bobby and Wanda, my brother, Michael, and my sister, Sharlene. Also to my wonderful colleagues at Baylor College of Medicine and Texas Children's Hospital. Most important, to the babies and families who have taught me the art of neonatal nursing.

MW

Contributors

Debra Armentrout, RNC, MSN, NNP
Assistant Professor, Pediatrics
University of Texas Health Science Center
Houston, Texas
Glucose Management

Debbie Fraser Askin, MN, RNC
Assistant Professor
Faculty of Nursing, University of Manitoba
Neonatal Nurse Practitioner
St. Boniface General Hospital
Winnipeg, Manitoba, Canada
Assisted Ventilation
Hematologic Disorders
Ophthalmologic and Auditory Disorders

Susan Bakewell-Sachs, PhD, RN, APRN, BC
Dean, School of Nursing
The College of New Jersey
Ewing, New Jersey
Pediatric Nurse Practitioner
The Children's Hospital of Philadelphia
Philadelphia, Pennsylvania
Nutritional Management

Linda K. Beauman, RNC, MSN, NNP
Neonatal Nurse Practitioner
The Children's Hospital
Denver, Colorado
Radiologic Evaluation

Kathleen Benjamin, RNC, MS, NNP
Neonatal Nurse Practitioner
Albany Medical Center Hospital
Albany, New York
Physical Assessment

Carol Botwinski, MS, ARNP
Neonatal Nurse Practitioner
All Children's Hospital
St. Petersburg, Florida
Renal and Genitourinary Disorders

S. Louise Bowen, RNC, CMTE, ARNP, MSN
Neonatal/Pediatric Transport Director
All Children's Hospital
St. Petersburg, Florida
Intrafacility and Interfacility Neonatal Transport

Amy Brandes, RD, LD, CLC
Clinical Dietician IV
Memorial Hermann Children's Hospital
Houston, Texas
Nutritional Management

Anne B. Broussard, CNM, DNS, FACCE
Professor, College of Nursing & Allied Health Professions
University of Louisiana at Lafayette
Lafayette, Louisiana
Antepartum-Intrapartum Complications

Carol Turnage Carrier, MSN, RN, CNS
Neonatal Clinical Nurse Specialist
Texas Children's Hospital
Houston, Texas
Developmental Support

Jane Deacon, RNC, MS, NNP
Neonatal Nurse Practitioner
The Children's Hospital
Denver, Colorado
Radiologic Evaluation

William Diehl-Jones, BSc, MSc, PhD, BScN, RN
Assistant Professor
Faculty of Nursing and Department of Zoology
University of Manitoba
Winnipeg, Manitoba, Canada
Assisted Ventilation
Hematologic Disorders
Ophthalmologic and Auditory Disorders

Susan Arana Furdon, MS, RNC, NNP
Neonatal Clinical Nurse Specialist/Nurse Practitioner
Neonatal Intensive Care Unit
Albany Medical Center
Albany, New York
Physical Assessment

Martha Goodwin, RNC, MS, NNP
Neonatal Nurse Practitioner
Children's Mercy Hospital
Kansas City, Missouri
Apnea

Karin Gracey, MSN, RNC, CNNP
Neonatal Nurse Practitioner
Hutzel Women's Hospital
Detroit Medical Center
Detroit, Michigan
Discharge Planning and Transition to Home Care

Brenda Hueske Halbardier, RN, BSN, MSN, NNP
Assistant Professor, Pediatrics
The University of Texas Health Science Center Medical School
Department of Pediatrics, Neonatal Division
Houston, Texas
Fluid and Electrolyte Management

Gina M. Heiss-Harris, RNC, MSN, NNP, CCRN
Neonatal Nurse Practitioner
Pediatrix Medical Group, Inc.
Austin, Texas
Common Invasive Procedures

Christine D. Hochwald, PharmD
Neonatal Clinical Pharmacist
Memorial Hermann Children's Hospital
Houston, Texas
Pharmacology

Kimberly M. Horns, PhD, NNP, RNC
Assistant Professor, Program Director
Neonatal Nurse Practitioner Program
College of Nursing, University of Utah
Neonatal Nurse Practitioner
Primary Children's Medical Center
Salt Lake City, Utah
Immunology and Infectious Disease

Helen M. Hurst, RNC, CNM, MSN
Instructor, Obstetrics and Women's Health
University of Louisiana at Lafayette
Lafayette, Louisiana
Antepartum-Intrapartum Complications

Carole Kenner, DNS, RNC, FAAN
Dean and Professor, College of Nursing
University of Oklahoma
Oklahoma City, Oklahoma
Families in Crisis

Nanette Landry, RN, MS, CNM
Certified Nurse Midwife
Aurora Nurse Midwives
Aurora, Colorado
Uncomplicated Antepartum and Intrapartum Care

Carolyn Houska Lund, RN, MS, FAAN
Neonatal Clinical Nurse Specialist
ECMO Coordinator
Children's Hospital Oakland
Oakland, California
Extracorporeal Membrane Oxygenation

Lynn Lynam, PhD, NNP
Clinical Research Manager
Ohmeda Medical
Laurel, Maryland
Neurologic Disorders

Denise Poirier Maguire, RN, C, PhD
Director of Nursing Education and Research
All Children's Hospital
St. Petersburg, Florida
Care of the Extremely Low Birth Weight Infant

Barbara Noerr, MSN, RNC, CRNP
Clinical Nurse Specialist—NICU
Penn State Children's Hospital
MS Hershey Medical Center
Hershey, Pennsylvania
Thermoregulation

Barbara Elizabeth Pappas, RNC, MSN, NNP
Neonatal Nurse Practitioner
Blank Children's Hospital—VCICN
Des Moines, Iowa
Neonatal Delivery Room Resuscitation

Kathleen Pitts, MSN, CPNP
Staff Pediatric Nurse Practitioner
Baylor College of Medicine
Texas Children's Hospital, Pediatric Otolaryngology Clinic
Houston, Texas
Perinatal Substance Abuse

Sharyl L. Sadowski, MS, APN, RNC, NNP
Neonatal Nurse Practitioner, Outreach Educator
Perinatal Center
University of Illinois
Chicago, Illinois
Cardiovascular Disorders

Julieanne Schiefelbein, MAppSc, MA(Ed), CNM, RNC, CPNP, NNP
Neonatal Nurse Practitioner, Pediatric Nurse Practitioner
Primary Children's Medical Centre
Salt Lake City, Utah
Genetics: From Bench to Bedside

Debora Simmons, RN, MSN, CCRN, CCNS
Senior Clinical Quality Analyst
The Institute for Healthcare Excellence
University of Texas MD Anderson Cancer Center
Houston, Texas
Patient Safety

Leann Sterk, MS, CNP, CNS
Certified Nurse Practitioner
Clinical Nurse Specialist
Rapid City Regional Hospital
Rapid City, South Dakota
Congenital Anomalies

Laura Stokowski, RN, MS
Registered Nurse
Inova Fairfax Hospital for Children
Falls Church, Virginia
Endocrine Disorders

Tanya Sudia-Robinson, RN, BSN, MN, PhD
Associate Professor, Center for Ethics
Emory University
Atlanta, Georgia
Ethical Issues

Diane M. Szlachetka, RNC, MSN, APRN
Neonatal Nurse Practitioner
Baystate Medical Center
Springfield, Massachusetts
Laboratory and Diagnostic Test Interpretation

Karen A. Thomas, RN, PhD
Professor, School of Nursing
University of Washington
Seattle, Washington
Research

M. Terese Verklan, PhD, RNC, CCNS
Associate Professor, Neonatal Clinical Nurse Specialist
University of Texas Health Science Center at Houston
Director, Clinical Research
Memorial Hermann Healthcare System
Houston, Texas
Adaptation to Extrauterine Life
Legal Issues
Neurologic Disorders

Marlene Walden, PhD, RNC, NNP, CCNS
Assistant Professor, Baylor College of Medicine
Neonatal Nurse Practitioner and Nurse Scientist
Texas Children's Hospital
Houston, Texas
Pain Assessment and Management

Brenda Walker, BSN, RNC
Pediatric Educator
Blank Children's Hospital
Des Moines, Iowa
Neonatal Delivery Room Resuscitation

Robin L. Watson, RN, MN, CCRN
Clinical Nurse Specialist, Neonatal/Pediatrics
Harbor—UCLA Medical Center
Torrance, California
Gastrointestinal Disorders

Catherine L. Witt, RNC, MS, NNP
Neonatal Nurse Practitioner
NNP Services of Colorado
P/SL Medical Center
Denver, Colorado
Neonatal Dermatology

Ksenia Zukowsky, PhD, CRNP
Neonatal Nurse Practitioner
Thomas Jefferson University Hospital
Philadelphia, Pennsylvania
Alfred I. duPont Hospital for Children
Wilmington, Delaware
Respiratory Distress

Reviewers

Hedy Cohen, RN, BSN, MS
Vice President
Institute for Safe Medication Practices
Huntingdon Valley, Pennsylvania

Sheryl J. Montrowl, ARNP, MSN
Clinical Coordinator, Pediatrics
University of Florida
Gainesville, Florida

Robin L. Watson, RN, MN, CCRN
Clinical Nurse Specialist, Neonatal/Pediatrics
Harbor—UCLA Medical Center
Torrance, California

Catherine L. Witt, RNC, MS, NNP
Neonatal Nurse Practitioner
NNP Services of Colorado
P/SL Medical Center
Denver, Colorado

Preface

The provision of intensive care to the high-risk neonate challenges every neonatal care provider. Research and refinements in technology have made "high-tech" modalities such as ECMO, nitric oxide, and hypothermia available to many more hospitals. The art and science of neonatal nursing is never stochastic. We learn from scientists, researchers, multidisciplinary colleagues, and of course, our infants and their families. At a minimum, we are expected to enhance our application of clinical knowledge by utilizing an evidence-based approach to improve patient outcomes. The role of the nurse is frequently to bring together all of the pieces of the puzzle to ensure comprehensive, clinically excellent, and compassionate care to sick newborns and their families.

This third edition of *Core Curriculum for Neonatal Intensive Care Nursing* is intended as a clinical resource. It is divided into sections and designed in outline format so that it can be used as an easy reference. The first section, *Antepartum, Intrapartum, and Transition to Extrauterine Life,* addresses clinical issues related to factors that affect the fetus and the neonate's ability to successfully adapt to postnatal life. Information is also presented as to how we can assist in the recognition of the high-risk fetus/neonate and plan interventions that support the physiologic demands of the neonate during transition. *Cornerstones of Clinical Practice* presents concepts common to the delivery of quality care to all high-risk newborns and families. New chapters have been added that provide the nurse with the latest information related to patient safety and organizational approaches to health care errors, as well as new data related to the human genome and up-to-date diagnostic testing for recognition of genetic abnormalities. The third section, *Pathophysiology: Management and Treatment of Common Disorders,* provides a systems approach to the assessment and management of disease processes high-risk neonates commonly present with. The last section, *Professional Practice,* focuses on the caregiver to strengthen competency with respect to research utilization, in addition to providing an overview of universal ethical and legal issues that may be encountered in the practice of neonatal nursing.

This text is the collaborative effort of the three major nursing specialty associations: the Association of Women's Health, Obstetric, and Neonatal Nurses (AWHONN), the American Association of Critical-Care Nurses (AACN) and the National Association of Neonatal Nurses (NANN). The book brings together experts in the care of the high-risk neonate, all having the common goal of providing a comprehensive resource for the management and care of sick newborns. We are honored to be the editors of such an outstanding collaborative effort.

M. Terese Verklan
Marlene Walden

Contents

SECTION ONE

ANTEPARTUM, INTRAPARTUM, AND TRANSITION TO EXTRAUTERINE LIFE

CHAPTER 1

Uncomplicated Antepartum and Intrapartum Care

NANETTE LANDRY

OBJECTIVES

1. Define term, preterm, and postterm pregnancy.
2. Describe the Nägele rule for estimated date of confinement.
3. Identify normal physiologic changes of each system in pregnancy.
4. Identify three methods of antepartum fetal surveillance.
5. Discuss the normal stages of labor.
6. Contrast low-risk intrapartum fetal monitoring management with high-risk fetal monitoring management.
7. Identify normal postpartum assessments and management.

Antepartum, intrapartum, and postpartum care is not usually thought of as within the practice parameters of the neonatal nurse. Yet an understanding of the normal processes of pregnancy provides a framework for beginning to understand factors that affect the developing fetus and the high-risk neonate. This chapter discusses uncomplicated antepartum, intrapartum, and immediate postpartum nursing care. In addition, an overview of the normal physiologic changes that can be expected in a healthy mother is included.

TERMINOLOGY

A. **Duration of gestation:** 280 days—40 postmenstrual weeks, or 10 lunar months.
B. **Trimesters:** division of gestation into three segments of approximately equal duration.
   1. First trimester: 0 to 12 weeks.
   2. Second trimester: 13 to 27 weeks.
   3. Third trimester: 28 to 40 weeks.
C. **Term pregnancy:** 38 to 42 weeks; preterm: less than 37 completed weeks; and postterm: longer than 42 weeks.

NORMAL PHYSIOLOGIC CHANGES OF SYSTEMS

Pregnancy affects all body systems. Some of the normal physiologic changes of systems include the following:

A. Alimentary tract.

1. There will be an increase in appetite of up to 300 kcal/day. The recommended caloric intake for the average woman in pregnancy is 2200 kcal/day. Pregnant teenagers need an additional 100 to 200 kcal/day.
2. Approximately 70% of pregnancies are affected by morning sickness from weeks 4 through 16.
3. The stomach loses tone and has delayed emptying time.
4. The gastroesophageal junction also relaxes and, in combination with increased intra-abdominal pressure, leads to reflux and resulting heartburn.
5. The small bowel has reduced motility. In the colon, constipation is a problem because of mechanical obstruction from the uterus, reduced motility, and increased water absorption.
6. The gallbladder empties much more slowly in the second and third trimesters, and high residuals increase the chance of gallstone formation from progesterone. High levels of estrogen lead to an increase in bile salts, linking pregnancy to cholestasis and pruritus gravidarum.
7. The liver remains unchanged in pregnancy as far as size and hepatic blood flow are concerned; however, some laboratory values, such as reduced serum albumin, elevated alkaline phosphatase, and elevated serum cholesterol, mimic liver disease. Prothrombin time and serum levels of bilirubin, aspartate aminotransferase, and alanine aminotransferase are unchanged in normal pregnancy.
8. As pregnancy progresses the stomach and intestines are displaced, causing the physical findings in certain disorders (e.g., appendicitis) to be altered.

B. Respiratory system.

1. Hypersecretion of mucus from the nasopharynx leads to nasal stuffiness and epistaxis during pregnancy.
2. The chest wall profile changes, resulting in an expansion of circumference and an increase in the subcostal margin angle. This results in the diaphragm's being elevated by 4 cm in the third trimester.
3. Up to 60% to 70% of all pregnant women have physiologic dyspnea, with increased tidal volume and reduced $Pa{CO_2}$ levels. Pulmonary function generally is not impaired. Respiratory diseases may be serious during pregnancy.

C. Skin (Cunningham et al., 2001).

1. Because of elevated levels of estrogen, spider angiomas (vascular red elevations with tiny vessels branching out from a central body) are frequently seen on the neck, face, throat, and arms. Palmar erythema—diffuse or blotchy spots on palms—is common in two thirds of white women and one third of black women.
2. Striae gravidarum, or "stretch marks," occur in women with a genetic predisposition to stretching of the skin or connective tissue.
3. Increased pigmentation is due to increased levels of estrogen, progesterone, and melanocyte-stimulating hormone. This is most marked on the nipples, areolas, perineum, and the midline of the lower portion of the abdomen (commonly called the linea nigra).
4. Sun-sensitive hyperpigmentation of the face, called chloasma or melasma and also referred to as the "mask of pregnancy," results in a dark, blotchy appearance of the face, forehead, and upper lip.
5. During gestation a greater percentage of the hair remains in the anagen (growth) phase, which decreases normal hair loss. Hair loss commonly

occurs between 2 and 4 months after delivery and is due to an increase in the telogen (resting) phase of hair growth. The hair returns to a normal growth phase within 6 months to 1 year (Gabbe et al., 2002).

D. Urinary system.

1. The kidneys enlarge and the ureters dilate. The consequences of these changes include:
   a. An increase in asymptomatic bacteriuria that may lead to cystitis and pyelonephritis.
   b. Difficulty in diagnosing obstruction on x-ray examination and interference with studies of glomerular filtration, renal blood flow, and tubular function.
2. The glomerular filtration rate increases in pregnancy by 50%, leading to:
   a. An increase in creatinine clearance and a decrease in nitrogen levels.
   b. Increased filtration of sodium, with increased reabsorption of sodium by renal tubules to balance the loss.
   c. A lower threshold at which glucose will be excreted by the kidneys, leading to:
      (1) Inability to use urine glucose measurements in management of pregnant women with diabetes mellitus.
      (2) Increase in susceptibility to urinary tract infections.

E. Cardiovascular system.

1. Cardiac output increases 30% to 50% in pregnancy and is highest in the second trimester.
2. By the third trimester of pregnancy the maternal heart rate increases by 15 to 20 beats above nonpregnant rates.
3. Because the heart is displaced leftward and upward by the enlarging uterus, the cardiac silhouette increases on x-ray films.
4. Altered cardiac sounds in pregnancy include splitting of the first heart sound, systolic flow murmurs (90% of pregnant women), and transient diastolic murmurs (20% of pregnant women).
5. Blood pressure remains normal (at the prepregnancy level) in the first trimester and drops during the second trimester, at approximately 24 weeks' gestation, by 5 to 10 mm Hg systolic and 10 to 15 mm Hg diastolic. It returns to normal prepregnancy levels at the end of pregnancy.
6. In late pregnancy, pressure obstruction of the inferior vena cava can occur in the supine position. The resulting 25% fall in cardiac output is called *supine hypotension*.
7. Blood stagnates in the lower extremities because of compression of the pelvic veins and the inferior vena cava. This contributes to dependent edema, varicosities of the legs and vulva, and hemorrhoid formation (Cunningham et al., 2001).

F. Breasts.

1. Early changes in the breasts (beginning by 4 weeks' gestation) include tingling, heaviness, tenderness, and enlargement. These symptoms usually subside at the end of the first trimester.
2. The areolas enlarge and darken.
3. Secretory glands called Montgomery glands appear on the areolas.
4. Colostrum may be expressed in late pregnancy.

G. Skeletal changes.

1. Compensating for the anteriorly positioned growing uterus, the lower portion of the back curves. This lordosis shifts the center of gravity backward over the lower extremities and causes low back pain, a common complaint in pregnancy.

2. Joints loosen during pregnancy because of the hormone relaxin.
3. These changes and an unsteady gait lead to falls, a common occurrence in pregnancy.
4. Numbness, tingling, weakness, and aching in the upper extremities are a result of marked lordosis. The resulting anterior flexion of the neck produces traction on the ulnar and median nerves.

H. **Hematologic changes.**
1. Plasma volume is increased by 50% at term.
2. The white blood cell count rises progressively during pregnancy and labor and then returns to normal pregnancy levels, ranging from 5000 to 12,000 cells/μl and increasing up to 25,000 cells/μl in labor and the early postpartum period.
3. The red blood cell count rises by 18% to 30% throughout pregnancy, and the plasma volume increases by 50%, reaching its peak at 30 to 34 weeks. This change in the ratio of red blood cells to plasma causes a drop in hematocrit, resulting in "physiologic anemia of pregnancy." The plasma volume increase levels off as the hematocrit begins to rise, resulting in a more normal ratio of red blood cells to plasma and a rise in hematocrit near term.
4. Platelet count decreases during pregnancy but remains within the normal range.
5. Pregnancy has been called a "hypercoagulable state." Fibrinogen is increased by 50%, and factors VII through X increase. Bleeding and clotting times remain normal. The incidence of thromboembolism increases during pregnancy and is greatest during the postpartum period.
6. Pregnancy is known to result in decreased immunologic function so that the "foreign fetus" is accommodated. This may also account for an abatement of certain autoimmune diseases in pregnancy and an increased susceptibility to certain infections.

ENDOCRINE AND METABOLIC CHANGES

A. **Thyroid.** The thyroid enlarges during pregnancy; however, there is little transplacental transfer of the hormones triiodothyronine (T_3) and thyroxine (T_4). Thyroid-binding globulin total (free and bound) serum T_4 and total T_3 all increase in the first trimester and plateau at approximately 18 to 20 weeks. There is an inverse relationship between the rise of chorionic gonadotropin concentrations and demonstrating thyrotropin concentrations. High serum chorionic gonadotropin levels are associated with decreased thyroid-stimulating hormone (TSH) levels. Fetal thyroid function appears to be independent of maternal thyroid function.

B. **Carbohydrate metabolism.**
1. Carbohydrate metabolism is significantly altered by human placental lactogen, and the effects are in direct proportion to placental mass.
2. The basal metabolic rate is increased by 25%.
3. Peripheral resistance to insulin is referred to as the "diabetogenic effect of pregnancy." The hormones responsible for this effect are human placental lactogen, progesterone, and estrogen.
4. Glucose is actively transported to the fetus; however, insulin and glycogen do not cross the placenta. Normal pregnancy is characterized by mild fasting hypoglycemia, postprandial hyperglycemia, and hyperinsulinemia. Levels of fatty acids, triglycerides, and cholesterol increase in the fasting pregnant woman. The switch in fuels from glucose to lipids is referred to as accelerated starvation, and ketonuria rapidly appears.

ANTEPARTUM CARE

A. Initial antepartum visit.

1. A thorough obstetric history should include:
   a. Gravidity—number of pregnancies; parity—number of births.
      (1) The obstetric history is often written as G3, P2, A0, L2, in which G is gravity, P is parity, A is the number of abortions, and L is the current number of living children.
      (2) Parity may be subdivided into term and preterm.
      (3) Abortions include all pregnancies terminated before 24 weeks—spontaneous and elective abortions, as well as ectopic pregnancies.
   b. Weeks of gestation achieved with each pregnancy.
   c. Hours of labor.
   d. Type of delivery (i.e., vaginal or operative).
   e. Size of newborns at birth.
   f. Any complications/transfusions.
2. Medical history of the patient and immediate family should include:
   a. Complete medical history.
   b. Infection history.
      (1) Hepatitis.
      (2) Human immunodeficiency virus (HIV).
      (3) Herpes.
      (4) Rubella.
      (5) Varicella.
      (6) Sexually transmitted diseases.
   c. Psychosocial risk assessment.
      (1) Drug or alcohol use.
      (2) Smoking.
      (3) Age.
      (4) Educational level.
      (5) History of emotional or abuse problems.
      (6) Support systems.
      (7) Attitude toward pregnancy.
3. Obtain a genetic background to identify factors that may lead to screening for Down syndrome, open neural tube defects (immediate family history), or any other possible genetic defects.
4. Obtain history of current pregnancy.
5. Perform a complete physical examination, including a complete pelvic examination.

B. Initial laboratory work.

1. Blood type and Rh status.
2. Antibody screening test.
3. Hematocrit and hemoglobin; complete blood cell count.
4. Papanicolaou smear.
5. Rubella titer.
6. Serologic tests.
7. Urinalysis for protein, glucose, and evidence of infections.
8. Hepatitis B surface antigen (HBsAg).
9. HIV, *Chlamydia*, and gonorrhea culture (depending on history and population).
10. Sickle cell screen, Tay-Sachs, Canavar, cystic fibrosis and α- and β-thalassemia screens for appropriate population (Gabbe et al., 2002).

C. Routine and diagnostic laboratory work and procedures (Table 1-1).

1. At 8 to 18 weeks: ultrasonography may be indicated to establish accurate dates or to detect genetic abnormalities.
2. Chorionic villus sampling at 9 to 11 weeks for chromosomal evaluation.
3. At 14 to 18 weeks: offer maternal serum alpha-fetoprotein (AFP) or maternal serum triple-screen measurements to screen for open neural tube defects, Down syndrome, and other potential problems with the pregnancy. Using the maternal serum triple-screen test enhances the detection rate of Down syndrome.
   a. The maternal serum AFP concentration is low in Down syndrome but elevated in neural tube defects.
   b. Human chorionic gonadotropin level is elevated in Down syndrome.
   c. Unconjugated estriol concentration is low in Down syndrome.
4. At 15 to 20 weeks: amniocentesis is used for genetic evaluation and measurement of AFP. Other studies, as suggested by the genetic history, may be performed.
5. At 24 to 28 weeks: a glucose screen for gestational diabetes is performed. A 50 g glucose load is given, and a plasma glucose concentration is determined 1 hour later. A level greater than 140 mg/dl is abnormal. Some use a level of 130 mg/dl.
   a. A glucose tolerance test is performed on all patients with an abnormal screen result. The test includes determination of a fasting plasma glucose concentration, as well as hourly values for 3 hours after a 100-g glucose load. The diagnosis of gestational diabetes is made if two values are elevated (plasma values: fasting, 105 mg/dl; at 1 hour, 190 mg/dl; at 2 hours, 165 mg/dl; and at 3 hours, 145 mg/dl).
6. At 28 weeks: obtain a repeated antibody titer for Rh-negative mothers; administer Rh immunoglobulin, 300 mg, if no anti-D antibody has been detected.
7. Early in the third trimester: obtain repeated hemoglobin and hematocrit determinations to recheck for anemia. Repeat at 36 weeks if anemia is detected.
8. At 36 to 40 weeks: ultrasonography may be indicated for serial growth evaluation, amniotic fluid volume testing, or placental assessment.
9. A repeat HIV, syphilis, gonorrhea, and chlamydia culture may be repeated at 36 weeks if indicated.
10. At 35 to 37 weeks obtain a vaginal/rectal group B streptococcus (GBS) culture.

MATERNAL INFECTIONS

A. TORCH infections (Table 1-2).

1. Acronym refers to syndrome of five infectious diseases: *t*oxoplasmosis, *o*ther infections (e.g., congenital syphilis), *r*ubella, *c*ytomegalovirus infection, and *h*erpes simplex.
2. All the infectious agents causing TORCH infections cross the placenta and may adversely affect the fetus.

B. Sexually transmitted diseases (Table 1-3).

1. These are transmitted during sexual intercourse.
2. Most cases occur in persons less than 25 years of age. A total of 12 million cases are reported each year.

Text continued on p.14.

TABLE 1-1
Prenatal Screening Tests

Test	Reason for Screening Test
Blood type, Rh status, antibody screen	Identifies fetuses at risk of isoimmune disease
Hemoglobin or hematocrit	Baseline laboratory studies: rule out anemia
Rubella antibody screen	Identifies women susceptible to acquiring rubella during pregnancy; susceptible women should be immunized *after* delivery
Tuberculin skin testing	Identifies infected women for treatment
Hepatitis B surface antigen	Identifies women whose offspring can be treated at birth to prevent hepatitis B infection
Serologic test for syphilis (VDRL or rapid plasmin reagin)	Treatment reduces fetal/neonatal morbidity; mandated by law in most states
Human immunodeficiency virus	Identifies women for treatment and perinatal therapy to decrease transmission to the fetus
Urinalysis	
Glucose, ketones, protein	Screen for diabetes, pregnancy-induced hypertension, renal disease
Red blood cells, white blood cells, bacteria	Possible urinary tract infection
Diabetes screen (24-28 weeks)	Fasting and glucose tolerance tests to rule out gestational diabetes
Papanicolaou smear	Identifies cervicitis and precancerous and cancerous lesions
Neisseria gonorrhoeae and *Chlamydia** cultures	Identify treatable sexually transmitted diseases, most of which can cause fetal or neonatal morbidity
Triple screen (maternal serum for AFP, human chorionic gonadotropin, estriol)	Tests done at 16 to 20 weeks at mother's discretion after counseling; AFP screens for neural tube defects, Down syndrome; combination of three tests very sensitive in identifying Down syndrome
Other†	

* Some centers also screen for *Mycoplasma hominis* and group B streptococcus colorization.

† Laboratory tests may vary from one center to another. Certain tests may be ordered if patient is at specific risk (i.e., hemoglobinopathy screen to rule out sickle cell disease in a black patient whose status is unknown or with a family history). Ultrasonography is considered by some to be a screening tool for congenital anomalies.

AFP, Alfa-fetoprotein; *VDRL,* Venereal Disease Research Laboratory.

Adapted from Clinic Protocol for Department of Obstetrics and Gynecology, University of Colorado Health Sciences Center. From O'Neill, P., Thureen, P.J., and Hobbins, J.: Maternal factors affecting the newborn. In P.J Thureen, J. Deacon, P. O'Neill, and J. Hernandez (Eds.): *Assessment and care of the well newborn.* Philadelphia, 1999, W.B. Saunders.

TABLE 1-2
TORCH Infections

Infection/Incubation	Transmission	Detection	Maternal Effects	Neonatal Effects	Incidence and Prevention
Cytomegalovirus Incubation: unknown	Intimate contact with infected secretions (breast milk, cervical mucus, semen, saliva, and urine) Transplacentally Organ transplantation	IgM titer	Clinically “silent”; only 1% to 5% acquire symptoms: low-grade fever, malaise, arthralgia, hepatomegaly	Infection is most likely to occur with maternal primary infection 90% of infected infants are free of symptoms at birth, but 5% to 15% of these may have long-term sequelae, 5% with severe involvement at birth: IUGR, microcephaly, periventricular calcification, deafness, blindness, chorioretinitis, mental retardation, hepatosplenomegaly	Primary occurs in 1% to 2% of pregnant women 90% of adult population in U.S. are seropositive Rigorous personal hygiene throughout pregnancy to prevent infection if not infected
Herpes simplex virus Incubation: 2 to 10 days	Intimate mucocutaneous exposure Passage through an infected birth canal Ascending infection, especially with rupture of membranes Transplacentally (rare) if initial infection occurs during pregnancy	Suspect with vesicles on cervix, vagina, or external genital area; painful lesions Presumptive diagnosis by fluorescent antibody or Papanicolaou smear on vesicular fluid Confirm diagnosis by vesicle culture	Painful genital lesions Primary infection commonly associated with fever, malaise, myalgias Numbness, tingling, burning, itching, and pain with lesions Lymphadenopathy Urinary retention	Rare transplacental transmissions have resulted in miscarriages Mortality rate of 5% to 60% if neonatal exposure is with active primary infection Neurologic or ophthalmic sequelae Disseminated infection in 70% of cases, with	Estimated 300,000 new cases per year 1:3000 to 20,000 live births with perinatal transmission Up to 80% of women delivering infected infants have no history of genital herpes; cesarean delivery if known active infection

				jaundice, respiratory distress, and CNS involvement	Avoid genital contact when male has penile lesions; use condoms
Rubella Incubation: 14 to 21 days	Nasopharyngeal secretions Transplacentally	Serologic antibody titer testing (IgG-specific rubella antibody) Virus isolation from throat	Pink maculopapular rash on face, neck, arms, and legs lasting 3 days Lymph node enlargement, fever, malaise, headache History of exposure 3 weeks earlier	Fetal infection rate greatest before 11 weeks, and after 35 weeks but severe sequelae occur with first-trimester infection; includes deafness (60%-70%), eye defects (10%-30%), CNS anomalies (10%-25%), congenital heart disease (10%-20%)	Since introduction of vaccine in late 1960s, rubella is rare Occurs more commonly in springtime Vaccine is contraindicated during pregnancy; vaccinate susceptible women postpartum
Toxoplasmosis (protozoa, *Toxoplasma gondii*) Incubation: 2 to 3 weeks	Eating raw meat containing *T. gondii* Ingesting *T. gondii* cysts secreted in feces of infected cats Transplacentally Impossible to transmit to others because the infecting organisms are tissue bound and are not secreted	Serologic antibody testing ELISA	90% of infected women have no symptoms Posterior cervical lymphadenopathy Malaise Premature labor and delivery	Severity varies with gestational age (usually, earlier infection results in more severe effects) Neurologic, ophthalmologic, and co-sequelae are variable IUGR Hydrocephalus Microcephaly	Incidence varies throughout world (1-4 infants per 1000 live births) 20% to 30% of U.S. women have been exposed Incidence of congenital toxoplasmosis infection in U.S. is 1:1000 to 8000 Reduce contact with cats during pregnancy

TORCH, Toxoplasmosis, *o*ther infections (e.g., congenital syphilis), *r*ubella, *c*ytomegalovirus infection, and *h*erpes simplex; CNS, central nervous system; *ELISA,* enzyme-linked immunosorbent assay; *IgG,* immunoglobulin G; *IgM,* immunoglobulin M; *IUGR,* intrauterine growth restriction

From O'Neill, P., Thureen, P.J., and Hobbins, J.: Maternal factors affecting the newborn. In P.J. Thureen, J. Deacon, P. O'Neill, and J. Hernandez (Eds.): *Assessment and care of the well newborn.* Philadelphia, 1999, W.B. Saunders.

TABLE 1-3
Sexually Transmitted Diseases

Infection/Agent/Incubation	Detection	Maternal Effects	Neonatal Effects	Incidence
Acquired immunodeficiency syndrome Human immunodeficiency virus Incubation: variable, months to years	ELISA for screening Western blot or indirect immunofluorescence assay p24 antigen for acute infection before seroconversion		30% chance of transmission from infected mother Syndrome develops in up to 65% of infected infants within a few months after birth	1991: estimated 200,000 cases in U.S.; 0.15% of all women who were delivered were infected
Chlamydiosis Bacterium: *Chlamydia trachomatis* Incubation: variable but more than 1 week	Culture of endocervical and urethral specimens ELISA or fluorescent antibody on swab specimen is less sensitive and specific	Most cases asymptomatic Mucopurulent cervicitis Frequently associated with other sexually transmitted diseases Occasionally premature rupture of membranes, preterm labor, IUGR, infertility, chorioamnionitis	30% to 40% of exposed infants have conjunctivitis 3% to 18% have pneumonia	Most common sexually transmitted disease Estimated 4 million cases occur annually in U.S., with prevalence rates in female patients 8% to 20% 70% of infections may be asymptomatic
Gonorrhea Bacteria: *Neisseria gonorrhoeae*, gram-negative diplococcus Incubation: 10 days	Endocervical, oral, or rectal cultures Genital or blood cultures Gram stain of lesions	60% to 80% of those infected are free of symptoms Occasionally pelvic peritonitis, premature rupture of membranes, postpartum endometritis, chorioamnionitis, increased infertility, ectopic pregnancy	Purulent conjunctivitis Sepsis or meningitis	More than 1 million cases are reported in U.S. each year Incidence in pregnancy ranges from 1% to 10%, depending on population
Human papillomavirus Incubation: unknown (3 months to years)	Single or multiple irregular painless papules in the genital or perianal area	Significant number of lesions enlarge during pregnancy Usually multicentric in pregnancy	Potential transmission of laryngeal papillomas Very rare (less than	Estimated 40 to 60 million people infected worldwide Viral lesions probably more

	Colposcopy used as adjunct in equivocal situations Cervical cytologic testing		1:1000-1500 pregnancies in which mothers have genital condyloma)	frequent in pregnant women because of increased hormone levels Increasing incidence noted in STD clinics and private offices Peak occurrence at ages 15 to 35 Associated with other STDs
Syphilis Spirochete: *Treponema pallidum* Incubation: 3 weeks on average	VDRL test Rapid plasma reagin test Fluorescent treponemal antibody absorption test	Primary chancre: painless ulcerative lesion Secondary syphilis: fever and malaise, red macules on palms or soles of feet Generalized lymphadenopathy Early latent (positive serologic finding <1 year's duration) syphilis Latent (cardiovascular) syphilis Neurosyphilis	Vary depending on gestation Stillbirth IUGR Nonimmune hydrops Premature labor	100,000 cases are reported in U.S. each year; 80% of these women are of reproductive age 3850 cases of congenital syphilis in 1992 70% to 100% fetal transmission rate in primary maternal disease
Trichomoniasis Protozoa: *Trichomonas vaginalis* Incubation: 4 to 20 days	"Wet prep" saline examination Papanicolaou smear Urinalysis	Malodorous, discolored vaginal discharge Dysuria	Infant contact through infected vagina Usually asymptomatic	Not reported to CDC but estimated in as many as 20% of pregnancies Estimates of 10% to 15% of all cases of vaginitis

CDC, Centers for Disease Control and Prevention; *ELISA,* enzyme-linked immunosorbent assay; *IUGR,* intrauterine growth retardation; *STD,* sexually transmitted disease; *VDRL,* Venereal Disease Research Laboratory.

From O'Neill, P., Thureen, P.J., and Hobbins, J.: Maternal factors affecting the newborn. In P.J. Thureen, J. Deacon, P. O'Neill, and J. Hernandez (Eds.): *Assessment and care of the well newborn.* Philadelphia, 1999, W.B. Saunders.

C. Other communicable diseases (Table 1-4).
 1. In all cases, both the fetus and the mother must be examined.
 2. Diseases of greatest concern are measles, chickenpox, mumps, mononucleosis, parvovirus infection, and influenza.

D. Chorioamnionitis.
 1. An infection of the chorion, amnion, and amniotic fluid that causes perinatal morbidity and death.
 2. Usually associated with ruptured membranes but can be found in women with intact membranes.
 3. Usually an ascending infection, commonly caused by *Escherichia coli*, group B streptococcus, anaerobic streptococci, and bacteroids.

E. Infection with group B streptococcus.
 1. Organism is cultured from the lower portion of the genital tract of 15% to 20% of all pregnant women between 23 and 26 weeks of gestation (Cunningham et al., 2001).
 2. Infection rate is 10 in 1000 infants born to colonized mothers; increases to 40 in 100 infants if there is premature labor and delivery, prolonged rupture of membranes, or intrapartum fever (American College of Obstetricians and Gynecologists [ACOG], 2002).
 3. All women should be screened at 35 to 37 weeks' gestation for anogenital group B streptococcus infection. Any woman with positive culture results should be offered chemoprophylaxis even if no risk factors are present (ACOG, 2002).
 4. Agreement concerning routine screening and treatment has not been achieved; however, in a consensus developed by the Centers for Disease Control and Prevention (CDC), ACOG, and American Academy of Pediatrics (AAP), the strategy of administering chemoprophylaxis to all women with risk factors is considered to be an acceptable practice. Risk factors include a previous infant with group B streptococcus, known infection with group B streptococcus in this pregnancy, delivery before 37 weeks' gestation, rupture of membranes 18 hours or more before birth, or an intrapartum temperature of 38° C or higher (ACOG, 2002).

ASSESSMENT OF GESTATIONAL AGE

A. Last menstrual period (LMP). Pregnancy may be detected by 5 to 6 weeks after the LMP. Estimating gestational age by counting from the LMP is a reliable method.
 1. A history should include:
  a. Duration of menstrual periods.
  b. Heaviness of menstrual flow.
  c. Menstrual history.
  d. Hormonal contraceptive use.
 2. Nägele rule determines the estimated date of confinement (EDC) or due date by the following formula: EDC = LMP – 3 months + 7 days + 1 year.

B. Pelvic examination and fundal height.
 1. Determination of the size of the uterus during an early examination (before 12 to 14 weeks) is relatively accurate if the mother is of normal height and not grossly obese. Fundal height measurements (in centimeters) are made from 16 to 35 weeks' approximate gestational age and are accurate within 3 weeks. The uterus is generally at the umbilicus at 20 weeks.
 2. Quickening is the first feelings of fetal movement.
  a. Primigravida: has quickening 18 to 20 weeks.
  b. Multigravida: has quickening 16 to 18 weeks.

TABLE 1-4
Other Communicable Diseases

Infection/Agent/Incubation	Mode of Transmission	Maternal Effects	Neonatal Effects	Incidence and Prevention
Influenza virus Incubation: 24 to 72 hours	Respiratory secretions	Usually brief but incapacitating disease Death occurs from secondary bacterial pneumonia	Any risk of malformation has been confined to first trimester Most studies fail to support teratogenicity	Killed virus vaccine Vaccine during pregnancy is indicated if mother is at medical risk because of other diseases
Mumps Paramyxovirus Incubation: 16 to 18 days	Respiratory secretions	Spontaneous abortion rate is increased twofold	Teratogenicity is unknown	Avoid pregnancy for 3 months after vaccination
Parvovirus B19 (fifth disease) DNA virus Incubation: 4 to 14 days	Respiratory secretions	Erythema Elevated temperature Arthralgia	Spontaneous abortions	Risk for women with primary infection during first 20 weeks of pregnancy is 15% to 17%
Hepatitis B	Sexually Perinatally Transplacentally Blood, stool, and saliva transmission	Fever, jaundice, malaise, hepatosplenomegaly Premature labor	Increased stillbirth rate Infected infants usually symptom-free at birth	200,000 to 300,000 cases in the U.S. each year One third of infants born to HBsAg-positive mother will have HBsAg/HBeAg positivity and anti-HBe negativity
Varicella (chickenpox) Varicella-zoster virus Incubation: 11 to 21 days	Probably by aerosolized respiratory droplets Portal of entry is respiratory tract Transplacentally	Severe in adults Risk of premature labor as a result of high temperature Risk of varicella pneumonia appears to be increased during pregnancy	2% of infants with maternal infection in first trimester have cutaneous scarring, eye abnormalities, and retardation At risk if maternal rash onset 5 days before to 2 days after delivery; severe disseminated neonatal disease may develop, and one third die	90% of women are immune In U.S. occurs in less than 0.1% of pregnancies

DNA, Deoxyribonucleic; *HBsAg,* hepatitis B surface antigen; *HBeAg,* hepatitis B "e" antigen.
From O'Neill, P., Thureen, P.J., and Hobbins, J.: Maternal factors affecting the newborn. In P.J. Thureen, J. Deacon, P. O'Neill, and J. Hernandez, J. (Eds.): *Assessment and care of the well newborn.* Philadelphia, 1999, W.B. Saunders.

C. **Fetal heart tones.** Can be detected by an electronic Doppler device as early as 9 weeks and commonly by 12 weeks, and may be auscultated with a fetoscope by 19 to 20 weeks.

D. **Ultrasonography.**
   1. Ultrasonography is most accurate in the first trimester (6 to 14 weeks), with crown-rump measurement accurately reflecting gestational age plus or minus 3 days.
   2. Fetal heart motion can be detected by real-time ultrasonography as early as 6 weeks' gestation by vaginal ultrasonography.
   3. Biparietal diameter is the most frequently used method of establishing gestational age; it is most accurate between 12 and 18 weeks (O'Neill et al., 1999).
   4. Abdominal circumference can be used to assess gestational age and intrauterine growth retardation. Combining biparietal diameter and abdominal circumference can give an estimate of fetal weight that is accurate within 10%.
   5. Fetal femur length may also be used to determine gestational age. Fetal weight within 7% to 10% can be determined by combining abdominal circumference and femur length.

E. **Laboratory assessments for documenting fetal lung maturity.**
   1. Lecithin/sphingomyelin (L/S) ratio greater than 2:1 occurs when fetal lung surfactant is present in amniotic fluid (at approximately 35 weeks). A level greater than or equal to 2:1 suggests that the newborn will not need respiratory support after birth.
   2. Phosphatidylglycerol (PG) is also present in amniotic fluid at around 35 weeks and increases rapidly at 37 weeks. Measurement of PG, a component of surfactant, is a more reliable test of lung maturity in mothers with diabetes than is measurement of the L/S ratio. PG is reported as present or not present.
   3. Fetal lung maturity assay is another test for lung maturity in the newborn infant that is growing in popularity. It is less expensive, is easier to perform, and has fewer false-negative results than the L/S ratio or PG measurement. Fetal lung maturity measures surfactant/albumin ratio in amniotic fluid. Results are reported as follows: 55 mg/g, mature lungs; greater than 39 to 55 mg/g, a 20% risk of respiratory distress in the neonate; and less than 39 mg/g, an 80% risk of respiratory distress in the neonate.

ANTEPARTUM VISITS

A. **Frequency.**
   1. In general, obstetric visits are recommended every 4 weeks until 28 weeks, then every 2 to 3 weeks until 36 weeks, and then weekly. Additional visits may be necessary around 18 to 20 weeks to establish the presence of heart tones with a fetoscope and the presence of quickening or to determine whether the pregnancy shows any signs of complications (Gabbe et al., 2002).

B. **Routine assessments.**
   1. Psychosocial assessments.
   2. Weight.
   3. Blood pressure.
   4. Urinary glucose and protein levels.
   5. Gestational age in weeks.

6. Fundal height in centimeters.
7. Presence of edema.
8. Fetal heart tones.
9. Fetal movement (after 20 weeks).
10. Fetal presentation.
11. Vaginal bleeding.
12. Prematurity signs and symptoms.
    a. Increased discharge/mucus show.
    b. Contractions, abdominal cramping, intestinal cramping.
    c. Dysuria, frequency of urination, and/or tenderness of costovertebral angle.
    d. Increased pelvic pressure.
13. Signs and symptoms of pregnancy-induced hypertension.
    a. Increased blood pressure, proteinuria, and edema.
    b. Epigastric pain.
    c. Nausea and/or vomiting.
    d. Hyperreflexia.
    e. Clonus.
    f. Visual disturbances.
    g. Headaches.
14. Warning signs to report: all of items 12 and 13, above; in addition:
    a. Chills and fever.
    b. Persistent vomiting.
    c. Abdominal pain.
    d. Leakage from vagina.
    e. Change in intensity or frequency of fetal movement.

ANTEPARTUM FETAL SURVEILLANCE

A. **Nonstress test (NST).** This is the most widely used screening method for fetal well-being.
   1. It is indicated for patients at risk of placental insufficiency and may be started as early as 30 to 32 weeks' gestation. Conditions that are of concern include the following:
      a. Postterm pregnancy.
      b. Diabetes mellitus.
      c. Hypertension.
      d. Previous stillbirths.
      e. Intrauterine growth restriction.
      f. Decreased fetal movements.
      g. Rh disease.
   2. Testing is repeated once or twice weekly. With a reactive test result, the perinatal death rate is approximately 5 in 1000.
   3. A reactive NST result is two or three fetal heart rate (FHR) accelerations (an FHR acceleration is defined as a 15-beat rise from baseline that lasts for at least 15 seconds with return to baseline) during a 20-minute period; a nonreactive test result is either no fetal movements after 40 minutes, in association with FHR accelerations, or no FHR accelerations in association with fetal movements.
   4. Whereas a reactive NST result is reassuring, a nonreactive result is an indication for further studies (O'Neill et al., 1999).

B. Contraction stress test (CST). CST, the first test of fetal well-being, evaluates the reserve function of the placenta. Indications for use are the same as for use of the NST; the CST is most often used after a nonreactive NST result.

1. CST can be achieved by the following:
   a. Spontaneous contraction test: three spontaneous contractions in a 10-minute period.
   b. Nipple stimulation test: naturally induced oxytocin by stimulation of nipples (endogenous).
   c. Oxytocin challenge test: artificially induced oxytocin by intravenous administration (exogenous).
2. The CST requires three contractions of moderate intensity lasting 40 to 60 seconds in a 10-minute period. This stimulates a labor pattern and allows the fetus to be stressed as in normal labor. The CST looks for decelerations, or decreases, in the FHR in relation to the onset of uterine contractions.
3. A positive CST result is defined as late decelerations of the FHR that are present with the majority (>50%) of contractions in a 10-minute window. Delivery should be considered with a positive CST result. Findings may also be considered suspect, equivocal, or unsatisfactory, or as showing hyperstimulation. These cases require retesting in the next 24 hours for adequate interpretation of fetal well-being.
4. Frequency of the CST is usually weekly, but the CST can be performed more frequently, as the fetus's condition warrants.

C. Biophysical profile.

1. The biophysical profile uses real-time ultrasonography to evaluate five parameters, each receiving either 0 or 2 points; the maximum score is 10 points.
   a. Fetal breathing movements.
   b. Gross body movements.
   c. Fetal tone.
   d. Quantitative amniotic fluid volume.
   e. NST.
2. Management is based on the assigned score:
   a. Score of 8 to 10 points: normal; weekly tests are indicated.
   b. Score of 6 points: requires repeated test in 4 to 6 hours or delivery if oligohydramnios is present.
   c. Score of 4 points: suspect chronic asphyxia; need for delivery will be determined on the basis of gestational age and lung maturity.
   d. Score of 2 points or less: strongly suspect chronic asphyxia; requires delivery regardless of gestational age (O'Neill et al., 1999).

NORMAL LABOR

A. Phases of labor. There are three phases of labor.

1. Latent phase: onset of labor to time when slope of cervical dilation changes.
2. Active phase: approximately 3 cm to complete cervical dilation.
3. Descent phase: coincides with second stage.

B. Seven cardinal movements of fetal head and body en route to delivery.

1. Engagement: the head enters the pelvis.
2. Descent: the head descends into the pelvis, past the pelvic brim.
3. Flexion: with flexion of the head, the narrowest diameter of the head is presented to the pelvis.
4. Internal rotation: the head enters the pelvis transversely and then rotates to an anteroposterior position.

5. Extension: the flexed head extends to be delivered.
6. External rotation: the head rotates back to the transverse position.
7. Expulsion: the body is expelled (Gabbe et al., 2002).

INTRAPARTUM LABOR MANAGEMENT

A. **Assessments.** Review the prenatal records and determine current status, including the following:
   1. Vital signs.
   2. Contraction pattern, intensity.
   3. Membrane status—intact, ruptured, or leaking.
   4. Fetal heart tones.
   5. Vaginal findings (if no bleeding or spontaneous rupture of membranes has occurred) to assess:
      a. Dilation of the cervix.
      b. Effacement, or thinning, of the cervix.
      c. Station, or position, of the presenting part in the pelvis. Station 0 represents entrance of the head into the pelvis. As descent occurs, the station is expressed as +1, +2, or +3 and descent is measured in centimeters.
      d. Presenting part.
      e. Position. The position of the head (i.e., anterior, posterior, or transverse) relative to the pelvis is assessed.

B. **Management of low-risk patient.** The patient should be identified as being at low or high risk on the basis of the available data. A patient determined to be at low risk during labor does not require continuous electronic fetal monitoring. According to ACOG *Technical Bulletin No. 207* (1995), auscultation should be performed at least every 30 minutes after a contraction for 30 seconds. In the second stage of labor, auscultation should be performed every 15 minutes. If electronic monitoring is used, evaluation should continue at the same intervals. Any detectable deceleration of the FHR should alert the nurse to apply the electronic fetal monitor to determine whether the FHR is reassuring (American Academy of Pediatrics [AAP]/ACOG, 2002).
   1. Auscultation. A nonreassuring FHR detected by auscultation for which electronic fetal monitoring should be performed is indicated by the following:
      a. A baseline FHR (average rate between contractions) of less than 100 beats per minute (bpm).
      b. An FHR of less than 100 bpm 30 seconds after a contraction.
      c. Unexplained baseline tachycardia of more than 160 bpm, especially with at-risk patients in whom the tachycardia persists through three or more contractions (10 to 15 minutes) despite corrective measures.
   2. Electronic fetal monitoring. This allows systematic evaluation of the FHR and labor. Contractions should be evaluated for polysystole (more than five contractions in 10 minutes), prolonged contractions lasting more than 90 seconds, and tetanic contractions. These conditions may cause increased stress for the fetus or mother. The baseline FHR should be observed for variability, periodic changes, and trends.
   3. FHR patterns reported to be associated with increased incidence of fetal compromise.
      a. Severe bradycardia: a rate less than 80 bpm for more than 3 minutes.
      b. Repetitive late decelerations: a symmetric fall in the FHR, beginning at or after the peak of the uterine contraction and returning to baseline only after the contraction has ended.

c. Undulating baseline: a pattern of rapid change between tachycardia (rates >160 bpm) and bradycardia (rates <100 bpm).
d. Any nonreassuring pattern associated with explained poor or absent baseline variability: a flat or nearly flat baseline.
e. Absence of accelerations.

PUERPERIUM: "FOURTH TRIMESTER"

The period from delivery through the sixth week is known as the "fourth trimester."

A. **Uterine involution.** Involution begins immediately after delivery; the fundus is at the level of the umbilicus.
B. **Placental site regeneration.** Process takes approximately 6 weeks after delivery.
C. **Lochia.** Postdelivery uterine discharge, with changes as follows:
   1. Lochia rubra: dark red or reddish brown; 3 to 4 days.
   2. Lochia serosa: pink or brown; 4 to 10 days.
   3. Lochia alba: yellow to white; approximately 10 days after delivery to 4 to 6 weeks after delivery.
D. **Breasts.** The breasts should be soft until the third or fourth postpartum day, when engorgement occurs. Engorgement resolves spontaneously within 24 to 36 hours. In non–breast-feeding mothers, lactation ceases within 1 week.
E. **Immunizations.**
   1. Rubella vaccination should be administered in the immediate postpartum period to all women who are not immune (Varney, 1997).
   2. Rh(D) immunoglobulin (300 μg given intramuscularly) is administered to the Rh negative mother within 72 hours of delivery to prevent sensitization from fetal-maternal transfusion of Rh-positive fetal erythrocytes (Varney, 1997).

REFERENCES

American Academy of Pediatrics and the American College of Obstetricians and Gynecologists: *Guidelines for perinatal care* (5th ed.). AAP/ACOG, Elk Grove Village, IL, 2002, pp. 133-134.

American College of Obstetricians and Gynecologists: Fetal heart rate patterns: Monitoring, interpretation and management. *Technical Bulletin No. 207,* Washington, DC, 1995, the College.

American College of Obstetricians and Gynecologists Committee on Obstetrics: Prevention of early onset perinatal group B streptococcal diseases in newborns. *Committee Opinion No. 279,* Washington, DC, December 2002, the College.

Cunningham, F.R., Leveno, K.J., Gant, N.F., et al.: *Williams' obstetrics* (21st ed.). New York, 2001, McGraw-Hill, pp. 172-175, 178, 181-182, 184-190, 192-194, 228-230.

Gabbe, S.G., Neibyl, J.R., and Simpson, J.L.: *Obstetrics: Normal and problem pregnancies* (4th ed.). New York, 2002, Churchill Livingstone, pp. 65, 71-82, 84, 86-87,142-147, 363-366.

O'Neill, P., Thureen, P.J., and Hobbins, J.: Maternal factors affecting the newborn. In P.J. Thureen, J. Deacon, P. O'Neill, and J. Hernandez (Eds.): *Assessment and care of the well newborn.* Philadelphia, 1999, W.B. Saunders, p. 7.

Thureen, P.J., Hall, D., Townsend, S., et al.: Fetal assessment, labor and delivery. In P.J. Thureen, J. Deacon, P. O'Neill, and J. Hernandez (Eds.): *Assessment and care of the well newborn.* Philadelphia, 1999, W.B. Saunders, p. 7.

Varney, H.: *Varney's midwifery* (3rd ed.). Sudbury, MA, 1997, Jones and Bartlett, pp. 340, 639-649.

CHAPTER 2

Antepartum-Intrapartum Complications

ANNE B. BROUSSARD AND HELEN M. HURST

OBJECTIVES

1. List maternal risk factors that may exist before pregnancy.
2. Discuss the effects of hypertension and diabetes on the maternal-placental-fetal complex.
3. Categorize intrapartum conditions that may result in complications for the newborn infant.
4. Assess the fetus/neonate for effects of tocolytic drugs.
5. Describe the effect on the fetus/neonate of these intrapartum crises: abruptio placentae, placenta previa, cord prolapse, and shoulder dystocia.
6. List neonatal complications associated with breech delivery.
7. Examine the effect of obstetric analgesia/anesthesia and cesarean delivery on the newborn infant.

An understanding of maternal complications enhances the ability of the nurse to anticipate and recognize neonatal complications and intervene appropriately. The purpose of this chapter is to provide a comprehensive view of possible neonatal complications resulting from maternal risk factors. These risk factors may exist before the pregnancy or develop during the antepartum and intrapartum periods (Table 2-1).

ANATOMY AND PHYSIOLOGY

A. **The fetus.** The fetus is a part of the maternal-placental-fetal complex.
B. **Conditions and substances that affect the pregnant woman.** These have the potential to affect placental functions of respiration, nutrition, excretion, and hormone production. Decreased placental function can in turn adversely affect the fetus.
C. **The placenta.** In addition, the traditional concept of the placenta as a barrier to noxious substances has long been superseded by the concept of the placenta as a sieve that permits transport of desirable *and* undesirable substances to the fetus. The placental membrane separating maternal and fetal circulations consists of four tissue layers; it thins to three layers after 20 weeks (Moore and Persaud, 1998).
D. **Placental transport mechanisms.** These mechanisms, including passive and facilitated diffusion, are affected by a number of factors (Moore and Persaud, 1998; Ross et al., 2002).

TABLE 2-1

Prenatal High-Risk Factors

Factor	Maternal Implications	Fetal/Neonatal Implications
SOCIAL-PERSONAL		
Low income level and/or low educational level	Poor antenatal care Poor nutrition ↑ Risk preeclampsia	Low birth weight IUGR
Poor diet	Inadequate nutrition ↑ Risk anemia ↑ Risk preeclampsia	Fetal malnutrition Prematurity
Living at high altitude	↑ Hemoglobin	Prematurity IUGR
Multiparity more than 3	↑ Risk antepartum/ postpartum hemorrhage	Anemia Fetal death
Weight less than 45.5 kg (100 lb)	Poor nutrition Cephalopelvic disproportion Prolonged labor	IUGR Hypoxia associated with difficult labor and birth
Weight more than 91 kg (200 lb)	↑ Risk hypertension ↑ Risk cephalopelvic disproportion	↓ Fetal nutrition
Age less than 16 years	Poor nutrition Poor antenatal care ↑ Risk preeclampsia ↑ Risk cephalopelvic disproportion	Low birth weight ↑ Fetal death
Age more than 35 years	↑ Risk preeclampsia ↑ Risk cesarean birth	↑ Risk congenital anomalies ↑ Chromosomal aberrations
Smoking 1 pack per day or more	↑ Risk hypertension ↑ Risk cancer	↓ Placental perfusion → ↓ O_2 and nutrients available Low birth weight IUGR Preterm birth
Use of addicting drugs	↑ Risk poor nutrition ↑ Risk of infection with intravenous drugs	↑ Risk congenital anomalies ↑ Risk low birth weight Neonatal withdrawal Lower serum bilirubin level
Excessive alcohol consumption	↑ Risk poor nutrition Possible hepatic effects with long-term consumption	↑ Risk fetal alcohol syndrome
PREEXISTING MEDICAL DISORDERS		
Diabetes mellitus	↑ Risk preeclampsia, hypertension Episodes of hypoglycemia and hyperglycemia ↑ Risk cesarean birth	Low birth weight Macrosomia Neonatal hypoglycemia ↑ Risk congenital anomalies ↑ Risk respiratory distress syndrome
Cardiac disease	Cardiac decompensation Further strain on mother's body ↑ Maternal death rate	↑ Risk fetal death ↑ Perinatal death
Anemia Less than 9 g/dl hemoglobin (white)	Iron deficiency anemia Low energy level ↓ oxygen-carrying capacity	Fetal death Prematurity Low birth weight

■ TABLE 2-1
■ ■ **Prenatal High-Risk Factors—cont'd**

Factor	Maternal Implications	Fetal/Neonatal Implications
Less than 29% hematocrit (white) Less than 8.2 g/dl hemoglobin (black) Less than 26% hematocrit (black)		
Hypertension	↑ Vasospasm ↑ Risk irritability of central nervous system → Convulsions ↑ Risk cerebrovascular accident ↑ Risk renal damage	↓ Placental perfusion → Low birth weight Preterm birth
Thyroid disorder	↑ Infertility	↑ Spontaneous abortion
Hypothyroidism	↓ Basal metabolic rate goiter, myxedema	↑ Risk congenital goiter Mental retardation → cretinism ↑ Incidence congenital anomalies
Hyperthyroidism	↑ Risk postpartum hemorrhage ↑ Risk preeclampsia Danger of thyroid storm	↑ Incidence preterm birth ↑ Tendency to thyrotoxicosis
Renal disease (moderate to severe)	↑ Risk renal failure	↑ Risk IUGR ↑ Risk preterm birth
Exposure to diethylstilbestrol	↑ Infertility, spontaneous abortion ↑ Cervical incompetence	↑ Spontaneous abortion ↑ Risk preterm birth
OBSTETRIC CONSIDERATIONS		
PREVIOUS PREGNANCY		
Stillborn	↑ Emotional/psychologic distress	↑ Risk IUGR ↑ Risk preterm birth
Habitual abortion	↑ Emotional/psychologic distress ↑ Possibility diagnostic study	↑ Risk abortion
Cesarean birth	↑ Possibility repeated cesarean birth	↑ Risk preterm birth ↑ Risk respiratory distress
Rh or blood group sensitization	↑ Financial expenditure for testing	Hydrops fetalis Icterus gravis Neonatal anemia Kernicterus Hypoglycemia
Large baby	↑ Risk cesarean birth ↑ Risk gestational diabetes	Birth injury Hypoglycemia
CURRENT PREGNANCY		
Rubella (first trimester)		Congenital heart disease Cataracts Nerve deafness Bone lesions Prolonged virus shedding

Continued

TABLE 2-1
Prenatal High-Risk Factors—cont'd

Factor	Maternal Implications	Fetal/Neonatal Implications
CURRENT PREGNANCY—cont'd		
Rubella (second trimester)		Hepatitis Thrombocytopenia
Cytomegalovirus		IUGR Encephalopathy
Herpesvirus type 2	Severe discomfort Concern about possibility of cesarean birth, fetal infection	Neonatal herpesvirus type 2 Hepatitis with jaundice Neurologic abnormalities
Syphilis	$\uparrow$ Incidence abortion	$\uparrow$ Fetal death Congenital syphilis
Abruptio placentae and placenta previa	$\uparrow$ Risk hemorrhage Bed rest Extended hospitalization	Fetal/neonatal anemia Intrauterine hemorrhage $\uparrow$ Fetal death
Preeclampsia/eclampsia (pregnancy-induced hypertension)	See "Hypertension"	$\downarrow$ Placental perfusion $\rightarrow$ Low birth weight
Multiple gestation	$\uparrow$ Risk postpartum hemorrhage	$\uparrow$ Risk preterm birth $\uparrow$ Risk fetal death
Elevated hematocrit More than 41% (white) More than 38% (black)	$\uparrow$ viscosity of blood	Fetal death rate 5 times normal rate
Spontaneous premature rupture of membranes	$\uparrow$ Uterine infection	$\uparrow$Risk preterm birth $\uparrow$ Fetal death

From Ladewig, P., London, M., and Olds, S.: *Maternal-newborn nursing care: the nurse, the family, and the community* (4th ed.). Boston, 1998, Addison-Wesley.

1. Placental area.
   a. To supply the increased growth needs of the fetus, the placenta normally increases in size as the pregnancy advances.
   b. A placenta that is not keeping pace with fetal growth or that has decreased functional area as a result of infarct or separation does not allow optimal transport of materials between fetus and mother.
   c. The outcome of decreased functional placental area can include a decrease in fetal growth, fetal or neonatal distress, and even fetal or neonatal death.
2. Concentration gradient.
   a. Passive and facilitated diffusion of unbound substances dissolved in maternal and fetal plasma occurs in the direction of lesser concentration.
   b. The greater the concentration gradient, the faster the rate of diffusion will be.
   c. Concentration gradients are maintained when dissolved substances are removed from the plasma by metabolism, cellular uptake, or excretion. For example, the excretion of CO_2 from the maternal lungs maintains the concentration gradient for CO_2, permitting fetal plasma CO_2 to cross from fetal plasma to maternal plasma. Inefficient maternal excretion of CO_2 may lead to maternal respiratory acidosis and fetal acidosis.

3. Diffusing distance.
   a. The greater the distance between maternal and fetal blood in the placenta, the slower the diffusion rate of substances will be.
   b. Any edema that develops in the placental villi increases the distance between the fetal capillaries within the villi and the maternal arterial blood in the intervillous spaces, thus slowing the diffusion rate of substances between the maternal and fetal circulations.
   c. Edema of villi may occur in:
      (1) Maternal diabetes.
      (2) Transplacental infections.
      (3) Erythroblastosis fetalis.
      (4) Twin-to-twin transfusion syndrome (donor twin).
      (5) Fetal congestive heart failure.
   d. Thinning of the placental membrane in the second half of pregnancy decreases diffusing distance, thus increasing functional efficiency of the placenta. However, this change also facilitates the passage of drugs in pregnancy and the intrapartum period.
4. Uteroplacental blood flow.
   a. At term, uterine blood flow is 750 cc per minute or more, representing 10% to 15% of the maternal cardiac output. Approximately 73% to 80% of uterine blood flow reaches the placenta.
   b. Decreased blood flow to the uterus or within the intervillous spaces will decrease the transport of substances to and from the fetus.
   c. Causes of decreased uteroplacental blood flow include:
      (1) Maternal vasoconstriction in hypertension, cocaine abuse, diabetic vasculopathy, and smoking.
      (2) Maternal vasodilatation caused by vasodilators, antihypertensives, and regional anesthetics with sympathetic blockade actions.
      (3) Decreased maternal cardiac output in supine hypotension.
      (4) Decreased maternal blood flow in intervillous spaces resulting from edema of placental villi.
      (5) Hypertonic uterine contractions.
      (6) Severe maternal physical stress.
      (7) Degenerative placental changes near term.
5. Fetal factors.
   a. Fetal tachycardia, often seen with fetal hypoxia, is analogous to an adult's "blowing off CO_2"; the increased heart rate increases the delivery of CO_2 to the placenta for diffusion to the maternal circulation.
   b. Conversely, fetal bradycardia resulting from hypoxia or anoxia causes an increased CO_2 level.
   c. Umbilical cord compression leads to CO_2 accumulation and acidosis.
   d. Fetal pH during labor is usually 0.1 to 0.15 unit less than the maternal pH; this difference increases the transport of acidophilic substances from the mother to the fetus and reduces albumin binding of drugs, resulting in more free drug in the fetal bloodstream.

CONDITIONS RELATED TO THE ANTEPARTUM PERIOD

Preeclampsia and Eclampsia

Hypertension in pregnancy, including acute gestational hypertension, preeclampsia, and chronic hypertension, is a major cause of maternal-fetal morbidity and death in the United States (Hallak, 2000). The main pathophysiologic events in preeclampsia are vasospasm, hematologic changes, and endothelial damage, leading to tissue hypoxia and multiple organ involvement (Shah, 2002).

A. **Incidence.** Incidence is 5% to 10% of all pregnancies (Reeder et al., 1997; Sibai, 2002).

B. **Etiology/predisposing factors.**
   1. The exact cause of preeclampsia and eclampsia has not been determined, although current theories involve an immunologic basis, dietary deficiencies or excesses, abnormal trophoblast invasion, alternations in coagulation, damage to vascular endothelium, and lack of cardiovascular adaptation (Sibai, 2002).
   2. Preeclampsia and eclampsia are associated with primigravidas, younger and older women, family history of preeclampsia or previous personal history of severe preeclampsia, low socioeconomic class, malnutrition and low weight gain in pregnancy, obesity, diabetes, chronic hypertensive or renal disease, thrombophilias, multifetal gestation or large fetus, hydatidiform mole, fetal hydrops, and trisomy 13. Other predisposing factors include placental abruption, fetal death, and intrauterine growth restriction (IUGR) in previous pregnancies (Reeder et al., 1997; Sibai, 2002; Varney, 1997).

C. **Clinical presentation.**
   1. A blood pressure (BP) of 140/90 mm Hg or above after week 20 of pregnancy. Severe preeclampsia is characterized by a BP of 160/110 or above.
   2. Edema due to salt retention and decreased plasma colloid osmotic pressure, evidenced by sudden and excessive weight gain, may or may not be present (33% of eclamptic women have not developed edema).
   3. Proteinuria due to decreased renal perfusion resulting in development of glomerular capillary endotheliosis.
   4. Other signs and symptoms: headache, hyperreflexia with clonus, visual and retinal changes, irritability, nausea and vomiting, epigastric pain, dyspnea, and oliguria.

D. **Potential complications.**
   1. Maternal.
      a. Mortality increasing with advancing maternal age (MacKay et al., 2001).
      b. Eclampsia (grand mal seizure).
      c. Cardiopulmonary failure and pulmonary edema.
      d. Hepatic rupture.
      e. Cerebrovascular accident.
      f. Renal cortical necrosis.
      g. Disseminated intravascular coagulation.
      h. HELLP syndrome (*h*emolysis, *e*levated *l*iver function test results, and *l*ow *p*latelet count).
      i. Retinal detachment.
   2. Placental/fetal.
      a. Premature placental aging, placental infarction, and decrease in amniotic fluid.
      b. Abruptio placentae in 2% to 10% of cases (Reeder et al., 1997).
      c. IUGR resulting from decreased placental blood flow.
      d. Fetal distress.
      e. Preterm birth.

E. **Assessment and management.**
   1. Severe preeclampsia.
      a. Primary goals of management include prevention of seizures (via limitation of stimuli and drug therapy), prevention of complications (via frequent systems assessments and lab studies), and birth of a live infant.

b. Seizure precautions.
c. Placental-fetal function tests: continuous electronic fetal monitoring; fetal movement; ultrasonography to determine fetal age and detect IUGR; serial nonstress tests, contraction stress tests, biophysical profile, and/or umbilical artery Doppler studies; and amniocentesis to determine fetal lung maturity.
d. Drugs.
   (1) Use of intravenous (IV) magnesium sulfate ($MgSO_4$) as a central nervous system (CNS) depressant to prevent seizures. A transient decrease in BP often occurs. Monitor fetal heart for decreased variability. Therapy is continued for at least 24 hours postpartum.
   (2) Use of antihypertensives is indicated when systolic BPs are greater than 180 or diastolic BPs are greater than 110:
      (a) Hydralazine (Apresoline). Monitor fetus for signs of hypoxia (tachycardia, bradycardia, late decelerations), which can occur with a sudden decrease in maternal BP.
      (b) Labetalol hydrochloride. Used to increase uteroplacental perfusion (Hallak, 2000). Monitor fetus for transient bradycardia (Murray, 1997).
   (3) Use of corticosteroids to increase fetal lung maturity when birth can be delayed for 48 hours and the woman is at less than 34 weeks' gestation.
e. Delivery by induction or cesarean if fetus is mature or if worsening maternal condition warrants.

2. Eclampsia.
   a. Immediate notification of physician or midwife.
   b. Bolus administration of IV $MgSO_4$.
   c. Safety measures for woman during and after seizures.
   d. Support of respirations with airway, oxygen, and suctioning.
   e. Monitor fetal heart for transient bradycardia, rebound tachycardia, decreased variability, and late decelerations (Murray, 1997; Sibai, 2002).
   f. Continuous maternal assessment, including assessment for abruptio placentae.
   g. Laboratory work: complete blood count (CBC), clot observation, serum creatinine, liver function tests, fibrinogen, arterial blood gases, and electrolytes (Sibai, 2002).
   h. Delivery by induction or cesarean based on the status of the maternal-placental-fetal complex.
3. Assessment of newborn infant for:
   a. IUGR.
   b. Preterm gestational age.
   c. Hypoxia and acidosis.
   d. Possible adverse drug effects on neonate:
      (1) Signs of hypermagnesemia when maternal administration of high doses of $MgSO_4$ occurs near the time of delivery: respiratory depression and neuromuscular depression, as evidenced by weakness, lethargy, hypotonia, flaccidity, and poor suck (Wilson et al., 2002).
      (2) Thrombocytopenia with daily maternal administration of hydralazine in the last trimester has been reported in a limited number of newborns (Briggs et al., 2002).
      (3) Hypotension, bradycardia, and hypoglycemia with maternal administration of labetalol (Poole, 1997).

Diabetes Mellitus

The woman with insulin-dependent diabetes who becomes pregnant and the pregnant woman in whom gestational diabetes mellitus (GDM) or type 1 diabetes develops are at risk during the antepartum period because of altered carbohydrate metabolism. The fetus/neonate is therefore also at risk. Strict control of maternal blood glucose concentration and anticipatory management of the newborn infant are important elements of perinatal care.

A. **Incidence.** Of all pregnancies, 2% to 5% are complicated by diabetes mellitus, and 2% to 3% by GDM (Pillitteri, 2003).

B. **Etiology and predisposing factors in gestational diabetes.**
   1. In the second half of pregnancy, secretion of estrogen, progesterone, and human placental lactogen increases cellular resistance to insulin. The pancreas of the woman who is predisposed to diabetes cannot meet the increased demand for insulin, and hyperglycemia results.
   2. Risk factors for GDM include maternal obesity; a family history of diabetes; age greater than 25 years; member of an ethnic group at risk for diabetes; and a history of having had an infant who was large for gestational age (LGA), who had a congenital anomaly, whose gestation resulted in hydramnios, or who was stillborn (National Institute of Child Health & Human Development, 2003).

C. **Clinical presentation and screening for gestational diabetes.**
   1. Much controversy exists about the association of abnormal blood values and poor fetal outcomes. No evidence exists that treatment of women with abnormal values results in improved perinatal outcomes (Enkin et al., 2000).
   2. Women at high risk for GDM should be screened at the first prenatal visit in addition to the routine testing at 26 to 28 weeks, because GDM may be asymptomatic or evidenced only by subtle changes (Landon et al., 2002).
   3. Women with average risk for GDM should be screened with a 1-hour glucose tolerance test, and an abnormally high value requires further testing (Landon et al., 2002).
   4. The American College of Obstetricians and Gynecologists (ACOG) now indicates that if a woman is considered to be low risk for GDM, glucose screening may not be required (ACOG, 2001).

D. **Potential complications.**
   1. Maternal.
      a. Hypoglycemic reactions in the first trimester.
      b. Ketoacidosis in the second and third trimesters.
      c. Progression of vasculopathy, nephropathy, and retinopathy with preexisting diabetes.
      d. Hydramnios.
      e. Pregnancy-induced hypertension.
      f. Anemia.
      g. Infections such as monilial vaginitis and urinary tract infections.
   2. Fetal/neonatal.
      a. Macrosomia (weight greater than 4000 g) with possible traumatic vaginal delivery such as with shoulder dystocia. IUGR when the mother has microvascular disease, hypertension, or nephropathy (Enkin et al., 2000).
      b. Fetal death.
      c. Respiratory distress syndrome.
      d. Hypoglycemia, hypocalcemia, and hypomagnesemia.
      e. Polycythemia, hyperviscosity, and hyperbilirubinemia.
      f. Cardiomyopathy with congestive heart failure.

g. Congenital malformation as a consequence of poorly controlled preexisting diabetes: renal anomalies such as Potter syndrome, polycystic kidneys, and double ureters; neural tube defects; skeletal defects such as caudal regression syndrome and spina bifida; cardiac anomalies such as patent ductus arteriosus, transposition of the great vessels, endocardial cushion defects, and ventricular septal defect; and gastrointestinal defects such as tracheoesophageal fistula, bowel atresia, and imperforate anus (Landon and Gabbe, 2000). The threefold increase in incidence of congenital anomalies can be reduced significantly by preconception control of blood glucose levels (Enkin et al., 2000).

E. Assessment and management.

1. In preexisting diabetes:
   a. Preconception counseling is provided, with optimal control of blood glucose levels. Insulin is considered the therapy of choice because oral antidiabetic agents can cause prolonged newborn hypoglycemia (Briggs et al., 2002). The woman should begin taking 4 mg of folic acid daily, and continue through the first trimester, to reduce the risk for neural tube defects (Landon and Gabbe, 2000).
   b. Glycosylated hemoglobin tests may be performed before conception and during the pregnancy to assess glucose control during the previous 1 to 2 months. Levels beyond the normal range are associated with increased congenital anomalies (Landon and Gabbe, 2000).
   c. Home blood glucose monitoring, diet, and either insulin pump therapy or several daily injections of insulin are prescribed to maintain tight control of the blood glucose concentration (101-121 mg/dl). Tight control is associated with decreased risk of macrosomia, respiratory distress syndrome, and perinatal death, as well as maternal urinary tract infection, preterm labor, and cesarean section (Enkin et al., 2000).
   d. Women are evaluated early in pregnancy for evidence of diabetic retinopathy and nephropathy (Landon and Gabbe, 2000).
   e. At 16 weeks' gestation, the woman should be offered maternal serum alpha-fetoprotein testing, accompanied by a comprehensive ultrasound at 18 to 20 weeks to assess for the presence of neural tube defects or other anomalies. Serial ultrasounds may be performed to evaluate fetal growth. Fetal echocardiography is also recommended (Landon and Gabbe, 2000).
   f. Weekly prenatal visits are made after 28 weeks, with fetal assessment by means of nonstress tests, biophysical profiles, and daily fetal movement counting.
   g. Before any decision is made about induction of labor, amniocentesis is performed to determine the lecithin/sphingomyelin (L/S) ratio and the presence of phosphatidylglycerol. Delivery is accomplished before term if maternal or fetal complications develop.
   h. Insulin is given IV during labor if blood glucose values are above 140 mg/dl (Landon and Gabbe, 2000). Glucose levels are monitored every hour to ensure optimum titration of insulin in order to decrease the risk of neonatal rebound hypoglycemia (Pillitteri, 2003).
2. In gestational diabetes (Landon et al., 2002; Landon and Gabbe, 2000):
   a. A 2000- to 2500-calorie diet with no simple carbohydrates is recommended.
   b. Fasting and 2-hour postprandial glucose levels are checked weekly.
   c. Maternal fetal movement counting begins at 28 weeks.
   d. Nonstress testing begins at 40 weeks in the well-controlled mother.

3. In neonate:
   a. Assess for gestational age and size (LGA or IUGR).
   b. Assess for:
      (1) Respiratory distress.
      (2) Hypoglycemia, hypocalcemia, and hypomagnesemia.
      (3) Polycythemia and hyperviscosity.
      (4) Complications resulting from decreased blood flow, erythrocyte hemolysis, and thrombosis.
      (5) Congenital malformations.
      (6) Birth injuries: fractured clavicles, intracranial bleeding, facial nerve paralysis, brachial palsy, and skull fractures.

CONDITIONS RELATED TO THE INTRAPARTUM PERIOD

Preterm Labor

The World Health Organization defines preterm labor as labor occurring at greater than 20 and less than 37 completed weeks of gestation (Goldenberg, 2002). If preterm labor is recognized in time, measures can be taken to stop the contractions. The prognosis for the fetus improves with each week of pregnancy gained.

A. **Incidence.** About 11% of all newborns in the United States are born before term, compared with 5% to 7% in Europe. The U.S. preterm birth rate has not declined in the past four decades (Goldenberg, 2002).

B. **Etiology/predisposing factors.**
   1. The exact cause of preterm labor is unknown, although chorioamnionitis and other genitourinary infections have been implicated in recent studies (Goldenberg, 2002; Von Der Pool, 1998).
   2. A number of maternal factors have been associated with an increased incidence of preterm labor: maternal age (<18 or >40), socioeconomic effects (lower socioeconomic status, nonwhite race, poor nutrition, inadequate prenatal care), medical/obstetric history (preterm labor or birth, one or more midtrimester pregnancy losses, short interpregnancy interval, uterine anomalies and incompetent cervix, systemic and genitourinary tract infections, polyhydramnios, immunologic factors, abruptio placentae, and placenta previa), and lifestyle factors (use of alcohol, cigarettes, and illicit drugs such as cocaine, and stressful work or personal situations) (Svigos et al., 2000; Varney, 1997; Von Der Pool, 1998).
   3. Fetal factors contributing to the development of preterm labor may include IUGR, congenital anomalies, intrauterine fetal death, and complications from multifetal gestation (Svigos et al., 2000).
   4. Risk scoring systems, designed to screen women during pregnancy, have a predictive value of only 17% to 34% (Svigos et al., 2000). Many women who give birth before term do not have any known risk factors.

C. **Clinical presentation.**
   1. Painless or painful uterine contractions.
   2. Low, dull, intermittent or constant backache.
   3. Intermittent or constant menstrual-like cramping.
   4. Intermittent pelvic pressure that may extend along the inner thigh.
   5. Abdominal cramps, which may be accompanied by diarrhea.
   6. Increased vaginal discharge, which may be mucoid, watery, or slightly bloody.
   7. Spontaneous premature rupture of membranes.
   8. A generalized feeling that something is wrong.
   9. Progressive cervical effacement and dilation unless intervention is performed.

D. Potential complications.

1. Maternal.
   a. No particular physical complications other than adverse reactions from tocolytic agents.
   b. Emotional stress and financial problems.
2. Fetal/neonatal.
   a. Preterm birth with an increase in neonatal morbidity and death.
   b. Adverse reactions to tocolytic agents (see a to e of the following section).

E. Assessment and management.

1. Screening of pregnant women at the first and subsequent prenatal visits for preterm labor risk factors.
2. Teaching *all* pregnant women the symptoms of preterm labor and the actions to take if they occur (lie down on the left side and drink several glasses of fluid; report to physician or midwife if contractions are still occurring after 1 hour).
3. Helping high-risk women modify their risk factors and take measures to prevent preterm labor (e.g., stop smoking, improve nutrition and hydration, treat infections, decrease work hours and stress, increase bed rest, and avoid nipple preparation that initiates signs of preterm labor).
4. Although weekly cervical examinations and ultrasonographic evaluation of the cervix are being performed by some providers, there is no compelling evidence that these interventions decrease the incidence of preterm birth (Enkin et al., 2000; Iams, 2002; Svigos et al., 2000).
5. Use of home contraction monitoring systems has not been proven effective in identifying women who will deliver preterm (Enkin et al., 2000; Iams et al., 2002).
6. Treatment decisions may be based on the results of a fetal fibronectin test performed on vaginal secretions. The test is valued more for its negative predictive value in symptomatic women than its low positive predictive value (Enkin et al., 2000; Svigos et al., 2000). The relatively high cost of this test and the potential legal implications of not treating symptomatic women with a negative test may have prohibited its widespread adoption.
7. While episodes of preterm labor are widely treated with hospitalization, hydration with IV fluid, bed rest in the left lateral position, and sedation, there is little evidence that these interventions are effective (Goldenberg, 2002). Corticosteroid therapy is recommended for women at risk of preterm delivery to reduce the incidence of neonatal morbidity and death from respiratory distress syndrome (National Institutes of Health, 2000).
8. When appropriate and not contraindicated, use of one of the following medications may prolong pregnancy 24 hours or more, allowing enough time for concurrent corticosteroid therapy to benefit the fetus and/or for transfer of the mother to a hospital with a level III nursery (Svigos et al., 2000).
   a. Ritodrine (Yutopar), given IV, inhibits uterine contractility. Potential fetal/neonatal side effects include tachycardia, cardiac septal hypertrophy, fetal hyperglycemia and neonatal hypoglycemia, pulmonary edema, cardiac failure, irritability, neonatal hyperbilirubinemia, hypotension, paralytic ileus, intraventricular hemorrhage, and death (Goldenberg, 2002; Iams, 2002).
   b. $MgSO_4$, given IV for uterine relaxation. Signs of hypermagnesemia in the neonate when maternal administration of high doses of $MgSO_4$ occurs near the time of delivery: respiratory depression and neuromuscular depression, as evidenced by weakness, lethargy, hypotonia, flaccidity, and poor suck (Wilson et al., 2002).

   c. Terbutaline (Brethine), given IV, subcutaneously, or via a subcutaneous pump. For long-term use at home, women can be taught to give themselves terbutaline in programmed continuous and bolus doses via a miniature subcutaneous automatic infusion pump, in conjunction with a home contraction monitoring system. Potential fetal/neonatal side effects are the same as for ritodrine.
   d. Indomethacin (Indocin) given prior to 32 weeks, either rectally or orally. Contraindications to its use include fetal anomalies, oligohydramnios, IUGR, chorioamnionitis, ductal dependent cardiac defects, and twin-to-twin transfusion syndrome (Iams, 2002). Fetal side effects include decreased renal blood flow, constriction of the ductus arteriosus, and neonatal pulmonary hypertension (Iams, 2002).
   e. Nifedipine (Procardia), a calcium channel blocker, is given orally. No major fetal side effects have been reported as yet (Goldenberg, 2002).
9. For women with preterm rupture of the membranes, cultures should be grown for group B streptococcus and antibiotics administered prophylactically to prevent infection with group B streptococcus in the newborn infant (Iams, 2002).
10. If the measures noted above are not successful, and the cervix continues to efface and dilate, the following measures are important:
   a. To allow the amniotic fluid to cushion the fetal skull, no rupture of the membranes is performed.
   b. The head is delivered in a slow, controlled fashion. Concerns about intracranial hemorrhage with a vaginal delivery of a preterm infant in the cephalic presentation are unfounded because intracranial hemorrhage may also occur in cesarean birth (Iams, 2002).
   c. Cesarean delivery is often suggested for the preterm fetus with a breech presentation because of the risk of cord prolapse and the potential risk of difficult delivery of the head (Iams, 2002).

Abruptio Placentae

In abruptio placentae the placenta separates suddenly, prematurely, and in varying degrees from the uterine wall during pregnancy or labor. It is a common cause of bleeding in the second half of pregnancy.

A. **Incidence.** In 2000, placental abruption occurred in 5.5 per 1000 births (0.5%) (Martin et al., 2002).
B. **Etiology/predisposing factors.**
   1. Although the cause of abruptio placentae has not been definitively established, there is a high correlation with hypertensive disorders during pregnancy, cocaine and crack use, trauma, placental abnormalities (circumvallate), and rupture of abnormally formed blood vessels (Chamberlain and Steer, 1999; Konje and Taylor, 2000).
   2. Additional predisposing factors include uterine leiomyomas or anomalies, polyhydramnios and multifetal pregnancy, increased parity, history of previous abruption, chorioamnionitis, external cephalic version, and maternal cigarette smoking and poor nutrition (Benedetti, 2002). Short cord is also considered a risk factor.
C. **Clinical presentation.**
   1. The abruption is classified as grade 1, 2, or 3 according to clinical findings and degree of coagulopathy (Benedetti, 2002; Corder-Mabe, 1998).
   2. Maternal signs and symptoms.

a. Mild labor pains with persistent cramping to sharp, continuous abdominal pain.
b. Boardlike and tender abdomen.
c. Dark or bright red vaginal bleeding (unless the bleeding is concealed behind the placenta), ranging from spotting to frank hemorrhage. In 20% of patients with abruption, there is no visible evidence of bleeding (Benedetti, 2002).
d. Uterine hyperactivity.
e. Enlargement of the uterus as blood accumulates, with increasing abdominal girth.
f. Fetal parts difficult to palpate (Chamberlain and Steer, 1999).

3. Fetal signs (Varney and Reedy, 1997).
   a. Loss of fetal heart tones or movement.
   b. Tachycardia.
   c. Late or variable decelerations.
   d. Decreased fetal heart rate variability.
   e. Sinusoidal fetal heart rate pattern.

D. Potential complications.

1. Maternal (Konje and Taylor, 2000).
   a. Anemia.
   b. Hypovolemic shock, sometimes resulting in anterior pituitary necrosis (Sheehan syndrome).
   c. Couvelaire uterus (blood forced between the muscle fibers of the uterus).
   d. Disseminated intravascular coagulation.
   e. Acute renal failure.
   f. Postpartum hemorrhage.
   g. Fetomaternal hemorrhage.
   h. Death.
2. Fetal/neonatal.
   a. Anemia.
   b. Hypoxia and asphyxia.
   c. Hypovolemia.
   d. Neurobehavioral problems such as cerebral palsy (Benedetti, 2002).
   e. 25% to 30% incidence of death (Benedetti, 2002).

E. Assessment and management.

1. Any episode of bleeding during pregnancy in an Rh-negative woman requires a Kleihauer-Betke test and the administration of Rh immunoglobulin (RhoGAM) (Enkin et al., 2000).
2. Assessment if fetus is stable and maternal hematologic status can be maintained:
   a. Ultrasonography to locate placenta and determine degree of placental separation and location of hematoma (Benedetti, 2002).
   b. Bed rest in left lateral position, close assessment of abdomen for rigidity and pain, and close assessment of vaginal bleeding.
   c. Monitoring of maternal vital signs and continuous monitoring of fetal heart for bradycardia, late decelerations, and prolonged decelerations (Murray, 1997).
   d. Placement of two IV lines with 16-gauge catheters for administration of fluids and blood products.
   e. CBC, coagulation studies, and type and cross-match for blood (Benedetti, 2002).
   f. Possible collection of urine for drug screening.
   g. Possible induction of labor and/or vaginal delivery.

3. Preparation for cesarean delivery if fetal distress or severe hemorrhage occurs:
   a. Inform and support parents and ensure that surgical consent is obtained.
   b. Laboratory tests as above.
   c. Prepare abdomen and insert indwelling urinary catheter.
   d. Notify neonatal intensive care unit (NICU) and neonatologist/pediatrician.

Placenta Previa

Placenta previa is a placenta that is implanted in the lower part of the uterus near the cervix (marginal) or in varying degrees (partial or total) over the cervix. Cervical dilation at or near term is accompanied by bleeding from the placenta. Placenta previa is a common cause of bleeding in the second half of pregnancy, when the lower uterine segment stretches and thins (Benedetti, 2002; Chamberlain and Steer, 1999).

A. **Incidence.** In 2000 the incidence was 3.2 per 1000 births (0.3%) in the United States (Martin et al., 2002).

B. **Etiology/predisposing factors.**
   1. The precise cause of placenta previa is unknown, but it occurs most frequently in multiparous and older women.
   2. Other associated and predisposing factors include previous placenta previa, history of low-segment cesarean delivery, history of myomectomy or postpartum endometritis, and increased placental size.

C. **Clinical presentation.**
   1. Bright red, painless vaginal bleeding. Although the first bleeding episode may be slight in amount, more blood is usually lost in subsequent episodes (Chamberlain and Steer, 1999).
   2. Uterine contractions in 20% of cases, but otherwise the uterus is usually soft and nontender (Benedetti, 2002).
   3. Finding on ultrasonography at 17 weeks' gestation in 5% to 15% of pregnant women, with resolution by term 90% of the time (Benedetti, 2002).
   4. Failure of presenting part of fetus to become engaged. Fetus may lie transversely or be in breech position (Chamberlain and Steer, 1999).

D. **Potential complications.**
   1. Maternal.
      a. Anemia.
      b. Hypovolemic shock.
      c. Endometritis.
      d. Decreased contractile strength of the lower uterine segment, which can lead to postpartum hemorrhage and need for hysterectomy (Chamberlain and Steer, 1999).
      e. Abnormal placental implantation (placenta accreta, percreta, and increta) (Benedetti, 2002).
   2. Fetal/neonatal.
      a. Hypoxia and asphyxia.
      b. IUGR.
      c. Fetal hemorrhage and death.
      d. Prematurity.
      e. Infection.

E. **Assessment and management.**
   1. Treatment and delivery decisions are based on amount of bleeding, gestational age, and condition and presentation of fetus (Benedetti, 2002). Any episode of bleeding during pregnancy in an Rh-negative woman

requires a Kleihauer-Betke test and the administration of RhoGAM (Enkin et al., 2000).

2. Marginal or partial placenta previa and low-lying placenta with minimal bleeding are managed conservatively:
   a. Ultrasonography to confirm diagnosis and to rule out IUGR.
   b. No vaginal examinations.
   c. Bed rest and activity level at home or in the hospital determined by clinical presentation.
   d. Avoidance of intercourse and orgasm, which can cause uterine contractions (Varney and Reedy, 1997).
   e. Amniocentesis for fetal lung maturity if there is any question about term status.
   f. If fetus is mature, vaginal delivery can be accomplished if placenta is anterior and bleeding continues to be minimal (with an anterior placenta, bleeding may be decreased due to compression of the placenta between the fetal head and the symphysis pubis) (Chamberlain and Steer, 1999).
3. Partial or total placenta previa with greater amounts of bleeding is handled as noted above, except that vaginal delivery may not be possible. In addition:
   a. Frequent assessment of vaginal bleeding, with pad counts and/or weighing of pads.
   b. Frequent assessment of maternal vital signs and fetal heart tones, and palpation of abdomen.
   c. Laboratory work: CBC, type and cross-match for possible blood transfusion.
   d. With significant bleeding, placement of IV lines with 16-gauge catheters for blood administration.
   e. Method of delivery.
      (1) Vaginal delivery may be performed if bleeding remains minimal and the placenta is anterior. Artificial rupture of membranes may be performed to allow presenting part of fetus to compress placental site (Chamberlain and Steer, 1999).
      (2) If bleeding is significant or the placenta is posterior, cesarean delivery is performed (Chamberlain and Steer, 1999).

Umbilical Cord Prolapse

Umbilical cord prolapse is an event that is life threatening to the fetus and requires immediate and effective management by the nurse. It occurs when the cord falls below the presenting part or is compressed between the presenting part and the pelvis or cervix.

A. **Incidence.** Less than 1 in 200 labors (0.5%) (Steer and Danielian, 2000).
B. **Etiology/predisposing factors.**
   1. The fetal presenting part does not fill the pelvic inlet well, and the cord slips past it, often when the membranes rupture.
   2. Predisposing factors include malpresentation (transverse lie and breech presentation), premature or small-for-gestational-age fetus, multifetal pregnancy, polyhydramnios, cephalopelvic disproportion that prevents fetal engagement, lack of engagement before the onset of labor (as is common with multiparous women), and abnormal placentation (Norwitz et al., 2002; Steer and Danielian, 2000).

C. **Clinical presentation.**
   1. Cord is protruding from vagina or is palpable on vaginal examination.
   2. In an occult prolapse, cord is not visible or palpable but is located between the presenting part and the pelvis or cervix.
   3. Station of presenting part is 0 to –4 cm, and membranes are often ruptured.
   4. Fetal heart changes can include increase in fetal heart rate, uniform accelerations, bradycardia, and variable decelerations (Murray, 1997).

D. **Potential complications.**
   1. Maternal.
      a. Trauma to the birth canal from rapid forceps delivery.
      b. General anesthesia resulting in uterine atony with subsequent postpartum bleeding.
      c. Blood loss from cesarean delivery.
   2. Fetal/neonatal.
      a. Perinatal mortality rate is 50% (Norwitz et al., 2002) and increases as increased time elapses between cord prolapse and birth.
      b. Fetal anoxia leading to long-range neurologic complications.
      c. Neonatal infection.

E. **Assessment and management.**
   1. Assessments on admission to labor and delivery.
      a. Presenting part and its station.
      b. Dilation of cervix.
      c. Status of membranes.
      d. Estimation of fetal weight and fetal heart rate.
   2. Assessment for presence of polyhydramnios or lack of engagement of presenting part. Ambulation during labor and artificial rupture of membranes may be contraindicated in these and other situations.
   3. Assessment after artificial or spontaneous rupture of membranes.
      a. Monitor fetal heart for changes as indicated above.
      b. Perform vaginal examination to detect prolapse if indicated.
   4. If prolapse has occurred:
      a. Keep examining hand in vagina to push presenting part away from cord until delivery of fetus. The provider may also attempt to replace the prolapsed cord into the uterus (Steer and Danielian, 2000).
      b. An alternative measure is to insert an indwelling catheter to fill the mother's bladder with sterile saline solution in order to elevate the fetal presenting part so that it is off the cord (Steer and Danielian, 2000).
      c. Have assistant help woman into knee-chest or steep Trendelenburg position, with hips elevated and head down (Steer and Danielian, 2000).
      d. Monitor fetal heart rate continuously and palpate cord lightly for continued pulsation. Administer oxygen to woman as indicated for fetal distress.
      e. Tocolytic agents such as terbutaline may be used.
      f. If the cervix is fully dilated and the fetal station is below the ischial spines, vaginal delivery may be expedited. Emergency cesarean delivery may be preferable, especially if cervix is not fully dilated and the fetus exhibits a nonreassuring heart rate pattern.

Shoulder Dystocia

Shoulder dystocia is an acute emergency in which the physician or midwife is unable to deliver the shoulders of the infant by the usual maneuvers after birth of the head.

A. **Incidence.** Incidence is 1% to 2% (Steer and Danielian, 2000).

B. **Etiology/predisposing factors.**
   1. The fetal shoulders are too broad to be delivered between the symphysis pubis and the sacrum.
   2. Predisposing factors include maternal obesity, excessive weight gain, fetus more than 4000 g, history of large siblings or previous shoulder dystocia, poorly controlled maternal diabetes, contracted pelvic outlet, and postdate pregnancy (Shua and Arulkumaran, 2000; Varney, 1997).

C. **Clinical presentation.**
   1. Slow active phase of labor.
   2. Second stage longer than 2 hours, with slow descent of head.
   3. After delivery of the head, it recoils against the perineum and restitution does not occur ("turtling"). The usual traction from below is not successful in delivering the neonate.

D. **Complications.**
   1. Maternal.
      a. Vaginal or perineal lacerations.
      b. Ruptured uterus.
      c. Postpartum hemorrhage or infection.
      d. Bladder trauma.
   2. Fetal/neonatal.
      a. Birth injuries such as brachial palsy, Erb palsy, facial nerve palsy, or fractured clavicle or humerus (Steer and Danielian, 2000).
      b. Anoxia, perinatal depression, hypoxic-ischemic encephalopathy .
      c. Intrapartum or neonatal death.

E. **Assessment and management.**
   1. Anticipate shoulder dystocia if descent of the head is slow and estimated weight is large. Make sure the woman's bladder is empty before birth occurs.
   2. If shoulder dystocia occurs, physician or midwife will (Lanni and Seeds, 2002; Steer and Danielian, 2000):
      a. Use the McRoberts maneuver (an exaggerated lithotomy position).
      b. Have the nurse perform firm suprapubic pressure to attempt to release the anterior shoulder.
      c. Perform or extend the episiotomy.
      d. If the above are not effective, perform other maneuvers to expedite delivery:
         (1) Turn the woman onto her side or pull the hips off the bed to free the sacrum.
         (2) Turn the woman on all fours to widen the pelvic outlet if this can be easily accomplished.
         (3) Manually rotate shoulders from the anteroposterior to the oblique diameter in the pelvis.
         (4) Use the Wood screw maneuver, in which both hands are inserted internally to rotate the posterior shoulder to the anterior position for delivery under the pubic bone, with the maneuver repeated for the other shoulder.
         (5) Extract posterior shoulder and arm.
         (6) Fracturing the clavicle to collapse the diameter of the shoulders may be necessary on rare occasions (Enkin et al., 2000).
         (7) The Zavanelli maneuver can be performed to push the fetal head back into the vagina so that a cesarean delivery can be done, but it is rarely used.

Breech Delivery

A. **Incidence.** Incidence is 25% at less than 28 weeks, 14% at 29 to 32 weeks, 2% to 3% at term, overall 3% to 4% of all labors (Lanni and Seeds, 2002; Penn, 2000). Incidence increases in multiple gestation and in preterm birth.

B. **Etiology/predisposing factors (Penn, 2000).**
   1. Maternal.
      a. Polyhydramnios or oligohydramnios.
      b. Uterine anomalies.
      c. Contracted pelvis.
      d. Use of anticonvulsant medications or alcohol abuse.
   2. Placental/fetal.
      a. Placenta previa.
      b. Multifetal gestation.
      c. IUGR or fetal anomalies, especially those related to CNS problems.
      d. Short cord.
      e. Large fetus or preterm fetus.
      f. Fetal death.

C. **Clinical presentation.**
   1. Woman feels fetus kicking in lower abdomen.
   2. Fetal heart sounds are heard loudest above umbilicus.
   3. Use of Leopold maneuvers indicates head is in fundal area and breech is in pelvis.
   4. On vaginal examination, it is found that the presenting part is soft, no fontanelles are felt, and the genitalia may be identified.

D. **Complications.**
   1. Studies have indicated no significant differences in neonatal outcomes between vaginal and cesarean delivery (Penn, 2000).
   2. Fetal/neonatal complications resulting from vaginal delivery.
      a. Prolapsed cord.
      b. Asphyxia from slow delivery of fetal head or from compression of umbilical cord between pelvis and head during delivery.
      c. Aspiration of amniotic fluid with potential for meconium aspiration syndrome.
      d. CNS injuries such as intracranial hemorrhage and severed spinal cord especially if fetal head is hyperextended (Penn, 2000).

E. **Assessment and management.**
   1. A procedure that may help the fetus turn from breech to cephalic presentation is postural exercise in which the woman assumes either the knee-chest or an elevated-hip posture several times a day until the fetus turns (Enkin et al., 2000).
   2. The physician may attempt external cephalic version after 37 weeks with or without the use of a uterine relaxant and, if the fetus remains in a cephalic presentation, vaginal delivery. However, in many cases the fetus reverts to breech (Enkin et al., 2000).
   3. Assessments on admission to labor and delivery:
      a. Perform Leopold maneuvers and vaginal examination to determine presentation.
      b. Report clinical findings immediately to physician or midwife.
   4. Ultrasonography may be ordered to confirm breech presentation, determine degree of flexion of fetal head, evaluate size of fetal head, estimate fetal weight, diagnose fetal anomalies, and locate placenta.

5. A trial of labor for vaginal delivery for the term breech may be attempted.
   a. The fetal position must be a frank or complete breech with the head flexed, and the pelvis must be adequate.
   b. The estimated fetal weight must be approximately 1500 to 3900 g (Penn, 2000), and no other indications for cesarean delivery must exist.
   c. The nurse should perform, at the time of rupture of the membranes, a vaginal examination to check for prolapsed cord and should monitor the fetal heart tones closely.
   d. Meconium in the amniotic fluid is not necessarily a sign of fetal hypoxia when the fetus is in a breech position. However, meconium aspiration at the time of delivery may be a serious complication.
   e. The woman may receive an episiotomy, and Piper forceps may be used to assist in delivery of the neonate's head. The nurse may be asked to perform suprapubic pressure to keep the neonate's head flexed while the physician or midwife performs certain maneuvers during the delivery.
6. Many physicians will perform cesarean delivery when the fetus is breech in these situations: preterm fetus, hyperextension of head, and footling breech (Lanni and Seeds, 2002). Other situations may include primigravidous state, small pelvis, premature rupture of membranes, and large fetus.
7. Assessment of the neonate may reveal:
   a. Edema of the external genitalia.
   b. A continuation of the frank breech position for a period of time after the birth.

OBSTETRIC ANALGESIA AND ANESTHESIA

Although maternal deaths have resulted from anesthesia complications, including those caused by poor technique or overdosage, it is not one of the major causes of maternal mortality (Johnson and Niebyl, 2002). Most anesthesiologists, obstetricians, and midwives would agree that there is no method of pharmacologic pain relief that is completely safe for all laboring women. In addition, side effects or adverse reactions in the woman affect the fetus to some degree. For this reason, nonpharmacologic methods of pain management (e.g., labor support, breathing techniques, massage, water immersion, transcutaneous electrical nerve stimulation [TENS], and subcutaneous sterile water injections in the back) should be as routinely provided as pharmacologic methods, and may provide sufficient pain relief for many women.

Obstetric Analgesia

Obstetric analgesia is given by either the intramuscular (IM) or the IV route and in as small a dose as possible. The most commonly used analgesics are butorphanol (Stadol) and nalbuphine (Nubain).

A. Potential side effects or complications.
1. Maternal.
   a. Respiratory depression.
   b. Nausea and vomiting.
   c. Orthostatic hypotension.
   d. Drowsiness and dizziness.
2. Fetal/neonatal.
   a. Decreased fetal activity and variability; sinusoidal pattern; late decelerations if mother experiences hypotension.

b. Neonatal respiratory depression and respiratory acidosis.
c. Thermoregulation problems related to lethargy and/or hypotonia.

B. Assessment and management.

1. Avoid administration of analgesics close to delivery if possible.
2. Administer IV analgesics slowly; give during a uterine contraction to minimize amount of drug the fetus receives.
3. Observe woman for side effects and monitor fetus continuously with electronic fetal monitor or periodic auscultation.
4. With maternal hypotension, turn woman onto her left side, increase IV infusion of fluids, and closely monitor fetal heart tones as well as woman's BP.
5. Have naloxone (Narcan), oxygen, and ventilatory equipment available for use with the newborn infant if respiratory depression occurs.
6. Document use of analgesic and transmit this information to nursery nurse.
7. In nursery, observe neonate for side effects of maternal analgesia.

Obstetric Anesthesia

Several types of anesthesia are used with women in labor and delivery. General anesthesia is used only for emergency cesarean deliveries and complicated vaginal deliveries when it is not possible to have immediate and effective regional anesthesia. Regional anesthesia includes continuous lumbar epidural, spinal, and pudendal block. Local anesthesia involves perineal infiltration prior to episiotomy, birth, and/or perineal repair.

A. Potential complications with general anesthesia.

1. Maternal.
   a. Vomiting and aspiration of gastric contents, with acid pneumonitis (Mendelson syndrome) as a consequence (Enkin et al., 2000).
   b. Respiratory depression.
   c. Cardiac irritability and arrest.
   d. Hypotension or hypertension.
   e. Tachycardia.
   f. Laryngospasm.
   g. Postpartum uterine atony.
2. Fetal/neonatal.
   a. Decreased fetal cardiac variability and movements.
   b. Neonatal respiratory depression and hypotonicity.
   c. Fetal depression in proportion to the amount of anesthesia.

B. Assessment and management with general anesthesia.

1. The woman must have nothing by mouth while in labor if there is a strong possibility that she will receive general anesthesia.
2. Note the time of her last meal.
3. Physician may order 30 ml of clear antacid to be administered before general anesthesia to increase the pH of the stomach contents in case of aspiration.
4. Endotracheal tube and cricoid pressure are techniques used by the anesthesiologist to prevent aspiration.
5. Place wedge under right hip to cause displacement of uterus from aorta and vena cava and to prevent supine hypotensive syndrome during surgery.
6. Monitor woman's cardiorespiratory status during and after surgery, and uterine bleeding postoperatively.
7. Monitor newborn infant after surgery for complications.

C. Potential complications with regional anesthetics.
- **1.** Maternal.
  - **a.** With spinal and epidural anesthesia:
    - (1) Hypotension due to sympathetic blockade (Hawkins et al., 2002).
    - (2) Allergic reaction to the injected anesthetic.
    - (3) Toxic reaction to overdose or intravascular injection, with seizure activity (Hawkins et al., 2002).
    - (4) Respiratory paralysis from inadvertent high spinal anesthesia.
    - (5) Headaches after spinal anesthesia.
    - (6) Failure of anesthetic to be effective.
    - (7) Urinary retention during labor and in postpartum period.
    - (8) Slowing of labor, with need to use oxytocin and forceps if anesthetic is given too early.
    - (9) Formation of a hematoma that compresses the spinal cord, with potential for permanent damage (Hawkins et al., 2002).
    - (10) Paralysis (rare).
  - **b.** With epidural anesthesia:
    - (1) Shearing off of epidural catheter.
    - (2) Trauma to spinal cord or nerve roots.
    - (3) Some evidence of increased malposition and instrumental delivery (Enkin et al., 2000).
    - (4) Long-term backache, chronic headache, and bladder dysfunction are possible complications; however, more study is needed (Enkin et al., 2000).
    - (5) "Epidural shakes" and "epidural fever" (involuntary shivering that leads to an elevated temperature) (Lieberman et al., 1997).
  - **c.** With pudendal block (London et al., 2003):
    - (1) Sciatic nerve trauma.
    - (2) Perforated rectum.
    - (3) Broad-ligament hematoma.
- **2.** Fetal/neonatal.
  - **a.** Toxic reaction from overdose or intravascular injection.
  - **b.** Fetal compromise with prolonged maternal hypotension, as evidenced by late decelerations, bradycardia, and either increased or decreased variability (Murray, 1997).
  - **c.** Hyperthermia with epidural anesthesia (Lieberman et al., 1997).

D. Assessment and management with regional anesthetics.
- **1.** Note history of allergies to local anesthetics.
- **2.** Prehydrate with 500 to 1000 ml IV fluid before spinal or epidural anesthesia to minimize hypotensive effects from sympathetic blockade.
- **3.** Position and reassure woman during administration of anesthetic. To prevent supine hypotension, a small roll may be placed under the right hip.
- **4.** Monitor woman's BP after administration of spinal or epidural anesthetic; monitor fetal heart after any type of regional anesthesia.
- **5.** Monitor bladder distention and catheterize if necessary.
- **6.** Complications and their management.
  - **a.** Hypotension.
    - (1) Signs and symptoms.
      - (a) Decreased baseline BP.
      - (b) Dizziness or affected vision.
      - (c) Nausea and vomiting.

(2) Management.
(a) Increase IV fluids.
(b) Displace uterus from aorta and vena cava.
(c) Administer oxygen and IV ephedrine as ordered.
(d) Monitor fetus for hypoxia and fetus/newborn for side effects of ephedrine (tachycardia, jitteriness, and increased muscular activity).

b. High spinal.
(1) Signs and symptoms.
(a) Breast numbness indicating a rising level of anesthesia.
(b) Sensation of inability to breathe.
(c) Respiratory arrest.
(2) Management.
(a) Notify anesthesia immediately.
(b) Maintain airway and ventilation.
(c) Monitor fetal heart tones.

c. Toxic reaction.
(1) Signs and symptoms.
(a) Metallic taste.
(b) Ringing in ears.
(c) Slurring of speech.
(d) Numbness of tongue and mouth.
(e) Seizures.
(f) Cardiovascular and respiratory depression.
(2) Management.
(a) Cardiorespiratory support.
(b) Drugs to control seizures.
(c) Monitor newborn infant for seizures, bradycardia, apnea, and hypotonia.

d. Allergic reaction.
(1) Signs and symptoms.
(a) Bronchospasm.
(b) Laryngeal edema.
(c) Urticaria.
(2) Management: use of IV antihistamine such as diphenhydramine (Benadryl).

Cesarean Delivery

A. Incidence. The cesarean delivery rate in the United States was 22.9% in 2000, the highest rate since 1989; reasons for this include an increase in the number of primary cesareans and a decrease in the number of vaginal births after cesarean section (VBACs) (Martin et al., 2002). The rate is as high as 40% in some institutions (Curtin and Kozak, 1997).

B. Indications.

1. Maternal.

a. Cephalopelvic disproportion.
b. Failure to progress in labor.
c. Previous classic (vertical) uterine cesarean incision.
d. Pregnancy-induced hypertension.
e. Cardiac disease.
f. Diabetes.

  - **g.** Premature rupture of membranes with failed induction.
  - **h.** Active herpes.
- **2.** Placental.
  - **a.** Abruptio placentae.
  - **b.** Placenta previa.
  - **c.** Placental insufficiency.
- **3.** Fetal.
  - **a.** Distress.
  - **b.** Breech or other malpresentation.
  - **c.** Multifetal gestation.
  - **d.** Preterm delivery.

C. Potential complications.

- **1.** Maternal.
  - **a.** Infection.
  - **b.** Anemia.
  - **c.** Hemorrhage.
  - **d.** Morbidity and death from anesthesia.
  - **e.** Inadvertent operative injuries.
  - **f.** Pulmonary embolus and atelectasis.
  - **g.** Thrombophlebitis.
- **2.** Fetal/neonatal.
  - **a.** Asphyxia.
  - **b.** Preterm birth.
  - **c.** Respiratory distress syndrome caused by retained fluid in the lungs.
  - **d.** Persistent pulmonary hypertension (Levine et al., 2001).
  - **e.** Anemia from blood loss caused by incision of placenta and lack of full placental transfusion.

D. Assessment and management.

- **1.** Perform usual interventions to prepare woman for operative delivery.
- **2.** Notify infant's physician per policy.
- **3.** Give antacid if ordered.
- **4.** Remove fetal scalp electrode before surgery.
- **5.** Place wedge under woman's right hip to displace uterus to left to avoid supine hypotension and fetal hypoxia.
- **6.** Follow Neonatal Resuscitation Program (NRP) protocols for neonatal care following delivery.

REFERENCES

American College of Obstetricians and Gynecologists: Pregnant women should be screened for gestational diabetes. *ACOG News Release*, August 31, 2001. Retrieved January 25, 2003 from www.acog.org/from_home/publications/press_releases/nr08-31-01.cfm.

Benedetti, T.: Obstetric hemorrhage. In S. Gabbe, J. Niebyl, and J. Simpson (Eds.): *Obstetrics: Normal and problem pregnancies* (4th ed.). New York, 2002, Churchill Livingstone, pp. 503-538.

Briggs, G., Freeman, R., and Yaffe, S.: *Drugs in pregnancy and lactation: A reference guide to fetal and neonatal risk* (6th ed.). New York, 2002, Lippincott Williams & Wilkins.

Chamberlain, G. and Steer, P.: ABC of labour care: Obstetric emergencies. *British Medical Journal, 318*:1342-1345, 1999.

Corder-Mabe, J.: Complications of pregnancy. In E. Youngkin and M. Davis (Eds.): *Women's health: A primary care clinical guide* (2nd ed.). Upper Saddle River, NJ, 1998, Appleton & Lange, pp. 533-600.

Curtin, S. and Kozak, L.: Cesarean delivery rates in 1995 continue to decline in the United States. *Birth: Issues in Perinatal Care, 24*(3):194-196, 1997.

Enkin, M., Keirse, M., Neilson, J., et al.: *A guide to effective care in pregnancy and childbirth* (3rd ed.). New York, 2000, Oxford University Press.

Goldenberg, R.: The management of preterm labor. *Obstetrics and Gynecology, 100*(5): 1020-1037, 2002.

Hallak, M.: Hypertension in pregnancy. In D. James, P. Steer, C. Weiner, and B. Gonik (Eds.): *High risk pregnancy: Management options* (2nd ed.). New York, 2000, W.B. Saunders, pp. 639-663.

Hawkins, J., Chestnut, D., and Gibbs, C.: Obstetric anesthesia. In S. Gabbe, J. Niebyl, and J. Simpson (Eds.): *Obstetrics: Normal and problem pregnancies* (4th ed.). New York, 2002, Churchill Livingstone, pp. 431-472.

Iams, J.: Preterm birth. In S. Gabbe, J. Niebyl, and J. Simpson (Eds.): *Obstetrics: Normal and problem pregnancies* (4th ed.). New York, 2002, Churchill Livingstone, pp. 755-826.

Iams, J., Newman, R., Thom, E., et al.: Frequency of uterine contractions and the risk of spontaneous preterm delivery. *New England Journal of Medicine, 346*(4):250-255, 2002.

Johnson, T. and Niebyl, J.: Preconception and prenatal care: Part of the continuum. In S. Gabbe, J. Niebyl, and J. Simpson (Eds.): *Obstetrics: Normal and problem pregnancies* (4th ed.). New York, 2002, Churchill Livingstone, pp. 139-159.

Konje, J. and Taylor, D.: Bleeding in late pregnancy. In D. James, P. Steer, C. Weiner, and B. Gonik (Eds.): *High risk pregnancy: Management options* (2nd ed.). New York, 2000, W.B. Saunders, pp. 111-128.

Landon, M., Catalano, P., and Gabbe, S.: Diabetes mellitus and other endocrine diseases. In S. Gabbe, J. Niebyl, and J. Simpson (Eds.): *Obstetrics: Normal and problem pregnancies* (4th ed.). New York, 2002, Churchill Livingstone, pp. 1081-1116.

Landon, M. and Gabbe, S.: Diabetes in pregnancy. In D. James, P. Steer, C. Weiner, and B. Gonik (Eds.): *High risk pregnancy: Management options* (2nd ed.). New York, 2000, W.B. Saunders, pp. 665-684.

Lanni, S. and Seeds, J.: Malpresentations. In S. Gabbe, J. Niebyl, and J. Simpson (Eds.): *Obstetrics: Normal and problem pregnancies* (4th ed.). New York, 2002, Churchill Livingstone, pp. 473-501.

Levine, E., Ghai, V., Barton, J., and Strom, C.: Mode of delivery and risk of respiratory diseases in newborns. *Obstetrics and Gynecology, 97*(3):439-442, 2001.

Lieberman, P., Lang, J., Frigoletto, F., et al.: Epidural analgesia, intrapartum fever, and neonatal sepsis evaluation. *Pediatrics, 99*(3):415-419, 1997.

London, M., Ladewig, P., Ball, J., and Bindler, R.: *Maternal-newborn and child nursing: Family-centered care.* Upper Saddle River, NJ, 2003, Prentice Hall.

MacKay, A., Berg, C., and Atrash, H.: Pregnancy-related mortality from preeclampsia and eclampsia. *Obstetrics and Gynecology, 97*(4):533-538, 2001.

Martin, J., Hamilton, B., Ventura, S., et al.: Births: Final data for 2000. *National Vital Statistics Reports, 50*(5):February 12, 2002. Retrieved February 24, 2003 from www.cdc.gov/nchs/data/nvsr50/nvsr50_05.pdf.

Moore, K. and Persaud, T.: *The developing human: Clinically oriented embryology* (6th ed.). New York, 1998, Saunders.

Murray, M.: *Antepartal and intrapartal fetal monitoring.* Albuquerque, NM, 1997, Learning Resources International, Inc.

National Institute of Child Health & Human Development: Understanding gestational diabetes: A practical guide to a healthy pregnancy. *NICHD—Publications On-line.* Retrieved February 26, 2003 from www.nichd.nih.gov/publications/pubs/gest1.htm.

National Institutes of Health: Antenatal corticosteroids revisited: Repeat courses. *NIH Consensus Statement Online 2000 August 17-18,* 17(2):1-10, 2000. Retrieved January 25, 2003 from http://consensus.nih.gov/cons/112/112_statement.htm.

Norwitz, E., Robinson, J., and Repke, J.: Labor and delivery. In S. Gabbe, J. Niebyl, and J. Simpson (Eds.): *Obstetrics: Normal and problem pregnancies* (4th ed.). New York, 2002, Churchill Livingstone, pp. 353-394.

Penn, Z.: Breech presentation. In D. James, P. Steer, C. Weiner, and B. Gonik (Eds.): *High risk pregnancy: Management options* (2nd ed.). New York, 2000, Saunders, pp. 1025-1050.

Pillitteri, A.: *Maternal and child health nursing: Care of the childbearing and childrearing family* (4th ed.). New York, 2003, Lippincott Williams & Wilkins.

Poole, J.: Aggressive management of HELLP syndrome and eclampsia. *AACN Clinical Issues: Advanced Practice in Acute and Critical Care, 8*(4):November, 1977. Retrieved February 24, 2003 from www.aacn.org/AACN/jrnlci.nsf/GetArticle/ArticleThree84?Open Document.

Reeder, S., Martin, L., and Koniak-Griffin, D.: *Maternity nursing: Family, newborn, and women's health care* (18th ed.). New York, 1997, W.B. Saunders.

Ross, M., Ervin, M., and Novak, D.: Placental and fetal physiology. In S. Gabbe, J. Niebyl, and J. Simpson (Eds.): *Obstetrics: Normal and problem pregnancies* (4th ed.). New York, 2002, Churchill Livingstone, pp. 37-62.

Shah, A.: Preeclampsia and eclampsia. *Emedicine,* January 4, 2002. Retrieved January 25, 2003 from www.emedicine.com/neuro/topic323.htm.

Shua, S. and Arulkumaran, S.: Poor progress in labor including augmentation, malpositions, and malpresentations. In D. James, P. Steer, C. Weiner, and B. Gonik (Eds.): *High risk pregnancy: Management options* (2nd ed.). New York, 2000, W.B. Saunders, pp. 1103-1119.

Sibai, B.: Hypertension in pregnancy. In S. Gabbe, J. Niebyl, and J. Simpson (Eds.): *Obstetrics: Normal and problem pregnancies* (4th ed.). New York, 2002, Churchill Livingstone, pp. 945-1004.

Steer, P. and Danielian, P.: Fetal distress in labor. In D. James, P. Steer, C. Weiner, and B. Gonik (Eds.): *High risk pregnancy: Management options* (2nd ed.). New York, 2000, W.B. Saunders, pp. 1121-1149.

Svigos, J., Robinson, J., and Vigneswaran, R.: Threatened and actual preterm labor including mode of delivery. In D. James, P. Steer, C. Weiner, and B. Gonik (Eds.): *High risk pregnancy: Management options* (2nd ed.). New York, 2000, W.B. Saunders, pp. 999-1013.

Varney, H.: *Varney's midwifery* (3rd ed.). Boston, 1997, Jones and Bartlett.

Varney, H. and Reedy, N.: Screening for and collaborative management of antepartal complications. In H. Varney, (Ed.): *Varney's midwifery* (3rd ed.). Boston, Jones and Bartlett, 1997, pp. 327-377.

Von Der Pool, B.: Preterm labor: Diagnosis and treatment. *American Family Physician, 57*(10): 2457-2470, 1998.

Wilson, B., Shannon, M., and Stang, C.: *Nurse's drug guide 2002*. Upper Saddle River, NJ, 2002, Prentice Hall.

CHAPTER

3 Perinatal Substance Abuse

KATHLEEN PITTS

OBJECTIVES

1. Describe three behavioral or psychologic signs of an infant exposed to cocaine in utero.
2. Describe the effects of cocaine, alcohol, and tobacco abuse on lactation.
3. Describe three physical characteristics of an infant with a diagnosis of fetal alcohol syndrome (FAS).
4. List six nonpharmacologic nursing interventions appropriate for withdrawing infants.
5. List four psychologic characteristics of women who abuse substances and/or alcohol.
6. Discuss three suggested nursing interventions to use when working with mothers who abuse substances and/or alcohol.
7. List the five areas used to categorize symptoms of an infant with neonatal abstinence syndrome (NAS).

INTRODUCTION

1. "In the United States illicit drug use is the ninth leading contributing cause of death" (Ebrahim and Gfroerer, 2003). The use and abuse of licit and illicit drugs in society have increased alarmingly during the past 25 to 30 years. Patterns of alcohol and substance abuse have also changed and polydrug use has become more prevalent. Perinatal exposure is associated with high morbidity and mortality rates, and as a consequence, substance and alcohol abuse in pregnancy is a problem with devastating social, medical, and economic implications.
2. Half of women who use illicit drugs are of childbearing age (15-44 years). Data collected from the National Hospital Discharge Survey in the United States, between 1979 and 1990, identified a 576% increase in the number of drug-using parturient women. Five and one half percent (5.5%) of pregnant women continue to use illicit drugs and prenatal episodes of substance and alcohol use are not declining significantly. From 1996 to 1998, 1 of 14 U.S. women of childbearing age reported using illicit drugs in the past month and only one quarter of them had abstained from illicit use during the third trimester (Ebrahim and Gfroerer, 2003). When urine and meconium analysis is utilized, a three- to sixfold increase over maternal self-report is reported (urine, 13%-18%; meconium, 31%) (Nordstrom-Klee et al., 2002).
3. Prenatal care, drug treatment programs, and coordinated aftercare can make a significant difference in improving pregnancy and childhood outcomes. Key points to be aware of when working with mothers with a substance abuse disorder and their infants are that:

a. Polydrug use is more common than use of a single substance or alcohol alone.
b. Research and statistics on incidence and outcomes of the substance-exposed infant remain conflicting and controversial.
c. Outcomes of the substance-exposed infant are based on a multifactorial perspective (genetic, biologic, environmental, and social areas).
d. Short-term deficits may not be representative of long-term outcomes.
e. The overall adverse drug effects infants present with are subtle. The four areas targeted in all prenatal exposed infants are affect, attention, arousal, and action—termed the "four A's" of infancy (Lester and Tronick, 1994).
f. Evidence-based research must be included at all levels of the neonatal intensive care unit (NICU) and each nurse plays a vital part in furthering research development with ideas and problem-solving strategies.
g. Opportunities for changing the addicted woman's behavior and her view of health care providers can be influenced by the care she and her infant receive while hospitalized.

The following chapter presents the illicit drugs used in pregnancy and the adverse effects they have on the pregnancy, fetus, and neonate. Management recommendations and nursing interventions for both prenatal and postnatal care of mother and neonate are outlined. Finally, a brief overview of the general and psychologic profile of the substance-using mother, gender-specific treatment and aftercare needs, and ethical and legal issues is presented.

DRUGS OF ABUSE

Categories of drugs presented in first section include those in Box 3-1.

Tobacco and Nicotine

A. **Incidence of smoking in pregnancy.**
   1. Ranges from 15% to 20%.
   2. More than half of pregnant women (54%) who admitted to using illicit drugs in 1996 through 1998 also used tobacco and alcohol (Bennett, 1999; Ebrahim and Gfroerer, 2003).
   3. Rate of tobacco use is second to alcohol use.
   4. Adolescents (12-17 years of age) who smoke cigarettes are 12 times as likely to use illicit drugs and 23 times as likely to consume heavy amounts of alcohol.
   5. Whites smoke more heavily than blacks and Hispanics.

BOX 3-1
CATEGORIES OF DRUGS

Cannabinoids	Inhalants
Designer/club drugs	Narcotics/opioids
Ethyl alcohol	Sedatives/hypnotics
Hallucinogens	Stimulants
	Tobacco/nicotine

6. Environmental tobacco smoke (ETS):
   a. Reduces birth weight (BW) in nonsmoking mothers (Dejmek et al., 2002).
   b. Can further compromise high-risk infants by increasing long-term respiratory problems.

B. Pharmacology.
1. Tobacco is a central nervous system (CNS) stimulant.
2. The active constituents of cigarette smoke are nicotine, tar, carbon monoxide, and cyanide (approximately 4000 compounds found in cigarette smoke).
3. Nicotine is water and lipid soluble and crosses the placenta.
4. Carbon monoxide combines with hemoglobin to form carboxyhemoglobin. It is this form that impairs oxygenation for both the mother and fetus, yielding profound fetal hypoxia. Other effects are placental vasoconstriction and vasospasm.
5. There is a dose-related response between the number of cigarettes smoked and neonatal effects.

C. Effects on pregnancy (Mahoney and Larig, 2001).
1. Spontaneous abortion.
2. Placenta previa.
3. Abruptio placentae.
4. Preterm labor.
5. Premature rupture of membranes (PROM).
6. Cesarean section.

D. Effects on the fetus and newborn infant.
1. Increase in intrauterine growth restriction
   a. Decrease in BW (it declines as tobacco exposure increases, but is not a linear relation) (England et al., 2002; Secker-Walker and Vacek, 2003).
   b. Decrease in head circumference.
   c. Decrease in length.
2. Small increased risk of congenital malformations, including CNS malformations, hypospadias, inguinal hernia, eye and ear malformations, polycystic kidneys, aortopulmonary septum defects, gastroschisis, and skull deformities (Haustein, 1999).
3. Neurobehavioral effects suggesting that children exposed to prenatal nicotine do less well on tests of cognitive, psychomotor, language, and in general academic achievement.
4. Sudden infant death syndrome (SIDS) increased:
   a. with the number of cigarettes smoked (dose-dependent relationship observed) (Golding, 1997);
   b. in households with exposure to tobacco smoke before or after birth; and
   c. in those families in which only paternal smoking occurred (Dybing and Sanner, 1999).
5. Increased cost of hospitalization. "The smoking attributable neonatal cost in the U.S. represent almost $367 million in 1996 dollars; these costs range from less than a million in smaller states to over $35 million in California alone. All of these costs are preventable" (Adams et al., 2002).
6. Perinatal mortality was seen with an increase of 150% in women who smoke (Andres and Day, 2000).

E. Nursing considerations.
1. Regular documentation of all growth parameters.
2. Education regarding risk factors associated with SIDS. Recommend and encourage:
   a. Supine or side-lying position (with dependent arm pulled forward) for sleep.
   b. Head to remain uncovered during sleep.
   c. Smoke-free environment for infant.
   d. Avoidance by smokers of sharing bed with infant.
   e. Provide mother opportunity to complete infant cardiopulmonary resuscitation (CPR).
   f. Encourage all efforts for smoking cessation.

Alcohol

A. Incidence of alcohol use in pregnancy.
1. Combined 1999 and 2000 numbers indicate that 12.4% of pregnant women ages 15 to 44 years, used alcohol and 3.9% were binge drinkers. The number has been reported to be as high as 20% to 24% (Office of Applied Studies [OAS], 2000).
2. In the United States, 1995 incidence was 16.3% (up from 1991 estimates of 3.5%) (Centers for Disease Control and Prevention [CDC], 1997).

B. Pharmacology.
1. Alcohol is an anxiolytic analgesic with a depressant effect on the CNS.
2. Alcohol is absorbed rapidly from the stomach (20%) and the intestines (80%). It is metabolized by the liver (95%) and eliminated by the kidneys and lungs (both total 5%). Fetal ethanol concentration is eliminated only by maternal hepatic biotransformation.
3. Ethanol reaches the fetus through diffusion across the placental membranes and impairs normal placental function by altering the transfer of essential nutrients to the fetus. Ethanol is metabolized into acetaldehyde then to acetate. Acetaldehyde is more toxic than ethanol.
4. Alcohol is a teratogen. Effects in infants are directly related to dose levels, chronicity of alcohol use, gestational stage (timing of use), and duration of exposure (Polygenis et al., 1998).

C. Dosage of alcohol.
1. No safe level of alcohol consumption has been established for pregnant women. The American Academy of Pediatrics (AAP) Committee on Substance Abuse and Committee on Children with Disabilities (2000) statement reads, "Because there is no safe amount of alcohol consumption during pregnancy, abstinence from alcohol for women who are pregnant or who are planning a pregnancy is recommended."
2. Risk to the fetus appears greatest with:
   a. 3 ounces of absolute alcohol per day (equivalent to six standard drinks).
   b. Binge drinking (equivalent to 5 ounces or more at one sitting).
3. With lower levels of alcohol consumption, the degree and severity of effect on an infant are variable.
4. Short- and long-term outcome is associated with both chronicity and quantity. The most affected children are born to women in the chronic stages of alcoholism. Long-term outcomes have shown significant negative input in learning and memory skills at a 10-year follow-up (Richardson et al., 2002).

D. Effects on pregnancy.

1. Increase in spontaneous abortion (twofold to fourfold in moderate and heavy drinkers).
2. Increased risk of abruptio placentae.
3. Breech presentation: 70% of FAS newborns are delivered breech.
4. Decrease in abnormalities and growth restriction, which can be prevented when drinking ceases during any period of the pregnancy.

E. Effects on the fetus and neonate.

1. FAS is the leading cause of mental retardation, and the only preventable cause.
2. Incidence:
   a. One of the *Healthy People 2010* objectives (objective 16-18) targets a reduction in the occurrence of FAS. The CDC and five states (Alaska, Arizona, Colorado, New York, and Wisconsin) have collaboratively developed the Fetal Alcohol Syndrome Surveillance Network (FASSNet). The goal of the project is to monitor occurrence of FAS and to evaluate prevention, education, and intervention methods (*Morbidity and Mortality Weekly Report [MMWR],* 2002).
   b. In the United States during the 1980s and 1990s, FAS was estimated to be 0.5 to 2 per 1000 live births (0.08 per 1000 live births reported in other countries) (May and Gossage, 2001; Riley et al., 2003).
   c. The incidence of fetal alcohol effects (FAE) is 4 per 1000 live births. The combined rate of FAS, FAE, alcohol-related neurodevelopmental disorder (ARND), and alcohol-related birth defects (ARBD) may be as high as 9.1 per 1000 live births (Jones and Bass, 2003). Prevalence rate is 2.5 to 5.6 per 1000 live births among Native Americans/Alaskan Natives from two states (*MMWR,* 2002; National Institute on Alcohol Abuse and Alcoholism, 1991, 1994).
   d. FAS occurs in all socioeconomic groups with a higher incidence in low socioeconomic groups.
   e. Firstborn children appear less likely to have FAS than subsequent offspring, and there is significant risk (increase of 406 times) of a sibling having FAS, with a documented case in the family.
   f. Maternal risk factors associated with FAS, FAE, ARBD, or ARND include:
      (1) Advanced maternal age.
      (2) Low socioeconomic status.
      (3) Frequent binge drinking.
      (4) Family and friends with problems with alcohol.
      (5) Poor social and psychologic indicators.
3. Five diagnostic categories are used to describe effects of alcohol exposure:
   a. FAS with a confirmed history of maternal alcohol intake.
   b. FAS with phenotypic features but no confirmed history of maternal alcohol intake.
   c. Partial FAS—confirmed history of maternal alcohol intake, some facial abnormalities, and one of the following: CNS abnormalities, growth restriction, or behavioral or cognitive disabilities.
   d. ARBD—some adverse birth outcomes related to prenatal alcohol exposure. Congenital anomalies may include:
      (1) Cardiac: atrial or ventricular septal defects, tetralogy of Fallot.
      (2) Skeletal.
      (3) Renal: aplastic or dysplastic kidneys; hydronephrosis.

(4) Ocular: strabismus, optic nerve hypoplasia, increased tortuosity of the retinal vessels, impaired vision (Stromland and Pinazo-Duran, 2002).
(5) Auditory: conductive or neurosensory hearing loss.

e. ARND—CNS abnormalities related to prenatal alcohol exposure. CNS neurodevelopmental abnormalities in one of the following:
(1) Decreased cranial size at birth.
(2) Structural brain abnormalities (e.g., microcephaly, agenesis of corpus callosum, cerebellar hypoplasia).
(3) Neurologic signs: as age appropriate (e.g., impaired fine motor skills, neurosensory hearing loss, poor eye-hand coordination) (Hannigan and Armant, 2000).
(4) Evidence of behavior or cognitive abnormalities that are inconsistent with developmental level and unexplained by hereditary or environmental factors alone.

F. Neonatal withdrawal from alcohol.

1. Withdrawal symptoms from alcohol are relatively mild in comparison with infant narcotic withdrawal.
2. Onset is between birth and 12 hours after birth.
3. Symptoms include the following:
   a. hypertonia;
   b. tremors;
   c. opisthotonos;
   d. weak suck and poor feeding pattern.
4. Infants sleep little, cry more, and often engage in exaggerated mouthing behavior.

G. Nursing considerations.

1. Careful and thorough assessment.
2. Documentation of growth parameters (to include head circumference, length, and birth weight).
3. Careful examination of facial features over a period of tim
4. Regular neurologic assessment for symptoms of neonatal withdrawal patterns.
5. Genetics consultation is indicated should FAS be suspected.
6. Family counseling and assessment of parenting skills.

STIMULANTS

This class of drugs include: amphetamines; caffeine; cocaine, dextroamphetamines; methamphetamines (MDMA) [ecstasy]; crystal meth); and methylphenidates (Ritalin).

Cocaine

A. Incidence of cocaine use in pregnancy. The National Institute on Drug Abuse conducted the National Pregnancy and Health Survey in 1992 to 1993 surveying 4 million women who gave birth. The statistics showed that 221,000 women used illegal drugs during their pregnancy and 45,000 reported using cocaine. The Maternal Lifestyle Study, which included 8627 mother-infant pairs from May 1993 to May 1995, showed that 49% of women ages 18 to 25 years, 44% of women 26 to 35 years, and 8% of those 36 to 49 years, 13% admitted to having used cocaine and 59% used cocaine during their pregnancy (Klitsch, 2002).

Data from the National Household Survey on Drug Abuse collected 1996 to 1998 showed that 6.4% of nonpregnant women of childbearing age and 2.8% of pregnant women reported using illicit drugs. Of those that used illicit drugs,

28% abstained from drug use during the first trimester and 93% abstained during the third trimester. Only 24% abstained during the postpartum period, and approximately one tenth of the illicit drug users were using cocaine.

Cocaine prevalence during pregnancy declined from 1.1% in 1991 to 0.3% in 2000-2001 ($p = .04$) as reported by Buchi and colleagues (2003).

B. Pharmacology.

1. Cocaine is a CNS stimulant taken for its mood-altering properties.
2. It is one of the most powerful addicting substances of abuse.
3. It may be taken orally, sublingually, intranasally, intravenously, or inhaled ("crack").
4. Cocaine is derived from the leaves of the South and Central American plant *Erythroxylon coca*.
5. Crack cocaine is made by mixing cocaine powder with ammonia, water, and baking soda. The resulting mixture cracks when heated and releases the cocaine vapor, which is inhaled. Smoking crack offers a peak effect within 60 to 90 seconds, a high lasting only 5 to 10 minutes, and is the most popular form.
6. Cocaine is fat soluble, with a relatively low molecular weight, making passage through the blood-brain barrier and across the placenta very easy.
7. Cocaine is metabolized and made water soluble by plasma and liver cholinesterases for excretion in the urine. Metabolism is slower in the fetus and newborn infant with metabolites persisting in the infant's urine for 4 to 14 days (metabolites in an adult can be detected up to 72 hours in urine).
8. Cocaine inhibits the reuptake of both norepinephrine and dopamine. "The resulting excess of these neurotransmitters at the postsynaptic receptor sites results in a prolonged stimulation" (Ostrea, Jr. et al., 1994). The stimulation is what gives the euphoric "high." The hypothalamus is affected by the diminished reuptake of norepinephrine, causing a lack of appetite.
9. Peripheral vasoconstriction, tachycardia, hypertension, and hyperthermia are side effects that can lead to acute myocardial infarction, cerebrovascular accident, pulmonary edema, and renal and bowel infarction if heavy use continues.
10. Cocaine is rarely used alone; it is associated with polydrug use and should be a red flag for all health care providers.

C. Effects on pregnancy.

1. Use is associated with little to no prenatal care, which contributes to the poor pregnancy outcomes. Women are fearful about the legal ramifications to themselves and their children (present or future) if they present in a clinic to a professional. Medical complications related to maternal cocaine use include:
   a. Anorexia (decreased uptake of norepinephrine acts through the hypothalamus to decrease appetite).
   b. Anemia.
   c. Cardiac disease.
2. Sexually transmitted diseases or infections may be present.
   a. Gonorrhea.
   b. Syphilis.
   c. Hepatitis B (HBV).
   d. Hepatitis C (HCV, 4%-7% per pregnancy) (Yeung et al., 2001) increases four- to fivefold with HBV coinfection.
   e. Human immunodeficiency virus (HIV) infection.

■ BOX 3-2
■ **OBSTETRIC EFFECTS OF COCAINE**

Abruptio placentae
Fetal hypoxia and stillbirth
Meconium staining
Precipitous delivery
Pregnancy-induced hypertension
Preterm labor
Spontaneous abortion

Two major side effects of cocaine use—vasoconstriction and hypertension—are responsible for most of the following adverse complications (Box 3-2):

D. Effects on the fetus and neonate.

1. Suggested that cocaine may be a teratogen with deformities cited including:
   a. Genitourinary tract abnormalities.
   b. Cranial defects.
   c. Cardiac anomalies, particularly ventricular septal defect.
   d. Bowel atresia (ileal).
   e. Terminal limb defects (upper limbs).
   f. Prune belly syndrome.
   g. Ambiguous genitalia (Church et al., 1998).
2. Intrauterine growth restriction resulting in low birth weight, decreased head circumference, and decreased length. Low birth weight more affected by heavier cocaine use (Hulse et al., 1997). A negative relationship is seen with the amount of cocaine used in the third trimester and infant head circumference and length (Eyler et al., 1998).
3. Fetal depression during labor may promote meconium aspiration or persistent pulmonary hypertension (PPHN) after delivery.
4. Cerebrovascular accident, intraventricular hemorrhage, and infarction due to precipitous labor and delivery.
5. Increased risk of SIDS.

E. Neonatal withdrawal from cocaine.

1. Signs of CNS irritability after birth are considered to be an effect of cocaine rather than withdrawal. Infants may be restless, irritable, tremulous, and hypertonic.
2. Following an initial hyperirritability period, infant may exhibit drowsiness and/or lethargy.
3. Changes in behavioral state displayed may include:
   a. Difficulty in responding to the human voice and face.
   b. Maintenance of alert states with difficulty, alternating between periods of sleep and agitation.
   c. Depressed interactive behaviors and poor responses to environmental stimuli.
   d. Poor response to comforting by caregivers.
   e. Startle that is easily elicited.
   f. Rapid change in state.
   g. Distressed easily (exhibited by rapid respirations, frantic gaze aversion, color changes, and/or disorganized motor activity
4. Neuromotor deficits may include hyper- or hypotonic muscle tone, abnormal movements, and abnormal suck-swallow pattern (causing poor feeding).

F. Limited follow-up studies.

1. Controversial research findings suggest that a high-risk environment may play more a role in cognitive and behavioral deficits than prenatal exposure (Keller and Snyder-Keller, 2000). Maternal psychologic function has been found to have influenced the overall functional outcome of the child (Accornero et al., 2002).
2. Improvement in state control abilities seen at 1 month.
3. Hypertonia may persist for up to 2 years. Infants with cocaine-related hypertonia exhibit lower cognitive scores.
4. Weight and length normalize at 1 year of age, but head circumference remains smaller throughout first 2 years of life.
5. Significant effects on cognitive development seen at 2 years; however, child is twice as likely to have significant delay. No significant motor delay seen (Singer et al., 2002).
6. No significant adverse effects based on level of cocaine exposure on the Mental Development Index (MDI), Psychomotor Development Index (PDI), or Infant Behavior Record of the Bayley Scales of Infant Development (Frank et al., 2002).

G. Nursing considerations.

1. Hospital costs for cocaine-exposed infants have been estimated to be $5200 more than for nonexposed infants.
2. Symptom management usually does not require pharmacologic intervention.
3. Address the needs of prematurity more than substance exposure.
4. Keep environmental stimuli to a minimum.
5. Provide swaddling and frequent small feeds as needed.
6. Arrange for supportive care for the mother prior to discharge.

Amphetamines (3,4-methylenedioxymethamphetamine [MDMA])

A. Incidence of amphetamine use in general population and pregnancy.
In the 1998 National Household Survey on Drug Abuse (NHSDA), it was reported that an estimated 1.5% (3.4 million) of Americans had used MDMA at least once during their lifetime. The heaviest use (5% or 1.4 million people) was reported for those between the ages of 18 and 25 years.

- MDMA has been shown to have steady growth in use (particularly in women) and popularity (eightfold increase of use in Canada since 1993).
- MDMA is inexpensive and easy to access.
- MDMA appeals to a younger age group of users.
- There is a high incidence of polydrug use in this population (tobacco, alcohol, binge drinking).

B. Pharmacology.

1. Amphetamines are a group of drugs that act as CNS stimulants. Sympathomimetic drugs usually are used for appetite suppression, weight loss, depression, hyperkinesis, and treatment of narcolepsy.
2. Consists of amphetamine, dextroamphetamine, methamphetamine, MDMA, ("ecstasy," Adam, bean, E, M, roll, X, XTC, and lovers' speed), crystal methamphetamine (batu, crystal, glass, hiropon, ice, shabu, shards, Tina, ventano, and vidrio), and methylphenidate (Ritalin).
3. Amphetamines can be inhaled, injected, smoked, or taken orally.
4. They are neurotoxic.
5. They cause vasoconstriction and hypertension.

6. Intense physical and psychologic exhilaration is produced. Duration of 2 to 14 hours is dependent on dose. Effects are similar to those of cocaine.
7. MDMA reclassified as a Schedule I drug in 1985 and is now a banned substance. (MDMA is an amphetamine that has hallucinogenic properties similar to mescaline).
8. Crystal methamphetamine is a colorless, odorless form of d-methamphetamine, also a powerful stimulant. Is often compared with crack cocaine because it produces similar physiologic effects. It may be inhaled or injected with the effect lasting up to 12 hours (U.S. Department of Justice, 2002).

C. **Effects on pregnancy.**
1. Prematurity, abruptio placentae, hypertension, cardiac arrhythmias, myocardial infarction, clefting, and fetal growth restriction deficits (Plessinger, 1998).
2. When teratogenicity has been produced in human studies, only a small increase was documented in the following: CNS and cardiac anomalies/defects (26 per 1000 life births), cleft palate, limb reduction and/or musculoskeletal anomalies (38 per 1000 life births), and congenital defects have been found (McElhatton et al., 1999).

D. **Effects on the fetus and neonate.**
1. Intrauterine growth restriction (low birth weight, length, and head circumference).
2. Animal studies have shown varying results that indicate some teratogenicity (CNS and cardiac defects) (Colado et al., 1997).
3. High incidence of retroplacental hemorrhage.

E. **Neonatal withdrawal from amphetamines.**
1. Characterized by abnormal sleep patterns, poor feeding, tremors, abnormal weight gains, and state disorganization.
2. Diaphoresis, episodes of agitation alternating with lassitude, miosis, and vomiting can occur shortly after birth.
3. Frantic fist sucking, high-pitched cry, loose stools, fever, yawning, hyperreflexia, and excoriation when both cocaine and amphetamines were used.

F. **Nursing considerations.**
1. Provide supportive care to the mother. Refer to social services to assist with underlying psychologic morbid issues.
2. Promote and facilitate frequent and positive visits with infant.

CANNABINOIDS

Marijuana

A. **Incidence of marijuana use.** The most commonly used illicit drug, and usually used in conjunction with other drugs or alcohol, with estimated overall incidence of 4.8% to 5.4% for the U.S. population.

B. **Pharmacology.**
1. Marijuana has both depressant and mild hallucinogenic effects on the CNS.
2. It is usually smoked in a cigarette or pipe; alternatively, can be cooked in biscuits or cakes.
3. It comes from dried leaves and flowering tops of the plant *Cannabis sativa*.
4. Hashish is more potent and is prepared by drying and compressing the resin of flowering tops and leaves of the female cannabis plant.

5. The psychoactive ingredient is tetrahydrocannabinol (THC), which has high affinity for lipids and accumulates in the fatty tissues throughout the body.
6. Placental transfer is highest in the first trimester of pregnancy.
7. Smoking marijuana increases the blood carbon monoxide level and may result in hypoxia.
8. The THC content in marijuana has changed from the 1960s by fifteenfold. Therefore the risks and consequences of this strength cannot be equated to studies performed in the past.

C. **Effects on pregnancy.**
1. Harm associated with the same adverse effects as those who use tobacco.
2. Effects are limited, inconsistent, and conflicting. Controversial issues relate to:
   a. Length of gestation (shortened).
   b. Duration of labor and outcome (preterm delivery).

D. **Effects on the fetus and neonate.**
1. Limited studies have been conducted with controversial findings including:
   a. Congenital anomalies.
   b. Intrauterine growth restriction due to increase in carboxyhemoglobin.
   c. Some evidence of neonatal withdrawal (tremulousness, alterations of sleep patterns, prolonged startle, high-pitched cry) but usually does not persist beyond 1 month.
   d. Significant association between SIDS and paternal marijuana use in all periods (Klonoff-Cohen and Lam-Kruglick, 2001).

NARCOTICS AND OPIOIDS

This class includes: (a) natural opioids: morphine and opium; (b) semisynthetic opioids: heroin, methadone; and (c) synthetic opioids: propoxyphene (Darvon), Dilaudid (hydromorphone hydrochloride), oxycodone (OxyContin).

A. **Incidence of opiate use in pregnancy.**
1. In 2000 heroin was ranked second to cocaine as the most serious drug problem by 20% of the Pulse Check sources (Pulse Check is a grouping of cities that are part of the Committee of Epidemiologic Workshop Group sponsored by National Institute on Drug Abuse (NIDA) investigating different aspects of substance use and trends).
2. Heroin increased from 22% in 1999 to 26% in 2000 as a serious drug problem.
3. There are no current national prevalence data that give accurate statistics on heroin drug use by pregnant women in the United States. However, it has been estimated that each year between 100,000 and 375,000 women use illicit drugs during pregnancy.
4. Among pregnant women ages 15 to 44 years, 3.3% reported using illicit drugs in the month prior to interview (based on the combined 1999 and 2000 NHSDA samples). This rate is significantly lower than the rate among nonpregnant women ages 15 to 44 years (7.7%). Among pregnant women ages 15 to 17 years, the rate of use was 12.9%, nearly equal to the rate for nonpregnant women of the same age (13.5%).
5. In California in 1992 1.1% of urine samples from pregnant women were positive for cocaine and 1.4% positive for opiates. Black women had the highest rates: 7.8% for cocaine and 2.5% for opiates. NIDA has reported that as of December 1999, data from 20 cities in the United States have shown a

trend in which marijuana and heroin abuse had increased (Office of Applied Studies [OAS], Samhsa, 2000).
6. In a 2001 report from the Substance Abuse and Mental Health Services Administration (SAMHSA), approximately 4% of pregnant women between the ages of 15 and 44 years reported being current users of illicit drugs. There was a nearly equal rate of drug use for pregnant and nonpregnant women ages 15 to 17 years of age (pregnant, 15.1% and nonpregnant, 14.1%).
7. Heroin and methadone are the two most commonly used narcotics in the United States.
8. There has been an increase in oxycodone use and emergency department visits in the United States (89% between 1993 and 1999; increase in 68% in 2000) (U.S. Department of Justice, 2001).

B. Pharmacology.

1. Opiates are CNS depressants.
2. They are derived from the opium poppy, *Papaver somniferum*.
3. Heroin is a semisynthetic opiate that may be sniffed, smoked, or injected.
4. Heroin is quick acting and produces a sense of euphoria within 10 seconds after injection.
5. Heroin is much stronger than morphine and readily crosses the placental barrier.
6. Methadone, a synthetic opiate, is usually taken orally but can be injected. Methadone also crosses the placental barrier.
7. Methadone is absorbed slowly and has a long duration of action, making it suitable for treatment of heroin addicts.
8. Methadone in pregnancy is preferred to heroin because:
   a. The drug level delivered to the fetus is more stable and reduces the risk of fetal withdrawal.
   b. There is less risk of infection from the use of contaminated needles.
9. Opiates interfere with the normal menstrual cycle, thereby reducing fertility. Many addicted women do not realize they are pregnant until between the fifth and seventh months.
10. Oxycodone is manufactured by modifying thebaine, an alkaloid found in opium. It is an opiate agonist, used for moderate to high pain relief and is highly addictive. (Trade names are Percocet, Percodan, Tylox, and OxyContin.)

C. Effects on pregnancy.

1. Pregnant addicts may present with a number of medical complications related to their drug use:
   a. Anorexia.
   b. Anemia.
   c. Cardiac disease.
   d. Thrombosis.
   e. Abscesses.
2. Sexually transmitted diseases or infections may also be present:
   a. Gonorrhea.
   b. Syphilis.
   c. Hepatitis B and C.
   d. HIV.
3. Women may be polydrug abusers.
4. Many of the effects of opiate use in pregnancy are correlated directly to the amount of prenatal care received and the maternal lifestyle, rather than to the drug itself.

5. Morbidity and mortality rates are lower in infants born to methadone-dependent women who have adequate prenatal care.
6. Spontaneous abortions are common.
7. Obstetric complications include (Box 3-3):

D. **Effects on the fetus and neonate.**
1. Hypoxia due to an unstable intrauterine environment and reduction in placental blood flow.
2. Lower Apgar scores.
3. NAS. Concern about the administration of naloxone, a narcotic antagonist for respiratory depression, has been raised. Rapid withdrawal and seizures may result, and urgent treatment for withdrawal may be needed (American Academy of Pediatrics Committee on Drugs, 1998).
4. Meconium aspiration and aspiration pneumonia.
5. Intrauterine growth restriction.
6. Lower incidence of respiratory distress syndrome.
7. Lower degrees of physiologic jaundice.
8. Congenital infections.
9. Increased incidence of SIDS.
10. Low birth weight.
11. Microcepahly.
12. Increased chromosomal aberrations (heroin-only exposed infants).

E. **Results of follow-up studies.**
Inconsistent. May be alterations in physical growth and in neurologic, behavioral, and cognitive functioning in early infancy and childhood (Hans and Jeremy, 2001; Kenner and D'Apolito, 1997).

F. **Comparison of methadone with heroin.**
1. With adequate prenatal care in a low-dose methadone program, perinatal outcome is improved in terms of prematurity, fetal loss, and medical complications (Dashe et al., 2002).
2. Both groups of infants present with low birth weight; however, methadone infants are generally larger (Hulse et al., 1997).
3. Infants exposed to both methadone and heroin may exhibit signs of NAS. However, NAS usually occurs later in infants exposed to methadone because it is stored in the fetal lung, liver, and spleen and metabolized after birth. Very little heroin is stored by the fetus (Weiner and Finnegan, 1998).

SEDATIVES/HYPNOTICS

This class of drugs includes barbituates (Seconal, Nembutal, Amytal, Tuinal, phenobarbital) and benzodiazepines (Valium, Librium, Xanax, Halcion, Ativan).

BOX 3-3
OBSTETRIC COMPLICATIONS OF METHADONE

Toxemia	Precipitous delivery
Abruptio placentae	Breech delivery
Premature labor	Fetal distress
Shorter than average labor	Stillbirth

Street names include downers, ludes, sopers, trenks, 714s, yellow jackets, reds, blues, rainbow.

A. **Incidence of sedative and hypnotic use.**
   1. Not generally the primary drug of abuse. Used to induce sleep or to decrease anxiety related to alcohol withdrawal or to accentuate effects of alcohol or other drugs.
   2. Popular to use and desired due to no outward signs of use; no odor detected.

B. **Pharmacology.**
   1. Benzodiazepines largely replaced short-acting barbituates in the 1960s. They are used in combination with alcohol for a sedative effect or to take the edge off withdrawal from cocaine.
   2. They act on the CNS but without significant CNS depression. Also they alter the balance of the neurotransmitter, gamma-aminobutyric acid (GABA), in the limbic system of the brain-regulating emotional state.
   3. Onset is 30 to 45 minutes and can last for 3 to 5 hours. Its half-life in adults is 20 to 60 hours and can be four times longer in neonates (mean plasma half-life in neonate is about 31 hours).
   4. They are highly addictive.

C. **Effects on pregnancy and effects on the fetus and neonate.**
   1. They are readily transmitted across the placenta; concentration in fetal blood is similar to maternal circulation due to high lipid solubility.
   2. Substantial accumulation may occur in adipose tissue; a high concentration also is present in the brain, lungs, and heart.
   3. Side effects may include abortion, malformations, intrauterine growth restriction (IUGR), functional deficits, carcinogenesis, and mutagenesis (Iqbal et al., 2002).
   4. Fetuses exposed to long-acting benzodiazepines on a long-term basis showed neonatal hypotonicity, failure to feed, and/or withdrawal syndrome (Perault et al., 2000).
   5. There is inconsistent research showing risk of congenital malformations.
   6. Regular use of benzodiazepines in mothers showed infants who had side effects similar to FAS.

INHALANTS

Examples of inhalants include benzene, Freon, gasoline and lighter fluid, and nitrous oxide, shoe polish, toluene, and typewriter correction fluid.

A. **Pharmacology.**
   1. Two main categories:
      a. volatile solvents and aerosols (solvents: glue [toluene], typewriter correction fluid, and gasoline; aerosols: spray paint and cooking sprays).
      b. nitrites (amyl nitrites [poppers, snappers], butyl nitrite, isopropyl nitrite [rush, locker room], and nitrous oxide [laughing gas, whippets].
   2. CNS depressants that cause alcohol-like intoxication symptoms.
   3. Short-acting heart stimulant and vasodilator. Nitrites decrease blood pressure, increase heart rate, and reduce oxygen flow to brain.
   4. Effects take place immediately (30-60 seconds) and can last 15 minutes to several hours.
   5. Readily cross the placenta.

B. Effects on pregnancy.

1. Long-term use results in:
   - **a.** accidents (due to memory loss, heightened sense of power, judgment problems).
   - **b.** tissue damage (permanent damage to brain, bone marrow, liver, kidneys, and other major organs).
   - **c.** sudden "sniffing" death (related to cardiac failure).
   - **d.** suffocation (when plastic bags are used to inhale solvent vapors).
2. Excessive use may cause glaucoma, blood cell damage (can trigger methemoglobinemia), acquired immunodeficiency syndrome (AIDS) and rupture of lungs (if high pressure tank is used).

C. Effects on the fetus and neonate.

1. Fetal dysmorphogenesis syndrome (similar to FAS) has been associated with these exposures.
2. High concentrations of *toluene* exposure have been reported to include the following deficits: small for gestational age (SGA), microcephalic, short palpebral fissures, deep-set eyes, small face, low-set ears, micrognathia, spatulate fingertips, small fingernails, developmental delay, language impairment, hyperactivity, and cerebellar dysfunction (Jones and Balster, 1997).

D. Neonatal abstinence syndrome (NAS). Neonatal abstinence is described as a generalized disorder characterized by 21 signs most commonly seen in withdrawing infants (Finnegan, 1990) (see Table 3-1).

1. More than two thirds of neonates born to opiate-dependent women will exhibit signs of NAS.

TABLE 3-1
Neonatal Signs of Withdrawal

System	Sign
Neurologic	Hypertonia
	Tremors
	Hyperreflexia
	Irritability and restlessness
	High-pitched cry
	Sleep disturbances
	Seizures
Autonomic	Yawning
	Nasal stuffiness
	Sweating
	Sneezing
	Low-grade fever
	Skin mottling
Gastrointestinal	Diarrhea
	Vomiting
	Poor feeding
	Regurgitation
	Dysmature swallowing
	Excessive sucking
Respiratory	Tachypnea
Miscellaneous	Skin excoriation
	Behavioral irregularities

2. Onset varies from shortly after birth to 2 weeks of age, depending on the type and quantity of substances used; timing and dose of drug(s) before delivery; nature of labor; type of anesthesia or analgesia during labor; and maturity and nutritional status of infant.
3. Majority of signs appear within 72 hours of birth (see Table 3-2).
4. Duration ranges from 8 to 16 weeks or longer.
5. Presentation of NAS is variable. It can be mild and transient, intermittent, delayed in onset, or waver between acute and subacute withdrawal.
6. Chronic drug users have more severe withdrawal.
7. The closer to delivery the drug is taken, the greater the delay of onset and the more severe the signs (Weiner and Finnegan, 1998).
8. NAS is milder in the preterm infant.

E. **Neonatal Abstinence Scoring System (Finnegan score).**
1. The Neonatal Abstinence Scoring System assists in the detection of the onset of withdrawal symptoms and charts the progression and response to therapeutic intervention (see Table 3-3).
2. The scoring system can be used to assess withdrawal from both opioid and nonopioid CNS depressants (Weiner and Finnegan, 1998).
3. Assess all high-risk infants 2 hours after birth and then every 4 hours.
4. If, at any point, the score is 8 or greater, the scoring should be initiated every 2 hours and should be continued for a minimum of 24 hours.
5. If pharmacotherapy is not required, the infant is scored for the first 96 hours of life.
6. If the infant scores 8 or higher on *three* consecutive scoring times, the infant should be evaluated for pharmacotherapy.
7. NAS symptoms often mimic common neonatal metabolic conditions (such as hypoglycemia, hypocalcemia, sepsis, and meningitis). A complete blood cell count and calcium and glucose levels are recommended before therapy is initiated.

F. **Pharmacologic treatment of NAS.**
1. Approximately 50% to 60% of infants exposed in utero to opiates will require pharmacologic intervention (Weiner and Finnegan, 1998).
2. Begin pharmacologic treatment only when withdrawal is not controlled by supportive measures.
3. Pharmacologic agents used to treat NAS are provided in Table 3-4.
4. Opiates are used for NAS due to opiate exposure; sedatives for nonopiate or polydrug exposure (Osborn et al., 2003).
5. Oral morphine is the opiate of choice. The second-line drugs are paregoric and tincture of opium (used less because of their high alcohol content).

TABLE 3-2
Onset of Drug Withdrawal Symptoms after Delivery

Drug	Onset of Withdrawal Symptoms after Delivery
Alcohol	3-12 hours after delivery
Narcotics (heroin, methadone)	48-72 hours; may be as late as 4 weeks
Barbiturates	4-7 days on average (1-14 days possible)
Cocaine	48-72 hours

Source: American Academy of Pediatrics Committee on Drugs: Neonatal drug withdrawal, *Pediatrics, 101*(6), pp. 1079-1088, 1998.

TABLE 3-3
Neonatal Abstinence Scoring System

	Score			
Signs	**0**	**1**	**2**	**3**
Tremors (muscle activity of limbs)	Normal	Minimally ↑ when hungry or disturbed	Moderate or marked ↑ when undisturbed, subside when fed or held snugly	Marked even when undisturbed, going on to seizurelike movements
Irritability (excessive crying)	None	Slightly ↑	Moderate to severe when disturbed or hungry	Marked even when undisturbed
Reflexes	Normal	Increased	Markedly increased	
Stools	Normal	Explosive, but normal frequency	Explosive, more than 8/day	
Muscle tone	Normal	Increased	Rigidity	
Skin abrasions	No	Redness of knees and elbows	Breaking of skin	
Respiratory rate/minute	<55	55-75	76-95	
Repetitive sneezing	No	Yes		
Repetitive yawning	No	Yes		
Vomiting	No	Yes		
Fever	No	Yes		

Scoring: Identification of newborn with narcotic withdrawal when score >17 (78% probability).
Source: Lipsitz, P.J.: A proposed narcotic withdrawal score for use with newborn infants: A pragmatic evaluation of its efficacy. *Clinical Pediatrics, 14*(6):592-594, 1975.

6. Opiates do not make the infant drowsy or interfere with infant feeding. They are effective for controlling a variety of gastrointestinal disturbances.
7. Once withdrawal is controlled, pharmacologic treatment can be gradually weaned.
8. Control is defined as meeting the following conditions:
   a. Scores of 8 or less.
   b. Infant is easily consoled.
   c. Infant maintains a rhythmic sleep and feeding cycle.
   d. Steady weight gain.

G. **Iatrogenic NAS.**
   1. Opiates are used extensively in the care of critically ill neonates and infants as analgesics and sedatives to assist in ventilation.
   2. Abrupt cessation of these drugs may result in signs of withdrawal following prolonged use.
   3. It is recommended to wean from opiates with the assistance of the same neonatal abstinence scoring system.

MANAGEMENT RECOMMENDATIONS

A. **Document maternal drug use.** Review history, drug of choice, and pattern during prenatal period.

■ TABLE 3-4
■ ■ **Drugs Used to Reduce Opioid Withdrawal in Neonates**

Name	Dosing	Recommendations
Tincture of opium	0.1 ml/kg or 2 drops/kg with feedings every 4 hours After 3 to 5 days stabilization, taper by decreasing dose without altering frequency	Preferred over paregoric; 25-fold dilution contains same concentration of morphine found in paregoric
Paregoric	0.1 ml/kg or 2 drops/kg with feedings every 4 hours; may be increased by 2 drops/kg every 3 to 4 hours until stabilized After 3 to 5 days stabilization, taper by decreasing dose without altering frequency	Infants have greater physiologic sucking and weight gain Use of paregoric declined because of potential toxic effects of ingredients
Morphine	Parenteral: 0.1 mg/kg Oral: 4 mg/ml	Oral route provides less analgesic than parenteral Respiratory depressant; can be life threatening
Methadone	0.05 to 0.1 mg/kg every 6 hours with increases of 0.05 mg/kg until stable After controlled, dose every 12 to 24 hours Discontinue after weaning to 0.05 mg/kg/day	Treat NAS from opioid withdrawal
Clonidine	Oral: 0.5 to 1.0 mg/kg single dose Maintenance: 3-5 mg/kg/day in divided doses every 4-6 hours	May have immediate reversal of symptoms Treatment shorter than phenobarbital Oral liquid not available
Chlorpromazine	IM/PO: 0.55 mg/kg every 6 hours	CNS and GI signs produced by withdrawal are controlled Multiple side effects
Phenobarbital	Loading dose: 16 mg/kg per 24 hours Maintenance: 2 to 8 mg/kg per 24 hours When stabilized, decrease by 10 to 25% per day Blood levels 24 to 48 hours after loading dose: 20 to 30 mg/ml	Good choice for nonnarcotic-related withdrawal signs Does not relieve GI symptoms
Diazepam	1 to 2;mg every 8 hours	Multiple side effects

NAS, Neonatal abstinence syndrome; *CNS,* central nervous system; *GI,* gastrointestinal; *IM,* intramuscular; *PO,* by mouth.
Source: Naegle, M.A. and D'Avanzo, M.A.: *Addictions and substance abuse: Strategies for advanced practice nursing.* Upper Saddle River, NJ, 2001, Prentice Hall, p. 244. Adapted from American Academy of Pediatrics Committee on Drugs: Neonatal drug withdrawal, *Pediatrics, 101*(6):1079-1088, 1998.

B. Obtain toxicology screening for all infants when there is a moderate to strong suspicion of use. For urine, obtain the earliest urine possible. Consent may be needed in some states. Follow the Health Insurance Portability and Accountability Act (HIPAA) guidelines set by your institution.

C. Consider HIV testing pending the mother's consent and your hospital's policy. If no prenatal care, HIV testing may be part of admission maternal serology panel.

D. **If a careful physical examination reveals abnormalities, investigate further.** Any malformations, growth restriction, or microcephaly noted is cause for additional screening for congenital infections and possible referral to genetics or dysmorphologist on staff.
E. **Obtain additional tests.** Follow unit protocol to obtain cranial and renal ultrasound, electroencephalogram (EEG), visual evoked response, ophthalmologic examination, and brainstem auditory evoked response prior to discharge.
F. **Observe carefully and monitor consistently** for signs of feeding intolerance and difficulty. Observe mother during feeding and offer helpful suggestions.
G. **Evaluate for signs of withdrawal** (see Table 3-3).
H. **Counsel and educate the mother regarding breast-feeding.** Provide lactation specialist referral in-house and support group contact numbers.
I. **Initiate a careful and comprehensive plan of care for discharge.** Attention to maintaining continuity of care after discharge for both mother and infant is imperative (Payot and Berner, 2000).
J. **Consult with social services and other health care providers (HCPs).** Make referrals to appropriate agencies or for foster care, if needed (this includes all cases of FAS/FAE). The mother must be clearly informed of all medical, social, and legal circumstances regarding her and the infant. Consider using a translation service (or designated person in the hospital—not a family member) if there is any doubt about language competency. This process needs to be well documented in the medical chart.

NURSING INTERVENTION

A. **The infant.** Each infant presents with a variable prenatal history, delivery scenario, and response to the environment. Table 3-5 provides strategies that the nurse and parent can use to help ease the prenatal exposure to drug sequelae in the neonatal nursery, newborn nursery, and at home.
B. **Mother-nurse interactions.**
   1. Nurses must confront their own feelings regarding these issues. Many nurses still harbor punitive and negative attitudes toward these mothers, rather than positive and supportive ones (Selleck and Redding, 1998).
   2. Addiction is a chronic disease requiring ongoing health care intervention. All patients should be treated in a professional manner. Nurses need to be knowledgeable about substance exposure and addiction theories to be effective change agents with mothers and the family.
   3. Develop a therapeutic relationship with the mother by establishing trust. Proceed slowly and take cues from the mother at a comfortable pace for her.
   4. Provide consistency in caregivers, preferably with a primary nurse or team. Provide support to the mother by being present during dialogs, rounds, and consults with neonatologists and other health care providers. Help her interpret what she heard in terms understandable to her.
   5. Provide clear information and specific guidelines for expected behavior of both mother and infant. Provide mother with realistic expectations of infant's behavior and progress. Be sensitive to the fact that repeated explanation of skills or information already presented in the past may be required.
   6. Present truthful information and education in a nonjudgmental manner while allowing opportunity for the mother's concerns, fears, and questions to be addressed.

TABLE 3-5

Strategies for Caring for Infants Prenatally Exposed to Drugs

Infant Behavior	Behavior Description	Strategies
Vomiting or poor feeding	Infants frequently display gastrointestinal difficulties throughout their first year of life. Vomiting is frequent during the first 6 to 9 months, as are intermittent constipation and diarrhea. These difficulties tend to increase irritability and discomfort. If allowed, some infants sleep up to 20 hours per day during the first 6 months of life and miss feedings. They are therefore at risk for inadequate nutrition and failure to thrive.	■ If necessary, wake infant for feeding. ■ Give small quantities of food. ■ Allow infant to rest frequently during feeding. ■ Have infant upright for feeding. After feeding, place infant in side-lying or prone position to prevent aspiration of milk. ■ If infant vomits, clean skin immediately to prevent irritation from stomach acid.
Uncoordinated sucking and swallowing	A variety of abnormal oral-motor behaviors have been observed, including a preemie-like suck pattern, poorly coordinated suck/swallow patterns, inability to stabilize tongue in midline, and (occasionally) tongue thrusting and tongue tremors. These abnormal patterns increase feeding time. Consequently, a great deal of infant energy is required, and stress and frustration may occur in mother and infant.	■ Hold infant in sitting position with arms forward in slight trunk flexion (curve) during feeding. ■ Keep infant's chin tucked downward. Infants prenatally exposed to drugs often push head back, which causes an abnormal swallow pattern. ■ If sucking is difficult for infant, support infant's chin or chin and cheeks with your hand. ■ Play soft, rhythmic music to help infant relax and to facilitate rhythmic sucking.
Weak pull-to-sit development	Infants often are slow learning pull-to-sit movement; frequently, it is accomplished with head lag or excessive effort after 6 months of age. (Infants normally pull-to-sit with no head lag by 4 months.) Some prenatally exposed to drugs who are able to pull-to-sit with no head lag may compensate by pulling their arms back into a strong *W* position. Usually pull-to-sit is accomplished with arms forward and some trunk flexion. The skill is a developmental milestone that indicates abdominal and neck muscle strength; it later affects the quality and endurance of balance, sitting, walking, and protective reflexes.	■ Move infant from supine to sitting position, supporting the head so that it does not lag. ■ While moving infant into sitting position, support shoulders close to infant's body with head forward (neck flexion). With infant semireclined (45° angle), encourage infant to assist with pull-to-sit. Give additional head support if needed to prevent head lag and bring infant's arms forward into midline position. ■ Place infant in supported sitting position, and move infant slowly backward within the range of head control. Then slowly rock or move infant back and forth to strengthen neck and abdominal muscles.
Irritability and difficulty sleeping	Exposure to drugs in utero can cause infant's state to vary from highly irritable to very passive. Most of these infants, however, are highly irritable and often have difficulty sleeping. Irritable infants can reach a frantic-cry state, which needs to be avoided. If infant is passive, interaction needs to take place during quiet alert, not hyperalert, states. Caregivers need to monitor their interactions by	■ Reduce noise in environment. ■ Turn down lights. ■ Swaddle infant in a cotton blanket in flexed position with arms close to body. ■ Hold swaddled infant close. ■ Put infant in bunting-type wrapper and carry close to body.

Continued

TABLE 3-5
Strategies for Caring for Infants Prenatally Exposed to Drugs—cont'd

Infant Behavior	Behavior Description	Strategies
	being alert to infant behavioral and psychological cues that indicate stress and adjust interactions appropriately. Caregivers will be affected by infant irritability, resulting in frustration and feelings of inadequacy in the mothering role and in infant/caregiver attachment. The caregiver needs to be made aware of behavior typical in infants prenatally exposed to drugs. Subsequently, the quality of their relationship will improve, negative judgments about infant will be reduced, and the likelihood of child abuse will be decreased.	■ Rock infant slowly and rhythmically, either horizontally or with head supported vertically, whichever soothes. ■ Place in a front-pack carrier. ■ Walk with infant. ■ Give child pacifier. ■ Provide hydrotherapy (warm bath). ■ Respond to stress cues by stopping activity with infant. This response will give infant a timeout. ■ Provide firm, calm touch to the mid-chest, back, or soles of infant's feet. ■ Play soft music or sing or hum quietly. ■ Provide background noise (for example, a hair dryer or vacuum cleaner), often called white noise, which may calm infant. ■ If all else fails, place infant in a quiet, darkened room with no outside stimulation. (Caregivers report this works with both premature and full-term infants exposed prenatally to drugs.)
Tremors, trembling, and extraneous movement	Tremors of the hands, arms, legs, chin, and tongue are commonly observed in infants prenatally exposed to drugs, although usually more pronounced and intense in younger infant. Tremors and tremulousness of movements have been observed in infants older than 1 year, but the intensity is diminished. In younger infants, tremors are primarily observed when infants are at rest. As they get older, fewer and less intense at-rest tremors occur, and intention tremors emerge. They tend to increase as the infant tires. Intention tremors occur when the infant is actively attempting a specific motor movement, for example, reaching for a toy. Intervention is often successful with intention tremors of arms and hands. Signs of stress often occur after persisting with an activity that elicits intention tremors because physical movements are difficult, and more energy and time are required to accomplish	■ Swaddling and holding infant close may be helpful for early at-rest tremors and extraneous movement. ■ Hold infant semireclined (almost sitting) with arms and shoulders forward to reduce the effort exerted by infant to maintain arm at midline while reaching for, holding, or manipulating toys. ■ Touch tremulous area firmly and calmly. Touch chest firmly and calmly.

	a task. Fine-motor development is at risk. Some infants prenatally exposed to drugs exhibit constant extraneous movements that make it difficult for them to soothe themselves. These extraneous movements slow acquisition of organized intentional motor control and visual-motor skills.	
Stiffness and rigidity	Stiffness and rigidity, or increased extensor tone, are often seen in infants prenatally exposed to drugs. The increased muscle tone, which causes these infants to frequently roll over at a few weeks of age, interferes with normal motor development, ability to cuddle, and pull-to-sit, and it delays control of arms at midline. Increased extensor tone in infants tends to diminish slowly. By 1 year of age, some degree of increased tone usually remains and diminishes the quality and smoothness of gross-motor patterns, as well as balance and protective reactions. These infants often arch their backs when held in a variety of positions, or when being fed. Arching occurs up to 12 months of age. More energy is used to accomplish fine- and gross-motor tasks; thus, some level of frustration is created.	■ Bathe infant in warm water. ■ Try gentle, calming massage. ■ Swaddle in flexion with shoulders and arms close to body. ■ Place infant in baby hammock to help ease rigidity, to maintain infant in slight spinal flexion, and to inhibit abnormal extension pattern. ■ Do not leave infant supine if the position maintains or increases stiffness, for example, head pushing back with scapular retraction (shoulder blades pinching together), or arms pushing into *W* position. Instead put infant in cloth, sling-style seat, as this position inhibits abnormal extension pattern. ■ Discourage the use of baby walkers, as they are known to further increase extensor tone.
Arms in W position	A large majority of infants prenatally exposed to drugs exhibit scapular retraction and/or resistance or weakness when attempting to bring arms to midline. When supine, arms are typically widespread and in a *W* position or one arm is in a unilateral *W* position. As these infants develop, difficulty continues in bringing arms to midline or sustaining a midline position. Younger infants compensate by locking their hands together, but when they release them, their arms snap backward into a *W* position, much like a rubberband effect. When infants are older, they can use their arms against increased extensor tone and, thus, use large amounts of active energy to maintain control. Fine-motor performance is compromised, and development of bimanual skills is difficult. Maintaining hands at midline is an important developmental step in acquiring fine-motor skills.	■ Swaddle infant with arms in midline position. ■ Carry or hold infant in a semireclining position with shoulders forward so that infant will experience arms at midline without excessive effort. ■ Place infant in cloth, sling-style infant seat. ■ Use reverse figure-eight strap to sustain arms in forward position while infant is in cloth, sling-style seat or in prone or sitting position. Infant can have successful experience without struggling for control. ■ Use a Forth infant feeder chair to position child and assist in keeping arms at midline. This strategy can be used for infants who cannot tolerate the reverse figure-eight strap.

Source: Lewis, K.D., Bennett, B., and Schmeder, N.H.: The care of infants menaced by cocaine abuse, *MCN American Journal of Maternal Child Nursing 14*(5):324-329, 1989.

7. Assist mothers to attach emotionally to their infants by encouraging and facilitating touch. Allow the mother to assist with caregiving skills and personalize her achievements.
8. Provide positive reinforcement and immediate feedback for all caretaking activities and interactions.
9. Parent education should be culturally sensitive, goal directed, and tailored to the mother's education level. Provide clear steps of the caretaking tasks and clinical milestones both mother and infant must meet before discharge.
10. Explain the infant's behavior in simple terms. Engage in discussion about the infant's oversensitivity to the environment and to excessive handling (stimulation).
11. Explain and reinforce repeatedly to the mother that the infant's behavior is not a rejection of her.
12. Teach mothers how to intervene early with crying infants by explaining that the infants are not yet able to quiet themselves. Dealing with stressful parenting situations are areas in which these women have difficulty in their daily lives. It is often this type of stress that has been, or can be, a trigger for continued substance use. Serving as a role model by talking and demonstrating ways to problem solve and reduce the stress may well serve the mother in future situations. They are not unlike other mothers that may need to share the issues that are causing them problems. Be open to allowing them to vent their frustrations then redirect their focus on the infant's progress or setbacks and needs today.
13. Provide and introduce kangaroo care (skin to skin) time if the mother desires.
14. Recognize that substance-using mothers and exposed infants require increased flexibility, intense commitment of energy and time, and patience.

DRUG SCREENING

A. **Policy.**

1. The American Academy of Pediatrics (AAP) considers the practice of performing drug screening unethical for the primary reason of detecting illegal use. AAP set forth a policy statement for neonatal drug withdrawal that includes guidelines for screening (AAP Committee on Drugs, 1998, www.aap.org/policy/re9746.html).

   Maternal characteristics that suggest screening include those in Box 3-4.
2. Drug screening during pregnancy must be accompanied with a reporting process that includes provision of rehabilitation and supportive services and long-term involvement of court or social services without criminal prosecution (for example, use of family drug courts) (MacMahon, 1997).

BOX 3-4

MATERNAL CHARACTERISTICS FOR DRUG SCREENING

No prenatal care
Previous unexplained fetal demise
Abruptio placentae
Hypertensive episodes
Severe mood swings
Myocardial infarction or cerebrovascular accident
Repeated spontaneous abortions

B. Method.

1. Accuracy of drug screening is dependent on
   a. laboratory used.
   b. test used.
   c. minimum drug in sample considered positive (see Table 3-6).
   d. reliability of the testing procedure.
   e. drug use pattern of person being tested (one-time dose, moderate use, etc.).
2. Thin-layer chromatography (TLC) is the most popular inexpensive method that hospitals use despite high false-negative rates and poor sensitivity in the detection of low quantities of marijuana, PCP, LSD, MDA, MDMA, mescaline, or fentanyl.
3. Enzyme immunoassay (EIA) (other types of this method called enzyme multiplied immunoassay test [EMIT]; radioimmunoassay [RIA]; fluorescent polarization immunoassay [FPIA); high-performance TLC [HPTLC]), and gas chromatography/mass spectrometry (GC/MS), available in larger hospitals, offer a 5- to 10-drug panel analysis.
4. All positive tests are confirmed by Western blot or another analysis run.

C. Urine.

1. Most common method used (inexpensive, rapid, and available in any hospital laboratory.
2. Can be collected noninvasively, stored, and frozen easily for long term.
3. Limitation is that it can only detect "recent" use (5 days after marijuana use, 3 days after cocaine use, 2 days after heroin use, and 12 hours after alcohol use).
4. Cannot measure quantity or frequency of drug use.

D. Blood.

1. Requires invasive collection.
2. Elimination half-life dependent on actual drug compound.

E. Meconium.

1. Meconium accumulates throughout pregnancy, therefore provides higher sensitivity (detects three times more drug users than urine) (Bar-Oz et al., 2003).
2. May detect second trimester drug exposure.
3. Limited availability in hospitals and more expensive.
4. Easy to obtain (collected noninvasively) and abundant quantity. Can provide an approximate 20-week historical snapshot of exposure (must be collected in the first 2 days of life).

TABLE 3-6
Basic Urine Drug Screen for Illicit Drug Use

Class	Screening Cutoff	Confirmation Cutoff
Amphetamines	1,000 ng/ml	Amphetamines, 500 ng/ml Methamphetamines, 500 ng/ml
Cannabinoids	50 ng/ml	THC-COOH, 15 ng/ml
Cocaine	300 ng/ml	Benzoylecgonine, 150 ng/ml
Opiates	300 ng/ml	Codeine, 300 ng/ml Morphine, 300 ng/ml
Phencyclidine	25 ng/ml	Phencydidine 25 ng/ml

Source: Naegle, M.A. and D'Avanzo, M.A.: *Addictions and substance abuse: Strategies for advanced practice nursing.* Upper Saddle River, NJ, 2001, Prentice Hall, p. 118.

F. **Neonatal hair and nails.**
1. Detects long-term drug use and can stay positive for up to 3 months after birth (Bar-Oz et al., 2003).
2. Three times more sensitive than urine screen.
3. Curly black hair has higher affinity for binding drug metabolites than brown hair.
4. Parents may be reluctant to provide sample of hair.

BREAST-FEEDING

Alcohol, caffeine, nicotine, and marijuana can all have a large effect on the production, volume, composition, and ejection of breast milk in addition to direct effects on infants (Liston, 1998).

A. **Nicotine and smoking.**
1. Elimination half-life of nicotine in milk ($t_{1/2}$ = 97 ± 20 minutes) slightly exceeds half-life of nicotine in serum ($t_{1/2}$ = 81 ± 9 minutes). Actual nicotine detected in milk is 1.5 to 3 times that found in maternal plasma (AAP Committee on Drugs, 2001).
2. No clear long-term effects of breast-feeding while smoking have been established.
3. Evidence demonstrates a less detrimental effect of respiratory illnesses in infants whose mothers smoked and breast-fed than for those mothers who smoked and bottle fed (AAP, 2001).
4. If mothers continue to smoke, recommend not smoking during nursing or directly in the infant's presence. Smoke immediately after breast-feeding or during an infant's long nap.
5. Mothers should be encouraged to decrease the number of cigarettes and to consider smoking cessation programs.

B. **Alcohol.**
1. Use of alcohol during lactation should be discouraged.
2. Moderate to heavy drinking has been shown to interfere with oxytocin release, causing inhibition of the letdown reflex.
3. Alcohol crosses into the breast milk, and changes in the infant's sleep-wake patterning and gross motor development have been demonstrated. Infants fall asleep sooner but sleep for shorter periods and spend less time in active sleep (Mennella and Garcia-Gomez, 2001; Mennella and Gerrish, 1998).

C. **Cocaine and amphetamines.**
1. Breast-feeding is contraindicated with active use.
2. Cocaine remains in the system for up to 60 hours after maternal ingestion.
3. Adverse effects seen may include cocaine intoxication, poor sleeping patterns, irritability, vomiting, diarrhea, tremulousness, and seizures.

D. **Marijuana.**
1. Breast-feeding is not recommended.
2. Impairment of deoxyribonucleic acid (DNA) and ribonucleic acid (RNA) formation and of use of essential proteins has been reported.
3. No long-term effect has been shown in research to date.

E. **Heroin.**
1. Heroin-dependent women should not breast-feed.
2. Adverse side effects include tremors, restlessness, vomiting, and poor feeding and sleep patterns.

F. **Methadone.**
1. In 2001 the AAP eliminated the dose restriction for methadone and stated that methadone is compatible with breast-feeding.

2. There is no clear indication of how much methadone is present in breast milk; transfer is considered minimal.
3. Women who are taking methadone and are breast-feeding should be educated about the effects of methadone and the use of illicit drugs.
4. Breast-feeding by a woman using methadone should not be stopped abruptly; the infant should be weaned gradually to prevent withdrawal.

G. **Sedatives/hypnotics.**
1. Long-term use of diazepam by women has been reported to cause sedation and lethargy in those neonates who are breast-fed. Effects may result in feeding difficulties or weight loss.
2. Recommend to discontinue breast-feeding in those infants that present with signs of weight loss or lethargy.

H. **Hepatitis B virus (HBV).**
1. Breast-feeding is not a contraindication.
2. HBV has been detected in breast milk of women who have tested positive for hepatitis B surface antigen (Gardner et al., 1998). An infant should receive hepatitis B immunoglobulin and vaccine as indicated by AAP and hospital guidelines.

I. **Hepatitis C virus (HCV).**
1. Research does not show breast-feeding as an important risk to HCV transmission when nipples are not traumatized (bleeding) and HCV is not active (Yeung et al., 2001).
2. Benefits and risks of breast-feeding should be explained to the mother to allow her to make an informed decision (AAP Committee on Infectious Diseases, 1998).

J. **HIV.**
1. It is recommended that women who are HIV seropositive be counseled not to breast-feed. The HIV antigen has been isolated in breast milk. "The probability of HIV-1 infection per liter of breast milk ingested by an infant is similar in magnitude to the probability of heterosexual transmission of HIV-1 unprotected sex acts in adults" (Richardson et al., 2003).
2. Women who are HIV seronegative but at high-risk for seroconversion should be given information concerning the transmission of HIV through breast milk and methods to reduce the risk of becoming infected.

PROBLEMS ASSOCIATED WITH MATERNAL DRUG USE

A. **Characteristics of women with a substance-use disorder** (see Box 3-5).

B. **Psychologic profile of women with a substance-use disorder** (see Box 3-6).

C. **Maternal-infant relationships.**
1. The attachment process between mother and infant is based on reciprocity. *Maternal* characteristics found to negatively impact the development of this relationship include:
   a. "More disengaged from their infants."
   b. "Display a higher degree of emotional instability" (inability to attach or securely attach to infant).
   c. "Unpredictable and unavailable in caregiving."
   d. "Display a lack of enjoyment and communication in interactions with infant."
   e. Possess "less sensitivity to identify cues that their infant displays" (Johnson, 2001).

BOX 3-5
CHARACTERISTICS OF WOMEN WITH A SUBSTANCE USE DISORDER

Family of origin is dysfunctional
Lack of a positive relationship with their own parents
Little to no positive parenting role models in their life
One or more parent that has a history of substance abuse
History of trauma as a child (physical, emotional, and/or sexual abuse)
Lack of education (less than 16 years of formal education)
Unemployed and poor vocational skills
Maintain chaotic lifestyle
Homeless or living in unstable or dangerous environment
Poor or lack of prenatal care (fear of legal reprisal)
Reliance of public assistance for health care during hospitalization
Lack network of social support (estranged from family members)
Single, divorced, or separated
Patterns of abuse by their spouses or significant others (domestic violence)
Biologic father of infant or partner often substance abuser; enables woman to maintain addiction and not involved in parenting
Lack of knowledge about child development and child-care skills

BOX 3-6
PSYCHOLOGIC PROFILE OF WOMEN WITH A SUBSTANCE USE DISORDER

Inability to ask for help
Lacks ability to establish positive personal relationships
Comorbidity (depression, anxiety, codependency, etc.)
Low self-esteem (high sense of guilt, shame, unworthiness; poor ego development and insecure)
Lacks coping mechanisms and skills. Impulsive: lacks ability to be future oriented

2. Factors in the *infant* that contribute to impaired maternal-infant interaction include:
   a. Extreme irritability, with arching and writhing behavior.
   b. Difficulty or resistance to being comforted.
   c. Rarely reaches alert state.
   d. Low threshold for stimulation, easily disturbed, and unable to transition well from state to state.
   e. Erratic sleep patterns, spending less time in active sleep.
   f. Difficult to feed and poor weight gain.

D. **Continuity of care and follow-up.**
   1. Develop a discharge plan that focuses on an interdisciplinary approach. Include short- and long-term follow-up. Areas that require attention include: abuse and neglect, attachment, and development, not just the immediate postnatal time period.
   2. Lack of continuity of care is often due to limited treatment and home visitation programs that accept both mothers and infants. Be aware of what resources are available in the community. This is an important first step toward advocating for the infant and ensuring future success of recovery for the mother.

3. Referrals should be made early to a local drug rehabilitation program and other appropriate community resources (for example, the Women, Infants, and Children program [WIC], lactation phone line support, nearby or hospital-based clinic, Planned Parenthood, and women's shelters and centers).

E. **Treatment, rehabilitation, and recovery.**
   1. "There are no simple predictors of women's substance abuse treatment outcomes" (Comfort et al., 2003).
   2. Abstinence is found to be related to length of stay in a treatment program.
   3. Treatment success may involve multiple treatment program attempts and completion as well as variety of types of treatment (outpatient vs. residential).
   4. Recovery is considered a long-term process.
   5. Definition of successful recovery is controversial.

F. **Gender-specific treatment needs.**
   1. Treatment programs that allow women to have infants or children with them are essential.
   2. Drug treatment should include a program that:
      a. Offers a multifaceted and integrative approach to recovery.
      b. Incorporates gender-based theories (women's psychosocial development) (Angove and Fothergill, 2003).
      c. Integrates parenting and child-rearing guidance and skill mastery.
      d. Directs and identifies children's behavior appropriately.
      e. Enhances self-esteem of women and relationship building.
      f. Offers supportive psychotherapy (group and individual).
      g. Provides anger control, conflict management and stress reduction skills.
      h. Offers a supportive environment that provides multiple role models.
      i. Supports a full range of ancillary services (child care services, social services, medical support, vocational, educational and aftercare).

ETHICAL AND LEGAL CONSIDERATIONS

A. **Ethical principles.** When interacting with women and substance use/abuse, consider:
   1. Justice: what is the equitable allocation of health, social resources, and treatment for women who use/abuse alcohol and substances?
   2. Beneficence: is one providing advocacy for what is best for the mother and child? That which is doing good can also include preventing harm that threatens someone.
   3. Nonmaleficence: not doing harm. (Although nonmaleficence and beneficence are closely related, it is still important that the requirement to avoid harm is much stronger than the requirement to do good.)
   4. Autonomy: the freedom to live your life. This becomes maternal autonomy vs. fetal rights when the woman is pregnant. To be autonomous one needs:
      a. liberty of action: no one is stopping you;
      b. freedom of choice: you have alternatives available
      c. effective deliberation: you are able to make a rational decision (Tiedje, 1998).

B. **Legal implications.**
   1. Legal statutes vary based on country and state of residence. "In March 2001, the Supreme Court determined that nonconsensual drug screening of pregnant women by clinicians in a public hospital violated the woman's

Fourth Amendment rights to be secure against unreasonable search and seizure" (Marshall et al., 2003).

2. No state has passed a law criminalizing pregnancy and drug use, but an estimated 250 women in more than 30 states have been prosecuted on the theory of "fetal abuse."
3. Most countries have mandatory laws obligating HCPs to report existing or suspected child abuse and neglect. Thus notification to the authorities may be necessary after delivery if HCPs are concerned about safety of the infant and/or the parents' ability to care for the infant.

C. **Criminal model vs. the harm-reduction model.**

1. Experts in the field of perinatal substance abuse believe that substance abuse is an illness and do not support prosecution of mothers (Catlin, 1997; Lowinson et al., 1997).
2. Fear of prosecution may deter women from seeking prenatal care and treatment for their drug problems. Lack of prenatal care is one of the major preventable factors that contribute to adverse pregnancy outcomes among pregnant drug users (Garcia, 1997). The harm-reduction model balances what is best for each individual with protection of the public good (Tiedje, 1998).
3. The rights and needs of the mother and those of the fetus require a view of being interrelated. In this manner solutions may be developed to support both.
4. Drug courts are an alternative to incarceration of women with a substance use disorder. There are 940 drug courts operating in 49 states, with 441 courts in the planning stages. The judges in these courts require abstinence, altered behavior through a combination of graduated sanctions, mandated drug testing, case management, and supervised treatment and aftercare programs.

RESOURCES

Al-Anon Family Group/Alateen
800-356-9996
www.al-anon.alateen.org
Alcoholics Anonymous
www.alcoholics-anonymous.org

Hazelden Foundation
P.O. Box 11, CO3, Center City, MN 55012-0011
800-257-7810
(651) 213-4000
info@hazelden.org
The International Nurses Network Interested in Alcohol, Tobacco & Drug Misuse (TINN)
www.tinnurses.org

International Nurses Society on Addictions (IntNSA)
Jim Scarborough, executive director
j.scarborough@mindspring.com
www.IntSNA.org

Latino Council on Alcohol and Tobacco Prevention (LCAT)
1875 Connecticut Avenue, NW, Suite 732, Washington, DC 20009
(202) 265-8054
lcat@nlcatp.org
www.nlcatp.org/

National Asian Pacific American Families Against Substance Abuse, Inc.
www.igc.apc.org/apiahf/napafasa.html

National Clearinghouse for Abused Drugs and Information (NCADI)
800-729-6686

National Institute on Drug Abuse (NIDA)
www.nida.nih.gov/

SMART Recovery
7537 Mentor Avenue, Suite #306, Mentor, OH 44060
(440) 951-5357; Fax: (440) 951-5358 contact your local SMART Recovery chapter.
www.smartrecovery.org

Substance Abuse and Mental Health Services Administration (SAMHSA)
Rm 12-105 Parklawn Building, 5600 Fishers Lane, Rockville, MD 20857
www.samhsa.gov/about/about.html

Women For Sobriety, Inc.
P.O. Box 618, Quakertown, PA 18951-0618
(215) 536-8026
www.womenforsobriety.org

FAS

Family Empowerment Network (FEN)
www.fammed.wisc.edu/fen
800-462-5254

*FAS Family Resource Institute (FAS*FRI)*
P.O. Box 2525, Lynnwood, WA 98036
800-999-3429
(253) 531-2878

National Organization on Fetal Alcohol Syndrome (NOFAS)
216 G Street NE, Washington, DC 20002
(202) 785-4585
800-66 NOFAS; Fax: 202-466-6456
www.nofas.org/main/index2.htm

REFERENCES

Accornero, V.H., Morrow, C.F., Bandstra, E.S., et al.: Behavioral outcome of preschoolers exposed prenatally to cocaine: Role of maternal behavioral health. *Journal of Pediatric Psychology*, *27*(3):259-269, 2002.

Adams, E.K., Miller, V.P., Ernst, C., et al.: Neonatal health care costs related to smoking during pregnancy. *Journal of the American Medical Association*, *287*(2): 195-202, 2002.

American Academy of Pediatrics Committee on Drugs (AAP): Neonatal drug withdrawal. *Pediatrics*, *101*(6):1079-1088, 1998.

American Academy of Pediatrics Committee on Drugs (AAP): The transfer of drugs and other chemicals into human milk. *Pediatrics*, *108*(3):776-789, 2001.

American Academy of Pediatrics Committee on Infectious Diseases (AAP): Hepatitis C virus infection. *Pediatrics*, *101*(3 Pt 1): 481-485, 1998.

American Academy of Pediatrics Committee on Substance Abuse and Committee on Children with Disabilities: Fetal alcohol syndrome and alcohol-related neurodevelopmental disorders. *Pediatrics*, *106*(2):358-361, 2000.

Andres, R.L. and Day, M.: Perinatal complications associated with maternal tobacco use. *Seminars in Neonatology*, *5*(3):231-241, 2000.

Angove, R. and Fothergill, A.: Women and alcohol: Misrepresented and misunderstood. *Journal of Psychiatric and Mental Health Nursing*, *10*(2):213-219, 2003.

Bar-Oz, B., Klein, J., Karaskov, T., and Koren, G.: Comparison of meconium and neonatal hair analysis for detection of gestational exposure to drugs of abuse. *Archives of Disease in Childhood: Fetal and Neonatal Edition*, *88*(2):F98-F100, 2003.

Bennett, A.D.: Perinatal substance abuse and the drug-exposed neonate. *Advanced Nurse Practitioner*, *7*(5):32-36, 1999.

Buchi, K.F., Zone, S., Langheinrich, K., and Varner, M.W.: Changing prevalence of prenatal substance abuse in Utah. *Obstetrics and Gynecology*, *102*(1):27-30, 2003.

Catlin, A.J.: Commentary on Deborah L. Burns' article. Positive toxicology screening in newborns: Ethical issues in the decision to legally intervene. *Pediatric Nursing*, *23*(1):76-78, 1997.

Centers for Disease Control and Prevention: Alcohol consumption among pregnant and childbearing-aged women—United States, 1991 and 1995: Behavioral Risk Factor Surveillance System. *Morbidity and Mortality Weekly Report (MMWR)*, *46*(16):346-350, 1997.

Church, M.W., Crossland, W.J., Holmes, P.A., et al.: Effects of prenatal cocaine on hearing, vision, growth and behavior. *Annals of the New York Academy of Sciences*, *846*(Jun 21):12-28, 1998.

Colado, M.I., O'Shea, E., Granados, R., et al.: A study of the neurotoxic effect of MDMA ("ecstasy") on 5-HT neurones in the brains of mothers and neonates following administration of the drug during pregnancy. *British Journal of Pharmacology*, *121*(4):827-833, 1997.

Comfort, M., Sockloff, A., Loverro, J., and Kaltenbach, K.: Multiple predictors of substance-abusing women's treatment and life outcomes: A prospective longitudinal study. *Addictive Behaviors*, *28(2)*: 199-224, 2003.

Dashe, J.S., Sheffield, J.S., Olscher, D.A., et al.: Relationship between maternal methadone dosage and neonatal withdrawal. *Obstetrics and Gynecology*, *100*(6):1244-1249, 2002.

Dejmek, J., Solansky, I., Podrazilova, K., and Sram, R.J.: The exposure of nonsmoking and smoking mothers to environmental tobacco smoke during different gestational phases and fetal growth. *Acta Paediatrica*, *91*(3), 323-328, 2002.

Dybing, E. and Sanner, T.: Passive smoking, sudden infant death syndrome (SIDS) and childhood infections. *Human Experiments in Toxicology*, *18*(4), 202-205, 1999.

Ebrahim, S.H. and Gfroerer, J.: Pregnancy-related substance use in the United States during 1996-1998. *Obstetrics and Gynecology*, *101*(2): 374-379, 2003.

England, I.J., Kendrick, J.S., Gargiullo, P.M., et al.: Measures of maternal tobacco exposure and infant birth weight at term. *European Journal of Pediatrics*, *161*(8): 445-448, 2002.

Eyler, F.D., Behnke, M., Conlon, M., et al.: Birth outcome from a prospective, matched study of prenatal crack/cocaine use: I. Interactive and dose effects on health and growth. *Pediatrics, 101*(2):229-237, 1998.

Finnegan, L.P. Neonatal abstinence syndrome. In N. Nelson (Ed). Current therapy in neonatal-parinatal medicine. 2nd ed. Ontario: BC Decker.

Frank, D.A., Augustyn, M., Knight, W.G., et al.: Growth, development and behavior in early childhood following prenatal cocaine exposure: A systematic review. *Journal of the American Medical Association, 285*(12):1613-1625, 2001.

Frank, D.A., Jacobs, R.R., Beeghly, M., et al.: Level of prenatal cocaine exposure and scores on the Bayley Scales of Infant Development: Modifying effects of caregiver, early intervention, and birth weight. *Pediatrics* 110(6);1143-1152, Dec, 2002.

Garcia, S: Ethical and legal issues associated with substances abuse by pregnant and parenting women. *Journal of Psychoactive Drugs, 29*(1), 101-111, 1997.

Gardner, S.L., Snell, B.J., and Lawrence, R.A: Breast feeding the neonate with special needs. In G.B. Merenstein and S.L. Gardner (Eds.): *Handbook of neonatal intensive care* (4th ed.). St Louis, 1998, Mosby, pp. 224-246.

Golding, J.: Sudden infant death syndrome and parental smoking—a literature review. *Peadiatric Perinatal Epidemiology, 11*(1), 67-77, 1997.

Hannigan, J.H. and Armant, D.R.: Alcohol in pregnancy and neonatal outcome, *Seminars in Neonatology, 5*(3):243-254, 2000.

Hans, S.I. and Jeremy, R.J.: Postneonatal mental and motor development of infants exposed in utero to opioid drugs. *Infant Mental Health Journal, 22*(3): 300-315, 2001.

Haustein, K.O: Cigarette smoking, nicotine and pregnancy. *Human Experiments in Toxicology, 18*(4): 202-205, 1999.

Hulse, G.K., Milne, E., English, D.R. and Holman, C.D.J.: The relationship between maternal use of heroin and methadone and infant birth weight. *Addiction, 92*(11):1571-1579, 1997.

Iqbal, M.M., Sobhan, T., and Ryals, T.: Effects of commonly used benzodiazepines in the fetus, the neonate and the nursing infant. *Psychiatric Service, 53*(1):39-49, 2002.

Johnson, M.O.: Mother-infant interaction and maternal substance use/abuse: An integrative review of research literature in the 1990s. *The Online Journal of Knowledge Synthesis for Nursing*, February *16*(8): 2, 2001.

Jones, H.E. and Balster, R.L.: Neurobehavioral consequences of intermittent prenatal exposure to high concentrations of toluene. *Neurotoxicology and Teratology, 19*(4):305-313, 1997.

Jones, M.W. and Bass, W.T.: Fetal alcohol syndrome. Neonatal network, 22(3):63-70. May, June, 2003

Keller, Jr., R.W., and Snyder-Keller, A.: Prenatal cocaine exposure. *Annals of the New York Academy of Sciences, 909*:217-232, 2000.

Kenner, C. and D'Apolito, K.: Outcomes for children exposed to drugs in utero. *Journal of Obstetric, Gynecologic, and Neonatal Nursing, 26*(5):595-603, 1997.

Klitsch, M.: Prenatal cocaine and opiate use are linked to a wide variety of health hazards. *Perspectives on Sexual and Reproductive Health, 34*(4), 2002. Retrieved on April 14, 2003 from www.guttmacher.org/pubs/journals/3421802.htm.

Klonoff-Cohen, H. and Lam-Kruglick, P.: Maternal and paternal recreational drug and sudden infant death syndrome. *Archives of Pediatrics & Adolescent Medicine, 155*(7):765-770, 2001.

Lester, B.M. and Tronick, E.: The effect of prenatal cocaine exposure and child outcome: Lessons from the past. *Infant Mental Health Journal, 15*(2): 107-120, 1994.

Liston, J.: Breastfeeding and the use of recreational drugs—alcohol, caffeine, nicotine, and marijuana, *Breastfeeding Review, 6*(2):27-30, 1998.

Lowinson, J.H., Ruiz, P., Millman, R.B., and Langrod, J.G. (Eds.): *Substance abuse: A comprehensive textbook* (3rd ed.). Baltimore, 1997, Williams & Wilkins.

MacMahon, J.R.: Perinatal substance abuse: The impact of reporting infants to child protective services. *Pediatrics, 100*(5):1-9, 1997.

Mahoney, D. and Larig, S.: Substance-related problems and childbearing. In M.A. Naegle and C.E. D'Avanzo (Eds.): *Addictions and substance abuse: Strategies for advanced practice nursing*. Upper Saddle River, NJ, 2001, Prentice Hall Health, pp. 221-270.

Marshall, M.F., Menikoff, J., and Paltrow, L.M.: Perinatal substance abuse and human subjects research: Are privacy protections adequate? *Mental Retardation and Developmental Disabilities Research Reviews*, *9*(1):54-59, 2003.

May, P.A. and Gossage, J.P.: Estimating the prevalence of fetal alcohol syndrome: A summary. *Alcohol Research and Health*, *25*(3):159-167, 2001.

McElhatton, P.R., Bateman, D.N., Evans, C., et al.: Congenital anomalies after prenatal ecstasy exposure. *Lancet*, *354*(9188): 1441-1442, 1999.

Mennella, J.A. and Garcia-Gomez, P.L.: Sleep disturbances after acute exposure to alcohol in mothers' milk. *Alcohol*, *25*(3), 153-158, 2001.

Mennella, J.A. and Gerrish, C.J.: Effects of exposure to alcohol in mother's milk on infant sleep. *Pediatrics*, *101*(5), e2, 1998.

Morbidity and Mortality Weekly Report (MMWR): Fetal alcohol syndrome—Alaska, Arizona, Colorado and New York, 1995-1997. *Morbidity and Mortality Weekly Report (MMWR)*, *51*(20):433-435, 2002.

National Institute on Alcohol Abuse and Alcoholism (NIAA): *Alcohol alert no. 13*, Rockville, MD, U.S. Department of Health and Human Services, 1991. Retrieved March 14, 2003, from www.niaaa.nih.gov/publications/aa13.htm.

National Institute on Alcohol Abuse and Alcoholism (NIAA): *Alcohol alert no. 23*, Rockville, MD, U.S. Department of Health and Human Services, 1994. Retrieved March 14, 2003, from www.niaaa.gov/publications/aa23.htm.

Nordstrom-Klee, B., Delaney-Black, V., Covington, C., et al.: Growth from birth onwards of children prenatally exposed to drugs: A literature review. *Neurotoxicology and Teratology*, *24*(4): 481-488, 2002.

Office of Applied Studies (OAS), Substance Abuse and Mental Health Administration (SAMHSA): *National Household Survey on Drug Abuse (NHSDA)*, 2000. Retrieved February 3, 2003, from www.samhsa.gov/oas/ p0000014.htm #NHSDA.

Osborn, D.A., Cole, M.J., and Jeffrey, H.E.: Opiate treatment for opiate withdrawal in newborn infants. *The Cochrane Database of Systematic Reviews*, *1*:1-23, 2003.

Ostrea, E.M., Jr., Lucena, J.L., and Silvestre, M.A.: The infant of the drug-dependent mother. In G.B. Avery, M.A. Fletcher, and M.G. Macdonald (Eds.): *Neonatology: Pathophysiology and Management of the Newborn*, Philadelphia, 1994, J.B. Lippincott, pp. 1300-1333.

Payot, A. and Berner, M.: Hospital stay and short-term follow-up of children of drug-abusing mothers born in an urban community hospital—A retrospective review. *European Journal of Pediatrics*, *159*(9):679-683, 2000.

Perault, M.C., Favreliere, S., Minet, P., and Remblier, C.: Benzodiazepines and pregnancy. *Therapie*, *55*(5):587-595, 2000.

Plessinger, M.A.: Prenatal exposure to amphetamines: Risks and adverse outcomes in pregnancy. *Obstetrics and Gynecology Clinics in North America*, *25*(1):119-138, 1998.

Polygenis, D., Wharton, S., Malmberg, C., et al.: Moderate alcohol consumption during pregnancy and the incidence of fetal malformations: A meta-analysis. *Neurotoxicology and Teratology*, *20*(1):61-67, 1998.

Richardson, B.A., John-Stewart, G.C., Hughes, J.P., et al.: Breast milk infectivity on human immunodeficiency virus type 1 infected mothers. *Journal of Infectious Diseases*, *187*(5):736-740, Epub, 2003.

Richardson, G.A., Ryan, C., Willford, J., et al.: Prenatal alcohol and marijuana exposure: Effects on neuropsychological outcomes at 10 years. *Neurotoxicology and Teratology*, *24*(3):309-320, 2002.

Riley, E.P., Guerri, C., Calhoun, F., et al.: Prenatal alcohol exposure: Advancing knowledge through international collaborations. *Alcoholism: Clinical and Experimental Research*, *27*(1):118-135, 2003.

Secker-Walker, R.H. and Vacek, P.M.: Relationships between cigarette smoking during pregnancy, gestational age, maternal weight gain, and infant birthweight. *Addictive Behaviors*, *28*(1):55-66, 2003.

Selleck, C.S. and Redding, B.A.: Knowledge and attitudes of registered nurses toward perinatal substance abuse. *Journal of Obstetric, Gynecologic and Neonatal Nursing*, 27(1):70-77, 1998.

Singer, L.T., Arendt, R., Minnes, S., et al.: Cognitive and motor outcomes of cocaine-exposed infants. *Journal of the American Medical Association, 287*(15): 1952-1960, 2002.

Stromland, K. and Pinazo-Duran, S.K.: Ophthalmic involvement in the fetal alcohol syndrome: Clinical and animal model studies. *Alcohol and Alcoholism, 37*(1):2-8, 2002.

Tiedje, L.B.: Ethical and legal issues in the care of substance-using women. *Journal of Obstetric, Gynecologic and Neonatal Nursing, 27*(1):92-98, 1998.

U.S. Department of Justice: Crystal methamphetamine, *Information Bulletin,* August. Johnstown, PA, 2002, National Drug Intelligence Center.

U.S. Department of Justice: Oxycontin diversion and abuse, *Information Bulletin,* August. Johnstown, PA, 2001, National Drug Intelligence Center.

Weiner, S.M. and Finnegan L.P.: Drug withdrawal in the neonate. In G.B. Merenstein, and S.L. Gardner (Eds.): *Handbook of neonatal intensive care.* (4th ed.) St Louis, 1998, Mosby.

Yeung, L.T., King, S.M., and Roberts, E.A.: Mother-to-infant transmission of hepatitis C virus. *Hepatology, 34*(2):223-229, 2001.

CHAPTER

4 Adaptation to Extrauterine Life

M. TERESE VERKLAN

OBJECTIVES

1. Identify primary features of fetal circulation.
2. Identify physiologic changes that occur during transition to extrauterine life.
3. Identify routine care considerations for a newborn infant during the transition period.
4. Identify signs and symptoms of common problems in the transition period.
5. Define the methods and intervention times for parental teaching.

The transition period is considered to be the first 6 to 10 hours of life, but more than a period of time, it is a process of physiologic change in the newborn infant that begins in utero as the child prepares for transition from intrauterine placental support to extrauterine self-maintenance. The fetus prepares for transition during the course of gestation in such ways as storing glycogen, producing catecholamines, and depositing brown fat. The neonate's ability to accomplish the transition to extrauterine life will depend on gestational age and the quality of placental support during gestation as well as any physical defects or anomalies that may affect major organ systems.

ANATOMY AND PHYSIOLOGY

Characteristics of Placental/Fetal Circulation

A. **Placenta.**
   1. Blood oxygenation and elimination of waste products of metabolism. Transfer of O_2 and CO_2 across the placenta is by simple diffusion.
   2. High rate of metabolism. Placenta uses one third of all the oxygen and glucose supplied to it by the maternal circulation for its own metabolic needs.
   3. Low-resistance circuit. Placenta receives approximately 50% of fetal cardiac output.
   4. Uterine venous blood has a P_{CO_2} of 38 mm Hg, P_{O_2} of 40 to 50 mm Hg, and pH of 7.36 as it enters the intervillous space.

B. **Fetal shunts/blood flow** (Fig. 4-1) **(Moore and Persaud, 2003).**
   1. Umbilical vein (P_{O_2} 32-35 mm Hg) carries oxygenated blood from the placenta to the fetus.
   2. Ductus venosus. Forty to sixty percent of the umbilical venous blood bypasses the liver through the ductus venosus to the inferior vena cava (IVC). The venous duct is a low-resistance channel that allows a significant

portion of relatively well-oxygenated blood to enter the heart directly; the other half passes through the liver and enters the IVC via the hepatic veins. This mixing of blood slightly lowers the Po_2.

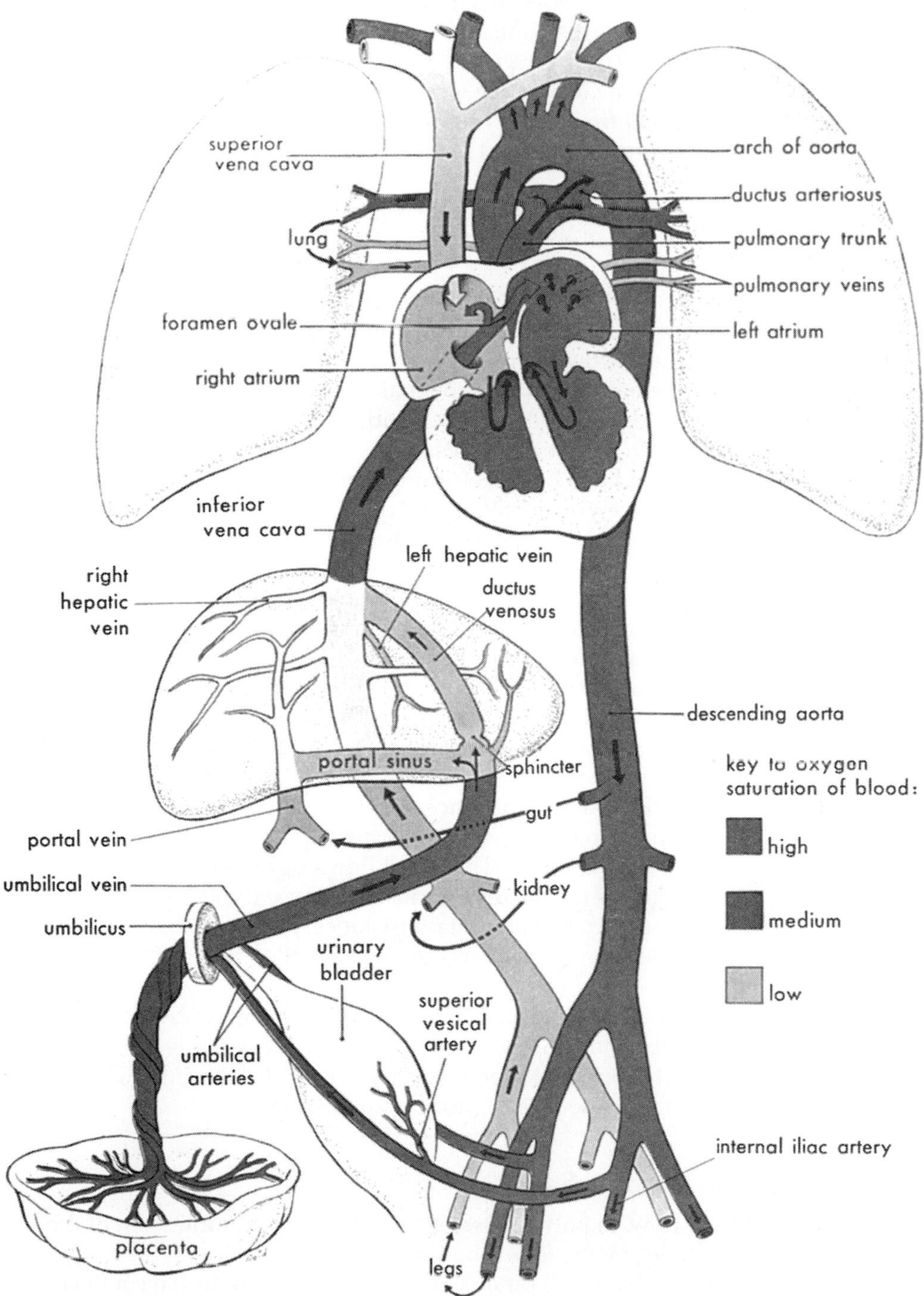

FIGURE 4-1 ■ Simplified scheme of fetal circulation. Shaded areas indicate oxygen saturation of the blood; arrows show course of fetal circulation. Organs are not drawn to scale. (From Moore, K.L. and Persaud, T.V.N.: *The developing human: Clinically oriented embryology* [7th ed.]. Philadelphia, 2003, Saunders.)

3. IVC blood and the blood from the coronary sinuses (Po_2 = 25-28 mm Hg). This blood is largely deflected across the right atrium, through the foramen ovale, and into the left atrium. In contrast, most of the blood from the superior vena cava (SVC), also returning to the right atrium, is deflected to the right ventricle (see item 6, below). The crista dividens (lower edge of the septum secundum) separates the flow of blood from the IVC into two streams, with 50% to 60% of the blood from the IVC being diverted across the foramen ovale into the left atrium (Blackburn, 2003) and the remainder of blood from the IVC remaining in the right atrium and mixing poorly oxygenated blood from the superior vena cava and coronary sinus.
4. Left atrium. Blood is received from the right atrium via the foramen ovale and mixes with a small amount of blood returning from the lungs via the pulmonary veins.
5. Left ventricular blood (Po_2 = 25-28 mm Hg). Virtually all this blood is from the IVC by way of the right atrium-foramen ovale–left atrium pathway. Left ventricular blood is pumped out through the aorta to the brain from the upper part of the aortic arch. Approximately 90% of the blood from the ascending aorta feeds the coronary, carotid, and subclavian arteries and thus the brain and upper extremities.
6. The SVC. Unoxygenated blood returning from the brain and upper extremities is received by the SVC. Ninety-seven percent enters the right atrium and flows to the right ventricle through the tricuspid valve; only 3% flows to the left atrium via the foramen ovale.
7. Right atrium. Some mixing occurs here between the unoxygenated SVC blood and the oxygenated IVC blood not shunted directly into the left atrium via the foramen ovale.
8. Right ventricle. The dominant ventricle (Po_2 = 19-22 mm Hg) ejects about 66% of the total cardiac output. Most of the blood is shunted across the ductus arteriosus, away from the lungs, and into the descending aorta to supply the kidneys and intestines. It then divides into two arteries, which subsequently return back to the placenta.
9. Ductus arteriosus. Equal in size to the aorta, it connects the pulmonary artery to the descending aorta. The blood flows right to left (pulmonary artery to aorta) across the ductus arteriosus because of high pulmonary vascular resistance and low placental resistance. Patency is maintained by the low oxygen tension in utero and by the vasodilating effect of prostaglandin E_2.
10. Low pulmonary blood flow (only 8%-10% of right ventricular output) results from high pulmonary vascular resistance.
11. Descending aorta supplies kidneys and intestines, divides into two arteries, and returns blood to the placenta for oxygenation.

Fetal Lung Characteristics

A. **Decreased blood flow.** In part the decrease is caused by compression of the pulmonary capillaries by the fetal lung fluid.
B. **Pulmonary arteries.** The small pulmonary arteries of the fetus have a thick, muscular medial layer; they are very reactive and are actively constricted by low Po_2 normally present during fetal life. Pulmonary vascular resistance increases throughout fetal life.

C. **Lung fluid secretion.** Fetal lungs actively secrete fluid; secretion of fluid is decreased near term. At term the lung contains 30 ml of plasma ultrafiltrate per kilogram of body weight. This is comparable to a postnatal thoracic gas volume of 25 ml/kg. An adequate fluid volume is necessary for lung development. Fluid moves into and out of the lungs through the trachea.

D. **Fetal breathing.** In utero fetal breathing movements have been detected as early as 11 weeks of gestation. They contribute to lung development.

E. **Surfactant.** Surfactant is secreted into the amniotic fluid by the fetal lung before 20 weeks of gestation. The absolute quantity of surfactant increases throughout gestation in both lung and amniotic fluid and can support extrauterine respiration at approximately 34 weeks of gestation.

Fetal Metabolism and Hematology

A. **Glucose.** Fetal blood glucose concentrations are 70% to 80% of maternal blood glucose concentrations. Glucose is exchanged via the placenta by facilitated diffusion.

B. **Glycogen.** Large glycogen stores (2-10 times that of an adult) provide large energy reserves to sustain the newborn infant through the transition period.

C. **Hemoglobin.** Fetal hemoglobin has an increased affinity for oxygen. Fetal hemoglobin is progressively replaced by adult hemoglobin from 32 to 36 weeks of gestation and is approximately 80% of total hemoglobin at term.

Labor

A. **Placenta.** Maternal placental perfusion ceases with uterine contractions.

B. **Stress hormones.** High concentrations of stress hormones (predominantly norepinephrine) are released as a direct effect of the resultant hypoxia on the adrenal medulla.

Cardiopulmonary Adaptation at Birth

A. **Cardiovascular adaptation** (Fig. 4-2) **(Moore and Persaud, 2003).**
   1. Umbilical cord is clamped.
      a. Placenta is separated from the circulation, and the umbilical arteries and veins constrict.
      b. As the low-resistance placental circuit is removed, there is a resultant increase in systemic blood pressure; the systemic vascular resistance then exceeds the pulmonary vascular resistance.
   2. The three major fetal shunts (ductus venosus, foramen ovale, and ductus arteriosus) functionally close during transition.
      a. Ductus arteriosus. The lungs now provide more efficient oxygenation of the blood, and the arterial oxygen tension rises. This rise in PO_2 is the most potent stimulus to constriction of the ductus arteriosus (Nelson, 1999). Removal of the placenta decreases prostaglandin levels, further influencing closure (Nelson, 1999).
      b. Foramen ovale. The fall in pulmonary vascular resistance results in a drop in right ventricular and right atrial pressure, and the increased systemic vascular resistance results in an increase in left atrial and left ventricular pressures, causing the foramen ovale to close.

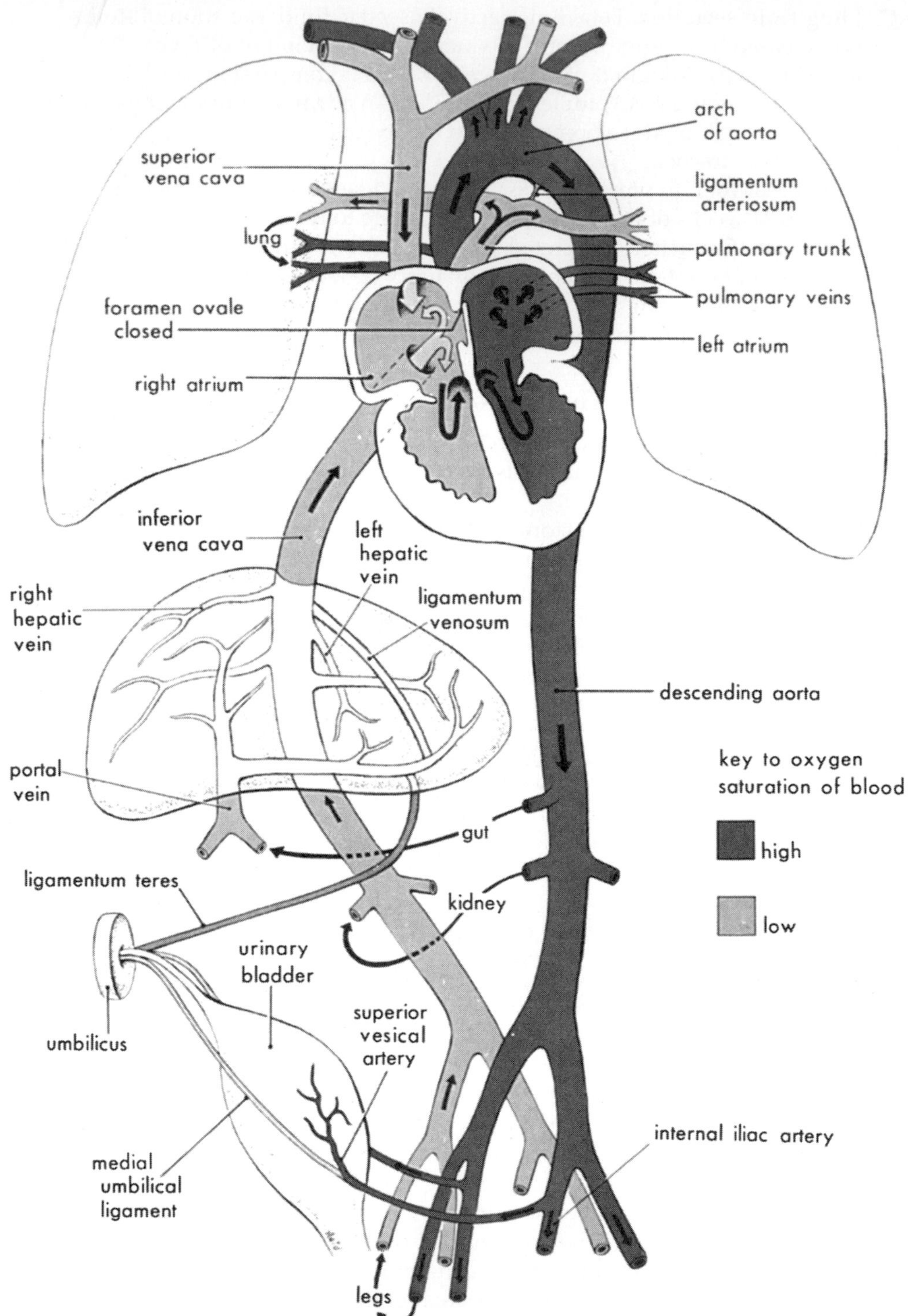

FIGURE 4-2 ■ Simplified representation of circulation after birth. Adult derivatives of fetal vessels and structures that become nonfunctional at birth are also shown. Arrows indicate course of neonatal circulation. Organs are not drawn to scale. (From Moore, K.L. and Persaud, T.V.N.: *The developing human: Clinically oriented embryology* [7th ed.]. Philadelphia, 2003, Saunders.)

(1) The foramen ovale becomes sealed by the deposit of fibrin and cell products during the first month of life.
(2) Until the foramen ovale is anatomically sealed, anything that produces a significant increase in right atrial pressure can reopen the foramen ovale and allow a right-to-left shunt.

c. Ductus venosus. Absent umbilical venous return leads to closure of the ductus venosus. It functionally closes within 2 to 3 days and becomes the ligamentum venosum.

3. Postnatal circulation (see Fig. 4-2) (Moore and Persaud, 2003).
   a. Systemic venous blood enters the right atrium from the SVC and the IVC.
   b. Poorly oxygenated blood enters the right ventricle and passes through the pulmonary artery into the pulmonary circulation for oxygenation.
   c. The oxygenated blood returns to the left atrium through the pulmonary veins.
   d. This blood passes through the left ventricle and into the aorta to supply the systemic circulation with oxygenated blood.

B. Pulmonary adaptation (Nelson, 1999).

1. The lungs as the organ of gas exchange. Intermittent breathing begins in utero long before delivery and, after birth, is a continuation of movements and reflexes that have been well established.
2. Stimuli for initiating respiration. The mild hypercapnia, hypoxia, and acidosis that result from normal labor are due partially to the intermittent cessation of maternal-placental perfusion with contractions. The decreased pH stimulates the respiratory center directly; the low Po_2 and high Pco_2 stimulate the respiratory center by means of central and peripheral chemoreceptors. Other stimuli include cold, light, noise, and touch.
3. Entry of air into lungs with the first breath.
   a. Aeration of the lungs drives fluid into the interstitium; it is then absorbed through the lymphatic and pulmonary circulation. The rate at which this process occurs is variable, and fine crackling rales may be audible throughout the lungs until this process is completed.
   b. The pulmonary vessels respond to the increase in Po_2 with vasodilation. Pulmonary vascular resistance progressively decreases until adult levels are reached at 2 to 3 weeks of age.
4. Inspiration of air and expansion of lungs. After the thoracic squeeze (during labor and vaginal delivery this empties the lungs of approximately one third of the fetal lung fluid), the subsequent recoil of the chest wall causes inspiration of air and expansion of the lungs. Negative intrathoracic pressures generated with the first breath may be as high as 40 to 80 cm H_2O because of the mechanical advantage created by the high resting level of the diaphragm in the nonaerated lung. Subsequent breaths in the normal newborn infant require 15 to 20 cm H_2O pressure.
5. Respiratory augmentation. Head's paradoxic reflex is a vagally mediated hyperinflation triggered by distention of stretch receptors in the large airways.
6. Work of inspiration. This is mainly (80%) devoted to overcoming the surface tension of the walls of the terminal lung units at the gas-tissue interface. On expiration, the ability to retain air depends on surfactant.
   a. Surfactant is a complete lipoprotein produced by type II alveolar pneumocytes; surfactant release increases in response to increased catecholamine levels at birth.

b. Surfactant has the ability to lower surface tension at an air-liquid interface.
c. As surfactant lowers surface tension in the alveolus at end-expiration, it stabilizes the alveoli and prevents collapse.

7. Increase in functional residual capacity with each breath. Less inspiratory pressure is thus required for subsequent breaths.
8. Lung compliance. This improves in the hours after delivery as a result of circulating catecholamines. The increased levels of catecholamines (especially of epinephrine) also clear the lungs by decreasing secretion of the lungs' fluids and increasing their absorption through the lymphatic system.

ROUTINE CARE CONSIDERATIONS IN THE TRANSITION NURSERY (Izatt, 2002; Lissauer, 2002)

A. Assessment/observation.

1. Body measurements. Head circumference, length, and weight are recorded.
2. Vital sign assessment. Vital signs recorded on admission will include heart rate, respiratory rate, and axillary temperature. Universal blood pressure screening in the well newborn infant is not warranted (American Academy of Pediatrics Policy Statement [AAP], 1993).
3. Gestational age assessment. Weight, head circumference, and length are graphed against the assessed gestational age and record (refer to Chapter 7).
4. Clinical changes. During the first hours of life vital signs stabilize and the newborn proceeds through sleep-wake cycles associated with readiness to feed behaviors (Verklan, 2002). The time sequence of changes is altered in infants with low Apgar scores, immaturity, maternal medications, and intrinsic disease (refer to Chapter 5).
5. Head-to-toe physical examination (refer to Chapter 7). The following findings seen during transition are within normal limits as the infant progresses through the physiologic changes described under cardiopulmonary adaptation, above.
   a. Skin.
      (1) Acrocyanosis. Vasoconstricted peripheral vessels result in a mottled appearance; peripheral pulses are decreased initially. (These findings are sequelae of catecholamine release, mild acidosis, and cold stress.)
      (2) Petechiae of the face and facial bruising. A vertex presentation, a rapid second stage of labor, or a tight nuchal cord may result in these skin changes. (With severe facial bruising, central color may be assessed by looking at the mucous membranes in the mouth.)
   b. Head.
      (1) The newborn infant's head is large relative to the body; during vaginal delivery, considerable molding of the skull bones may take place to facilitate passage through the birth canal. Molding resolves during the first hours and days.
      (2) Caput succedaneum (edema of the presenting part of the scalp, caused by pressure that restricts the return of venous and lymph flow during vaginal delivery), may be present.
   c. Respirations/breath sounds.
      (1) Initially, coarse rales and moist tubular breath sounds. These breath sounds may continue until clearing of lung fluid is complete.
      (2) Prolonged expiratory phase.

(3) Respiratory rate, 30 to 60 breaths per minute.
(4) Grunting and retracting (intercostal and substernal). These findings may be present during the first hours of life as lung fluid is cleared.

d. Heart sounds.
(1) Second heart sound may be loud during first 2 hours; splitting of the second heart sound is usually detectable at 2 to 4 hours of age and increases during the next 12 hours (pulmonic ahead of aortic component).
(2) Soft grade 2/6 systolic murmur may be present; represents a left-to-right shunt across the ductus arteriosus before its closure.

e. Heart.
(1) Normal heart rate 120 to 160 beats per minute (bpm); increased initially, with mean peak of 180 bpm, and then decreased or irregular.
(2) Consistently high or low heart rate suggests a pathologic condition.

f. Intestines.
(1) Blood flow is reduced initially.
(2) As the bowel begins to fill with air, normal motility and bowel sounds are present within 15 minutes.
(3) The normal term neonate passes meconium within the first 24 hours after birth. If a term neonate has not passed meconium by 48 hours after birth, the lower gastrointestinal tract may be obstructed (AAP and ACOG, 2002.)

g. Urinary function.
(1) Urine is normally passed within the first 24 hours after birth.
(2) Failure to void within the first 24 hours may indicate genitourinary obstruction or abnormality (AAP and ACOG, 2002).

h. Extremities. Findings may include deformities resulting from intrauterine position.

B. Thermoregulation considerations in the nursery (Blake and Murray, 2002). The admission assessment and observation should be done in a controlled environment, such as a radiant warmer or incubator, that both provides warmth and prevents heat loss so that the infant maintains a normal temperature without increasing oxygen consumption, using glucose stores, or exceeding brown fat stores in the process of nonshivering thermogenesis (mediated by norepinephrine released by cold stress). Normal ranges are 36.5° to 37° C (axillary) and 36.0° to 36.5° C (skin). Hypothermia and hyperthermia occur when the infant's attempts to maintain a normal temperature fail, which has serious metabolic consequences for the newborn infant (refer to Chapter 6, Thermoregulation).

1. Monitor temperature. Check axillary temperature every 30 minutes to 1 hour during transition while the infant is under a radiant warmer. Avoid hyperthermia (skin temperature greater than 37° C or axillary temperature greater than 37.5° C). NOTE: Monitoring the axillary temperature allows time for successful intervention before a fall in core temperature indicates failure of the body's heat-regulation mechanism.
2. First bath. Delay bath until body temperature has stabilized and is within normal limits. Check temperature 30 minutes after the bath and 1 hour after transfer to open crib.
3. Temperature. Check temperature at least every 4 hours until infant's condition is stable, and then every 8 hours until discharge.
4. Environmental temperature (incubator or warmer). Record environmental temperature with temperature checks of the infant to monitor his or her

environmental requirements. NOTE: These requirements can be checked against the normal ranges of neutral thermal environmental temperature needs as a tool in evaluating an infant's condition.

C. **Transition nursery medications (Izatt, 2002).**
   1. Eye care. Administered to both eyes before 1 hour of age in infants born by cesarean delivery, as well as those delivered vaginally.
      a. Recommendation. Apply two drops of 1% silver nitrate solution or a 1-to 2-cm ribbon of sterile ophthalmic ointment containing 0.5% erythromycin or 1% tetracycline for prophylaxis of ophthalmia neonatorum due to *Neisseria gonorrhoeae*. Prophylaxis for *Chlamydia trachomatis* requires erythromycin or tetracycline (AAP and ACOG, 2002).
      b. Procedure. Instill medication into conjunctival sac within 1 hour of birth; medication should not be flushed from the eye after application. A new tube is used for each infant.
      c. Side effects. Sensitivity reaction may be seen. Chemical conjunctivitis can be observed after silver nitrate instillation.
   2. Vitamin K_1 (phytonadione). Administer vitamin K within 1 hour of birth.
      a. Recommendation. Every neonate should receive a single parenteral 0.5 to 1-mg dose of natural vitamin K (phytonadione) (AAP and ACOG, 2002). Administer 0.5 mg if infant weighs less than 1.5 kg or 1 mg if infant weighs more than 1.5 kg. NOTE: Vitamin K may be given orally in 1 or 2 mg dose; the oral route was recommended as an alternative by the British Paediatric Association in 1992 but is not recommended by the AAP because oral administration of vitamin K has not been shown to be as efficacious as parenteral administration (AAP and ACOG, 2002).
      b. Risk of deficiency. Maternal dietary inadequacy of vitamin K, hepatic immaturity, reduced liver stores, and absence of intestinal flora predispose the child to deficiency of vitamin K; gut bacteria are a substantial source. Vitamin K is needed to promote the hepatic biosynthesis of vitamin K–dependent clotting factors, including prothrombin (factor II), proconvertin (factor VII), plasma thromboplastin component (factor IX), and Stuart factor (factor X). Deficiency results in hemorrhagic disease of the newborn (HDN).
         (1) Classic HDN. The disease occurs at 1 to 7 days of life. The infant is healthy at birth but develops cutaneous or gastrointestinal (GI) bleeding. Other sites of bleeding include nasal bleeding or bleeding after circumcision. Classic HDN can be prevented with vitamin K prophylaxis.
         (2) Early HDN. Maternal exposure to drugs, including warfarin, anticonvulsants, and antituberculosis drugs, may affect coagulation. Severe or life-threatening hemorrhage may occur during delivery or in the first day of life. Intracranial hemorrhage is a common complication. Early HDN is the only type that cannot be prevented by vitamin K prophylaxis.
         (3) Late HDN. The late form of HDN may occur between 1 and 3 months of life. Acute intracranial hemorrhage is the most common initial finding and is often fatal or neurologically devasting. Other findings include gastrointestinal or mucous membrane bleeding. Late HDN can be prevented by vitamin K prophylaxis.
   3. Hepatitis vaccine and hepatitis B immunoglobulin (HBIG) (also see Appendix B, Recommended Childhood and Adolescent Immunization Schedule).

a. Rate of infection. Approximately one third of infants born to hepatitis B surface antigen (HBsAg)-positive mothers will be HBsAg positive, with rates as high as 70% to 90% if mothers are HBeAg positive and anti-HBeAg negative (Thureen and Abzug, 1999).
b. Chronicity. Ninety percent of infected infants will become chronic hepatitis B virus (HBV) carriers (Burchett, 1998).
c. Maternal HbsAg-positive treatment recommendations:
   (1) Child is bathed as soon as temperature is stable.
   (2) Hepatitis B vaccine (Engerix-B, 10 µg or Recombivax-HB, 5 µg) and HBIG, 0.5 ml IM (prepared from plasma to contain a high titer of antibody against HBsAg), should be administered before 12 hours of age (AAP, 1997); may be given concurrently at different sites; 85% to 95% effective in preventing both HBV infection and the chronic carrier state.
   (3) Remaining doses of hepatitis B vaccine are given at 1 and 6 months of age.
d. Maternal HBsAg negative–treatment recommendations:
   (1) Hepatitis B vaccine should be administered to all infants, including those born to HBsAg-negative mothers.
   (2) Hepatitis B vaccine (Engerix-B, 10 µg or Recombivax-HB, 5 µg) is administered prior to discharge from the hospital. The second dose is administered at 1 to 2 months of age and the third dose at 6 to 18 months of age.
e. Unknown maternal HBsAg status at delivery. Follow schedule for maternal HBsAg positive. Additional HBIG administration will depend on results of maternal serologic screening done within 12 hours after delivery.
f. Premature infants with birth weight less than 2 kg born to HBsAg-negative mothers should receive the vaccine just before hospital discharge if the infant weighs more than 2 kg or dose is delayed until 2 months of age when other routine immunizations are given. All premature infants born to HBsAg-positive mothers should receive immunoprophylaxis (HBIG) and vaccine beginning as soon as possible after birth, followed by appropriate postvaccination testing (AAP Committee on Infectious Diseases, 2000).

D. Glucose needs/first feeding (Kalhan and Price, 2001).

1. The stress of delivery causes increased conversion of fats and glycogen to glucose for the increased energy needs of temperature maintenance, skeletal muscles, and breathing and crying. Breakdown products of this conversion are glucose, free fatty acids, and glycerol.
2. Hepatic glycogen is mobilized immediately after birth in response to the increased catecholamines to provide a continuing source of glucose to the brain in the absence of placental supply; in a healthy term infant, up to 90% of the hepatic glycogen stores may be consumed by 3 hours of life.
3. Blood glucose concentration at birth is about 85% of the maternal level. The last maternal meal, the duration of labor, the mode of delivery, the type and amount of IV fluids administered to the mother, and medications given to the mother all influence the actual concentration of glucose. The glucose level then falls for 1 to 2 hours, followed by an increase and stabilization at mean levels of 65 to 71 mg/dl by the age of 3 to 4 hours in healthy, nonstressed infants (Wilker, 1998).
4. A screening blood glucose test (on capillary whole blood) should be performed in infants with risk factors at 30 minutes to 1 hour of age.

A glucose level less than 40 mg/dl at any time in any newborn infant is an indication for evaluation and treatment (Wilker, 1998). The goal is to maintain the glucose value at greater than 40 mg/dl in the first day and greater than 40 to 50 mg/dl thereafter. NOTE: The whole-blood glucose level on the screening test is usually 10% to 15% lower than the corresponding serum or plasma level because the erythrocytes will continue to metabolize the glucose in the sample. Risk factors include:

a. Asphyxia, cold stress, increased work of breathing, and sepsis, which lead to an increased metabolic response and increased use of glucose.

b. Reduced stores of glucose in premature and small-for-gestational-age infants.

c. Hyperinsulinemia in infants of mothers with diabetes or gestational diabetes and in large-for-gestational-age infants, resulting in rapid removal of glucose from the circulation.

d. Any symptoms of a low blood glucose level. An infant may have jitteriness, irritability, seizures, hypothermia, temperature instability, lethargy, poor feeding, emesis, apnea, pallor, cyanosis, and weak or high-pitched cry. (See also Common Problems and Clinical Presentation, item F: Metabolic Problems, on p. 96.) NOTE: Capillary samples from an unwarmed heel may lead to a falsely low glucose value because of stasis of blood and ongoing transfer of glucose to the cells.

5. Early, frequent feedings should be given on demand; frequency is not to exceed 4 hours between feedings (maximum of 3 hours between feedings for infants weighing <2.5 kg). Allow the infant to begin feeding when he or she is demanding nutrition and when evaluation findings are within normal limits; nursing or formula feeding can be used (type of formula is by family's or physician's choice).

a. Evaluation before feeding.

(1) Physical examination. Bowel tones are normal, and abdomen is soft and nontender. Sucking reflex is normal, with no excessive mucus. Passage of an orogastric tube is indicated before feeding if questions exist regarding esophageal patency. Anus and nares are patent. Respiratory rate is less than 70 breaths per minute, and pattern of breathing is normal.

(2) Contraindications to nippling the feeding or to breast-feeding (consider gavage feeding for these infants).

(a) Choanal atresia.

(b) Respiratory rate greater than 70 breaths per minute without other signs of respiratory distress.

(c) Weak suck.

(d) Absent coordination of suck and swallow.

(3) Contraindications to any enteral feedings.

(a) Cyanosis.

(b) Severe birth asphyxia.

(c) Shock.

(d) Increased work of breathing and oxygen requirement.

(e) Suspicion of gastrointestinal obstruction.

b. Sterile-water "test" feeding. It is difficult to evaluate an infant's ability to suck and swallow with sterile water because most infants do not like the taste and on occasion will refuse to suck or swallow; therefore it is advisable to forgo "sips of water" in favor of a thorough evaluation before feeding.

c. Dextrose 5%. Use of dextrose 5% is not indicated as a "test" feeding because studies show that it is as irritating to lungs after

aspiration as is formula (Sun et al., 1998). Not indicated after feeding unless:
(1) Ordered by a physician.
(2) Requested by mother (e.g., at one night feeding in the nursery or if infant does not settle down after effective nursing).

d. Guidelines for feeding in transition nursery for transient asymptomatic hypoglycemia:
(1) May breast-feed or be offered formula (by nipple or gavage) if there are no contraindications to enteral feedings (see Contraindications, item a[3], on p. 90), and the infant is active and vigorous.
(2) Check glucose level 1 hour after feeding is given.

e. Indications for IV glucose infusion (see Initial Stabilization of the Sick Newborn Infant, on p. 97):
(1) Hypoglycemia is persistent and symptomatic.
(2) Enteral feedings are contraindicated.
(3) Oral feedings do not maintain normal glucose levels.
(4) Initial glucose screening level is less than 40 mg/dl.

E. Ongoing teaching in the transition nursery.

1. Discuss with family the infant's ability to see and hear, with a preference for black-white contrast initially, and the sound of a higher-pitched voice.
2. Demonstrate or point out infant's response to stimuli (tactile, visual, auditory): self-consolability, body movements, gaze, head turning.
3. Discuss physical findings.
   - **a.** Transient: head molding, acrocyanosis, birth trauma, positional deformities.
   - **b.** Permanent: congenital anomalies, birthmarks.
4. A stable infant may stay with the family from birth through recovery to postpartum period with appropriate observation and teaching provided by all staff members in contact with the family unit.

F. Transfer of infant from transition nursery when the following are stable.

1. Temperature, heart rate, respiratory rate.
2. Glucose level.
3. Normal physical assessment findings, or abnormal findings that do not require continuous observation or immediate intervention or treatment.

RECOGNITION OF THE SICK NEWBORN INFANT

Review of Perinatal History (Fanaroff et al., 2001)

A. Ultrasonographic-biophysical profile: estimated date of confinement, evidence of congenital anomalies, twins, breech, preterm, intrauterine growth restriction.

B. Medications or history of substance abuse: alcohol, nicotine, cocaine, opiates, marijuana, amphetamines, tocolytics, anticonvulsants, anticoagulants, and analgesics/anesthetics.

C. Maternal illnesses: pregnancy-induced hypertension, diabetes, intrapartum fever/infection (e.g., with group B streptococcus, genital herpes simplex virus, human immunodeficiency virus, varicella), HBsAg positive, thyroid disease, inherited disorders, cardiac disease.

D. Perinatal fetal distress, delivery complications: abnormal fetal heart rate pattern, meconium staining of the amniotic fluid, rapid delivery, difficult delivery, rupture of membranes more than 18 hours before delivery.

E. Cesarean delivery and indications: breech presentation, fetal distress, placenta previa, abruptio placentae, cephalopelvic disproportion, failure to progress in labor.

Physical Assessment

A. **Skin.**
   1. Cyanotic.
   2. Pale.
   3. Mottled.
   4. Cool to touch.
   5. Poor perfusion.

B. **Respiratory system.**
   1. Poor color.
   2. Tachypnea.
   3. Decreased air entry.
   4. Increased work of breathing: grunting, flaring, retracting.
   5. Apnea.
   6. Unequal breath sounds.
   7. Oxygen requirement.

C. **Cardiovascular system.**
   1. Abnormal heart sounds such as murmur.
   2. Weak, absent, or unequal pulses.
   3. Hepatosplenomegaly.

D. **Central nervous system.**
   1. Hypertonic or hypotonic.
   2. Jitteriness; tremors.
   3. Lethargy.
   4. Bulging fontanelle (record baseline head circumference).
   5. Seizures.
   6. Irritability; high-pitched cry.

E. **Morphologic features.**
   1. Congenital anomalies (e.g., abdominal wall defects, imperforate anus).
   2. Severe birth trauma.
   3. Absent or decreased limb movement.
   4. Asymmetry.

F. **GI tract.**
   1. Abdominal distention (measure baseline abdominal girth).
   2. Increased gastric contents on aspiration.
   3. Inability to pass an orogastric tube.
   4. Excessive mucus.
   5. Emesis soon after birth or after first feeding.

Diagnostic Tools (Pierce and Turner, 2002)

A. **Pulse oximetry (peripheral monitoring of oxygen saturation).**
   1. Oxygen saturation (SaO_2) of blood is that percentage of the total hemoglobin concentration that is chemically combined with oxygen.
   2. A baseline PaO_2 value should be obtained to confirm the infant's oxygen level.
   3. For hyperoxic study, administer 100% oxygen to differentiate between pulmonary and cardiac disease. (In infants with pulmonary disease, saturation will improve, whereas in infants with cyanotic heart disease, little or no change will occur. Use caution to avoid exposing the ductus arteriosus to high oxygen levels in ductal-dependent cardiac lesions.)

B. **Arterial blood gas determinations.** If oxygen requirement persists, pulse oximetry saturations in room air are decreased and cyanosis is present.
C. **Chest x-ray examination.** Anteroposterior and lateral views are needed if respiratory distress is present or cardiac disease is suspected.
D. **Transillumination.** Use a high-intensity light placed over the side of the chest in question if pneumothorax or pneumomediastinum is suspected.
E. **Whole-blood glucose screening test or serum glucose determination if indicated by history or assessment results** (see Routine Care Considerations in the Transition Nursery, item D: Glucose Needs/First Feeding, on p. 89).
F. **Hematocrit determination.**
   1. History of blood loss.
   2. Plethoric or pale infant.
   3. Twins (to rule out twin-to-twin transfusion).
   4. Heel-stick (capillary) samples tend to have higher results of approximately 10%.
   5. Hematocrit variations. Highest hematocrit is at 2 to 4 hours of age and then progressively falls due to the beginning of red blood cell breakdown and the cessation of erythropoiesis in response to a comparatively oxygen-enriched environment.
G. **Complete blood cell count with differential examination of the white blood cells.**
   1. As part of a sepsis diagnostic evaluation.
   2. To screen for normal and abnormal hematologic indices.
H. **Blood culture as part of a diagnostic evaluation for sepsis.**
I. **Urine sample collection.**
   1. Urinalysis.
   2. Screening test for drugs of abuse.
J. **Lumbar puncture.** Performed at the discretion of the physician as part of a diagnostic evaluation for sepsis.
K. **Ultrasonography, computed tomography, magnetic resonance imaging.**
   1. Cranial evaluation for abnormal central nervous system (CNS) findings.
   2. Abdominal examination if history of two-vessel cord to rule out renal anomalies.
L. **Echocardiography and electrocardiography.** As part of a diagnostic study for a congenital cardiac defect.
M. **Passage of orogastric tube.**
   1. To check patency of esophagus in infants with excessive pooling of mucus in oropharynx.
   2. To decompress a distended abdomen.
   3. To measure and assess gastric contents (>25 ml and/or significant bile in the stomach indicates obstruction).

Common Problems and Clinical Presentation

A. **Birth trauma (refer to Chapter 2).**
B. **Birth asphyxia (Phibbs, 1999; Vannucci, 2002).**
   1. Birth asphyxia is defined as interference with gas exchange resulting in compromised oxygen delivery, accumulation of CO_2, and a switch to anaerobic metabolism.
   2. Fetal distress is indicated by abnormal fetal heart rate pattern, meconium staining of the amniotic fluid, scalp pH less than 7.20, and Apgar scores less than 5 at 1 minute of age and less than 7 at 5 minutes of age.

3. Pathophysiologic sequelae include:
   a. Decreasing Po_2. The tissue hypoxia that ensues leads to anaerobic metabolism with release of lactic acid into the circulation.
   b. Respiratory acidosis from elevated levels of a carbon dioxide.
   c. Metabolic acidosis.
      (1) Results in high pulmonary vascular resistance.
      (2) Leads to decreased surfactant release.
   d. Hypoxic-ischemic damage to less vital organs such as kidney and gut after redistribution of blood to vital organs.
   e. The myocardium depends on its stored reserves of glycogen for energy as its supply of oxygen falls. Eventually this reserve is consumed and the myocardium is simultaneously exposed to progressively lower Po_2 and pH levels. The combined effects lead to reduced myocardial function with decreased blood flow to vital organs (Phibbs, 1999).
4. All newborn infants have some degree of respiratory acidosis and hypoxia during labor and vaginal delivery; a healthy term infant has increased tolerance and reserves. The asphyxiated newborn infant has more prolonged hypoxia and respiratory acidosis and may have additional metabolic acidosis, hypothermia, and hypoglycemia.
5. Clinical findings.
   a. Mild to moderate perinatal asphyxia.
      (1) Extended awake, alert state (45 minutes to 1 hour).
      (2) Dilated pupils.
      (3) Normal muscle tone.
      (4) Active suck.
      (5) Regular or slightly increased respiratory rate.
      (6) Normal or slightly increased heart rate.
   b. Moderate to severe perinatal asphyxia.
      (1) Hypothermia.
      (2) Hypoglycemia.
      (3) Pupils constricted.
      (4) Respiratory distress manifested by grunting, flaring, retracting, tachypnea, and oxygen requirement.
      (5) Seizures (subtle and multifocal clonic; 12-24 hours of age).
      (6) Acute tubular necrosis following reduced blood flow to the kidneys.
      (7) Hypotonia initially; lethargy.
      (8) Bradycardia.
   c. Severe perinatal asphyxia, which requires constant monitoring in a level II (intermediate care) or level III (intensive care) nursery.
      (1) Pale; poor perfusion.
      (2) Cerebral edema.
      (3) Seizures.
      (4) Apnea.
      (5) Intracranial hemorrhage.

C. **Pulmonary problems (Miller et al., 2002).**
   1. Pneumothorax (2% of all births); pneumomediastinum.
      a. Tachypnea, unequal breath sounds, shift of heart tones, distant heart tones.
      b. Transillumination of chest is positive for free air.
   2. Retained lung fluid, respiratory distress syndrome (RDS) (because of prematurity or birth asphyxia), pneumonia.
      a. Decreased air entry with RDS and pneumonia.
      b. Increased work of breathing: grunting, flaring, retracting.

c. Tachypnea, apnea.
d. Decreased saturations (SaO_2), cyanosis, continued oxygen requirement.
3. Aspiration syndromes (meconium, blood).
a. Coarse rales.
b. Tachypnea.
c. Barrel chest.
4. Upper airway obstruction (e.g., choanal atresia or micrognathia).
5. Extrapulmonary (e.g., phrenic nerve injury with resultant diaphragmatic paralysis or eventration of the diaphragm).

D. Cardiovascular problems (Brook et al., 2001).
1. Congenital heart disease.
a. Acyanotic lesions.
(1) Patent ductus arteriosus with a left-to-right shunt.
(2) Ventricular septal defect.
(3) Atrial septal defect.
(4) Endocardial cushion defect or atrioventricular canal defects.
b. Obstructive lesions.
(1) Aortic stenosis.
(2) Coarctation of the aorta.
(3) Pulmonary valve stenosis or atresia.
(4) Hypoplastic left heart syndrome.
c. Admixture of lesions.
(1) Normal or increased pulmonary blood flow.
(a) Complete transposition of the great vessels.
(b) Truncus arteriosus.
(c) Anomalous venous connections of the pulmonary veins.
(2) Decreased pulmonary blood flow.
(a) Tetralogy of Fallot.
(b) Tricuspid valve atresia.
2. Persistent fetal shunts.
a. Patent ductus arteriosus with right-to-left shunt.
b. Persistent pulmonary hypertension.
3. Clinical findings.
a. Cyanosis with or without increased work of breathing; decreased oxygen saturations. NOTE: Absence of any signs of abnormal respiratory function in the presence of cyanosis suggests congenital heart disease.
b. Unequal or absent pulses, bounding pulses, decreased blood pressure in the lower extremities, decreased perfusion.
c. Increased precordial activity, shift of point of maximal impulse (PMI) of heart tones to right, murmur.
d. Congestive heart failure, indicated by tachypnea, moist breath sounds, tachycardia, peripheral edema, cardiomegaly, and hepatomegaly.

E. Hemodynamics.
1. Acute hypovolemic shock.
a. Internal hemorrhage resulting from birth trauma; intracranial hemorrhage.
b. External hemorrhage resulting from placenta previa or abruptio placentae; cord accident; fetal-maternal or twin-to-twin transfusion.
c. Respiratory distress, pallor, poor perfusion, hypotension, weak or absent pulses, anemia.
2. Polycythemia.
a. Plethoric, cyanotic, or excessively flushed with crying.
b. Hypoglycemia.
c. CNS symptoms including jitteriness, hypotonia, lethargy, seizures.

3. Anemia.
   a. Acute or chronic blood loss.
   b. Hemolysis from sepsis or ABO/Rh blood group incompatibilities.
   c. Reduced red blood cell production, manifested by severe asphyxia, sepsis, aplastic anemia.
   d. Pale skin, murmur, tachypnea, normal arterial blood pressure, signs of congestive heart failure including hepatosplenomegaly and increased vascular markings on x-ray film.

F. Metabolic problems.

1. Hypoglycemia.
   a. Observed in infants who are large or small for gestational age, infants of diabetic mothers, premature infants, and stressed infants such as those with sepsis, cold stress, or respiratory distress.
   b. Clinical findings:
      (1) Jitteriness, irritability.
      (2) Seizures.
      (3) Hypothermia, temperature instability.
      (4) Lethargy.
      (5) Poor feeding, emesis.
      (6) Apnea.
      (7) Cardiorespiratory distress, cyanosis, oxygen requirement.
      (8) Pallor.
      (9) Tachycardia.
      (10) Weak or high-pitched cry.
2. Adverse effects of maternal medications; maternal use of illicit drugs.
   a. Magnesium sulfate. Infants present with respiratory depression, decreased muscle tone, decreased serum calcium concentration.
   b. Tocolytics. Infants may present with hypoglycemia.
   c. Narcotics. Infants present with apnea, respiratory depression, periodic breathing.
   d. Cocaine. Infants may present with apnea, poor muscle tone initially and then irritability and agitation, tremors, feeding difficulties.
   e. Marijuana or methadone. Infants present with hyperthermia, agitation, diarrhea.
   f. Alcohol. Infants have fetal alcohol syndrome with dysmorphic and behavioral abnormalities.

G. Infection (see also Chapter 31).

1. Generalized bacterial or viral disease; acquired in utero or nosocomial.
2. Clinical findings. NOTE: Nearly 90% of neonates with early-onset group B streptococcus have signs of infection within 12 hours of birth (Mitchell et al., 1997).
   a. Temperature instability.
   b. Tachypnea, apnea.
   c. Respiratory distress, cyanosis.
   d. Tachycardia.
   e. Cool, mottled skin; weak pulses; capillary refill lasting longer than 2 seconds; hypotension.
   f. Disseminated intravascular coagulation.
   g. Hepatosplenomegaly.
   h. Unexplained jaundice.
   i. Purpura, petechiae.
   j. Hypoglycemia or hyperglycemia.

k. Poor feeding, emesis, abdominal distention.
l. Lethargy, poor muscle tone.

3. In utero viral infection. Infant may be small for gestational age with microcephaly.

H. **Congenital anomalies** (frequently obvious on gross examination).
1. Diaphragmatic hernia.
   a. Immediate onset, at birth, of significant respiratory distress.
   b. Shift in heart tones, decreased or unequal breath sounds, bowel tones heard in chest, scaphoid abdomen, cyanosis.
2. Esophageal atresia with or without tracheoesophageal fistula.
   a. Excessive amniotic fluid.
   b. Increased pooling of secretions in oropharynx, respiratory distress; unable to place orogastric tube.
3. Abdominal wall defects: omphalocele, gastroschisis.
4. Limb anomalies: amniotic banding, talipes equinovarus, polydactyly, syndactyly.
5. Neural tube defects.
6. Intestinal obstructions.
7. Chromosomal abnormalities such as trisomy 21 or trisomy 18.
8. Urogenital abnormalities: exstrophy of bladder, hypospadias, epispadias, ambiguous genitalia.

Initial Stabilization of the Sick Newborn Infant

A. **Short-term observation in transition nursery to monitor trends before infant's transfer to neonatal intensive care unit (NICU).**
1. Infant may be capable of resolving the problem on his or her own if given time (e.g., correction of mild acidosis from asphyxia, clearing of lung fluid, stabilization of blood glucose concentration, stabilization of blood pressure).
2. Monitor and record trends (i.e., improved respiratory rate toward normal, improved perfusion, normal glucose screens).

B. **Avoid excessive handling.**
1. Organize care and interventions to avoid frequent, unnecessary stimulation of an already stressed infant.
2. Use pulse oximeter or cardiorespiratory monitor to reduce hands-on determination of vital signs.
3. Reduce background stimulation such as loud noises or bright lights.
4. Use nonnutritive sucking to lower activity levels and reduce energy needs.
   a. Infant may be more comfortable in a prone position.
   b. Crying can be stressful and is similar to a Valsalva maneuver, with prolonged exhalation, obstructed venous return, quick inspiratory gasp, and right-to-left shunting at the foramen ovale.
   c. Crying depletes energy reserves and increases oxygen consumption.

C. **Provide a neutral thermal environment (refer to Chapter 6).**
1. Observe infant for apnea and hypotension during warming.
2. Avoid hyperthermia.

D. **Supply glucose.**
1. Oral administration of glucose for a blood glucose level of 30 to 40 mg/dl in an otherwise healthy asymptomatic neonate; early, frequent feedings by nipple, gavage, or nursing.

a. Give at least 0.5 to 1 ounce of formula by nipple or gavage if there are no contraindications to enteral feedings and the infant is free of symptoms (see Routine Care Considerations in the Transition Nursery, on p. 86). If condition is stable, infant may be allowed to nurse 5 to 10 minutes on each breast.
b. Begin maintenance formula at 50 to 70 kcal/kg/day or breast-feed on demand every 2 to 3 hours.
c. Check blood glucose 30 minutes to 1 hour after feeding.
d. Consider giving a formula designed for premature infants.
   (1) These formulas provide 50% of carbohydrate in the form of glucose polymers that are easily absorbed; salivary amylase retains its activity in the infant's stomach because of increased gastric pH and is effective in digestion of glucose polymers (Blackburn, 2003).
   (2) Approximately 50% of the fats are provided as medium-chain triglycerides (MCTs). MCTs are absorbed from the stomach; they may also increase the level of plasma ketones, which can be used as an alternative substrate to glucose for brain metabolism (Blackburn, 2003).
   (3) The process of absorbing fat (fatty acid oxidation and ketogenesis) spares glucose for brain energy needs; free fatty acids and ketones promote glucose production by providing essential gluconeogenic cofactors.
   (4) Healthy newborn infants respond to a protein meal by preferentially increasing glucagon, which elicits a glycemic response.

2. Intravenous administration of glucose for hypoglycemia (see Routine Care Considerations in the Transition Nursery, item D: Glucose Needs/First Feeding on p. 89) is as follows:
   a. Provide bolus (2 ml/kg) of 10% dextrose in water ($D_{10}W$), followed by an infusion of 6 to 8 mg/kg/minute; $D_{10}W$ = 100 mg/ml.
   b. Monitor therapy with frequent glucose checks and titrate infusion rate and concentration to meet the infant's needs. NOTE: Do not administer an IV bolus of glucose greater than 25% dextrose in water because of reactive hypoglycemia and hypertonicity of the solution. Always follow a glucose bolus with a continuous infusion of glucose.

E. **Supply oxygen;** assess needs with a pulse oximeter or arterial blood gas determinations and close observation.
   1. Extended oxygen use in the transition nursery requires notification of the physician and transfer to a level II or III setting.
   2. Provide warmed, humidified oxygen by oxygen hood, continuous positive airway pressure by nasal prongs, or assisted ventilation by endotracheal tube according to the infant's needs (refer to Chapter 25).
   3. Monitor oxygen provided with an oxygen analyzer. Record blow-by oxygen as liters per minute and distance from infant's face.

F. **Supply volume expanders, including blood and normal saline solution.**
   1. For hypotension and blood loss.
   2. Requires IV line placement and transfer to level II nursery for continued management and observation, including cardiorespiratory monitoring and blood pressure checks to adjust therapy as necessary.

G. **Naloxone hydrochloride (Narcan).**
   1. Administer drug for severe respiratory depression in delivery room and history of maternal narcotic administration within past 4 hours.
   2. Do *not* use naloxone if mother has history of opioid dependency: *may precipitate acute withdrawal symptoms.*

H. **Antibiotics.**
   1. As indicated by history, current status of the infant, and initial results of sepis evaluation.
   2. Administer via peripheral IV or heparin-lock IV line.

PARENT TEACHING

Before Delivery

A. **History.** Review obstetric history; anticipate needs of infant at delivery.
B. **Complications.** If there are expected complications (preterm delivery, congenital anomalies) and time permits, discuss anticipated plan of care with the family.
   1. Discuss plans for managing the infant, including plans for transfer to a level II or III nursery and any special equipment that may be used (oxygen hood, incubator, ventilator, monitors).
   2. Allow the parents to tour the NICU if possible.
C. **Parental support.** Encourage parents to express their feelings, fears, misgivings; involve support people.

At Delivery

A. **Place infant on mother's abdomen when possible with uncomplicated deliveries; use family's birth plan as much as possible.**
B. **After delivery room assessment, return infant to family if infant's condition is stable.**
C. **Answer questions regarding acrocyanosis, Apgar scores, morphologic findings.**
D. **Allow parents time to visit, breast-feed, see extended family.**

During Transition

A. **"Introduce" newborn to family by noting unique features (dimples, long eyelashes, hair color).**
B. **Encourage support person to touch and talk to the infant.**
C. **Discuss physical findings such as caput succedaneum, head molding, positional deformities, birthmarks.**
D. **Discuss infant's sensory capabilities, including seeing, hearing, smell.**
E. **Listen to the parents.** Allow them to express their reactions as they compare their "dream" infant with the real infant they now have (too tiny, not the right sex, deformed, premature).
F. **After completion of admission procedures, the infant is returned to the family for feeding and visiting.**
G. **Allow family to participate in the infant's care, such as giving the first bath or first feeding.**

Postpartum Period (Early Discharge)

A. **Parental involvement.** Involve the parents in evaluation of their learning needs; begin teaching as soon as delivery occurs.
B. **Short hospital stays and family instruction.** With shorter hospital stays, there is less time available for teaching and an increased importance of teaching. This may be the only information many families receive on care of a newborn infant.
   1. Classes; videotaped lectures.
      a. Cardiopulmonary resuscitation; safety.
      b. Breast-feeding.

c. Childbirth preparation.
d. Developmental milestones.

2. Follow-up visits by nurse to the home and phone calls from postpartum nurses. Encourage families to call the nursery if they have questions about their newborn's care.
3. Follow-up visit with primary care provider. Encourage family to select a primary care provider and assist in making an appointment for the first visit.
4. Return visit for newborn screening if needed.

Transfer to Level II or III Setting

A. **Provide prenatal teaching—if possible, with visits to NICU.**
B. **Provide information booklets, with location, phone numbers, visiting regulations, parent-to-parent groups, necessary support personnel.**
C. **Bring mother to infant's bedside if infant is unable to return to mother after delivery.** Allow family members to be near infant as much as possible and encourage them to see past the equipment to the infant and his or her special needs (gentle touch, stroking, soft voice, a familiar person).
D. **When infant is stable, allow family members to visit in the privacy of their postpartum room or a parent room if condition warrants;** for example, an infant with a heparin lock for antibiotics might go to the mother's room to nurse.
E. **Provide a picture and footprints of the infant for the family.** This is especially important if transfer to a level II or III nursery will be to another facility.
F. **Facilitate family in keeping in contact with the transfer facility, and be available to explain information given to the family.**

REFERENCES

American Academy of Pediatrics Policy Statement: Routine evaluation of blood pressure, hematocrit, and glucose in newborns (RE9322). *Pediatrics, 92*(3): 474-476, 1993.

American Academy of Pediatrics: *Report of the committee on infectious disease* (25th ed.). Elk Grove Village, IL, 2000, Authors.

American Academy of Pediatrics and American College of Obstetricians and Gynecologists: *Guidelines for perinatal care* (5th ed.). Elk Grove Village, IL, and Washington, DC, 2002, Authors.

American Academy of Pediatrics Committee on Infectious Diseases: Update on timing of hepatitis B vaccine for premature infants and for children with lapsed immunizations. *Pediatrics, 94*(3):403-404, 2000.

Blackburn, S.T.: *Maternal, fetal, and neonatal physiology: A clinical perspective* (2nd ed.). St Louis, 2003, Saunders, pp. 413-414, 420.

Blake, W.W. and Murray J.A.: Heat balance. In G. B. Merenstein and S.L. Gardner (Eds.): *Handbook of neonatal intensive care* (5th ed.). St Louis, 2002, Mosby, pp. 102-116.

Brook, M.M., Heymann, M.A., and Teitel, D.F.: The heart. In M.H. Klaus and A.A. Fanaroff (Eds.): *Care of the high-risk neonate* (5th ed.). Philadelphia, 2001, Saunders, pp. 393-424.

Burchett, S.K.: Viral infections. In J.P. Cloherty and A.R. Stark (Eds.): *Manual of neonatal care* (4th ed.). Philadelphia, 1998, Lippincott-Raven, pp. 265-269.

Fanaroff, A.A., Kiwi, R., and Shah, D.M.: Antenatal and intrapartum care of the high-risk neonate. In M.H. Klaus and A.A. Fanaroff (Eds.): *Care of the high-risk neonate* (5th ed.). Philadelphia, 2001, Saunders, pp. 1-44.

Izatt, S.D.: Care of the newborn. In A.A. Fanaroff and R.J. Martin (Eds.): *Neonatal-perinatal medicine: Diseases of the fetus and infant* (7th ed.). St Louis, 2002, Mosby, pp. 450-459.

Kalhan, S.C. and Price, P.T.: Nutrition and selected disorders of the gastrointestinal tract. In M.H. Klaus and A.A. Fanaroff (Eds.): *Care of the high-risk neonate* (5th ed.). Philadelphia, 2001, Saunders, pp. 147-194.

Lissauer, T.: Physical examination of the newborn: In A.A. Fanaroff and R.J. Martin (Eds.): *Neonatal-perinatal medicine: Diseases of the fetus and infant* (7th ed.). St Louis, 2002, Mosby, pp. 441-450.

Miller, M.M., Fanaroff, A.A., and Martin, R.J.: Respiratory disorders in preterm and term infants. In A.A. Fanaroff and R.J. Martin (Eds.): *Neonatal-perinatal medicine: Diseases of the fetus and infant* (7th ed.). St Louis, 2002, Mosby, pp. 1025-1049.

Mitchell, A., Steffenson, N., Hogan, H., and Brooks, S.: Neonatal group B streptococcal disease. *MCN American Journal of Maternal Child Nursing*, 22(5):249–253, 1997.

Moore, K.L. and Persaud T.V.N.: *The developing human: Clinically oriented embryology* (7th ed.). Philadelphia, 2003, W.B. Saunders, pp. 366-374.

Nelson, N.: Physiology of transition. In G.B. Avery, M.A. Fletcher, and M.G. MacDonald (Eds.): *Neonatology: Pathophysiology and management of the newborn* (4th ed.). Philadelphia, 1999, J.B. Lippincott, pp. 257-278.

Phibbs, R.H.: Delivery room management of the newborn. In G.B. Avery, M.A. Fletcher, and M.G. MacDonald (Eds.): *Neonatology: Pathophysiology and management of the newborn* (4th ed.). Philadelphia, 1999, J.B. Lippincott, pp. 279-300.

Pierce, J.R. and Turner, B.S.: Physiologic monitoring. In G.B. Merenstein and S.L. Gardner (Eds.): *Handbook of neonatal intensive care* (5th ed.). St Louis, 2002, Mosby, pp. 117-131.

Sun, Y., Awnetwant, E.L., Collier, S.B., et al.: Nutrition. In J.P. Cloherty and A.R. Stark (Eds.): *Manual of neonatal care* (4th ed.). Philadelphia, 1998, Lippincott-Raven, pp. 120-121.

Thureen, P.T. and Abzug, M.J.: Viral infections. In P.J. Thureen, J.M. Deacon, P. O'Neill, and J. Hernandez (Eds.): *Assessment and care of the well newborn.* Philadelphia, 1999, Saunders, p. 324.

Vannucci, R.C.: Perinatal asphyxia. In A.A. Fanaroff and R.J. Martin (Eds.): *Neonatal-perinatal medicine: Diseases of the fetus and infant* (7th ed.). St Louis, 2002, Mosby, pp. 867-879.

Verklan, M.T.: Physiologic variability during transition to extrauterine life. *Critical Care Nursing Quarterly*, 24(4):41-56, 2002.

Wilker, R.E.: Metabolic problems. In J.P. Cloherty and A.R. Stark (Eds.): *Manual of neonatal care* (4th ed.). Philadelphia, 1998, Lippincott-Raven, p. 545

CHAPTER

5 Neonatal Delivery Room Resuscitation

BARBARA ELIZABETH PAPPAS AND BRENDA WALKER

OBJECTIVES

1. Describe three anatomically unique features of the neonate that require special consideration during resuscitation.
2. Compare three physiologic characteristics of the neonate that make neonatal resuscitation different from adult resuscitation.
3. List three antepartum, intrapartum, and postpartum factors that indicate the neonate may be at risk of developing asphyxia.
4. Identify the equipment needed for neonatal resuscitation.
5. Review the components of neonatal resuscitation as outlined by the American Heart Association/American Academy of Pediatrics' Neonatal Resuscitation Program.
6. Recognize three neonatal disease states or congenital malformations that may alter the resuscitation process.
7. Describe three potential complications of neonatal resuscitation.
8. Discuss the postresuscitative needs of the neonate.
9. Verbalize three risk factors that may leave the neonate at risk for cardiopulmonary arrest after the initial period of stabilization.
10. Recall two experimental therapies relating to neonatal resuscitation.

Few newly born infants require resuscitation at birth. The risk for cardiopulmonary arrest in the immediate period following birth most frequently arises from respiratory depression and insufficiency. Most often, the newly born infant requires basic stabilization including thermoregulation and airway management. Infants at higher risk benefit from prompt, organized, and efficient interventions tailored to their needs and response. The overall goal of resuscitation should be to minimize the effects of hypoxia and promote stabilization and recovery for optimal outcome.

DEFINITIONS

Newly born: time of the infant's life from birth to first hours after birth.
Neonate: refers to the first 28 days of the infant's life.
Infant: neonatal period extending through the first 12 months of life.

ANATOMY AND PHYSIOLOGY

A. **Physiologic and anatomic characteristics.** Normal characteristics specific to the neonate differ from the adult, leaving the neonate at significant risk for compromise. A thorough understanding of the uniqueness of the neonate often allows anticipation and intervention before the neonate is compromised to the point of cardiac failure. Unique characteristics specific to the neonate include:

1. Large head in proportion to body size. At risk for:
   a. Insensible water loss (IWL).
   b. Heat loss: no insulating fat layer.
   c. Minimal insulation from hair.
2. Large surface area/body size ratio. At risk for:
   a. IWL.
   b. Heat loss.
3. Decreased muscle mass. At risk for:
   a. Increased potential for heat loss through external gradient.
   b. Decreased ability to flex body to conserve heat.
   c. Decreased ability to generate heat.
4. Decreased subcutaneous fat (premature birth, intrauterine growth restriction). At risk for:
   a. Decreased heat production (from brown fat metabolism).
   b. Increased heat loss (from lack of insulation).
5. Thinner epidermal layer.
   a. Increased IWL; the more premature the greater the loss.
   b. Decreased support of internal gradient to maintain heat.
   c. Increased risk for breakdown and injury can contribute to increased IWL.
6. Immature systems.
   a. Central nervous system (CNS): impaired ability to regulate vasomotor stability resulting in impaired perfusion and poor autoregulation of blood pressure and temperature regulation.
   b. Neuromuscular system: neonate is unable to shiver and generate heat.
   c. Liver: ability to metabolize drugs and mobilize glucose stores is decreased.
   d. Kidneys: risk for decreased perfusion with compromise, ability to excrete drugs and fluids is impaired.
   e. Gastrointestinal tract (GI): gastric distention and respiratory compromise related to decreased GI motility and forced air entry with bag-and-mask ventilation.
   f. Metabolism: decreased stores, decreased ability to convert stored glucose, and increased utilization of glucose results in hypoglycemia.
   g. Respiratory system: decreased surface area for gas exchange, decreased availability of surfactant, and increased risk for aspiration from gastric distention.
   h. Immune system: increased predisposition to infection.
7. Glottis positioned anteriorly in hypopharynx.
   a. Intubation may be difficult.
   b. Neonate is predisposed to airway compromise from positioning.
8. Short neck.
   a. Lack of clarity in identifying landmarks contributes to difficulty in intubation.
   b. Tendency for hyperextension and flexion of neck.
9. Preferential nasal breathing.
   a. Preferential nose breather; patency is essential to airway maintenance.
   b. Anatomic patency must be confirmed.

10. Venous access.
    a. Small and superficial veins: access is difficult, vessels fragile.
    b. Access difficult with altered perfusion.
    c. Umbilical access. Normal cord includes two arteries and one vein. Inadvertent cannulization of the portal vein with umbilical vein catheterization can lead to liver damage with chemical resuscitation.

RISK FACTORS

Risk factors are warning signs that alert the perinatal team to the possibility of a crisis and the need for anticipatory preparation of neonatal resuscitation.

A. **Prepartum period (maternal risk factors):** conditions during pregnancy that predispose mother and fetus to stress and can interfere with successful transition of the fetus to extrauterine life.
   1. Maternal age more than 35 years or less than 16 years.
   2. Maternal diabetes.
   3. Hemorrhage, anemia.
   4. Maternal substance abuse.
   5. Maternal drug therapy.
   6. No or limited prenatal care.
   7. Polyhydramnios or oligohydramnios.
   8. Maternal cardiac, renal, pulmonary, thyroid, or neurologic disease.
   9. Premature rupture of membranes.
   10. Anatomic abnormalities of the uterus.
   11. Isoimmunization, Rh, or ABO (blood group) incompatibilities.
   12. Hypertension (toxemia, chronic).
   13. Multiple gestation.
   14. Previous pregnancy complication or fetal loss.
   15. Maternal infection.

B. **Intrapartum period:** conditions that predispose the fetus to difficult transition to extrauterine life or signs that the fetus is not tolerating the stresses of labor. Unsuccessful transition may ensue.
   1. Abnormal fetal positioning or presentation (e.g., breech position).
   2. Cesarean delivery.
   3. Fetal heart rate abnormalities.
   4. Size-date discrepancies.
   5. Maternal or fetal intrapartum blood loss.
   6. Maternal sedation, anesthesia, or analgesia.
   7. Maternal fever or infection (e.g., chorioamnionitis).
   8. Prolonged or difficult labor (>24 hours or second stage >2 hours).
   9. Premature labor.
   10. Precipitous delivery.
   11. Prolonged rupture of membranes (>18 hours).
   12. Prolapse of the umbilical cord.
   13. Fetal anomalies.
   14. Meconium-stained amniotic fluid.
   15. Instrument-assisted delivery (e.g., vacuum or forceps).

C. **Postpartum period:** signs or conditions in the delivery room or during the transitional period that indicate the neonate is having difficulty making all the physiologic changes needed for successful adaptation from intrauterine to extrauterine life.

1. Congenital defects (e.g., cardiac, respiratory, gastrointestinal, neurologic).
2. Cardiac arrhythmia or murmur (e.g., tachycardia or bradycardia).
3. Extreme color change (e.g., cyanosis, plethora, pallor).
4. Prolonged or delayed capillary refill time.
5. Respiratory distress (e.g., apnea, tachypnea, grunting, altered breath sounds).
6. Temperature instability.
7. Hypertonia/hypotonia.
8. Hypotension.
9. Seizures.
10. Hypoglycemia.
11. Prematurity.
12. Postmaturity.
13. Feeding difficulty or intolerance.

ANTICIPATION OF AND PREPARATION FOR RESUSCITATION

Anticipation and preparation for resuscitation requires a comprehensive and multidisciplinary approach that integrates national regulatory and institutional guidelines, protocols, and procedures. The International Liaison Committee on Resuscitation (ILCOR) formulates evidence-based recommendations on resuscitation. Based on these recommendations, the Neonatal Resuscitation Program (NRP), designed by the American Heart Association and the American Academy of Pediatrics, is an internationally accepted program that provides education for health care professionals on resuscitation of the newborn infant and neonate. All units and facilities caring for newborn infants and neonates must be adequately staffed, prepared, and equipped to deliver resuscitative care when anticipated or unexpected resuscitation needs arise.

A. General preparation.

1. Educate and maintain skill levels of staff. At a minimum, annual competency evaluation and review is recommended. Review prior to anticipated need if possible (including drug doses, concentrations, side effects, and handling equipment).
2. Evaluate and update equipment needs frequently.
3. Arrange for periodic evaluation and maintenance of electrical equipment by the biomedical engineering department on a regularly scheduled basis.
4. Schedule periodic evaluation and maintenance of all respiratory equipment.
5. Formulate supply replacement procedures. Evaluate and replace supplies as quickly as possible after use (use equipment checklist).
6. Test alerting system for rapid, consistent response of personnel.

B. Delivery room preparation.

1. Promote effective communication between personnel, departments, and institutions that encourages identification and notification of high-risk situations and preparedness.
2. Prewarm room to minimize thermal losses in the newly born infant.
3. Assemble equipment in organized, easily available system. Check function of equipment routinely and prior to use.
4. Ensure safety of team members and utilization of standard precautions.

5. Preheat warmer, hat, blankets and nest (blanket rolls or bendable positioning device). Approximately 15 minutes (heat output set on high) is required to thoroughly warm the mattress on a radiant warmer bed. Assemble alternative heat sources to bedside as needed (i.e., warming pad, heating lamps).
6. Identify and assemble available team members and designate roles.
7. Position resuscitation algorithms and charts easily within view of the resuscitative area.
8. Promote family-centered care through active family communication and involvement in decision making.

C. **Personnel roles.**
1. Personnel roles should be defined by institutional policies and job descriptions in addition to state laws, license regulations, and scope of practice definitions.
2. Preparedness for resuscitation should exist at every delivery. Every delivery should be attended by at least one person skilled in neonatal resuscitation who is solely responsible for management of the newly born infant, with additional qualified personnel available for more complex situations.
3. A family-centered approach should include a designated support and communication liaison to the family. Family support should not be left unassigned.

D. **Nondelivery room preparation.** As with delivery room resuscitation, being prepared for unforeseen events throughout the entire infant's hospitalization can facilitate success in a time of crisis. Unlike delivery room events, nondelivery room resuscitation is often unpredictable and risks ill preparedness. The following events may precipitate respiratory or circulatory compromise:
1. Apnea.
2. Choking or aspiration (i.e., feedings).
3. Unwitnessed cardiac arrest.
4. Seizure.
5. Hypoxia or airway obstruction.
6. Infection.
7. Postoperative period.
8. Air leak syndromes.
9. Severe anemia.

EQUIPMENT FOR NEONATAL RESUSCITATION

Not every item on the equipment list (Box 5-1) will be used, but it is important to have appropriate sizes and supply quantities to support a prolonged effort. Ensuring that equipment is functional and up to date is vital to a successful resuscitation. It is important that staff members be familiar with the equipment they will be using and practice with it frequently.

DECISION-MAKING PROCESS

For many years delivery room resuscitation decisions were based on Apgar scores (Table 5-1). Current recommendations discourage the use of the Apgar score for decision making in resuscitation. Components of the Apgar score are used for assessment and reassessment of resuscitative progress (Covey and Butterfield, 1962) (Box 5-2).

BOX 5-1
NEONATAL RESUSCITATION EQUIPMENT LIST

- Radiant warmer with firm mattress and/or other heat source
- Warmed linen and hat
- Cardiac monitor or pulse oximeter (optional)
- Mechanical suction with tubing
- Suction catheters: 5F or 6F, 8F, 10F or 12F
- Bulb syringe
- 8F feeding tube and 20-ml syringe
- Meconium aspiration device
- Resuscitation bag: flow-inflating or self-inflating, 750 ml or less, with pressure-release valve or pressure manometer capable of delivering 90% to 100% oxygen
- Face mask: premature and newborn sizes
- Oxygen source: flow rate up to 10 ml/min
- Oxygen tubing
- Air source (tank or wall) for blended oxygen
- Stethoscope: neonatal size
- Clock with second hand and timer (optional)
- Standard Precautions supplies: gloves, barrier gown, mask, eye protection
- Laryngoscope with straight blade, No. 0 (premature), No. 1 (term) to No. 00 (ELBW) optional
- Extra batteries and bulbs for laryngoscope
- Endotracheal tubes: 2 (optional), 2.5, 3, 3.5, 4 mm
- Stylet (optional)
- Scissors
- Tape or securing device for endotracheal tube, latex free preferred
- Normal saline for endotracheal tube instillation or flushing
- Alcohol swabs
- Skin preparation or pectin skin barrier (approved for neonate)
- Carbon dioxide detector (optional)
- Laryngeal mask airway (optional)
- Oral airways: size 000, 00, and 0 or 30, 40, and 50 mm lengths
- Epinephrine 1:10,000 (0.1 mg/ml)
- Normal saline for IV infusion, volume expansion
- Lactated Ringer's
- Sodium bicarbonate 4.2% (0.5 mEq/ml)
- Naloxone hydrochloride (0.4 mg/ml or 1 mg/ml)
- Dextrose 10% water for IV infusion, 250 or 500 ml
- Surfactant (optional)
- 5F or 6F feeding tube
- Syringes: 1, 3, 5, 10, 20 ml
- Needles: 25, 21, 18 gauge or needleless system puncture device
- Dextrose 5% water or normal saline for IV flush
- Medication and syringe labels
- Umbilical catheterization supplies
- Umbilical catheters: 3.5F and 5F
- Three-way stopcock
- Supplies for blood gas evaluation

ELBW, Extremely low birth weight; *IV,* intravenous.

Interventions should never be delayed pending the 1-minute Apgar score. Decisions about resuscitation interventions are based on quick and frequent assessment and evaluation of the newborn. Follow-up assessment and evaluation of the effectiveness of the action are made frequently throughout the resuscitation and continued intervention are based on the neonate's status and response.

NEONATAL RESUSCITATION "ABCs"

The steps taken to rescue or resuscitate a neonate are best remembered with the familiar "ABCs" of resuscitation used in all resuscitation programs of the American Heart Association.

TABLE 5-1
Apgar Score

The Apgar score is a method of evaluating a newborn infant's condition at birth on the basis of five characteristics: heart rate, respiratory effort, muscle tone, reflex irritability, and color. For each parameter the infant receives a score of 0 if it is absent, 1 if it is present but abnormal, and 2 if it is normal. Traditionally scores are assigned at 1 and 5 minutes, but in prolonged resuscitation a score can be assigned at any time to reflect the condition of the infant and the response to resuscitative efforts. With perinatal depression, the Apgar characteristics generally disappear in a predictable manner: first the pink coloration is lost, next the respiratory effort, and then tone, followed by reflex irritability and, finally, heart rate. Return of the characteristics with recovery is not in the same order with tone returning last.

	Score		
Sign	**0**	**1**	**2**
Heart rate	Absent	Less than 100 beats per minute (bpm)	More than 100 bpm
Respiratory effort	Absent	Weak, irregular	Good, crying
Muscle tone	Flaccid	Some flexion of extremities	Well flexed
Reflex irritability (catheter in nose)	No response	Grimace	Cough or sneeze
Color	Blue, pale	Body pink, extremities blue	Completely pink

A. ABCs defined.
1. Preparation for ABCs. Ask the following questions:
   - **a.** Is the amniotic fluid clear? Is there meconium present?
   - **b.** Is the neonate breathing? Does the neonate cry?
   - **c.** Is the neonate's muscle tone appropriate for gestational age?
   - **d.** What is the neonate's color? Does the neonate have central cyanosis?
   - **e.** Is the neonate term?
2. A = Airway.
3. B = Breathing.
4. C = Circulation.
5. D = Drugs/medications.
6. E = Environment.

BOX 5-2
PRACTICAL EPIGRAM OF THE APGAR SCORE

Sign
A = Appearance (color)
P = Pulse (heart rate)
G = Grimace (reflex irritability response to stimulation of sole of foot)
A = Activity (muscle tone)
R = Respiration (respiratory effort)

From Covey, M.J. and Butterfield, L.J.: Practical epigram of the Apgar score (letter), *Journal of the American Medical Association 181*:353, 1962.

B. Initial steps. At most deliveries, the following five steps are the only interventions necessary. Initial steps should not take longer than approximately 30 seconds unless managing the infant that is depressed with meconium.

1. Prevent hypothermia, which may increase metabolic requirements and contribute to respiratory distress, metabolic acidosis, and hypoglycemia.

a. Place and keep neonate in preheated environment (radiant heat source or incubator). Supplement environmental support with:

(1) Warmed linens and towels.

(2) Warmed hat.

b. Avoidance of drafts, e.g., sidewalls up on radiant warmer; limit door open and closing; keep bed away from ventilation drafts.

2. Open the airway.

a. Position infant on the back or side, with neck slightly extended.

(1) Care should be taken to avoid hyperextension or flexion of the neck (Fig. 5-1).

(2) A shoulder pad may help maintain the correct airway position.

(3) When supine, the infant's head may be turned to the side without airway compromise.

b. Suction the mouth before the nose.

(1) Use bulb syringe or wall suction. The suction pressure should be approximately 80 to 100 mm Hg for the term neonate and 60 to 80 mm Hg for the preterm neonate.

(2) Vigorous or prolonged deep suctioning can result in bradycardia or apnea induced by stimulation of the posterior pharynx and vagus nerve.

(3) When meconium-stained fluid is present and the neonate is not vigorous (heart rate less than 100, apneic or gasping, poor muscle tone), intubate the trachea and perform direct tracheal suctioning.

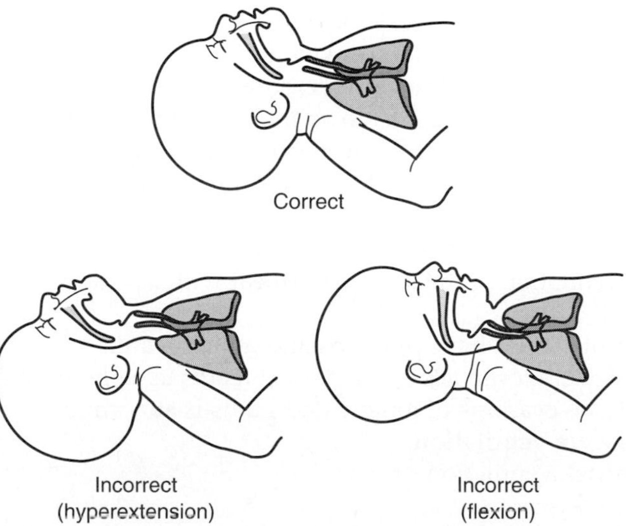

FIGURE 5-1 ■ Correct and incorrect head positions for airway management. (From Kattwinkel, J. (Ed.): *Textbook of neonatal resuscitation* [4th ed.]. Elk Grove Village, IL, 2000, American Academy of Pediatrics/American Heart Association.)

Repeat intubation and suctioning until clear of meconium or heart rate indicates continued deterioration.

(4) A vigorous neonate born through meconium-stained fluid may not require intubation and visualization of the vocal cords for the presence of meconium. Clinical judgment must be used.

3. Continued thermal and airway support.

a. Maintain dry, warm environment.

(1) Dry thoroughly.

(2) Remove wet linen immediately after drying infant and replace with dry linen.

(3) Place warmed, dry hat.

(4) Provide additional heat source as necessary. Use of warm water gloves may contribute to increased heat loss as water in gloves cools and neonate conducts heat to the gloves.

b. Reposition airway.

4. Stimulate respirations.

a. Gently slap or flick the soles of the infant's feet.

b. Gently rub the back, trunk, and extremities.

c. Attempts to stimulate should be brief, no more than two attempts. If respirations do not begin, proceed to bag-and-mask ventilation (unless diaphragmatic hernia is suspected, in which case intubate the trachea and ventilate the infant through the endotracheal tube with the resuscitation bag).

5. Begin blow-by oxygen at any time if central cyanosis is present, heart rate is greater than 100 beats per minute (bpm), and respirations are adequate.

a. Provide 100% oxygen at 5 to 10 L/minute. Deliver by oxygen mask, cupped hand holding oxygen tubing over infant's face, or through flow-inflating bag and mask via the reservoir tail. Deliver oxygen close to the face, allowing some oxygen to escape the mask and preventing a buildup of pressure within the bag-and-mask system.

b. Continue oxygen delivery until infant pinks and then slowly withdraw, ensuring adequate delivery for infant to remain pink.

6. Evaluate the infant's condition frequently.

a. Airway: assess for alignment, secretions, inadvertent extubation.

b. Respiratory effort: rate, breath sounds, work of breathing (grunting, flaring, retracting, depth), symmetry of chest movement.

c. Heart rate: count for 6 seconds and multiply by 10. Obtain heart rate by:

(1) Palpation at the base of the umbilical cord stump.

(2) Auscultation of the apical heartbeat with a stethoscope.

d. Color.

(1) Infant should have pink lips and a pink trunk.

(2) Peripheral cyanosis of hands and feet is usually normal.

(3) Central cyanosis of tongue and gums is abnormal.

C. Positive-pressure ventilation.

1. Bag-and-mask ventilation.

a. Initiate when:

(1) Apnea or gasping respirations.

(2) Inadequate ventilatory effort.

(3) Heart rate is less than 100 bpm.
(4) Color remains cyanotic despite 100% blow-by oxygen.
(5) Need for continued ventilation is determined by frequent assessment of the infant's response to interventions.

b. Equipment.
(1) Self-inflating bags must have a reservoir to deliver high concentrations of oxygen, and should have a pressure gauge and a pressure-release valve.
(2) Flow-inflating (anesthesia) bags must have a pressure gauge and flow control valve.
(3) The size of the resuscitation bag should be no larger than 750 ml.
(4) Bag, mask, and tubing should always be connected to 100% oxygen source at 5 to 10 L of flow.
(5) Mask of proper size should be used to obtain adequate seal. Appropriate sizing should have the mask covering the chin, mouth, and nose, but not the eyes.
(6) Equipment should always be present, ready for use, and checked before each use, as well as at least once per shift. Preset equipment with equipment check prior to use.

c. Procedure.
(1) Assemble, set, and test the equipment.
(2) Position the neonate as in "Initial Steps," item B, Open the Airway under Neonatal Resuscitation "ABCs," page 109.
(3) Apply mask and ensure proper seal. Be careful not to apply too much pressure to the neonate's face or neck.
(4) Observe for easy chest rise and fall. Rate of ventilation is 40 to 60 breaths per minute. Approximate pressure required for the lung inflation should be:
(a) Initial breath: 30 to 40 cm H_2O pressure.
(b) Normal lungs: 15 to 20 cm H_2O pressure.
(c) Diseased lungs: 20 to 40 cm H_2O pressure.
(5) If necessary, pause to check 6-second heart rate. Continue ventilation until neonate begins spontaneous effective breathing and the heart rate is greater than 100 bpm.
(6) If bag-and-mask ventilation is ineffective or if there is need for prolonged ventilation, endotracheal intubation should be performed.

d. Exceptions.
(1) Meconium-stained fluid and nonvigorous neonate. If thick particulate meconium or thin meconium and depressed respirations are present, intubate the trachea for suctioning prior to initiating bag-and-mask ventilation.
(2) If a diaphragmatic hernia is present or is suspected, perform intubation, give bag-to-tube ventilation, and place orogastric tube for gastric decompression.

e. Oral gastric tube placement.
(1) Ventilation for more than several minutes (with or without compressions) can cause air to accumulate in the stomach.
(2) Ensure the tube is placed through the mouth rather than the nose to maximize ventilation through the nose.
(3) Secure in place and leave open to air.

2. Ventilation by bag to endotracheal tube.
   a. Indications.
      (1) The neonate does not respond to bag-and-mask ventilation, as evidenced by inadequate chest expansion, lack of spontaneous respirations, continued heart rate less than 100, diminished muscle tone, or persistent central cyanosis.
      (2) Diaphragmatic hernia is suspected or confirmed.
      (3) Prolonged ventilation is required.
      (4) Tracheal suctioning is required.
      (5) Extreme prematurity.
      (6) Surfactant administration.
      (7) Chemical resuscitation.
      (8) Administration of chest compression to facilitate coordination of compressions and ventilation, maximize efficiency of ventilation.
   b. Equipment.
      (1) Laryngoscope, batteries, bulbs, and size 00, 0, and 1 blades (straight preferred).
      (2) Noncuffed endotracheal tubes, with vocal cord guide, in a variety of sizes (two each): sizes 2.0 (optional), 2.5, 3.0, 3.5, and 4.0.
      (3) Endotracheal tube stylets (optional).
      (4) Suction equipment with catheters in sizes 5F, 6F, 8F, and 10F or larger (two each).
      (5) Shoulder roll for positioning.
      (6) Adhesive tape and scissors.
      (7) Resuscitation bag (less than 750 L), manometer, and masks.
      (8) Oxygen source, flowmeter, and tubing.
      (9) Stethoscope.
   c. Procedure (see Chapter 15).
      (1) Should be a clean procedure.
      (2) Perform intubation.
      (3) Confirm placement of endotracheal tube.
      (4) Secure tube.
      (5) Observe for dislocation of endotracheal tube or unplanned extubation.

D. Chest compressions.

1. Chest compressions should be initiated when the heart rate is less than 60 bpm after 15 to 30 seconds of ventilation with 100% oxygen.
2. Use one of the following two methods (Fig. 5-2):
   a. Thumb technique.
      (1) Place both thumbs over the lower third of the infant's sternum above the xiphoid process.
      (2) Encircle the infant's torso with hands and provide support for the back. If hands are too small, ensure that the infant is on a firm surface.
   b. Two-finger technique.
      (1) Place the tips of the middle finger and either the index finger or the ring finger of one hand over the lower third of the infant's sternum.
      (2) Place other hand under the infant's back to provide support.

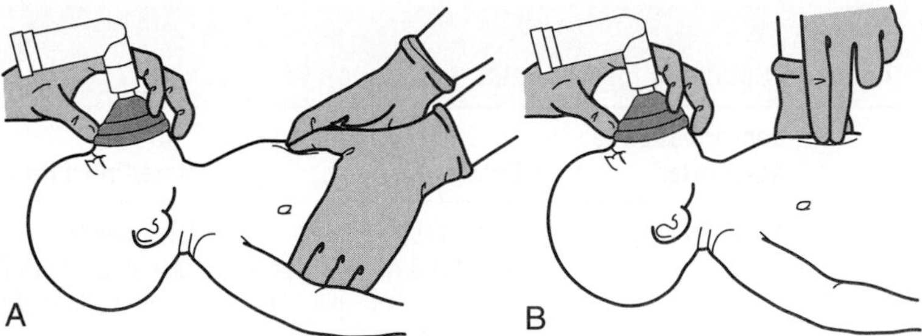

FIGURE 5-2 ■ Two techniques for providing chest compressions. (From Kattwinkel, J. (Ed.).: *Textbook of neonatal resuscitation* [4th ed.]. Elk Grove Village, IL, 2000, American Academy of Pediatrics/American Heart Association.)

(3) Compressions should squeeze the heart between the spinal column and the sternum.
  (a) Force of compression should be straight down to minimize rib or lung damage.
  (b) Depress the sternum approximately one third of the anterior-posterior diameter of the chest.
  (c) Fingers or thumbs should remain in contact with the chest at all times, both during compression and release. Lack of contact with chest wall increases risk for complications and wastes time relocating landmarks for compression area.

(4) Compression:ventilation ratio: 1:3.
  (a) Provide three compressions, pause for a single ventilation. This will equal 30 ventilations and 90 compressions, or 120 events per minute.
  (b) Optimally the neonate's trachea should be intubated during compressions.
  (c) Reevaluate respiratory effort and heart rate every 30 seconds during compressions and ventilations.

(5) Indications for discontinuing chest compressions.
  (a) Heart rate greater than 60 bpm, and increasing.
  (b) After 10 minutes of asystole or 15 to 20 minutes of absent heart rate in spite of full resuscitation measures.

E. **Chemical resuscitation.** Most neonatal resuscitations do not require medications or volume expanders. An umbilical catheter or peripheral intravenous (IV) line will need to be placed to administer medications or volume expanders (see Chapter 15). Epinephrine and naloxone hydrochloride (Narcan) may be administered through the endotracheal tube until IV access is established.

1. Indications.
   a. Stimulate the heart.
   b. Increase tissue perfusion.
   c. Correct metabolic acidosis.
   d. Failure of infant to improve despite adequate ventilation with 100% oxygen and chest compressions.

TABLE 5-2
Medications and Solutions for Neonatal Resuscitation

Medication	Concentration to Administer	Dosage/Route	Rate/Precautions
Epinephrine	1:10,000	0.01 to 0.03 mg/kg 0.1 to 0.3 ml/kg IV or ET	Give rapidly May dilute with 0.5 to 1 ml normal saline if per ETT May flush with 0.5 to 1 ml normal saline if undiluted
Volume expanders	Normal saline Lactated Ringer's Whole blood	10 ml/kg IV	Give over 5 to 10 minutes
Sodium bicarbonate	4.2% solution or 0.5 mEq/ml	2 mEq/kg (4 ml/kg) IV only	Give slowly—not faster than 1 mEq/kg/min (2 ml/kg/min) Ensure adequate ventilation prior to administration
Naloxone hydrochloride	1 mg/ml	0.1 mg/kg IV, ET preferred IM, SQ acceptable	Give rapidly

ET, Endotracheal; *ETT*, endotracheal tube; *IM*, intramuscular; *IV*, intravenous; *SQ*, subcutaneous.

2. Medications and solutions (Table 5-2).
 a. Epinephrine, a cardiac stimulant, increases the heart rate and strength of contractions and causes peripheral vasoconstriction.
  (1) Indications for use:
   (a) Heart rate is less than 60 bpm after ventilation with 100% oxygen, endotracheal tube, and chest compressions.
   (b) Heart rate is undetectable while ventilations and compressions are being started.
  (2) Concentration: 1:10,000.
  (3) Dose: 0.1 to 0.3 ml/kg, given rapidly.
  (4) Route: peripheral IV infusion, through endotracheal tube, or through umbilical catheter (venous catheter preferred).
  (5) When given through endotracheal tube, the dose may be diluted in 1 ml of normal saline solution or flushed in with 0.5 to 1 ml normal saline solution to ensure delivery.
  (6) Response: effect should be evident within 30 seconds of administration. Dosing may be repeated every 3 to 5 minutes.
 b. Volume expanders are fluids that increase the neonate's circulating blood volume to correct hypovolemia and facilitate tissue perfusion.
  (1) Indicated when there is suspected or documented blood loss with signs of hypovolemia or shock, or if the infant fails to respond to resuscitation efforts.
   (a) Weak or absent peripheral pulses.
   (b) Low blood pressure.
   (c) Persistent bradycardia or tachycardia.

(d) Pale or mottled skin despite good oxygenation.
(e) Diminished or limp muscle tone.
(f) Continued respiratory depression or apnea.

(2) Solutions.
(a) Normal saline solution (preferred).
(b) Lactated Ringer's solution.
(c) Whole blood (type O-negative, cross-matched to the mother if time permits).

(3) Dose: 10 ml/kg in 5 to 10 minutes.

(4) Route: peripheral IV line or through umbilical catheter (venous preferred).

(5) Response: increase in blood pressure, improvement of skin perfusion, and increase in the intensity of pulses should occur within minutes. Procedure may be repeated if necessary.

c. Sodium bicarbonate, a base buffer, raises the pH of the blood.

(1) Adequate ventilation required prior to use. Sodium bicarbonate breaks down into water and carbon dioxide, which will conjugate to form carbonic acid if the carbon dioxide is not effectively removed via ventilation.

(2) Indications for use:
(a) Documented or suspected metabolic acidosis.
(b) Evidence of prolonged asphyxia.

(3) Concentration: 4.2% solution, 0.5 mEq/ml.

(4) Dose: 2 mEq/kg, slow IV push (do not exceed 1 mEq/kg/minute).

(5) Route: peripheral IV infusion or through umbilical catheter (venous preferred). Sodium bicarbonate can be very damaging to lung tissue and should not be given per endotracheal tube.

(6) Response: pH should change and tone and respirations improve.

d. Naloxone hydrochloride (Narcan), a short-acting narcotic antagonist, displaces narcotics from receptor sites and reverses the physiologic depressant effects of the narcotic.

(1) Indications for use.
(a) Not the first intervention for respiratory depression. Use should follow ventilatory support and other initial steps of resuscitation.
(b) Respiratory depression in a neonate whose mother (known not to be addicted to narcotics or on methadone therapy) was given a narcotic within 4 hours prior to birth.

(2) Concentration: 1.0 mg/ml.

(3) Dose: 0.1 mg/kg given rapidly.

(4) Route: peripheral IV line, umbilical catheter or endotracheal preferred. Subcutaneous or intramuscular is acceptable but absorption may be delayed, especially in the depressed neonate.

(5) Response.
(a) Respiratory depression should decrease within seconds or minutes (depending on route) after administration. Duration of action is widely variable (1 to 4 hours). Monitor closely for return of respiratory depression. May be repeated several times if needed.
(b) If given to a neonate of a mother who is narcotic addicted or on methadone maintenance, naloxone may precipitate immediate and severe withdrawal, including seizures or cardiorespiratory arrest.

UNUSUAL SITUATIONS

A. Pulmonary hypoplasia.

1. Definitions and characteristics.
   a. Underdeveloped lungs resulting from insufficient space within the thoracic cavity for normal development.
   b. Associated with Potter syndrome, dysplastic renal conditions, chronic oligohydramnios, and diaphragmatic hernia.
2. Clinical presentation: deterioration may be acute.
   a. Inability to ventilate lungs adequately exhibited by poor chest movement, decreased breath sounds, and cyanosis.
   b. Very high pressures required to expand small, stiff lungs.
   c. High risk of pulmonary air leak.
   d. Low and/or descending Apgar.
   e. Poor perfusion.
   f. Diminished muscle tone.
3. Management.
   a. Intubate.
   b. Ventilate with 100% oxygen and as much pressure as necessary to expand the lungs (i.e., adequate chest rise and fall).
   c. Transilluminate and auscultate chest frequently, assessing for pulmonary air leaks.
   d. Place orogastric tube as soon as possible to prevent gastric and intestinal inflation, which could compromise diaphragmatic excursions.

B. Abdominal wall defects.

1. Definition and characteristics.
   a. Gastroschisis: herniation of stomach, liver, or intestines through a defect next to the umbilical cord, usually to the right of the cord.
   b. Omphalocele: midline herniation of the bowel into the umbilical cord.
   c. Exstrophy of the bladder: externalization and aversion of the bladder, urethra, or ureteral orifices through a defect in the lower portion of the abdominal wall.
2. Clinical risks.
   a. Fluid and heat loss through exposed viscera (exposure increases surface area).
   b. Potential for visceral damage from drying or trauma.
   c. Increased risk of infection.
3. Management.
   a. Handle the defect gently and use sterile technique.
   b. Position infant to allow adequate visceral perfusion.
      (1) Position infant supine with lateral support to keep defect in midline position, promoting optimal blood flow of the superior mesenteric artery. If defect lies even slightly to the side, superior mesenteric artery may kink and perfusion may be compromised.
      (2) Position infant on right side to prevent kinking of the superior mesenteric artery where it exits the abdomen.
   c. Cover defect. Use of sterile gauze on the defect may be controversial.
      (1) Place infant in sterile bowel bag from axillary region down.
      (2) Wet gauze may cool and exaggerate hypothermia.
      (3) Gauze may stick to the intestinal surface and cause damage when removed.

d. Ensure neutral thermal environment.
e. Observe for hypovolemia. Provide adequate fluid support and maintenance. Fluid losses will be higher than normal.
f. Place orogastric tube to intermittent suction to prevent gastric and intestinal inflation, which would complicate repair.

C. Neural tube defects.

1. Most common types and characteristics.
   a. Anencephaly: most severe form, in which neural tube failed to close and brain is exposed. Death most common in newborn period.
   b. Encephalocele: defect in closure of the neural tube at proximal end, with outpouching of brain tissue through or at the base of the skull.
   c. Myelomeningocele: defect in closure of the neural tube at the distal end, with exposure of the neural tube. Occurs at any level of the spinal column.
2. Acute clinical problems.
   a. Heat and fluid losses through open defect.
   b. Increased risk of infection.
   c. Potential for damage of exposed nervous system tissue as a result of trauma.
   d. Difficulty in handling infant because of exposed tissue.
   e. Ethical and legal questions of viability or organ donation from infants with anencephaly.
3. Management.
   a. Initiate latex precautions immediately to minimize risk of development of latex allergies.
   b. Cover defect with sterile, saline solution–soaked sponges and a plastic barrier to prevent heat and fluid losses.
   c. Maintain neonate in a neutral thermal environment.
   d. Keep neonate on side or prone.
   e. Assisted ventilation may be given with the neonate in side-lying or prone position as necessary.
   f. Manage all defects in the same manner, no matter how severe. Discuss viability issues after resuscitation and stabilization.

D. Choanal atresia/upper airway obstruction.

1. Definitions and characteristics.
   a. Bony or soft tissue obstruction of the posterior nares; may be bilateral or unilateral.
   b. Respiratory distress may be present immediately after birth because of blockage of the primary airway, the nose.
   c. May present with cyanosis when quiet or at rest, pinks with crying.
   d. Inability to pass small-gauge suction catheter or nasogastric tube may be an indicator of choanal atresia.
2. Management.
   a. Stimulate neonate to cry, thereby using the secondary airway (mouth) for ventilation.
   b. Insert an oral airway.
   c. Administer oxygen if needed.
   d. Suction secretions as needed.
   e. Infants with more complicated craniofacial malformations may require endotracheal intubation.

E. Congenital diaphragmatic hernia.

1. Definitions and characteristics (see Chapter 28).
   - a. Herniation of the abdominal contents into the chest cavity early in gestational development.
   - b. Pulmonary hypoplasia arises secondary to compression from abdominal organs and limited capacity for growth in the thoracic cavity.
   - c. Most commonly occurs on the left.
   - d. May present with a scaphoid abdomen.
   - e. Severity of symptoms is associated with the amount of lung compression. May present with rapid respiratory distress and descending Apgars near the time of delivery or respiratory distress later in life.
   - f. Breath sounds absent or decreased on side of defect.
   - g. Bowel sounds audible in chest.
   - h. Heart sounds may be audible on right side if left-sided defect.
   - i. Prenatal diagnosis possible through ultrasound. Polyhydramnios often present.
2. Management.
   - a. Consider immediate endotracheal intubation and ventilation to minimize overdistention of the stomach resulting from bag-and-mask ventilation.
   - b. Provide gastric decompression per oral or nasogastric tube.
   - c. Systemic hypotension and respiratory or metabolic acidosis commonly occur. Aggressive management necessary to minimize pulmonary hypertension.
   - d. Extracorporeal membrane oxygenation (ECMO) and nitric oxide may be used for infants not responding to conventional therapies.

F. Esophageal atresia/tracheoesophageal fistula.

1. Definitions and characteristics.
   - a. Failure of the trachea to differentiate and separate appropriately from the esophagus during gestational development (see Chapter 28).
   - b. Copious secretions present at birth. May cause airway obstruction, aspiration, and respiratory distress.
   - c. Failure to pass oral or nasogastric tube.
2. Management.
   - a. Oral or nasogastric decompression of esophageal pouch to decrease risk of aspiration.
   - b. Position prone or side lying to facilitate secretion drainage.

G. Hydrops fetalis.

1. Definition and characteristics.
   - a. Generalized subcutaneous edema usually accompanied by ascites and pleural or pericardial effusion (see Chapter 28).
2. Management.
   - a. Maintain airway through positioning and endotracheal intubation.
   - b. Thoracentesis or paracentesis may be required to improve ventilation and oxygenation.
   - c. Volume expansion may be necessary due to extravascular fluid shift.

H. Congenital heart disease.

1. Definition and characteristics.
   - a. Cardiac anomalies causing respiratory or cardiac decompensation.
   - b. Persistent cyanosis despite adequate ventilation with 90% to 100% oxygen.
   - c. Murmur may be present.

2. Management.
   a. Cardiorespiratory support as symptoms indicate.
   b. Presentation in the delivery room may range from mild respiratory distress to severe shock and cardiorespiratory arrest.

I. **Multiple gestation.**
1. Definitions and characteristics.
   a. May be small for gestational age or intrauterine growth restricted.
   b. Compression deformations may be present.
   c. Distress may be related to placental abnormalities, compromise of cord blood flow, or mechanical complications during delivery.
2. Management.
   a. Delivery of multiples may be unexpected. Ensure adequate supplies and equipment are available to manage multiple prolonged resuscitative efforts.
   b. Twin-to-twin transfusion may require volume resuscitation.
   c. Premature delivery common.
   d. Systematic and planned approach for mobilizing extra resuscitative teams is necessary to ensure appropriate resuscitation of unexpected multiples.
   e. Always have enough equipment and supplies available, in addition to back-up supplies, to allow for multiple prolonged resuscitative efforts.

J. **Extremely low birth weight infant.**
1. Definitions and characteristics.
   a. Multisystem immaturity.
   b. Fragile skin.
   c. Susceptible to trauma from resuscitative intervention.
   d. Susceptible to infection and thermal instability.
2. Management.
   a. Elective endotracheal intubation.
   b. Utilize additional heat sources to maintain thermal neutral environment (i.e., use circulating water heating pad in addition to radiant heat).
   c. Administration of surfactant.
   d. Provide developmental care to promote physiologic stability.
   e. If at all possible, the family and the primary care physician, along with the neonatal team, should explore viability issues and expected outcome before the birth.
   f. Be as gentle as possible with the tiny neonate (i.e., drying, ventilating, cardiopulmonary resuscitation [CPR]).

COMPLICATIONS OF RESUSCITATION

A. **Trauma.**
1. Skin: bruises and abrasions from chest compressions, handling, and tape application and removal.
2. Mucosa: laryngoscopy and intubation can cause trauma to and bleeding of gums, lips, pharynx, and trachea.
3. Internal organ damage from chest compressions.

B. **Pulmonary air leaks.**
1. Pneumothorax.
2. Pneumomediastinum
3. Pneumopericardium.

C. **Complications related to use of umbilical vessel catheters.**
1. Vessel perforation.
2. Accidental blood loss.

3. Thrombus and emboli.
4. Organ and vessel endothelial damage from infusion of hypertonic solutions.
5. Organ ischemia from blockage of major vessels by the catheter tip.
6. Sepsis.

D. **Intracranial hemorrhage.**
1. Subarachnoid.
2. Periventricular.
3. Intraventricular.

POSTRESUSCITATION CARE

The goal of postresuscitation care is to evaluate the infant's condition for complications, avoid intensifying conditions that may impair outcome (i.e., hypothermia, hypoglycemia), and help diagnose and treat underlying disease.

A. **Assess oxygenation, ventilation, and acid-base balance.**
1. Check arterial blood gas concentrations.
2. Correlate findings with neonate's clinical condition.
3. Correlate findings with transcutaneous and/or pulse oximetry–monitoring devices.
4. Adjust neonate's respiratory support as needed.

B. **Monitor glucose concentrations to ensure normoglycemia.**
1. Serial screening of blood glucose.
2. Treat hypoglycemia and adjust maintenance dextrose infusion if IV fluids required. Bolus infusions ($D_{10}W$, 2 ml/kg) may be required to elevate serum glucose in addition to maintenance infusion.
3. Feeding may not be recommended depending on infant's status.
4. Perform follow-up blood glucose checks as necessary.

C. **Volume and electrolyte support.**
1. Assess perfusion and evaluate for anemia, polycythemia, and hypovolemia.
2. Calculate fluid volume received during resuscitation and estimate volume deficiencies.
3. Determine amount needed (in milliliters per kilogram per day).
4. Adjust IV rate as needed.
5. Monitor urine output. Keep accurate account of intake.

D. **Chest and abdominal x-ray examination for pneumothorax, pneumomediastinum, pneumopericardium, and pneumoperitoneum.**
1. Assess endotracheal tube position.
2. Assess position of umbilical catheters.
3. Evaluate for lung and cardiac disease.
4. Rule out fractures and anomalies.

E. **Monitor vital signs.**
1. Provide a neutral thermal environment to prevent the sequelae of hypothermia.
2. Continue assessment of perfusion and capillary refill in seconds.
3. Monitor blood pressure, preferably arterial.
4. Continuous cardiorespiratory monitoring is recommended. Assess heart rate and respiratory rate as needed.
5. Monitor for seizure activity.

F. **Screen for infection.**
1. Evaluate maternal history: titers, cultures, pretreatment, and risk factors.
2. Obtain a complete blood cell count, differential cell count, platelet count, and C-reactive protein.

3. Obtain blood and viral cultures and for sensitivity testing as indicated.
4. If index of suspicion is high and neonate's condition is stable, lumbar puncture may be performed for cerebral spinal fluid analysis.

G. **Support family.**
1. Provide a family-centered approach to care.
2. Report neonate's condition to mother and significant others.
3. Make appropriate referrals to ancillary support services.

H. **Documentation.**
1. Accurate charting including descriptive and often minute-by-minute documentation reveals the events, interventions, and infant responses to the resuscitative efforts.
2. Include pertinent perinatal factors, physical findings, procedures and care performed, infant response, and team communication.
3. Vital signs, medications, laboratory findings, and other factual data should also be included.
4. Developmental support and infant's behavioral response to care should be integrated into resuscitation and stabilization documentation.

I. **Ethics.**
1. Noninitiation or discontinuation of resuscitation may be appropriate in the delivery room when extreme prematurity or severe congenital anomalies are involved (i.e., confirmed trisomy 13 or 18, gestational age <23 weeks or birth weight <400 g).
2. Information at or around the time of delivery is often incomplete. Resuscitative options may include initiation of therapy and reevaluation of treatment decision making after more information is available.
3. Collaboration with the family is essential with all decision making.

J. **Potential new therapies in resuscitation.**
1. Room air versus 100% oxygen in positive-pressure ventilation.
2. Cerebral hypothermia after perinatal asphyxia.
3. Laryngeal mask airway (LMA).
4. End-tidal CO_2 monitoring for endotracheal confirmation.

REFERENCES

Behar, P.M. and Todd, N.W.: Resuscitation of the newborn with airway compromise. *Clinics in Perinatology, 26*(3):717-732, 1999.

Blackburn, S.T.: *Maternal, fetal, and neonatal physiology: A clinical perspective* (2nd ed.). St Louis, 2003, Saunders.

Chahine, A.A. and Ricketts, R.R.: Resuscitation of the surgical neonate. *Clinics in Perinatology, 26*(3):693-715, 1999.

Covey, M.J. and Butterfield, L.J.: Practical epigram of the Apgar score. *Journal of the American Medical Association,* 181: 353, 1962.

Ginsberg, H.G. and Goldsmith, J.P.: Controverises in neonatal resuscitation. *Clinics in Perinatology, 25*(1):1-15, 1998.

Kattwinkel, J. (Ed.): *Textbook of neonatal resuscitation* (4th ed.). Elk Grove Village, IL, 2000, American Academy of Pediatrics and American Heart Association.

Thigpen, J.: Developmental considerations for resuscitation of the VLBW infant. *Neonatal Network, 21*(4):21-26, 2002.

SECTION TWO

Cornerstones of Clinical Practice

CHAPTER

6 Thermoregulation

BARBARA NOERR

OBJECTIVES

1. Define specific concepts of thermoregulation.
2. Describe differences in thermoregulation between neonates and adults.
3. List guiding concepts for nursing care related to heat transfer mechanisms.
4. Outline effects of neonatal thermal instability.
5. Identify strategies to limit hypothermia and hyperthermia.

Thermoregulation is imperative for optimal physiologic functioning and survival of the neonate (Blackburn, 2003). Although the use of incubators for infants was described in 1722, it was a French physician, Pierre Budin, who first associated a low neonatal body temperature with decreased survival rates (Cone, 1985). Budin's text *The Nursling* described better survival rates for neonates whose rectal temperatures were maintained between 36° and 37°C (96° and 98.6° F). Subsequently, Martin Couney, a student of Budin's, used "modern" incubators from 1932 to 1933 to display preterm neonates at fairs and carnivals, emphasizing that proper care increased the likelihood of survival (Cone, 1985).

Maintenance and ongoing assessment of neonatal thermal stability is critical. Neonates with poor thermoregulatory control are more likely to have poorer outcomes than peers who maintain temperature stability (Blackburn, 2003). Thus a comprehensive understanding of neonatal thermoregulation is the basis of optimal neonatal nursing care. This chapter will outline concepts of neonatal thermoregulation and nursing interventions to support these principles.

CONCEPTS OF THERMOREGULATION

A. **Homeotherm:** animal (e.g., human) able to maintain body temperature within narrow range of environmental temperatures by balancing heat loss and heat production (Blake and Murray, 2002).

B. **Neutral thermal environment (NTE)** (aka thermal neutrality): ideal environmental temperature in which body temperature is maintained within the normal range while metabolic rate, and thus oxygen and glucose consumption, is minimal (Blackburn, 2003) (Table 6-1).

C. **Thermoneutral state:** circumstances in which the neonate is neither gaining nor losing heat and oxygen and glucose consumption are minimal; gradient between skin and core temperature is small (Blackburn, 2003).

D. **Thermogenesis:** heat production.

■ TABLE 6-1
■ ■ **Neutral Thermal Environmental Temperatures**

Age and Weight	Range of Temperature (°C)	Age and Weight	Range of Temperature (°C)
0-6 hours		72-96 hours	
<1200 g	34-35.4	<1200 g	34-35
1200-1500 g	33.9-34.4	1200-1500 g	33-34
1501-2500 g	32.8-33.8	1501-2500 g	31.1-33.2
>2500 g	32-33.8	>2500 g	29.8-32.8
6-12 hours		4-12 days	
<1200 g	34-35.4	<1500 g	33-34
1200-1500 g	33.5-34.4	1501-2500 g	31-33.2
1501-2500 g	32.2-33.8	>2500 g	
>2500 g	31.4-33.8	4-5 days	29.5-32.6
12-24 hours		5-6 days	29.4-32.3
<1200 g	34-35.4	6-8 days	29-32.2
1200-1500 g	33.3-34.3	8-10 days	29-31.8
1501-2500 g	31.8-33.8	10-12 days	29-31.4
>2500 g	31-33.7	12-14 days	
24-36 hours		<1500 g	32.6-34
<1200 g	34-35	1501-2500 g	31-33.2
1200-1500 g	33.1-34.2	>2500 g	29-30.8
1501-2500 g	31.6-33.6	2-3 weeks	
>2500 g	30.7-33.5	<1500 g	32.2-34
36-48 hours		1501-2500 g	30.5-33
<1200 g	34-35	3-4 weeks	
1200-1500 g	33-34.1	<1500 g	31.6-33.6
1501-2500 g	31.4-33.5	1501-2500 g	30-32.7
>2500 g	30.5-33.3	4-5 weeks	
48-72 hours		<1500 g	31.2-33
<1200 g	34-35	1501-2500 g	29.5-32.2
1200-1500 g	33-34	5-6 weeks	
1501-2500 g	31.2-33.4	<1500 g	30.6-32.3
>2500 g	30.1-33.2	1501-2500 g	29-31.8

Adapted from Scopes, J.W, and Ahmed, I.: Range of critical temperatures in sick and premature babies. *Archives of Disease in Childhood 41*:417, 1966. For their table, Scopes and Ahmed had the walls of the incubator 1 to 2 degrees warmer than the ambient air temperatures.

Generally speaking, the smaller infants in each weight group will require a temperature in the higher portion of the temperature range. Within each time range, the younger the infant, the higher the temperature required. All infants who weighed more than 2500 g were born at more than 36 weeks of gestation.

From Klaus, M.,H., Fanaroff, A.,A., and Martin, R.J.: In M.H. Klaus and A.A. Fanaroff (Eds.): *Care of the high-risk neonate* (3rd ed.). Philadelphia, 1986, W.B. Saunders, pp. 96-112.

PHYSIOLOGIC DIFFERENCES AFFECTING THERMOREGULATION

Differences between neonates and adults lead to increased risk for thermoregulation problems in neonates. Relative to heat loss, heat production is low in neonates. Heat production in the body results from an aerobic (oxygen requiring) metabolic/chemical process via the metabolism of substrate (e.g., glucose, fats, and proteins).

Maintenance of a constant body temperature depends on activity, state, health status, and environmental temperature (Blackburn, 2003).

A. **Shivering is the mainstay of additional heat production in adults.** Although neonates rarely shiver (Blake and Murray, 2002), they may use shivering and increased muscular activity to some extent to generate heat, but the shivering threshold is likely at a lower body temperature than in the adult (Blackburn, 2003). Shivering is a late event in neonates, noted after prolonged cold stress. Preterm neonates have little ability to produce heat via shivering (Kenner, 2003).

B. **Neonates rely on nonshivering thermogenesis for heat production via metabolism of brown adipose tissue (BAT).**

C. **Heat transfer from neonatal organs to skin surface is increased compared with adults due to the neonate's decreased subcutaneous (SQ) fat and large body surface area to weight ratio.**
   1. SQ fat accounts for only 16% of body fat in neonates compared with approximately 30% in adults (Blackburn, 2003).
   2. Term neonates have three times the surface area to weight ratio as an adult, which increases to five times in preterm neonates and even higher in extremely low birth weight (ELBW) neonates (Blackburn, 2003). An increased surface area to weight ratio allows for increased transfer of heat from the body to the environment.
   3. Full-term neonates can decrease heat loss from exposed body surfaces by assuming a flexed position, but preterm neonates have a limited ability to maintain body flexion (Kenner, 2003).
   4. Critically ill neonates often lie outstretched unless positioned by caregivers.

D. **Preterm neonates have increased heat loss via evaporation due to increased total body water and thin skin.**

CONTROL OF BODY TEMPERATURE

A. **Heat production.**
   1. Thermoregulation is controlled by the hypothalamus.
      a. External thermal stimuli on the skin surface provide the preoptic nucleus of the anterior hypothalamus information for setting a temperature threshold that maintains the body core temperature within a narrow range.
      b. The posterior hypothalamus is the central control for heat response—production or dissipation of heat in response to stimuli from central and peripheral receptors in the skin, abdomen, spinal cord, and internal organs.
      c. During cold stress heat is conserved via vasoconstriction of skin blood vessels and heat is generated via nonshivering thermogenesis.
      d. Heat stress results in an increase in evaporative loss, peripheral vasodilation, and respiration (Blackburn, 2003).
      e. Neurologic abnormalities (e.g., hypoxia, central nervous system depression from drugs, meningitis, intraventricular hemorrhage) that affect the hypothalamus may interfere with heat balance (Blake and Murray, 2002).

B. **Brown adipose tissue/metabolism.**
   1. The sympathetic nervous system (SNS) initiates nonshivering thermogenesis via BAT in the neonate when the mean skin temperature falls between 35°

and 36°C (95° and 96.9° F) (Blackburn, 2003). Characteristics of BAT include (Blackburn, 2003):

a. Major function is heat production.
b. Found in the mediastinum, around the great vessels, kidneys, adrenal glands, axilla, nape of the neck, and between the scapulas.
c. Production begins at 26 to 28 weeks' gestation.
d. Stores increase until 3 to 5 weeks postnatal unless depleted by cold stress.
e. Reduced quantity in preterm and very low birth weight (VLBW) infants.
f. Cannot be replenished once used.
g. High degree of metabolic activity.

2. **BAT metabolism key points** include (Blackburn, 2003):
   a. Instigated by thermal receptor stimulation in the skin (prominent over facial trigeminal area).
   b. Regulated by specific protein—thermogenin, located in mitochondria of BAT.
   c. Directed by SNS via norepinephrine release, which frees BAT lipase and triglyceride breakdown into glycerol and nonesterified fatty acids (NEFAs), which release heat into circulation
   d. Requires oxygen and glucose.

C. **Heat loss.**

1. **Fetal thermoregulation.**
   a. Fetal temperature control is dependent, coupled with maternal temperature.
   b. During normal conditions fetal temperature is 0.5° C (0.9° F) higher than maternal.
   c. Risk of fetal hyperthermia during maternal infection, dehydration, exercise, or increases in environmental temperatures (e.g., saunas, hot tubs).
   d. Potential untoward effects on the fetus from maternal hyperthermia include hypoxia due to maternal and fetal tachycardia, teratogenesis, and preterm labor likely stemming from the underlying maternal infection (Blackburn, 2003).
2. **Four heat transfer mechanisms occur between the neonate and the environment (Blake and Murray, 2002; Hackman, 2001):**
   a. Conduction: heat transfer via direct contact.
      (1) Heat loss occurs when neonates come in contact with any cold surface (e.g., mattress, x-ray plate, scale).
      (2) Heat gain occurs when neonates come in contact with surfaces warmer than body temperature (e.g., warming mattress, warm blankets).
      (3) Heat transfer rate varies directly with size of temperature gradient; increasing surface area contact with object will increase rate of heat transfer. An object's conductive property influences heat transfer (e.g., heat loss is greater via metal than from fabric or skin).
   b. Convection: heat transfer via air currents.
      (1) Amount of heat transferred depends on temperature gradient, airflow (velocity), and surface area exposed to the air. Increasing the temperature gradient, airflow, and surface area will increase heat transfer (Kim et al., 2002).
      (2) Mode of heat transfer for heat gain in incubators.

c. Radiation: heat transfer of radiant energy without direct contact through absorption and emission of infrared rays (Blackburn, 2003).
   (1) Transfer depends on temperature gradient, surface absorptive properties and amount and angle of skin surface area facing the object (Blackburn, 2003).
   (2) Transfer is independent of ambient temperature, airflow, and other heat loss mechanisms.
   (3) Accounts for *major* source of incubator heat loss (neonate will lose heat via radiation if incubator walls are cooler than body temperature despite warm ambient incubator air temperature).
   (4) "Greenhouse" effect can occur if an incubator is placed near sunlight (or other bright heat source such as bank phototherapy) with transmission of heat from the sun through incubator walls with potential for neonatal overheating.
   (5) Mode of heat transfer via radiant warming bed while increasing insensible water loss (IWL) (Flenady and Woodgate, 2002).
d. Evaporation: heat loss by conversion of liquid (e.g., water) into vapor.
   (1) Depends on air speed and relative humidity (increased humidity decreases evaporative heat loss).
   (2) Accounts for 25% of neonatal heat loss at delivery resulting in 3° C decrease in temperature over 10 minutes (Blackburn, 2003).
   (3) Includes heat loss across skin and via respiratory tract (IWL).
   (4) Corresponds to gestational age with greatest loss in ELBW neonates due to dermal immaturity, with transepidermal water loss 6 times higher in VLBW neonates compared with term neonates (Blackburn, 2003). High total body water content enhanced by relatively large body surface area to weight ratio in preterm neonates increases loss.
   (5) Increased activity, tachypnea, radiant warming beds, and bank phototherapy augment loss.
e. Nursing interventions to prevent heat loss based on heat transfer mechanisms are presented in Box 6-1.

3. **Weaning from incubator to open crib**
   a. Weaning the preterm neonate to an open crib is an essential stride in preparation for discharge to home.
   b. Successful weaning is likely to be accomplished if the neonate weighs at least 1500 g, has had at least five consecutive days of weight gain, is tolerating feedings, and is free of major medical conditions (Blake and Murray, 2002).
   c. Proceed with weaning over at least a day, fully dressing and swaddling the neonate inside the incubator while decreasing the incubator temperature. Assess the neonate's temperature frequently.
   d. Once weaned to an open crib keep the neonate away from drafts and monitor body weight daily.

D. **Thermal instability.** Thermal instability is defined when the neonate's temperature is outside of the expected normal ranges.

1. **Expected normal range (Blackburn, 2003; Blake and Murray, 2002; Hackman, 2001; Sinclair, 2002).**
   a. Axillary temperature 36.5° to 37.5° C (97.9°-99.7° F) for term, 36.3° to 36.9° C (97.4°-98.4° F) for preterm neonates.
   b. Skin temperature 36° to 36.5° C (96.8°-97.7° F) for term, 36.2° to 37.2° C (97.2°-99° F) for preterm neonates.

BOX 6-1
NURSING INTERVENTIONS TO DECREASE HEAT LOSS

Conduction: Use warm blankets at delivery, preheat surfaces for delivery room resuscitation, warm cold scales or use warmed cover on scales, cover x-ray plates with warmed linen, warm incubator mattress prior to use, use appropriately warmed chemical activated mattress or heated water pads on transport (L'Herault et al., 2001) or during special procedures (avoid placing neonate directly on warming surface to prevent burns), warm large-volume intravenous fluids prior to administration, warm stethoscope and hands prior to examining the neonate or performing care, and consider parental skin-to-skin care while closely monitoring neonate's response (Bohnhorst et al., 2001; Ludington-Hoe, et al., 2000; Mellien, 2001).

Convection: Keep ambient temperature of nursery/neonatal intensive care unit (NICU) warm (72°-76° F [22.2°-24.4° C]), consider use of hybrid beds (radiant warming bed and incubator are combined into one unit) for extremely low birth weight (ELBW) neonates, transfer ELBW neonates from radiant warming bed to incubator once admission procedures are complete, transport neonates in enclosed incubator to procedures in other areas of hospital, work inside incubator via portholes, use plastic sleeves on incubator if recommended by manufacturer, bundle/nest with warm blankets or developmental positioning aids when inside incubator (Short, 1998), avoid drafts and air vents, use transparent plastic across radiant warming bed sides to decrease airflow across bed, place knit cap on neonate in delivery room once head is thoroughly dry (standard stockinette material is relatively ineffective, use thick material [Blake and Murray, 2002]), and warm all gas sources (e.g., oxygen).

Evaporation: Thoroughly dry neonate at delivery, replacing wet towels with warm, dry ones; monitor body temperature and delay initial bath until temperature has stabilized (Glass, 1999; Varda and Behnke, 2000), consider "dry bath" in ELBW neonate initially, provide additional heat source during bath (e.g., use heat lamps with caution, monitor body temperature frequently), bathe only in draft-free area; bathe one body part, dry it, then proceed to another body part; humidify oxygen, consider increased incubator humidity for ELBW neonate for first 7 to 10 days of life; use head covering at delivery after head is thoroughly dried and warmed, replace cap if damp because wet material will increase heat loss (Kenner, 2003); examine use of skin-protective barriers (e.g., paraffin, barrier creams) to decrease ELBW transepidermal water/heat loss (Kenner, 2003), and consider occlusive wrapping (polyethylene) of VLBW neonate at delivery (Vohra et al., 1999).

Radiation: Keep ambient temperature of nursery/NICU warm (72°-76° F; 22.2°-24.4° C), do not place incubators/beds near cold outer walls, consider thermal window blinds and incubator covers (Fig. 6-1), use double-walled incubators, cover transport incubator with thermal shield (Fig. 6-2), consider thermal heat shields for use inside incubator, avoid heat shield use with radiant warming bed or cold-stressed neonates (Kenner, 2003), and use clothing inside incubator to decrease exposed surface area and provide external thermal insulation.

Note: Nursing interventions are listed in relation to the underlying heat transfer mechanism.

Sources: Blackburn, S.T.: Thermoregulation. In *Maternal, fetal, and neonatal physiology: A clinical perspective* (2nd ed.). Philadelphia, 2003, W.B. Saunders, pp. 707-730; Blake, W. and Murray, J: Heat balance. In G.B. Merenstein and S.L. Gardner (Eds.): *Handbook of neonatal intensive care* (5th ed.). St Louis, 2002, Mosby, pp. 102-116; Hackman, P.: Recognizing and understanding the cold-stressed term infant. *Neonatal Network, 20*(8):35-41, 2001.

2. **Accurate temperature measurements.**
   a. **Deep body (core) temperature** is measured in the esophagus and tympanic membrane. Both are difficult to obtain and impractical.
   b. **Infrared tympanic thermometry** is not recommended for use in neonates (Blake and Murray, 2002).

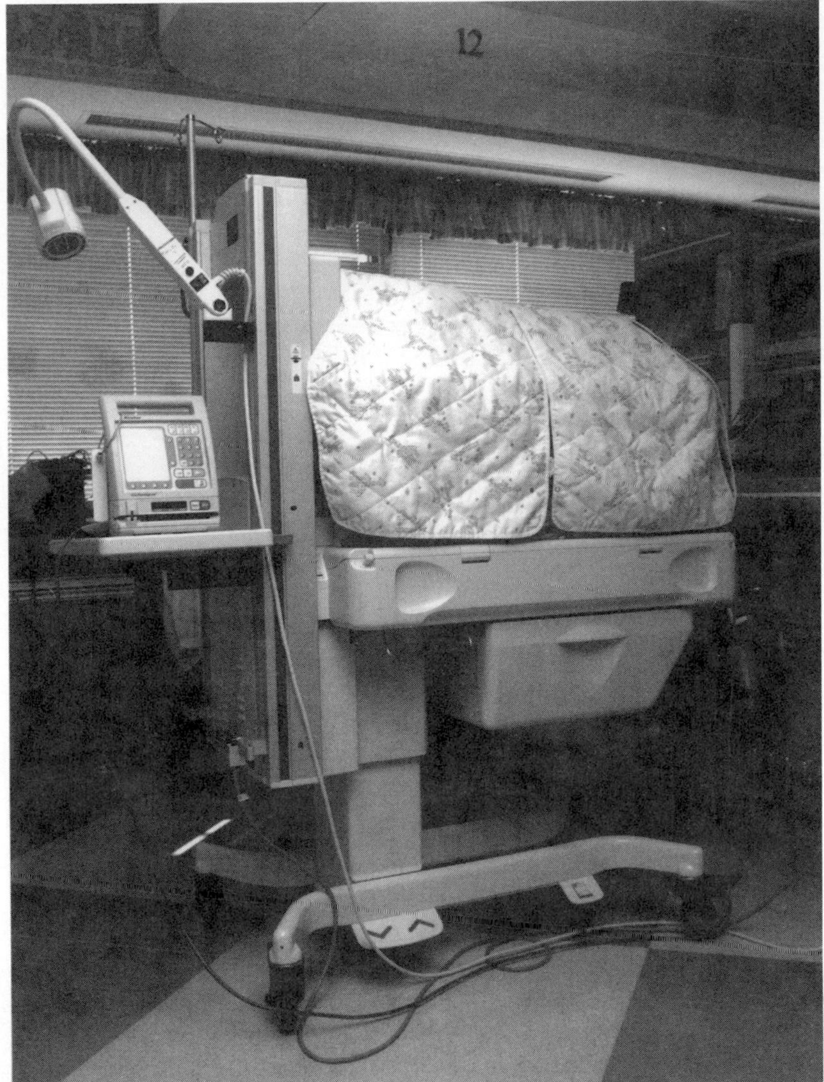

FIGURE 6-1 ■ Incubator with cover. Covering the incubator decreases radiant heat loss, a major factor in incubator use. (Courtesy Barbara Noerr, Palmyra, Pa.)

c. **Rectal temperatures** should not be taken routinely due to the risk of perforation. Flexible thermistors would need to be inserted at least 5 cm into the rectum for accurate measurements (Blake and Murray, 2002).
d. **Normal skin or core temperature is not a sensitive indicator of thermal neutrality** because the neonate may be increasing the metabolic rate to maintain adequate body temperature (Blackburn, 2003).
e. **Continuous skin temperature** is required for neonates using servo-controlled mode on an incubator or radiant warming bed.
   (1) Attach skin thermistors to the abdomen with insulated probe covers in a manner that allows for neonatal position change without readjustment of the probe.

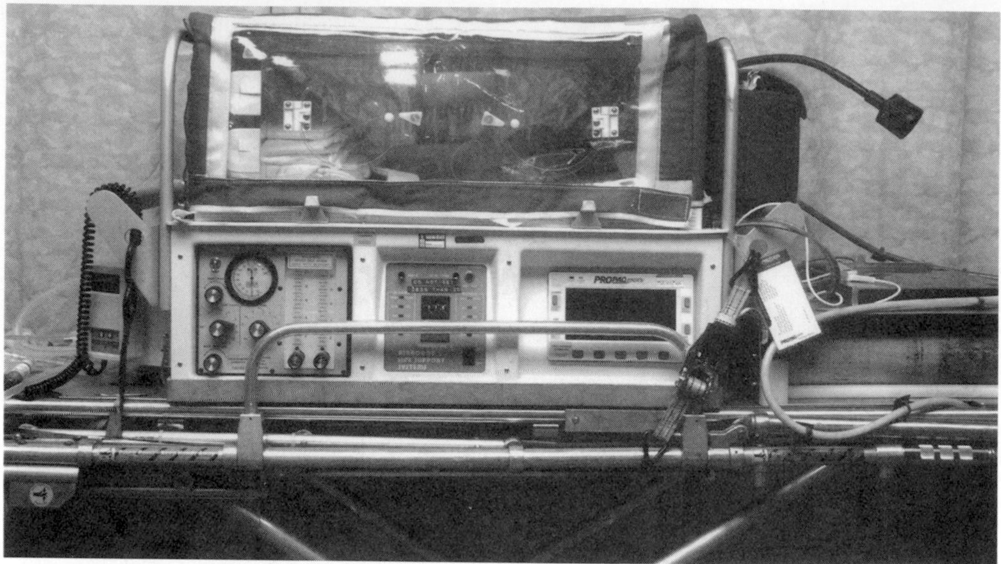

FIGURE 6-2 ■ Thermal cover on a neonatal transport incubator. The thermal cover decreases radiant heat loss. Prevention of radiant heat loss is important during external transports in cold climates. (Courtesy Barbara Noerr, Palmyra, Pa.)

(2) The neonate should not lie on the probe. Avoid placing thermistors in areas of BAT (e.g., axilla) due to likely increase in temperature providing false information to incubator or radiant warmer bed controls (Blake and Murray, 2002).

(3) Document incubator or radiant warming bed temperature simultaneously with all body temperature assessments (Blake and Murray, 2002).

f. **Ill neonates** need axillary temperature measurement every 1 to 4 hours, in addition to continuous skin temperature monitoring.

(1) **Axillary temperatures** are safe, easy, and accurate when done correctly. Hold the thermometer in midaxillary space in compliance with manufacturer's recommendation to ensure accuracy.

(2) **Assess neonatal temperature every 30 minutes to 1 hour during transition period, with subsequent assessment at least every 2 to 4 hours** until stable (Glass, 1999).

(a) Preterm neonates often require assessment every hour until stable.

(b) Full-term healthy neonates may be accurately assessed every 8 hours.

(3) **Use of external heat sources** (e.g., phototherapy, heat lamps) mandates frequent assessment of temperature (Blake and Murray, 2002). Sunlight, blankets, and added clothing can increase risk of hyperthermia.

3. **Hypothermia (<36.2° C [97.2° F]).**

a. Cold stress leads to a series of events in neonates initiated by norepinephrine release.

(1) Peripheral vasoconstriction occurs in an attempt to decrease heat loss.

(2) Thermogenesis is initiated, consuming BAT, glycogen stores, and oxygen, with resultant increase in lactic acid production.

(3) Metabolic acidosis leads to pulmonary vasoconstriction and decreased blood flow to other vital organs.
(4) BAT metabolism releases nonesterified fatty acids (NEFAs) that compete with bilirubin for albumin binding sites, increasing the risk of hyperbilirubinemia.

4. Neonates at risk for hypothermia (Blackburn, 2003):
   a. Preterm or small for gestational age.
   b. Central nervous system (CNS), endocrine, or cardiorespiratory abnormalities.
   c. Hypoglycemia, electrolyte imbalances, nutritional problems.
   d. Congenital anomalies (e.g., abdominal wall defects, neural tube defects).
   e. Sedation (e.g., maternal analgesia).

5. Treatment of neonatal hypothermia should be initiated promptly.
   a. Begin by providing a heat-gaining environment (e.g., increasing incubator/radiant warmer temperature gradually until the NTE is reached).
   b. Minimize factors contributing to heat loss (e.g., cool drafts).
   c. Continually monitor the neonate's response to both hypothermia and rewarming efforts. Severe hypothermia may necessitate more rapid methods such as use of a heated mattress.

6. Clinical manifestations of thermal instability, including hypothermia and hyperthermia are presented in Box 6-2.

7. Hyperthermia (>37.5° C).
   a. Neonates are at amplified risk for hyperthermia compared with older persons due to decreased ability for heat storage, large surface area to body weight, and a more narrow thermal neutral state (Blackburn, 2003).
   b. Neonates at risk (Blackburn, 2003):
      (1) Environmental overheating.
      (2) Hypermetabolism (e.g., sepsis, cardiac problems, drug withdrawal).
      (3) Dehydration.
      (4) Medication effects (e.g., prostaglandin administration).
      (5) CNS injury (e.g., intraventricular hemorrhage [IVH], birth trauma).

BOX 6-2
CLINICAL MANIFESTATIONS OF NEONATAL THERMAL INSTABILITY

Hypothermia: apnea, bradycardia, central cyanosis, signs of respiratory distress, irritability, hypoglycemia, pulmonary vasoconstriction, peripheral vasoconstriction, acidosis, hypoxia, lethargy, hypotonia, increased metabolic rate, weak cry or suck, increased gastric residuals, abdominal distention, emesis, shivering (mature neonates in presence of severe hypothermia), poor weight gain (chronic hypothermia).

Hyperthermia: warm to touch, flushed/red skin, sweating (term neonates), irritability, lethargy, apnea, weak or absent cry, poor feeding, tachypnea, tachycardia, increased insensible water loss, central nervous system depression.

Sources: Blackburn, S.T.: Thermoregulation. In *Maternal, fetal, and neonatal physiology: A clinical perspective* (2nd ed.), Philadelphia, 2003, W.B. Saunders, pp. 707-730; Blake, W. and Murray, J. Heat balance. In G.B. Merenstein and S.L. Gardner (Eds.): *Handbook of neonatal intensive care* (5th ed.). St Louis, 2002, Mosby, pp. 102-116; Hackman, P.: Recognizing and understanding the cold-stressed term infant. *Neonatal Network, 20*(8):35-41, 2001.

c. Treatment of hyperthermia is cooling, accomplished via lessening of heat sources (e.g., decrease the incubator temperature, limit direct sunlight) and removal of anything that blocks heat loss (e.g., extra blankets and clothing) (Blake and Murray, 2002).

REFERENCES

Blackburn, S.T.: Thermoregulation. In *Maternal, fetal, and neonatal physiology: A clinical perspective* (2nd ed.). Philadelphia, 2003, W.B. Saunders, pp. 707-730.

Blake, W. and Murray, J: Heat balance. In G.B. Merenstein and S.L. Gardner (Eds.): *Handbook of neonatal intensive care* (5th ed.). St Louis, 2002, Mosby, pp. 102-116.

Bohnhorst, B., Heyne, T., Peter, C., and Poest, C.: Skin-to-skin (kangaroo) care, respiratory control, and thermoregulation. *Journal of Pediatrics, 138*(2):193-197, 2001.

Cone, T.: *History of the care and feeding of the premature infant*, Boston, Little, Brown, 1985.

Flenady, V. and Woodgate, P.: Radiant warmers versus incubators for regulating body temperature in newborn infants. *Cochrane Database of Systematic Reviews, 2*:CD000435, 2002.

Glass, S.: Routine care. In P. Thureen, J. Deacon, P. O'Neill, and J. Hernandez (Eds.): *Assessment and care of the well newborn*. Philadelphia, 1999, Saunders, pp. 189-195.

Hackman, P.: Recognizing and understanding the cold-stressed term infant. *Neonatal Network, 20*(8):35-41, 2001.

Kenner, C.: Resuscitation and stabilization of the newborn. In C. Kenner and J. Lott (Eds.): *Comprehensive neonatal nursing: A physiologic perspective* (3rd ed.). Philadelphia, 2003, Saunders, pp. 210-227.

Kim, Y., Kwon, C., and Yoo, S.: Experimental and numerical studies on convective heat transfer in a neonatal incubator. *Medical & Biological Engineering & Computing, 40*(1):114-121, 2002.

L'Herault, J., Petroff, L., and Jeffrey, J.: The effectiveness of a thermal mattress in stabilizing and maintaining body temperature during the transport of very-low-birth weight newborns. *Applied Nursing Research, 14*(4):210-219, 2001.

Ludington-Hoe, S., Nguyen, N., Swinth, J., and Satyshur, R.: Kangaroo care compared to incubators in maintaining body warmth in preterm infants. *Biological Research for Nursing, 2*(1):60-73, 2000.

Mellien, A.: Incubators versus mothers' arms: Body temperature conservation in very-low-birth-weight premature infants. *Journal of Obstetric, Gynecologic, and Neonatal Nursing, 30*(2):157-164, 2001.

Short, M.: A comparison of temperature in VLBW infants swaddled versus unswaddled in a double-walled incubator in skin control mode. *Neonatal Network, 17*(3):25-31, 1998.

Sinclair J.: Servo-control for maintaining abdominal skin temperature at 36C in low birth weight infants. *Cochrane Database of Systematic Reviews, 1*:CD001074, 2002.

Varda, K. and Behnke, R.: The effect of timing of initial bath on newborn's temperature. *Journal of Obstetric, Gynecologic, and Neonatal Nursing, 29*(1):27-32, 2000.

Vohra, S., Frent, G., Campbell, V., et al.: Effect of polyethylene occlusive skin wrapping on heat loss in very low birth weight infants at delivery: A randomized trial. *Journal of Pediatrics, 134*(5):547-551, 1999.

CHAPTER 7

Physical Assessment

SUSAN ARANA FURDON AND KATHLEEN BENJAMIN

OBJECTIVES

1. Review key aspects of the perinatal history as it relates to physical assessment of the newborn.
2. Describe methods of determining gestational age.
3. Relate growth pattern and maturity to classification of newborns by gestational age and weight.
4. Describe a systematic approach in the examination of the newborn infant.

A comprehensive newborn physical examination requires a synthesis of perinatal and neonatal risk factors with a systematic approach to the examination. An understanding of growth, maturity, and gestational age risk factors provides a framework for defining wellness or subsequent problems. The nurse is in a unique position of providing a detailed observation and description within the context of these factors.

PERINATAL HISTORY (See Chapters 1, 2, 3 and 4)

Elements of a perinatal history focus on relationship of maternal medical condition and the overall growth and maturity of the infant. Communication from obstetric staff to pediatric staff of fetal anomaly(s) and risk factors for abnormal growth or fetal well-being is essential.

A. **Family history.**
   1. Known inherited disease: cystic fibrosis, Down syndrome, sickle cell anemia, and phenylketonuria.
   2. Chronic disorders or disabilities: diabetes, hypertension, mental retardation, cardiac lesions, and seizures.

B. **Maternal medical history.**
   1. General health: age, physical activity, diet, exposure to potential teratogens.
   2. Chronic illness: diabetes, hypertension, asthma, thyroid disorder, and anxiety disorder.
   3. Surgical procedures and hospitalizations.
   4. Medications before and during pregnancy.

C. **Obstetric history.**
   1. History of infertility: abnormal uterine structure, hormonal imbalance and treatment.
   2. Previous pregnancies (gravida): number of live born, term versus preterm, spontaneous or elective abortions.
   3. Birth weight(s) of live born and neonatal problems identified.
   4. Neonatal death(s): age of infant and reason for death.

D. **Social history: early identification of family stressors or support and barriers to teaching.**
   1. Marital status and consanguinity.
   2. Financial support, socioeconomic status (SES), and education level.

3. Tobacco, alcohol, and recreational drug use.
4. History of depression.
5. Domestic violence.
6. Religious and cultural considerations.
7. Factors affecting teaching.
   a. Primary language.
   b. Sensory deficits.

E. **Pregnancy history.**
1. Prenatal care: timing of first visit; compliance to follow-up.
2. Estimated date of confinement (EDC).
   a. Last menstrual period (LMP).
   b. Ultrasound dating.
   c. Birthdate calculator (wheel).
3. Single vs. multiple gestation.
4. Weight gain and nutritional status.
5. Risk for blood group incompatibility: Rh, ABO.
6. Congenital infection: rubella, syphilis, cytomegalovirus (CMV), hepatitis, human immunodeficiency virus (HIV), human papillomavirus (HPV), and chlamydia.
7. Maternal diabetes.
8. Abnormal fetal growth: fundal height; serial ultrasounds.
9. Intrauterine growth restriction (IUGR) factors (Doctor et al., 2001; Southgate and Pittard, 2001).
   a. Age greater than 45 or less than 15 years; single marital status.
   b. Low prepregnancy weight; low pregnancy weight gain.
   c. Unexplained history of miscarriage or stillbirth greater than 20 weeks' gestation.
   d. Multiple gestation.
   e. Smoking.
      (1) Nicotine releases catecholamines; reduces prostacycline synthesis.
      (2) Vasoconstriction and increased vascular resistance decreases placental delivery of nutrients and oxygen.
      (3) Associated with placental abruption and late fetal death.
      (4) Intrauterine growth restriction rates 3 to 4.5 times nonsmokers.
   f. Hypertensive/vascular disorders causing placental insufficiency.
      (1) Chronic hypertension.
      (2) Preeclampsia.
      (3) Advanced diabetes mellitus.
      (4) Placental or umbilical cord disruption.
   g. Chronic renal failure.
   h. Congenital infections: CMV most common association.
   i. Congenital malformations and chromosomal abnormalities.
10. Fetal anomaly: ultrasound, fetal echocardiography (ECHO), and amniocentesis.
11. Placenta or vascular abnormality: abnormal cord insertion, reverse end-diastolic flow, and twin-to-twin transfusion.
12. Amniotic fluid volume: polyhydramnios and oligohydramnios.

F. **Labor and delivery.**
1. History of presenting problem: preterm labor (PTL) and abruption.

2. Infection risks: maternal temperature and preterm premature rupture of membranes (PPROM) and Group B streptococcus (GBS) (Guinn and Gibbs, 2002).
3. Fetal lung maturity (FLM).
   a. Less than 5% risk of respiratory distress syndrome (RDS) if mature FLM test after 34 weeks' gestation (American Academy of Pediatrics and the American College of Obstetricians and Gynecologists [AAP/ACOG], 2002).
   b. Optimal benefit of glucocorticosteroid: 24 hours after administration up to 7 days.
4. Spontaneous vs. induced labor.
5. Cord prolapse.
6. Fetal distress and nonreassuring fetal heart tracing.
7. Analgesic and anesthetic prior to and at delivery.
8. Mode of delivery: vaginal, cesarean, assisted, forceps, and vacuum.
9. Appearance of amniotic fluid.
   a. Clear: normal.
   b. Green: meconium stained.
   c. Yellow: old meconium, old blood, and sepsis.
   d. Cloudy: sepsis.

G. Newborn resuscitation (see Chapter 5).

GESTATIONAL AGE INSTRUMENTS

The principal basis for use of gestational age instruments is that fetal maturity follows a predictable, organized course and that characteristics are common to a given gestational age (Sansoucie and Cavaliere, 2003).

A. General considerations.

1. Use from birth to 5 days, before physical characteristics change.
2. Perform within 48 hours of birth for highest accuracy.
3. Consider lack of accurate tools for less than 28 weeks' gestation when making treatment or withdrawal of care decisions for extremely premature infants (Donovan et al., 1999).

B. Most common tools.

1. Dubowitz: clinical assessment of gestational age (Dubowitz et al., 1970).
   a. Scores criteria: 10 neurologic and 11 external (physical).
   b. Combined total score correlated to weeks of gestation.
   c. Combined score has higher correlation (±2 weeks, 95% confidence) than either component separately.
   d. Small for gestational age (SGA) infants: external signs underscored and neurologic signs overscored; combined score reliable.
2. Ballard: newborn maturity rating.
   a. Simplified system based on Dubowitz's method; less time to use.
   b. Eliminates active tone scoring; passive tone more useful than active tone.
   c. Six neurologic and six physical criteria; scores totaled.
   d. Gestational age (GA) maturity rating assigned using form chart.
3. New Ballard Score (Ballard et al., 1991).
   a. Modified to assess gestational age 20 to 44 weeks.
   b. Accurate within 2 weeks of gestation; sick or well infants.
   c. For 20 to 26 weeks' gestation: most accurate when scored within first 12 hours of life.

d. Limitations.

(1) Examination should be done twice by two different examiners for objectivity.

(2) Infant must be in a quiet, alert state.

(3) Scoring affected by:

(a) Breech and positional deformities.

(b) Neurologic disorders and asphyxia.

(c) Infants affected by maternal medications.

(4) Inaccurate for infants less than 28 weeks' gestation (Donovan et al., 1999).

4. Embryonic vessels on the lens: from 27 to 34 weeks' gestation, examination of the anterior vascular capsule of the lens is helpful in determining gestational age by examining the level of remaining embryonic vessels on the lens (Fig. 7-1).

C. Gestational age examination (Fig. 7-2). Use the chart for scoring each criterion.

1. Technique for assessment of neurologic criteria.

a. Posture.

(1) Evaluates degree of arm and leg flexion and extension and leg abduction.

(2) Flexion and hip adduction increases with increasing gestational age.

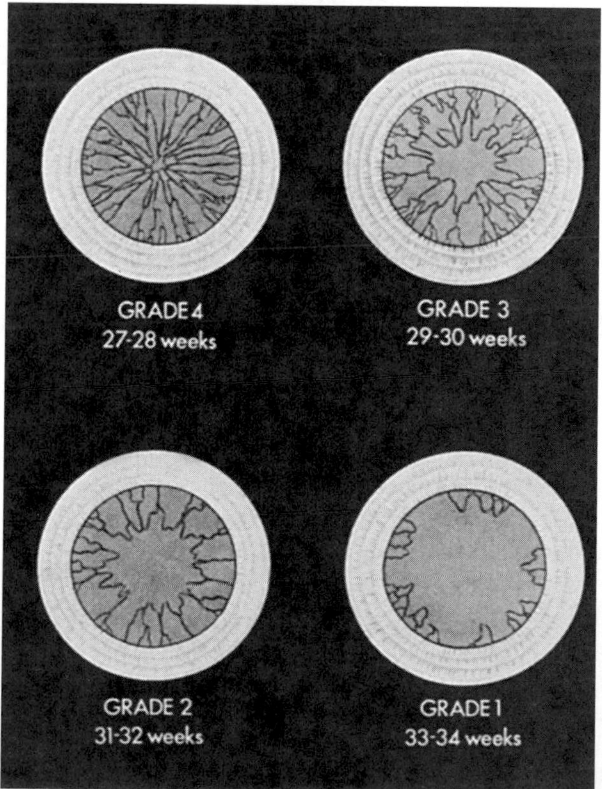

FIGURE 7-1 ■ Grading system for assessment of gestational age by examination of anterior vascular capsule of lens. (From Hittner, H.M., Hirsch, N.J., and Rudolph, A.J.: Assessment of gestational age by examination of the anterior vascular capsule of the lens. *Journal of Pediatrics, 91*[3]:455-458, 1977.)

(3) Early in gestation the infant's resting posture is hypotonic.
(4) Observe infant's posture while supine and quiet.

b. Square window.
(1) Evaluates flexion when the wrist is at a right angle to the forearm.
(2) Angle decreases with increasing gestational age due to influence of maternal hormones at end of pregnancy.

NEUROMUSCULAR MATURITY

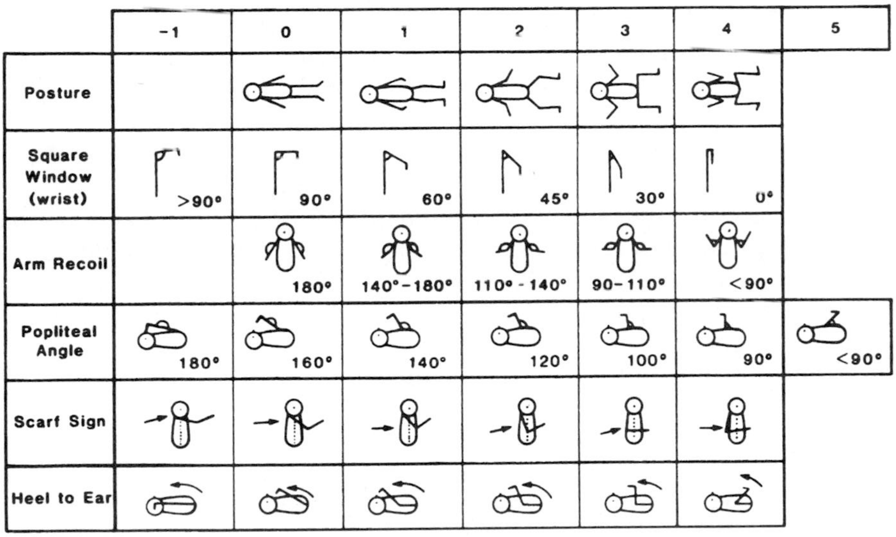

	−1	0	1	2	3	4	5
Posture							
Square Window (wrist)	>90°	90°	60°	45°	30°	0°	
Arm Recoil		180°	140°−180°	110° - 140°	90−110°	<90°	
Popliteal Angle	180°	160°	140°	120°	100°	90°	<90°
Scarf Sign							
Heel to Ear							

SCORE
Neuro-muscular ______
Physical ______
Total ______

PHYSICAL MATURITY

Skin	sticky friable transparent	gelatinous red, translucent	smooth pink, visible veins	superficial peeling &/or rash, few veins	cracking pale areas rare veins	parchment deep cracking no vessels	leathery cracked wrinkled
Lanugo	none	sparse	abundant	thinning	bald areas	mostly bald	
Plantar Surface	heel–toe 40–50 mm: −1 <40 mm: −2	>50 mm no crease	faint red marks	anterior transverse crease only	creases ant. 2/3	creases over entire sole	
Breast	imperceptible	barely perceptible	flat areola no bud	stippled areola 1–2 mm bud	raised areola 3–4 mm bud	full areola 5–10 mm bud	
Eye/Ear	lids fused loosely: −1 tightly: −2	lids open pinna flat stays folded	sl. curved pinna; soft; slow recoil	well-curved pinna; soft but ready recoil	formed & firm instant recoil	thick cartilage ear stiff	
Genitals male	scrotum flat, smooth	scrotum empty faint rugae	testes in upper canal rare rugae	testes descending few rugae	testes down good rugae	testes pendulous deep rugae	
Genitals female	clitoris prominent labia flat	prominent clitoris small labia minora	prominent clitoris enlarging minora	majora & minora equally prominent	majora large minora small	majora cover clitoris & minora	

MATURITY RATING

score	weeks
−10	20
−5	22
0	24
5	26
10	28
15	30
20	32
25	34
30	36
35	38
40	40
45	42
50	44

FIGURE 7-2 ■ New Ballard Score, expanded to include extremely premature infants. (From Ballard, J.L., Khoury, J.C., Wedig, K., et al.: New Ballard Score, expanded to include extremely premature infants. *Journal of Pediatrics, 119*[3]:417-423, 1991.)

(3) Findings do not change after birth.
(4) Flex infant's hand on the forearm between examiner's thumb and index finger. Use sufficient pressure to get full flexion. Visually measure angle between hypothenar eminence and ventral aspect of forearm.

c. Arm recoil.
(1) Evaluates degree of arm flexion and the strength of recoil.
(2) Place infant supine, flex arms for 5 seconds, then fully extend arms by pulling the hands downward, then release.

d. Popliteal angle.
(1) The angle decreases with increasing gestational age.
(2) Position infant supine, pelvis flat on surface; hold thigh in knee-chest position with left index finger and thumb. Place right index finger behind infant's ankle and extend leg with gentle pressure.
(3) Measure angle between the lower leg and thigh, posterior to the knee.

e. Scarf sign.
(1) Position infant supine; take hand and pull across chest and around neck as far posterior as possible toward the opposite shoulder. Assist maneuver by lifting elbow across body.
(2) Observe the position of the elbow to the midline of the infant's body.

f. Heel to ear.
(1) Position infant supine, pelvis flat on the bed. Draw foot to head as near as it will extend without force.
(2) Observe distance between the foot and head and the degree of knee extension. Knee is left free and may draw down alongside abdomen.

2. Physical examination criteria: observe and grade according to Figure 7-2.

a. Skin.
(1) With increasing gestational age, transparency decreases and more texture develops, vessels become obscured.
(2) As gestation progresses beyond 38 weeks, subcutaneous tissue decreases, causing wrinkling and desquamation.

b. Lanugo.
(1) Fine, downy hair that covers the body of the fetus from 20 to 28 weeks.
(2) At 28 weeks it begins to disappear around the face and anterior aspect of the trunk.
(3) At term a few patches may be present over the shoulders.

c. Plantar creases.
(1) Creases first appear on the anterior portion of the foot, between 28 and 30 weeks' gestation, and extend toward the heel as gestation progresses.
(2) An infant with IUGR and early loss of vernix caseosa may have more plantar creases than expected for size.
(3) After 12 hours skin begins to dry and plantar creases are no longer a valid indicator of gestational age.

d. Breast development.
(1) Nipple size and amount of breast tissue are examined.
(2) A 1- to 2-mm nodule of breast tissue is palpable by about 36 weeks and grows to approximately 10 mm by 40 weeks' gestation.

e. Eyes and ears.
(1) Evaluated for fused eyelids.
(2) At 26 to 30 weeks' gestation, fused eyelids open.

(3) Assess ear formation and amount of pinna cartilage.
(4) Inward curving of the upper pinna usually begins by 34 weeks' gestation and by 40 weeks extends to the lobe.
(5) Before 34 weeks the pinna has little cartilage and will stay folded on itself.
(6) By 36 weeks there is some cartilage, and the pinna will spring back from being folded.

f. Genitalia.
(1) Female infant: evaluate development of the labia minora and majora and prominence of the clitoris.
(a) Early in gestation the clitoris is prominent, with small, widely separated labia.
(b) By 40 weeks, fat deposits have increased in size in the labia majora, so that the labia majora completely cover the labia minora.
(2) Male infant: evaluate presence of testes, degree of descent into scrotum, and development of rugae on the scrotum.
(a) The testes begin to descend from the abdomen at 28 weeks.
(b) At 37 weeks the testes can be palpated high in the scrotum.
(c) At 40 weeks the testes are completely descended and the scrotum is covered with rugae.
(d) As gestation progresses the scrotum becomes more pendulous.

D. Clinical estimate of GA (AAP/ACOG, 2002).
1. Determination of GA on all newborns is recommended.
2. Assign GA after review of all history and examination findings.
3. Document marked discrepancy between data.
4. Classify.
   a. Preterm: infant born before completion of 37 weeks of gestation.
   b. Term: infant born from first day of 38th week through 42 weeks.
   c. Postterm: infant delivered after completion of 42 weeks of gestation.

CLASSIFICATION OF GROWTH AND MATURITY

The intrauterine growth pattern reflects fetal well-being. This pattern is influenced by maternal health or disease, placental function, medications, nutrition, and smoking. There are multiple reasons to classify growth and maturity of the newborn infant.

- Assist in identification of the most commonly occurring problems in the newborn period.
- Estimate dating if there is no prenatal care.
- Examine discrepancy between weight and GA.
- Standardize reports of health statistics.

A. Measurement.
1. Comparison of newborn's measurements should be of population-based growth curves, representing the patient in gender, race, geographic region for altitude, and other environmental variances.
2. For clinical purposes, use of 10th and 90th percentile range is reasonable (Fletcher, 1998).

B. Obtain measurements.
1. Type.
   a. Normal-appearing infants: weight, length, head circumference, and abdominal circumference.
   b. Dysmorphic appearance: may require more extensive measurements.

2. Birth weight.
   a. Obtain as soon as possible after delivery.
   b. Express in grams.
   c. Weigh unclothed infant when quiet: weight can be falsely increased with significant motion (Fletcher, 1998).
   d. Classifications (regardless of gestational age) (AAP/ACOG, 2002).
      (1) Low birth weight: less than 2500 g birth weight.
      (2) Very low birth weight: less than 1500 g birth weight.
      (3) Extremely low birth weight: less than 1000 g birth weight.
3. Length: crown-to-heel measurement.
   a. Most variable measurement: requires full extension of normally flexed infant.
   b. Measure length with infant supine and leg extended, head to heel.
   c. Accuracy facilitated by use of measurement board.
   d. Use crown-to-rump measurement to establish proportionality when length falls below norms (referenced data in *Smith's Recognizable Patterns of Human Malformation* [Jones 1997]).
      (1) Congenital dwarfism.
      (2) When lower extremity anomalies make crown-to-heel measurement unreliable.
4. Head circumference (HC): indication of normal brain growth.
   a. Measurement of largest occipitofrontal circumference (OFC).
   b. Apply paper measurement tape firmly around head above the eyebrow ridges, from most prominent frontal to occipital areas.
   c. OFC may be erroneous: significant cranial molding, craniosynostosis, caput, cephalohematoma need to be noted along with the measurement.
   d. Consider parent head size vs. intracranial pathology when head size is of concern.

C. Plot newborn's weight, length, and head circumference by gestational age on standardized growth charts.

1. Centers for Disease Control and Prevention (CDC) national reference for term infants: www.cdc.gov.growthcharts.
2. Commonly used charts: Colorado Intrauterine Growth Chart (Fig. 7-3) (Lowdermilk and Perry, 2004).
   a. Colorado growth charts developed in 1960s.
   b. Other limitations of Lubchenco data (Thomas et al., 2000).
      (1) Charts developed at mile-high elevation (Denver); 10th percentile is lower than data from centers at sea level.
      (2) Overestimates number of infants greater than 90th percentile and less than 10th percentile.
      (3) Population sample only whites and primarily low socioeconomic groups.
      (4) Leads to inaccurate classification of SGA and large for gestational age (LGA) that is gender and race specific.
3. Pediatrix Medical Group Inc. Growth Chart (Thomas et al., 2000) (Fig. 7-4).
   a. Gestational age had largest influence on each growth parameter (head circumference, birth weight, length).
      (1) Infants less than 30 weeks: overall lower growth parameters, compared with Lubchenco chart.
      (2) Infants greater than 36 weeks: larger and heavier.
   b. Gender and race differences found in 1996 to 1998 population data.
      (1) Females smaller than males.
      (2) Black infants smaller than Hispanic and white infants at each GA.
   c. Revised charts reflecting race, gender, gestational age, and multiple birth differences are needed.

CLASSIFICATION OF NEWBORNS—
BASED ON MATURITY AND INTRAUTERINE GROWTH
Symbols: X - 1st Examination O - 2nd Examination

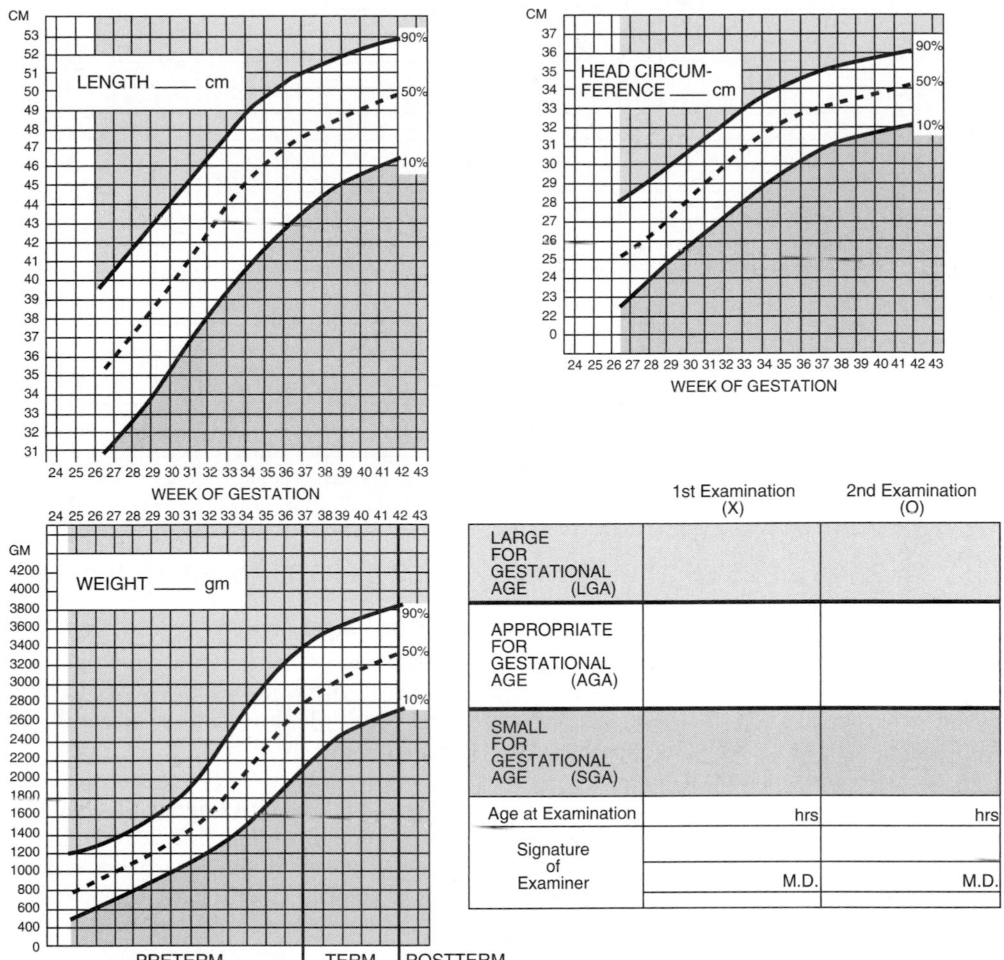

FIGURE 7-3 ■ Estimating gestational age: newborn classification based on maturity and intrauterine growth. (In Lowdermilk, D.L. and Perry, S.E.: *Maternity & women's health care* [8th ed.]. St Louis, 2004, Mosby; modified from Lubchenco, L., et al.: Intrauterine growth in length and head circumference as estimated from live births at gestational ages from 26 to 42 weeks. *Journal of Pediatrics, 37*:403, 1966; Battaglia, F. and Lubchenco, L.: A practical classification of newborn infants by weight and gestational age. *Journal of Pediatrics 71*[2]:159-163, 1967.)

D. Compare weight with gestational age to determine size classification (weight compared with established norm).
   1. SGA: birth weight less than 10th percentile.
   2. Appropriate for gestational age (AGA): birth weight within 10th to 90th percentiles.
   3. LGA: birth weight greater than 90th percentile.

E. Compare all growth parameters (head circumference, birth weight, and length) with gestational age.
   1. IUGR.
      a. Process of slowing of intrauterine growth rate.
      b. IUGR infants may or may not be SGA.

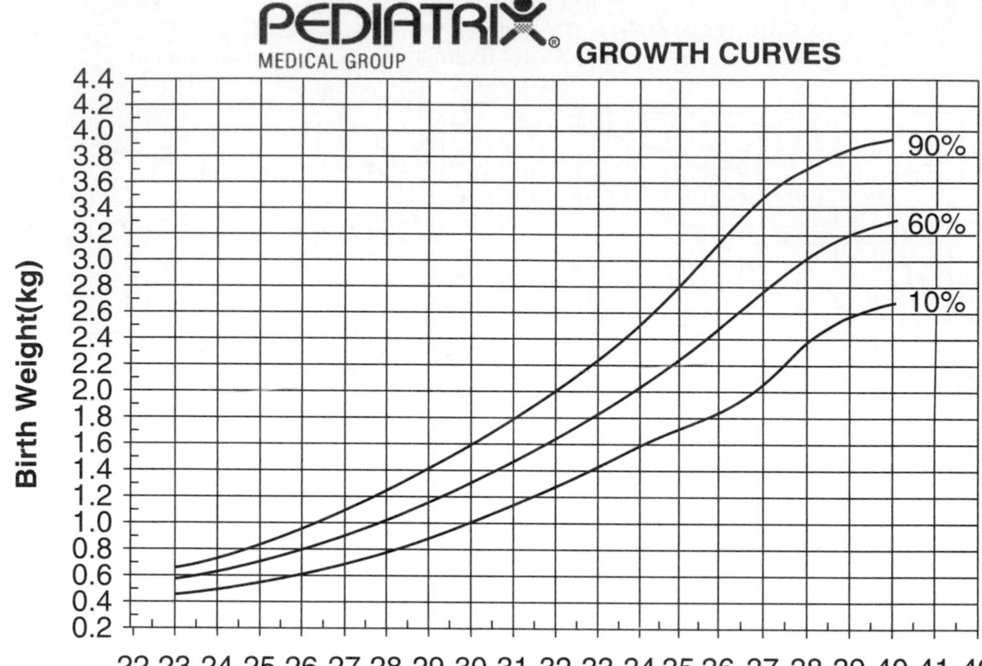

FIGURE 7-4 ■ These growth curves represent an estimate of intrauterine growth based on data from 80,011 neonates admitted to 114 NICUs (birth weight above 0.25 kg and gestational ages of 22-42 wks). Gender, race, and multiple births had a small but significant effect on each parameter (see the Clinical Research Center at Pediatrix U™ www.pediatrixu.com/clinical_research_center.asp). These curves are a reference for the clinician to assess neonates' intrauterine and postnatal growth. The CDC national references (http://www.cdc.gov/growthcharts/) may also be used for term infants. © 2001 Pediatrix Medical Group, Inc. Reproduction of this material by any means without the express written permission of Pediatrix Medical Group, Inc. is prohibited. Reprinted with permission.

- **c.** Below expected norms for weight and length at birth based on GA, race, and gender.

2. Classifications (Britton, 2001).

- **a.** Symmetric.
  - (1) Proportional decreased growth.
  - (2) Measurements for weight, length, and HC all within same growth curve, all less than 10th percentile.
  - (3) Etiology: decreased growth potential or reduced fetal cells.
    - (a) Intrauterine congenital infection.
    - (b) Congenital malformation.
    - (c) Chromosomal disorder.
- **b.** Asymmetric (head-sparing IUGR).
  - (1) Disproportionate reduction in weight and length at birth compared with head circumference.
  - (2) Weight below expected norms for GA, race, and gender.
  - (3) Etiology: normal number of cells; reduced cell size.
    - (a) Uteroplacental insufficiency.
    - (b) Maternal malnutrition.
    - (c) Extrinsic factors occurring late in pregnancy.

F. Determine neonatal mortality risk based on classification of newborns by standardized birth weight norms and gestational age.

1. Morbidity and mortality statistics: standardized reporting of reproductive health statistics.
2. Establishment of level of risk for short- and long-term complications.
   a. Higher morbidity and mortality if term infants at or below 3rd percentile of weight for GA (McIntire et al., 1999).
   b. Preterm infants: no specific birth weight thresholds for morbidity and mortality.
3. Mortality risk (Fig. 7-5).
4. Morbidity risk by birth weight and GA (Fig. 7-6).

G. Identify infants at risk for respiratory disease, hypoglycemia, and thermal instability based on classification(s):

1. Preterm: problems with immaturity of body systems: respiratory distress syndrome (RDS), necrotizing enterocolitis (NEC), and patent ductus arteriosus (PDA).
2. Postterm: problems associated with placental insufficiency: asphyxia and meconium aspiration.
3. IUGR.
   a. Typical appearance of infant (Southgate and Pittard, 2001).
      (1) Head disproportionately large for trunk.
      (2) Extremities appear wasted.
      (3) Facial appearance: "wizened old man."
      (4) Large anterior fontanelles with cranial sutures wide or overlapping.
      (5) Thin umbilical cord, diminished Wharton's jelly.
      (6) Scaphoid abdomen.

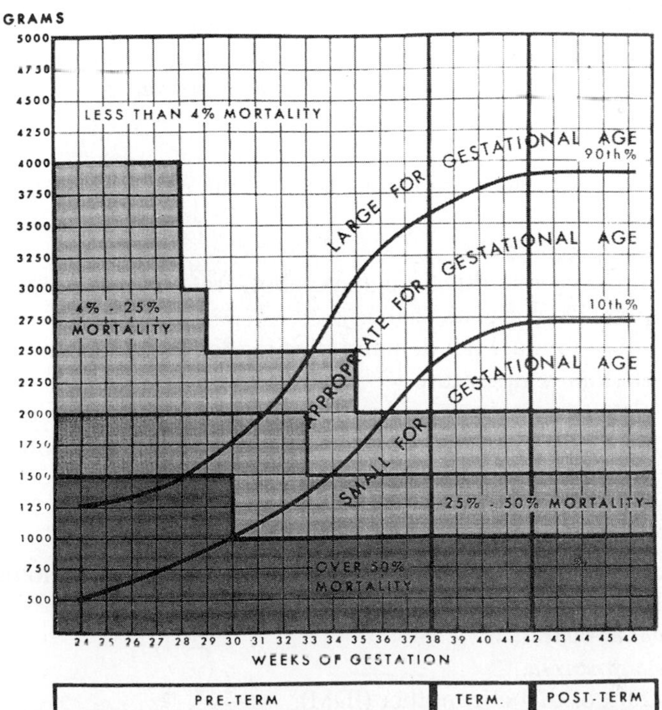

FIGURE 7-5 ■ University of Colorado Medical Center classification of newborns by birth weight and gestational age and by neonatal mortality risk. (From Battaglia, F. and Lubchenco, L.: A practical classification of newborn infants by weight and gestational age. *Journal of Pediatrics, 71*[2]:159-163, 1967.)

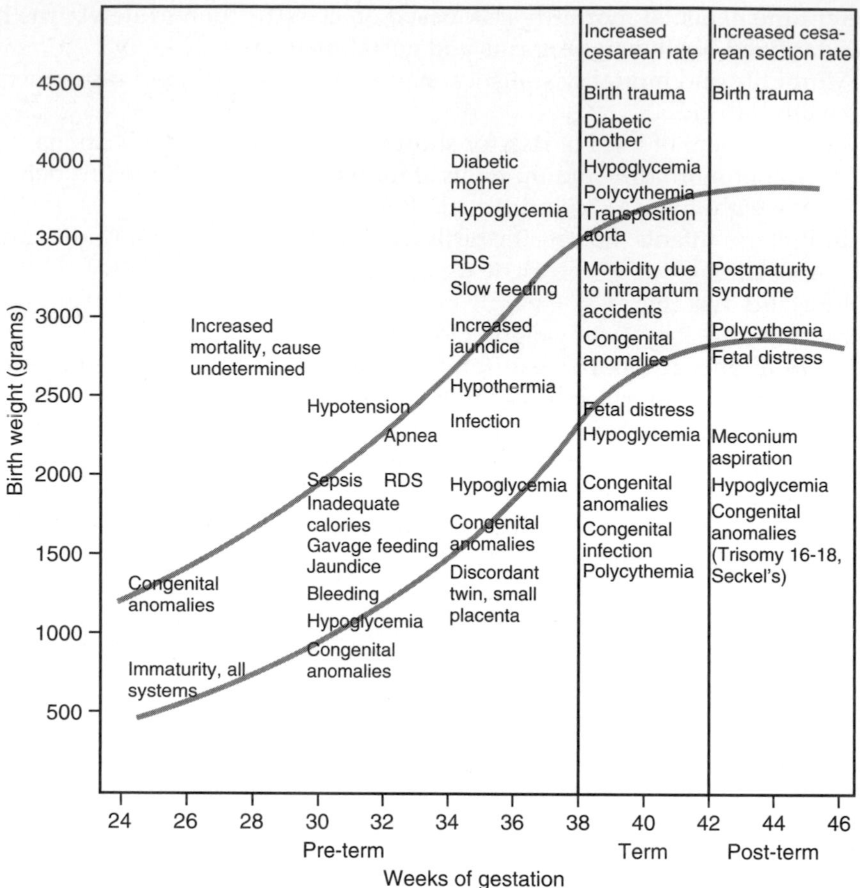

FIGURE 7-6 ■ Specific neonatal morbidity by birth weight and gestational age. (From Lubchenco, L.O.: *The high-risk infant*. Philadelphia, 1976, Saunders.)

(7) Skin: loose, decreased subcutaneous fat, dry, flaky, little or no vernix caseosa.

b. Potential problem list.

(1) Hypoglycemia due to high metabolic rate and decreased glycogen stores (Doctor et al., 2001).

(2) Hypothermia: high demand plus inadequate adipose tissue to maintain temperature.

(3) Polycythemia: increased red blood cell production in utero caused by chronic hypoxia or endocrine/metabolic or chromosomal disorder.

(4) Hypoxia: birth asphyxia and meconium aspiration.

(5) Infection.

(6) Problems related to etiology of growth restriction.

(7) Long-term morbidity and mortality dependent on etiology.

4. LGA infant.

a. Typical appearance.

(1) Macrosomia.

(2) Infant of diabetic mother (IDM).

(a) Hairy ear (Clark, 2000).

(b) Characteristic large body with head circumference within normal limits for gestational age (insulin does not cross blood-brain barrier).

b. Potential problem list.
  (1) Abnormal glucose metabolism after birth; hyperinsulinemia and hypoglycemia.
  (2) Birth trauma from difficult extraction (fractured clavicle, brachial plexus injury) or asphyxia.
  (3) Complications from operative or assisted delivery: respiratory distress, adverse effects of anesthesia.
  (4) Iatrogenic prematurity: overestimation of fetal GA.
  (5) Association with other problems related to infant of diabetic mother: RDS, hypoglycemia, hypocalcemia, polycythemia, hyperbilirubinemia, and congenital anomalies.
  (6) Pulmonary hypertension.
  (7) Poor feeding.
  (8) Thermal instability as result of central nervous system (CNS) trauma or infection.

PHYSICAL EXAMINATION

A systematic approach to the physical examination of the newborn prevents pertinent omissions and provides a detailed description that can be utilized in communication of alterations in anatomic structure or changes in physiology or function. These observations ultimately must be made within the context of the patient's history and GA. Communication to the primary care provider is essential for further evaluation and prompt treatment.

A. Assessment techniques.
  1. Examine in well-lit room; direct light should not be in infant's face.
  2. Warm hands and equipment.
  3. Keep infant warm by using overhead heat source or uncovering small areas at a time to prevent hypothermia.
  4. Complete detailed observations prior to physical contact.
  5. Order of examination:
    a. Depends on the purpose of the examination and the current state of the infant (Fletcher, 1998).
    b. Generally: least invasive observations to most disturbing techniques.
    c. Observe skin throughout the examination.
    d. Evaluate neurobehavior within context of infant's behavioral state.
  6. Document physical examination in patient care record inclusive of description of abnormalities and vital signs.

B. Timing of examinations (AAP/ACOG, 2002).
  1. Recognize life-threatening symptoms and address those prior to comprehensive examination.
  2. Modify elements of examination based on infant's state or illness.
  3. Initial examination in delivery room.
    a. Apgar scoring.
    b. Inspection for birth injury or major congenital malformation.
    c. Evaluation of pulmonary and cardiovascular adjustment to extrauterine life.
    d. Notification of primary care provider.
      (1) Apgar less than 5.
      (2) Maternal fever.
      (3) Abnormal examination findings.
      (4) Evidence of or suspected substance abuse.

4. Comprehensive newborn examination.
   a. Within 24 hours of life: evaluation of size, growth and GA, transition to extrauterine life, and congenital anomalies.
   b. Discharge examination: focus on problem(s) during hospitalization, problems with feeding and weight gain, and ability of parent(s) to meet infant's needs.

C. **General appearance: initial impression.**
1. State: indicator of well-being.
   a. Sleep states: deep sleep and light sleep.
   b. Awake states: quiet alert, actively alert, and crying.
2. Color (Spilman and Furdon, 1998).
   a. Most reliable indicator of color: mucous membranes. Other areas include conjunctiva, nailbeds, lips, buccal mucosa, earlobes, and soles of feet.
   b. Lighting and color of blankets can affect perception of color.
   c. Central cyanosis.
      (1) Recognition influenced by hematocrit (Hct), temperature, and environmental factors.
      (2) Central cyanosis: superficial capillaries exceed 5 g/dl unsaturated hemoglobin (Hgb) (Roberton, 2000).
      (3) Variety of etiologies: cardiac, pulmonary, infection, metabolic, neurologic, and hematologic.
   d. Acrocyanosis.
      (1) Suggests instability of peripheral circulation.
      (2) Cyanosis limited to hands, feet, and circumoral area.
      (3) May be result of cold, stress, shock, and polycythemia.
      (4) May be normal finding for 24 to 48 hours after birth.
   e. Pallor: pale, white appearance.
      (1) Reflects poor perfusion and circulatory failure or acidosis.
      (2) With bradycardia indicates anoxia or vasoconstriction found in shock, sepsis, or severe respiratory distress.
      (3) With tachycardia can indicate anemia.
   f. Plethora: ruddy or red appearance.
      (1) May indicate polycythemia.
   g. Jaundice: yellow pigmentation in skin or conjunctiva due to deposition of bilirubin.
      (1) Abnormal in the first 12 hours of life.
      (2) Cephalocaudal progression.
   h. Mottling: checkerboard red and white pattern.
      (1) May be normal.
      (2) May be seen in cold stress, hypovolemia, and sepsis.
   i. Harlequin sign: distinct midline demarcation.
      (1) Pale on one side and red on opposite side.
      (2) Due to immature autoregulation of blood flow.
3. Respiratory effort.
   a. Rate.
      (1) Normal 40 to 60 respirations per minute.
      (2) Rate can vary with activity of infant.
   b. Quality: absence of "work of breathing."
      (1) Retractions: occur more often in premature due to highly compliant chest wall (Bates and Balistreri, 2002).
      (2) Nasal flaring: diameter of nares increased as mechanism to decrease airway resistance.

(3) Expiratory grunting: increase in intrathoracic pressure to prevent volume loss during expiration as a result of alveolar collapse.

4. Wheezing: due to increased airway resistance. High-pitched rhonchi heard more loudly on expiration.
5. Stridor: partially obstructed airway.
6. Nutritional status.
   a. Well nourished: increased subcutaneous fat, without loose skin.
   b. Growth restricted: thin and wasted appearance, no subcutaneous fat, loose skin.
7. Tone.
   a. Based on GA expectations.
   b. Degree of flexion and amount of resistance demonstrated with examiner's extension of extremities.
   c. Decreased flexion (hypotonia) or increased flexion (hypertonia) should be evaluated further.
8. Congenital defects.
   a. Determine if malformation (abnormal shape or structure) or deformation (fully formed but influenced by in utero environment).
   b. Describe anatomic structures fully: size, number, shape, position, color, texture, continuity, and alignment (Fletcher, 1998).
9. Temperature (see Chapter 6).

D. Skin.

1. General considerations.
   a. Findings differ with GA, especially with extremely low birth weight (ELBW).
   b. Indicators of underlying illness: petechiae, pigmentation, rashes, and pustules.
   c. Congenital lesions may not be apparent at birth; influenced by maternal hormones.
   d. Differentiate between findings at birth vs. injury after birth (medical interventions).
   e. Use basic descriptors: color quantity, size, shape, pattern of distribution, and texture (Fletcher, 1998).
2. Skin is soft, smooth, and opaque and should be warm to the touch; cold clammy skin may indicate shock.
3. Inspect lesions, rashes, bruises, and birthmarks.
4. Palpate for texture (raised, flat) unless lesion is open.
5. Vernix caseosa.
   a. White or yellow material on the skin; discolored with postmaturity, hemolytic disease, and meconium staining.
   b. Sebaceous gland secretions and exfoliated skin cells.
   c. Presents during third trimester and decreases with increasing gestational age.
6. Erythema toxicum (newborn rash).
   a. Erythematous macules, each containing central papule (yellow or white).
   b. Papules contain eosinophils in a fluid that is sterile.
   c. Persist for several days and then resolve spontaneously.
   d. Most often located on trunk, arms, and perineal areas.
   e. Never located on soles of feet or palms of hands.
7. Ecchymosis: nonblanching blue or black area.
   a. Extravasation of blood into tissue.
   b. Related to trauma of blood vessels.

8. Petechiae.
   a. Tiny red or purple nonblanching pinpoint macules.
   b. Benign when found on presenting part.
   c. Require further evaluation when progressive (Fletcher, 1998).
9. Vascular nevi.
   a. Common cutaneous malformation(s) that can occur anywhere on body.
   b. May present at birth or may develop in early infancy.
   c. Types.
      (1) Nevus simplex or capillary hemangiomas (stork bite).
         (a) Macular patches with diffuse borders.
         (b) Found on forehead, nape of neck, glabella, and eyelids.
         (c) Blanch when pressure is applied.
         (d) Resolve spontaneously.
      (2) Nevus flammeus (port wine stain).
         (a) Flat, sharply defined lesion.
         (b) Most common on back of neck.
         (c) If present over the face following branches of trigeminal nerve (forehead and upper eyelid), may be associated with Sturge-Weber syndrome.
         (d) Will not blanch with pressure.
         (e) May fade with time but will not resolve.
10. Café au lait spots.
   a. Light tan or brown macules with well-defined borders.
   b. Deeper pigmentation than surrounding skin.
   c. Six or more may be pathologic.
11. Strawberry hemangioma(s).
   a. Red, raised, circumscribed, and compressible.
   b. Can occur anywhere on the body.
   c. Proliferate: increase in size and number.
   d. Most involute spontaneously.
   e. No treatment is required unless they affect vital function.
   f. Occur with increasing frequency with decreased GA.
12. Epidermolysis bullosa.
   a. Blistering internally and externally.
   b. May be either autosomal dominant or recessive.
13. Staphylococcal scalded skin syndrome.
   a. Skin response to *Staphylococcus aureus*.
   b. Scalded skin appearance.

E. **Head.**
1. General considerations.
   a. Up to 90% of the congenital malformations present at birth are apparent on the head and neck (Fletcher, 1998).
   b. Review perinatal history, abnormal ultrasound findings, and mode of delivery.
   c. Many variations are transient or racial, sexual, or familial traits.
2. Obtain HC.
   a. Measurement reflects brain growth.
   b. Predictable measurement: follows norms for GA and weight.
   c. Usually HC falls on same percentile curve as length. Determine etiology of abnormal growth if length and HC differ by greater than one quartile (Fletcher, 1998).
   d. HC should be 2 cm larger than the chest circumference. N = 32 to 38 cm for full-term AGAs.

(1) Microcephalic: poor brain growth, atrophy, or premature cranial synostosis.
(2) Macrocephalic: familial (follows persistently higher but consistent growth curve) and pathologic (hydrocephalus: increase in cerebrospincal fluid [CSF] results in increasing HC).

3. Observe shape and symmetry; may reflect affect of birth process or in utero position or significant anatomic defect.

a. Molding.
(1) Occurs with vaginal delivery from a vertex position; adaptive mechanism to facilitate passage through birth canal.
(2) Elongation of head with prominence of occiput and overriding sagittal suture line.
(3) Resolution in first week of life.
(4) Not uncommon for overriding sutures to persist longer than 1 week in the ELBW infant.

b. Rounded head occurs with delivery by cesarean section without labor; flat head with increased anterior-posterior diameter occurs with breech delivery.

c. Abnormal prominence, depressions, or flattening.

d. Abnormal shape of skull.
(1) Plagiocephaly: asymmetric appearance of head; flattened on one side.
(2) Craniosynostosis: premature closing of one or more of cranial sutures.
(3) Anencephaly: failed closure of neural tube without skull formation.

4. Palpate sutures and fontanelles (Fig. 7-7).

a. Sutures: check for mobility of sutures by placing thumb on opposite sides of suture and alternately pushing (gently).
(1) Well approximated.
(2) Overriding.
(a) Molding.
(b) Fused suture: premature synostosis.
(3) Wide sutures.
(a) May be wide in the absence of increased intercranial pressure.
(b) Widened lambdoid suture: indicates increased pressure.
(c) Sagittal and metopic sutures normally wider in black infants (Fletcher, 1998).
(4) Craniotabes: soft demineralized area typically found in parietal and occipital regions along the lambdoidal suture line.
(a) Under gentle pressure the area will collapse and then recoil.
(b) Infant engaged in vertex position for prolonged period.
(c) Pressure of skull against maternal pelvis results in delayed ossification or reabsorption of bone.

b. Anterior fontanelle.
(1) Location: junction of sagittal and coronal sutures.
(2) Shape: diamond.
(3) Size: measures 4 to 6 cm at largest diameter (bone to bone).
(4) Normally closes at 18 months.

c. Posterior fontanelle.
(1) Location: junction of lambdoidal and sagittal sutures.
(2) Shape: triangular.
(3) Size: usually fingertip.
(4) Normally closes by 2 months of age.

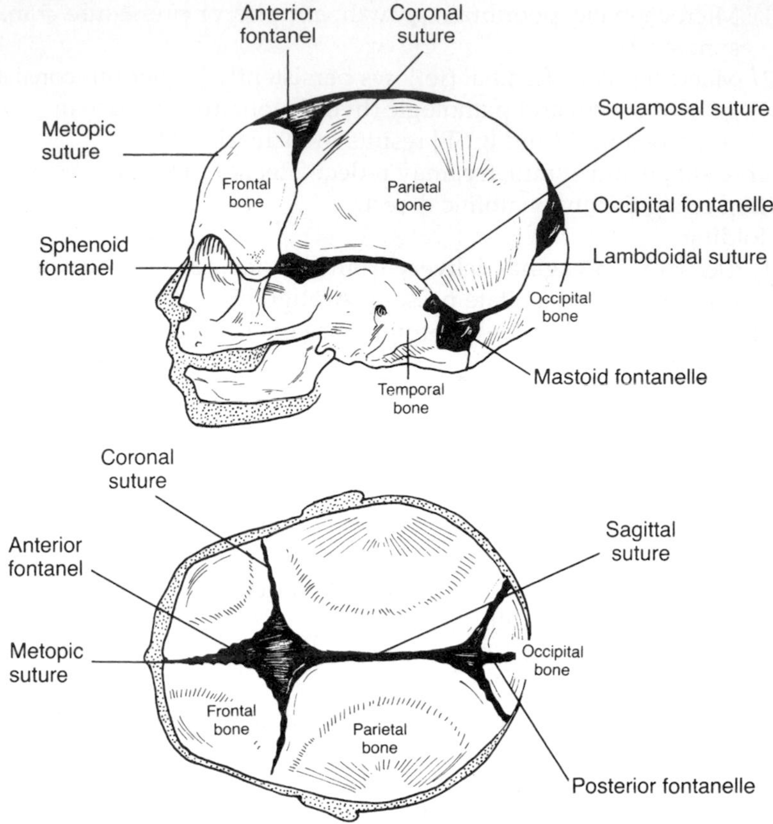

FIGURE 7-7 ■ Two views of skull, showing fontanelles and sutures.

- **d.** Abnormal findings.
  - (1) Third fontanelle: between anterior and posterior fontanelles along sagittal suture (may be associated with congenital anomalies).
  - (2) Size: large fontanelle considerable racial variations; not pathognomonic for any condition (Fletcher, 1998).
  - (3) Closed fontanelles with immobile, rigid sutures suggest premature synostosis.
  - (4) Bruit over temporal, frontal, or occipital area associated with high output cardiac failure and arteriovenous malformation.
  - (5) Abnormal tension.
    - (a) Bulging, tense, full fontanelle: associated with increased intracranial pressure secondary to hydrocephalus, birth injury, bleeding, or infection.
    - (b) Depressed fontanelle: associated with dehydration.

5. Palpate soft tissue findings on scalp, face, and neck (Furdon and Clark, 2001).
- **a.** Caput succedaneum: common finding in infants born in vertex position due to compression of local blood vessels.
  - (1) Maximal swelling present at birth.
  - (2) Edema extends across suture lines and has poorly defined borders.
  - (3) Edema can shift to dependent position.
  - (4) +/– ecchymosis, petechiae, or purpura.
  - (5) Disappears within 24 to 48 hours.

b. Cephalohematoma: subperiosteal hemorrhage due to traumatic delivery.
   (1) Typically not present at birth; increases in size over first day of life.
   (2) Unilateral; fixed, firm, palpable mass.
   (3) Swelling does not cross suture lines.
   (4) Often no ecchymosis.
   (5) Poor tone, feeding, and decreased activity may be indication of underlying skull fracture.
   (6) Resolution may not occur for several months, often leaving a calcified "knot."

c. Subgaleal hemorrhage: due to forces that compress and drag the head through the pubic outlet.
   (1) Is a clinical emergency.
   (2) Ballotable scalp mass present at birth that is mobile; not fixed.
   (3) Swelling crosses suture lines and fontanelles; poorly defined margins.
   (4) Rapidly can increase in size and shape with significant acute blood loss resulting in shock as the presenting symptom.
   (5) Bleeding, seen as swelling, can expand to orbital ridges, around the ears and dissect along tissue planes into the neck.
   (6) Least common of the birth injuries; however, has the greatest potential for complications.

6. Inspect the scalp.
   a. Intact skin; normal hair pattern (direction of growth) and distribution.
   b. Abnormal findings.
      (1) Lacerations or abrasions as the result of instruments at delivery or scalp electrode.
      (2) Vesicles: electrode site and behind the ears.
      (3) Cutis aplasia: localized absence of skin associated with trisomy 13.
      (4) Hair whorls: spiral hair growth pattern; multiple hair whorls or abnormal placement may represent abnormal brain growth or development.
      (5) Anterior hairline well onto the forehead.

7. Note position infant holds head at rest.
   a. Reflects fetal position.
   b. Usual position: anterior neck flexion.
   c. Observe for full range of motion.

F. Face.

1. Observe for symmetry and location of eyes, nose, and mouth.
   a. Divide the face into thirds for inspection: one third, forehead; one third, eyes and nose; and one third, mouth and chin.
   b. At rest and with crying or sucking.
   c. Asymmetry when infant crying: facial palsy.

2. Observe relationship and location of eyes, nose, and mouth.
   a. Eyes.
      (1) Spacing and size.
         (a) Space between inner and outer canthus of one eye approximates the width between the two inner canthi.
         (b) Hypertelorism (widened distance between orbits); hypotelorism (decreased distance between orbits) associated with various syndromes.
      (2) Number: anophthalmos (absent); cyclopia (one).
      (3) Conjunctiva and sclera.
         (a) Subconjunctival hemorrhage: result from pressure on fetal head during delivery.

(b) Sclera color usually white.
(c) Blue sclera: extreme prematuriy, osteogenesis imperfecta, other chromosomal associations.
(d) Yellow sclera: jaundiced.
(4) Cornea, iris, and pupils.
(a) Cornea relatively cloudy at birth:
(i) Term infant: cloudiness resolves within a few days.
(ii) Asymmetric or dense cloudiness: abnormal.
(iii) Infantile cataracts: rubella, CMV, familial association, and chromosomal defect.
(b) Iris: dark blue until 3 to 6 months of age, then eye color may change.
(i) Brushfield's spots: speckled appearance; occurs in 75% of infants with trisomy 21; also normal (Fletcher, 1998).
(ii) Coloboma: cleft-shaped fissure (keyhole shape); can be sporadic or in association with trisomy 13 or choanal atresia, posterior coloboma, heart defect, choanal atresia, retardation, genital and ear abnormalities (CHARGE) sequence.
(c) Pupils.
(i) PERL (pupils equal, round, and react to light).
(ii) White color: abnormal.
(d) Red reflex: reflection of ophthalmoscope's light on the retina.
(e) Color range: red (light-skinned infant) to yellow (dark-skinned infant).
(i) White: congenital cataracts.
(ii) Absence: retinoblastoma, glaucoma, or hemorrhage.
(5) Symmetry of eye movements.

b. Nose.
(1) Shape and size.
(a) Positional deformities often due to birth process; resolve without treatment.
(b) Abnormal shape: may be associated with a congenital syndrome.
(c) Abnormal: flat, broad nasal bridge.
(2) Patency of nostrils.
(a) Place a cold, metal object under each nostril and observe for fogging: presence of airflow.
(b) Causes of nasal obstruction.
(i) Choanal atresia or stenosis: membranous or bony obstruction; unilateral or bilateral.
(ii) Iatrogenic: swollen mucosa from suction catheters.
(iii) Inflammation and secretions.

c. Mouth, tongue, and perioral region.
(1) Mouth should be symmetric and positioned in the midline:
(a) Microstomia: very small mouth; may be associated with trisomy 18.
(b) Macrostomia: large mouth; often associated with mucopolysaccharidosis, Beckwith syndrome, or hypothyroidism.
(c) Suck and swallow develops at 32 to 34 weeks, and root and gag response at 36 weeks. They should be elicited during the examination.

(2) Cleft upper lip: can vary from a niche in the lip to a complete separation extending up onto the floor of the nose.
(3) Thin upper lip in association with flat philtrum: fetal alcohol syndrome.
(4) Soft and hard palate should be examined for the presence of submucous or membranous clefts.
(5) Mucosal cysts.
   (a) Epithelial or Epstein's pearls: small, white epidermal cysts commonly found on the hard and soft palates and on gum margins and disappear after a few weeks.
   (b) Bohn nodule: equivalent to milia on the skin.
   (c) Gingival or alveolar cysts.
(6) Dental eruptions and neonatal teeth.
   (a) If mobile or poor root formation: generally removed.
   (b) Consult with pediatric dentist; may be primary teeth.
(7) Frenulum.
   (a) Small lingual frenulum normal ("tongue tied").
   (b) Short frenulum that limits tongue movement: abnormal; tip of tongue will form inverted V shape.
(8) Tongue.
   (a) Large tongue (macroglossia): generally part of syndrome (Beckwith-Wiedemann).
   (b) Large tongue can obstruct airway.
   (c) Protruding tongue: trisomy 21 and Beckwith-Wiedemann.
(9) Thrush: oral moniliasis: usually contracted from mothers with vaginal moniliasis at time of delivery.
   (a) Lacy white material present on surface of oral mucous membranes.
   (b) Does not wipe away with a cotton-tipped swab.

3. Observe other facial features.

a. Eyelids.
(1) Should open to above midpoint of pupil when the eye is in a neutral position.
(2) Edema: related to birth process or chemical irritation with eye prophylaxis.
(3) Fused eyelids: extreme prematurity; generally not fused by 28 weeks' gestation; should not be used as an indicator of viability or nonviability.
(4) Ptosis: abnormal drooping of one or both eyelids.

b. Palpebral fissures.
(1) Slant is primarily racially determined.
(2) Variations typical of several syndromes.

c. Epicanthal folds.
(1) Vertical fold of skin at inner canthus on either side of the nose.
(2) Common in trisomy 21.
(3) Manifestation of in utero compression (Potter facies).

d. Eyelashes, eyebrows.
(1) Appear at 20 to 23 weeks.
(2) Abnormalities.
   (a) Absent lashes or long lashes.
   (b) High-arched eyebrows or synophrys (meeting of eyebrows in middle).

e. Nasolacrimal ducts.
(1) Tears are rare until 2 to 4 months of age.
(2) Obstruction: visible mass.

4. Inspect facial skin.
a. Milia: 1-mm white or yellow papules without erythema; resolve spontaneously within first weeks of life.
b. Miliaria: clear, thin vesicles 1 to 2 mm that develop in sweat glands; primarily seen on forehead, scalp, and creases.
c. Lacerations, ecchymosis, abrasions from forceps.
d. Petechiae over head and neck: typically from nuchal cord, rapid second stage of labor.
e. Pits or sinus: facial cleft syndromes.

5. Observe for size of jaw and relationship to maxilla.
a. Micrognathia: abnormally small jaw with normal size tongue.
(1) May present serious airway problem.
(2) Seen in Pierre Robin, Treacher Collins, and de Lange syndromes.

G. Ears (Spilman, 2002).

1. Note presence or absence of external ear.
2. Determine position and rotation.
a. Helix attaches to scalp at a point horizontal to the inner canthus of the eye.
b. Normal: 30% of pinna above imaginary line drawn from the inner canthi of the eyes toward the occiput and tragus (cartilaginous projection in front of the external meatus of the ear).
c. Cranial molding may distort landmarks; ears may appear low-set.
d. Low-set ears may be associated with various syndromes and chromosomal abnormalities.

3. Check for presence of ear canals; visualization of eardrums not typically necessary.
4. Examine for abnormal findings.
a. Microtia: disorganized or dysplastic ear.
(1) Associated with atresia of auditory meatus and conductive hearing loss.
(2) Variations.
(a) Lop ear: helix folded downward because of inadequate development of the antihelix.
(b) Cup ear: small cup-shaped ear.
b. Preauricular pits and sinus.
(1) Pinpoint openings at base of helix or front of tragus.
(2) Increased risk of congenital deafness and renal abnormalities.
c. Preauricular ear appendages (tags).
(1) Single or multiple; vary in size.
(2) Differentiate from accessory auricle or tragus.
(3) Consistently seen in Goldenhar syndrome: syndrome with wide range of facial, ear, and vertebral defects (Jones, 1997).
(4) Associated with urinary tract abnormalities (Kohelet and Arbel, 2000) and other brachial arch abnormalities: cleft lip, cleft palate, and hypoplasia of mandible.

H. Neck and clavicles.

1. Inspect and palpate neck.
a. Mass: note location.
(1) Most common: cystic hygroma.

(a) Multiloculated cyst arising from lymphatic channels typically located posterior to the sternocleidomastoid muscle and extending into the scapula and axillary and thoracic compartments.
(b) Can distort anatomy of airway.
(2) Thyroglossal duct cyst or branchial cleft cyst.
b. Webbing.
(1) Excessive skinfold extending from mastoid process to shoulders.
(2) Associated with Turner and Noonan syndromes and trisomy 21.
c. Torticollis: rotation limited due to constant position of head to one side.
2. Gently palpate neck and clavicles.
a. Crepitus: due to fractured bone ends rubbing together.
(1) Swelling, discoloration, or tenderness associated with fractured clavicle.
(2) Observe for asymmetric arm movement with the Moro reflex or signs of pain with manipulation.

I. Chest and lungs.
1. Review influencing factors: GA, timing of examination, intrapartum and delivery history, maternal drugs, and cool environment.
2. Inspect the shape and size of the chest (Fig. 7-8).
a. Compare size relationship of the thorax and abdomen.
b. Normal: round symmetric shape with the anterior-posterior diameter approximately the same as the transverse diameter.
c. Large or barrel-shaped chest: associated with air trapping and hyperinflation.
d. Pigeon chest or protrusion of sternum: associated with Marfan syndrome.
e. Chest wall itself depressed or funnel shaped: pectus excavatum; no clinical significance.
f. Short sternum: associated with trisomy 18.
g. Rib margins apparent in premature infants: thinner layers of muscle and fat.
3. Observe.
a. Color: refer to C. General Appearance: Initial Impression, p. 148.
b. Respiratory rate and pattern.
(1) Should be evaluated at rest and before any manipulation.
(2) Rate: normal: 40 to 60 breaths per minute; easy; unlabored and typically abdominal or diaphragmatic.
(3) Tachypnea: rate greater than 60 breaths per minute: lung pathology, cardiac disease, infection, overheating, fever, and pain.
(4) Bradypnea or shallow respirations: CNS depression.
(5) Periodic breathing: 5- to 20-second pauses without changes in color, tone, or heart rate.
(6) Apnea: cessation of breathing for more than 20 seconds. May be accompanied by bradycardia, change in muscle tone, or color change; apnea of prematurity, infection, respiratory insufficiency, gastroesophageal reflux (GER).
(7) Slow, gasping respirations: respiratory failure and acidosis.
c. Depth and ease of respirations.
(1) Normal: irregular and varying depth.
(2) Chest pulled inward as abdomen rises with inspiration due to normal diaphragmatic excursion.
(3) Retractions: accessory muscles used.
(a) Note depth (minimal, marked).

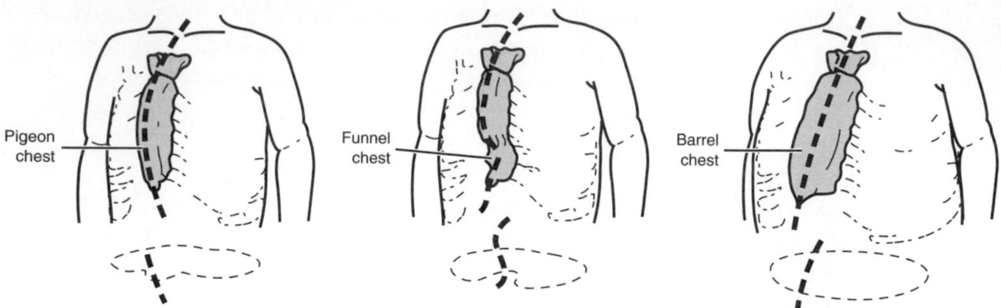

FIGURE 7-8 ■ Different chest shapes. (Adapted from Alexander, M.M. and Brown, M.S.: *Pediatric history taking and physical diagnosis for nurses* [2nd ed.]. St Louis, 1979, Mosby.)

(b) Subcostal, substernal: common after birth. Persistence may indicate respiratory problems.
(c) Intercostal.
(4) Nasal flaring retractions, tachypnea, and grunting: symptomatic of respiratory distress.

4. Auscultate breath sounds.
 a. Compare and contrast each side of chest.
 b. Presence of air entry: normal, fair, or poor.
 c. Asymmetric breath sounds: pneumothorax, cystic adenomatoid malformation (CAM), or congenital diaphragmatic hernia (CDH).
 d. Normal breath sounds: clear; little differentiation between inspiration and expiration.
 e. Adventitious breath sounds.
  (1) Crackles: fine or coarse; lower pitched; fine crackles heard on inspiration; often present after birth due to clearing lung fluid.
  (2) Wheeze: high pitched usually heard on exhalation; reactive airway.
  (3) Rhonchi: low pitched; arise from partial obstruction by mucus or secretions.
  (4) Stridor: rough, harsh sound worse during inspiration; caused by reduced airway diameter (edema, mass, vascular ring).
  (5) Diminished breath sounds: atelectasis, effusion, decreased air entry, poor respiratory effort.
  (6) Peristaltic sounds: bowel sounds indicate CDH.
  (7) Friction rub: pleural effusion.

5. Inspect breasts and nipples.
 a. Size.
  (1) Based on gestational age.
  (2) Enlarged breasts: effects of maternal estrogen; transient.
  (3) Unilateral redness or firmness indicates sepsis.
 b. Location and symmetry: widespread nipples: distance between nipples more than 25% of full chest circumference; may indicate variety of conditions (Hernandez and Hernandez, 1999).
 c. Number: supernumerary nipples; small, raised, pigmented areas vertical with main nipple line 5 to 6 cm below normal nipple; familial.
 d. Discharge.
  (1) Witch's milk.
   (a) Milky discharge produced in response to maternal hormones.
   (b) Lasts for several weeks to months.
  (2) Purulent: mastitis due to staphylococcal infection.

J. Heart and cardiovascular system.

1. General considerations: congenital heart defects are associated with other congenital malformations, chromosomal defects, maternal medication or substance use (phenytoin [Dilantin], alcohol), maternal health or illness (diabetes), viral illness, and familial association.
2. Observe color.
3. Heart rate: normal range 120 to 160 beats per minute (bpm) varies with infant behavioral state.
   a. Bradycardia: rate less than 100 bpm.
      (1) May be associated with apnea, cerebral defects, vagal response, congenital heart block.
      (2) Term infant in deep sleep can have heart rate of 80 to 90 bpm; should increase as infant awakens.
   b. Tachycardia: more than 160 bpm sustained.
      (1) May be associated with respiratory distress, anemia, congestive heart failure, hyperthermia, shock, and supraventricular tachycardia (SVT).
   c. Brief irregularities are common; identification of abnormality cannot be made by auscultation alone.
4. Location of point of maximal intensity (PMI).
   a. Normal: lateral to midclavicular line at 4th intercostal space.
   b. Shift in location can indicate tension pneumothorax.
   c. Right side location: dextrocardia, CDH.
   d. Observe precordial activity.
      (1) Within 6 hours of birth may be visible along left sternal border (Southgate and Pittard, 2001).
      (2) Visible for longer periods in premature infants.
      (3) Associated with congestive heart failure, heart disease, and fluid overload.
5. Auscultate heart sounds.
   a. First heart sound.
      (1) Accentuated at birth.
      (2) Increase in intensity: PDA, ventricular septal defect (VSD), tetralogy of Fallot, anemia, hyperthermia, and arteriovenous fistula.
   b. Second heart sound.
      (1) Sound produced by closure of aortic and pulmonary valves.
      (2) No splitting of heart sound: pulmonary atresia, transposition of the great artery (TGA), or truncus arteriosus.
   c. Muffled heart sounds: may indicate pneumopericardium, pneumomediastinum, or CDH.
6. Auscultate murmur: turbulence in blood flow (Fig. 7-9).
   a. Can be innocent or pathologic (underlying cardiovascular disease).
   b. Timing of appearance.
      (1) First 48 hours of life: can be related to cardiovascular transition; should be followed up.
      (2) Audible after transition complete: VSD, turbulence in pulmonary arteries secondary to obstruction; severe outflow tract obstruction.
   c. Location and radiation.
      (1) Describe as interspace, midclavicular, midsternal, or axillary.
      (2) Transmission: auscultate back or axilla.
   d. Timing within cycle.
      (1) Continuous: extends beyond second heart sound into diastole.
      (2) Systolic ejection murmur: occurs before the first heart sound; ends at or before second heart sound; flow across pulmonary valve.

e. Loudness or quality.
   (1) Grade 1: barely audible.
   (2) Grade 2: soft but easily audible.
   (3) Grade 3: moderately loud but no thrill.
   (4) Grade 4: loud with thrill.
   (5) Grade 5: loud; audible with stethoscope placed lightly on chest.
   (6) Grade 6: loud; audible with stethoscope placed near chest.

7. Palpate pulses: strength and equality (upper to lower and side to side).
   a. Brachial, radial, and palmar.
   b. Femoral, popliteal, posterial tibial, and dorsalis pedis.
   c. Grading scale (Vargo, 1996).
      0: not palpable.
      +1: very difficult to palpate; weak, thready, easily obliterated with pressure.
      +2: difficult to palpate; may be obliterated with pressure.
      +3: easy to palpate; not easy to obliterate with pressure; found in normal pulses.
      +4: strong and bounding; not obliterated with pressure; associated with PDA.
   d. Absent femoral: associated with coarctation of aorta.
8. Assess capillary refill or perfusion.
   a. Press and release skin over abdomen until area blanches.
   b. Count number of seconds until color returns to area.
   c. Normal: less than or equal to 3 seconds.

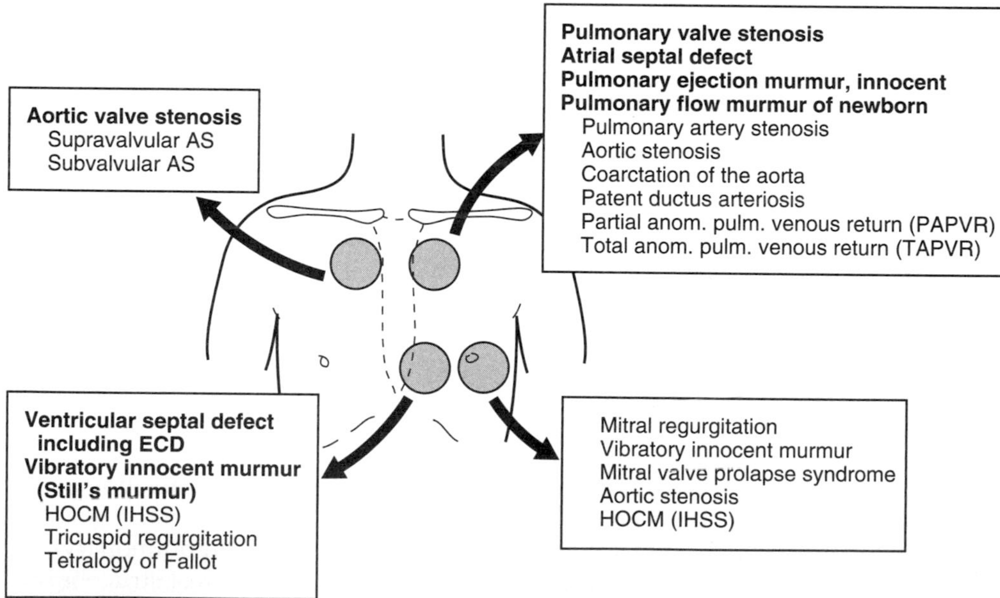

FIGURE 7-9 ■ Diagram showing systolic murmurs audible at various locations. Less common conditions are shown in lighter type. *AS,* Aortic stenosis; *ECD,* endocardial cushion defect; *HOCM,* hypertrophic obstructive cardiomyopathy; *IHSS,* idiopathic hypertrophic subaortic stenosis. (From Park, M.K.: *Pediatric cardiology for practitioners* [3rd ed.]. St Louis, 1995, Mosby.)

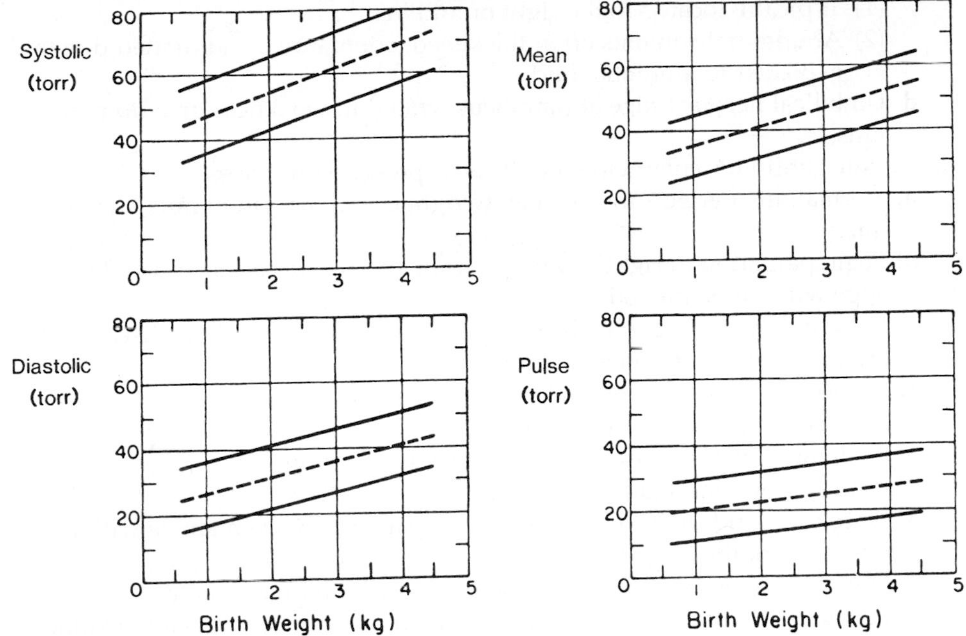

FIGURE 7-10 ■ Blood pressure by birth weight. (From Versmold, H.T., Kitterman, J.A., Phibbs, R.H., et al.: Aortic blood pressure during the first 12 hours of life in infants with birth weight 610 to 4200 grams. *Pediatrics, 67*[5]:607-613, 1981.)

9. Blood pressure (Fig. 7-10).
   a. Depends on gestational age and chronologic age.
   b. Differential greater than 20 mm Hg between upper and lower extremity blood pressure indicates obstruction (coarctation of aorta).
   c. Blood pressure (BP) in lower extremities should be slightly higher than in the upper extremities.

K. Abdomen.

1. General considerations: review history for feeding intake, emesis, stooling, maternal medications affecting bowel function, maternal blood type, and intrauterine infection.
2. Observe abdomen: slightly rounded, soft, and symmetric.
   a. Scaphoid abdomen: abdominal contents in chest (diaphragmatic hernia). May appear slightly concave at birth, but will become distended as bowel fills with air.
   b. Decreased abdominal tone or muscles in abdominal wall (prune belly syndrome).
   c. Distention: obstruction, infection, masses, or enlargement of an abdominal organ.
3. Observe for abdominal wall defect (Reu Donlon et al., 2002).
   a. Etiology: disruption in migration of abdominal contents from umbilical cord and defect in development of abdominal wall musculature.
   b. Omphalocele: abdominal contents usually covered with a membrane; commonly associated with cardiac lesions, trisomy 13, trisomy 18, Beckwith-Wiedemann syndrome.
   c. Gastroschisis: abdominal wall defect resulting in protrusion of abdominal contents not covered with a membrane.

(1) Typically located to the right of midline.
(2) Abdominal contents often thickened, edematous, and matted due to exposure to amniotic fluid.

d. Umbilical hernia: bulge at umbilicus related to weakness in abdominal muscle.

4. Palpate gently for enlargement in liver or presence of masses.

a. Normal: liver edge 1 to 2 cm below right costal margin in midclavicular line.
b. Begin palpation in right lower quadrant and progress upward so liver edge will not be missed.
c. Enlarged liver: congenital heart disease, infection, hemolytic disease, and arteriovenous (AV) malformation.
d. A normal spleen is rarely palpable; palpable spleen more than 1 cm below left costal margin is abnormal.
e. Abdominal mass: most often of urinary tract origin.

5. Palpate kidneys and bladder.

a. Place one hand under the flank and palpate gently from above with the fingertips of the other hand.
b. Normal kidney in term infant is 4.5 to 5 cm from pole to pole.
c. Further evaluation needed: absence of palpable kidney or enlarged kidneys.
d. Bladder can be palpated 1 to 4 cm above pubic symphysis when urine present.

6. Ausculate for bowel sounds.

a. Absent or hyperactive bowel sounds may indicate obstruction.

7. Inspect the umbilical cord (Reu Donlon et al., 2002).

a. Important clues to fetal growth, development, and well-being.
b. Normal: bluish white, moist, and gelatinous.
c. Diameter of cord varies and is related to Wharton jelly.
(1) Supportive covering protecting the cord vessels from compression or occlusion.
(2) Increases with GA.
(3) Thin cord may reflect placental insufficiency and intrauterine growth retardation.
d. Total length of cord: normal 30 to 90 cm.
(1) Length determined by intrauterine space and fetal activity.
(2) Infants with limited fetal activity (Down syndrome, congenital neuromuscular disorders) have short cords.
e. Presence of knots.
f. Color: green or yellow (meconium); red (blood); depth of staining correlates with duration of exposure.
g. Number of vessels.
(1) Normally contains two arteries and one vein.
(2) Single umbilical artery may be associated with renal anomalies.
h. Urine draining from umbilicus: patent urachus (embryologic communication between bladder and umbilicus).

L. Genitalia and anus.

1. General considerations.

a. Review pertinent history.
(1) Gestational age; appearance changes with gestational age (see Gestational Age Assessment: Physical Criteria on p. 140).
(2) Oligohydraminos or polyhydraminos: possible renal/urinary anomaly.
(3) Family history: associated genetic predisposition.

b. Congenital defects are relatively rare but highly stressful to parents.
c. Normal variations are more common than pathologic conditions.
d. Genitourinary anomalies are highly associated with other system disorders (see Chapter 32).
e. Breech deliveries can cause significant bruising and edema of genitalia and perineum.
f. No circumcision should be done in infants with epispadias, hypospadias, or chordee.

2. General inspection and palpation: position infant supine for examination.
   a. Gender identification: if not clearly distinguishable, do not assign sex until further evaluation. Inform parents of ambiguity and need for further testing.
   b. Anus: locate position in relation to genitalia and determine patency.
      (1) Anal opening: approximately midline.
      (2) Slightly more anterior to genitalia in females.
      (3) Check for anal wink in any infant suspected of neural tube defect; stroke anal opening lightly; observe positive constriction.
   c. Passage of meconium; ensures open communication only.
      (1) Fistulas: anterior or posteriorly placed; may be accompanied with bowel distention
         (a) Rectovaginal fistula (female) or rectoperineal fistula (male).
      (2) Constant dribbling of loose stool: suspect neural tube defect.
   d. Inguinal area (Benjamin, 2002).
      (1) Assess for hernia(s) when inguinal mass observed.
      (2) Groin bulge: may be unilateral or bilateral; increase in size with crying or straining or spontaneously reduce.
      (3) Palpate from lower abdomen along inguinal canal to labia or scrotum.
      (4) Attempt to gently compress bowel back toward abdomen. Irreducible hernias are at high risk for incarceration and subsequent necrosis.
3. Male.
   a. Penis: inspect size, appearance, and foreskin.
      (1) Normal.
         (a) Straight, may be erect.
         (b) Size proportionate to body, average term length 2.5 to 3.5 cm from pubic bone to glans tip (Hernandez and Hernandez, 1999).
         (c) Glans covered by prepuce (foreskin) in uncircumcised infant.
         (d) Physiologic phimosis: tight, nonretractable foreskin; does not retract until 2 to 3 years of age.
         (e) Small, white epithelial cysts on distal prepuce.
      (2) Abnormal.
         (a) Chordee: curving or bowing of penis.
         (b) Micropenis: less than 2.5 cm.
   b. Determine position of urinary meatus.
      (1) Normal: midline at glans tip.
      (2) Abnormal.
         (a) Hypospadias: urethral opening located at ventral surface of penis; associated with chordee, meatal stenosis, inguinal hernia, and undescended testes.
         (b) Epispadias: urethral opening located on dorsal surface of penis.
   c. Urine: observe strength, direction of stream, and color.
      (1) Normal.
         (a) Straight, forceful, and continuous stream.

(b) Most newborns void within first 24 hours of birth.
(c) Uric acid crystals (flaky, rust colored) are a normal variant.
(2) Abnormal.
(a) Altered stream direction may indicate urinary obstruction; urine from perineum or abdomen indicates urinary fistula.
(b) Abnormal color: red (hemoglobin or myoglobin); brown (bilirubin); brown-yellow (concentrated).

d. Scrotum and testes: inspect for size, symmetry, color, presence of rugae, and location of testes.
(1) Normal.
(a) Firm, smooth testes of equal size palpable in scrotal sac; undescended testes in inguinal canal normal for preterm infants.
(b) Darker skin pigmentation.
(2) Abnormal: scrotal swelling or discoloration; nonpalpable testes.
(a) Cryptorchidism, extrascrotal testes position: needs further investigation with ultrasound and karyotyping.
(b) Nonpalpable testes: if not detected in phenotypic male, evaluate for virilizing adrenal hyperplasia.
(c) Bifid scrotum.
(d) Hydrocele: unilateral or bilateral fluid collection in scrotal sac, + transillumination.
(e) Testicular torsion: blue discoloration, palpable firm mass, tender or nontender; – transillumination. May be surgical emergency.

4. Female.

a. Labia and clitoris: separate labia and exert gentle downward traction to evaluate structures.
(1) Normal: smooth, wrinkling with weight loss, hyperpigmented from hormonal influence.
(2) Edematous at birth due to maternal hormones.
(3) Perineum is smooth, no dimpling; fingertip width.
(4) Abnormal.
(a) Labia bulge may indicate inguinal hernia or ectopic ovary.
(b) Labioscrotal fusion; female virilization.
(c) Cliteromegaly; pseudohermaphroditism.
(d) Genitourinary (GU) anomalies: abnormal spacing between orifices.
(e) Rugae: ambiguous genitalia.

b. Vagina.
(1) Normal: pink, patent.
(a) White or blood-tinged discharge due to hormonal influence (pseudomenstruation); can persist 2 to 4 weeks.
(b) Redundant hymen tissue and vaginal skin tags are common.
(2) Abnormal.
(a) Rectovaginal fistula: feces from vagina; indicates rectovaginal fistula.
(b) Imperforate hymen: secretions pool in vagina; can be confused with enlarged Bartholin cysts.
(c) Hydrometracolpos: membrane covering vaginal opening causes uterine enlargement and pooling of vaginal secretions; seen as perineal or suprapubic mass.

c. Urethral meatus.
(1) Normal position: below clitoris; often obscured by hymen.
(2) Abnormal: anterior displacement.

M. Back, spine, and extremities.

1. General considerations.
   a. Influencing factors: gestational age, maternal hormones, in utero position, delivery mode/history, and timing of examination.
   b. Many abnormalities are deformations from compression and contracture in utero rather than congenital defects.
   c. Review for relevant history.
      (1) Elevated maternal alfa-fetoprotein (AFP) (neural tube defects).
      (2) Maternal diabetes mellitus (sacral agenesis).
      (3) Decreased fetal movement (congenital neuromuscular disorders).
      (4) Postnatal *S. aureus* sepsis (risk for osteomyelitis).
      (5) Family history (hip dysplasia).
2. Observe infant at rest: appropriate number of limbs and digits; size and symmetry of upper and lower extremities; movement, position of comfort, range of motion, and trauma.
3. Palpate for joint or bone swelling, tenderness, or crepitus.
4. Back: position infant prone.
   a. Inspect for symmetry of sides, scapula position and symmetry, spine alignment and integrity, and presence of dermal lesions over spine or masses.
   b. Inspect skin.
      (1) Mongolian spots.
         (a) Normal variant; macular gray-blue lesions from melanocyte concentration in dermis.
         (b) Most commonly in lumbosacral region but can be found on legs, back, and shoulders.
         (c) Occurs more often in black, Hispanic, Asian, and Native American infants.
         (d) Benign; fade during childhood.
      (2) Subtle findings can indicate hidden spinal defects; observe for sacral dimples, sacral tracts (pilonidal cysts), hair tufts, hemangiomas, or lipomas.
   c. Congenital spine defects.
      (1) Neural tube defect.
         (a) Failure of posterior neural tube closure (see Chapters 33 and 34).
         (b) Defect can be open with spine and nerves exposed or covered with skin or tissue.
      (2) Sacrococcygeal teratoma: tumor (mainly benign).
      (3) Scoliosis: lateral spine curvature; evaluate for associated GU tract anomalies.
5. Extremities.
   a. Upper extremities.
      (1) Absent humerus, radius, or ulna: associated with syndromes.
      (2) Clavicle or humerus fractures: associated with birth injury or osteogenesis imperfecta.
      (3) Blisters on hands or forearms: in utero sucking.
      (4) Brachial plexus injury: stretching or tearing of nerve roots by lateral traction on shoulder during birth (Volpe, 2001); or pressure from the maternal sacral promontory during fetal descent (Jennet et al., 2002).
         (a) Erb palsy paralysis of arm with intact grasp; asymemetric Moro reflex.
         (b) Klumpke paralysis: forearm paralysis with absent grasp.
         (c) Total brachial plexus injury: because the neonate can't move the shoulder, the arms remain extended and turned inward, with the flaccid hand suggesting a "waiter's tip" hand.

(5) Observe hands for shape and of digits.
   (a) Syndactyly: webbing between adjacent digits of hands.
   (b) Polydactyly: supernumerary digits.
   (c) Clinodactyly: congenital deviation of digits.
   (d) Brachydactyly: shortened digit from shortened finger joint; normal variant; associated with achondroplasia and trisomy 21.
(6) Simian crease: single palmar crease; normal variant , positive finding in less than 50% of trisomy 21 infants (Fletcher, 1998).
(7) Nails: yellowing from meconium or postmaturity; dysplasia with chromosomal defects.

b. Buttocks.
(1) Observe for blanching or cyanosis of extremities or buttocks while umbilical catheters in use; indicates circulation compromise and potential necrosis.
(2) Dimple on buttocks can indicate congenital anomaly of femur (Fletcher, 1998).

c. Hips.
(1) Positional hip abduction: persistent joint flexion or contraction with knee extension resulting from prolonged breech position in utero.
(2) Developmental dysplasia of the hip (DDH) (French and Dietz, 1999).
   (a) Asymmetric creases of buttocks and thighs due to shortened adductor muscles.
   (b) Uneven knee level (positive Galeazzi sign) when positioned prone with feet level and knees at 90-degree angle.
   (c) Ortolani maneuver: detects dislocated hips.
   (d) Barlow maneuver: determines dislocatable hips (Fig. 7-11).

d. Lower extremities.
(1) Legs normally slightly bowed with everted feet.
(2) Genu recurvatum: knee hyperextension; related to breech position.
(3) Limb or digit amputation (amniotic band syndrome).
   (a) Strands of amnion can wrap around any digit or more frequently, a limb.
   (b) Causes constriction and amputation.
(4) Metatarsus adductus (Furdon and Reu Donlon, 2002).
   (a) May be positional or structural.
   (b) Convex shape to lateral border of foot (C shaped).
   (c) Adduction at tarsal metatarsal joint; wider space between first and second toes.
(5) Talipes equinovarus (TEV); clubfoot.
   (a) May be positional or structural.
   (b) Inversion deformity of heel (sole points medially), forefoot incurving and ankle in equinus posture (toes pointing down and heel pointing up).
(6) Talipes calcaneovalgus: related to intrauterine position; sole of foot is flattened against uterine wall.
(7) Rocker bottom feet: arch looks like rocker bottom.

N. Neurologic examination.

1. General considerations.

a. Repeat examination of abnormal findings; assess changes over time.

b. Review history: familial, genetic, or neurologic diagnosis, birth trauma, difficult delivery, perinatal depression, maternal medication/alcohol/drugs.

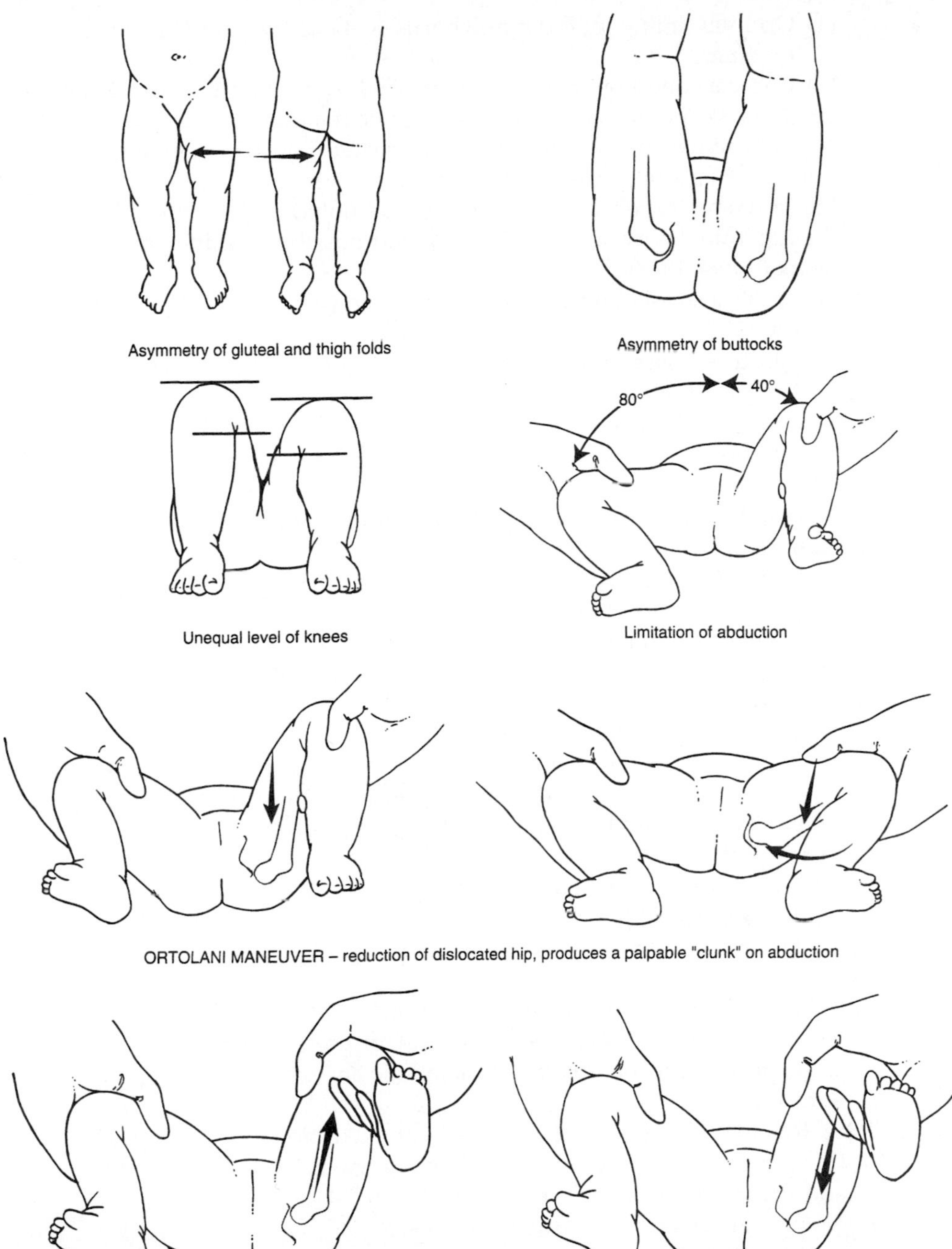

FIGURE 7-11 ■ Assessment of newborn infant for dislocated or unstable hip includes gluteal and thigh folds, buttocks, knees, abduction, Ortolani maneuver, and Barlow maneuver. (From Nichols, F.H. and Zwelling, E.: *Maternal-newborn nursing: Theory and practice.* Philadelphia, 1997, Saunders.)

c. Gestational age is an important consideration; responses of preterm infant are immature.

d. Timing and sequence of examination may alter the neurologic examination (Dubowitz et al., 1999).

(1) Optimal timing for older newborns is about two thirds between feedings.
(2) Clinical condition may necessitate exclusion of parts of examination.

2. Observe for skin lesions related to neurologic disorders.
   a. Neurofibromatosis: café au lait spots, greater than 1.5 cm in length or in numbers of six or greater (Jones, 1997).
   b. Sturge-Weber syndrome: nevus flammeus noted unilaterally, following the trigeminal nerve tract on the face and possibly involving the upper trunk (Jones, 1997).
   c. Tuberous sclerosis: areas of hypopigmented (white) macules on the skin (Jones, 1997).
3. Assess posture: assess infant in quiet awake, quiet active, or light sleep state(s); unswaddled; position supine with head midline.
   a. Term infant lies with arms adducted, hips abducted and partially flexed, moderate flexion of all extremities, and with loosely clenched fists.
   b. Preterm infant becomes more hypotonic with decreasing gestational age.
   c. Abnormal.
      (1) Persistent neck extension (opisthotonos).
      (2) Obligate thumb flexion (cortical thumb).
      (3) Elbow flexion with dorsum of hands on bed.
      (4) Frog-leg position greater than 36 weeks' gestation.
4. Observe spontaneous movement.
   a. Term infant moves limbs smoothly.
   b. Preterm infant's movements may be jittery and jerky, with tremors.
   c. Environmental stimuli or discomfort produces mass movements.
   d. Coarse tremors and brief chin trembling are normal.
   e. Jittery: rhythmic movements of equal intensity.
      (1) Occurs more after startle or crying.
      (2) Distinguish between tonic-clonic seizures using gentle restraint: tremors will stop; seizures will continue.
5. Cry.
   a. Lusty, with normal pitch: normal term infant.
   b. Weak or monotonous cry: depressed, ill, or preterm infant.
   c. High-pitched cry: neurologic or metabolic abnormalities, drug withdrawal.
6. Tone. Refer to Gestational Age Assessment: Neurologic Criteria, p. 138.
   a. Preterm infants can be difficult to distinguish between random movement and true recoil (Dubowitz et al., 1999).
   b. Note weak, absent, or unequal responses.
   c. Assess resistance to movement (passive tone).
      (1) Limb recoil, heel-to-ear, scarf sign.
      (2) Tendon reflex: only patellar reflex is reliable at birth; note sustained clonus.
   d. Assess resistance to gravity (active tone).
      (1) Traction response: pull-to-sit, ventral suspension; note degree of resistance.
      (2) Ventral and horizontal suspension.
7. Reflexes.
   a. Developmental reflexes (primitive reflexes): should be elicited in the normal term infant. Note any exaggerated or absent responses.
      (1) Sucking reflex: gently stimulate lips; infant opens mouth and begins to suck.

(a) Evaluate the coordination and strength of the suck with a gloved finger.
(b) Present at birth even in the premature infant, although it is not as strong as at term.

(2) Rooting reflex: stroke cheek: infant turns head and opens mouth toward the stimulated side.

(3) Palmar grasp: stroke the infant's palm with finger; infant will grasp the finger.
(a) Attempts to remove the finger will elicit a tighter grasp.
(b) Grasp should be equal bilaterally.

(4) Tonic neck reflex (fencing position).
(a) Position the infant supine. Turn the infant's head to one side.
(b) The infant will extend the upper extremity on the side where the head is turned and flex the opposite upper extremity.

(5) Moro reflex (startle reflex). "Head drop" method preferred depending on the infant's condition (Dubowitz et al., 1999). The high-risk neonate can be startled by making a loud noise close to the ear and noting the response.
(a) Hold infant supine in a neutral position several inches off the bed.
(b) Hold one hand behind the upper back and other supporting head. Infant's arms should cover chest.
(c) Head is held midline and dropped back 10 degrees with supportive hand.
(d) Infant will partially abduct shoulder, extend, and then smoothly adduct arms.
(i) Evaluate arm responses only.
(ii) Repeat two or three times as needed for detailed observation.
(iii) Asymmetric response may indicate brachial plexus injury.

(6) Stepping reflex. Hold the infant upright, allowing the soles of the feet to touch a flat surface; infant will alternate stepping movements.

(7) Babinski reflex.
(a) Stimulate sole of foot; infant will either flex or extend toes.
(b) Persistent absence of reflex can indicate CNS depression or spinal nerve dysfunction.

b. Spinal reflexes.

(1) Truncal incurvation reflex (Galant reflex).
(a) Hold infant in ventral suspension.
(b) Apply firm pressure along the side parallel to spine.
(c) Infant should flex pelvis toward the stimulated side.
(d) Indicates T2-S1 innervation.

(2) Anocutaneous reflex (anal wink).
(a) Stimulate perianal skin.
(b) External sphincter constricts.
(c) Indicates S4-5 innervation.

8. Cranial nerves.

a. Olfactory (I).
(1) Not usually assessed in newborns.
(2) Can attempt in infants with strong scents such as clove or peppermint placed under nose; evaluate for sniffing, grimace, or startle reflex.

b. Optic (II).
(1) Evaluate visual acuity and fields by using tracking methods.
(2) Watch for wandering or persistent nystagmus.
(3) Check pupils for size and constriction in response to light.

c. Oculomotor (II), trochlear (IV), and abducens (VI) nerves: supply pupils and extraocular muscles.
   (1) Observe pupil response to light.
   (2) Evaluate eye size and symmetry.
   (3) "Doll's-eyes" test (vestibular response): move infant's head from side to side, eyes should move away from the direction of rotation.
   (4) Fixed position or movement in same direction may indicate brainstem or oculomotor dysfunction.

d. Trigeminal nerve (V): supplies sensory nerves of jaw and face.
   (1) Touch the cheek; infant will demonstrate rooting reflex.
   (2) Place a gloved finger in the infant's mouth to evaluate sucking and biting reflex.

e. Facial nerve (VII): controls facial expression.
   (1) Observe for symmetric movement of the face.
   (2) Inability to wrinkle brow or close eyes with crying indicates injury.

f. Auditory nerve (VIII): tested only grossly without proper auditory equipment (see 9. Sensory Function responses).

g. Glossopharyngeal nerve (IX): evaluate and inspect tongue movements and elicit gag reflex.

h. Vagus nerve (X): supplies soft plate, pharynx, and larynx.
   (1) Listen to cry: determine the presence or absence of stridor, hoarseness, or aphonia.
   (2) Evaluate infant's ability to swallow.

i. Accessory nerve (XI): supplies neck muscles (sternocleidomastoid and trapezius).
   (1) Turn infant's head from midline to one side.
   (2) Infant should attempt to bring head back to midline.

j. Hypoglossal nerve (XII): supplies tongue muscles. Evaluate suck, swallow, and gag reflexes.

9. Sensory function responses.
   a. Touch.
      (1) Painful stimulus to a foot elicits a withdrawal reflex.
      (2) Touch sole of the foot with a pin to provoke flexion of the limb and extension of the contralateral limb.
      (3) Absence of flexion in the stimulated leg is abnormal.
   b. Light: shining a penlight into the infant's eye results in eyelid closure.
   c. Sound.
      (1) Ring a bell sharply within a few inches of the infant's ear while the infant is lying supine.
      (2) Response is based on observable attentiveness to the sound.
      (3) A brainstem auditory evoked response (BAER) is recommended in the newborn period for all infants.

REFERENCES

American Academy of Pediatrics and American College of Obstetricians and Gynecologists. *Guidelines for perinatal care* (5th ed.). Elk Village Grove, IL, 2002, AAP/ACOG.

Ballard, J.L., Khoury, J.C., Wedig, K., et al.: New Ballard Score, expanded to include extremely premature infants. *Journal of Pediatrics, 119*(3):418, 1991.

Bates, M.D. and Balistreri, W.F.: The neonatal gastrointestinal tract: part one: Development of the human digestive system. In A.A. Fanaroff and R.J. Martin (Eds.): *Neonatal-perinatal medicine: Diseases of the fetus and infant* (7th ed.). St Louis, 2002, Mosby.

Benjamin, K.: Scrotal and inguinal masses in the newborn period. *Advances in Neonatal Care,* 2(3):140-148, 2002.

Britton, B.A.: Intrauterine growth retardation: A review and update. *Central Lines, 17*(5):16-23, 2001.

Clark, D.A.: *Atlas of neonatology*. Philadelphia, 2000, W.B. Saunders.

Doctor, B.A., O'Riordan, M.A., Kirchner, H.L., et al.: Perinatal correlates and neonatal outcomes of small for gestational age infants born at term gestation. *American Journal of Obstetrics and Gynecology, 185*(3):652-659, 2001.

Donovan, E.F., Tyson, J.E., Ehrenkranz, R.A., et al.: Inaccuracy of Ballard scores before 28 weeks' gestation. National Institute of Child Health and Human Developmental Neonatal Research Network. *Journal of Pediatrics, 135*(2 Pt 1):147-152, 1999.

Dubowitz, L.M.S., Dubowitz, V., and Goldberg, C.: Clinical assessment of gestational age in the newborn infant. *Journal of Pediatrics, 77(1)*:1-10, 1970.

Dubowitz, L.M.S., Dubowitz, V., and Mercuri, E.: *The neurological assessment of the newborn, preterm, and full-term infant.* London, 1999, MacKeith Press.

Fletcher, M.A.: *Physical diagnosis in neonatology.* Philadelphia, 1998, Lippincott-Raven.

French, L.M. and Dietz, F.R.: Screening for developmental dysplasia of the hip. *American Family Physician, 60*(1):177-184, 1999.

Furdon, S.A. and Clark, D.A: Differentiating scalp swelling in the newborn. *Advances in Neonatal Care,* (1): 22, 2001.

Furdon, S.A. and Reu Donlon, C.: Examination of the newborn foot: Positional and structural abnormalities. *Advances in Neonatal Care,* 2(5):248-258, 2002.

Guinn, D. and Gibbs, R.: Infection-related preterm birth: A review of the evidence. *Neoreviews* 3(5):E86, 2002.

Hernandez, P.W. and Hernandez, J.A: Physical assessment of the newborn. In P.J. Thureen, J. Deacon, P. O'Neill, and J.A. Hernandez (Eds.): *Assessment and care of the well newborn.* Philadelphia, 1999, Saunders.

Jennet, R.J., Tarby, T.J., and Krauss, R.L.: Erb's palsy contrasted with Klumpe's and total palsy: Different mechanism are involved. *American Journal of Obstetrics and Gynecology, 186*(6):112-116, 2002.

Jones, K.L: Facial features as major feature. In K.L. Jones (Ed.): *Smith's recognizable patterns of human malformation* (5th ed.). Philadelphia, 1997, Saunders, p. 250.

Kohelet, D. and Arbel, E.: A prospective search for urinary tract abnormalities in infants with isolated preauricular tags. *Pediatrics, 105(5)*:e61, 2000.

Lowdermilk, D.L. and Perry, S.E.: *Maternity & women's health care* (8th ed.). St Louis, 2004, Mosby.

McIntire, D.D., Bloom, S.L., Casey, B.M., and Leveno, K.J.: Birth weight in relation to morbidity and mortality among newborn infants. *New England Journal of Medicine, 340*(16):1234-1238, 1999.

Pediatrix Growth Curves; retrieved March 5, 2003 from www.natalu.com.

Reu Donlon, C., Furdon, S., and Clark, D.A.: Look before you clamp: Delivery room examination of the umbilical cord. *Advances in Neonatal Care,* 2(1):19-26, 2002.

Roberton, N.R.C.: Clinical examination. In S.K. Sinha and S.M. Donn (Eds.): *Manual of neonatal and respiratory care* Armonk, NY, 2000, Futura Publishing, p. 45.

Sansoucie, D.A. and Cavaliere, T.A.: Newborn and infant assessment. In C. Kenner, and J.W. Lott (Eds.): *Comprehensive neonatal nursing: A physiologic perspective* (3rd ed.). Philadelphia, 2003, Saunders, p. 308.

Southgate, W.M. and Pittard, W.B.: Classification and physical examination of the newborn infant. In M.H. Klaus and A.A. Fanaroff (Eds.): *Care of the high-risk neonate* (5th ed.). Philadelphia, 2001, Saunders, p. 100.

Spilman, L.: Examination of the external ear. *Advances in Neonatal Care* 2(2):72-80, 2002.

Spilman, L.J. and Furdon, S.A.: Recognition, understanding and current management of cardiac lesions with decreased pulmonary blood flow. *Neonatal Network,* 17(4):7-18, 1998.

Thomas, P., Peabody, J., Turnier, V., and Clark, R.H.: A new look at intrauterine growth and the impact of race, altitude, and gender. *Pediatrics, 106*(2), 2000. Retrieved March 5, 2003 from www.pediatrics.org/cgi/content/full/106/2/e21.

Vargo, L.: Cardiovascular assessment of the newborn. In E. Tappero and M. Honeyfield (Eds.): *Physical assessment of the newborn* (2nd ed.). Petaluma, CA, 1996, NICU Ink, pp. 81, 87, 90.

Volpe, J.H.: *Neurology of the newborn* (4th ed.). Philadelphia, 2001, Saunders.

CHAPTER

8 Fluid and Electrolyte Management

BRENDA HUESKE HALBARDIER

OBJECTIVES

1. Identify the influences on fluid and electrolyte homeostasis in the newborn infant.
2. Describe fluid and electrolyte management in the neonate.
3. Compare fluid and electrolyte management of the full-term infant and the prematurely born newborn.
4. Discuss acid-base balance in the neonatal period.

An essential part of the successful transition to extrauterine life is the achievement of fluid, electrolyte, and acid-base homeostasis and control. Because mature control of these processes may not occur for days to weeks after birth, premature and other stressed neonates can have transient disturbances of fluid, electrolyte, and acid-base balance.

FLUID BALANCE

Physiologic and Assessment Considerations

A. **Fluid homeostasis in the fetus and neonate.**
   1. Body water distribution. Water, the most abundant component of the body, is distributed in two main compartments: intracellular fluid (ICF) and extracellular fluid (ECF); the latter is composed of intravascular and interstitial spaces. As gestation progresses, the fetus undergoes changes in total body water (TBW) and its distribution:
      a. Early in gestation, water makes up 95% of total body weight, with the majority in ECF compartments.
      b. By term, water makes up 75% of body weight and a greater proportion has shifted from ECF to ICF compartments. These changes are largely due to increases in body fat content.
   2. Fluid adjustments after birth.
      a. An acute increase in intravascular volume occurs after birth. Timing of cord clamping can influence the volume increase.
      b. A physiologic contraction of ECF volume occurs with diuresis in the first week of life resulting in postnatal weight loss. This is reflected in weight loss of 5% to 10% in term infants and up to 20% in preterm infants. This may be related to levels of circulating atrial natriuretic peptide (Modi et al., 2000).

B. **Regulation of fluid balance.**
   1. Renal mechanisms.
      a. Because water and electrolyte balance is regulated by the placenta, the role of the fetal kidneys is primarily to maintain amniotic fluid volume.

Fetal nephrons are functional but immature until 34 weeks. Renal blood flow, renal tubular function, and glomerular filtration rate (GFR) are all immature in the fetus and in the extremely premature infant (Vogt et al., 2001).

b. After birth, renal blood flow increases as renal vascular resistance falls. Improved renal function in the days after birth from increased GFR is more pronounced in the term than in the preterm infant.

c. Both term and preterm infants can dilute urine; however, when faced with a rapid fluid load, the preterm infant may have a delayed response, resulting in fluid retention.

d. Reabsorption of sodium, bicarbonate, and glucose is limited in the newborn infant.

e. The use of antenatal steroids has been associated with decreased insensible water losses (IWLs), less frequent incidence of hypernatremia, and an earlier diuresis. The exact mechanism of action is not known (Omar et al., 1999).

2. Hormonal mechanisms.

a. Antidiuretic hormone (ADH) is released by the posterior pituitary in response to a variety of stimuli including hypotension and hyperosmolality. ADH influences water balance by stimulating the kidneys to conserve water. In the absence of ADH, the distal tubules remain impermeable to water, which is excreted as urine.

b. Because of decreased responsiveness to ADH, neonates cannot efficiently concentrate urine in response to fluid deprivation.

C. **Fluid losses in the neonatal period**.

1. Renal losses. Urine output ranges from 1 to 4 ml/kg/hour. Highest flow rates occur during the physiologic reduction in ECF.

2. IWLs. IWL are the nonmeasurable losses that occur through the skin and respiratory system. Factors influencing IWLs are summarized in Box 8-1.

a. Transepidermal water loss (TEWL). TEWL occurs as body water diffuses through the immature epidermis and is lost to the atmosphere. Skin

BOX 8-1
ENVIRONMENTAL INFLUENCES ON INSENSIBLE WATER LOSS (IWL)

Factors That May Increase IWL:	Factors That May Decrease IWL:
Extreme prematurity	Increasing gestation
Postnatal age less than 1 week	Increasing postnatal age
Low relative ambient humidity	High relative ambient humidity
Radiant warmer use	Incubator use
High ambient temperature	Neutral thermal environment
Hyperthermia	Heat shields/plastic blankets
Convection; drafts	Humidification of inspired gases
Ventilation with dry gases	Ointments or transparent dressings on skin
High minute ventilation	Clothing
Phototherapy	
Activity	

features such as poor keratinization, high water content, low subcutaneous fat, large surface area, and high degree of skin vascularity all predispose the premature infant to high evaporative losses.

(1) TEWL increases with decreasing gestational age (Agren et al., 1998).

(2) TEWL is the major source of IWL in very premature infants.

(3) TEWL is highest on the first day after birth, decreasing on subsequent days as the barrier function of the skin improves. This improvement slows with decreasing gestational age, taking several weeks for the development of a fully functional stratum corneum in the extremely premature infant (Agren et al., 1998; Kalia et al., 1998).

(4) TEWL is closely related to ambient relative humidity. TEWL increases with decreasing ambient humidity.

(5) TEWL does not appear to be influenced by antenatal steroids or gender (Jain et al., 2000).

(6) Failure to account for TEWL increases the possibility of inaccurate estimates of fluid needs with resultant fluid and electrolyte imbalances.

b. Respiratory losses: roughly 0 to 10 ml/kg/day; related to temperature and humidity of inspired gases and to minute ventilation.

3. Stool losses: estimated to be 5 ml/kg/day in the first week of life, increasing to 10 ml/kg/day thereafter.

4. Other losses are possible. These include but may not be limited to gastric drainage, enterostomies, surgical wounds, and pleural fluid drainage.

D. Fluid therapy.

1. Goal of fluid therapy. The goal is to permit physiologic, adaptive fluid and electrolyte changes to occur appropriately (Davis and Avner, 2002; Lorenz, 1997).

2. General principles guiding fluid volume decisions. No fixed fluid administration schedules are appropriate for all infants.

a. During the first 3 to 5 days after birth, fluid intake should be at a level to allow a reasonable weight loss yet avoid intracellular dehydration. Provision of 60 to 100 ml/kg/day, depending on the degree of control over IWL, is a typical starting point. Extremely premature infants require more fluid relative to body weight because of larger IWL. Fluids given to correct shock, hypoglycemia, or acidosis must be taken into account.

b. Fluid intake is gradually increased on subsequent days to 150 to 175 ml/kg/day, although fluids may be restricted longer for infants with severe cardiorespiratory disorders, renal failure, and postasphyxial syndrome.

c. Infants with ongoing fluid losses (chest tube drainage, gastric drainage, enterostomy drainage, diarrhea) may need replacement of these volumes with appropriate fluids.

d. It is generally recommended to use birth weight, rather than current body weight, to calculate fluids on a per-kilogram basis early in life.

3. Fluid constituents.

a. Dextrose 10% in water is most commonly used for initial fluid therapy. Decreasing dextrose concentrations may be prescribed initially for infants who weighed less than 1 kg at birth, because of the incidence of hyperglycemia in this population.

b. Electrolytes are not usually added to maintenance intravenous (IV) fluids for the first 24 to 48 hours after birth. Serum electrolyte levels and urine output are used to determine when to add these electrolytes to IV fluids.

E. **Assessment of fluid balance.** Quantifying fluid requirements in extremely preterm infants is difficult. Fluid restriction places the infant at risk for dehydration, whereas fluid excess places the infant at risk for intravascular fluid overload (Davis et al., 2002). Close monitoring of hydration status is imperative, with some infants requiring assessment of their fluid balance as often as every 6 to 8 hours.
   1. Body weight. Weight changes with alterations in fluid balance only if there is a net change in TBW; internal shifts of body fluid may not be detected by weight alone. Because the procedure for weighing the ELBW infant is prone to errors and a significant source of stress for the infant, some neonatal intensive care units (NICUs) have abandoned weighing these infants in the first few days after birth. In-bed electronic scales may be used; however, weights obtained in this manner can be affected by the amount of equipment attached to the infant and how it is handled during weighing.
   2. Urine volume. For greatest possible accuracy, urine output must be measured right after it occurs; urine collected onto diapers lying under radiant warmers may evaporate before the diapers are weighed for determination of output.
   3. Specific gravity of urine: an indirect measure of urine osmolality. Normal values (1.002-1.012) reflect a normal urine osmolality (100-300 mOsm/L). Specific gravity is an unreliable predictor of urine osmolality if glucose, blood, or protein is present.
   4. Assessment parameters: quality of skin turgor, mucous membranes, presence of edema, appearance of eyes, and level of anterior fontanelle. Hemodynamic assessment includes pulse quality, blood pressure, and perfusion (capillary refill time, temperature, and acid-base balance).
   5. Laboratory evaluation of hydration status: serum sodium level, osmolality, blood urea nitrogen (BUN), creatinine, and/or hematocrit.

DISORDERS OF FLUID BALANCE

Disorders of fluid balance in the newborn infant do not always fit neatly into categories such as "fluid depletion" or "fluid excess"; some involve elements of both. One such disorder is septic shock, in which low intravascular volume (a fluid deficit) can coexist with interstitial and cellular edema (a fluid surplus). For simplicity an attempt is made here to group clinical conditions according to the primary effect on TBW (e.g., decreased, as in dehydration, or increased, as in congestive heart failure), even though overlap may exist.

Fluid Depletion

A. **Pathophysiology.** Fluid can be lost from the body acutely or gradually. Sudden loss of body fluid can result in signs and symptoms of shock. If lost fluid is not restored, the body will attempt to compensate by retaining sodium and water. Gradual or chronic fluid loss, even though central blood pressure may be maintained, can result in serious metabolic disturbances.

B. **Causes and precipitating factors.**
   1. Extreme prematurity (<28 weeks' gestation, <800 g). The large TEWL and rapid contraction of the ECF result in a sodium excess that cannot be excreted efficiently by the kidneys. If fluid intake is inadequate, hyperosmolar hypernatremic dehydration ensues.

2. Acute blood loss/hypovolemia: hemorrhagic losses at birth, postnatal internal hemorrhage, surgical blood loss, or the removal of large volumes for laboratory tests.
3. Diarrhea.
4. Diabetes insipidus (pure renal water loss from failure to secrete or respond to ADH). This condition is treated with intranasally administered arginine vasopressin (DDAVP).
5. Abdominal or pleural cavity exposure during surgery.
6. Unreplaced losses from gastric suction.
7. Medications that may cause diuresis: caffeine and theophylline.
8. Breast-feeding malnutrition: inadequate intake in a breast-fed infant with a cycle of reduced milk production and decreasing demand, resulting in severe malnutrition, dehydration, and hypernatremia.

C. **Clinical presentation and assessment.**
1. Weight loss if net reduction in TBW.
2. Low urine output (<0.5 ml/kg/hour); possibly high specific gravity. Urine output may be normal or even high in the ELBW infant during postnatal diuresis.
3. Poor skin turgor (gently pinched skin is slow to retract) and dry skin and mucous membranes.
4. Hemodynamic changes: tachycardia or decreased pulses with peripheral vasoconstriction (pale, cool, mottled skin with prolonged capillary filling time) increased core-peripheral temperature differential, central blood pressure either normal or low.
5. In breast-feeding malnutrition, possible excessive sleepiness, disinterest in feeding, or irritability.

D. **Diagnostic studies.**
1. Serum sodium can be low, normal, or high, depending on the cause of dehydration/fluid loss.
2. With dehydration, BUN and creatinine may be elevated.
3. Hematocrit may be increased or decreased with blood loss.
4. Blood gas values may reveal metabolic acidosis in the infant with hypovolemia.

E. **Patient care management.**
1. Hypovolemic states (shock, hemorrhage) are managed acutely with volume replacement and vasoactive inotropic agents, as described elsewhere in this text.
2. The type of fluid given to replace other fluid deficits depends on the constituents of lost fluid (e.g., free water loss, electrolyte loss) and the infant's electrolyte levels. Determination of the fluid constitution can be guided by evaluating the electrolyte composition of the fluid being lost.
3. Management of severe dehydration involves replacing the free water deficit slowly over several days to avoid a rapid fall in serum osmolality.

F. **Fluid management of hypernatremic hyperosmolar dehydration in the preterm infant.**
1. Prevention of TEWL is more effective than replacing these losses. This is because fluid lost is mostly solute free, whereas replacement fluids contain solutes that can aggravate hyperosmolality.
2. The single method or combination of methods most effective in reducing TEWL has yet to be proved. Each of the following strategies will decrease TEWL to some degree.

a. Use of incubators rather than radiant warmers. TEWL is higher under radiant warmers because of the lower ambient relative humidity and increased air currents on the radiant warmer.
b. Supplemental humidity. Devices to saturate the air immediately surrounding the infant can be used with both incubators and radiant warmers. Humidifier temperature, airflow setting, and seasonal ambient relative humidity variations can significantly affect the achievable humidity level.
c. Heat shields or plastic film "blankets" increase ambient humidity by using the infant's own trapped evaporative losses.
d. Semipermeable dressings (adhesive or nonadhesive) may help reduce TEWL.
e. Topical preservative-free ointment reduces TEWL (Soll and Edwards, 2003).

3. Reduce respiratory water losses by using humidified gas mixtures.
4. Even with maximal reductions in IWL, fluid intake must occasionally be increased, especially in ELBW infants. Giving too much fluid in response to hypernatremic dehydration can aggravate hyperglycemia and increase the risk of heart failure, pulmonary edema, and central nervous system (CNS) injury. It is usually recommended to give just enough fluid to maintain the serum sodium in the high normal range (145-150 mEq/L) during the first 24 to 72 hours of life (Costarino and Baumgarten, 1998).
5. Restrict sodium (unless the infant is hyponatremic), adding gradually when serum sodium level decreases and diuresis begins.
6. Monitor hydration closely. Weight loss may be accepted if other parameters indicate adequate hydration.

G. **Complications.**
1. Excessive weight loss.
2. Hypotension; tissue damage; metabolic acidosis from hypoperfusion.
3. Impaired excretion of drugs when urine output is minimal.
4. Electrolyte imbalances from slow excretion of daily solute load.
5. Renal failure and vascular thrombosis: possible result of severe dehydration.

Fluid Excess

A. **Pathophysiology.** The spectrum of disease that can cause body fluid excess in the neonate is broad. Many of the disorders are characterized by edema, which is the abnormal accumulation of ECF within the interstitial spaces. Edema can be caused by:
1. Low colloid osmotic pressure (decreased plasma protein concentration).
2. Increased capillary permeability to water and protein (may be secondary to tissue hypoxia).
3. Increased hydrostatic pressure within the capillaries.
4. Impaired lymphatic drainage of interstitial fluids and proteins.

With some of the disorders associated with these pathologic processes, a combination of venous congestion, renal failure, and edema suggests a state of fluid overload even when circulating blood volume is low.

B. **Etiologies and precipitating factors.**
1. Cardiac dysfunction: congenital heart disease, congestive heart failure, patent ductus arteriosus (PDA).

2. Respiratory distress syndrome and bronchopulmonary dysplasia (BPD). Therapeutic use of oxygen and positive-pressure ventilation causes endothelial injury with subsequent fluid leakage. In the first few days after birth increased lung fluid complicates the picture of respiratory distress and failure to clear the fluid adds to possibility of developing BPD (Adams et al., 2000; Adams et al., 2002).
3. Perinatal asphyxia.
4. Sepsis; necrotizing enterocolitis.
5. Hydrops fetalis.
6. Renal failure.
7. Miscalculation of fluid needs or provision of too much fluid (possibly from failure to account for all sources of fluid such as flush solutions, medications, colloids).
8. Use of neuromuscular blocking agents.
9. Syndrome of inappropriate antidiuretic hormone (SIADH): usually associated with CNS infection or injury. ADH secretion is inappropriate to usual osmotic and volume stimuli. The result is fluid retention with hyponatremia, low serum osmolality, and high urinary sodium loss.

C. **Clinical presentation and assessment.**
1. Weight gain, if there is a net increase in TBW.
2. Urine output: possible decrease.
3. Edema: peripheral, generalized, pulmonary.
4. Hemodynamic changes: dependent on intravascular volume status. When increased, there may be symptomatic PDA, tachycardia, and increased pulses or blood pressure. With congestive heart failure, venous filling pressure is high.

D. **Diagnostic studies.**
1. Serum osmolality is low (<280 mOsm/L); urine osmolality is normal.
2. In SIADH, osmolalities and sodium levels of urine and serum are diagnostic (urine output is low with high specific gravity and high sodium levels; serum has low sodium level and low osmolality).

E. **Patient care management.** In addition to therapy aimed at the underlying disease process:
1. Precise fluid management with fluid restriction is necessary. Daily fluid calculations must take into account renal function and extra fluids given to administer medications and flush intravascular catheters.
2. Diuretics may be useful.
3. Infants with severe edema and low intravascular volume (shock) present a challenge. Maintenance of an adequate circulating blood volume may require volume expansion and vasoactive agents while minimizing maintenance fluid administration.
4. Edema may predispose the infant to necrotic injury of the skin. The skin must be protected from pressure with careful repositioning, support, and the use of a nonrigid sleeping surface, such as a gel- or water-filled mattress.

F. **Complications.**
1. Fluid sequestration in static body fluid compartments ("third spacing") can result in a loss of effective blood volume, compromising delivery of oxygen and nutrients to tissues throughout the body. This can lead not only to serious metabolic imbalances but also permanent tissue damage.
2. Excessive fluid administration early in life has been associated with worsening of respiratory distress syndrome and development of BPD, symptomatic PDA, and necrotizing enterocolitis.

ELECTROLYTE BALANCE AND DISORDERS

Sodium

A. Sodium homeostasis.

1. Functions of sodium (Na). Na, the major extracellular cation, is closely involved in water balance. Na and other electrolytes are found in varying concentrations in all body fluid compartments. Electrolytes determine the tonicity of the fluid compartment and influence the passage of water through the vascular and cell membranes, thereby controlling the osmotic equilibrium between compartments. With a surplus of Na, blood becomes hypertonic, causing a shift of fluid from intracellular to extracellular spaces, which results in cellular dehydration. A deficit of Na causes hypotonicity and fluid shifts into the cells (cellular edema).
2. Regulation of Na. Cellular transport of Na is achieved by the sodium-potassium pump, which maintains the electrochemical sodium and potassium gradients across the cell membrane. Renal (GFR, tubular function) and hormonal (aldosterone, ADH) mechanisms influence the body content of Na. Although preterm infants can excrete sodium, low GFR early in life may hamper this ability. In addition, minimal responsiveness to aldosterone and ADH contributes to a baseline salt-wasting tendency.
3. Positive Na balance. Na intake greater than Na losses. This is a prerequisite for the growth of new tissue.

B. Hyponatremia.

1. Pathophysiology. A low serum Na reflects either an excess of body water relative to normal body Na content or a primary Na depletion. When urinary Na wasting occurs, a proportionate loss of water (isotonic dehydration) can reduce ECF volume and lead to oliguria.
2. Causes and precipitating factors.
   - **a.** Prematurity (renal and hormonal immaturity, with tendency to excrete Na). Preterm infants are most vulnerable to hyponatremia just after the period of postnatal extracellular volume contraction (Modi, 1998).
   - **b.** Conditions associated with low intravascular volume (e.g., shock). Baroreceptor stimulation of ADH results in reduced renal water excretion and a dilutional hyponatremia.
   - **c.** Dilutional hyponatremia from excessive free water intake.
   - **d.** Renal losses related to medications (furosemide, methylxanthines).
   - **e.** Inadequate Na intake during period of rapid growth, especially in preterm infants fed exclusively human milk. Called "late hyponatremia" because it occurs after the first week of life.
3. Clinical presentation and assessment.
   - **a.** Usually asymptomatic, but apnea, irritability, twitching, or seizures can occur if Na drops acutely or falls to less than 115 mEq/L.
   - **b.** Infants with late hyponatremia may fail to gain weight.
4. Diagnostic studies.
   - **a.** Serum Na low (<130 mEq/L) and osmolality low (<280 mOsm/L). Serum Na can be factitiously low in the presence of hyperlipidemia.
   - **b.** Urine Na excretion rate to rule out excessive Na losses.
5. Patient care management.
   - **a.** Provide Na supplementation after postnatal diuresis begins (usually on day 2). Maintenance Na requirement is 1 to 4 mEq/kg/day and is usually given as sodium chloride, though Na-acetate or Na-bicarbonate may be used if the infant has metabolic acidosis. In very small infants, early Na supplementation has been associated with increased risk of BPD (Hartnoll et al., 2000).

b. A chronic hyponatremic state is corrected gradually over 48 to 72 hours to prevent injury to brain cells (Modi, 1998).
c. Monitor weight, urine output, parameters of hydration, and adequacy of intravascular volume (monitoring of central venous pressure, capillary refill time, and core-peripheral temperature differential).
d. When hyponatremia is associated with an excess of body water, fluids are restricted. True SIADH is managed with fluid restriction and monitoring of Na, osmolality, and urine output.
e. Commercial preparations designed to fortify human milk supply additional dietary sodium for this population.

6. Complications.
a. Acute drops in the serum Na can lead to a shift of fluid into brain cells and cellular edema. This may result in apnea and seizures.
b. The degree to which the infant's brain may be able to adapt to chronic hyponatremia is not known; however, chronic hyponatremia does impair skeletal and tissue growth.

C. **Hypernatremia.**

1. Pathophysiology. Hypernatremia usually reflects a deficiency of water relative to total body Na content and thus is actually a disorder of water balance rather than one of Na balance.
2. Causes and precipitating factors.
a. Excessive IWL with insufficient fluid intake (even without added Na).
b. High inadvertent Na intake (saline infusions in arterial catheters, sodium bicarbonate [$NaHCO_3$], medications) or early addition of maintenance sodium chloride (NaCl).
c. Breast-feeding malnutrition in term infants. Elevated human milk Na content accompanying insufficient lactation and decreased amount of free water contribute to the hyperosmolar state.
d. Diabetes insipidus: deficiency of pituitary-secreted ADH, causing loss of water in excess of loss of Na.
3. Clinical presentation and assessment.
a. Signs of dehydration may be present.
b. In severe hypernatremia, high-pitched cry, lethargy, irritability, and apnea can progress to seizures and coma.
4. Diagnostic studies: serum Na (>150 mEq/L) and osmolality (>300 mOsm/L).
5. Patient care management.
a. Gradually restrict Na to avoid sudden fall in plasma osmolality. If maintenance Na administration has not been started, it is usually delayed.
b. Recalculate fluid intake. Fluids may have been restricted too much in light of insensible losses.
c. Prevent hypernatremia in ELBW infants. Na supplementation may be withheld longer than usual after birth if serum Na level remains normal. This approach has been shown to reduce the need for additional fluids during the first days of life (Costarino et al., 1998). In addition, measures to reduce TEWL will aid in the prevention of hypernatremia.
d. The need for saline solutions to maintain catheter patency presents a dilemma. Attempts to lower the infused Na concentration too far result in administration of hypotonic solutions, with risk of hemolysis.
6. Complications. As hypernatremia develops, intracellular water can be drawn out, causing cells to shrink. If this process is rapid, this can affect the brain. Sudden increases in plasma osmolality can also contribute to intraventricular hemorrhage.

Potassium

A. Potassium homeostasis.

1. Functions of potassium (K). The major cation in ICF, K contributes to intracellular osmotic activity and in part determines ICF volume. K plays a fundamental role along with Na in regulating cell membrane potential.
2. Regulation of K. K is distributed both intracellularly and extracellularly. The distribution of K between ICF and ECF is regulated by the sodium-potassium pump and is influenced by acid-base balance, insulin, and glucagon. The excretion of K from the body depends on kidney function, GFR, urine flow rate, and aldosterone sensitivity.

B. Hypokalemia.

1. Pathophysiology. Because K is 90% intracellular, it is assessed indirectly by measuring the quantity in the serum. A subnormal serum K implies insufficient K within the cells, which may impede their function. Muscle cells of the gastrointestinal (GI) system and the heart can be affected.
2. Causes and precipitating factors.
   a. Loss of K in the urine (kaliuresis) during postnatal diuresis, before K supplementation is begun.
   b. Inadequate K intake.
   c. Increased GI losses from an enterostomy or nasogastric tube.
   d. Metabolic alkalosis. A high serum pH drives K into cells, resulting in a low serum K.
   e. Medications including bicarbonate, diuretics, and insulin. Insulin increases cellular uptake of K through stimulation of activity of the sodium-potassium pump.
3. Clinical presentation and assessment. Cardiac effects (flattened T waves, prominent U waves, ST depression), hypotonia, abdominal distention, and ileus.
4. Diagnostic studies: serum K (<3.5 mEq/L).
5. Patient care management.
   a. Begin K supplementation when urine output is well established, usually on the second or third day of life. The maintenance K requirement is 2 to 3 mEq/kg/day.
   b. Correction of hypokalemic states must be done cautiously, with continuous cardiac monitoring.
6. Complications.
   a. Rapid administration of K to correct hypokalemia can lead to fatal arrhythmias.
   b. Hypokalemia potentiates digitalis toxicity.

C. Hyperkalemia.

1. Pathophysiology. In the ELBW infant, the normal postnatal shift of K from the intracellular to the extracellular compartment is intensified. During the prediuretic phase, this excess K is not efficiently excreted secondary to a low GFR and a low Na excretion rate (Lorenz et al., 1997).
2. Causes and precipitating factors.
   a. Extreme prematurity (nonoliguric, hyperkalemia).
   b. Endogenous release of K from tissue destruction, hypoperfusion, hemorrhage, and bruising.
   c. Metabolic acidosis. A low serum pH shifts K out of cells.
   d. Renal failure, with decreased K clearance.
   e. Adrenal insufficiency.
   f. Transfusion with blood stored longer than 3 days.

3. Clinical presentation and assessment. Cardiac effects may be seen: ventricular tachycardia, peaked T wave, widened QRS complex.
4. Diagnostic studies.
   a. Serum K (>6.5 mEq/L) from venipuncture or arterial line. Heel-stick samples are often hemolyzed, rendering results unreliable.
   b. Tests of renal function: BUN, creatinine.
   c. Electrocardiogram (ECG) to detect cardiac arrhythmias.
   d. Serum ionized calcium, because hypocalcemia may potentiate cardiac toxicity from hyperkalemia.
5. Patient care management.
   a. For prevention of hyperkalemia, K is withheld from early IV fluids. Serum K is monitored as diuresis (and K excretion) begins; K is added when serum K stabilizes in the 4 to 4.5 mEq/L range.
   b. Acidosis is corrected.
   c. Diuretics and low-dose dopamine therapy may improve renal excretion of K. Dopamine also enhances K uptake by stimulation of activity of the sodium-potassium pump.
   d. Temporary measures may be needed to reduce the effects of circulating K until the total body K level can be reduced.
      (1) Administration of calcium gluconate will lower the cell membrane threshold transiently, antagonizing the effects on the heart muscle.
      (2) Glucose/insulin infusion to enhance cellular uptake of K.
      (3) $NaHCO_3$ (metabolic alkalosis shifts K into cells).
   e. When other measures fail to normalize K:
      (1) Cation exchange resin. Kayexalate (Sodium Polystyrene Sulfonate). Na is exchanged for K in the intestine to increase excretion of K. Because the onset of action is within 2 to 24 hours, treatment with this medication alone may not be sufficient to rapidly correct severe hyperkalemia (Taketamo et al., 2002).
      (2) Exchange transfusion.
      (3) Peritoneal dialysis or continuous arteriovenous hemofiltration for severe, intractable hyperkalemia.
6. Complications.
   a. Hyperkalemia is life threatening because of the risk of cardiac arrest.
   b. Kayexalate (Sodium Polystyrene Sulfonate) can cause hypocalcemia, hypomagnesemia, and hypernatremia.

Calcium

A. Calcium homeostasis.

1. Functions of calcium (Ca). Ca plays a central role in many physiologic processes, maintaining cell membrane permeability and activating enzyme reactions for muscle contraction, nerve transmission, and blood clotting. Ca is vital for normal cardiac function and development of the skeleton, where 99% of the body's Ca is stored.
2. Regulation of Ca.
   a. Parathyroid hormone (PTH) increases serum Ca by mobilizing Ca from bone and intestines and reducing renal excretion of Ca. PTH is stimulated by low serum Ca and magnesium (Mg) levels and is suppressed by high Ca and Mg levels.

b. Vitamin D acts with PTH to restore Ca to normal levels by increasing absorption of Ca and phosphorus from the intestines and bone.
c. Calcitonin, a Ca counterregulatory hormone secreted from thyroid C cells, lowers Ca levels by antagonizing the Ca, which mobilizes the effects of PTH.
d. Phosphorus (P) also inhibits the absorption of Ca (the higher the P, the lower the absorption of Ca).

3. Serum Ca is transported in three forms:
   a. Protein-bound calcium, accounting for 40% of total serum Ca.
   b. Inactivated Ca (complexed with anions such as bicarbonate, lactate, and citrate), accounting for 10% of total serum Ca.
   c. Free ionized calcium (iCa), the physiologically active form that can cross the cell membrane, accounting for 50% of the total serum Ca. Blood pH influences the amount of iCa: acidosis increases iCa, and alkalosis decreases iCa.

B. **Fetal Ca metabolism.** Fetal Ca needs are met by active transport of Ca across the placenta. Ca accretion increases during the last trimester as Ca is incorporated into newly forming bones. Because maternal PTH and calcitonin do not cross the placenta, the fetus is relatively hypercalcemic, which suppresses fetal PTH and stimulates fetal calcitonin.

C. **Neonatal Ca metabolism.** When the supply of Ca ceases at birth, the neonate depends on stored and dietary Ca to avoid hypocalcemia. After birth, the Ca level declines to its nadir by 24 hours of age, but PTH activity remains low. By 48 to 72 hours, PTH and vitamin D levels rise and the calcitonin level declines, allowing Ca to be mobilized. The serum Ca level returns to normal despite a low Ca intake. A recent review has reported 16% of infants born less than 32 weeks' gestation develop nephrocalcinosis in the face of normal serum Ca levels (Narendra et al., 2001). Development is multifactorial, but is associated with increased furosemide use, increased gentamicin levels, and extreme prematurity.

D. **Hypocalcemia.**

1. Pathophysiology. Failure to achieve Ca homeostasis after birth can result from inadequate Ca stores, immature hormonal control, inability to mobilize Ca, or interference with Ca use. Hypocalcemia increases cellular permeability to Na ions and increases cell membrane excitability.
2. Causes and precipitating factors.
   a. "Early" hypocalcemia.
      (1) Prematurity: reduced Ca stores and relative hypoparathyroidism (blunted PTH response to hypocalcemia).
      (2) Infant of a diabetic mother (IDM): prolonged delay in PTH production by infant after birth.
      (3) Placental insufficiency: reduced Ca stores.
      (4) Perinatal asphyxia and stress, which precipitate a surge in calcitonin that suppresses Ca. In addition, tissue damage and glycogen breakdown release phosphorus into the circulation, which decreases Ca uptake.
      (5) Maternal anticonvulsant therapy, which affects hepatic enzymes involved in vitamin D metabolism.
      (6) Low intake of Ca.
      (7) Factors that may decrease iCa even when the total serum Ca is normal: exchange transfusion, intravenous administration of lipid emulsion, alkalosis, or alkali therapy for acidosis.

b. "Late" hypocalcemia.
   (1) Hypomagnesemia.
   (2) Transient congenital hypoparathyroidism or secondary hypoparathyroidism from maternal hyperparathyroidism. An increased PTH level in the mother raises the fetal Ca level and suppresses the fetal parathyroid gland. After birth, the suppressed gland cannot maintain a normal Ca level.
   (3) DiGeorge syndrome; absence of thymus and parathyroid glands.
   (4) High-phosphate formulas or cereals. The neonate cannot excrete the excess phosphate; the hyperphosphatemia suppresses Ca.
   (5) Intestinal malabsorption.
3. Clinical presentation and assessment.
   a. Early hypocalcemia is usually asymptomatic; signs of neuromuscular excitability (jitteriness, twitching) may be present.
   b. Severe hypocalcemia (neonatal tetany) is rare and presents with jitteriness, seizures, high-pitched cry, laryngospasm, stridor, prolonged QT interval.
4. Diagnostic studies.
   a. Serum total calcium (<7 mg/dl) or ionized Ca (<4.4 mg/dl). The proportion of iCa cannot be reliably predicted from total serum Ca levels.
   b. Magnesium and phosphorus levels; acid-base balance.
5. Patient care management.
   a. Monitor serum Ca of infants at risk: premature, IDM, asphyxiated.
   b. Early, mild hypocalcemia often resolves without treatment.
   c. Serious hypocalcemia is treated with boluses and/or continuous infusions of calcium gluconate (can also be given orally).
   d. Treatment of late hypocalcemia depends on the underlying cause.
6. Complications.
   a. Rapid infusion of Ca can cause bradycardia or cardiac arrest. Infusions for rapid correction of hypocalcemia should be administered slowly, over 20 to 30 minutes by syringe pump, while the heart rate is monitored.
   b. Tissue necrosis and calcifications can result from extravasated Ca.
   c. Intestinal necrosis and liver necrosis have been reported with Ca infusion given via umbilical catheter.

E. Metabolic bone disease.

1. Pathophysiology of metabolic bone disease (MBD). Infants born prematurely can miss all or most of the period of greatest intrauterine mineral accretion, which places them at risk of having inadequate postnatal bone mineralization. The primary cause of MBD is inadequate Ca and P intake, rather than vitamin D deficiency.
2. Causes and precipitating factors.
   a. Prematurity: the more immature the infant, the higher the MBD rate.
   b. Parenteral nutrition: low Ca and P intakes.
   c. Unsupplemented human milk feeding (inadequate Ca and P content) or use of formulas not designed for the preterm infant.
   d. BPD secondary to fluid restriction and use of diuretics, with renal Ca wasting.
3. Clinical presentation and assessment.
   a. MBD is asymptomatic; it is often detected initially on routine x-ray examination.
   b. Skeletal fractures may be seen in the thoracic cage or extremities.
   c. Other reported presentation is late-onset respiratory distress from "softening" of the ribs.
   d. Pain may occur with handling; close monitoring of response is necessary.

4. Diagnostic tests.
   a. Serum: normal Ca, low P, high alkaline phosphatase, and high 1,25-dihydroxyvitamin D levels. Ca and P levels alone are not good indicators of metabolic bone disease.
   b. Urine: low or absent P excretion; increased urinary Ca.
   c. Radiologic bone examinations. Wrist x-ray films at age 6 to 8 weeks are used to monitor for MBD. Early evidence can be difficult to discern because bone mineral content must decrease by 30% to be visible. Photon absorptiometry may be done in centers where the necessary equipment is available.
   d. X-ray examination. Findings may include "washed out" (undermineralized) bones, known as osteopenia, or epiphyseal dysplasia and skeletal deformities, known as rickets (Faerk et al., 2002; Huttner, 1998).
5. Patient care management and prevention of MBD.
   a. Maintain Ca:P ratio in parenteral nutrition at 1.3:1 to 1.7:1.
   b. For enteral feeding, use preterm formulas or human milk supplementation.
   c. Direct supplementation of Ca and P may be needed. Ca given without P will be inadequately used, resulting in hypercalciuria and possibly nephrocalcinosis.
   d. Gentle handling of infants at risk and avoidance of chest physiotherapy are warranted to prevent fractures.

F. Hypercalcemia.

1. Pathophysiology. A rise in the serum Ca level can rapidly overwhelm the infant's compensatory mechanisms for Ca equilibrium. An excess supply of Ca has multiple effects and is potentially lethal.
2. Causes and precipitating factors.
   a. Iatrogenic: overtreatment with Ca or vitamin D.
   b. Hyperparathyroidism: primary neonatal disorder or secondary to maternal hypoparathyroidism, with chronic stimulation of the fetal parathyroid gland.
   c. Phosphate depletion: caused by low dietary intake; may be associated with low phosphate content in human milk.
   d. Subcutaneous fat necrosis: found over the back and limbs; associated with difficult delivery, hypothermia, and maternal diabetes. Pathogenic mechanism is unknown.
   e. Familial infantile hypercalcemia.
   f. Hypervitaminosis D: excessive maternal intake of vitamin D.
3. Clinical presentation and assessment.
   a. Hypotonia, weakness, irritability, and poor feeding, all from a direct effect of Ca on the CNS.
   b. Bradycardia.
   c. Constipation.
   d. Polyuria, dehydration (associated with severe hypercalcemia).
4. Diagnostic studies.
   a. Serum Ca (>11 mg/dl); iCa (>5.8 mg/dl).
   b. In hyperparathyroidism the serum Ca level is high, phosphate levels may be low, and urinary Ca and phosphate excretion are high.
5. Patient care management.
   a. Hydrate infant and promote excretion of Ca (furosemide has calciuretic action).
   b. Restrict Ca and vitamin D intake; increase phosphate intake.

6. Complications.
   a. Nephrocalcinosis from hypercalciuria, but may be seen with normal serum Ca levels.
   b. Metastatic calcification of damaged cells/tissues throughout the body, including the brain.
   c. Cardiac effects: bradycardia and arrhythmias.

Magnesium

A. Magnesium homeostasis.

1. Functions of magnesium (Mg). Mg is a catalyst for many intracellular enzyme reactions, including muscle contraction and carbohydrate metabolism and is critical for normal parathyroid function and bone-serum Ca homeostasis. Mg is regulated primarily by the kidneys.
2. Fetal and neonatal Mg homeostasis. The fetus receives its supply of Mg by active transport across the placenta. Maternal health and diet can influence the amount of Mg accrued by the fetus. After birth, Mg level falls along with Ca level, then rises to normal within 48 hours.
3. Serum total Mg versus the ionized form. Ionized Mg (iMg) is the biologically active fraction of Mg. Total Mg concentration in the serum does not necessarily reflect iMg activity.
4. Concurrent use of Mg and gentamicin potentiates the neuroblocking effect of the Mg, which may result in apnea. Clinical status must be monitored closely. Slow infusion times for the gentamicin are indicated (Taketamo et al., 2002).

B. Hypomagnesemia.

1. Pathophysiology. A low neonatal Mg level is directly related to the maternal level before birth. Although an acute decline in Mg stimulates PTH release, chronic Mg deficiency suppresses PTH and blocks the hormone's actions on the bone and kidneys. Hypocalcemia ensues.
2. Causes and precipitating factors.
   a. Decreased Mg supply: prematurity, placental insufficiency and intrauterine growth restriction (IUGR), low dietary intake.
   b. Increased Mg losses: renal and intestinal disorders, including renal tubular acidosis, diarrhea, short bowel syndrome.
   c. Endocrine causes: neonatal hypoparathyroidism, maternal hyperparathyroidism.
3. Clinical presentation and assessment.
   a. Tremors, irritability, and hyperreflexia, progressing to seizures.
   b. Failure to respond to therapy for hypocalcemia: hypomagnesemia a possibility.
4. Diagnostic studies: serum Mg level (<1.5 mg/dl).
5. Patient care management.
   a. If hypomagnesemia is severe, administration of magnesium sulfate may be necessary to relieve symptoms until Ca balance is restored.
   b. Seizures are usually unresponsive to anticonvulsant agents.
6. Complications. Overtreatment with magnesium sulfate can result in hypotonia and respiratory depression, hypotension, and cardiac arrhythmias.

C. Hypermagnesemia.

1. Pathophysiology. An excess of Mg is slow to be excreted by the neonatal kidneys. Very high Mg levels can cause CNS and neuromuscular depression.

2. Causes and precipitating factors.
   a. Excessive Mg load: magnesium sulfate treatment in labor, excess administration of Mg to neonate.
   b. Reduced excretion of Mg: renal failure, oliguria.
3. Clinical presentation and assessment (may be asymptomatic).
   a. Respiratory depression, apnea.
   b. Neuromuscular depression: lethargy, poor suck, loss of reflexes, flaccidity, hypotonia.
   c. Gastrointestinal hypomotility, abdominal distention.
4. Laboratory and diagnostic studies: high serum Mg (>2.5 mg/dl).
5. Patient care management.
   a. Prepare to resuscitate infants born to mothers receiving large doses of magnesium sulfate.
   b. Hypermagnesemia usually resolves with adequate hydration and urine output. Mg excretion can be increased with furosemide.
   c. If infant is unresponsive to treatment, exchange transfusion may be necessary.
6. Complications. Cardiac arrest and respiratory failure are possible.

ACID-BASE BALANCE AND DISORDERS

Acid-Base Physiology

A. **pH.** Acid-base balance is normal when the pH of the blood is between 7.35 and 7.45. The pH is determined by the hydrogen ion (H^+) concentration in the ECF. An acid is an H^+ donor; a base is an H^+ receptor. A complex system of buffers, compensation, and excretion regulates the H^+ concentration, thus keeping the pH in the normal range.

B. **Buffering system.** This is the first line of defense against excess H^+ concentration. Buffers, including bicarbonate (HCO_3^-), plasma proteins, and hemoglobin, act rapidly to pick up excess H^+. The major buffer, HCO_3^-, teams with H^+ to form carbonic acid, which dissociates into water and CO_2 to be eliminated. The normal HCO_3^- level in the neonate is 18 to 21 mEq/L, lower than in the adult.

C. **Lung regulation.** The lungs act to lower the H^+ level in the blood by removing CO_2, which is produced as a waste product of cellular metabolism. It is then transported to the lungs, where it is removed from the body by ventilation. The rate of CO_2 removal can be increased or decreased by altering minute ventilation.

D. **Kidney regulation.** The kidney acts to maintain equilibrium between acids and bases in the body by reabsorbing HCO_3^- and other buffers and by excreting H^+ and other acids. In this way the body eliminates the daily load of nonvolatile acids produced by normal metabolism.

E. **Compensation.** When one or more of the body's regulatory systems fail, other systems have a limited ability to maintain the acid-base equilibrium. When the pH is outside the normal range (<7.35 or >7.45), compensation has failed.
   1. An acid-base deviation is *respiratory* if it is due to an abnormal Pco_2 and *metabolic* if it is due to an abnormal level of plasma HCO_3^-.
   2. The lungs attempt to compensate for a metabolic aberration, and the kidneys for a respiratory aberration. The result is a change in pH toward normal despite an abnormal blood Pco_2 or HCO_3^-. The lungs compensate much more quickly than the kidneys; however, neither can totally normalize the pH unless the underlying disorder is corrected.

Disorders of Acid-Base Balance

Only those disorders classified as primary metabolic problems are discussed here.

A. **Metabolic acidosis.**

1. Pathophysiology. A pH of less than 7.35 can result from the loss of HCO_3^- (buffering capacity) or from excess acid production. The immature kidneys contribute to acidosis by failing both to reabsorb HCO_3^- and to excrete H^+ when faced with an acid load. When cells do not receive enough oxygen (because of low blood oxygen levels or diminished perfusion), they must use anaerobic metabolism to meet energy needs. This results in the accumulation in the body of lactic acid (lactate), the level of which reflects the severity of tissue oxygen deficiency. Blood lactate may be a more sensitive indicator of tissue hypoxia than pH and base-excess values (Deshpande and Ward Platt, 1997).
2. Causes and precipitating factors.
   a. Loss of HCO_3^-: normal anion gap.
      (1) Prematurity: poor renal conservation of HCO_3^-.
      (2) Renal tubular acidosis: decreased proximal reabsorption.
      (3) Severe diarrhea or ileal drainage.
   b. Excess acid load: ingestion or endogenous production of acid, greater than the ability to excrete it; increased anion gap.
      (1) Lactic acidosis from conditions resulting in hypoxia or hypoperfusion: respiratory distress, congenital heart disease, PDA, sepsis, asphyxia, shock/hypovolemia.
      (2) Inborn errors of metabolism: disorders of organic acid and carbohydrate metabolism.
      (3) Caloric deprivation: catabolism of protein or fat for energy.
      (4) Parenteral amino acid solutions.
      (5) "Late metabolic acidosis" of prematurity, caused by intolerance of cow's milk protein.
3. Clinical presentation and assessment.
   a. Metabolic acidosis occurring early in life is primarily related to systemic illness (e.g., respiratory, cardiac); thus the signs and symptoms are those of the underlying condition(s).
   b. Late metabolic acidosis may present at 1 to 3 weeks of age by poor growth, hyponatremia, and persistent renal acid excretion (urinary pH <5).
   c. Infants with profound acidosis (metabolic defects such as congenital lactic acidosis) may have respiratory compensation (tachypnea, hyperpnea) or neurologic depression (seizures, coma) reflecting CNS acidosis.
4. Diagnostic studies.
   a. Blood pH less than 7.35: acidemia.
   b. Serum HCO_3^- level less than 18 mEq/L.
   c. Anion gap to differentiate between excess acid and insufficient HCO_3^- as cause of acidosis: anion gap = (serum Na + K) – (serum Cl + HCO_3^-). Usual range is 8 to 16 mEq. If high (>20 mEq), acidosis is due to excess acid. If normal with elevated chloride level, acidosis is due to loss of HCO_3^-.
   d. Urinary pH greater than 7 with systemic acidosis: suggests renal tubular acidosis. If low (<5), kidneys are excreting acid.
   e. Plasma lactate level greater than 2.5 mmol/L: may be elevated in some conditions, such as early sepsis, even when the pH is normal.
5. Patient care management.
   a. Treat underlying cause of acidosis.
   b. Correction of severe acidosis (pH <7.2) is usually with $NaHCO_3$ (concentration of 0.5 mEq/ml), in a 1 to 2 ml/kg dose. Administer slowly

by syringe pump or continuous drip; rapid increase in osmolality and pH may be dangerous.

c. Late metabolic acidosis, if not self-correcting, is sometimes treated with oral $NaHCO_3$.

6. Complications.
   a. Severe acidosis: may depress myocardial contractility and cause arteriolar vasodilation, hypotension, and pulmonary edema.
   b. Impaired surfactant production.
   c. Electrolyte imbalance: decreased iCa, hyperkalemia.
   d. Adverse effects of $NaHCO_3$: cerebral hemorrhage or edema related to wide swings in plasma osmolality. $NaHCO_3$ can also worsen acidosis by rapidly increasing CO_2 if lung disease is present and ventilation is inadequate. $NaHCO_3$ can aggravate hypernatremia and cause tissue injury in extravasation.
7. Outcome. In follow-up studies, metabolic acidosis was correlated with poor developmental outcome in VLBW infants (Goldstein et al., 1995).

B. Metabolic alkalosis.

1. Pathophysiology. Metabolic alkalosis results from an excess of HCO_3^- or from a loss of acid.
2. Causes and precipitating factors.
   a. Gain of HCO_3^- from overcorrection of acidosis with $NaHCO_3$.
   b. Loss of H^+ during vomiting or nasogastric suction.
   c. Increased renal acid loss from diuretic therapy.
   d. Rapid ECF reduction (contraction alkalosis).
3. Diagnostic studies: blood pH (>7.45: alkalemia); HCO_3^- (>26 mEq/L).
4. Patient care management.
   a. Decrease $NaHCO_3$ intake if alkali therapy is cause of alkalosis.
   b. Restoring fluid and electrolyte balance is critical.
5. Complications. Severe alkalosis causes tissue hypoxia, neurologic damage, and electrolyte disturbances (increased iCa, hypokalemia).

REFERENCES

Adams, E., Counsell, S.J., Hajnal, J.V., et al.: Investigation of lung disease in preterm infants using magnetic resonance imaging. *Biology of the Neonate, 77*(Suppl 1):17-20, 2000.

Adams, E., Counsell, S.J., Hajnal, J.V., et al.: Magnetic resonance imaging of lung water content and distribution in term and preterm infants. *American Journal of Respiratory and Critical Care Medicine, 166*(3):397-402, 2002.

Agren, J., Sjors, G., and Sedin, G.: Transepidermal water loss in infants born at 24 and 25 weeks of gestation. *Acta Paediatrica, 87*(11):1185-1190, 1998.

Costarino, A. and Baumgarten, S.: Neonatal water metabolism. In R.M. Cowett (Ed.): *Principles of perinatal-neonatal metabolism* (2nd ed.). New York, 1998, Springer.

Davis, I.D. and Avner, E.D.: Fluid, electrolytes, and acid-base homeostasis. In A.A. Fanaroff and R.J. Martin (Eds.): *Neonatal-perinatal medicine: Diseases of the fetus and infant* (7th ed.). St Louis, 2002, Mosby.

Deshpande, S.A. and Ward Platt, M.P.: Association between blood lactate and acid-base status and mortality in ventilated babies. *Archives of Disease in Childhood, Fetal Neonatal Edition, 76*(1): F15-F20, 1997.

Faerk, J., Peitersen, B., and Michaelson, K.F.: Bone mineralisation in premature infants cannot be predicted from serum alkaline phosphatase or serum phosphate. *Archives of Disease in Childhood, Fetal Neonatal Edition, 87*(2):F133-F136, 2002.

Goldstein, R.F., Thompson, R.J., Oehler, J., et al. Influence of acidosis, hypoxemia, and hypotension on neurodevelopmental outcome in very low birthweight infants, *Pediatrics,* 95:238-243, 1995.

Hartnoll, G., Betremieux, P., and Modi, N.: Randomised controlled trial of postnatal sodium supplementation on oxygen dependency and body weight in 25-30 week gestational age infants. *Archives of Disease in Childhood, Fetal Neonatal Edition, 82*(1):F19-F23, 2000.

Huttner, K.M.: Metabolic bone disease of prematurity. In J.P. Cloherty and A.R. Stark (Eds.): *Manual of neonatal care.* Philadelphia, 1998, Lippincott-Raven.

Jain, A., Rutter, N., and Cartlidge, P.: Influence of antenatal steroids and sex on maturation of the epidermal barrier in the preterm infant. *Archives of Disease in Childhood, Fetal Neonatal Edition, 83*(2):F112-F116, 2000.

Kalia, Y., Nonato, L.B., Lund, C.H., and Guy, R.H.: Development of skin barrier function in premature infants. *Journal of Investigative Dermatology, 111*(2):320-326, 1998.

Lorenz, J.M.: Assessing fluid and electrolyte status in the newborn. *Clinical Chemistry, 43*(1):205-210, 1997.

Lorenz, J.M., Kleinman, L.I., and Markarian, K.: Potassium metabolism in extremely low birth weight infants in the first week of life. *Journal of Pediatrics, 131*(1 Pt 1):81-86, 1997.

Modi, N.: Hyponatremia in the newborn. *Archives of Disease in Childhood, Fetal Neonatal Edition, 78*(2):F81-F84, 1998.

Modi, N., Betremieux, P., Midgley, J., and Hartnoll, G.: Postnatal weight loss and contraction of the extracellular compartment is triggered by atrial natriuretic peptide. *Early Human Development, 59*(3):201-208, 2000.

Narendra, A., White, M.P., Rolton, H.A., et al.: Nephrocalcinosis in preterm babies. *Archives of Disease in Childhood, Fetal Neonatal Edition, 85*(3):F207-F213, 2001.

Omar, S., DeCristofaro, J.D., Agarwal, B.I., and La Gamma, E.F.: Effects of prenatal steroids on water and sodium homeostasis in extremely low birth weight neonates. *Pediatrics, 104*(3 Pt 1):482-488, 1999.

Soll, R.F. and Edwards, W.H.: Emollient ointment for preventing infection in preterm infants. *Cochrane Database of Systematic Reviews*, Issue 2, 2003.

Taketamo, C.K., Hodding, J. H., and Kraus, D.M.: (2002). Pediatric Lexi-Comp Drugs. (On-line). Available at www.lexi.com.

Vogt, B.A., Davis, I.D., and Avner, E.D.: The kidney. In M. Klaus and A. Fanaroff (Eds.): *Care of the high-risk neonate* (5th ed.). Philadelphia, 2001, W.B. Saunders.

CHAPTER

9 Glucose Management

DEBRA ARMENTROUT

OBJECTIVES

1. Describe mechanisms of glucose homeostasis in the fetus and newborn.
2. Discuss hypoglycemia and hyperglycemia in the neonate.
3. Discuss infants of diabetic mothers.
4. Differentiate neonatal diabetes from hyperglycemia.

Organ systems, especially the human brain, are primarily dependent on glucose as their major energy source. Compared with adults, infants have a higher brain to body weight ratio, resulting in a higher glucose demand in relation to glucose production capacity. Cerebral glucose utilization accounts for 90% of the neonate's total glucose consumption. Continuous glucose and energy delivery to the fetus is provided from the maternal circulation via the placenta so there is no need for fetal glucose production in utero. An essential part of the neonate's successful transition to extrauterine life therefore is the maintenance of euglycemia. Whereas most infants are indeed able to readily adapt to the metabolic demands of extrauterine life, newborns in general remain extremely susceptible to any condition that may impair their ability to establish normal glucose homeostasis during this transition process (McGowan, 1999; Sunehag and Haymond, 2002).

GLUCOSE HOMEOSTASIS

Glucose is vital for cellular metabolism throughout the body. Blood glucose concentration is determined by the balance between intake/production of glucose and glucose use by the body.

A. **Glucose production.**
   1. Glucose intake not required for immediate energy needs is converted to *glycogen* via *glycogenesis* and stored in the liver, heart, and skeletal muscles. During fasting, glycogen is broken down to re-form glucose that is then released from the liver in a process known as *glycogenolysis*. The infant's ability for glycogenolysis varies according to fetal growth and maturity.
   2. The other main source of glucose is *gluconeogenesis:* production of glucose and glycogen in the liver by means of nonglucose precursors such as lactate, pyruvate, glycerol (fat), and amino acids (Haninger and Farley, 2001; Kalhan and Parimi, 2000).

B. **Glucose metabolism.** Glucose can be metabolized in the body in several ways: production of energy, storage as glycogen, and conversion to gluconeogenic precursors. In the brain, however, because glucose is the primary source of fuel, it is completely oxidized to provide 99% of cerebral energy production (Halamek and Stevenson, 1998). This process is dependent on a number of important enzymes and reactions.

1. Glucose molecules are transported across the blood-brain barrier and into brain cells by glucose transporter (GLUT) proteins (Noerr, 2001).
2. Within the cytoplasm, glucose is metabolized by *glycolysis* to pyruvate. Pyruvate is then oxidized to *acetyl-coenzyme A* (acetyl-CoA), which is transported to the mitochondrion for entry into the citric acid cycle. The end products are carbon dioxide, water, and energy released in the generation of *adenosine triphosphate* (ATP).
3. Of importance to the neonate is that during hypoglycemia other substrates (ketone bodies, lactate, glycerol, and amino acids) can also be converted to pyruvate, enter the citric acid cycle, and produce ATP, thus serving as a source of energy for the brain (Noerr, 2001).

C. **Hormonal regulation of glucose homeostasis.**

1. Insulin. Secreted by the pancreatic β-cells in response to an increase in plasma glucose, insulin decreases the blood glucose level by promoting glycogen formation, suppressing hepatic glucose release, and driving peripheral uptake of glucose. Insulin does not control entry of glucose into the brain or liver.
2. Glucagon. Secreted by the pancreatic α-cells when blood glucose levels decrease, glucagon promotes glycogenolysis and gluconeogenesis. Glucagon is called a *counterregulatory hormone* because it opposes the effect of insulin by raising the blood glucose level. Other counterregulatory hormones include catecholamines, cortisol, and growth hormone. Although these hormones may not be important regulators in the fast-feed cycle of healthy neonates, minimum basal levels may be needed to maintain euglycemia (Hawdon and Aynsley-Green, 1999a).

D. **Fetal glucose homeostasis.**

1. Glucose reaches the fetus by facilitated diffusion across the placenta at a concentration of about 60% to 80% of the mother's (Noerr, 2001).
2. Glycogen storage for postnatal energy needs begins early in gestation, with most glycogen accumulating during the third trimester.
3. Fetal insulin, with its apparently more important role in fetal growth than in fetal metabolic control (Hawdon and Aynsley-Green, 1999a), is detectable early in gestation, but the response to a glucose load is not fully developed even at term.
4. The fetus is capable of gluconeogenic activity, using substrates such as lactate if needed to meet metabolic demands in utero.

E. **Neonatal glucose homeostasis.** With the loss of the maternal glucose source, the neonate must assume control of glucose homeostasis and regulate it during the fast-feed cycle while still ensuring an adequate supply of fuel for the brain and other organs. Early events in this process:

1. After cord clamping, the neonate's blood glucose concentration falls, reaching a nadir at 1 to 2 hours of age.
2. In the first postnatal hours, the neonatal brain metabolizes lactate, which is abundant, so that even though the glucose concentration is low, the brain is not fuel deficient.
3. The neonate gradually mobilizes glucose to meet energy needs by secreting glucagon and catecholamines and suppressing insulin release. Thus even if a healthy term newborn infant is not fed soon after birth, blood glucose levels rise at 3 to 4 hours of age.

4. Hepatic glycogen, however, is rapidly depleted if feeding is not established early and the infant is dependent on gluconeogenesis and lipolysis as the primary modes of maintaining euglycemia (Sunehag and Haymond, 2002).

HYPOGLYCEMIA

A. Definition of hypoglycemia.

1. Ongoing advances in perinatal care have led to the current recommendations for upward modifications in the definition of neonatal hypoglycemia. No single value divides "normal" from "low" blood glucose concentrations in all infants. Most clinicians believe that rather than a specific value neonatal hypoglycemia lies on a continuum of low blood glucose values of varied duration and severity that is influenced by a number of different factors. These factors include conceptual and postnatal age, adequacy of gluconeogenic pathways, general health status, and presence or absence of symptoms (Cornblath and Ichord, 2000).
   a. Statistical norms provide a starting point in defining hypoglycemia, but the critical threshold of blood glucose concentration needs to be individualized according to the neonate's clinical status. A widely used cutoff point for *plasma glucose concentration* is 40 mg/dL. This remains the typical threshold for intervention in both premature and term neonates.

B. Incidence.

1. Overall incidence is 1 to 5/1000 live births.
2. The incidence in at-risk infants may be as high as 30%, occurring in 8% of large for gestational age (LGA) infants and in 15% of premature and small for gestational age (SGA) infants (McGowan, 1999).

C. Pathophysiology.

1. The immediate postnatal drop in the blood glucose concentration is physiologic. Failure to increase glucose concentrations after 4 hours is pathologic. Subsequently, hypoglycemia is usually a result of inadequate hepatic glucose production that cannot meet peripheral demand or excessive insulin production (Cowett and Loughead, 2002).
2. Glucose delivery is dependent on blood glucose concentration and blood flow rate. During hypoglycemia, the brain increases blood flow to improve glucose delivery that may predispose the neonatal brain to hemorrhagic and hyperoxic injury if there is diminished cerebral autoregulatory ability (Halamek and Stevenson, 1998).
3. When glucose consumption exceeds delivery, the brain uses alternate fuels such as ketone bodies, lactic acid, free fatty acids, and glycerol if they are available. The production of energy from these sources involves the use of brain structural components such as proteins and phospholipids that may play a contributory role in neuronal damage (Halamek and Stevenson, 1998; Noerr, 2001; Vannucci and Vannucci, 2000).
4. Lactic acid becomes elevated in late fetal and early postnatal life and healthy term infants produce ketones effectively on days 2 and 3 of life, thus protecting their brains from fuel deficiency if the blood glucose level falls while feeding becomes established. However, the ability of preterm infants and of infants who are SGA to mount a counterregulatory ketogenic response at any time is severely limited, so these infants are heavily dependent on an adequate glucose supply (Cowett and Loughead, 2002; Vannucci and Vannucci, 2000).

5. Prolonged hypoglycemia, when not compensated by a supply of alternative fuels, induces biochemical changes at the cell level that may damage the neuronal and glial cells of the brain. It is believed that an accumulation of excitatory amino acids, especially glutamate, during hypoglycemia leads to prolonged cellular depolarization with entry of water and calcium into the cell, first impairing neuronal growth and eventually causing cell death (McGowan, 1999). In addition, the hypoglycemic brain may be more vulnerable to the damaging effects of ischemia. Degrees of ischemia and hypoglycemia that alone would not result in brain injury might do so in combination (Noerr, 2001).

D. **Etiologies and precipitating factors.** Various classification systems have been developed to categorize the various causes of neonatal hypoglycemia. All classifications essentially describe two main categories: (1) conditions with diminished/inadequate production or substrate delivery and (2) conditions with excess utilization or hyperinsulinism. Some conditions involve a combination of the two etiologies.

1. Inadequate production or supply of glucose accounts for the more common causes of neonatal hypoglycemia. These conditions involve decreased substrate (glycogen, lactate, glycerol, amino acids) availability, immature or altered enzyme pathways, or altered responses to neural or hormonal factors (Cornblath and Ichord, 2000; Cowett and Loughead, 2002).
   a. Prematurity: possible diminished oral and parenteral intake, immature counterregulatory response to low glucose concentration, insufficient glycogen stores and release (Cowett and Loughead, 2002; Noerr, 2001).
   b. Intrauterine growth restriction: low glycogen and fat stores, increased substrate utilization (Cowett and Loughead, 2002).
   c. Delayed feedings, insufficient breast-feeding, or fluid restriction (Cornblath and Ichord, 2000).
   d. Inborn errors of metabolism: defective gluconeognesis and/or glycogenolysis (e.g., galactosemia, amino acid disorders, organic acid deficiencies) (Cowett and Loughead, 2002).
   e. Glycogen storage disease: autosomal recessive defects characterized by a deficient or abnormally functioning enzyme involved with formation or degradation of glycogen in the liver (Sunehag and Haymond, 2002).
   f. Perinatal stress/hypoxia, respiratory distress, hypothermia, polycythemia/hyperviscosity, infection, adrenal hemorrhage, congestive heart failure (Cowett, 1998; Cowett and Loughead, 2002).
2. Increased uptake of glucose related to hyperinsulinism.
   a. Infant of the diabetic mother (IDM) (see p.199).
   b. Persistent neonatal hyperinsulinism and nesidioblastosis: autosomal recessive disorders thought to be caused by regulatory defects in β-cell function. Surgical exploration may be necessary for definitive diagnosis with subtotal pancreatectomy the required therapeutic measure (Cowett, 1998; Cowett and Loughead, 2002).
   c. Beckwith-Wiedemann syndrome: of unknown cause; characterized by omphalocele, macroglossia, visceromegaly and hypoglycemia. Pancreatic islet cell hyperplasia noted. The resultant hypoglycemia may be quite profound and difficult to treat (Cowett, 1998; Cowett and Loughead, 2002).
   d. Rh incompatibility: severe cases can have associated β-cell hypertrophy and hyperinsulinemia (Cowett, 1998; Cowett and Loughead, 2002).
   e. High glucose infusion and tocolytics used before delivery. β-adrenergic agonists such as terbutaline can stimulate fetal pancreatic β-cells (Cowett and Loughead, 2002).

f. Iatrogenic: position of tip of umbilical artery catheter near the pancreas can cause glucose to be directly delivered to the pancreas via the celiac artery, resulting in excessive insulin secretion (Cowett and Loughead, 2002).

E. Clinical presentation and assessment.

1. Most neonates are free of symptoms. Signs often linked with hypoglycemia are nonspecific and may occur in conjunction with other clinical conditions, making them unreliable markers for hypoglycemia. In addition these clinical signs may be present at varying blood glucose concentrations in different infants or they may not be evident at all even though the infant is experiencing severe hypoglycemia. Signs/symptoms of hypoglycemia include:
   a. Tremors; jitteriness; irritability; exaggerated Moro reflex.
   b. Abnormal cry: high pitched or weak.
   c. Respiratory distress: apnea, irregular respirations, tachypnea, cyanosis.
   d. Stupor, hypotonia, lethargy, refusal to feed.
   e. Hypothermia, temperature instability.
   f. Seizures (Cowett and Loughead, 2002; Eidelman, 2001; Noerr, 2001).
2. For clinical signs and symptoms to be attributed to hypoglycemia, Whipple's triad must be met:
   a. A reliable low blood glucose.
   b. Signs and symptoms consistent with hypoglycemia must be evident.
   c. Signs and symptoms resolve after euglycemia is achieved (Cornblath and Ichord, 2000).
3. Growth is discordant with gestational age: small or large for gestational age.
4. Some disorders have recognizable features at presentation:
   a. Beckwith-Wiedemann syndrome: macroglossia, abdominal wall defect, ear pit.
   b. Hypopituitarism: microphallus, midline facial defect.

F. Diagnostic studies.

1. Point-of-care blood glucose screening.
   a. Common bedside methods, used for speed and convenience, use whole blood, an enzymatic reagent strip, and a color chart or reflectance meter. Their reliability is questioned because:
      (1) They may underestimate the true glucose level because whole blood gives a reading 10% to 15% lower than the plasma value.
      (2) They may fail to detect clinically important hypoglycemia because of unpredictable measurement error.
      (3) They are sensitive to error from technical and operator variables such as timing, blotting, and distribution of blood droplets.
   b. Newer devices have been shown to approximate laboratory values more closely, with fewer errors. These include absorption photometry with enzymes to hemolyze erythrocytes before analysis and electrochemical glucose meters (Dollberg et al., 2001; Innanen et al., 1997; Noerr, 2001).
   c. Subcutaneous microdialysis is a potential method of long-term glucose monitoring of high-risk infants that also decreases blood sampling and its associated stress and pain (Baumeister et al., 2001). A microdialysis catheter is inserted into the infant's subcutaneous adipose tissue of the lateral thigh, where it mimics a blood capillary. The microdialysis catheter contains a semipermeable membrane that is continuously perfused with a liquid (usually a sterile Ringer's solution) that equilibrates with the surrounding interstitial fluid. Dialysate samples can be collected for several days after insertion of the microdialysis catheter.

2. All current techniques require laboratory confirmation for the establishment of the diagnosis of neonatal hypoglycemia. Appropriate interventions should be initiated promptly and not wait on laboratory confirmation (McGowan, 1999; Noerr, 2001). Blood samples should be analyzed within 30 minutes of drawing to prevent continued metabolism of glucose by blood cells.
3. In suspected hyperinsulinism, testing may include concurrent insulin and glucose levels (insulin level will be inappropriately elevated), ketone and free fatty acid levels (which will be low because release of these fuels is suppressed by hyperinsulinism), and cortisol and growth hormone levels.

G. **Patient care management.** Four principles govern the clinical management of neonatal hypoglycemia: (1) high-risk infants need to be monitored; (2) there is confirmation that the plasma glucose level is indeed low; (3) clinical manifestations resolve after euglycemia is achieved; and (4) events are carefully observed and documented (Cornblath and Ichord, 2000).

1. Identify infants at risk with perinatal history, physical examination, body measurements (weight, length, and head circumference), and gestational age assessment (Cowett and Loughead, 2002).
2. Prevent hypoglycemia in infants at risk by providing glucose substrate through early enteral feedings (human milk or formula) or intravenous (IV) glucose at 4 to 6 mg/kg/minute. When tolerated, feedings are preferred over parenteral glucose because milk provides more energy than the equivalent volume of IV fluid and may contribute more essential nonglucose substrate. However, when maintenance of euglycemia requires an administrative rate of 6 mg/kg/minute, oral feedings alone will probably not be sufficient to prevent hypoglycemia (Cowett, 1998).
3. Assess glucose status with blood glucose screening.
   a. Perform blood glucose screening test on infants at risk on admission and before the first three or four feedings or at 2, 4, 6, 12, 24, and 48 hours of age if the infant is not being fed. In addition, screening should occur after changes to the feeding or IV regimen (Cornblath and Ichord, 2000).
   b. Clinically unstable infants and any infant with signs of a possible low blood glucose concentration require regular monitoring.
   c. Early and exclusive breast-feeding will meet the nutritional and energy needs of healthy full-term infants, and routine blood glucose screening of these infants is not presently recommended (Cornbalth and Ichord, 2000; Eidelman, 2001; Haninger and Farley, 2001).
4. If hypoglycemia persists despite feeding, correction is with IV glucose infusion. A minibolus (dextrose 10% in water, 2 ml/kg), followed by continuous infusion at a rate of 6 to 8 mg/kg/minute, rapidly raises the blood glucose level but does not treat the underlying hormonal and metabolic causes of the hypoglycemia (Cornblath and Ichord, 2000; Cowett and Loughead, 2002; Noerr, 2001).
5. Monitoring of blood glucose levels must then continue, for documentation of the resolution of hypoglycemia with IV therapy and subsequently during the transition to full enteral feedings. Oral feedings should be initiated once clinical symptoms have resolved (Cornblath and Ichord, 2000).
6. Persistent hypoglycemia raises the possibility of hyperinsulinism, although some infants without biochemical hyperinsulinism also have transiently high glucose requirements. Those with true hyperinsulinism may require:
   a. High IV glucose infusion rates (12-16 mg/kg/minute). Delivery of concentrated glucose (>12.5%) requires a central line for safe administration.

b. Hormonal therapy, which may include glucagon, diazoxide, and somatostatin. Glucagon stimulates glycogen release from the liver and can be used to determine if the liver contains adequate stores. SGA infants and IDMs as well as some normal infants may not respond to smaller doses (30 μg/kg). Higher doses (300 μg/kg) result in a prolonged and sustained hyperglycemia. Glucagon, however, may also stimulate insulin release, so its use requires the presence of an IV glucose infusion (Cowett and Loughead, 2002). Glucagon is mainly used as a temporizing measure until IV access is achieved (McGowan, 1999).

Diazoxide (10-15 mg/kg/day) suppresses pancreatic insulin secretion. Its use is reserved for situations of profound hyperinsulinism that have failed other therapies. It has been used for prolonged periods (years) without significant side effects noted (Cowett, 1998; Cowett and Loughead, 2002; Noerr, 2001).

Somatostatin suppresses insulin and glucagon secretion; however, its use is limited by its extremely short half-life (Cowett and Loughead, 2002).

c. Corticosteroids stimulate gluconeogenesis from noncarbohydrate (protein) sources. Hydrocortisone (5 mg/kg/day IV or orally every 12 hours) or prednisone (2 mg/kg/day orally) may be used when parenteral glucose therapy is greater than 15 mg/kg/minute. Gradual decreases in corticosteroid dosage and decreases in parenteral glucose concentrations are required as oral intake is increased (Cornblath and Ichord, 2000; Cowett, 1998; Cowett and Loughead, 2002).

d. Subtotal or total pancreatectomy may be required if severe, persistent hyperinsulinism is unresponsive to medical therapy.

H. Complications.

1. Hypoglycemia will often recur when a bolus of glucose is not followed by a continuous infusion.
2. Extravasations of peripheral glucose infusions may cause necrosis of skin and other tissue. If available, hyaluronidase can be injected subcutaneously around the periphery of any extravasation site to prevent/limit tissue injury. Elevation of the affected area, if an extremity, may limit the damage. The use of a topical antimicrobial ointment may be indicated if tissue damage is evident. The use of a petrolatum-impregnated gauze may facilitate healing. Skin injury may be prevented by making multiple puncture holes over the involved area and allowing the infiltrated fluid to leak out (Lund and Kuller, 2003).
3. Reactive hypoglycemia with return of symptomatology may occur if the intravenous glucose infusion infiltrates or is stopped abruptly.

I. Outcome. Because glucose is essential for cerebral metabolism, a serious potential consequence of hypoglycemia is neurologic impairment, including both intellectual and motor deficits. Studies have reported associations with neonatal hypoglycemia and neurologic handicaps. However, these studies are limited and may suffer from methodologic limitations, making causal relationships difficult to establish (Cornblath and Ichord, 2000; Noerr, 2001). Radiologic studies (head ultrasound [HUS]), magnetic resonance imaging [MRI], and positron emission tomography [PET] scans) have shown brain abnormalities in infants that experienced neonatal hypoglycemia. Further follow-up, however, is needed to determine the long-term implications of these findings (Kinnala et al., 1999; Kinnala et al., 2000). Outcome is primarily dependent on proper assessment, diagnosis, and intervention to correct the hypoglycemia and then to maintain euglycemia (Marks and Maisels, 1997).

1. In a sample of SGA infants followed for 5 years postbirth, recurrent episodes of hypoglycemia were strongly correlated with persistent neurodevelopmental and physical growth deficits (Duvanel et al., 1999).
2. In general, outcome studies show that neonates with seizure-associated hypoglycemia have the worst neurologic prognosis (Halamek and Stevenson, 1998).
3. Follow-up of infants that experienced persistent neonatal hyperinsulinism suggests that early events were responsible for the subsequent mental retardation (Menni et al., 2001).

INFANT OF DIABETIC MOTHER (IDM)

A. **Incidence.** 100,000 per year in the United States (Cordero et al., 1998).

B. **Pathophysiology.** The hormonal and metabolic changes that complicate diabetic pregnancy can adversely affect the developing fetus and neonate in a number of ways.

1. Early in gestation during organogenesis, the abnormal metabolic milieu is teratogenic, resulting in a higher incidence of congenital malformations.
2. Throughout pregnancy and particularly in the third trimester, the pregnant diabetic woman is increasingly insulin resistant and often has hyperglycemia and hyperaminoacidemia. Excess glucose and amino acids are freely delivered to the fetus, but maternal insulin is not. These nutrients stimulate the fetal pancreas to produce insulin to use the excess fuels resulting in β-cell hyperplasia and hyperinsulinemia. This fetal hyperinsulinemia, in turn, stimulates protein, lipid, and glycogen synthesis, causing a high rate of fetal growth, increased deposition of fat and visceral enlargement (especially heart and liver), and subsequent macrosomia. This fetal macrosomia does not involve the brain or kidneys (Cowett, 1998; McGowan, 1999).
3. After birth the neonate's pancreas continues to produce insulin, and available glucose is rapidly used. The infant's ability to mobilize glycogen stores is decreased (Noerr, 2001). The IDM may exhibit an exaggerated and persistent hypoglycemia. Maternal glucose homeostasis during pregnancy as well as maternal glycemia during delivery influence the degree of neonatal hypoglycemia (Cowett, 1998).
4. The IDM is at risk of having neural impairment because, even with plentiful adipose tissue, ketogenesis and lipolysis are suppressed by hyperinsulinemia, leaving the brain without a supply of alternative fuels for metabolism during hypoglycemia.

C. **Clinical presentation and assessment.**

1. Hypoglycemia: may occur immediately after birth without symptoms. In one large retrospective series, hypoglycemia (defined as serum glucose <40 mg/dl) occurred in about one third of IDMs. The majority of those responded rapidly to treatment, but 10% had persistent hypoglycemia despite treatment (Cordero et al., 1998).
2. Macrosomia/LGA (≈35% of IDMs) (Cordero et al., 1998). Some infants are SGA because of placental insufficiency in advanced stages of diabetes.
3. Increase in preterm births in association with diabetic pregnancy. Hyperbilirubinemia in IDMs may be secondary to prematurity.
4. Respiratory distress syndrome and other conditions such as transient tachypnea of the newborn infant. Fetal hyperinsulinemia may retard the maturation of various aspects of the pulmonary surfactant system and not

just inhibit surfactant production, delaying lung maturation (Hawdon and Aynsley-Green, 1999b).

5. Polycythemia (venous hematocrit >65%). The insulin-induced high glucose uptake and high metabolic rate causes a cellular hypoxia leading to an elevated erythropoieten level (Hawdon and Aynsley-Green, 1999b). Newborns with polycythemia do not always look plethoric, so the hematocrit must be measured.
6. Hypocalcemia, hypomagnesemia believed to result from a functional hypoparathyroidism due to maternal magnesium loss (Hawdon and Aynsley-Green, 1999b).
7. Cardiomyopathy, visceromegaly possibly related to maternal diabetes control and to fetal/neonatal hyperinsulinemia (Hawdon and Aynsley-Green, 1999b).
8. Congenital malformations. Cardiac defects (especially transposition), neural tube defects, sacral agenesis, and caudal regression are two to four times more frequent than in the general population. The anomalies are believed to be due to the diabetic intrauterine environment during organogenesis frequently before the pregnancy is recognized and prenatal diabetic treatment initiated (Hawdon and Aynsley-Green, 1999b).

D. Diagnostic studies.

1. Blood glucose screening with laboratory confirmation of plasma glucose.
2. Other laboratory analyses, including calcium and magnesium levels and venous hematocrit.
3. X-ray examination if fractures from traumatic delivery are suspected.
4. Echocardiography.

E. Patient care management.

1. The main goal of the treatment of gestational diabetes is to achieve and maintain euglycemia. Tight control of intrapartum glucose levels may reduce the incidence of neonatal complications (Cordero et al., 1998; Hawdon and Ansley-Green, 1999b).
2. Anticipate problems of IDM before delivery; prompt recognition and treatment of neonatal morbidities postdelivery (Cordero et al., 1998).
3. Provide early feeding of human milk or formula, orally or via gavage tube if the infant does not feed well. IV administration of glucose is necessary for infants too small or sick to tolerate enteral feeding (Cordero et al., 1998).

F. Complications.

1. Seizures resulting from cerebral fuel deficiency.
2. Shoulder dystocia. Macrosomic infants delivered with forceps or vacuum extraction may have brachial plexus injury (Erbs palsy) or fractures.
3. Renal vein thrombosis (secondary to polycythemia/hyperviscosity).
4. Development of juvenile insulin dependent diabetes with a 2% transmission risk for female IDM, and 6% for male IDM (Schwartz and Terano, 2000).

G. Outcome.

1. Increased perinatal mortality rate results from relatively high rates of congenital malformations, stillbirths, and premature delivery.
2. Morbidities associated with IDM include neurologic sequelae, developmental delay, behavioral differences, obesity, and diabetes.
3. Maternal complications, including poor glycemic control, vascular disease, infection, and pregnancy-induced hypertension, are associated with poorer perinatal outcome. Improved outcomes are seen in IDMs when the maternal diabetes is metabolically controlled.

4. The outcomes for SGA infants born to women receiving intensive therapy for gestational diabetes may be worse than those of appropriate for gestational age (AGA) or LGA infants (Garcia-Patterson et al., 1998).

HYPERGLYCEMIA

A. **Definition.** Whole blood glucose concentration greater than 120 to 125 mg/dl or a plasma glucose concentration greater than 150 mg/dl (Hemachandra and Cowett, 1999).

B. **Incidence.** Prevalence of 29% to 86% in low birth weight infants overall (Hawdon and Aynsley-Green, 1999a); 2% of infants weighing more than 2000 g; 45% of infants less than 1000 g; and up to 80% of infants weighing less than 750 g (Hemachandra and Cowett, 1999).

C. **Pathophysiology.** The glucose intolerance occasionally seen in the extremely low birth weight (ELBW) infant is not fully understood. Normally an infant responds to an exogenous glucose supply with a rise in insulin, suppressing endogenous glucose production and enhancing peripheral uptake of glucose. Though clinically stable ELBW infants may be able to regulate glucose in this manner, many of them become hyperglycemic. Hepatic glucose production in this latter group continues in the presence of hyperglycemia and circulating insulin. This represents a failure of glucose autoregulation involving both the pancreas and liver of infants with hyperglycemia. Corticosteroid therapy stimulates glycogenolysis and gluconeogenesis and may block insulin secretion as well as inhibit its peripheral action (Hawdon and Aynsley-Green, 1999a).

D. **Etiologies and precipitating factors.**
   1. Low birth weight, extreme prematurity, and intrauterine growth restriction (IUGR).
   2. Excessive glucose load (>6-8 mg/kg/minute) with 50% of infants receiving a glucose infusion rate (GIR) of 11 mg/kg/minute and all infants receiving a GIR of 14 mg/kg/minute developing hyperglycemia (Hemachandra and Cowett, 1999).
   3. Stress related to clinical problems such as sepsis or infection.
   4. Transient/permanent neonatal diabetes mellitus (see p. 202).
   5. Dexamethasone therapy for chronic lung disease.
   6. Lipid infusion, which may contribute to hyperglycemia.
   7. Post anesthesia/surgical procedures.

E. **Clinical presentation and assessment.** Onset can be as early as 24 hours of age; usually before 3 days of life. There is no characteristic clinical presentation although dehydration, weight loss, failure to thrive, fever, glycosuria, ketosis, and metabolic acidosis may be seen (Hemachandra and Cowett, 1999). Diagnosis is usually determined by measuring blood glucose concentration.

F. **Diagnostic studies.**
   1. Serum or plasma blood glucose levels greater than 125 mg/dl or 150 mg/dl, respectively.
   2. Urinary glucose. Very low birth weight (VLBW) infants have a low renal threshold for glucose and may spill sugar at blood glucose levels as low as 80 to 100 mg/dl.
   3. Investigation for possible underlying cause (sepsis workup to rule out infection or insulin level to rule out neonatal diabetes mellitus).

G. **Patient care management.**
   1. Monitor blood glucose of infants at risk of developing hyperglycemia, particularly when fluid intake is increased on day 2 or 3 of life.

2. Decrease glucose load as able to allow the blood glucose level to stabilize in a normal range (<125 mg/dl or plasma glucose <150 mg/dl) (Sunehag and Haymond, 2002).
3. Monitor weight, urine output, fluid intake, GIR, electrolytes, acid-base balance.
4. Insulin is sometimes administered to ELBW infants along with parenteral nutrition in an attempt to normalize blood glucose levels without reducing caloric intake. Insulin is also used to treat transient neonatal diabetes. Insulin normalizes blood glucose by suppressing hepatic glucose production and by increasing peripheral glucose utilization. However, premature infants have a very small mass of insulin-dependent tissue with only 10% of their glucose utilization being insulin dependent (Sunehag and Haymond, 2002). Hemachandra and Cowett (1999) advise reserving insulin therapy until plasma glucose concentration exceeds 300 to 400 mg/dl.
5. Begin enteral feedings when feasible because the subsequent release of gut hormones may promote insulin secretion, allowing for improved blood glucose control (Hawdon and Aynsley-Green, 1999a; Hemachandra and Cowett, 1999).

H. **Complications.**
1. Neonatal hyperglycemia may be accompanied by urinary loss of glucose and an osmotic diuresis with its risk of dehydration. In addition, possible resultant hyperosmolarity of extracellular fluid in the brain may increase the premature infant's chance for intraventricular hemorrhage (Sunehag and Haymond, 2002).
2. Insulin management may be difficult in the ELBW infant; blood glucose levels can fluctuate widely. A precisely controlled continuous infusion pump is essential. Priming of the tubing is required because insulin tends to stick to the catheters. Whether insulin therapy promotes linear growth or just converts glucose into fat is not yet fully understood.
3. Electrolyte abnormalities, elevated CO_2 retention, elevated triglyceride level (Hemachandra and Cowett, 1999).

I. **Outcome.** Controversy exists concerning the outcome of neonatal hyperglycemia. Hay (1999) and Hemachandra and Cowett (1999) support that a strong association exists between neonatal hyperglycemia and increased mortality rates/poor neurodevelopmental outcomes among survivors. Hawdon and Aynsley-Green (1999a) contend that neonatal hyperglycemia is usually self-limiting and not associated with adverse outcomes.

TRANSIENT OR PERMANENT NEONATAL DIABETES

A. **Definition.** Hyperglycemia requiring insulin therapy occurring within the first month of life and lasting at least 2 weeks to several months (Cashin and Briars, 1999).

B. **Incidence.** 1:500,000. Predominantly occurring in SGA infants, with 46% developing permanent diabetes in the neonatal period, 23% in childhood or adolescence; 31% resolved in the neonatal period (Hawdon and Aynsley-Green, 1999b).
1. 75% of transient neonatal diabetes present in the first 10 days of life (Hemachandra and Cowett, 1999).
2. A family history of diabetes is found in one third of cases of transient neonatal diabetes, with increased occurrence among siblings or between mothers and offspring (Hemachandra and Cowett, 1999). A high incidence of diabetes is also found in cases of permanent neonatal diabetes, with a high

incidence between siblings, parents of affected infants, and close family relations (Soliman et al., 1999).

C. **Pathophysiology.** Both transient and permanent neonatal diabetes mellitus (NDM) are due to a failure of pancreatic β-cells causing an endogenous insulin deficiency with the exact pathogenesis involved not yet fully understood (Hemachandra and Cowett, 1999). Soliman and colleagues (1999) propose the etiology to be a recessively inherited disorder that leads to a failure in β-cell development. The IUGR seen with many affected infants may result in a maturational delay of the β-cells so that they do not respond appropriately (Cashin and Briars, 1999).

D. **Etiologies.**
   1. Prematurity, ELBW, SGA, IUGR.

E. **Clinical presentation.**
   1. Hyperglycemia (frequently >600 mg/dl), polyuria, glycosuria, weight loss, dehydration, fever, failure to thrive, ketosis, and metabolic acidosis may or may not be evident, low levels of C-peptide and plasma insulin (Cashin and Briars, 1999; Hemachandra and Cowett, 1999; Soliman et al., 1999).
   2. Transient neonatal diabetes does not usually resolve for several weeks to months and is typically indicated by a rise in C-peptide levels (Hemachandra and Cowett, 1999).

F. **Management.**
   1. Restore intravascular volume.
   2. Replace fluid and electrolyte losses as indicated and provide for ongoing needs.
   3. Correct the hyperglycemia; monitor glucose levels.
   4. Provide adequate nutrition for growth and development.
   5. Usually a daily dose of 0.2 to 3 units/kg/day of insulin is necessary to achieve plasma glucose levels of 100 to 180 mg/dl; however, individualization of insulin requirement is needed.
   6. Average length of insulin therapy varies from 2 weeks to 18 months. Tapering of insulin dose as requirement decreases lessens the risk of recurrent hyperglycemia (Cashin and Briars, 1999).

G. **Complications.** See hyperglycemia above.

H. **Outcomes.** Soliman and colleagues (1999) reported infants with permanent neonatal diabetes treated with insulin with normal developmental milestones and improved growth despite being IUGR at birth. Despite permanent/prolonged remissions, late complications such as retinopathy and nephropathy are rarely reported in people with NDM even after 20 years of treatment (Cashin and Briars, 1999).

REFERENCES

Baumeister, F.A., Rolinski, B., Busch, R., and Emmrich, P.: Glucose monitoring with long-term subcutaneous microdialysis in neonates. *Pediatrics, 108*(5):1187-1192, 2001.

Cashin, K.M. and Briars, R.L.: Neonatal diabetes: A case study. *Pediatric Nursing, 25*(3):271-277, 1999.

Cordero, L., Treuer, S.H., Landon, M.B., and Gabbe, S.G.: Management of infants of diabetic mothers. *Archives of Pediatrics and Adolescent Medicine, 152*(3):249-254, 1998.

Cornblath, M. and Ichord, R.: Hypoglycemia in the neonate. *Seminars in Perinatology, 24*(2):136-149, 2000.

Cowett, R.M.: Hypoglycemia and hyperglycemia in the newborn. In R.A. Polin and W.W. Fox (Eds.): *Fetal and neonatal physiology, Volume I.* Philadelphia, 1998, Saunders, pp. 596-608.

Cowett, R.M. and Loughead, J.L.: Neonatal glucose metabolism: Differential diagnoses, evaluation, and treatment of hypoglycemia. *Neonatal Network, 21*(4): 9-19, 2002.

Dollberg, S., Bauer, R., Lubetzky, R., and Momouni, F.F.: A reappraisal of neonatal blood chemistry reference ranges using Nova M electrodes. *American Journal of Perinatology, 18*(8):433-439, 2001.

Duvanel, C.B., Fawer, C-L., Cotting, J., et al.: Long-term effects of neonatal hypoglycemia on brain growth and psychomotor development on small-for-gestational age preterm infants. *Journal of Pediatrics, 134*(4):492-498, 1999.

Eidelman, A.I.: Hypoglyemia and the breastfed neonate. *Pediatric Clinics of North America, 48*(2):377-387, 2001.

Garcia-Patterson, A., Corcoy, R., Balsells.M., et al.: In pregnancies with gestational diabetes mellitus and intensive theory, perinatal outcome is worse in small-for-gestational-age newborns. *American Journal of Obstetrics and Gynecology, 179*(2):481-485, 1998.

Halamek, L.P. and Stevenson, D.K.: Neonatal hypoglycemia, part II. Pathophysiology and therapy. *Clinical Pediatrics, 37*(1):11-16, 1998.

Haninger, N.C. and Farley, C.L.: Screening for hypoglycemia in healthy term neonates: Effects on breastfeeding. *Journal of Midwifery and Women's Health, 46*(5):292-301, 2001.

Hawdon, J.M. and Aynsley-Green, A.: Disorders of blood glucose homeostasis in the Neonate. In J.M. Rennie and N.R.C. Roberton (Eds.): *Textbook of neonatology.* London, 1999a, Churchill Livingstone, pp. 939-956.

Hawdon, J.M. and Aynsley-Green, A.: The infant of a diabetic mother. In J.M. Rennie and N.R.C. Roberton (Eds.): *Textbook of neonatology.* London, 1999b, Churchill Livingstone, pp. 401-405.

Hay, W.W.: Addressing hypoglycemia and hyperglycemia. *Pediatrics in Review, 20*(7): E4-E5, 1999. Retrieved August 10, 1999, from www.pedsinreview.org/.

Hemachandra, A.H. and Cowett, R.M.: Neonatal hyperglycemia. *Pediatrics in review, 20*(7): E16-E24, 1999. Retrieved August 10, 1999, from www.pedsinreview.org/.

Innanen, V.T., Deland, M.E., deCampos, F.M., and Dunn, M.S.: Point of-care glucose testing in the neonatal intensive care unit is facilitated by the use of the Ames Glucometer Elite electrochemical glucose meter. *Pediatrics, 130*:151-155, 1997.

Kalhan, S. and Parimi, P.: Gluconeogenesis in the fetus and neonate. *Seminars in Perinatology, 24*(2):94-106, 2000.

Kinnala, A., Korvenranta, H., and Parkkola, R.: Newer techniques to study neonatal hypoglycemia. *Seminars in Perinatology, 24*(2):116-119, 2000.

Kinnala, A., Rikalainen, H., Lapinleimu, H., et al.: Cerebral magnetic resonance imaging and ultrasonography findings after neonatal hypoglycemia. *Pediatrics, 103*(4 Pt 1): 724-729, 1999.

Lund, C.H. and Kuller, J.M.: Assessment and management of the integumentary system. In C. Kenner and J.W. Lott (Eds.): *Comprehensive neonatal nursing: A physiologic perspective.* Philadelphia, 2003, Saunders, pp. 700-724.

Marks, K.H. and Maisels, M.J.: Critical neonatal illnesses. In R.A. Hoekelmen (Ed.): *Primary pediatric care.* St Louis, 1997, Mosby, pp. 550-560.

McGowan, J.E: Neonatal hypoglycemia. *Pediatrics in Review, 20*(7):E6-E15, 1999. Retrieved August 10, 1999, from www.pedsinreview.org/.

Menni, F., de Lonlay, P., Sevin, C., et al.: Neurologic outcomes of 90 neonates and infants with persistent hyperinsulinemic hypoglycemia. *Pediatrics, 107*(3): 476-479, 2001.

Noerr, B.: State of the science; neonatal hypoglycemia. *Advances in Neonatal Care, 1*(1):4-21, 2001.

Schwartz, R. and Terano, K.A.: Effects of diabetic pregnancy on the fetus and newborn. *Seminars in Perinatology, 24*(2): 120-135, 2000.

Soliman, A.T., ElZalabany, M.M., Bappal, B., et al.: Permanent neonatal diabetes mellitus: Epidemiology, mode of presentation, pathogenesis and growth. *Indian Journal of Pediatrics, 66(3)*:363-373, 1999.

Sunehag, A.L. and Haymond, M.W.: Glucose extremes in newborn infants. *Clinics in Perinatology, 29(2)*:245-260, 2002.

Vannucci, R.C. and Vannucci, S.J.: Glucose metabolism in the developing brain. *Seminars in Perinatology, 24*(2):107-115, 2000.

CHAPTER

10 Nutritional Management

SUSAN BAKEWELL-SACHS AND AMY BRANDES

OBJECTIVES

1. Describe the effects of prematurity on the physiology of digestion and absorption.
2. Identify nutritional deficiencies most common in preterm and term infants.
3. Describe basic nutritional requirements for term and preterm infants and factors that influence these requirements.
4. Describe the standards used to assess growth in preterm infants.
5. Identify nutritional components, uses, methods of delivery, complications, and nursing care issues for parenteral nutrition.
6. Describe assessment of an infant's readiness for enteral nutrition.
7. Describe minimal enteral feedings and their use in preterm infants.
8. Review the use of human milk feedings for preterm infants and related nursing care issues.
9. Review the use of commercial premature infant formulas for enteral nutrition management.
10. Describe the various methods for enteral feedings and the advantages and disadvantages of each.
11. Describe assessments used to determine infant nutritional status.
12. Describe risks and interventions for feeding intolerances and nutritional deficiency states in preterm infants.

Neonatal nurses face challenges in helping to meet the basic nutritional requirements and supporting the growth needs of high-risk and preterm infants. Tremendous advances in technology and pharmacology permit the survival of extremely prematurely born infants, who require intensive and specialized care and support for immature body systems. Nutritional care is of vital importance for these preterm infants, who have been deprived of transplacentally acquired nutrient stores and who have rapid extrauterine growth rates. Other high-risk infants have special needs related to illness-associated metabolic demands and physiologic instability.

Neonatal nurses with knowledge of the effects of prematurity on gastrointestinal functioning, the special nutritional needs of preterm infants, and methods of delivering nutritional support can better assess infant status and contribute to nutritional management. This chapter reviews the nutritional requirements of preterm and high-risk infants, methods for providing parenteral and enteral nutrition, and nursing interventions for optimal nutritional care.

ANATOMY AND PHYSIOLOGY OF THE PRETERM INFANT'S GASTROINTESTINAL TRACT

A. Anatomic and functional development of the gastrointestinal (GI) tract.

1. Anatomic development. GI tract resembles that of a term newborn infant by 20 weeks' gestation (Blackburn, 2003).
2. Functional development.
   a. Limited before 26 weeks' gestation and continues after birth (Carver and Barness, 1996).
   b. Sucking movements occur in utero as early as 13 to 15 weeks' gestation, but functional coordination of suck, swallow, and breathing is not developed before 31 to 34 weeks (Simpson, et al. 2002) with complete synchrony expected by 36 to 38 weeks (Blackburn, 2003).
   c. By 28 weeks the fetus has the biochemical and physiologic capacities for limited digestion and absorption (Carver and Barness, 1996).
   d. Preterm infants have limited lactase levels, which rise postnatally but should be adequate to handle slowly initiated lactose-containing enteral feedings (Neu and Koldovsky, 1996). Lactase reaches mature levels around 36 to 40 weeks (Kien, 1996). Other carbohydrate-digesting enzymes, disaccharidases, are functionally active after 27 to 28 weeks' gestation (Blackburn, 2003).
   e. Fat digestion begins in the stomach, where a portion of milk fat is digested and partial hydrolysis occurs as a prerequisite to intestinal fat digestion. Gastric lipase activity is already high at 25 weeks' gestation, remains constant up to 34 weeks, when it peaks, and then decreases slightly before term. Gastric fat digestion is greater in preterm infants fed mother's milk (25%) than in those fed formula (14%), likely because of the bile salt–dependent lipase of human milk (Hamosh, 1996; 2001).
   f. Pancreatic lipase has a limited contribution to fat digestion in neonates compared with that in adults. Pancreatic lipase activity is lower in preterm than in term infants and is lower in preterm infants who are small for gestational age (SGA) than in those who are appropriate in size for gestational age (Lebenthal and Lebenthal, 1999).
   g. Protein enzyme activity increases rapidly after birth in premature and term infants (Hamosh, 1996).
   h. Preterm infants have limited production of gut digestive enzymes and growth factors (Blackburn, 2003).
   i. Immature motor function limits the ability to move nutrients through the GI tract and is evidenced by lack of sucking coordination, decreased esophageal sphincter tone, delayed gastric emptying, and slow intestinal transit (Berseth, 1996). Peristalsis and intestinal motility begin to mature after 30 to 32 weeks but remain less organized until near term (Blackburn, 2003).

B. Postnatal development of the GI tract.

1. GI motility is the main limiting factor in providing enteral nutrition to preterm infants (Berseth, 1996).
2. Diet is a major factor in the regulation of GI growth and function (Carver and Barness, 1996).
   a. Oral nutrients can have direct or indirect effects through stimulation of hormone secretion.
   b. Vitamins and minerals, such as iron and zinc, are growth factors.
   c. Folic acid and vitamin B_{12} are necessary for deoxyribonucleic acid (DNA) synthesis.
   d. Vitamin D hydroxylation influences calcium and phosphorus absorption.

e. A variety of amino acids are essential for growth.
f. Diet composition influences enzyme activities and gut flora, which may then affect GI development and function.
g. Increased oral nutrient intake and increased rate of weight gain lead to earlier maturation of the small intestine epithelium.

3. Systemically administered growth factors (e.g., by means of parenteral nutrition) can stimulate GI growth and maturation.

C. Nutrient store deficiencies of preterm infants.

1. Energy.
   a. Fat provides 9 kcal/g and is therefore the major energy source for neonates (Hamosh, 1996). Significant fat accretion occurs in the fetus between 24 weeks and 40 weeks. At 24 weeks the body composition is less than 2% stored fat, at 32 weeks 5%, and at 40 weeks 15%. Essential fatty acids are important for brain and retinal growth and function (Heird et al., 1997; Innis et al., 2002).
      (1) Sources of fat for the newborn infant include:
         (a) Release of free fatty acids stored in adipose tissue.
         (b) Absorption of fat from human milk or formula (approximately 50% of calories from fat).
         (c) Intravenous (IV) lipids.
      (2) Preterm infants have low adipose tissue stores at birth.
   b. Carbohydrate is the second major energy source for neonates. The human neonate's brain is glucose dependent, accounting for 75% of fetal glucose consumption. During the third trimester, glucose is stored as glycogen in the liver.
      (1) Term infants have sufficient energy stores in the form of glycogen and fat for use during the relative starvation state that normally occurs during the first few days of life.
      (2) Preterm infants have limited fat and glycogen stores and will quickly exhaust endogenous energy sources if sufficient exogenous energy is not provided. Nutritional support should ideally begin as soon as medically appropriate to give enough nonprotein and protein calories to prevent existing tissue catabolism. (Rivera et al., 1993; Thureen et al., 2000; Van Goudoever et al., 1995). Dextrose alone will result in muscle catabolism for energy (Thureen and Hay, 1993).
2. Vitamins and minerals.
   a. Nutrients such as vitamins A and E, and minerals and trace elements, such as calcium, phosphorus, iron, copper, zinc, selenium, chromium, manganese, molybdenum, cobalt, fluoride, and iodine, normally accumulate at an appreciable rate, predominantly in the third trimester of pregnancy. These nutrients play an essential role in promoting normal tissue growth and repairing injured tissue. Trace elements also play an important role in numerous metabolic pathways (Zlotkin et al., 1995).
3. Inadequate quantities of many essential nutrients. Prevention of further depletion of reserves and achievement of comparable intrauterine accretion rates are difficult and sometimes not possible.
4. Inadequate nutrition affects all organs.

STANDARDS FOR ADEQUATE GROWTH

A. Intrauterine growth curves.

1. Widely accepted as basis for assessing growth in the newborn period.

2. Standard for adequate growth: normal fetus at postconceptional age similar to that of preterm newborn infant.
3. May be an inappropriate standard for adequate growth for preterm infants for the following reasons:
   a. Because of immature organ systems of the preterm infant, it is impossible, even with total parenteral nutrition (TPN) and commercially prepared preterm infant formulas, to match the transplacental provision of nutrients.
   b. As gestational age decreases, extrauterine provision of comparable nutrients becomes increasingly difficult and may be undesirable in extremely low birth weight (ELBW) or critically ill infants.
   c. Severe illness affects both nutrient demands and nutrient use (Wahlig and Georgieff, 1995).
   d. Overly aggressive attempts to attain comparable intrauterine growth may result in the following:
      (1) Acidosis.
      (2) Fluid overload and patent ductus arteriosus (PDA).
      (3) Increased risk of bronchopulmonary dysplasia (BPD) secondary to PDA.

B. Postnatal growth curves for preterm infants.
1. Weight, length, and head circumference are based on birth gestational age.
2. Growth curves attempt to account for early postnatal weight loss.
3. Growth curves reflect a slower growth velocity than is seen with intrauterine growth curves.
4. Clinicians must bear in mind that definitive criteria for adequate growth remain controversial.
5. Anthropometric measurements and standardized growth curves are necessary tools for assessing growth and nutrition.
6. The National Institute of Child Health and Development (NICHD) Neonatal Research Network has developed postnatal growth curves for infants with birth weights between 500 and 1500 g based on growth of multiple network centers. These growth curves also relate growth velocity to several common major morbidities. These growth curves can be accessed at http://neonatal.rti.org (Ehrenkranz et al., 1999).

NUTRITIONAL REQUIREMENTS AND ENTERAL FEEDING FOR TERM INFANTS

A. Caloric and fluid requirements.
1. Healthy newborn infants require approximately 98 to 108 kcal/kg/day for adequate growth and development (American Academy of Pediatrics Committee on Nutrition [AAP-CON], 1998a).
2. Adequate caloric intake is generally achieved by intake of 150 to 180 ml/kg/day when formula with 20 kcal per ounce or human milk is used.

B. Protein, fat, and carbohydrate.
1. Total caloric intake should be represented by the following:
   a. Protein: 7% to 12%.
   b. Fat: 35% to 55%.
   c. Carbohydrate: 35% to 55%.
2. Human milk and standard commercial infant formulas supply these nutrients within acceptable ratios. Infant formulas are designed to approximate the nutrients in human milk.

3. Vitamins, minerals, and trace elements.
   a. Vitamin deficiency in healthy term infants is rare.
   b. Human milk and standard formulas provide adequate amounts of most vitamins to meet the needs of infants. However, supplements of fluoride, vitamin D, and iron are often recommended for breast-fed infants.
   c. Recommended daily requirements and intakes are described elsewhere (Moran and Greene, 1998) and are available at www.nap.edu.
4. Human milk and term-infant formulas.
   a. Human milk is the ideal food for term infants. All healthy mothers should be encouraged to breast-feed their infants for the first 12 months of life (AAP Workgroup on Breastfeeding, 1997).
      (1) Vitamin B_{12} may be deficient in the milk of strictly vegetarian women who do not take supplements.
      (2) The unique absorption of iron and zinc from human milk results in only rare deficiencies of these minerals, despite their low content in human milk. Supplemental feedings, however (i.e., formula, cereal, fruit), decrease iron and zinc absorption from human milk.
   b. Commercial formulas for term infants are cow milk or soy based. Although both types support adequate weight gain for term infants, cow milk formulas are recommended unless the infant has galactosemia, primary lactase deficiency, or immunoglobulin E (IgE)–mediated cow milk allergy (AAP-CON, 1998b).
5. Supplements. Controversy exists regarding supplementation of human milk or formulas with additional vitamins and minerals. Some recommendations for supplementation are as follows:
   a. Iron.
      (1) Iron supplementation may be beneficial for exclusively breast-fed infants beginning at 4 months of age.
      (2) Iron supplements may be given in the form of ferrous sulfate, multivitamins with iron, iron-fortified formula, or iron-fortified cereal.
   b. Vitamin D.
      (1) Adequate amounts are supplied in formula when intake is adequate.
      (2) The American Academy of Pediatrics (AAP) recommends vitamin D supplementation (200 IU/day) for all infants who are exclusively breast-fed (AAP-CON, 2003).
   c. Fluoride.
      (1) Fluoride supplementation is recommended after age 6 months, when the concentration of fluoride in the drinking water is less than 0.3 ppm.
      (2) For ages 6 months to 3 years, the dose is 0.25 mg/day (Orth, 1997).
      (3) In areas where drinking water is adequately treated with fluoride, breast-fed infants may not require supplementation (Slusser and Powers, 1997).
      (4) If fluoride in the local water supply is less than 0.3 ppm, the supplementation recommendation is 0.25 mg/day.
      (5) If the fluoride content in the local water supply is more than 0.3 ppm, no supplementation is recommended.
   d. Vitamin B_{12}. Supplementation in the amount of 0.3 to 0.5 μg/day is recommended for infants whose mothers eat no animal products and take no vitamin B_{12} supplements (Slusser and Powers, 1997).

NUTRITIONAL REQUIREMENTS FOR PRETERM INFANTS

A. General considerations.

1. Recommendations for nutritional requirements and advisable intakes must be used as guidelines for meeting nutritional requirements.
2. Individual infant nutritional needs may be highly variable.
3. Gestational age and birth weight influence nutrient body stores at birth, as well as digestive, absorptive, and metabolic capabilities.
4. Estimated requirements vary for parenteral and enteral routes.
5. Day-to-day clinical status of the infant will determine nutrient requirements.
6. Recommendations for parenteral and enteral nutritional needs for premature infants are presented in Table 10-1.

B. Specific recommendations.

1. Water.
   a. Requirement = amount of water lost from insensible water loss + fecal and urine water + amount retained in newly synthesized tissue.

TABLE 10-1
Daily Nutritional Requirements for Premature Infants

Nutrient	Parenteral (per kg)	Enteral (per kg)
Energy	80-90 + kcal	105-130 kcal
Protein	2.7-3.8 g	3-4 g
Carbohydrate	6-12 mg/kg/min	10.8-16.8 g
Fat	0.5-3 g	5.4-7.2 g
Sodium	2-4 mEq	2-3.5 mEq
Potassium	2-3 mEq	2-3 mEq
Chloride	2-3 mEq	2-3 mEq
Vitamin A	280 μg	90-1500 IU
Vitamin D	4 μg	150-400 IU
Vitamin E	2.8 mg	1.3-12 IU
Vitamin K	80 μg	4.8-10 μg
Vitamin C	32 mg	18-24 mg
Thiamine	0.48 mg	48-240 μg
Riboflavin	0.56 mg	72-360 μg
Niacin	6.8 mg	0.3-4.8 mg
Vitamin B_6	0.4 mg	42-210 μg
Folate	56 μg	25-50 μg
Vitamin B_{12}	0.4 μg	0.18-0.3 μg
Pantothenic acid	2 μg	0.36-1.8 mg
Biotin	8 μg	1.8-6 μg
Calcium	60-100 mg	120-230 mg
Phosphorus	43-70 mg	60-140 mg
Magnesium	3-7.2 mg	7.9-15 mg
Iron	—	2-4 mg
Zinc	400 μg	600-1000 μg
Copper	20 μg	108-125 μg
Selenium	1.5-2 μg	1.3-3 μg
Chromium	0.05-0.2 μg	0.1-0.5 μg
Manganese	1 μg	6.0-7.5 μg
Molybdenum	0.25 μg	0.3 μg
Iodine	1 μg	6-60 μg

Adapted from Anderson, D.M.: Nutrition for premature infants. In P.Q. Samour, K.K. Helm, and C.E. Lang (Eds.): *Handbook of pediatric nutrition* (2nd ed). Gaithersburg, MD, 1999, Aspen, pp. 43-63.

b. Actual requirements are highly variable and are dependent on the clinical status of the infant.
c. Minimum requirement is approximately 120 to 150 ml/kg/day for a growing preterm infant receiving 110 to 120 kcal/kg/day with enteral feedings or approximately 120 to 150 ml/kg/day for an infant receiving parenteral fluids (Tsang et al., 1993).
d. Factors that increase fluid requirements include:
   (1) Abnormal fluid losses (ileostomy, colostomy, chest tubes).
   (2) Diarrhea, vomiting.
   (3) Increase in activity level.
   (4) Labile body temperature, fever, cold stress.
   (5) Low environmental humidity.
   (6) Phototherapy.
   (7) Prematurity.
   (8) Radiant warmers.
   (9) Renal dysfunction (glycosuria, acute tubular necrosis).
   (10) Third spacing.
e. Factors that result in decreased fluid requirements include:
   (1) Hypoxic ischemic encephalopathy.
   (2) BPD.
   (3) PDA.
   (4) Postoperative status.
   (5) Congestive heart failure.
   (6) Meningitis.
   (7) Renal failure.

2. Calories.
   a. Energy intake = energy stored + energy expended + energy excreted.
   b. Generally, fortified human milk or premature formula at 120 kcal/kg/day will meet the requirements of stable, growing preterm infants (Tables 10-1 and 10-2). Some premature infants may require as much as 150 kcal/kg/day for catch-up growth.
   c. Parenteral requirements are about 20% less than enteral requirements, or about 80 to 90 kcal/kg/day.
   d. Adequate caloric intake should be assessed on the basis of appropriate daily weight gain, or 10 to 20 g/kg/day for preterm infants (Ehrenkranz et al., 1999; Putet, 1993).

TABLE 10-2
Estimation of Caloric Requirements for the LBW Infant (kcal/kg/day)

Physiologic Activity	Kcal/kg/day
Energy expended	40-60
Resting metabolic rate	40-50
Activity	0-5
Thermoregulation	0-5
Fecal losses	15
Specific dynamic action (energy cost of digestion and metabolism)	15
Growth	20-30
TOTAL	90-120

Adapted from American Academy of Pediatrics Committee on Nutrition: *Pediatric nutrition handbook* (4th ed.). Elk Grove Village, IL, 1998, American Academy of Pediatrics, p. 57.

e. Factors that increase caloric requirements are as follows:
   (1) Acute or chronic respiratory disease.
   (2) Fluctuations of ambient temperature outside the limits of neutral thermal range.
   (3) Hypothermia, hyperthermia.
   (4) Increased cardiac output; left-to-right shunting.
   (5) Increased muscular activity, agitation, and pain.
   (6) Infection.
   (7) Malabsorption of prematurity.
   (8) Short gut syndrome or other malabsorption syndromes.
   (9) SGA.
   (10) Periods of rapid growth.

3. Protein.
   a. Necessary for cell growth and synthesis of enzymes and hormones.
   b. Requirement = growth needs + losses through skin, urine, and feces.
   c. Precise requirements are not available, and there are several formulas for estimation.
   d. Protein intake of 3 to 3.8 g, with protein intake being 7% to 12% of total caloric intake, is generally recommended (Micheli and Schutz, 1993).
   e. For proper protein utilization, about 24 to 32 nonprotein kilocalories must be delivered for each gram of protein administered.
   f. Must consider amino acid constituents.
      (1) In addition to the eight essential amino acids necessary for cell growth, preterm infants require four conditionally essential amino acids: histidine, taurine, cysteine, and tyrosine (Blackburn, 2003; Pereira, 1995).
      (2) Recent studies have studied the safety and benefit of adding glutamine to the amino acid solution. Supplementation with this amino acid appears safe; however, clinical benefits have yet to be seen (Poindexter et al., 2003).
      (3) Preterm infants have a limited ability to use excess amino acid and, with unbalanced amino acid intake, are at risk for hyperammonemia, azotemia, metabolic acidosis, and altered plasma amino acid profiles.
      (4) Amino acid requirements for extremely preterm infants range from 2.5 to 3.5 g/kg/day, with higher amounts being used for the smallest preterm infants during active growth (Pereira, 1995).
      (5) The essential and conditionally essential amino acids are present in immature human milk and preterm infant formulas in adequate amounts. Cysteine has poor solubility in aqueous solutions, so minimal amounts are present in commercial parenteral amino acid preparations. However, cysteine can be added to the parenteral solution separately.
   g. Whey-predominant formulas are better suited metabolically for preterm infants and are provided in preterm infant formulas (60:40) to resemble human milk more closely. Human milk has a whey:casein ratio of 70:30, whereas the whey:casein ratio of cow's milk is 18:82 (Schanler, 1995).
   h. Adequate protein intake is not achievable with unfortified human milk, especially if the infant is fluid restricted or very small (<1200 g).

4. Fat.
   a. Fat is a major source of energy for growing preterm infants and necessary for transport of fat-soluble vitamins.

b. Guidelines for fat intake are as follows:
   (1) The AAP Committee on Nutrition (AAP-CON, 1998a) recommends 4.5 to 6 g of fat per 100 kcal of enteral intake for stable, growing preterm infants. For preterm infants weighing less than 1000 g, enteral fat intake should be 3 to 4 g/kg/day (Pereira, 1995).
   (2) Intake should be approximately 35% to 55% of total caloric intake.
c. Good source of energy because of high caloric content and lack of osmolality; however, not all fats are well absorbed by preterm infants.
d. Human milk provides about 50% of energy from fat; commercial formulas provide 40% to 50%.
e. Because of fatty acid composition, organization of the human fat milk globule, and presence of bile salt–stimulated lipase, the fat of human milk is easier to digest and absorb by low birth weight infants than is fat derived from cow's milk. The lipase in human milk is heat labile and inactivated when pasteurized (63° C) (Innis, 1993). Combining fresh human milk (40%) with formula (60%) has been shown to result in an increase in fat absorption in low birth weight infants, in comparison with use of formula alone (Schanler, 1995).
f. Medium-chain triglycerides (MCTs) are easier to absorb than long-chain fatty acids; MCTs are absorbed by passive diffusion and do not require bile salts.
g. Premature infant formulas use a combination of MCTs and shorter-chain vegetable fatty acids from vegetable oil.
h. Linoleic acid is an essential fatty acid and should account for at least 3% of total calories (0.4+ g/100 kcal) (AAP-CON, 1998a). This amount is achieved with adequate intake of human milk and commercial premature infant formulas. Linolenic acid is also an essential fatty acid for preterm infants; recommended intake for stable, growing premature infants is 0.11 to 0.44 g/100 kcal (Tsang et al., 1993).
i. Research has emphasized the importance of very long-chain fatty acids—arachidonic acid and docosahexaenoic acid—which are derivatives of linoleic and linolenic acids and are found in human milk but not cow's milk. These fatty acids have been associated functionally with cognition and vision (Schanler, 1995).

5. Carbohydrates.
   a. Glucose is essential for brain function.
   b. Glucose intake must be adequate to maintain serum levels greater than 40 mg/dl. Glucose can be manufactured from other carbohydrates, protein, and fats, so there is not an absolute intake requirement. The usual dose of glucose provided parenterally during the transitional neonatal period is 4 to 6 mg/kg/minute and can be met by 10% dextrose at infusion rates of 60 to 90 ml/kg/day (Shaffer and Weismann, 1992). Preterm infants rapidly become hypoglycemic with inadequate glucose intake. Hyperglycemia can also be a problem with extremely premature infants. Hyperglycemia contributes to hyperosmolality and may be a risk factor for intracranial hemorrhage in those infants.
   c. Carbohydrate intake should provide 35% to 55% of total calories. Lactose, or a combination of lactose and other sugars, is the preferred carbohydrate for enteral nutrition.
   d. Lactose is the carbohydrate in human milk and is the predominant carbohydrate in most milk-based formulas for term infants. The lactose content of human colostrum is lower than that of mature milk.

e. Lactose may promote the growth of nonpathogenic lactobacillus, which may be somewhat protective against pathogens such as *Klebsiella, Escherichia coli*, and *Enterobacter* (Neu and Koldovsky, 1996).
f. Low intestinal mucosal lactase activity in preterm infants may affect digestion of lactose and may result in the slow advance of feedings, especially in small infants. Concern regarding lactase deficiency should not be used to support the use of elemental formulas rather than human milk.
g. It is uncertain whether the addition of glucose polymers facilitates better tolerance by preterm infants than 100% lactose.
h. A combination of lactose and glucose polymers, sucrose, or other partially hydrolyzed starches is used as a carbohydrate source in many preterm infant formulas.

6. Electrolytes.
   a. Sodium, potassium, and chloride are necessary for growth and play a significant role in water and acid-base balance.
   b. Preterm infants, especially very low birth weight (VLBW) infants, have increased urine sodium and obligatory water loss during the transitional neonatal period. Fluid therapy management during the first week must account for this, otherwise there is increased risk for fluid overload (Blackburn, 2003; Oh, 1997).
   c. After reduction of the extracellular fluid, loss of body weight slows and urinary excretion of sodium chloride decreases. The sodium requirement for stable, growing preterm infants is 2 to 4 mEq/kg/day (Brandes, 2003; Pereira, 1995).
   d. Factors that influence electrolyte balance include:
      (1) Abnormal or immature renal function.
      (2) Diuretic therapy.
      (3) Increased GI losses from diarrhea, vomiting, or gastric suction.
      (4) Gestational age.
      (5) Sepsis.
      (6) Insensible water losses.
   e. Preterm infant formulas provide higher amounts of sodium, potassium, and chloride than term infant formulas and are generally sufficient for growing preterm infants.
   f. Preterm human milk has higher sodium and chloride levels than mature human milk (after 4 weeks), but levels may still be insufficient to meet infant needs; close monitoring of electrolyte levels is therefore warranted.
7. Vitamins and minerals.
   a. Exact requirements of vitamins and trace minerals by preterm infants have not been established. Preterm infant formulas provide greater amounts than term infant formulas to prevent deficiencies, provide stores equivalent to those accumulated by a term infant, and avoid toxic effects of excess amounts (Moran and Greene, 1998; Zlotkin et al., 1995).
   b. Preterm infants require more of some vitamins and minerals than term infants because of preterm infants' diminished nutrient stores at birth and the rapid growth that occurs once preterm infants are stable and well.
   c. Table 10-1 provides advisable enteral intakes of vitamins and minerals for preterm infants. Vitamin and mineral supplements are generally unnecessary for preterm infants on fortified breast milk or preterm formula.

d. Vitamin A (fat soluble).
   (1) Low vitamin A levels have been noted in infants with BPD (Shenai, 1993).
   (2) Studies show intramuscular supplementation of vitamin A will slightly decrease the risk of chronic lung disease in premature infants less than 1000 g (Tyson et al., 1999)

e. Vitamin K (fat soluble).
   (1) Necessary for manufacturing several clotting factors (e.g., prothrombin and factor VII).
   (2) All newborn infants, term and preterm, require 0.5 to 1 mg vitamin K, given intramuscularly, at birth.
   (3) Deficiency may result in hemorrhagic disease of the newborn infant (see Chapter 4).

f. Calcium, phosphorus, and magnesium.
   (1) Necessary for tissue structure and function, particularly bone mineralization.
   (2) Low stores at birth make the preterm infant susceptible to rickets if adequate intakes are not provided during growth.
   (3) Calcium and phosphorus retention and absorption are interdependent.
   (4) Alkaline phosphatase levels greater than 500 to 700 mg/dl or radiologic evidence of rickets indicates a possible need to increase calcium and phosphorus intake. However, the amount of calcium and phosphorus that can be added to parenteral nutrition is limited by the possibility of precipitation.
   (5) Calcium, phosphorus, and alkaline phosphatase levels should be monitored periodically to assess bone mineralization status. Decreased calcium and phosphorus levels or increased alkaline phosphatase levels may indicate bone demineralization (Frentner, 1995).
   (6) Human milk and standard term infant formulas provide inadequate amounts of calcium and phosphorus for growing preterm infants.
   (7) Human milk fortifiers (Enfamil Human Milk Fortifier, Similac Human Milk Fortifier, and Similac Natural Care) can supplement human milk to supply adequate amounts of calcium and phosphorus.
   (8) Preterm infant formulas (Similac Special Care and Enfamil Premature Lipil) have increased amounts of calcium, phosphorus, and magnesium and appear to be adequate for most preterm infants. Neosure Advance and Enfacare provide more calories (22 calories per ounce), calcium, phosphorus, and magnesium than standard term infant formulas but less than preterm infant formulas and are designed for use after hospital discharge. Studies vary as to how long to continue using the follow-up formulas (Carver et al., 2001; Lucas et al., 1992).
   (9) Hypophosphatemia (serum concentration >4 mg/dl) is common in premature infants fed human milk without fortification and should be considered an early warning sign of decreased bone mineralization.

g. Iron.
   (1) Important for synthesis of hemoglobin, myoglobin, and iron-containing enzymes.
   (2) Difficult to provide extrauterine iron to achieve fetal accretion rates because of poor enteral absorption.
   (3) Early physiologic anemia of prematurity is not benefited by iron therapy.

(4) Iron supplementation.
   (a) AAP-CON (1998a) recommends iron supplementation of 2 mg/kg/day for all preterm infants by the age of 2 months or when birth weight is doubled. Iron supplementation has been shown to reduce the incidence of iron deficiency anemia significantly at 6 and 11 months of age (Pereira, 1995).
   (b) Vitamin E supplementation may be needed for premature infants receiving iron supplementation beyond the amount in human milk or formula.
   (c) At this time only one human milk fortifier contains a significant amount of iron (Enfamil Human Milk Fortifier). Premature infants on fortified human milk without significant amounts of iron will need additional iron supplementation.
   (d) Iron supplementation is required for infants being treated for early physiologic anemia of prematurity with erythropoietin.

PARENTERAL NUTRITION

Parenteral nutrition (PN) is indicated for initiation of nutrition support for preterm neonates and can be used in conjunction with enteral nutrition to provide partial daily requirements for certain infants.

A. Indications for PN in the neonatal period.
   1. Surgical gastrointestinal disorders (e.g., gastroschisis, tracheoesophageal fistula, malrotation, intestinal obstruction).
   2. Short bowel syndrome.
   3. Serious acute alimentary diseases (e.g., necrotizing enterocolitis [NEC]).
   4. Congenital anomalies.
   5. Renal failure.
   6. Special circumstances (e.g., cystic fibrosis, cardiac cachexia, hepatic failure, sepsis).
   7. Birth weight less than 1500 g and gestational age less than 32 weeks.
   8. Insufficient caloric or nitrogen content of enteral feeds.
   9. Severe respiratory or cardiac disease.

B. PN administration.
   1. Peripheral route.
      a. Should be used to provide nutritional support when enteral intake is not possible or does not provide sufficient caloric requirements.
      b. Is less invasive than central administration, but IV access may become problematic if PN is required for several weeks or more.
      c. Requires that dextrose concentrations be limited to 12.5% or less to prevent irritation of small peripheral veins.
      d. Can provide up to about 90 kcal/kg/day with combination dextrose and lipid emulsions.
   2. Central route.
      a. Dextrose concentrations are not restricted in comparison with peripheral route; therefore more adequate nutritional support may be achieved.
      b. Increased risk of the following:
         (1) Mechanical complications.
         (2) Sepsis.
         (3) Thrombosis of large vessels.
      c. Percutaneous central venous catheters are commonly being used in neonatal intensive care units (NICUs). They provide long-term venous

access and may be placed at the bedside by specially trained NICU nurses, advanced practice nurses or medical staff (Chathas and Paton, 1997).

d. Surgically placed central venous catheters (i.e., Broviac or Hickman) provide long-term venous access but have risks of surgery and anesthesia; they may be more stable than percutaneous central venous catheters because of the sutured cuff.

3. General considerations for PN.

a. Because of the lack of digestive losses and energy expenditure for food digestion in the GI tract, nutrient intakes for PN are different from those for enteral nutrition.

b. Assessment of nutritional status and complications related to PN differ from those associated with enteral nutrition. Table 10-3 provides a suggested nutritional assessment monitoring schedule for infants receiving PN.

TABLE 10-3
Commonly used Commercial Infant Formulas

Product/Calories per Ounce	Manufacturer	Comments
MILK-BASED FORMULAS FOR FULL-TERM INFANTS		
Enfamil with iron, 20	Mead Johnson	Routine feeding for term infants greater than 2000 g.
Enfamil Lipil		Contains essential fatty acids DHA and ARA for early brain and eye development.
Similac with iron, 20	Ross	Routine feeding for term infants greater than 2000 g.
Similac Advance		Contains DHA and ARA.
MILK-BASED FORMULAS FOR PRETERM INFANTS		
Enfamil Premature Lipil, 24 Similac Special Care, 24	Mead Johnson Ross	Growing LBW infant (<2000 g) feeding Increased energy, higher concentration of whey-predominant protein, decreased lactose load, blend of medium-chain triglycerides, higher concentration vitamins, minerals, and trace elements. Contain DHA and ARA.
Neosure Advance, 22 Enfacare, 22	Ross	Growing VLBW (<1500 g) and LBW infant feeding for up to first year of life, posthospital discharge. Increased energy and minerals compared with term but less than preterm infant formulas. Contain DHA and ARA.

Continued

■ TABLE 10-3
■ ■ **Commonly used Commercial Infant Formulas—cont'd**

Product/Calories per Ounce	Manufacturer	Comments
Enfamil Human Milk Fortifier Similac Human Milk Fortifier	Mead Johnson Ross	Powdered human milk fortifiers. Increase caloric, protein, and mineral content. Usual dilution: 4 packages fortifier per 100 ml expressed mother's milk.
Similac Natural Care	Ross	Liquid human milk fortifier. Increases caloric, protein, and mineral content. Designed to be mixed with expressed mother's milk or fed alternatively with breast milk.
SOY-BASED FORMULAS		
Similac Isomil, 20 Similac Isomil Advance, 20 Enfamil Prosobee, 20 Enfamil Prosobee Lipil, 20 Alsoy, 20 i-Soyalac, 20	Ross Ross Mead Johnson Mead Johnson Carnation LomaLinda	Recommended for term infants with IgE-mediated reaction to cow's milk protein, for those with lactase deficiency or galactosemia, and for use by vegetarians. Has been demonstrated to be nutritionally equivalent to milk-based formulas in supporting weight gain. Not recommended for preterm infants born weighing less than 1800 g.
PROTEIN HYDROLYSATE-BASED FORMULAS		
Pregestimil, 20 and 24	Mead Johnson	Indicated for use in infants with cow's milk and soy protein allergies and for those with malabsorption due to gastrointestinal or hepatobiliary disease. Protein, fat, and carbohydrate modified. Iron fortified. Available in powder for easy caloric concentration or as ready to feed.
Alimentum, 20	Ross	Complete elemental formula for infants. Protein, fat, and carbohydrate modified (see Pregestimil).
Nutramigen, 20	Mead Johnson	Protein-modified, lactose-free formula. Indicated for protein allergy or sensitivity, severe or persistent diarrhea. Iron fortified. Available in powder or as ready to feed. Generally not used for preterm infants
AMINO ACID–BASED HYPOALLERGENIC FORMULAS		
Neocate, 20	SHS	Amino acid–based formula for the management of cow's milk allergy, short bowel syndrome, and multiple food protein intolerance. Sucrose-, lactose- and galactose-free.
Elecare, 20	Ross	

Data from American Academy of Pediatrics Committee on Nutrition: *Pediatric nutrition handbook* (4th ed.). Elk Grove Village, IL, 1998, American Academy of Pediatrics; and from manufacturer information brochures from Mead Johnson, Ross, Carnation, SHS, and LomaLinda.

ARA, Arachidonic acid; *DHA,* docosahexaenoic acid; *IgE,* immunoglobulin E; *LBW,* low birth weight; *VLBW,* very low birth weight.

C. Guidelines for determining appropriate intake, compositions of available preparations, and guidelines for IV administration.
  1. Calories. Parenteral requirements are about 20% less than enteral intake, or about 90 kcal/kg/day.
    a. Caloric values must be adjusted to meet activity levels, body temperature, and degree of stress.
    b. Activity and catabolic states can cause a 25% to 75% increase in metabolic demands.
  2. Water.
    a. Minimum requirement approximately 100 to 150 ml/kg/day.
    b. Water requirement varies with gestational and postnatal age and environmental conditions, such as incubator versus radiant heat source and phototherapy. Incubators and heat shields can reduce insensible water losses, whereas radiant warmers and phototherapy increase these losses.
  3. Nutrients (see Table 10-1).
    a. Protein.
      (1) Available preparations:
        (a) Pediatric crystalline amino acid solutions.
          (i) Require no further metabolism before protein utilization.
          (ii) Amount of amino acids needed ranges from 2 to 4 g/kg/day.
        (b) Amino acids (4 kcal/g).
      (2) Formula for calculating amount of protein an infant is receiving: Protein dose = weight (in kilograms) × % amino acid/dl IV fluid × number of 100 ml increments of IV fluid received (LeFrak-Okikawa, 1988).
    b. Fat.
      (1) Available preparations:
        (a) 10% lipid preparations: 1.1 kcal/ml.
        (b) 20% lipid preparations: 2.2 kcal/ml.
        (c) Soybean oil–based lipid emulsions: recommended over safflower oils because of potential risk of development of linolenic acid deficiency and hypertriglyceridemia with safflower oils (Pereira, 1995).
        (d) Lipid emulsions (0.5-1 g/kg/day), for prevention of deficiency of essential fatty acids. For maintenance of energy balance, IV lipid, 0.5 to 1 g/kg/day, should be introduced as component of PN by 24 to 48 hours of age. That dose can be increased by 0.5 to 1 g/kg/day in progressive daily or alternate-day steps, as tolerated, up to 3 g/kg/day, based on serum triglyceride clearance (Van Aerde et al., 1998).
        (e) A 20% lipid emulsion is preferred over a 10% emulsion in neonates. Although both emulsions contain the same amount of phospholipid by volume, the 20% emulsion has less phospholipid per gram of fat. High amounts of phospholipid have been associated with increased triglyceride, cholesterol and low-density lipoprotein levels in neonates (Haumont et al., 1989).
      (2) Guidelines for parenteral fat administration:
        (a) To calculate amount of fat an infant is receiving, use the following formula: Lipid dose = milliliters of fat per day ÷ 10 or 5 ÷ weight (in kilograms) (NOTE: divide by 10 if 10% preparation is used; divide by 5 if 20% preparation is used) (LeFrak-Okikawa, 1988).

(b) Lipid tolerance may be enhanced by adding 1 U heparin per milliliter of infusate (0.5 U/ml for VLBW premature infants). Heparin enhances the release of lipoprotein and hepatic lipases into the circulation (Kilbride et al., 2002).

(c) 20% preparations are commonly used and are generally well tolerated. They are especially useful for infants requiring a great caloric intake but are fluid restricted (e.g., infants with BPD).

c. Carbohydrates.

(1) Carbohydrate source: glucose monohydrate (dextrose), 3.4 kcal/g.

(a) Dextrose preparations are made according to the infant's tolerance.

(b) Standard dextrose concentrations are available in 5% or 10% solutions (percentage: grams of dextrose per deciliter of solution). Other concentrations may be tailored to the individual needs of the infant.

(2) Guidelines for carbohydrate administration:

(a) Glucose infusion rates of 4 to 6 g/kg/day are necessary for minimal caloric intake, protein metabolism, and growth.

(b) Dextrose concentrations may be increased by 1 to 2 mg/kg/minute each day (until the maximal percentage is obtained for the route being used), as long as serum glucose remains at less than 150 mg/dl and urinary glucose at less than 0.5%. The maximal glucose infusion rate is 12 to 14 mg/kg/minute—the rate of glucose oxidation by the liver. Higher rates increase the risk of fatty infiltration of the liver.

(c) In some ELBW infants, severe hyperglycemia may present and continue despite reduced carbohydrate intakes. A continuous insulin infusion may be used. Routine use is NOT advised due to side effects. The usual infusion of insulin is 0.01 to 0.1 unit/kg/hour (Farrag and Cowett, 2000).

d. Calcium and phosphorus.

(1) PN preparations for infants receiving fluids of at least 120 to 150 ml/kg/day should contain 60 to 100 mg of calcium and 43 to 70 mg of phosphorus per kilogram per day (Brandes, 2003).

(2) Because of the precipitation of minerals in parenteral fluids, it is not possible to supply the extremely premature infant with adequate amounts of parenteral calcium and phosphorus to meet in utero fetal accretion rates.

e. Vitamins and minerals (see Table 10-1).

D. Complications associated with PN administration.

1. Potential complications associated with protein administration.

a. Excessive protein intake is associated with metabolic disturbances (hyperammonemia, metabolic acidosis, azotemia, and hyperaminoacidemia).

b. Cholestasis and cholestatic jaundice (direct bilirubin >2 mg/dl) may occur as a result of excessive protein intake or PN for more than 2 weeks. Factors that may increase the risk of cholestasis and jaundice include:

(1) Prolonged periods without enteral feeding and conditions that contribute to ineffective utilization and metabolism of protein.

(2) Hepatitis.

(3) GI surgery.

(4) Viral infections (e.g., infection with cytomegalovirus).

2. Potential complications associated with fat administration.
   a. Inadequate fat intake may lead to deficiency of essential fatty acids and may be evidenced by the following:
      (1) Dry, scaly skin.
      (2) Poor growth.
      (3) Poor platelet aggregation.
      (4) Thrombocytopenia.
      (5) Deficiencies of fat-soluble vitamins.
   b. IV lipids may be contraindicated for infants with severe hyperbilirubinemia because fatty acids compete with bilirubin for binding sites on plasma albumin.
   c. Assessment of triglyceride levels is necessary for all jaundiced infants receiving IV lipids.
3. Potential complications associated with carbohydrate administration.
   a. Hyperosmolarity.
   b. Hyperglycemia (serum glucose >150 mg/dl) or glucosuria (urinary glucose >0.5%); frequently seen in VLBW infants and infants with sepsis.
   c. Hypoglycemia resulting from insufficient glucose administration or excessive insulin administration.
4. Additional complications associated with PN.
   a. Dehydration caused by hyperglycemia.
   b. Vitamin imbalance.
      (1) Vitamin A. In parenteral solutions, decreases significantly within 24 hours because of adherence to infusion-pump tubing and photodegradation (Blackburn, 2003).
      (2) Riboflavin. Destroyed by exposure to light; half may be lost in a 24-hour period, with greater loss during phototherapy.
   c. Inadequate calcium and phosphorus intake, leading to increased risk of rickets.
   d. Trace element deficiency.
   e. Extravasation of IV site, complications related to central lines.
   f. Infection; contributing factors:
      (1) Indwelling venous catheter.
      (2) Preterm infant's limited immunologic response to infection.
      (3) Excellent medium for bacterial and fungal growth provided by lipid preparation.
5. Measures to prevent or minimize complications associated with PN.
   a. Standardized procedures/policies should be developed to facilitate a consistent methodology to prevent and/or minimize complications.
   b. Use volumetric chamber for 4-hour aliquots of PN to avoid overhydration in the event of infusion-pump malfunction.
   c. Record intake and assess IV site hourly.
   d. Readjust fluid volume, dextrose concentration, protein and/or fat intake, and insulin supplementation as soon as problems are identified.
   e. PN should be decreased and enteral feedings initiated to stimulate bile production as soon as possible.
   f. Pharmacy preparation of PN under laminar airflow hood. Nothing should be added to TPN solution once it leaves the pharmacy.
   g. Filter central PN with an in-line filter.
   h. Wash hands scrupulously before handling any PN tubing or IV sites.
   i. Use sterile technique for all dressing changes.

j. If alkaline phosphatase levels exceed 500 mg/dl:
   (1) Verify calcium and phosphorus is maximized.
   (2) Begin enteral feedings as soon as possible.

ENTERAL FEEDINGS: HUMAN MILK AND COMMERCIAL FORMULAS

A. Human milk.

1. Term infants.
   a. Human milk is the ideal food for term and near-term infants.
2. Preterm infants.
   a. Human milk may have to be fortified to provide adequate calories and certain nutrients for preterm infants.
      (1) Human milk alone, both mature and preterm, cannot meet the additional calories, protein, sodium, calcium, and phosphorus for the growing preterm infant. Preterm milk has greater protein (total nitrogen content) content for the first several weeks after birth (Hall and Carroll, 2000; Schanler, 1995).
      (2) Fat, protein, and sodium content of human milk decreases during lactation.
   b. Fortified mother's milk may be the optimal food for preterm infants.
      (1) Commercially prepared human milk fortifiers (Enfamil Human Milk Fortifier, Similac Human Milk Fortifier, Similac Natural Care) enhance protein, calories, vitamin, and mineral content of mother's milk (see Table 10-3).
      (2) Premature infant formulas can also be mixed with human milk as a means of nutrient fortification.
      (3) To minimize fat losses from adherence to infusion tubing, use a short length of tubing, use bolus feeds, and position the syringe upright. The fat will rise to the top of the syringe and be infused first.
3. Advantages of human milk (over formula).
   a. Host resistance factors and antiinfective properties.
   b. Enhanced fat, amino acid, and carbohydrate absorption and digestion compared with cow's milk formula.
   c. Improved gastric emptying with human milk, along with many factors that may stimulate GI growth and motility and enhance maturation of the GI tract.
   d. Very long-chain fatty acids, which may be important for cognition, growth, and vision.
   e. Increased absorption of zinc and iron.
   f. Low renal solute load.
   g. Optimal distribution of calories for term infants: 7% provided as protein, 55% as fat, and 38% as carbohydrate.
   h. Presence of thyroid hormones, which may delay onset of hypothyroidism.
   i. Maternal involvement in care of infant.
   j. Enteromammary immune system. The mother produces secretory IgA antibody after exposure to foreign antigens and is stimulated to make specific antibodies that are then delivered in her milk, which may improve host defenses in her preterm infant in the NICU (Schanler, 1995). Skin-to-skin contact between mother and infant may enhance this activity.
4. Considerations with human milk (compared with formula).
   a. Risk of transmission of infection (e.g., human immunodeficiency virus [HIV], miliary tuberculosis).
   b. Maternal drug use and some maternal medications.

c. Protein, calcium, phosphorus, and some vitamins may need to be supplemented for the growing premature infant.
d. Adequate technique for expression, collection, and storage of milk to prevent bacterial colonization.
5. Establishment and maintenance of adequate milk supply.
 a. Most mothers of preterm or acutely ill infants must establish lactation by expressing milk with a breast pump for several weeks to several months before their infants are able to nurse.
 b. Nurses can play a key role in helping mothers successfully initiate and maintain an adequate supply of milk for their infants.
  (1) A lactation specialist or a breast-feeding support and education group, composed of nurses, physicians, and dietitians, can provide consistent, up-to-date educational and clinical information to staff and families.
  (2) Mothers often need help with obtaining an electric pump for home use, learning how to use the pump, and learning how to collect and store the breast milk. Additionally, mothers need a great deal of ongoing emotional support and follow-up.
  (3) Institutional standards of care for all mothers who wish to breast-feed need to be established, making certain that barriers are not created by policies and attitudes (Meier, 2001).
  (4) The significant benefits of human milk for preterm infants warrant encouraging and actively supporting mothers to pump and provide milk for their infants (Schanler, 1995; Schanler et al., 1999).

B. Commercially prepared formulas (see Table 10-3).

1. Recommendations and standards for commercially prepared formulas were first developed in the 1940s by the U.S. Food and Drug Administration.
2. Soon after, the AAP-CON developed a recommended range of nutrient composition for infant formulas.
3. In 1980 the U.S. Congress passed the Infant Formula Act, which codified the recommendations of AAP-CON and required that all commercially prepared infant formulas meet these standards. The standards were revised in 1986 (AAP-CON, 1998a).
4. Formulas can be classified as milk based, soy based, or elemental (i.e., protein, fat, or carbohydrate modified).
 a. Milk-based formulas.
  (1) Appropriate for most infants.
  (2) Term infant formulas, designed to approximate micronutrient content of human milk.
  (3) Promotes rapid growth during the first 6 months of life similar to human milk.
  (4) Preterm infant formulas.
   (a) Provide added calories, protein, vitamins, and minerals to meet the needs of growing low birth weight infants.
   (b) Modifications in fat, protein, and carbohydrate sources enhance the digestibility and absorption of nutrients for infants with immature GI function (Ernst and Gross, 1998).
    (i) Fat: MCTs (25%-50%), with vegetable oils.
    (ii) Protein: whey 60%, casein 40%, nonfat cow's milk, and demineralized whey.
    (iii) Carbohydrate: reduced amount of lactose (40%-50%) compared with term formulas; glucose polymers (corn syrup solids or hydrolyzed cornstarch) to maintain low osmolality.

b. Soy-based formulas.
   (1) Lactose free.
   (2) Not appropriate for infants less than 1800 g (AAP-CON, 1998b).
   (3) Appropriate for infants with galactosemia.

c. Elemental formulas. Appropriate for infants with:
   (1) Protein (cow's milk and soy) allergy/intolerance.
   (2) Fat malabsorption.

5. Several forms of formula exist, including ready to feed, powdered, and liquid concentrate.
   a. Powdered formula is not recommended for premature infants because it is not sterile.
   b. An association exists between premature infants who received powdered formula and those who are infected with *Enterobacter sakazakii* (www.pediatricnutrition.org).

ENTERAL FEEDING METHODS

Enteral feedings are achieved via several routes, including oral, nasogastric tube, and orogastric tube. The infant's gestational age, clinical condition, and ability to feed orally are factors used to determine the method of enteral feeding (AAP-CON, 1998a).

A. **Minimal enteral feedings or trophic feedings** (before 2 weeks of age) have significant long-term advantages for preterm infants (Berseth, 1995). Minimal enteral or trophic feedings are tube feedings given simultaneously with PN. PN supplies the majority of the infant's nutrient intake and the small-volume enteral feedings stimulate growth and maturation of the GI tract. As such, minimal enteral feedings are used not to provide nutrition but encourage functional development of the gut. Minimal enteral feedings varying from 12 to 24 ml/kg/day result in a shorter time required to achieve full enteral nutrition, a lower incidence of feeding intolerance, and a possible decrease in incidence of necrotizing enterocolitis (Berseth et al., 1995; Berseth et al., 2003; Premji, 1998; Schanler et al., 1999, Tyson and Kennedy, 2001).
   1. Promotion of gut mucosal development.
   2. Stimulation of intestinal motor activity.
   3. Increased secretion of GI hormones and peptides.
   4. Colonization of the gut with normal flora. Normal flora reduce the possibility of translocation of pathogenic bacteria and resulting infection. Human milk stimulates colonization with lactobacilli and *Bifidobacterium*, which limits colonization by other pathogenic organisms.
   5. Improvement in metabolic status.
   6. Reduction in the liver enzyme abnormalities associated with PN methods. Decreases the incidence of cholestasis and lowers serum bilirubin and alkaline phosphatase levels.
   7. May decrease the incidence of NEC (Berseth et al., 2003).
   8. Improvement of lactase activity (Shulman et al., 1998).

B. **When to initiate feedings and what method to use are controversial issues.** Several criteria that are applied in making feeding decisions are as follows:
   1. Episodes of apnea and bradycardia are not necessarily contraindications for enteral feedings, but feedings may need to be postponed or withheld if apnea-bradycardia and/or desaturation episodes become acutely severe or frequent.

2. GI peristalsis must be confirmed and assessed by auscultating bowel sounds, monitoring stooling patterns, and measuring abdominal girth.
3. GI perfusion is decreased with PDA. Feedings may be postponed until PDA is closed.

C. **Oral feedings are initiated after careful assessment.**

1. Indications for oral feedings. Nurses often have input into assessing readiness for oral feedings (Kinneer and Beachy, 1994). How to assess readiness systematically has not been determined, however, and the process of transitioning infants to oral feedings is often not evidence based (Kinneer and Beachy, 1994; McCain et al., 2001; Siddell and Froman, 1994). Additionally, research has demonstrated differences in terms of successful breast-feeding vs. bottle feeding, with competency in breast-feeding occurring at a younger postconceptional age than in bottle feeding (Meier et al., 1993). Consequently there is great variation in oral feeding practices across the United States. Gestational age and weight are traditional criteria used to determine readiness for oral feedings, with behavioral cues more recently included as criteria. One published care map includes evaluation of oral motor readiness at 32 to 34 weeks' postconceptional age (Tobin et al., 1998).
   a. Infant should be free of signs and/or symptoms of respiratory distress (e.g., respiratory rate <60 breaths per minute; blood gas values within normal limits); clinicians may modify these criteria for infants with chronic lung disease.
   b. Infant demonstrates suck-swallow-breathe coordination with an intact gag reflex (Shaker, 1990). Sucking and swallowing appear to be coordinated by approximately 32 to 34 weeks' gestation, but the ability to suck, swallow, and breathe may not be well coordinated until an infant reaches 37 weeks' gestation (Bu'Lock et al., 1990). All infants need to be assessed individually.
   c. Neonatal behavioral profile that is predictive of oral feeding success does not exist; however, assessment of infant behavioral cues and status and provision of individualized developmental care have been demonstrated to facilitate the transition to oral feeding (Als et al., 1994; Anderson et al., 1990; McCain, 1995; McCain et al., 2001). Infant sucking behaviors, such as on fingers and pacifiers, are also reportedly used by nurses to assess readiness for oral feeding (Siddell and Froman, 1994).
2. Oral feeding routine.
   a. Oral feedings are the feeding method of choice for most infants born at greater than 34 weeks' gestation.
   b. A healthy infant born at more than 34 weeks' gestation may have feedings initiated as soon after birth as indicated. Factors to be considered include infant behavior, maternal preference for breast-feeding or bottle feeding, and results of hypoglycemia screening of infants who are SGA or large for gestational age (LGA) or whose mothers are diabetic.
   c. For infants born at 32 to 34 weeks' gestation and/or infants who are in transition from gastric gavage (bolus) feeding:
      (1) Feedings should be offered as oral feedings in a progressive fashion; use of infant state assessment has been shown to facilitate semi-on-demand feedings with more rapid progression to full feedings (McCain et al., 2001).
      (2) Careful monitoring must take place during feedings to ensure safe intake without complications of aspiration, desaturation (or increased

requirement for fractional inspired oxygen), apnea, and bradycardia. Such complications have been reported to occur less frequently during breast-feeding than bottle feeding (Meier and Pugh, 1985; Meier et al., 1993).

3. Advantages of oral feeding.
   a. Facilitates the infant's total digestive capacity.
   b. Allows the infant to self-regulate feeding.
   c. Social behavior states of infants are promoted, especially when there is parental involvement.
   d. Complications of indwelling feeding tubes (e.g., perforation) are avoided.
   e. Parents are not forced to adapt to an invasive care routine in the home setting.
4. Disadvantages of oral feeding.
   a. May be associated with an exaggerated vagal response in preterm infants who are in transition from gavage to bottle feedings.
   b. Increased risk of aspiration in infants who do not coordinate sucking, swallowing, and breathing during oral feeding.
5. Disadvantage of bottle feeding: greater decrease in infant oxygenation during and after feeding, in comparison with breast-feeding (Meier, 1988; Meier and Anderson, 1987).
6. Technique for putting preterm infants to breast.
   a. Preterm infants have been able to breast-feed successfully as early as 32 weeks' gestation and may establish mature suck-swallow-breathe coordination earlier with breast-feeding than with bottle feeding (Meier, 1991).
   b. Breast-feeding may be less physiologically stressful to preterm infants than bottle feeding (Meier, 1988; Meier, 2001; Meier and Anderson, 1987). This may be related to the intermittent nature of breast-feeding, which permits an intermittent sucking pattern and better regulation of breathing in the preterm infant (Shiao, 1997).
   c. Test-weighing of infants (before and after breast-feeding) with an electronic scale has been shown to be a reliable method of determining infant intake of human milk from the breast (Meier et al., 1990).

D. Gavage feedings.

1. Enteral feeding of infants born at less than 32 weeks' gestation and infants who are unable to feed orally with safety.
2. Orogastric versus nasogastric gavage feedings. Four studies suggest that the use of indwelling nasogastric tubes results in respiratory compromise in VLBW preterm infants (Greenspan et al., 1990; Shiao, 1997; Shiao et al., 1995; Van Someren et al., 1984). Shiao and colleagues (1995) reported lower minute ventilation and tidal volume, in addition to lower oxygen saturation, pulse rate, and less forceful sucking during attempts at oral feedings with the tube in place.
3. PN, if necessary, to supplement enteral intake when feedings are being initiated.
4. Intermittent intragastric gavage feeding routine.
   a. A size 5F to 8F feeding tube is inserted by a standard measuring technique: from the nose to the ear to the lower end of the sternum and adding 1 cm, or from the ear to the nose to a point midway between the xiphoid process and the umbilicus (Weibley et al., 1987). Orogastric tube measurement is from the mouth to the ear to the lower end of the sternum (Anderson et al., 2002). Size 5F is desirable for nasally placed tubes (Lefrak-Okikawa and Meier, 1993).

b. The tube should be secured in place with tape.
c. Proper placement should be assessed after insertion and before each feeding, or at predetermined intervals for infants receiving continuous feedings.
d. A polyvinyl chloride (PVC) tube may be left in place for 24 to 72 hours or may be removed after each feeding, depending on clinical preferences and manufacturers' recommendations. Long-term polyurethane nasal feeding tubes should be discarded/replaced after 4 weeks or as per manufacturer's instructions (Anderson et al., 2002), or if placed nasally, changed to the opposite nare weekly.
e. Most nurses check for residual before each feeding; however, practice regarding refeeding or not refeeding is inconsistent (Hill and Rath, 1993; Hodges and Vincent, 1993). Residuals of 2 to 4 ml/kg or a 1-hour volume if the infant is on continuous feedings are considered normal and should generally be returned to the infant (Anderson et al., 2002). If the residuals are routinely discarded, monitor the infant for signs and symptoms of electrolyte imbalance and metabolic complications (Premji, 1998).
f. Administer feedings by gravity or pump within 15 to 30 minutes; gravity allows for a natural "burp" through the tube and avoids direct, forceful pressure into the GI tract.
g. During a feeding the infant should be observed for intolerance and complications (e.g., oxygen desaturation, emesis, bradycardia, apnea).
h. Nonnutritive sucking on a pacifier should be offered during the feeding (Bernbaum et al., 1983; Measel and Anderson, 1979).
i. After a feeding the tube should be cleared with air or sterile water and then capped off to air. A tube that is to be removed after each feeding is removed by pinching it off and withdrawing it quickly.

5. Possible indications for continuous gavage feedings (at least one randomized controlled clinical trial has demonstrated that bolus feedings are associated with less feeding intolerance and better weight gain) (Schanler et al., 1999).
   a. VLBW infants whose gastric capacity is limited, infants receiving minimal enteral feedings, and infants who require a steady influx of glucose (e.g., infant with severe hypoglycemia and diabetic mother).
   b. Infants with malabsorptive syndromes (e.g., short bowel syndrome, post-NEC, neonatal abstinence syndrome).
   c. Severe gastroesophageal reflux.
6. Continuous nasogastric feeding routine.
   a. See previous discussion in section 4, "Intermittent intragastric gavage feeding routine," items a. through f; p. 226-227.
   b. A 4-hour feeding volume should be aseptically prepared and purged through the appropriate infusion-pump tubing. (Syringe infusion pumps are recommended because of their low priming volume and low cost.) Nurses must be vigilant in avoiding inadvertent infusion into an IV site.
   c. For human milk feedings, infusion-pump tubing should be changed every 4 hours (i.e., with each 4-hour feeding volume setup) to eliminate exponential bacterial growth in expressed mother's milk (Lefrak-Okikawa and Meier, 1993; Lemons et al., 1983; Meier and Brown, 1996). Placing the pump so that the syringe is vertical, with the tubing coming from the top and below level of the infant, will facilitate improved fat delivery because fat rises to the surface of the milk (Schanler, 1995).

d. After insertion, taping, and assessment for proper placement, the infant's feeding tube is connected to the infusion-pump tubing.
e. The infusion pump is programmed to deliver the appropriate volume to the infant at the appropriate rate.
f. Hourly enteral feeding intake should be recorded.
g. Assess every 2 to 4 hours (Norris and Steinhorn, 1994):
(1) Gastric residuals may be normal if there are no other signs of feeding intolerance.
(2) Abdominal girth.
(3) Bowel sounds. Hyperactive bowel sounds may indicate intolerance.
(4) Infant's behavior. Agitation may indicate abdominal discomfort.

7. Advantages of gavage feedings. Infants who are unable to feed orally with safety are given the benefits of enteral nutrition (e.g., stimulation of bile flow and feeding-induced hormones, improved weight gain).
8. Disadvantages of gavage feedings.
a. Possible bacterial inoculation of the GI tract via feeding tube and milk.
b. Potential risks associated with improper placement of feeding tube.
c. No possibility of self-regulated feeding.
d. Limited parental involvement in some nursery settings.
9. Disadvantages of continuous (vs. intermittent) gavage feedings.
a. Higher risk of aspiration when infant is unattended.
b. Gastric readiness for bolus feedings not promoted (i.e., stomach capacity remains small).
c. Alteration of enteric gut hormone secretion because cyclic surges in gut hormones are not accommodated.
d. Takes longer to reach full feeds (Premji and Chessell, 2001).
e. Higher incidence of feeding intolerance.
10. Possible disadvantages of intermittent bolus gavage feedings.
a. Impaired pulmonary function after feeding (Blondheim et al., 1993).
b. Decreased mean cerebral blood flow velocity (Nelle et al., 1997).
11. Note of caution: Infants must be observed individually for subtle physiologic changes during feedings.

E. **Transpyloric feedings.**
1. Not recommended for routine use because feedings bypass the stomach and may result in fat malabsorption (Pereira, 1995).
2. Transpyloric feedings are associated with greater risks and no identifiable benefits of growth rate (McGuire and McEwan, 2003).
3. Recommended for infants who are at great risk of aspiration (e.g., infants with severe gastroesophageal reflux). Risk is minimized because the end of the tube is located beyond the pyloric sphincter.
4. Transpyloric feeding routine.
a. Nasojejunal tube (Silastic or polyurethane) is inserted by using a standard measuring technique (i.e., from the tip of the infant's nose to the knee).
b. Placement is assessed by checking pH of aspirated fluid (pH of 5-7 indicates transpyloric placement). X-ray confirmation may also be indicated (Hill and Rath, 1993).
c. Infusion pump and tubing should be prepared and connected to the feeding tube as outlined previously in section D, "Gavage feedings," subsection 4, a-i, p. 226-227. "Intermittent intragastric gavage feeding routine." Transpyloric feedings are administered only continuously and deliver a small volume to the narrow lumen of the duodenum or jejunum (AAP-CON, 1998a).

5. Advantage of transpyloric (vs. gastric gavage) feedings: potentially less chance of aspiration because feedings are administered below the pyloric sphincter.
6. Disadvantages of transpyloric (vs. gastric) feedings.
   a. Increased risk of intestinal perforation from the tubing, although this risk is reduced with the use of silicone tubes, which are soft (AAP-CON, 1998a; Hill and Rath, 1993).
   b. May require tube verification by x-ray examination, as well as increased nursing time to place the tube; both are costly.
   c. May induce symptoms of fat malabsorption (i.e., frequent stooling and increased excretion of fat and potassium) because the stomach enzymes are not able to aid in the digestive process.
   d. Increased mortality (McGuire and McEwan, 2003).

F. **Gastrostomy feedings.**
1. Indications for gastrostomy feedings.
   a. Congenital anomalies of the GI tract requiring surgical intervention.
   b. Inability to suck and swallow (e.g., because of severe neurologic insult).
   c. Need for long-term gavage feedings.
2. Gastrostomy feeding routine.
   a. Residuals are assessed before each feeding by unclamping and lowering the gastrostomy tube or by aspirating gastric contents.
   b. Feedings are administered by gravity or pump for 15 to 30 minutes or may be delivered by continuous drip or infusion.
   c. Tube should be cleared with water or air after feeding is finished.
   d. Tube may be left unclamped after feedings at a level of 10 to 12 cm above the patient for "burping" or clamped after feeding, depending on infant's tolerance and comfort.
   e. Tube migration should be evaluated with any sign of feeding intolerance.
   f. Gastrostomy site should be assessed regularly for leakage around the tube and cleaned daily.
3. Advantages of gastrostomy feedings.
   a. Maintenance of enteral feedings if oral or gavage routes are not feasible (e.g., esophageal atresia, feeding disorder).
   b. More comfortable feeding method than gavage feedings for infants with long-term oral feeding problems.
4. Disadvantages of gastrostomy feedings.
   a. Infant may not be provided with the opportunity to develop suck-swallow-breathe coordination and oral motor development. Nonnutritive sucking and introduction of oral feedings as indicated permits development.
   b. See previous discussion in section D, "Gavage feedings," subsection 8, "Disadvantages of gavage feedings," items a. through d, p. 228.

NUTRITIONAL ASSESSMENT

A. **Anthropometric measurements.**
1. Monitor at following intervals:
   a. Weight: daily during acute phase, unless condition is too medically unstable. Infant may be weighed less frequently toward end of hospitalization.
   b. Length and head circumference: weekly.
2. Plot weight, head circumference, and length on growth curves weekly.

3. Monitor intake.
   a. Fluid, protein, and caloric intake should be calculated daily.
   b. Laboratory values should be monitored at regular intervals (Berry et al., 2002). Growing preterm infants may require weekly measurement of electrolytes, calcium, phosphorus, total protein, albumin, and hemoglobin, and twice-monthly measurement of alkaline phosphatase activity. (See Table 10-4 for suggested laboratory monitoring while the infant is receiving PN.)

B. **Feeding tolerance.**
   1. Premature infants are at risk of having a variety of problems related to enteral feedings as a result of the physiologic limitations of the preterm infant's GI tract (see "Anatomy and Physiology of the Preterm Infant's Gastrointestinal Tract" at the beginning of this chapter).

TABLE 10-4
Sample Monitoring Schedule for Infants Receiving Parenteral Nutrition

Parameter	Initial	Daily	Weekly	As Needed
ANTHROPOMETRIC				
Weight	X	X		
Length	X		X*	
Head circumference	X		X*	
Metabolic (blood or plasma)				
Sodium/potassium/chloride	X		X†	
Bicarbonate	X		X†	
Glucose	X		X†	
BUN/creatinine	X		X†	
Calcium/phosphorus	X		X†	
Magnesium	X		X	
Triglycerides	X		X‡	
Albumin/total protein	X		X	
Liver function studies (include SGPT and alk phos)	X		X	
Bilirubin (total and direct)	X		X	
Hgb/Hct	X		X	X
Platelets, PT, PTT	X			X
WBC count and differential				X
Prealbumin				X
Copper/zinc				X
Iron studies				X
Ammonia				X
Vitamin E				X
pH				X
Cultures				X
URINE				
Glucose	X	X		X
Ketones	X	X		X

From Groh-Wargo S, Thompson M, Cox JH, eds. *Nutritional care for high-risk newborns.* Chicago, Ill, 2000, Precept Press; 101.

*Until 3 months corrected age, then monthly thereafter.

†Daily until stable, then twice weekly.

‡Initially and before each IV lipid increase. Once IV lipids are maximized, weekly determinations are adequate. If an infant becomes septic, a triglyceride level should be assessed, since lipid intolerance is often present during sepsis.

2. During the initiation of feedings and until full feedings are maintained and well tolerated, the nurse should assess the following before each feeding or every 2 to 4 hours during continuous feedings:
   a. Presence of bowel sounds.
   b. Correct placement of gastric or transpyloric tube, if present (see previous sections on gavage and transpyloric feeding methods, p. 226-227).
   c. Gastric residuals.
   d. Abdominal girth measurement: compare with previous measurements.
   e. Observation of distended bowel loops on abdominal surface.
3. Frequency, amount, and consistency of stools must be noted with each stool and documented.
   a. Slow GI motility may lead to constipation and result in gastric distention, gastric residual, and possibly vomiting.
   b. Glycerin suppositories may be needed to facilitate stooling.
4. Periodically stools may be checked for occult blood once feedings are started; however, there is no data that demonstrates routine use of this test is predictive of NEC or decreases the disease severity (Pinheiro et al., 2003).
   a. If result of test for occult blood is positive, further evaluation is needed. Occult blood may be present if maternal blood was swallowed, if meconium stools are still being passed, after esophageal or gastric irritation from feeding tubes, and if infant has rectal fissures.
   b. Reducing substance in stools may signify carbohydrate malabsorption but may also be a normal finding in infants who are breast-fed.
      (1) Results of tests for reducing substance are accurate only when fresh stool is used because bacteria in stool decrease the sugar content within minutes.
      (2) Carbohydrate malabsorption has been detected in infants with NEC and may represent an early predictor of the infant's risk of NEC.
         (a) In tests for reducing substances with a Clinitest tablet, a finding of 3+ for three consecutive stools is significant (LaGamma and Browne, 1994).
         (b) In the absence of significant indicators of NEC, a reduction in the concentration of carbohydrate or in feeding volumes may alleviate the problem until GI function matures.

NURSING INTERVENTIONS TO FACILITATE TOLERANCE OF ENTERAL FEEDINGS

A. Nonnutritive sucking during gavage feedings (Medoff-Cooper and Ray, 1995).
   1. May accelerate maturation of the sucking reflex and facilitate more rapid transition from gavage to oral feedings.
   2. May improve weight gain.
   3. Lessens behavioral distress caused by stressors (DiPietro et al., 1994).
   4. Results in pleasurable facial and oral stimulation (e.g., firm facial stroking during bathing and after tube changes can help to decrease oral defensiveness) (Cox, 1997).

B. Position of infant during and after feedings.
   1. Position achieved by elevating the head of the bed by 30 degrees may lessen gastric emptying time.

C. Assessment of infant readiness (state) before or during feedings.
   1. May enhance infant feeding.
   2. Promotes infant behavior conducive to social interaction.

REFERENCES

Als, H., Lawhon, G., Duffy, F., et al.: Individualized developmental care for the very low-birth-weight preterm infant: Medical and neurofunctional effects. *Journal of the American Medical Association, 272*(11):853-858, 1994.

American Academy of Pediatrics Committee on Nutrition: *Pediatric nutrition handbook* (4th ed.). Elk Grove Village, IL, 1998a, the Academy.

American Academy of Pediatrics Committee on Nutrition: Soy protein-based formulas: Recommendations for use in infant feeding. *Pediatrics, 101*:148-153, 1998b.

American Academy of Pediatrics Committee on Nutrition: Prevention of rickets and vitamin D deficiency: New guidelines for vitamin D intake. *Pediatrics, 111*(4 Pt 1): 908-910, 2003.

American Academy of Pediatrics Workgroup on Breastfeeding. Breastfeeding and the use of human milk. *Pediatrics, 100*(6):1035-1039, 1997.

Anderson, G.C., Behnke, M., Gill, N.E., et al.: Self-regulatory gavage to bottle feeding for preterm infants: Effect on behavioral state, energy expenditure, and weight gain. In S.G. Funk, E.M. Tornquist, M.T. Champagne, et al. (Eds.): *Key aspects of recovery: Nutrition, rest, and mobility*. New York, 1990, Springer, pp. 83-97.

Anderson, M.S., Johnson, C.B., Townsend, S.F., and Hay, W.W.: Enteral nutrition. In G.B. Merenstein and S.L. Gardner (Eds.): *Handbook of neonatal intensive care* (5th ed.). St Louis, 2002, Mosby, pp. 314-340.

Bernbaum, J.C., Pereira, G.R., Watkins, J.B., and Peckham, G.: Nonnutritive sucking during gavage feeding enhances growth and maturation in preterm infants. *Pediatrics, 71*(1):41-45, 1983.

Berry, D.B., Adcock, E.W., and Starbuck, A.: Fluid and electrolyte management. In G.B. Merenstein and S.L. Gardner (Eds.): *Handbook of neonatal intensive care* (5th ed.). St Louis, 2002, Mosby, pp. 283-298.

Berseth, C.: Minimal enteral feedings. *Clinics in Perinatology, 22*(1):195-205, 1995.

Berseth, C.: Gastrointestinal motility in the neonate. *Clinics in Perinatology, 23*(2): 179-190, 1996.

Berseth, C., Bisquera J.A., and Paje, V.U.: Prolonging small feeding volumes early in life decreases the incidence of necrotizing enterocolitis in very low birth weight infants. *Pediatrics, 111*(3):529-534, 2003.

Blackburn, S.: *Maternal, fetal, and neonatal physiology: A clinical perspective* (2nd ed.). Philadelphia, 2003, W.B. Saunders.

Blondheim, O., Abbasi, S., Fox, W., and Bhuthani, V.: Effect of enteral gavage feeding rate on pulmonary functions of very low birth weight infants. *Journal of Pediatrics, 122*(5 Pt 1):751-755, 1993.

Brandes, A.: Nutrition management of the preterm infant. In N.L. Nevin-Folino (Ed.): *Pediatric manual of clinical dietetics* (2nd ed.). Chicago, 2003, American Dietetic Association, pp. 515-527.

Bu'Lock, F., Woolridge, M.W., and Baum, J.D.: Development of coordination of sucking, swallowing and breathing: Ultrasound study of term and preterm infants. *Developmental Medicine and Child Neurology, 32*(8):669-678, 1990.

Carver, J.D. and Barness, L.A.: Trophic factors for the gastrointestinal tract. *Clinics in Perinatology, 23*(2):265-285, 1996.

Carver, J.D., Wu, P.Y., Hall, R.T., et al.: Growth of preterm infants fed nutrient-enriched or term formula after hospital discharge. *Pediatrics, 107*(4):683-689, 2001.

Chathas, M.K. and Paton, J.B.: Meeting the special nutritional needs of sick infants with a percutaneous central venous catheter quality assurance program. *Journal of Perinatal and Neonatal Nursing, 10*(4):72-87, 1997.

Cox, J.H.: Bronchopulmonary dysplasia. In J. Cox (Ed.): *Nutrition manual for at-risk infants and toddlers*. Chicago, 1997, Precept Press, pp. 158-166.

DiPietro, J., Cusson, R., Caughy, M., and Fox, N.: Behavioral and physiologic effects of nonnutritive sucking during gavage feeding in preterm infants. *Pediatric Research, 36*(2):207-214, 1994.

Ehrenkranz, R.A., Younes, N., Lemons, J.A., et al.: Longitudinal growth of hospitalized very low birth weight infants. *Pediatrics, 104*(2 Pt 1):280-289, 1999.

Ernst, J. and Gross, S.: Types and methods of feeding for infants. In R. Polin and W. Fox (Eds.): *Fetal and neonatal physiology*

(2nd ed.). Philadelphia, 1998, W.B. Saunders, pp. 363-383.

Farrag, H.M. and Cowett, R.M.: Glucose homeostasis in the micropremie. *Clinics in Perinatology, 27*(1):1-22, 2000.

Frentner, S.: Metabolic bone disease. *Central Lines, 11*:1, 4, 16, 1995.

Greenspan, J., Wolfson, M., Holt, W., and Shaffer, T.: Neonatal gastric intubation: Differential respiratory effects between nasogastric and orogastric tubes. *Pediatric Pulmonology, 8*(4):254-258, 1990.

Hall, R.T. and Carroll, R.E.: Infant feeding. *Pediatrics in Review, 21*(6):191-199, 2000.

Hamosh, M.: Digestion in the newborn. *Clinics in Perinatology, 23*(2):191-209, 1996.

Hamosh, M.: Bioactive factors in human milk. *Pediatric Clinics of North America, 48*(1):69-86, 2001.

Haumont, D., Deckelbaum, R.J., Richelle, M., et al.: Plasma lipid and plasma lipoprotein concentrations in low birth weight infants given parenteral nutrition with twenty or ten percent lipid emulsion. *Journal of Pediatrics, 115*(5 Pt 1):787-793, 1989.

Heird, W.C., Prager, T.C., and Anderson, R.E.: Docosahexaenoic acid and the development and function of the infant retina. *Current Opinion in Lipidology, 8*(1):12-16, 1997.

Hill, A. and Rath, L.: The care and feeding of the low-birth-weight infant. *Journal of Perinatal and Neonatal Nursing, 6*:56-68, 1993.

Hodges, C. and Vincent, P.A.: Why do NICU nurses not refeed gastric residuals prior to feeding by gavage? *Neonatal Network, 12*(8):37-40, 1993.

Innis, S.: Fat. In R.C. Tsang, A. Lucas, R. Uauy, and S. Zlotkin (Eds.): *Nutritional needs of the preterm infant: Scientific basis and practical guidelines*. Baltimore, 1993, Williams & Wilkins, pp. 65-86.

Innis, S.M., Adamkin, D.H., Hall, R.T., et al.: Docosahexaenoic acid and arachidonic acid enhance growth with no adverse effects in preterm infants fed formula. *Journal of Pediatrics, 140*(5):547-554, 2002.

Kien, C.L.: Digestion, absorption, and fermentation of carbohydrates in the newborn. *Clinics in Perinatology, 23*(2): 211-228, 1996.

Kilbride, H.W., Leick-Rude, M.K., and Allen, N.H.: Total parenteral nutrition. In G.B. Merenstein and S.L. Gardner (Eds.): *Handbook of neonatal intensive care* (5th ed.). St Louis, 2002, Mosby, pp. 341-357.

Kinneer, M. and Beachy, P.: Nipple feeding premature infants in the neonatal intensive-care unit. *Journal of Obstetric, Gynecologic, and Neonatal Nursing, 23*(2):105-112, 1994.

LaGamma, E.F. and Browne, L.E.: Feeding practices for infants weighing less than 1500 g at birth and the pathogenesis of necrotizing enterocolitis. *Clinics in Perinatology, 21*(2):271-306, 1994.

Lebenthal, A. and Lebenthal, E.: The ontology of the small intestinal epithelium. *Journal of Parenteral and Enteral Nutrition, 23*(5 Suppl):S3-S6, 1999.

Lefrak-Okikawa, L.: Nutritional management of the very low birth weight infant. *Journal of Perinatal and Neonatal Nursing, 2*(1):66-77, 1988.

Lefrak-Okikawa, L. and Meier, P.: Nutrition: Physiologic basis of metabolism and management of enteral and parenteral nutrition. In C. Kenner, A. Brueggemeyer, and L. Gunderson (Eds.): *Comprehensive neonatal nursing*. Philadelphia, 1993, W.B. Saunders, pp. 414-433.

Lemons, P.M., Miller, K., Eitzen, H., et al.: Bacterial growth in human milk during continous feeding. *American Journal of Perinatology, 1*(1):76-80, 1983.

Lucas, A., Bishop, N.J., King, F.J, and Cole, T.J.: Randomised trial of nutrition for preterm infants after discharge. *Archives of Disease in Childhood, 67*(3):324-327, 1992.

Macdonald, P.D., Skeoch, C.H., Carse, H., et al.: Randomised trial of continuous nasogastric, bolus nasogastric, and transpyloric feeding in infants of birth weight under 1400 g. *Archives of Disease in Childhood, 67*(4 Spec No.):429-431, 1992.

McCain, G.C.: Promotion of preterm infant nipple feeding with nonnutritive sucking. *Journal of Pediatric Nursing, 10*(1):3-8, 1995.

McCain, G.C., Gartside, P.S., Greenberg, J.M., and Lott, J.W.: A feeding protocol for healthy preterm infants that shortens time to oral feeding. *Journal of Pediatrics, 139*(3):374-379, 2001.

McGuire, W. and McEwan, P.: Transpyloric versus gastric tube feeding for preterm infants (Cochrane Review). In: *The Cochrane Library*, Issue 2, 2003. Oxford: Update Software.

Measel, C.P. and Anderson, G.C.: Nonnutritive sucking during tube feedings: Effect on clinical course in premature infants. *Journal of Obstetric, Gynecologic, and Neonatal Nursing, 8*:265-272, 1979.

Medoff-Cooper, B. and Ray, W.: Neonatal sucking behaviors: State of the science. *Image*, *27*(3):195-200, 1995.

Meier, P.: Bottle and breastfeeding: Effects on transcutaneous oxygen pressure and temperature in preterm infants. *Nursing Research*, *37*(1):36-41, 1988.

Meier, P.: Nursing management of breastfeeding for preterm infants. In S.G. Funk, E.M. Tornquist, M.T. Champagne, et al.: (Eds.): *Key aspects of recovery: Nutrition, rest, and mobility*. New York, 1990, Springer.

Meier, P.: Breast feeding the premature infant. Clinical Update '91: Gastrointestinal Dysfunction. Denver, Conference of the National Association of Neonatal Nurses, 1991.

Meier, P. and Anderson, G.C.: Responses of small preterm infants to bottle- and breast-feeding. *American Journal of Maternal-Child Nursing*, *12*(2):97-105, 1987.

Meier, P. and Brown, L.: State of the science: Breastfeeding for mothers and low birth weight infants. *Nursing Clinics of North America*, *31*(2):351-365, 1996.

Meier, P., de Monterice, D., Crichton, C., and Mangurten, H.: Suck-breath patterning during breast and bottle feeding for preterm infants. Symposium presentation in Medoff-Cooper, B. (Chair): Toward an objective measure of feeding readiness in preterm infants. Proceedings of ANA Council of Nurse Researchers: 1993 Scientific Session (p. 462). Washington, DC, American Nurses Association, 1993.

Meier, P. and Pugh, E.J.: Breastfeeding behavior of small preterm infants. *MCN American Journal of Maternal-Child Nursing*, *10*(6):396-401, 1985.

Meier, P.P.: Part 2: The management of breastfeeding; breastfeeding in the special care nursery. *Pediatric Clinics of North America*, *48*(2): 425-442, 2001.

Meier, P.P., Lysakowski, T.Y., Engstrom, J.L., et al.: The accuracy of test-weighing for preterm infants. *Journal of Pediatric Gastroenterology and Nutrition*, *10*(1):62-65, 1990.

Micheli, J.-L. and Schutz, Y.: Protein. In R.C. Tsang, A. Lucas, R. Uauy, and S. Zlotkin (Eds.): *Nutritional needs of the preterm infant: Scientific basis and practical guidelines*. Baltimore, 1993, Williams & Wilkins, pp. 29-46.

Moran, J.R. and Greene, H.L.: Vitamin requirements. In R. Polin and W. Fox (Eds.): *Fetal and neonatal physiology* (2nd ed.). Philadelphia, 1998, W.B. Saunders, pp. 344-353.

Nelle, M., Hoecker, C., and Linderkamp, O.: Effects of bolus tube feeding on cerebral blood flow velocity in neonates. *Archives of Disease in Childhood, Fetal Neonatal Edition*, *76*(1):F54-F56, 1997.

Neu, J. and Koldovsky, O.: Nutrient absorption in the preterm neonate. *Clinics in Perinatology*, *23*(2):229-243, 1996.

Norris, M.K. and Steinhorn, D.M.: Nutritional management during critical illness in infants and children. *AACN Clinical Issues*, *5*(4):485-492, 1994.

Oh, W.: Fluid, electrolyte and acid-base homeostasis. In A.A. Fanaroff and R.J.Martin (Eds.): *Neonatal-perinatal medicine: Diseases of the fetus and infant* (6th ed.). St Louis, 1997, Mosby.

Orth, A.M.: Dental health. In J.A. Fox (Ed.): *Primary health care of children*. St Louis, 1997, Mosby, pp. 235-243.

Pereira, G.: Nutritional care of the extremely premature infant. *Clinics in Perinatology*, *22*(1):61-75, 1995.

Pinheiro J.M., Clark, D.A., and Benjamini, K.G.: A critical analysis of the routine testing of newborn stools for occult blood and reducing substances. *Adv Neonatal Care*, 3(3):133-138, 2003.

Poindexter, B.B., Ehrenkranz, R.A., Stoll, B.J., et al.: Effect of parenteral glutamine supplementation on plasma amino acid concentration in extremely low birth weight infants. *American Journal of Clinical Nutrition*, *77(3)*:737-743, 2003.

Premji, S.: Ontogeny of the gastrointestinal system and its impact on feeding the preterm infant. *Neonatal Network*, *17*(2):17-24, 1998.

Premji, S. and Chessell, L.: Continuous nasogastric milk feeding versus intermittent bolus milk feedings for premature infants less than 1500 grams (Cochrane Review). In *The Cochrane Library*, Issue 1, 2001. Oxford: Update Software.

Putet, G.: Energy. In R.C. Tsang, A. Lucas, R. Uauy, and S. Zlotkin (Eds.): *Nutritional needs of the preterm infant: Scientific basis and practical guidelines*. Baltimore, 1993, Williams & Wilkins, pp. 15-28.

Rivera, A., Bell, E.F., and Bier, D.M.: Effect of intravenous amino acids on protein metabolism of preterm infants during the first three days of life. *Pediatric Research*, *33*(2):106-111, 1993.

Schanler, R.: Suitability of human milk for the low birthweight infant. *Clinics in Perinatology, 22*(1):207-222, 1995.

Schanler R.J., Shulman R.J., Lau C., et al.: Feeding strategies for premature infants: randomized trial of gastrointestinal priming and tube-feeding method. *Pediatrics, 103*(2):434-439, 1999.

Shaffer, S. and Weismann, D.: Fluid requirements in the preterm infant. *Clinics in Perinatology, 19*(1):233-250, 1992.

Shaker, C.S.: Nipple feeding premature infants: A different perspective. *Neonatal Network, 8*(5):9-17, 1990.

Shenai, J.: Vitamin A. In R.C. Tsang, A. Lucas, R. Uauy, and S. Zlotkin (Eds.): *Nutritional needs of the preterm infant: Scientific basis and practical guidelines.* Baltimore, 1993, Williams & Wilkins, pp. 87-100.

Shiao, S.-Y.: Comparison of continuous versus intermittent sucking in very-low-birth-weight infants. *Journal of Obstetric, Gynecologic, and Neonatal Nursing, 26*(3):313-319, 1997.

Shiao, S.-Y., Youngblut, J.M., Anderson, G.C., et al.: Nasogastric tube placement: Effects on breathing and sucking in very-low-birth-weight infants. *Nursing Research, 44*(2):82-88, 1995.

Shulman, R.J., Schanler, R.J., Lau, C., et al.: Early feeding, feeding tolerance, and lactase activity in preterm infants. *Journal of Pediatrics, 133*(5):645-649, 1998.

Siddell, E. and Froman, R.: A national survey of neonatal intensive-care units: Criteria used to determine readiness for oral feedings. *Journal of Obstetric, Gynecologic, and Neonatal Nursing, 23*(9):783-789, 1994.

Simpson, C., Schandler, R.J., and Lau, C.: Early introduction of oral feeding in preterm infants. *Pediatrics, 110*(3):517-522, 2002.

Slusser, W. and Powers, N.: Breastfeeding update. Part 1. Immunology, nutrition, and advocacy. *Pediatrics in Review, 18*(4):111-119, 1997.

Thureen, P. and Hay, W.: Conditions requiring special nutritional management. In R.C. Tsang, A. Lucas, R. Uauy, and S. Zlotkin (Eds.): *Nutritional needs of the preterm infant: Scientific basis and practical guidelines.* Baltimore, 1993, Williams & Wilkins, pp. 243-265.

Thureen, P., Melara, D., Fennessey, P., and Hay, W.: Effect of low versus high intravenous amino acid intake on very low birth weight infants in the early neonatal period. *Pediatric Research, 53*(1): 24-32, 2000.

Tobin, C.R., Sabatte, E., Sandhu, A.S., and Penafiel, E.: A neonatal care map based on gestational age. *Neonatal Network, 17*(2):41-51, 1998.

Tsang, R., Lucas, A., Uauy, R., and Zlotkins, S.: *Nutritional needs of the preterm infant: Scientific basis and practical guidelines.* Baltimore, 1993, Williams & Wilkins.

Tyson J.E. and Kennedy K.A.: Minimal enteral nutrition for promoting feeding tolerance and preventing morbidity in parenterally fed infants (Cochrane Review). In *The Cochrane Library,* Issue 1, 2001. Oxford: Update Software.

Tyson, J.E., Wright, L.L., Oh, W., et al.: Vitamin A supplementation for extremely low birth weight infants. *New England Journal of Medicine, 340*(25):1962-1968, 1999.

Van Aerde, J.E., Feldman, M., and Clandinin, M.T.: Accretion of lipid in the fetus and newborn. In R. Polin and W. Fox (Eds.): *Fetal and neonatal physiology* (2nd ed.). Philadelphia, 1998, W.B. Saunders, pp. 458-477.

Van Goudoever, J.B., Colen, T., Watttimena, J.L.D., et al.: Immediate commencement of amino acid supplementation in preterm infants: Effect on serum amino acid concentrations and protein kinetics on the first day of life. *Journal of Pediatrics, 127*(3):458-465, 1995.

Van Someren, V., Linnett, S., Stothers, J., and Sullivan, P.G.: An investigation into the benefits of resisting nasoenteric feeding tubes. *Pediatrics, 74*(3):379-383, 1984.

Wahlig, T. and Georgieff, M.: The effects of illness on neonatal metabolism and nutritional management. *Clinics in Perinatology, 22*(1):77-96, 1995.

Weibley, T.T., Adamson, M., Clinkscales, N., et al.: Gavage tube insertion in the premature infant. *American Journal of Maternal-Child Nursing, 12*(1):24-27, 1987.

Zlotkin, S., Atkinson, S., and Lockitch, G.: Trace elements in nutrition for premature infants. *Clinics in Perinatology,* 22(1):223-240, 1995.

CHAPTER

11 Developmental Support

CAROL TURNAGE CARRIER

OBJECTIVES

1. Apply four (4) standards of developmental care to guide practice in the neonatal intensive care unit (NICU).
2. Assess physiologic and behavioral organization of preterm and ill newborn infants using the neurobehavioral subsystems from Als' Synactive Framework.
3. Design a developmental care plan that respects and supports each infant's unique needs as related to the environment, direct caregiving, parent support, and consistency of care.

Developmental support in the NICU integrates the developmental needs of infants within the context of medical care. The developmental continuum nature designed is disrupted through parent-infant separation and the complex, atypical environment of the NICU. Randomized controlled trials have shown positive benefits of developmental care and clinical, neurobehavioral, cost, and parent outcomes (Als et al., 1986; Als et al., 1994; Buehler et al., 1995; Fleisher et al., 1995; Westrup et al., 2000). Developmental support in the NICU is expected and not regarded as optional. Although developmental care continues to be defined, theory and research are available to guide practice. Developmental care is a philosophy of practice that is integrated into everyday routine, family-staff relationships, policy, and the overall NICU culture. It is a model of delivering individualized care to newborns within a family context.

BARRIERS TO INFANT DEVELOPMENT IN THE NICU SETTING

A. **The NICU environment lacks the developmentally nurturing physical and social components that normally occur for the maturing fetus and term newborn (Als, 1998; Anand, 2000; Glass, 1999; Goldberger and Wolfer, 1991).** Challenges in the NICU to developing preterm and newborn infants include some or all of the following (list not exclusive):
   1. Numerous caregivers—possibly as many as 30 to 40 nurses when primary teams or nurses are not provided.
   2. Medically necessary equipment such as endotracheal tubes, intravenous lines, arterial lines, drains, and monitor leads.
   3. Unpredictable schedules based on caregiver convenience for touch, care, and procedures.
   4. No sleep/wake cycle or routine.

5. Pain and discomfort.
6. Separation from parents, minimal touch policies.
7. Continuous sensory stimulation.
8. Restraint, confinement.
9. Alternative feeding practices without pleasure/enjoyment.
10. Medications that cause sedation or irritability and agitation.

B. Evaluating the challenges in each NICU allows for proactive changes in policy and practice that support a developmental philosophy for care delivery.

DEVELOPMENTAL CARE STANDARDS

A. Four standards of developmental care (Als and Gilkerson, 1997; Robison, 2003). Based on intervention research, these standards provide the foundation for a successful developmental program and guidance for evaluating individual practice and program implementation.

1. **Standard 1:** Caregiving is flexible and individualized based on observation and continuous feedback related to each infant's abilities, sensitivities, and thresholds of autonomic, motor, and state subsystem functioning.
2. **Standard 2:** A developmentally supportive environment is provided for every infant and family based on continuous assessment and interaction.
3. **Standard 3:** Parents are viewed as the most important relationship with continual support of this bond starting with the birth of the infant(s).
4. **Standard 4:** Collaborative and consistent caregiving is considered necessary for clinical and developmental support of infants and families.

Standard 1. Caregiving is flexible and individualized based on observation and continuous feedback related to each infant's abilities, sensitivities, and thresholds of autonomic, motor, and state subsystem functioning.

A. In order to provide flexible, individualized caregiving, the caregiver must accurately assess infant behavior. The framework for understanding premature infant behavior is based on work by Heidelise Als (Als, 1995; 1998; Als and Gilkerson, 1997). Five subsystems within three channels of communication include observable behaviors in the autonomic, motor, and state systems. These five subsystems as defined in detail in Table 11-1 are used as a systematic assessment. Basic premises of the model are that:

1. Infants continually strive to function in the smoothest manner at their current level of functioning.
2. Competence is seen in a hierarchic integration of subsystem competence:
   a. Stabilization of physiologic functioning.
   b. Restabilization of physiologic, motor, or state functioning as new skills or levels of functioning emerge.
   c. Gradual development of a full range of behavioral (sleep/wake) states.
   d. Attaining alert states that are clear and robust; sustained alerting with the ability to interact with people and the environment without compromise or physiologic instability.

B. Assessment is the key element for formulating moment-to-moment, as well as more global, changes (formal care plan) in care to meet the needs of individual infants. Data on autonomic, motor, and state functioning are collected before, during, and after care or procedures and to gain perspective on the infant's abilities, sensitivities, thresholds, and unique communication repertoire.

■ TABLE 11-1
■ ■ **Synactive Theory of Development: Neurobehavioral Subsystems**

Subsystem	Signs of Stress	Signs of Stability
AUTONOMIC	**PHYSIOLOGIC INSTABILITY**	**PHYSIOLOGIC STABILITY**
Respiratory	Tachypnea, pauses, gasping, sighing	Smooth, stable respirations, regular rate and pattern
Color	Mottled, flushed, dusky, pale or gray	Pink, stable color
Visceral	Hiccups, gagging, choking, spitting up, grunting, and straining as if having a bowel movement. Coughing, sneezing, yawning	Absence of hiccups, gagging, spitting up, etc.
Autonomic	Tremors, startles, twitches	Absence of tremors, startles, twitches, etc.
MOTOR	**Fluctuating tone, lack of control over movement, activity, and posture**	**Consistent tone, controlled or improved movement, activity, and posture**
Flaccidity	Low tone in trunk, limp/floppy upper and lower extremities, limp drooping jaw (gape face)	Tone consistent and appropriate for postconceptional age Well-maintained posture
Hypertonicity	Arm and/or leg extensions, arm(s) outstretched with fingers splayed in salute gesture, fingers stiffly outstretched, trunk arching, neck hyperextended	Smooth, controlled movements
Hyperflexion	Trunk, extremities, fisting	Successful motor strategies for self-regulation (see Self-Regulation)
Activity	Squirming, frantic diffuse activity, or little or no activity or responsiveness	
STATE	**Disorganized quality to state behaviors including range of available states, maintenance of state control, and transition from one state to another**	**Easy to read state behaviors that are maintained; calm, focused alertness; well-modulated sleep**
Sleep	Whimpering sounds, facial twitching, irregular respirations, fussing, grimacing, appears restless	Clear, well-defined sleep states, periods of quiet, restful sleep
Awake	Glazed, unfocused look, staring, worried or pained expression. Hyperalert or panicked appearance, eye roving, crying, cry-face, actively averting gaze or closing eyes, irritability, prolonged awake periods, inconsolability, frenzy	Alert with bright, shiny eyes, focused attention on object or person, animated expression (e.g., cheek softening, frowning, "ooh face," cooing, smiling) Robust crying Good calming, consolability
	Abrupt and/or rapid state changes	Smooth changes between states Full range of sleep/wake states

■ TABLE 11-1
■ ■ **Synactive Theory of Development: Neurobehavioral Subsystems—cont'd**

OTHER STATE-RELATED BEHAVIORS:		
Attention-Interaction	**Efforts to attend and interact with environmental stimulation elicits signs of stress and disorganized subsystem functioning**	**Responsive to auditory, visual, and social stimuli**
Autonomic	Physiologic instability of varying degrees with autonomic, respiratory, color, and visceral responses	Responsiveness to stimuli is well maintained and prolonged
Motor	Fluctuating tone, increased motor activity, progressively frantic diffuse activity if stimulation continues	Actively seeks auditory stimulus, minimal motor activity
State	Roving eyes, gaze averting, glazed-unfocused look or worried, panicked expression, weak cry, cry-face, irritability	Bright, shiny-eyed alert and attentive expression
	Closed eyes and sleep-like withdrawal	
	Abrupt state changes	Sustained awake and alert state
	Signs of stress when presented with more than one type of stimulus at a time	Shifts attention smoothly to more than one type of stimulation

Self-Regulation: Infant's efforts to achieve, maintain, or regain a balanced, stable, and relaxed state of subsystem functioning and integration. Success of these efforts will vary among infants depending on maturity, available self-regulatory skills, and overall subsystem organization. Examples of self-regulatory strategies include:

Motor — foot bracing against a boundary or blanket nest, hand holding, grasping hands together, hand to mouth or face, grasping blanket, tubing, etc., tucking trunk, sucking, position changes

State — lowers state from high arousal to quiet alert or sleep state, releases energy by rhythmic, robust crying, focused attention, and orientation

Facilitation by caregivers through environmental modifications or developmental care techniques can aid the infant's own self-regulatory abilities when environmental challenges exceed the infant's capabilities.

Modified from Als, H.: Toward a synactive theory of development: promise for the assessment and support of infant individuality. *Infant Mental Health Journal, 3*:229-243, 1982; Als, H.: A synactive model of neonatal behavior organization: Framework for the assessment of neurobehavioral development in the premature infant and for support of infants and parents in the neonatal intensive care environment. *Physical and Occupational Therapy in Pediatrics, 6:3*-55, 1986; Hunter, J.G.: The neonatal intensive care unit. In J. Case-Smith, A.S. Allen, and P.N. Pratt (Eds.): *Occupational therapy for children.* St Louis, 2001, Mosby, p.593; Carrier C.T., Walden, M., and Wilson, D.: The high-risk newborn and family. In M.J. Hockenberry, (Ed.): *Wong's nursing care of infants and children,* ed 7, St. Louis, 2003, Mosby.

1. Neurobehavioral subsystems (see Table 11-1) provide information regarding the infant's vulnerabilities, thresholds, strengths, and abilities and are placed within a context whether it is during care, procedures, nurturing by parents, or when the infant is alone.

2. Newborn state system provides the context for any interaction between infant and environment; used by the infant to control the amount and kind of input received from the environment.

a. Six sleep/wake states with the (A) subdivision relating to immature preterm behavioral states and (B) associated with robust states of a more mature infant (Als, 1995).

All infants are developing organized sleep during the first year of life. Full-term newborn infants sleep from 16 to 18 hours, whereas preterm infants spend about 75% of their time in light sleep (Als, 1995; 1998; Als and Gilkerson, 1997; Holditch-Davis et al., 2003; Thoman et al., 1987).

(1) *State 1A:* infant in deep sleep with momentary regular breathing, eyes closed, and no eye movements under closed lids; relaxed facial expression; no spontaneous activity, oscillating fairly rapidly with isolated startles, jerky movements or tremors and other behavior characteristics of State 2 (light sleep).

(2) *State 1B:* infant in deep sleep with predominantly regular breathing, eyes closed, no eye movements under closed lids; relaxed facial expression; no spontaneous activity except isolated startles.

(3) *State 2A:* light sleep with eyes closed; rapid eye movements can be observed under closed eyelids; low activity level with diffuse or disorganized movements; irregular respirations, with many sucking and mouthing movements, whimpers, facial twitching, and much grimacing; the impression of a "noisy" state is given.

(4) *State 2B:* light sleep, with eyes closed; rapid eye movements observable under closed lids; low activity level, with movements and dampened startles; movements likely to be of lower amplitude and more monitored than in State 1. Infant responds to various internal stimuli with dampened startle. Respirations are more irregular; mild sucking and mouthing movements can occur off and on; and one or two whimpers, as well as an isolated sigh or smile, may be observed.

b. Transitional states.

(1) *State 3A:* drowsy or semidozing; eyes may be open or closed, eyelids fluttering or exaggerated blinking; if eyes open, infant has glassy, veiled look. Activity level is variable, with or without interspersed, mild startles from time to time. Diffuse movement occurs, with fussing and/or much vocalization, with whimpers, facial grimacing, and so forth.

(2) *State 3B:* drowsy; same as above but with less discharge of vocalization, whimpers, facial grimacing, and so forth.

c. Awake states. Awake states must be carefully observed for quality to determine appropriate timing of any interaction. Low-level alerting and hyperalert states are often mistaken as opportunities for interaction. Infant cues to terminate sensory input must be recognized and respected before stress results in a physiologic cost.

(1) *State 4:* alert.

(a) *State 4AL:* awake and quiet, with minimal motor activity; eyes half open or open but with glazed or dull look, giving impression of little involvement and distance; or eyes focused, yet infant seems to look through, rather than at, object or examiner; or the infant is clearly awake and reactive but has eyes open intermittently.

(b) *State 4AH:* awake and quiet, minimal motor activity, eyes wide open, "hyperalert" or giving the impression of panic or fear; may appear to be hooked by the stimulus, seems to be unable to modulate or break the intensity of the fixation.

(c) *State 4B:* alert with bright, shiny look; seems to focus attention on source of stimulation and appears to process information actively and with modulation; motor activity is at a minimum.

(2) *State 5:* active.

(a) *State 5A:* eyes may or may not be open, but infant clearly awake and aroused, as indicated by motor arousal, tonus, and mildly distressed facial expression, grimacing, or other signs of discomfort; diffuse fussing.

(b) *State 5B:* eyes may or may not be open, but infant is clearly awake and aroused, with considerable well defined motor activity. Infant is also clearly fussing but not crying.

(3) *State 6:* crying.

(a) *State 6A:* intense crying, as indicated by intense grimace and cry-face; yet cry sound may be very strained or very weak or even absent.

(b) *State 6B:* rhythmic, intense crying that is robust, vigorous, and strong in sound.

C. **Individualized developmental care includes both the moment-to-moment caregiver adaptations while in interaction with an infant and the formal plans based on infant assessment that provide overall guidance for care of that particular infant.** Both are flexible, in that changes may need to be made based on infant responses at any given moment.

1. Direct care adjustments and modified techniques are based on each infant's response to touch, handling, and routine care and procedures. This component may include therapeutic handling techniques; repositioning methods; nurturing; facilitation during exams, procedures (routine or painful); care clusters; timing of care; and recovery time or time-out techniques. This component is dependent on the caregiver being completely in tune and in interaction with the infant rather than performing care on the infant.

2. Developmental plans reflect all four developmental standards (environment and direct care, parent/family, collaborative practice, and consistency) and:

   a. Allow infant's family and primary nurse to make specific recommendations regarding environmental modifications, positioning techniques, calming measures, and the promotion of self-quieting abilities.

   b. Should incorporate input from appropriate members of the multidisciplinary team: parents, medicine, nursing, occupational therapy, physical therapy, respiratory therapy, child life and social services.

   c. Communicate the plan developed between the family and health care providers that outlines environmental, direct care, parent, and consistency required by an individual infant for optimal behavioral organization and neurodevelopmental growth. The formal plan is communicated in writing and through direct report during medical and nursing rounds, shift report, and in family conferences.

3. Questions to consider when assessing an infant's level of behavioral stability or organization and planning developmental support include:

   a. How does the infant respond to the daily caregiving routine? How can the family be as involved in daily caregiving as they are comfortable?

   b. What therapeutic handling and positioning techniques best support this infant?

c. What, if anything, in the environment has a negative impact on the infant?
d. How much stimulation can the infant tolerate before losing the ability to stay organized?
e. What facilitation or environmental support is necessary to help the infant maintain stability?
f. Can the timing and organization of medical and nursing procedures be altered to help decrease the infant's level of stress and increase his or her organization?
g. What is missing from the infant's environment and experiences that typically support stability and the natural developmental progression in utero or at home (e.g., dim light, touch, parent smell, breast, milk odor, and taste)?

D. **Intervention strategies that can be used to help individual infants cope with NICU stress and support neurobehavioral organization must be carefully considered with the understanding that in developmental care "an intervention does not necessarily fit all."** Although intervention research is accumulating, the evidence base should be examined in light of its quality and strength before applying any practice in the NICU that has potential significant short- and long-term effects. There are available criterion lists for evaluating research (Philbin and Klaas, 2000a). In general, the nurse should think in terms of the most biologically relevant interventions based on the infant's stage of development (e.g., 26 weeks vs. 32 weeks) and experiences expected at that developmental and maturational level.

E. **Routine care.**

1. Providing a momentary time-out from incoming stimuli when an infant is stressed and disorganized allows him or her time to draw fully on self-regulatory abilities.
2. Observe for avoidance behaviors (e.g., gaze aversion, regurgitation, crying, increased extension patterns) in response to movement transitions or particular positions. Such patterns of behavior suggest repetitive responses that may evolve into heightened reactivity and agitation especially in infants with prolonged NICU stays or chronic conditions. These infants may need a referral for occupational therapy or an infant developmental specialist evaluation and intervention.
3. Simple modifications to routine care practices may be used to minimize stress for preterm infants such as swaddled bathing (Fern et al., 2002) or swaddled weighing (Neu and Browne, 1997).
4. "Clustered care" has been recommended to allow longer rest periods by clustering several routine or nursing care events together rather than spacing them out over time. Careful monitoring by staff during care clusters must take place to avoid overwhelming an immature or ill infant with too long or intense an episode of care (Peters, 1999).
5. Respect infant's sleep states as an important part of maturation and make every attempt not to disrupt sleep and provide care during naturally occurring awake periods.
6. Even when infants are lying alert in their beds, it is important to let them know care or touch is about to begin by soft speech, calling their name, smell, and finally touch so as not to startle them and elicit a disorganized response.
7. If an infant is motorically stressed, help him or her to reorganize by gently supporting extremities in flexion close to body with warmed hands until infant is calm, thereby decreasing unnecessary energy expenditure and encouraging self-regulation.

8. Containment by blanket swaddling or nesting is reported to decrease physiologic and behavioral stress cues during routine care such as eye examinations, weighing, or heel lance (Corff et al., 1995; Fearon et al., 1997; Graven, 2000; Peters, 1992; Slevin et al., 1999).

F. **Touch and handling.** With physiologically unstable high-risk infants, handling must be kept to a minimum to avoid further medical compromise and to help the infant conserve energy. The amount, type, and timing of touch require staff to consider each infant's current age, medical status, and sensitivity to stimulation and choose the most appropriate approach based on available evidence (Browne, 2000; Harrison and Woods, 1991; Harrison et al., 1991; Harrison et al., 1996).

1. Stroking infants who are not physiologically stable has been shown to elicit gasping, grunting, averted gaze, and decreased transcutaneous oxygen levels (Browne, 2000; Harrison et al., 1991; Harrison et al., 1996; Harrison and Woods, 1991).
2. Therapeutic touch may include a variety of types of tactile sensation that includes:
   a. Gentle human touch (GHT) or hand containment. GHT is the gentle placement of warmed hands on the head and lower back or buttocks applying supportive containment for about 15 minutes. A few studies have shown GHT may be soothing and without risk, but no long-term evidence is available. It is recommended that close monitoring accompany any touch or handling of a NICU infant (Harrison et al., 1991; Harrison et al., 1996; Harrison et al., 2000; Modrcin-Talbott et al., 2003).
   b. Conventional holding involves holding clothed infants in the traditional semi-upright position while supporting extremities and head close to the caregiver's body; often used when infants are stable enough to transfer from bed to parent's arms.
   c. Kangaroo care (KC) or skin-to-skin holding (Charpak et al., 2001; Feldman and Eidelman, 2003; Feldman et al., 2002a; McGrath and Brock, 2002). NICU parents perform skin-to-skin contact with their diaper-clad infant who is resting prone and semi-upright against the mother or father's bare chest covered by a blanket. Warmth, rise and fall of the chest (vestibular), tactile sensation of skin to skin, smell of parents (olfactory) and maternal breast, and the parent's tender, quiet, vocalizations, breathing sounds, and heartbeat (auditory) comprise the sensory modalities stimulated during KC. This intervention provides low-intensity stimulation to the earlier developing senses and is most appropriate for the NICU infant.
      (1) Controversial use with extremely premature infants during acute illness phase.
      (2) Maintaining physiologic and behavioral stability during transfer from bed to parent and back remains a challenge (Neu et al., 2000).
      (3) Positive benefits of KC include decreased incidence and severity of infections; longer duration of breast-feeding; increased weight gain; shorter length of stay; increased maternal milk volume; less variable heart rate and oxygenation levels; decreased apnea and bradycardia; less crying; and increased frequency/duration of quiet sleep (Acolet et al., 1989; Anderson, 1991; Bauer et al., 1996; Bauer et al., 1997; Chwo et al., 2002; Conde-Agudelo et al., 2000; Feldman and Eidelman, 2003; Fohe et al., 2000; Ludington-Hoe et al., 1999; McGrath and Brock, 2002; Messmer et al., 1997; Roberts et al., 2000; Tornhage et al., 1999).

Positive benefits of KC on preterm infant development include (Feldman and Eidelman, 2003; Feldman et al., 2002a; Feldman et al., 2002b):

(a) Better arousal modulation at 3 months when presented with increasingly complex stimulation.

(b) Higher scores at 6 months on Bayley Scales of Infant Development mental and psychomotor index than controls without KC.

(c) Improved state organization with longer quiet sleep, quiet alerting, and decreased amounts of active or light sleep.

(d) Improved habituation and orientation skills.

d. Massage. Positive benefits of massage such as weight gain, more active alert periods, more mature orientation, habituation, motor, and range of state behaviors on the Brazelton's Newborn Behavior Assessment Scale (BNBAS) have been reported in older, stable preterm infants greater than 31 weeks' gestation (Browne, 2000; Field et al., 1986; Vickers et al., 2000). Massage has also been shown to improve weight gain, decrease stress behaviors, reduce postnatal complications, and improve motor performance in infants prenatally exposed to cocaine (Wheeden et al., 1993).

(1) Smaller, fragile preterm infants are at risk for physiologic compromise during massage.

(2) Consider teaching parents rather than using a therapist to provide massage to older, stable preterm or term infants.

(3) Determine infant eligibility for massage on an individual basis in consultation with care team.

(4) Parent teaching should be performed only by certified infant massage therapists working in the NICU such as occupational therapists or neonatal child life specialists.

e. Other considerations for touch and handling in the NICU (Browne, 2000).

(1) Synchronize touch with sleep/wake behavior.

(2) Consider the risks/benefits of any touch or handling.

(3) Balance aversive touch with therapeutic touch opportunities.

(4) Consistent caregivers to provide nurturing touch.

(5) Continually monitor autonomic and behavioral responses and modify or stop interaction as appropriate.

(6) Consider parents the most appropriate providers of therapeutic touch.

(7) Teach parents to evaluate their infant's responses to touch and handling and how to intervene as necessary.

(8) Update knowledge with current literature on touch, massage, and KC.

3. The literature is insufficient to support specific recommendation for vestibular stimulation alone (Symington and Pinelli, 2002). In theory it is reasonable to believe that vestibular input is important to the developing preterm infant. Skin-to-skin care has a vestibular component of the rise and fall of mother's chest during breathing. Gentle vestibular stimulation may be tolerated by stable infants with gentle swaying or rocking.

4. Repositioning has been associated with significant physiologic stress responses (Evans, 1991); therefore sudden postural changes should be avoided. The impact of this procedure can be reduced by slowly repositioning while containing infant in a gentle, tucked midline position.

G. Positioning and containment. Provision of developmentally supportive positioning and containment interventions may promote a calm state, physiologic stability, and prevent position-related deformities in the high-risk infant.

1. Sequential patterns of neuromotor maturation (not timing, which is individual) are identified by examining the following (Sweeney and Gutierrez, 2002):
   a. Muscle development.
      (1) Muscle fiber development incomplete until term.
      (2) Lower ratio of type 1 muscle fibers (high oxidative type) to type 2 fibers (low oxidative) predisposes preterm infants to muscle fatigue (includes respiratory muscles).
   b. Muscle tone and reflex development proceeds caudocephalad (lower to upper extremities) and centripetal (distal to proximal).
   c. Skeleton and joint articulation.
      (1) Restricted movement and positioning in the NICU produce joint compression and poor refinement of mechanical receptors; these factors predispose fragile infants to skeletal deformation, shortening of muscles, and contractures.
      (2) Poor ossification and density of bone establish susceptibility to rib fractures.

H. **Common "acquired positioning malformations"** occur in preterm infants related to maturational hypotonia unless appropriate positioning interventions take place (Sweeney and Gutierrez, 2002). Common positioning deformities include hip adduction and external rotation (frog leg); shoulder retraction and scapular adduction (W position of arms); neck extension; arching postures; and abnormal head molding.

I. **Prevention of positioning deformities** requires specialized knowledge, careful thought and planning, skilled use of positioning aids/supports, and adequate monitoring of infants following any change in position.
   1. General considerations for positioning in the NICU:
      a. Provide support for breathing and ventilation.
      b. Promote skin integrity.
      c. Provide proprioceptive input to facilitate containment and security as needed.
      d. Facilitate developing flexion in both posture and movement.
      e. Provide opportunities for midline skill development (hand to face or mouth).
      f. Encourage alignment and symmetry.
      g. Support rest/calming/comfort and neurobehavioral organization.
      h. Counteract emerging stereotypical or abnormal postures.
      i. Offer a variety of well-supported and tolerated positions.
      j. Assist in the progression toward balanced flexor/extensor tone and movement.
   2. Monitor the infant's physiologic and behavioral response to positioning because benefits to motor and state control may be counterbalanced by destabilization of physiologic parameters (heart rate, breathing pattern, blood pressure, etc.).
   3. Intentional movement by infants enhances neuromotor development and stability. Regulatory efforts such as pushing against boundaries is one example of such movement. Containment or nests should not restrict movement that is necessary for growth and development of the neuromotor system. Restraint should be avoided unless absolutely necessary and then should be used only for a short period of time.
   4. General guidelines for positioning (Boxes 11-1 and 11-2).

■ BOX 11-1
■ **GENERAL CONSIDERATIONS FOR POSITIONING**

- Neutral or slightly flexed neck
- Gently rounded shoulders (no flattened posture against bed as in supine or prone positions)
- Elbow flexion
- Hands to face or midline as position allows
- Trunk slightly rounded with pelvic tilt
- Hips partially flexed and adducted to near midline (not medial or neutral alignment) and knee flexion (no frog leg or externally rotated hips flat against bed)
- Secure lower boundary for foot-bracing

Modified from Biber P., et al.: When to seek consultation. In P.J. Creger and J.V. Browne (Eds.): *Developmental interventions for preterm and high-risk infants: Self study modules for professionals.* Tucson, 1995, Therapy Skill Builders; Carrier, C.T., Walden, M., and Wilson, D.: The high-risk newborn and family. In M.J. Hockenberry, (Ed.): *Wong's nursing care of infants and children,* ed 7, St. Louis, 2003, Mosby.

5. Occupational and physical therapists (OT and PT) can offer treatment for muscle toning, increasing touch and handling tolerance, improving oral-motor function, movement and motor patterns, equilibrium, relaxation, sensory integration, and in some units teach massage to parents.

J. **Positioning for home.** The American Academy of Pediatrics (AAP) recommends the supine position as the preferred sleep position during infancy (AAP, 2000). Since 1992 and this change in sleeping pattern by many parents, the incidence of sudden infant death syndrome (SIDS) has been reduced by 40% (AAP, 2000). Prone positioning is recommended when infants are awake and being observed to promote acquisition of developmental milestones and prevent positional plagiocephaly. Parent teaching prior to discharge should include the AAP's recommendations and other recommended modifications identified by the AAP task force on infant sleep position and SIDS that include avoiding (AAP, 2000):
   1. Use of soft/loose bedding or objects such as pillows, quilts, comforters, sheepskins, stuffed toys.
   2. Use of waterbeds, sofas, or soft mattresses as a bed.
   3. Bed sharing or co-sleeping even with siblings.
   4. Overheating by too many clothes and overly warm bedroom temperature.

Standard 2. A developmentally supportive environment is provided for every infant and family based on continuous assessment and interaction.

A. **Environmental modifications are made according to the infant's responses, vulnerabilities, and thresholds and includes lighting, sound, activity around the bedside, bedding, positioning aids, and other environmental inputs.**

B. **Visual system.** Animal models have shown that early stimulation to an immature visual system can alter the developmental trajectory of the visual and other sensory systems resulting in atypical behavioral responses (Banker and Lickliter, 1993; Casey and Lickliter, 1998; Foushee and Lickliter, 2002; Honeycutt and Lickliter, 2001; Lickliter, 2000b, Sleigh et al., 1996; Sleigh and Lickliter, 1995, 1998).

BOX 11-2
POSITIONING GUIDELINES

1. Bedding and positioning aids must be individually determined to meet the needs of the infant. Soft bedding, such as sheepskin, secure nesting, and boundaries or swaddling, is used for those infants requiring such devices to maintain comfortable positioning and to prevent skin problems. Waterbeds (Fowler et al., 1997), or gel or water pillows (Marsden, 1980) are recommended to avoid abnormal head molding.
2. Calm, organized behavior may be improved by use of the following strategies:
   a. Prone position to facilitate improved oxygenation and ventilation.
   b. Side-lying position, well supported with swaddling, commercial containment devices or a heavy blanket roll surrounding the infant's flexed back, to promote midline hands-together or hands-to-face movements.
   c. Swaddling to provide the most secure containment and to be used in combination with other positioning devices as needed.
3. Repositioning is usually indicated every 2 to 3 hours or when care must be provided. An infant may demonstrate behavioral cues that suggest discomfort and the need for positional change.
4. Oversized diapers may result in hips maintained in the externally rotated and abducted "frog leg" posture. Appropriately sized commercial diapers are available and should be used to preserve normal hip alignment.
5. Tension from lines or tubing such as endotracheal tubes, naso- or orogastric tubes, cardiac leads, or intravenous lines may result in deforming pressures or postures and should be avoided.
6. Repositioning is often stressful for sick or preterm infants. Caregivers can reduce the stress of this necessary procedure with slow, gentle rolling of the infant while containing the extremities and providing a pacifier for a brief time after moving the infant.
7. Once repositioned, the infant's breathing pattern, color, oxygen saturation, heart rate, respiratory rate and pattern, behavioral cues, and stability of position should be monitored and noted whether positioning principles have been followed.
8. Finally, a very important consideration is that caregivers continually observe each infant's emerging capabilities to determine appropriate positioning and bedding options. Infants who begin to fight containment or boundaries or those who have matured beyond the need for positioning devices and can maintain a flexed posture unassisted should be allowed to do so. Transitioning infants out of boundaries and positioning aids is required before discharge. Slow transition will ease the process and prepare infants for being without aids once they are home.
9. Daily physical activity has been shown to enhance bone growth and development in low birth weight (LBW) preterm infants (Moyer-Mileur et al., 2000). It is important to avoid restrictive swaddling or nesting that inhibits infants from all movement or pushing against their boundaries. Such practice could prove detrimental to motor development.
10. Supine positioning at least 2 weeks before discharge should be initiated so that infants can adjust to the home sleeping position.

Modified from Hunter, J.: The neonatal intensive care unit. In J. Case-Smith (Ed.): *Occupational therapy for children* (4th ed.). St Louis, 2001, Mosby. Carrier C.T., Walden, M., and Wilson D: The high-risk newborn and family. In M.J. Hockenberry., (Ed.): *Wong's nursing care of infants and children,* ed 7, St. Louis, 2003, Mosby; Fowler, K., Kum-Nji, P., Wells, P.J., and Mangrem, C.L.: Water beds may be useful in preventing scaphocephaly in preterm very low birthweight neonates. *J Perinatology 17*(5):397, 1997. Marsden, D.J. Reduction of head flattening in preterm infants. *Developmental Medicine and Child Neurology 22*(4):308-314, 1980; Moyer-Mileur, L.J., Brunstetter, V., McNaught, T.P., et al: Daily physical activity program increases bone mineralization and growth in preterm very low birthweight infants. *Pediatrics 106*(5):1088-1092, 2000.

1. Although light has not been related to the development of retinopathy of prematurity (ROP), it remains to be seen what role early exposure to light may play in the development of cortical processes and visual-motor performance (Kennedy et al., 2001; Reynolds et al., 1998).
2. Studies using reduced lighting for premature infants have shown no negative visual impact or differences in medical outcomes and may be a safer, more conservative approach until more is known concerning the impact of illumination on early developing visual systems (Kennedy et al., 1997; Kennedy et al., 2001; Roy et al., 1999).
3. Phototherapy (Fielder and Moseley, 2000) is a known hazard that can negatively affect the visual system. The light exposure ranges from 200 to 280 foot-candles (ftc) (2400-3000 lux) with small amounts of ultraviolet radiation (UV) from 330 to 400 nanometers (nm) that can damage the retina. Careful monitoring to ensure eye patches are in place will reduce about 90% of the phototherapy light exposure and minimize the risk of visual impairment.
4. Preterm infants cared for with day/night cycled lighting have shown (Brandon et al., 2002) significantly faster weight gain; lower heart rate and activity during the reduced light cycle (Blackburn and Patterson, 1991); increased sleep time, improved feeding efficiency, and faster weight gain at 6 and 12 weeks after discharge (Mann et al., 1986); less time to oral feeding; and fewer ventilator days (Miller et al., 1995). None of the studies report visual function or long-term visual performance when cycled lighting is introduced at an earlier stage of development.

C. **Auditory environment.** Studies show that exposure to sound in the NICU can disrupt sleep patterns and alter physiologic and behavioral responses of premature and term infants (Anderssen, 1993; Gadeke, 1969; Long, et al., 1980; Morris, 2000; Zahr and Balian, 1995). The NICU sound environment must be evaluated in order to make the acoustic and personnel behavior changes that support sleep, normal development, and optimal parent-infant interaction. Auditory intervention in the NICU consists of reduction of ambient noise levels, provision of appropriate auditory stimulation, and screening/treatment for hearing loss (see Chapter 36).

1. Physiologic responses to acoustic stimulation are reported as early as 23 to 25 weeks' gestation in the developing fetus (Abrams and Gerhardt, 2000; Crade and Lovett, 1988; Hall, 2000).
2. The intrauterine influence on the preterm infant's auditory system is primarily made up of sounds emanating from the mother, the most important being the mother's voice (Abrams and Gerhardt, 2000; Gerhardt and Abrams, 2000; Graven, 2000; Moon and Fifer, 2000).
3. The fetal sound experience is important to the normal development of the auditory system. The preterm infant developing in the NICU is subjected to an atypical sound environment that may influence later postnatal language perception and acquisition (Graven, 2000; Jennische and Sedin, 1998; Lickliter, 2000a; Moon and Fifer, 2000; Robertson et al., 1999b; Robertson et al., 2001).
4. Undesirable effects associated with sudden, loud noise in the NICU have been reported in both term and preterm infants including increased heart rate; agitation, crying, and irritability; increased anterior fontanelle pressure; sleep disruption, irregular respirations, decreased oxygen saturation; mottling, apnea, and bradycardia; and increased motor activity (Anderssen et al., 1993; Gadeke et al., 1969; Graven, 2000; Morris et al., 2000; Philbin, 2000; Philbin and Klaas, 2000b; Wharrad and Davis, 1997; Zahr and Balian, 1995).

5. Speech delay, articulation, comprehension, receptive and expressive language, auditory memory, and processing problems have been reported at increased rates in preterm infants compared with full-term infants (Byrne et al., 1993; Davis et al., 2001; Jennische and Sedin, 1999; 2001; Whitfield et al., 1997).
6. Whether the NICU environment is directly related to later speech and language problems remains to be seen; however, the concern is that NICU noise can disrupt normal language development and communication processing by distorting socially relevant sounds during critical periods of speech and language development (Byrne et al., 1993; Davis et al., 2001; Dupin et al., 2000; Graven, 2000; Jennische and Sedin, 1999; 2001; Wharrad and Davis, 1997).
7. Quiet times scheduled in a NICU have been shown to increase duration of deep sleep (85% vs. 34%) and decrease crying (14% vs. 2%) in infants during "quiet hour" compared with control periods (Strauch et al., 1993). A general overall respect of the infant's sound environment is important at all times, keeping the noise levels low as to not disturb infant rest and providing stimulation at a level for infants who need it at a level that does not disturb infants nearby.
8. Structural modifications with acoustics designed to support noise abatement in the NICU setting have been successful (Philbin and Gray, 2002; Robertson et al., 1998; Robertson et al., 1999a; Smith, 1999; Strauch et al., 1993; Walsh-Sukys et al., 2001). Recommended changes to the environment include increased size of bed space and sound-absorbent surfacing for floors, walls, and ceiling. The evaluation and recommendations of an acoustical engineer are valuable when renovating or designing new NICUs (Philbin and Gray, 2002).
9. There is little evidence in the literature that supports the need for supplemental auditory stimulation beyond that provided naturally by parents and family. In a report by the Sound Study Group of the National Resource Center of The Physical and Developmental Environment of the High Risk Infant, recommendations for the NICU sound environment based on available evidence are as follows (Graven, 2000):
   a. NICUs should create and maintain a program for controlling noise within specified noise criteria guidelines for continuous sound in the infant's surroundings. Sound criteria limitations are:
      (1) maintenance of hourly loudness equivalent (Leq) of 50 decibels (dB),
      (2) hourly L10 of 55 dB (L10 is the level of sound exceeded 10% of the measurement interval and is a measure of how loud the unit is over that period of time.)
      (3) 1 second Lmax not to exceed 70dB (Lmax is the maximum sound level recorded during the smallest measurement interval and is related to the human perception of sound intensity or loudless)
      (4) measurements must be A-weighted on a slow response dosimeter (noise meter) setting
   b. Parents and infants should be afforded opportunities for interaction in a quiet, ambient environment that does not interfere or mask speech sounds.
   c. The use of earphones placed in or over the ear is not recommended.
   d. Recorded music or speech is not supported in the available research evidence and not recommended. Provision of recorded sound should not replace the interactive experience provided by parents necessary for speech and language development.

Standard 3. Parents are viewed as the most important relationship with continual support of this bond starting with the birth of the infant(s).

A. **Parental support strategies.** The key to supporting mutually satisfying parent-infant interaction is to establish a family-centered approach on admission that will empower the parents to assume the natural parental role of advocating for their child's needs and desires and become the primary nurturer to their infant. Supporting the parents' ability to understand their infant's level of communication through the infant's behavior will place the parents in a better position to respond to and interact with their infant in a developmentally supportive manner.

1. Establish an atmosphere in the NICU that is welcoming to parents and does not treat them as "visitors" but as parents who deserve respect as important members of their infant's care team.
2. Help parents identify the most effective techniques for interacting with their infant (e.g., recognizing stress and time-out signs). Include information on temperament differences in infants and ways to modify daily interactions to support varying temperament traits (Carey, 1998).
3. Place parents in situations in which they will succeed in interacting positively with their infant.
4. Help parents identify both the consoling measures unique to their infant and how their child is providing feedback concerning the consoling measures.
5. Have the caregiving team work with the parents to plan specific activities (i.e., KC or skin-to-skin holding, biologically meaningful smells/tastes, verbal interaction, eye contact, use of toys, therapeutic touch) for parental interaction when appropriate (McGrath and Brock, 2002; Porter and Winberg, 1999).
6. Encourage parents to assume caregiving responsibilities when appropriate.
7. Discuss parents' expectations and goals for themselves and their infant. Encourage families to write down these expectations and goals. Writing down these dreams and goals or journaling will be the beginning of a lifelong care plan.
8. Encourage the parents to use their child's medical record as a communication tool.
9. Be aware of and involve the family's support system. Encourage parent-to-parent support if possible, either in a formal or an informal manner. Reports by families show that attending a parent support group helps them cope with their circumstances by feeling supported, learning about infant development, and understanding how to use the hospital and community resources. When unit staff have participated in these groups, they expressed gaining insights that influenced their interactions with parents and behaviors in the NICU (Pearson and Andersen, 2001).
10. Studies have shown three areas of parenting influenced by cultural differences: parents' emotional responses and understanding of their infant's condition, utilization of resources by minority cultures, and interaction with health professionals (Bracht et al., 2002).
11. Consider implementing a "Parent Buddy Program" with identified parents of different cultures/backgrounds who have experienced having a child in the NICU to serve as a resource for parents who are not represented by support programs and educational opportunities already available (Bracht et al., 2002).
12. Request a qualified interpreter to assist with language and cultural implications whenever needed to reduce the impact of language barriers and cultural differences.

13. Document the family's goals and the interventions necessary to help them reach their objectives in an individualized family support plan (IFSP) (Robison, 2003).
14. As a professional caregiver, staff are accountable for incorporating the interventions from the IFSP or care plan with infants and families (Robison, 2003).
15. Recognize that the parents are the constant in the child's life and that the various health professionals will come and go. Family factors are more predictive of school performance at 10 years of age than perinatal conditions of low birth weight infants (Gross et al., 2001).

B. **Feeding within a developmental framework for nutrition and parent-infant interaction.** The goal of feeding is more than an infant ingesting an adequate volume of food. A key concept is recognizing the difference between a successful feeding (volume and duration of feeding) and a successful feeder (infant competence and enjoyment). Within this context lies the difference between task-oriented or procedural feedings and a developmental feeding philosophy.
1. The framework for a developmental feeding involves three concepts (Ancona et al., 1998).
   a. Physiologic, motor, and state behavioral assessment before, during, and after feeding.
   b. Individualized feeding approach based on specific infant cues.
   c. Fostering parent competence, confidence, and enjoyment while feeding the infant.
2. Nurse's role in preparing infants for transition to oral feeding (Hunter, 2001)
   a. Support sleep/wake behavioral organization.
   b. Provide therapeutic positioning to promote neuromuscular control and postural alignment necessary for suck, swallow, and breathing (prevent hyperextended neck or trunk and shoulder retraction).
   c. Protect against aversive oral stimulation.
   d. Provide pleasurable oral experiences.
   e. Offer opportunities to smell breast milk or formula depending on parent choice of food type.
   f. Offer a pacifier for pleasure and not just as comfort during routine care or uncomfortable/painful procedures.
3. The nurse's role in feeding is not just to ensure safe and adequate transition to oral feeding. It is as important that consistent caregivers develop a relationship with infant and parents to gain familiarity that aids in guiding and monitoring feeding skill and progression.
   a. Recognize feeding readiness behaviors (Hunter, 2001).
      (1) Medical status.
      (2) Energy for feeding.
      (3) Capable of quiet, alert state behavior.
      (4) Gag response with orogastric tube insertion.
      (5) Rooting and sucking behaviors.
      (6) Functional sucking reflex.

C. **Nonnutritive sucking (NNS).** A metaanalysis of NNS literature demonstrated a significant effect on length of hospital stay for infants receiving NNS. No negative outcomes were observed in the 13 randomized, controlled trials reviewed in the metaanalysis. With such a small number of studies for each outcome, the results are inconclusive (Pinelli and Symington, 2000). More studies are needed; however, the positive cues provided by the infant as to enjoyment make this a valuable intervention.

D. Nutritive sucking (Carrier et al., 2003; Hunter, 2001).

1. Greater coordination of the suck-swallow-breathe sequence is required than in NNS.
2. To encourage as normal a suck-swallow pattern as possible while infant maintains physiologic, motor, and state stability, it is very important to hold the nipple still and allow the infant to pace the feeding. Allow rest between suck bursts. Manage environmental distractions so the infant can focus on the task of learning to feed.
3. Monitor infant for fatigue, especially with first oral feeding trials; forced feeding after an infant is tired may lead to:
   a. Prolonged feeding duration.
   b. Increased energy expenditure.
   c. Poor weight gain.
   d. Increasing incoordination during the feeding.
   e. Higher risk of aspiration.
   f. Deglutition apnea (deglutition is the sequence of moving a liquid or solid bolus in the mouth, through the pharynx and into the esophagus).
   g. Oxygen desaturation.
   h. Bradycardia.
   i. Oral aversion and defensiveness.
4. Intervene with infants who become fatigued by oral feeding:
   a. Stop feeding when infant shows fatigue.
   b. Continue feeding by nasogastric (NG) or orogastric (OG) tube to provide adequate intake.
   c. Decrease number of oral feedings per day or feeding duration per each feed.
   d. If feeding fatigue persists, discuss with care team for further evaluation and planning.

E. Maturation and coordination of suck, swallow, and breathing in preterm infants (Lau et al., 2000; Mizuno and Ueda, 2003).

1. There is a significant correlation in the maturity of the infant's sucking ability and postconceptional age (PCA).
2. Neurobehavioral maturation is a developmental sequence that supports feeding progression/abilities.
3. Coordination of suck, swallow, and respiration is seen by 34 weeks' PCA.
4. Maturation of the swallowing-respiratory pattern is not fully established even at 36 weeks' PCA.
5. Sucking pressure, frequency, and duration are related to maturation.
6. Milk flow volume is related to nipple hole size (Hill, 2002).
7. Restricted milk flow facilitates oral feeding in preterm infants (Lau et al., 1997), allowing rest between suck and swallow with adequate time for bursts of respiration. Rapid flow nipples may overwhelm preterm infants with milk flow they cannot handle resulting in interference with respiration and stressful feeding.
8. Increased milk consumed per feeding, duration of oral feedings, efficiency of feeding, and percentage of successful feedings are enhanced with the use of a vacuum-free bottle that eliminates both hydrostatic pressure and vacuum within the bottle, allowing the preterm infant at 34 to 35 weeks (26-29 weeks at birth) to self-pace initial bottle feedings by allowing milk to flow only during sucking (Lau and Schanler, 2000).
9. Nipples advertised for use with premature infants are softer and allow for higher milk flow that is inappropriate considering the immature ability, and increase the risk of choking, coughing, and aspiration (Ross and Browne, 2002).

10. Changing nipples frequently may affect feeding organization and adaptation; identifying an appropriate nipple and using it regularly as long as an infant is successfully feeding may be more supportive.
11. Studies (Arvedson et al., 1994; Comrie and Helm, 1997) have shown that around 94% of aspiration in infants and children evaluated by video fluoroscopy is "silent" (without clinically observable signs).
12. In general, gut motility follows the same sequence as oral-motor development and is improved by around 35 weeks (Lemons, 2001).
13. Feeding success is directly related to an infant's ability to maintain physiologic stability, a flexed posture, and an alert state while feeding (Lemons, 2001).
14. Infants with medical complications may achieve full oral feedings 2 to 5 weeks later than other hospitalized infants.
15. Chronic lung disease from prematurity is the most common medical condition that affects feeding.
16. Breast milk odor may increase NNS during gavage feedings (Bingham et al., 2003).
17. Infants provided 5 minutes of NNS prior to feeding demonstrate more alert and quiet awake states during feeding than those who do not receive the intervention; the NNS infants also demonstrated higher oxygen saturation levels before and after feeding (Hill, 2002; Pickler et al., 1996).
18. Ross and Browne (2002) suggest that oral cheek and jaw support removes the infant's own ability to pace the feeding and also increases milk volume; both experiences may lead to negative feedback during a feeding and ultimately increase the risk of oral defensiveness or aversion.
19. In a randomized, controlled trial, preterm infants (32 to 34 weeks' PCA) receiving NNS prior to feeding, oral feedings based on feeding readiness cues, and amount by demand achieved full oral feeding an average of 5 days earlier than a control group on a standard time–based protocol (McCain et al., 2001).
20. Pacing is thought to support feeding success by regulating breathing breaks to slow sucking or successive swallowing and allow adequate breathing opportunity for infants who are having difficulty with stability during a feeding. Pacing is achieved by tilting the bottle slightly so that milk drains out of the nipple and does not continue to flow. This method is preferred to removing the nipple from the infant's mouth, resulting in frequent attempts to reestablish an appropriate latch onto the nipple.
21. Preterm infants randomized to receive early oral stimulation provided by occupational therapists attained full oral feeding about 7 days earlier than those who did not get the intervention. Overall volume and milk transfer rate was significantly greater in the experimental group (Fucile et al., 2002). Authors suggest that both nurses and parents can be taught to provide the oral stimulation to enhance feeding efficiency and performance.
22. Sucking rhythms become increasingly stable from 32 to 40 weeks and are comparable to term sucking patterns.
23. In a prospective study of weekly observations of infants around 35 to 36 weeks, infants with chronic lung disease demonstrated unstable sucking rhythms, decreased aggregation and duration of sucking bursts, and decreased percentage and duration of swallows compared with their healthy preterm counterparts (Gewolb et al., 2001). These infants will require carefully monitored feedings and may need consultation from feeding experts to assist development of oral feeding skills.

F. **Assessment. Feeding the preterm infant requires close monitoring and documentation of meaningful information to be used in planning the progression and nature of feedings (Ancona et al., 1998; Hunter, 2001; Ross and Browne, 2002).** Physiologic stability provides the safe foundation for feeding with the overall integration of physiologic, motor, and state systems working together to support success. If the feeding experience is overwhelming to an infant, both motor and state disruption may occur rapidly and lead to physiologic compromise. Repeated negative feeding experiences may manifest in oral defensiveness or aversion.

1. The new demand of feeding may result in instability of the physiologic, motor, and state systems.
2. As the infant restabilizes and integrates new information, the caregiver must observe cues and pace feedings accordingly.
3. Physiologic assessment includes heart rate, respiratory pattern, oxygenation, color, vigor, and stable digestion.
   a. Physiologic stability while managing oral feeding.
   b. Maintenance of stability following feeding.
   c. Choking or gagging during feeding.
   d. Apnea or bradycardia.
   e. Oxygen saturation and work of breathing.
   f. Signs of fatigue.
   g. Weight gain with adequate caloric intake.
4. Motor assessment includes:
   a. General tone and posture.
   b. Changes in muscle tone, posture, and movements with handling.
   c. Quality and strength of suck.
   d. Maturity of sucking pattern (rhythmic and efficient).
   e. Coordination of suck/swallow, breathing (breathing pauses are adequate).
   f. Control of the milk bolus (no significant loss of milk from mouth).
5. Behavioral state assessment includes:
   a. Timing, duration, and quality of arousal.
   b. Sensitivity to environment and/or stimulation (shutdown or hyperalerting).
   c. Response to touch, handling, and position changes.
   d. Interest in feeding by facial expression or stress evidenced by frown, grimace, slack or limp jaw.
   e. State transitions (rapidity, frequency).
   f. Signs of "shutdown" closed eyes, generally unresponsive, appearance of sleep.
6. Endurance.
   a. Volume taken.
   b. Time frame for feeding.
   c. Vigor during feeding.
7. Evaluation of a successful feeding.
   a. Physiologic and behavioral cost of feeding is minimal (vital signs are maintained with good oxygenation, muscle tone stable/relaxed, and predominant state is quiet, alert, and interested).
   b. Little or no recovery time required for physical and behavioral return to baseline.
   c. Energy and vigor maintained during and after feeding.
   d. Infant participates in feeding experience with interest, energy, and enjoyment.

e. Adequate intake by mouth and/or by mouth/gavage.
f. Adequate weight gain.
g. Tolerance of feeding observed by minimal residuals, soft abdomen with audible bowel sounds, and regular elimination.

G. **Interventions for oral feeding are** based on available evidence and clinical report using the four standards of developmental care as a guide (Ancona et al., 1998; Case-Smith and Humphrey, 1996; Comrie and Helm, 1997; Daley and Kennedy, 2000; Hunter, 2001; Pinelli and Symington, 2000; Premji et al., 2002a; Premji et al., 2002b; Ross and Browne, 2002) (Box 11-3).

BOX 11-3
FEEDING FACILITATION TECHNIQUES FOR PRETERM INFANTS

Environment
- Prepare calm, quiet area with dim lighting and no distractions.
- Ensure restful environment between feeding.

Direct Care
- Begin preparing for oral feeding by providing NNS and milk odors with gavage feedings.
- Avoid trial po feeds after stressful procedures.
- Allow adequate time for rest between caregiving and before feedings.
- Provide feedings on semi-demand or demand basis depending on institutional feeding practices.
- Choose slightly firmer nipple with slower flow rather than a "premie" nipple that may result in rapid milk flow (infant will gain strength of suck over time) that the infant cannot manage.
- Be prepared to focus on the infant and feeding with ongoing observation and adaptation.
- Gently arouse to alert state; may use NNS prior to feeding.
- Swaddle in gentle flexion with hands midline toward face.
- Support positioning with infant cradled close to body in semi-upright or upright position with neck in neutral to slightly flexed position.
- Continually observe physiologic, behavioral, and oral-motor functioning, careful to respond when subtle cues are demonstrated indicating the need for modification or termination of the feeding.
- Provide adequate breathing/rest periods for infants who cannot pace themselves by either gently removing nipple or if that is too stressful, tip bottle gently downward to drain milk from nipple.
- Provide gentle jaw and cheek support discriminately only when problems occur with latching onto nipple, weak seal, or loss of milk bolus and after determining whether infant is really ready for oral feeding because this intervention may be aversive and disable the infant's own control and pacing of the feeding.
- Institute "developmental burping" on shoulder with postural support and gentle back rubbing in an upward motion to stimulate burp; avoid sitting infant upright and leaning forward or patting the back because this is an unstable position with tactile stimulation that is often disorganizing for the preterm infant with immature motor subsystems.
- Recognize infant's limits and when to stop feeding to avoid potential fatigue, aversion, physical compromise, and aspiration (infant cues guide all feedings and progression of feedings).
- Gavage the rest of the feeding as needed based on infant cues.
  - Reduce energy expenditure.
  - Promote a positive feeding experience and minimize feeding aversion.

Continued

BOX 11-3
FEEDING FACILITATION TECHNIQUES FOR PRETERM INFANTS—cont'd

Direct Care—cont'd

- Schedule plenty of undisturbed rest between feedings.
- Evaluate feeding tolerance.
  - Soft abdomen without distention.
  - Normal bowel sounds.
  - Minimal or no gastric residual.
  - Usual frequency, color, and consistency of stools.
  - Little or no spitting or regurgitation.
  - Interest and pleasure in feeding observed.
  - Maintains quiet, awake state for most of feeding.
  - Stable physiologic, motor, and state functioning throughout and postfeeding.
  - Manages liquid without drooling or leaking.
  - Coordinated oral-motor abilities (suck/swallow/breathing).
  - Adequate growth for age on standard growth curve, length, and frontal-occipital circumference measurements.
- Document volume, duration of feeding, feeding behaviors (autonomic, state, and motor) and interventions required.
  - Avoid subjective qualifiers such as "infant fed well, fair, or poor."
  - Record stress/stability signs and predominant infant state during feeding.
  - Note type of nipple.
  - Identify nursing support needed by infant (pacing, rest, swaddling).
  - Describe specific feeding problems demonstrated by infant (fatigue, coordination of suck/swallow/breathing, leakage of milk, tongue thrust, loss of muscle tone, etc.).
  - Describe rationale for stopping a feeding (choking, fatigue, leakage, facial and body tone, coughing, color change, breathing pauses, etc.).
  - Report any signs of feeding intolerance.
  - Note duration of feeding and volume taken by mouth and by gavage if needed.
- Collaborate with team on feeding plan to make feeding both a pleasant, learning experience and maintain adequate nutrition.
  - Decrease number of oral feedings per day or limit feeding duration each feed based on infant responses.
  - Complement feeding with gavage to preserve adequate nutrition rather than "force feed" infant.
  - Follow occupational therapist's plan (when involved) to promote therapeutic goals.
  - Ensure consistency with core team of nurses working with infants as individuals.

Family Support and Education

- Model appropriate feeding techniques.
- Discuss cultural preferences for feeding experiences and incorporate when possible.
- Provide ample opportunities for feeding practice (starting with feeding preparation with kangaroo or skin-to-skin care and milk odor if family desires).
- Educate on infant cues and measuring feeding success.
- Identify both enjoyment and adequate nutrition as feeding goals.

Consistency of Care

- Same caregivers consistently feed infant.
- Consistent feeding techniques are used between caregivers.
- Consistent use of appropriate feeding equipment.

Modified from Hunter, J.: The neonatal intensive care unit. In J. Case-Smith (Ed.): *Occupational therapy for children* (4th ed.). St Louis, 2001, Mosby; Carrier, C.T., Walden, M., and Wilson, D.: The high-risk newborn and family. In M.J. Hockenberry (Ed.): *Wong's nursing care of infants and children* (7th ed.). St Louis, 2003, Mosby.

H. Parents and feeding (Thoyre, 2001). Safe oral feeding techniques and infant assessment are essential information required by parents prior to discharge. Ample opportunity to observe infant feeding behaviors and practice in an environment of nursing/health provider support can facilitate success, confidence, competence, and enjoyment.

I. Breast-feeding the preterm infant (AAP, 1997; Lau, 2001; Lau and Hurst, 1999; Meier, 2001; Reynolds, 2001; Schanler, 2001). An important antecedent to breast-feeding is the opportunity for skin-to-skin holding or KC that includes eye contact, containment, olfactory, tactile, vestibular motion from rhythmic maternal respirations, and mother's voice that integrate the sensory components necessary for nonnutritive then nutritive breastfeeding. The American Academy of Pediatrics (AAP) recommends human milk for all infants including premature and sick newborn infants except in rare circumstances (AAP, 1997). They also acknowledge that the choice of breast- or bottle feeding is within the parents' right to choose and as such, they should be provided with accurate and current information on the benefits and techniques of breastfeeding. Developmentally, breast-feeding follows the natural course for promoting the connection between mother and child along with advantages related to immunity, improved digestion and absorption, gastrointestinal (GI) function, neurodevelopmental outcomes, maternal psychological health, and emotional bonding/attachment.

1. Support for the breast-feeding mother and infant (Lau and Hurst, 1999).
   - **a.** Privacy and comfort of both infant and mother with the use of screens, comfortable chairs, pillows to support the infant, dim lighting, minimal activity around mother-infant dyad, decreased noise, and bottled water or fluids to quench thirst. Arm, back, and neck support with pillows and a footstool can help the mother relax during the breast-feeding session.
   - **b.** Easy access to pumping equipment and breast milk storage.
   - **c.** Lactation consultants available for education, evaluation, and personal support during breast-feeding.
   - **d.** Training in proper breast-feeding positions.
     - (1) Cradle—classic holding with infant's head at mother's elbow.
     - (2) Clutch—infant's body rests across mother's chest or is tucked (football style) underneath her arm with the infant's head gently held in mother's hand; very effective when the infant needs guidance and support in attaching to the breast.
     - (3) Infant position—comfortable alignment, gentle flexion of extremities, and slight extension of neck for full jaw excursion; well-supported flexion and containment.
   - **e.** Share feeding readiness cues and prepare the mother for assessing stability and stress cues throughout a feeding; discuss and model appropriate interventions as indicated.
   - **f.** Allow plenty of time because breast-feeding sessions are generally longer than bottle-feeding sessions. Avoid rushing or appearing hurried so as not to influence mother's attitude or perception.
   - **g.** The most common problem observed in preterm infants is the difficulty in maintaining secure attachment to the nipple and areola. Lau and Hurst (2001) report successful use of silicone nipple shields over the breast to help the infant latch on and successfully maintain attachment (Lau and Hurst, 1999).

h. Methods of measuring milk intake: accurate measurement by test-weighing in which the clothed infant is weighed before and after feeding under the same conditions (no diaper or clothing changes) using electronic scales provide mothers with an objective assessment that may alleviate more anxiety concerning milk intake than subjective estimates.
i. Assist mother in evaluating breast-feeding success with objective rather than subjective measures that may leave her discouraged.
j. Prompt evaluation and correction of inadequate positioning or latch-on is recommended to facilitate breast-feeding success.

2. Prescribing feeding volumes over an identified time interval (e.g., ≥50 ml over 4 hours) may be an appealing compromise when cue-based, demand feedings cannot be achieved due to the preterm infant's inconsistent cues or demand behaviors. This method will also allow time for demand feeding cues to emerge without being suppressed by rigid schedules (Meier, 2001).

J. **Alternative feeding modalities** include gavage or gastrostomy feeding by gravity or by syringe pump. Developmental inputs associated with normalized feeding are extremely important for enhancing the pleasure of feeding associated with the feeling of fullness and stomach filling. Ways to enhance these alternative feeding methods include:
1. Environmental modification to minimize stress.
2. Nonnutritive sucking opportunity during feeding.
3. Human contact through holding and/or containment.
4. Olfactory stimulation from breast milk or formula as appropriate.
5. Feeding during KC or skin to skin.
6. Continual monitoring of infant cues during feeding by alternative methods.

Standard 4. Collaborative and consistent caregiving is considered necessary for clinical and developmental support of infants and families.

A. **Collaboration fosters care that is consistent between caregivers.** Consistency and collaboration by caregivers who establish familiarity and predictable routine support trust with both infant and family.
1. Consistency of care is a continuum that requires documentation of individual stress and stability cues, written plans of care based on individual assessment of each infant's response to the environment, care, procedures, and medical treatments.
2. Communication through the medical record, easily accessible assessment and care plans, and direct communication between and among caregivers at shift report or daily medical/nursing rounds foster collaborative practice and enhance consistent care.
3. A familiar group of people that care for individual infants provide reassurance that establishes trust and builds a partnership that is rewarding to the entire team, especially the family.

REFERENCES

Abrams, R.M. and Gerhardt, K. J.: The acoustic environment and physiological responses of the fetus. *Journal of Perinatology, 20*(8 Pt 2):S31-S36, 2000.

Acolet, D., Sleath, K., and Whitelaw, A.: Oxygenation, heart rate and temperature in very low birthweight infants during skin-to-skin contact with their mothers. *Acta Paediatrica Scandinavica, 78*(2):189-193, 1989.

Als, H.: *Manual for the naturalistic observation of newborn behavior: Newborn individual-*

ized developmental care and assessment program, Harvard Medical School, 1995, Boston.

Als, H.: Developmental care in the newborn intensive care unit. *Current Opinion in Pediatrics, 10*(2):138-142, 1998.

Als, H. and Gilkerson, L.: The role of relationship-based developmentally supportive newborn intensive care in strengthening outcome of preterm infants. *Seminars in Perinatology, 21*(3): 178-189, 1997.

Als, H., Lawhon, G., Brown, E., et al.: Individualized behavioral and environmental care for the very low birth weight preterm infant at high risk for bronchopulmonary dysplasia: Neonatal intensive care unit and developmental outcome. *Pediatrics, 78*(6):1123-1132, 1986.

Als, H., Lawhon, G., Duffy, F.H., et al.: Individualized developmental care for the very low-birth-weight preterm infant. Medical and neurofunctional effects. *Journal of the American Medical Association, 272*(11):853-858, 1994.

American Academy of Pediatrics: Breastfeeding and the use of human milk. *Pediatrics, 100*(6):1035-1039, 1997.

American Academy of Pediatrics: Changing concepts of sudden infant death syndrome: Implications for infant sleeping environment and sleep position (RE9946). *Pediatrics, 105*(3):650-656, 2000.

Anand, K.J.: Effects of perinatal pain and stress. *Progress in Brain Research, 122*:117-129, 2000.

Ancona, J., Shaker, C.S., Puhek, J., and Garland, J.S.: Improving outcomes through a developmental approach to nipple feeding. *Journal of Nursing Care Quality, 12*(5):1-4, 1998.

Anderson, G.C.: Current knowledge about skin-to-skin (kangaroo) care for preterm infants. *Journal of Perinatology, 11*(3):216-226, 1991.

Anderssen, S.H., Nicolaisen, R.B., and Gabrielsen, G.W.: Autonomic response to auditory stimulation. *Acta Paediatrica, 82*:913-918, 1993.

Arvedson, J.C., Rogers, B., Buck, G., et al.: Silent aspiration prominent in children with dysphagia. *International Journal of Pediatric Otorhinolaryngology, 28*(2-3): 173-181, 1994.

Banker, H. and Lickliter, R.: Effects of early and delayed visual experience on intersensory development in bobwhite quail chicks. *Developmental Psychobiology, 26*(3):155-170, 1993.

Bauer, J., Sontheimer, D., Fischer, C., and Linderkamp, O.: Metabolic rate and energy balance in very low birth weight infants during kangaroo holding by their mothers and fathers. *Journal of Pediatrics, 129*(4):608-611, 1996.

Bauer, K., Uhrig, C., Sperling, P., et al.: Body temperatures and oxygen consumption during skin-to-skin (kangaroo) care in stable preterm infants weighing less than 1500 grams. *Journal of Pediatrics, 130*(2):240-244, 1997.

Bingham, P.M., Abassi, S., and Sivieri, E.: A pilot study of milk odor effect on nonnutritive sucking by premature newborns. *Archives of Pediatrics and Adolescent Medicine, 157*(1):72-75, 2003.

Blackburn, S. and Patterson, D.: Effects of cycled light on activity, state, and cardiorespiratory function in preterm infants. *Journal of Perinatal and Neonatal Nursing, 4*(4):47-54, 1991.

Bracht, M., Kandankery, A., Nodwell, S., et al.: Cultural differences and parental responses to the preterm infant at risk: Strategies for supporting families. *Neonatal Network, 21*(6):31-37, 2002.

Brandon, D.H., Holditch-Davis, D., and Belyea, M.: Preterm infants born at less than 31 weeks' gestation have improved growth in cycled light compared with continuous near darkness. *Journal of Pediatrics, 140*(2):192-199, 2002.

Browne, J.V.: Considerations for touch and massage in the neonatal intensive care unit. *Neonatal Network, 19*(1):61-64, 2000.

Buehler, D.M., Als, H., Duffy, F.H., et al.: Effectiveness of individualized developmental care for low-risk preterm infants: Behavioral and electrophysiologic evidence. *Pediatrics, 96*(5 Pt 1):923-932, 1995.

Byrne, J., Ellsworth, C., Bowering, E., and Vincer, M.: Language development in low birth weight infants: The first two years of life. *Journal of Developmental and Behavioral Pediatrics, 14*(1):21-27, 1993.

Carey, W.B.: Communicating with parents and community involvement: Teaching parents about infant temperament. *Pediatrics, 102*(5):1311-1316, 1998.

Carrier, C.T., Walden, M., and Wilson, D.: The high-risk newborn and family. In M.J. Hockenberry (Ed.): *Wong's nursing care of infants and children* (7th ed.). St Louis, 2003, Mosby, pp. 333-414.

Case-Smith, J. and Humphrey, R.: Feeding and oral motor skills. In J. Case-Smith (Ed.): *Occupational therapy for children*. St Louis, 1996, Mosby, pp. 430-460.

Casey, M.B. and Lickliter, R.: Prenatal visual experience influences the development of turning bias in bobwhite quail chicks *(Colinus virginianus). Developmental Psychobiology, 32*(4):327-338, 1998.

Charpak, N., Ruiz-Pelaez, J.G., Figueroa de, C.Z., et al.: A randomized, controlled trial of kangaroo mother care: results of follow-up at 1 year of corrected age. *Pediatrics, 108*(5):1072-1079, 2001.

Chwo, M.J., Anderson, G.C., Good, M., et al.: A randomized controlled trial of early kangaroo care for preterm infants: Effects on temperature, weight, behavior, and acuity. *Journal of Nursing Research, 10*(2):129-142, 2002.

Comrie, J.D. and Helm, J.M.: Common feeding problems in the intensive care nursery: maturation, organization, evaluation, and management strategies. *Seminars in Speech and Language, 18*(3):239-60; quiz 261, 1997.

Conde-Agudelo, A., Diaz-Rossello, J.L., and Belizan, J.M.: Kangaroo mother care to reduce morbidity and mortality in low birthweight infants. *Cochrane Database of Systematic Reviews*, (4):CD002771, 2000.

Corff, K.E., Seideman, R., Venkataraman, P.S., et al.: Facilitated tucking: A nonpharmacological comfort measure for pain in preterm neonates. *Journal of Obstetric, Gynecologic, and Neonatal Nursing, 24(2):*143-147, 1995.

Crade, M., and Lovett, S.: Fetal response to sound stimulation: Preliminary report exploring use of sound stimulation in routine obstetrical ultrasound examinations. *Journal of Ultrasound in Medicine, 7*(9):499-503, 1988.

Daley, H.K. and Kennedy, C.M.: Meta analysis: Effects of interventions on premature infants feeding. *Journal of Perinatal and Neonatal Nursing, 14*(3):62-77, 2000.

Davis, N.M., Doyle, L.W., Ford, G.W., et al.: Auditory function at 14 years of age of very-low-birthweight. *Developmental Medicine and Child Neurology, 43*(3): 191-196, 2001.

Dupin, R., Laurent, J.P., Stauder, J.E., and Saliba, E.: Auditory attention processing in 5-year-old children born preterm: Evidence from event-related potentials. *Developmental Medicine and Child Neurology, 42*(7):476-480, 2000.

Evans, J.C.: Incidence of hypoxemia associated with caregiving in premature infants. *Neonatal Network, 16*(3):33-40, 1991.

Fearon, I., Kisilevsky, B.S., Hains, S.M., et al.: Swaddling after heel lance: Age-specific effects on behavioral recovery in preterm infants. *Journal of Developmental and Behavioral Pediatrics, 18*(4):222-232, 1997.

Feldman, R. and Eidelman, A.I.: Skin-to-skin contact (kangaroo care) accelerates autonomic and neurobehavioural maturation in preterm infants. *Developmental Medicine and Child Neurology, 45*(4):274-281, 2003.

Feldman, R., Eidelman, A.I., Sirota, L., and Weller, A.: Comparison of skin-to-skin (kangaroo) and traditional care: Parenting outcomes and preterm infant development. *Pediatrics, 110*(1 Pt 1):16-26, 2002a.

Feldman, R., Weller, A., Sirota, L., and Eidelman, A.I.: Skin-to-skin contact (kangaroo care) promotes self-regulation in premature infants: Sleep-wake cyclicity, arousal modulation, and sustained exploration. *Developmental Psychology, 38*(2):194-207, 2002b.

Fern, D., Graves, C., and L'Huillier, M.: Swaddled bathing in the newborn intensive care unit. *Newborn and Infant Nursing Reviews, 2*(1):3-4, 2002.

Field, T.M., Schanberg, S.M., Scafidi, F., et al.: Tactile/kinesthetic stimulation effects on preterm neonates. *Pediatrics, 77*(5): 654-658, 1986.

Fielder, A.R. and Moseley, M.J.: Environmental light and the preterm infant. *Seminars in Neonatology, 24*(4):291-292, 2000.

Fleisher, B.E., VandenBerg, K., Constantinou, J., et al.: Individualized developmental care for very-low-birth-weight premature infants. *Clinical Pediatrics (Phila), 34*(10):523-529, 1995.

Fohe, K., Kropf, S., and Avenarius, S.: Skin-to-skin contact improves gas exchange in premature infants. *Journal of Perinatology, 20*(5):311-315, 2000.

Foushee, R.D. and Lickliter, R.: Early visual experience affects postnatal auditory responsiveness in bobwhite quail *(Colinus virginianus). Journal of Comparative Psychology, 116*(4):369-380, 2002.

Fucile, S., Gisel, E., and Lau, C.: Oral stimulation accelerates the transition from tube to oral feeding in preterm infants. *Journal of Pediatrics, 141*(2):230-236, 2002.

Gadeke, R., Doring, B., Keller, F., Vogel, A..: The noise level in a children's hospital and the wake-up threshold in infants. *Acta Paediatrica Scandinavica, 58*:164-170, 1969.

Gerhardt, K.J. and Abrams, R. M.: Fetal exposures to sound and vibroacoustic stimulation. *Journal of Perinatology, 20*(8):S21-S30, 2000.

Gewolb, I.H., Bosma, J.F., Taciak, V.L., and Vice, F.L.: Abnormal developmental patterns of suck and swallow rhythms during feeding in preterm infants with bronchopulmonary dysplasia. *Developmental Medicine and Child Neurology, 43*(7):454-459, 2001.

Glass, P.: The vulnerable neonate and the neonatal intensive care environment. In M.G. MacDonald (Ed.): *Neonatology: Pathophysiology and management of the newborn*. Philadelphia, 1999, Lippincott Williams & Wilkins.

Goldberger, J. and Wolfer, J.: An approach for identifying potential threats to development in hospitalized toddlers. *Infants and Young Children, 3*(3):74-83, 1991.

Graven, S.N.: Sound and the developing infant in the NICU: Conclusions and recommendations for care. *Journal of Perinatology, 20*(8 Pt 2):S88-S93, 2000.

Gross, S.J., Mettleman, B.B., Dye, T.D., et al.: Impact of family structure and stability on academic outcome in preterm children at 10 years of age. *Journal of Pediatrics, 138*(2):169-175, 2001.

Hall, J.I.: Development of the ear and hearing. *Journal of Perinatology, 20*(8):S12-S20, 2000.

Harrison, L., Olivet, L., Cunningham, K., et al.: Effects of gentle human touch on preterm infants: Pilot study results. *Neonatal Network, 15*(2):35-42, 1996.

Harrison, L.L., Leeper, J., and Yoon, M.: Preterm infants' physiologic responses to early parent touch. *Western Journal of Nursing Research, 13*(6):698-707; discussion 708-713, 1991.

Harrison, L.L., Williams, A.K., Berbaum, M.L., et al.: Physiologic and behavioral effects of gentle human touch on preterm infants. *Research in Nursing and Health, 23*(6):435-446, 2000.

Harrison, L.L. and Woods, S.: Early parental touch and preterm infants. *Journal of Obstetric, Gynecologic, and Neonatal Nursing, 20*(4):299-306, 1991.

Hill, A.S.: Toward a theory of feeding efficiency for bottle-fed preterm infants, *Journal of Theory Construction & Testing, 6*(1):75-81, 2002.

Holditch-Davis, D., Blackburn, S.T., and VandenBerg, K.A.: *Newborn and infant neurobehavioral development*. St Louis, 2003, Saunders.

Honeycutt, H. and Lickliter, R.: Order-dependent timing of unimodal and multimodal stimulation affects prenatal auditory learning in bobwhite quail embryos. *Developmental Psychobiology, 38*(1):1-10, 2001.

Hunter, J.: The neonatal intensive care unit. In J. Case-Smith (Ed.): *Occupational therapy for children, ed 4*, St Louis, 2001, Mosby, pp. 636-707.

Jennische, M. and Sedin, G.: Speech and language skills in children who required neonatal intensive care. I. Spontaneous speech at 6.5 years of age. *Acta Paediatrica, 87*(6):654-666, 1998.

Jennische, M. and Sedin, G.: Speech and language skills in children who required neonatal intensive care: Evaluation at 6.5 y of age based on interviews with parents. *Acta Paediatrica, 88*(9):975-982, 1999.

Jennische, M. and Sedin, G.: Linguistic skills at 6½ years of age in children who required neonatal intensive care in 1986-1989. *Acta Paediatrica, 90*(2):199-212, 2001.

Kennedy, K.A., Fielder, A.R., Hardy, R.J., et al.: Reduced lighting does not improve medical outcomes in very low birth weight infants. *Journal of Pediatrics, 139*(4):527-531, 2001.

Kennedy, K.A., Ipson, M.A., Birch, D.G., et al.: Light reduction and the electroretinogram of preterm infants. *Archives of Disease in Childhood, Fetal and Neonatal Edition, 76*(3):F168-F173, 1997.

Lau, C.: Effects of stress on lactation. *Pediatric Clinics of North America, 48*(1):221-234, 2001.

Lau, C., Alagugurusamy, R., Schanler, R.J., et al.: Characterization of the developmental stages of sucking in preterm infants during bottle feeding. *Acta Paediatrica, 89*(7):846-852, 2000.

Lau, C. and Hurst, N.: Oral feeding in infants. *Current Problems in Pediatrics, 29*(4):105-124, 1999.

Lau, C. and Hurst N.: *Oral feeding of the preterm infant*. Nutrition Conference, Texas Children's Hospital, Houston, TX, Nov. 15, 2001.

Lau, C. and Schanler, R.J.: Oral feeding in premature infants: Advantage of a self-paced milk flow. *Acta Paediatrica, 89*(4):453-459, 2000.

Lau, C., Sheena, H.R., Shulman, R.J., et al.: Oral feeding in low birth weight infants. *Journal of Pediatrics, 130*(4):561-569, 1997.

Lemons, P.K.: From gavage to oral feedings: Just a matter of time. *Neonatal Network 20*(3):7-14, 2001.

Lickliter, R.: Atypical perinatal sensory stimulation and early perceptual development: Insights from developmental psychobiology. *Journal of Perinatology 20*(8 Pt 2):S45-S54, 2000a.

Lickliter, R.: The role of sensory stimulation in perinatal development: Insights from comparative research for care of the high-risk infant. *Journal of Developmental and Behavioral Pediatrics, 21*(6):437-447, 2000b.

Long, J.G., Lucey, J.F., and Philip, A.G.: Noise and hypoxemia in the intensive care nursery. *Pediatrics* 65(1):143-145, 1980.

Ludington-Hoe, S.M., Anderson, G.C., Simpson, S., et al.: Birth-related fatigue in 34-36-week preterm neonates: Rapid recovery with very early kangaroo (skin-to-skin) care. *Journal of Obstetric, Gynecologic, and Neonatal Nursing, 28*(1):94-103, 1999.

Mann, N.P., Haddow, R., Stokes, L., et al.: Effect of night and day on preterm infants in a newborn nursery: Randomised trial. *British Medical Journal (Clinical Research Edition), 293*(6557): 1265-1267, 1986.

McCain, G.C., Gartside, P.S., Greenberg, J.M., et al.: A feeding protocol for healthy preterm infants that shortens time to oral feeding. *Journal of Pediatrics, 139*(3):374-379, 2001.

McGrath, J.M. and Brock, N.: Efficacy and utilization of skin-to-skin care in the NICU. *Newborn and Infant Nursing Reviews, 2*(1):17-26, 2002.

Meier, P.P.: Breastfeeding in the special care nursery. Prematures and infants with medical problems. *Pediatric Clinics of North America, 48*(2):425-442, 2001.

Messmer, P.R., Rodriguez, S., Adams, J., et al.: Effect of kangaroo care on sleep time for neonates. *Pediatric Nursing, 23*(4): 408-414, 1997.

Miller, C., White, R., Whitman, T., et al.: The effects of cycled versus noncycled lighting on growth and development in preterm infants. *Infant Behavioral Development, 18*:87-95, 1995.

Mizuno, K. and Ueda, A.: The maturation and coordination of sucking, swallowing, and respiration in preterm infants. *Journal of Pediatrics, 142*(1):36-40, 2003.

Modrcin-Talbott, M.A., Harrison, L.L., Groer, M.W., and Younger, M.S.: The biobehavioral effects of gentle human touch on preterm infants. *Nursing Science Quarterly, 16*(1):60-67, 2003.

Moon, C.M., and Fifer,W.P.: Evidence of transnatal auditory learning. *Journal of Perinatology, 20*(8):S37-S44, 2000.

Morris, B.H., Philbin, M.K., and Bose, C.: Physiological effects of sound on the newborn. *Journal of Perinatology, 20*(8 Pt 2):S55-S60, 2000.

Neu, M. and Browne, J.V.: Infant physiologic and behavioral organization during swaddled versus unswaddled weighing. *Journal of Perinatology, 17*(3):193-198, 1997.

Neu, M., Browne, J.V., and Vojir, C.: The impact of two transfer techniques used during skin-to-skin care on the physiologic and behavioral responses of preterm infants. *Nursing Research, 49*(4):215-223, 2000.

Pearson, J. and Andersen, K.: Evaluation of a program to promote positive parenting in the neonatal intensive care unit. *Neonatal Network, 20*(4):43-48, 2001.

Peters, K.: Infant handling in the NICU: Does developmental care make a difference? An evaluative review of the literature. *Journal of Perinatal and Neonatal Nursing, 13*(3):83-109, 1999.

Peters, K.L.: Does routine nursing care complicate the physiologic status of the premature neonate with respiratory distress syndrome? *Journal of Perinatal and Neonatal Nursing*, 6(2):67-84, 1992.

Philbin, M.K.: The influence of auditory experience on the behavior of preterm newborns. *Journal of Perinatology, 20*(8 Pt 2):S77-S87, 2000.

Philbin, M.K. and Gray, L.: Changing levels of quiet in an intensive care nursery. *Journal of Perinatology, 22*(6):455-460, 2002.

Philbin, M.K. and Klaas, P.: Evaluating studies of the behavioral effects of sound on newborns. *Journal of Perinatology, 20*(8 Pt 2):S61-S67, 2000a.

Philbin, M.K. and Klaas, P.: Hearing and behavioral responses to sound in full-term newborns. *Journal of Perinatology, 20*(8 Pt 2):S68-S76, 2000b.

Pickler, R.H., Frankel, H.B., Walsh, K.M., and Thompson, N.M..: Effects of nonnutritive sucking on behavioral organization and feeding performance in preterm infants. *Nursing Research, 45*(3):132-135, 1996.

Pinelli, J. and Symington, A.: How rewarding can a pacifier be? A systematic review of nonnutritive sucking in preterm infants. *Neonatal Network, 19*(8):41-48, 2000.

Porter, R.H. and Winberg, J.: Unique salience of maternal breast odors for newborn infants. *Neuroscience and Biobehavioral Reviews, 23*(3):439-449, 1999.

Premji, S., Paes, B., Jacobson, K., et al.: Evidence-based feeding guidelines for very-low-birthweight infants. *Advances in Neonatal Care, 2*(1):5-18, 2002a.

Premji, S.S., Chessell, L., Paes, B., et al.: A matched cohort study of feeding practice guidelines for infants weighing less than 1500 g. *Advances in Neonatal Care, 2*(1):27, 2002b.

Reynolds, A.: Breastfeeding and brain development. *Pediatric Clinics of North America, 48*(1):159-171, 2001.

Reynolds, J.D., Hardy, R.J., Kennedy, K.A., et al.: Lack of efficacy of light reduction in preventing retinopathy of prematurity. Light Reduction in Retinopathy of Prematurity (LIGHT-ROP) Cooperative Group. *New England Journal of Medicine, 338*(22):1572-1576, 1998.

Roberts, K.L., Paynter, C., and McEwan, B.: A comparison of kangaroo mother care and conventional cuddling care. *Neonatal Network, 9*(4):31-35, 2000.

Robertson, A., Cooper-Peel, C., and Vos, P.: Contribution of heating, ventilation, and air conditioning airflow and conversation to the ambient sound in a neonatal intensive care unit. *Journal of Perinatology, 19*(5):362-366, 1999a.

Robertson, A., Cooper-Peel, C., and Vos, P.: Sound transmission into incubators in the neonatal intensive care unit. *Journal of Perinatology, 19*(7):494-497, 1999b.

Robertson, A., Kohn, J., Vos, P., et al.: Establishing a noise measurement protocol for neonatal intensive care units. *Journal of Perinatology, 18*(2):126-130, 1998.

Robertson, A., Stuart, A., and Walker, L.: Transmission loss of sound into incubators: Implications for voice perception by infants. *Journal of Perinatology, 21*(4):236-241, 2001.

Robison, L.D.: An organizational guide for an effective developmental program in the NICU. *Journal of Obstetric, Gynecologic, and Neonatal Nursing, 32*(3): 379-386, 2003.

Ross, E.S. and Browne, J.V.: Developmental progression of feeding skills: An approach to supporting feeding in preterm infants. *Seminars in Neonatology, 7*(6):469-745, 2002.

Roy, M.S., Caramelli, C., Orquin, J., et al.: Effects of early reduced light exposure on central visual development in preterm infants. *Acta Paediatrica, 88*(4):459-461, 1999.

Schanler, R.J.: The use of human milk for premature infants. *Pediatric Clinics of North America, 48*(1):207-219, 2001.

Sleigh, M.J., Columbus, R.F., and Lickliter, R.: Type of prenatal sensory experience affects prenatal auditory learning in bobwhite quail *(Colinus virginianus). Journal of Comparative Psychology, 110*(3):233-242, 1996.

Sleigh, M.J. and Lickliter, R.: Augmented prenatal visual stimulation alters postnatal auditory and visual responsiveness in bobwhite quail chicks. *Developmental Psychobiology, 28*(7):353-366, 1995.

Sleigh, M.J. and Lickliter, R.: Timing of presentation of prenatal auditory stimulation alters auditory and visual responsiveness in bobwhite quail chicks *(Colinus virginianus). Journal of Comparative Psychology, 112*(2):153-160, 1998.

Slevin, M., Murphy, J.F.A., Daly, L., et al.: Retinopathy of prematurity screening, stress related responses, the role of nesting. *British Journal of Ophthalmology, 81(9)*:762-764, 1999.

Smith, D.: Facility profile. Noises off: Nursery pumps down the volume. *Health Facilities Management, 12*(5):20-21, 1999.

Strauch, C., Brandt, S., and Edwards-Beckett, J.: Implementation of a quiet hour: Effect on noise levels and infant sleep states. *Neonatal Network, 12*(2):31-35, 1993.

Sweeney, J.K. and Gutierrez, T.: Musculoskeletal implications of preterm infant positioning in the NICU. *Journal of Perinatal and Neonatal Nursing, 16*(1): 58-70, 2002.

Symington, A. and Pinelli, J.: Distilling the evidence on developmental care: A systematic review. *Advances in Neonatal Care,* 2(4):198-221, 2002.

Thoman, E.B., Davis, D.H., and Denenberg, V.H.: The sleeping and waking states of infants: Correlations across time and person. *Physiology and Behavior,* 41(6):531-537, 1987.

Thoyre, S.M.: Challenges mothers identify in bottle feeding their preterm infants. *Neonatal Network,* 20(1):41-50, 2001.

Tornhage, C.J., Stuge, E., Lindberg, T., et al.: First week kangaroo care in sick very preterm infants. *Acta Paediatrica,* 88(12):1402-1404, 1999.

Vickers, A., Ohlsson, A., Lacy, J.B., et al.: Massage for promoting growth and development of preterm and/or low birth-weight infants. *Cochrane Database of Systematic Reviews,* (2):CD000390, 2000.

Walsh-Sukys, M., Reitenbach, A., Hudson-Barr, D., et al.: Reducing light and sound in the neonatal intensive care unit: An evaluation of patient safety, staff satisfaction and costs. *Journal of Perinatology,* 21(4):230-235, 2001.

Westrup, B., Kleberg, A., von Eichwald, K., et al.: A randomized, controlled trial to evaluate the effects of the newborn individualized developmental care and assessment program in a Swedish setting. *Pediatrics,* 105(1 Pt 1):66-72, 2000.

Wharrad, H.J. and Davis, A.C.: Behavioural and autonomic responses to sound in pre-term and full-term babies. *British Journal of Audiology,* 31(5): 315-329, 1997.

Wheeden, A., Scafidi, F.A., Field, T., et al.: Massage effects on cocaine-exposed preterm neonates. *Journal of Developmental and Behavioral Pediatrics,* 14(5): 318-322, 1993.

Whitfield, M.F., Grunau, R.V., and Holsti, L.: Extremely premature (< or = 800 g) schoolchildren: Multiple areas of hidden disability. *Archives of Disease in Childhood, Fetal Neonatal Edition,* 77(2):F85-F90, 1997.

Zahr, L.K. and Balian, S.: Responses of premature infants to routine nursing interventions and noise in the NICU. *Nursing Research,* 44(3):179-185, 1995.

CHAPTER

12 Pharmacology

CHRISTINE D. HOCHWALD

OBJECTIVES

1. Define the concepts of (a) pharmacology, (b) pharmacodynamics, and (c) pharmacokinetics.
2. Describe the developmental changes that affect medication absorption, distribution, metabolism, and elimination.
3. Identify specific considerations when one is administering medications of the following types to a neonate: (a) antimicrobial agents, (b) cardiovascular agents, (c) central nervous system agents, (d) diuretics, and (e) immunizations.
4. Describe nursing responsibilities and interventions when administering medications to the neonate.

The study and clinical application of neonatal pharmacology can facilitate safe medication administration in the neonate. The application of pharmacologic principles involves evaluating existing knowledge related to the pharmacodynamic and pharmacokinetic responses of the neonate to specific medications. This knowledge must be considered relative to gestational and chronologic age, weight, fluid status, and the health-illness state of individual organ systems. The decision to administer a medication should be evaluated for desired response and potential for undesirable reaction. The nurse is in the ideal position to observe and evaluate both response and reaction and to intervene if necessary.

This chapter provides pharmacologic information specific to the neonate. Information on medication dosages and implications for medication administration is provided in individual clinical chapters. Additional current reference materials should also be available in the neonatal intensive care unit (NICU).

PRINCIPLES OF PHARMACOLOGY

Terminology

A. **Pharmacology:** the science of the properties of medications and their effects in the body.
   1. **Pharmacotherapy:** the administration of a medication to a patient with the intent of preventing, diagnosing, or treating disease.
   2. **Medication:** any substance or mixture of substances intended to be used for the cure, mitigation, or prevention of disease in human beings or animals.
   3. **Pharmacodynamics:** the relationship between medication concentrations at the site of action and the pharmacologic response (intensity and time course of therapeutic and adverse effects). This is what the drug does to the body.
   4. **Pharmacokinetics:** the fate of a medication in the body from the time it enters until it and all of its metabolites are removed. This includes medication absorption, distribution, metabolism, and excretion. It is also the

specialized study of the mathematical relationship between a medication dosage regimen and the resulting serum concentration. This is what the body does to the drug.

5. **Bioavailability:** the portion of the administered dose that reaches the site of action in the body. This is usually the amount entering the circulation and may be low when medications are given by mouth.
6. **Therapeutic range:** a range of medication concentrations within which the probability of the desired clinical response is relatively high and the probability of unacceptable toxicity or subtherapeutic response is relatively low.

B. **Therapeutic drug monitoring (TDM):** determinations of plasma medication concentrations to optimize medication therapy. TDM is valuable when:
   1. A good correlation exists between the pharmacologic response and plasma concentration.
   2. Wide intersubject variation in drug plasma levels results from a given dose.
   3. The medication has a narrow therapeutic range.
   4. The medication's desired pharmacologic effects cannot be readily assessed by other simple means.
   5. **Steady state:** a term used to refer to a situation in which the amount of medication administered is equal to the amount of medication eliminated. When steady state is reached in a patient, the blood concentrations remain "steady." Therefore at steady state, all peak drug levels and all trough drug levels should be the same.
   6. **Half-life:** the time necessary for a measured medication concentration to fall to half its original value. A medication's duration of action is often related to its half-life and may also indicate when another dose should be given. It takes approximately five half-lives to reach steady state.
   7. **Peak level:** a drug level that is drawn after the dose is given and after adequate time is allowed for the drug to distribute throughout the body. The time for the drug to distribute varies with each medication and the route of administration.
   8. **Trough level:** a drug level that is drawn just prior to the dose.
   9. **Random level:** a drug level that is drawn at any time after a dose is given. These levels are often used to follow drug levels in patients with changing renal function or changing volume status.

PHARMACODYNAMICS

A. **Receptor concept.** The principle that medications act by forming a complex with a specific macromolecule in a way that produces a given response. This response may include inhibition or potentiation of the macromolecule's activity to create the desired medication effect. Receptor effects are as follows:
   1. The medication's affinity for binding to the receptor plays a large part in the determination of the concentration of the medication required to achieve the desired response.
   2. The individual characteristics of the receptor are responsible for the selective nature of medication response.
   3. Receptor theory of medication action allows an explanation of medication antagonists. The antagonist medication may alter the characteristics of the receptor molecule in a way that limits or inhibits the response to the original medication (e.g., naloxone and morphine) or stimulus (e.g., a β-blocker such as propranolol).

4. Some medications do not appear to act through receptors. Their action is related to a direct response in the recipient.

B. General mechanisms of medication action.

1. Based on the nature of the receptor/medication complex.
2. Types of receptor/medication complexes.
   a. Receptor/medication complexes that regulate gene expression.
      (1) One common class of medications acts by mediating a response that ultimately involves gene expression and new protein synthesis.
      (2) These medications generally do not have a rapid effect after initial administration (e.g., epoetin alfa).
   b. Receptor/medication complexes that change cell membrane permeability.
      (1) Many clinically useful medications act by changing the cell membrane permeability and therefore altering membrane characteristics.
      (2) These medications may have a relatively short lag time between administration and response (e.g., penicillin).
   c. Receptor/medication complexes that increase the intracellular concentration of a second messenger molecule.
      (1) These medications increase production and activity of enzyme systems within the cell.
      (2) These medications may stimulate a rapid response in changing cell characteristics (dopamine).

C. Relationship between medication dose and clinical response.

1. Individuals in a population receiving a medication may have a wide range of responses to a medication dose. An idiosyncratic medication response is an abnormal response to a medication that is not usually observed. These unpredictable responses include the following:
   a. Low sensitivity: a patient who, on receiving the usual medication dose, exhibits a clinical or biologic response that is less intense than expected (e.g., inadequate pain relief with usual doses of analgesic medications).
   b. Extreme sensitivity: a patient whose response to a medication is more intense than is expected (e.g., severe hypotension from an antihypertensive agent).
   c. Unpredictable adverse reaction: a patient whose medication reaction is substantially different from what would have been predicted; for example, the patient's physiologic response to a particular medication may differ from the usual response in most patients.
   d. Tolerance: a diminished response to a given medication dose that is related to long-term administration of a medication (e.g., morphine doses must be increased as the length of therapy increases to achieve the same effects).
   e. Tachyphylaxis: a rapidly diminished medication response without a medication dosage change. This may be caused by any of a number of factors, including a limited number of receptor sites or limited numbers of transmitter chemicals (e.g., response to albuterol may diminish if given frequently).
2. Factors that may affect individual medication response are:
   a. Alterations in medication concentration: a change from the expected norm in the amount of medication that reaches the receptor molecule.
   b. Variation in amounts of antagonistic substances: an unusually large or limited amount of antagonistic substances that alter receptor molecule response.

c. Alterations in numbers or function of receptor molecules: an increased or diminished number of receptor molecules changes the number of potential medication/receptor complexes.
d. Changes in concentration of molecules other than receptor molecules: if medication response is ultimately dependent on an effect on molecules other than those of the medication/receptor complex, medication response may be limited by the amount of the third molecule type (e.g., prodrugs such as fosphenytoin).

D. Desired versus undesired effects of medications.

1. No medication causes only one effect; all medications have several effects, which can be divided into four groups:
   a. Desired, or therapeutic, effects: those effects that are the desired outcome of the medication administration (e.g., reduction in apnea episodes with theophylline treatment).
   b. Subtherapeutic effect: those effects that are less than the desired outcome of the medication administration (e.g., continued apnea episodes with low theophylline levels).
   c. Side effects: those medication effects that result from medication administration and that are in addition to the desired effects. All medications have some side effects, varying from minor and clinically insignificant to major side effects that are sufficiently adverse to require discontinuation of the medication therapy (e.g., tachycardia with theophylline treatment).
   d. Toxic effects: medication response that results from a medication overdose or unexpected high serum medication concentrations (e.g. seizures from a high theophylline level).
2. It is the responsibility of the health care provider to weigh the benefits of the therapeutic effect against the risk of undesirable side effects and toxic effects or subtherapeutic responses and make adjustments accordingly.

PHARMACOKINETICS

A. Principles of medication absorption (Fig. 12-1).

1. General principles of medication absorption.
   a. The movement of a medication from the site of administration to the bloodstream.
   b. Regardless of the route of administration, most medications must cross cell membranes to reach their site of action.
      (1) Most medications cross cell membranes by passive diffusion. Physiochemical properties of the medication molecule have a major impact on the ease of diffusion.
      (2) Medications may also enter the cell through other mechanisms, such as active transport or facilitated diffusion.
   c. The absorption of a medication is dependent, in large part, on the route of administration. The common sites of administration are:
      (1) Gastrointestinal (GI): commonly used because of convenience.
         (a) Surface and absorption area: structurally the neonatal GI tract has a greater ratio of surface area to body mass. This provides a more absorptive surface area (Nagourney and Aranda, 1998).
         (b) Gastric emptying and intestinal transit times: prolonged and irregular; approaches adult values at 6 to 8 months of age. Gastric and intestinal motility are reduced with prematurity, asphyxia,

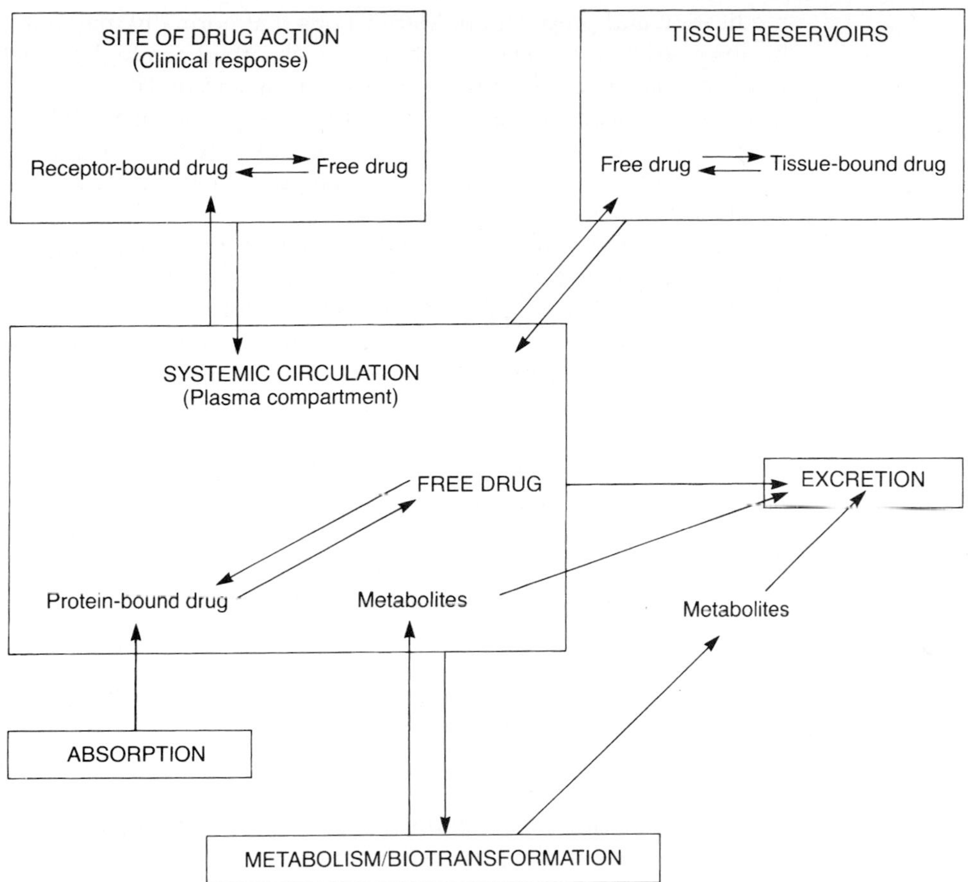

FIGURE 12-1 ■ Principles of medication absorption. From Aranda, J.V., Hales, B.F., and Reider, M.F.: Developmental pharmacology. In A.A. Fanaroff and R.J. Martin (Eds.): *Neonatal-perinatal medicine: Diseases of the fetus and infant* (6th ed.). St Louis, 1997, Mosby.

gastroesophageal reflux, and respiratory distress syndrome. The net effect of prolonged GI transit times appears to be, in most cases, increased absorption, in comparison with that of adults (Nagourney and Aranda, 1998). Administration of hypocaloric feeds, human milk or prokinetic agents such as metoclopramide or bethanechol can increase motility. Prolonged transit times and enterohepatic recirculation may also increase the bioavailability and pharmacologic effect of some substances (Chemtob, 1998). However, the bioavailability of the medication may decrease because of increased first-pass loss, increased GI destruction of medication or shortened transit times from diarrhea or emesis.

(c) GI tract acidity: presence of marked changes in pH from the stomach through the distal portion of the GI tract may affect absorption. The pH of the GI tract is nearly neutral at birth due to the presence of residual amniotic fluid. The stomach pH gradually decreases to adult values by the second year of life (Stewart and Hampton, 1987). The net effect of GI acidity on the absorption of medications is dependant on the pH characteristics of the medication and preparation. Medications that normally may not be absorbed well in the stomach may be absorbed at a higher rate in the neonate because of decreased stomach acidity. The absorption of acidic drugs will be reduced (e.g., phenobarbital, phenytoin) and the absorption of basic drugs will be enhanced (e.g., penicillin, erythromycin) as compared with adults (Kraus and Pham, 2001).

(d) GI enzyme activity: neonates are deficient in pancreatic enzymes at birth. This deficiency may inhibit absorption of some medications that require pancreatic enzymes for efficient absorption. One compensating mechanism that neonates have is an increased β-glucuronidase secretion. This is an enzyme produced by organisms normally present in the small intestine that are capable of metabolizing some medications. It is up to seven times the adult amounts.

(e) Bacterial flora: composition and rate of colonization of the GI tract by the normal bacterial flora may affect both GI tract motility and the metabolism of some medications. Colonization is dependent on oral intake, antibiotic administration, or disease states such as necrotizing enterocolitis or infectious gastroenteritis. Normal colonization in vaginally born term neonates occurs by 4 to 6 days of age. Intestinal flora are required for the production of vitamin K (Nagourney and Aranda, 1998).

(f) GI tract perfusion: in very ill neonates, hypoperfusion of the gut may decrease medication absorption.

(g) Underlying disease states: underlying disease states such as diarrhea, emesis, or the presence of nasogastric suction may reduce the time available for medication absorption. Diseases of genetic (e.g., cystic fibrosis) or circulatory (e.g., necrotizing enterocolitis) origin will alter pancreatic enzymes or intestinal mucosa, decreasing GI absorption.

(2) Rectal: may be a very rapid and efficient means of medication administration.

(a) Useful when rapid IV access is not available (e.g., patients in status epilepticus in need of anticonvulsant agents).

(b) Serum levels of some medications may be as high as levels obtained through the IV route of administration (Kraus and Pham, 2001).

(c) The routine administration by rectal route is discouraged. Relative volume and fragility of the neonatal rectum must be considered.

(d) The retention time is the rate-limiting step.

(3) Inhalation: useful for gaseous or easily vaporized medications.

(a) Absorption is favored due to large surface area of the alveolar membranes and the generous blood flow. Medication response may be very rapid.

(b) Medications administered by this route have a particular advantage when the site of desired action is the tracheobronchial tree (e.g., albuterol, terbutaline).

(c) There is a potential for fewer side effects when medications are administered this way, because much of the medication may not be systemically absorbed.

(d) Most frequently used in neonatal intensive care for the administration of various surfactant preparations.

(e) Certain medications (e.g., epinephrine, atropine, and lidocaine) can be given through the endotracheal tube in emergency situations when IV access is not readily available.

(f) This route may be less effective in a neonate with pulmonary hypertension and poor or abnormally distributed pulmonary blood flow.

(4) Topical/percutaneous: utility is limited to medications whose absorptive characteristics allow permeation through the skin or mucous membranes. Percutaneous absorption has particular advantages and risks in the newborn infant.

(a) The rate of absorption is inversely related to skin thickness and directly related to skin hydration. With increasing gestational age, skin thickness increases and water content decreases thus reducing the amount of absorption from this route. Maturation of the epidermis occurs between 23 and 33 weeks' gestation. In the extremely premature neonate, the stratum corneum is almost absent, but forms during the first 2 to 3 weeks after birth. Formation of this layer of the skin greatly decreases the permeability of the skin to water and other substances (Nagourney and Aranda, 1998). This allows much more efficient percutaneous absorption of medications in neonates of lower birth weight and younger gestational age. However, this poses a particular hazard in care, because substances that may be safely applied to the skin of a more mature patient may be absorbed in dangerous amounts in the immature neonate (Nahata and Taketomo, 2002).

(b) The ratio of body surface area to body weight is higher in neonates than adults, providing a relatively larger absorptive surface in comparison with body mass.

(c) The absorptive response time is variable and may be limited to the local area of application; however, some topically applied medications (e.g., nitroglycerin) can have a systemic effect. As a result, products that contain alcohol and hexachlorophene skin washes should be avoided. Any treatment with topical steroids should be limited to less than 2 weeks to prevent adrenal suppression. Antibiotic ointments will be more readily absorbed to treat infections, povidone-iodine (Betadine) absorption can prevent iodine deficiency, and topical safflower oil may prevent essential fatty acid deficiency.

(d) Occlusive dressings will increase the extent of absorption.

(5) Intramuscular/subcutaneous: administration into muscle or subcutaneous tissue.

(a) Minimal subcutaneous tissue and muscle mass significantly limit these two routes of administration, particularly in the low birth weight neonate.

(b) These routes are limited to medications that do not cause tissue damage at the administration site and are soluble at physiologic pH.

(c) These routes will achieve slower responses as compared with the IV route because of the lag time between administration and achievement of blood concentration.

(d) Response time is dependent on blood flow to muscle and may be greatly delayed in hypoperfused tissue. Poor peripheral blood flow and low blood pressure are common in neonates. These problems become less common with increasing gestational age but can occur in the presence of many neonatal disease states. Poor cardiac output frequently occurs with many illness states in the neonatal period. Subsequent increases in the peripheral perfusion after resolution of the primary illness states may put the neonate at risk of having an increase in the rate and amount of medication absorption.

(e) Diminished muscle activity in the ill neonate decreases muscle perfusion and consequently may limit absorption of medications administered by this route.

(6) Intravenous: direct administration into the bloodstream.

(a) Bypasses all absorptive barriers.

(b) Most effective and reliable method of medication administration because the medication is delivered directly to the circulating plasma volume.

(c) Significant medication serum concentrations are reached rapidly, allowing for immediate medication response. This includes both desired and undesired or toxic reactions.

(d) Adequate and equal distribution to all organs or compartments is not guaranteed. Characteristics of some biologic membranes may limit medication distribution to body compartments (e.g., blood-brain barrier with meningitis).

(e) Rapid achievement of potentially dangerous serum medication concentrations may require administration of the intravenous medication over a prolonged period (e.g., vancomycin, amphotericin, and aminoglycosides).

B. Principles of medication distribution.

1. Distribution: movement of the medication to and through various body compartments. The extent of this movement, the "size" of the compartment, the number and character of the binding sites, and the amount of the medication administered determine the amount of medication at the desired site of action. When medication movement reaches a steady state, the volume of distribution is defined as the hypothetical volume of body fluid that would be required to dissolve the total amount of medication as found in the serum. This volume is sometimes described as apparent volume of distribution. This volume may be larger than the total body volume if the medication is highly protein- or tissue-bound.

2. Body compartments.

a. Total body water: as age increases, total body water, as a percentage of total body mass, decreases. Total body water in adults compromises approximately 55% of total body weight; in term infants it is 75%, and in preterm infants it is 85% (Berry et al., 2002).

(1) As body water increases, as a percentage of body mass, water-soluble medications have a larger volume of distribution.

(2) Because of increased total body water, a less mature neonate may require a larger per-kilogram dose to achieve the same peak medication concentration and effect as an older patient (e.g., aminoglycosides).

(3) In the first several days after birth, neonates may have rapid changes in volume of distribution for water-soluble medications, in relation to normal physiology and illness states.

(4) Body water loss is divided into two main categories: sensible and insensible. Sensible losses can be measured and quantified. In term

neonates, insensible losses occur in a strong relationship to metabolism. In extremely premature neonates, insensible losses occur primarily through evaporative loss, independent of metabolic rate. Insensible losses are difficult to quantify (Chemtob, 1998).

(5) Medications frequently administered to the neonate (e.g., diuretics, indomethacin) may have a major impact on body water volume and, as a side effect, may alter volume of distribution (Chemtob, 1998).

(6) Neonates with disease states that alter water excretion (e.g., primary renal disease, secretion of inappropriate antidiuretic hormone [SIADH], congestive heart failure, capillary leak syndromes) may have expansion of body water as a result of this dysfunction.

(7) The preceding alterations make dosing medications that are primarily distributed in body water (e.g., aminoglycoside antibiotics such as gentamicin) difficult.

(8) Frequent monitoring of medication levels may be required as the mentioned changes in body compartment volumes occur.

b. Fat: wide variability of neonatal values, based on gestational age, intrauterine, and postnatal growth patterns. This percentage increases from 1% of body weight at 28 weeks' gestation to approximately 15% in a term neonate (Chemtob, 1998; Nagourney and Aranda, 1998).

(1) Medications with more lipid solubility have affinity for this tissue.

(2) Reduced amounts of the percentage of body fat may make the volume of distribution smaller for medications distributed primarily in fatty tissue. Hence the plasma levels of these medications will be higher because less drug will be bound in the fat tissue, resulting in a greater potential for side effects and toxicity (e.g., morphine, lorazepam).

c. Blood components: potential sites for medication binding.

(1) Erythrocytes: neonates contain 2.5 times more binding sites for digoxin as compared with the erythrocytes in adults. This results in the need for much higher doses per total body weight in neonates than adults (Stewart and Hampton, 1987).

(2) Plasma protein concentrations: medications may form a complex with large circulating molecules (usually proteins).

(a) The amount of medication that binds to these sites has a direct effect on the amount of medication available for the desired pharmacologic effect. This binding may result in a limited medication response because only the unbound medication can be distributed to active receptor sites. The more of the medication that is protein-bound, the less is available for the desired medication effect: serum concentration = protein-bound medication + unbound medication.

(b) The primary binding protein for acidic medications in the serum is albumin (e.g., phenytoin, indomethacin, and furosemide) (Nagourney and Aranda, 1998).

(c) Serum albumin levels may be markedly decreased in the ill extremely low birth weight neonate.

(d) The primary binding protein for basic molecules are lipoproteins, glycoproteins, and β-globulins (e.g., lidocaine, propranolol) (Chemtob, 1998).

d. Unconjugated bilirubin: many neonates have increased plasma unconjugated bilirubin levels. Fetal albumin has an increased affinity for bilirubin and a decreased affinity for medications. This causes the unconjugated bilirubin to displace some medications from the albumin-binding sites, allowing more free medication available for action. In contrast, some medications (e.g., ceftriaxone, sulfonamides) may displace unconjugated bilirubin from albumin-binding sites. This may lead to the deposition of unconjugated bilirubin in the neonatal brain causing kernicterus (Stewart and Hampton, 1987). These medications should be avoided if possible in patients younger than 2 months of age or in patients with high unconjugated bilirubin levels.

e. Free fatty acids: increased serum-free fatty acid concentrations have been shown to displace some medications from plasma albumin-binding sites (Chemtob, 1998).

f. Blood pH: acidosis is a common finding associated with many neonatal disorders. Changes in blood pH have been shown to change albumin-binding characteristics. This may cause medication displacement from albumin. Changes in blood pH may also cause medications to displace unconjugated bilirubin (see above).

g. Blood-brain barrier: incomplete in the newborn causing a greater permeability to lipophilic medications (e.g., phenytoin, benzodiazepines). This incomplete barrier may be beneficial when treating neonatal meningitis because the antibiotics penetrate the cerebrospinal fluid more readily (Kraus and Pham, 2001).

3. Medication movement: an important part of medication distribution involves medication movement from the site of administration to sites throughout the body. It is dependent on the blood flow and medication solubility.

a. Blood flow: amount and distribution of blood flow to the target organ or cell affect the delivery of a medication absorbed into the bloodstream. Continued adequate blood flow and serum medication concentration are required to maintain an adequate concentration of the medication at the target organ. Several neonatal conditions affect blood flow:

(1) Hypotension: may affect peripheral medication absorption and/or distribution.

(2) Distributive shock: caused by inappropriate vasodilatation; seen with sepsis. Medication distribution to specific organs may be limited by local hypoperfusion.

(3) Pulmonary hypertension: may impede medication delivery to pulmonary vascular bed.

(4) Patent ductus arteriosus: blood flow may be distributed preferentially to either the pulmonary or systemic circulation, depending on pressure differential.

(5) Congestive heart failure: may affect peripheral medication absorption or distribution.

b. Medication solubility: in biologic tissues, the relative ability of the medication to dissolve in biologic fluids.

(1) Medications with low lipid solubility do not distribute well through lipid membranes, though they may be distributed well through the body water spaces. Highly lipid-soluble medications are distributed readily through most lipid membranes but are not distributed well through body water spaces.

(2) The relative medication solubility may make some medication use inappropriate. A medication with low lipid solubility may not reach therapeutic concentrations in an organ that is primarily fat tissue.

C. **Principles of medication metabolism.**

1. General principles of medication metabolism. Many medications must be converted into more water-soluble compounds before they can be removed from the body. Metabolism (biotransformation) is the *chemical change* of a medication into another form. This transformed medication may be pharmacologically active or inactive. The liver, kidney, gastrointestinal tract, lung, adrenal gland, blood, and skin are tissues capable of biotransformation of certain compounds. Of these sites, the liver is the principal organ for medication metabolism.

   a. Liver.

   (1) Metabolic activity is divided into two main types.

   (a) Phase I (nonsynthetic) metabolism of medications: primarily oxidation, reduction, hydrolysis, or demethylation reactions, which generally occur in the smooth endoplasmic reticulum of the hepatocyte. The function of these enzymes in the full- and preterm neonate is approximately 50% to 70% of adult values (Stewart and Hampton, 1987). Maturation occurs as a function of chronologic rather than postconceptional age, with a wide range of variability. Maturation of nonsynthetic enzyme systems during the first several days of life requires careful monitoring of serum levels of some classes of medications (e.g., anticonvulsants). For instance, at term gestation, neonates have approximately 30% of adult ability to metabolize phenytoin. Hence the half-life is significantly prolonged. Within several weeks of medication exposure, metabolic enzyme activity for phenytoin surpasses adult activity.

   (b) Phase II (synthetic) metabolism of medications: primarily involves the acetylation, methylation, or conjugation of the medication with another substance. The function of these enzymes is also immature, and they may not reach adult levels in concentration and function until well after the neonatal period.

   (2) Hepatic uptake of the medication is dependent on the concentration of the medication in the liver (dependent on hepatic blood flow) and the hepatocyte concentration of ligandin (Y-protein). This protein is responsible for substrate uptake by hepatic cells.

   (3) In the first-pass effect, hepatic biotransformation may markedly alter medication availability by directly metabolizing medications absorbed from the GI tract, before those medications reach other organs. Slow GI motility may increase the potential for first-pass effect. Prolonged GI transit times may increase potential for hepatic metabolism and eventual excretion of orally administered medications.

   (4) Certain medications (e.g., phenobarbital) are thought to induce enzyme maturity in the fetus and neonate resulting in increased rates of medication elimination. This is the basis for the administration of phenobarbital as an adjunct treatment or as prophylaxis for hyperbilirubinemia (Nagourney and Aranda, 1998).

   (5) Both hepatic enzyme systems may be vulnerable to hypoxic/ischemic insult.

   (6) Maturational changes in medication metabolism can have a major clinical significance. Careful monitoring of serum levels of some medication classes (e.g., anticonvulsants, methylxanthines) is necessary in the first weeks of life.

D. Principles of medication excretion.

1. General principles of medication excretion. Excretion is the final elimination of medication from the body. The process of excretion begins with administration of the medication and ends when the medication is completely eliminated from the body. There are several important organs of excretion:
   - **a.** Salivary, sweat, and mammary glands: small amounts of medications may be excreted through these minor organs. Very limited sweat production makes excretion by this mode insignificant in the neonate.
   - **b.** Lungs: the lungs are an important route of excretion of gaseous anesthetics but are relatively less important for other medications. Excretion by the lungs is not well studied in the neonatal population. Because lung disease is common in newborn infants, adult data indicate that this may affect or limit the ability to excrete medications by this method.
   - **c.** GI tract: the large, lipid-soluble surface of the GI tract allows diffusion of medications into the bloodstream. The limited motility in neonates affects excretion and increases the potential for reabsorption of medications or metabolites back into the circulation.
   - **d.** Liver: the most important site of medication biotransformation also serves as an important site of medication excretion. The excretion of bile is an important means of medication elimination.
     - (1) Limited oral intake, long-term parenteral nutrition, or intrinsic hepatic disease may reduce bile flow. This may reduce the efficacy of this route of elimination.
     - (2) Metabolite or medication elimination in bile is dependent on solubility characteristics of that substance in bile.
   - **e.** Kidneys: the most important site for medication excretion.
     - (1) Renal blood flow:
       - (a) Clamping of the umbilical cord is a significant event that signals a major increase in renal blood flow.
       - (b) As a percentage of cardiac output, renal blood flow is limited in neonates in comparison with older children and adults. Limited renal blood flow as an absolute value and as a percentage of cardiac output restricts medication or metabolite delivery to the kidney for excretion.
       - (c) Renal blood flow increases with increasing gestational and postnatal age.
       - (d) High umbilical artery catheter placement may reduce the renal blood flow.
     - (2) Glomerular filtration rate (GFR): the removal, by passive filtration, of small unbound medication molecules at the glomerulus. Glomerular filtration is dependent on renal blood flow, the characteristics of the glomerular membranes, and the water solubility of the medication.
       - (a) The GFR function is extremely limited in neonates as compared with adult values (30% of adult values, per unit of body surface area; reaches adult values by 3 to 5 months of age) (Nagourney and Aranda, 1998).
       - (b) GFR is related to gestational age; the lower the gestational age, the lower the GFR. Neonates born at less than 34 weeks' gestation have fewer glomeruli, with total glomerular mass proportional to gestational age (John and Guignard, 1998). Nevertheless,

glomerular filtration has been shown to mature with postnatal age, independent of gestational age at birth.
(c) GFR can be further compromised with asphyxia, hypoxia, or indomethacin treatment. Limited glomerular filtration reduces removal of medications or metabolites at the glomerulus.
(d) Medication excretion dependent on glomerular filtration includes indomethacin, digoxin, aminoglycosides, and vancomycin.
(3) Tubular secretion: the active secretion of molecules into the tubular urine. Tubular secretion is dependent on the efficiency of tubular function.
(a) Neonates have a relatively small mass of functional tubular cells, as well as an immaturity of tubular function. This functional limitation is thought to be caused in part by a decrease of renal blood flow to the renal tubular region and by shortened renal tubules (John and Guignard, 1998; Nagourney and Aranda, 1998).
(b) The limitation in tubular mass and function causes poor excretion of medications and metabolites removed by this method.
(c) Tubular secretion matures much more slowly than glomerular filtration.
(d) Tubular secretion is also vulnerable to hypoxic-ischemic insult.
(e) Medications dependent on tubular secretion for excretion include penicillins, morphine, and thiazide diuretics.
(4) Tubular reabsorption: reabsorption, for some medications, back into the circulating plasma.
(a) May occur through either passive diffusion or active transport.
(b) Passive diffusion appears to be the most important process.
(c) Tubular reabsorption matures much more slowly than glomerular filtration.
(d) Substances dependent on tubular reabsorption include caffeine, glucose, phosphate, and sodium.
(5) Urinary output:
(a) Because of changes in renal blood flow, glomerular filtration, and tubular secretion in the neonate, urinary output is not a reliable sign of renal excretion of medications.
(b) Blood level monitoring is required to ensure safe serum levels of renally excreted medications.

MEDICATION CATEGORIES

Antimicrobial Agents

A. Introduction. The use of a larger variety of antimicrobial agents in the newborn population has occurred in the past several years because of advancing clinical sophistication in the use of antimicrobial medications as well as an expanding body of knowledge on the use of such agents in the newborn population.

B. Definitions.

1. Antimicrobial medications: medications that inhibit the growth of or kill microorganisms such as bacteria, fungi, viruses, protozoa, and amebae.

a. Bacteriostatic medications: agents that inhibit the growth of microorganisms, preventing their growth and allowing normal body defense mechanisms to control spread of the organism (e.g., clindamycin, fluconazole).

b. Bactericidal medications: agents that kill microorganisms. At lower concentrations they may be bacteriostatic (e.g., aminoglycosides, penicillin, cephalosporins).

2. Minimal inhibitory concentration (MIC): the lowest concentration of a medication that stops visible organism growth in a laboratory setting. In the body this cannot be directly measured and is dependent upon achieved tissue concentration and bacterial count. This is easily measured in the microbiology laboratory and is used to measure the susceptibility of the microorganism to antimicrobial agents.
3. Minimal bactericidal concentration (MBC): the lowest concentration of a medication that results in an equal to or more than 99.9% decline in microbial number, measured in the laboratory setting. It is useful when compared with known potential toxic concentration levels to choose the antimicrobial regimen that does the greatest good with the fewest adverse or toxic effects.
4. Resistance: the ability of microorganisms to counteract the bacteriostatic or bactericidal effects of an antimicrobial agent.
   a. Resistance interferes with the medication's action either through changes in the microorganism's cellular structure or through production of enzymes that reduce antimicrobial activity.
   b. Microorganisms develop resistance by:
      (1) Enzymes: microorganisms produce various enzymes to inactive antimicrobial agents (e.g., β-lactamase inactive penicillins and cephalosporins).
      (2) Decreased cellular penetration: microorganisms alter their cell wall permeability to prevent penetration of antimicrobial agents into the cell (e.g., *Pseudomonas aeruginosa* alters porin channels to decrease entry of ceftazidime, imipenem-cilastatin).
      (3) Altered target proteins: microorganisms change target proteins so that antimicrobial agents cannot bind and elicit antimicrobial activity (e.g., *Streptococcus pneumoniae* resistance to penicillin).
      (4) Efflux pump: microorganisms pump antimicrobial agents out of the cell before the antimicrobial agent can kill the microorganism (e.g., *S. pneumoniae* resistance to erythromycin).

C. **Basic principles of antimicrobial use.**
1. Antibiotics must reach the target tissue in a concentration adequate to inhibit the growth of or to kill the desired microorganism. This concentration:
   a. Ideally would be such that it would have limited side effects or toxic effects on target tissues or the patient as a whole.
   b. Must be readily achievable and sustainable for the desired duration of antimicrobial therapy.
2. The choice of antimicrobial agent(s) must take into account:
   a. Microorganism susceptibility to available antimicrobial agents.
   b. Relative permeability of the target tissue to agent of choice (e.g., blood-brain barrier).
   c. Bioactivity of chosen antimicrobial agent in target tissue (e.g., bactericidal or bacteriostatic).
   d. Known MIC/MBC in relation to existing body of knowledge concerning side effects and toxic effects in the specific population.
   e. Specific characteristics of the individual patient in relation to the chosen antimicrobial's toxicities (e.g., the blood levels of a nephrotoxic antimicrobial such as gentamicin should be closely monitored in patients with impaired renal function).

D. Specific considerations in the neonatal population.

1. Pharmacodynamics.
   a. Tissue concentration of medication may be altered by clinical and physiologic conditions that may increase or decrease bioavailability of the medication in the target tissue. (For example, cerebrospinal fluid penetration by antibiotics may be excellent early in meningitis. As meningeal inflammatory response subsides, penetration into the cerebrospinal fluid diminishes.)
   b. Differences in response or potential for toxic effects may result from immaturity and/or illness state.
2. Pharmacokinetics.
   a. In seriously ill neonates, greater consideration must be made for clinical status than for gestational or chronologic age. To optimize the probability of response to antibiotics, the unpredictable pharmacokinetic influences should be minimized, hence the intravenous (IV) route is preferred for septic patients.
   b. Absorption.
      (1) Changes in GI tract pH affect absorption of oral medication: may be increased or decreased (e.g., oral penicillin G is absorbed better in neonates than in older infants and children because of increased gastric pH).
      (2) Changes in skin permeability in the extremely immature neonate may allow topically applied antimicrobial agents to be absorbed systemically.
      (3) Blood flow changes may affect absorption and distribution of antimicrobials administered intramuscularly or subcutaneously (e.g., repeated intramuscular administration of aminoglycosides to premature neonates may result in local tissue damage and unacceptably variable rates of absorption).
   c. Distribution. Decreasing body water and increasing body fat concentration in more mature neonates affect the volume through which the antimicrobial agent is distributed. This may make dosage adjustments necessary in the first days of life.
   d. Metabolism. Limited hepatic function, because of immaturity or illness state, may affect dosage regimen of some antibiotics, requiring smaller or less frequent doses of some antibiotics (e.g., nafcillin, erythromycin).
   e. Excretion. Limited renal function with lower gestational age may prolong half-life of antimicrobials excreted by the kidneys (e.g., aminoglycosides, cephalosporins, penicillins). This limited renal function (GFR and tubular secretion) commonly improves significantly in the first few days of life and with advancing chronologic age. For this reason, serum antibiotic levels must be monitored closely and dosage adjustments made accordingly.

Cardiovascular Agents

A. Introduction.

1. A broad group of medications that affect the regulation, inhibition, or stimulation of the cardiovascular system.
2. The use of cardiovascular agents is increasing in the care of neonates.

B. Basic principles of cardiovascular medication use.

1. The wide range of pharmacologic actions of this class of medications requires specific in-depth knowledge about each medication and about concurrent medication therapy.
2. Knowledge of the pathophysiologic basis of neonatal cardiovascular disease is necessary to ensure proper application of this class of medications.
3. Many of these medications have overlapping or synergistic effects. This overlap in clinical response makes the optimal choice of a medication and dose difficult.
4. Extensive knowledge and application of invasive and noninvasive cardiovascular monitoring techniques in the neonatal population are necessary to allow titration of the medication dose to the clinical response.

C. Types of cardiovascular medications.

1. Inotropic/vasopressive agents.
   a. Includes a broad range of medications that act to improve cardiac output by increasing the heart rate (chronotropic effect), increasing the force of myocardial contraction (inotropic effect), and increasing vascular tone.
   b. Used both for cardiovascular resuscitation and long-term support of the myocardium.
   c. Specific inotropic agents:
      (1) Digitalis glycosides (e.g., digoxin). Inhibits the sodium/potassium pump to increase intracellular calcium thus increasing myocardial contractility. It also decreases conduction through the sinoatrial (SA) and atrioventricular (AV) nodes to slow the ventricular rate in tachyarrhythmias.
      (2) Sympathomimetic amines (e.g., epinephrine, dopamine, dobutamine, isoproterenol).
         (a) Clinical responses stimulated by this group of medications are classified according to effects on "receptors" in the body. These receptors are categorized as either α- or β-types and are further subcategorized as α_1 or α_2 and β_1 or β_2.
            (i) α_1-adrenergic receptor response: contractions of vascular smooth muscle and constriction of blood vessels.
            (ii) α_2-adrenergic receptor response: activation of central nervous system (CNS) receptors in the brain to suppress outflow of sympathetic nervous system activity from the brain. Results in decreased motility and tone of intestine and stomach.
            (iii) β_1-adrenergic receptor response: increased strength and rate of myocardial contraction.
            (iv) β_2-adrenergic receptor response: vascular smooth muscle dilation and bronchial muscle relaxation.

         For example epinephrine increases blood pressure by stimulating the α_{1-} and β_1-receptors. Dobutamine increases cardiac output by stimulating the β_1- and β_2-receptors.
         (b) Response to each of these medications depends on relative amounts of α- and β-effects.
         (c) Prolonged administration of sympathomimetic amines may result in diminished clinical efficacy secondary to diminished responses of α- and β-receptors, referred to as tachyphylaxis.
2. Antihypertensives/vasodilators.
   a. Used to normalize blood pressure in patients with hypertension, reduce vascular resistance in patients with poor myocardial function, and reduce

pulmonary vascular resistance in conditions associated with pulmonary hypertension.
- **b.** May be used to inhibit pathophysiologic changes that cause increased blood pressure (e.g., captopril, propranolol) or directly reduce blood pressure through changes in intravascular volume (e.g., diuretics) or vascular resistance (e.g., hydralazine, nitroprusside).

3. Antiarrhythmics.
   - **a.** Used to treat cardiac dysrhythmias causing adverse effects on cardiovascular stability.
   - **b.** Includes adenosine, digoxin, esmolol, and lidocaine.

D. Specific considerations in the neonatal population.

1. Pharmacodynamics.
   - **a.** Specific in-depth knowledge about neonatal cardiovascular physiology and pathophysiology is required to determine the need for these medications.
   - **b.** Cardiovascular medications are commonly used in conjunction with other medications that may affect the neonate's response to the medication regimen (e.g., the digoxin-furosemide combination may result in electrolyte loss with the diuretic, which in turn may potentiate a toxic response to the digoxin).
2. Pharmacokinetics.
   - **a.** Absorption. Many cardiovascular medications cannot be given effectively through any significant absorptive barrier. For this reason, IV administration is necessary in many cases (e.g., pressors, inotropes).
   - **b.** Distribution.
     - (1) Poor cardiac output/shock states may affect distribution of medication to all tissues.
     - (2) Medication administered for a desired response to one target organ may cause an undesirable systemic response (e.g., dobutamine increases cardiac output but may cause decreased blood pressure, furosemide reduces pulmonary edema but may decrease blood pressure).
     - (3) Some cardiovascular medications are highly albumin-bound; this raises the possibility of unconjugated bilirubin displacement from albumin.
   - **c.** Metabolism.
     - (1) Hepatic metabolic activity may markedly affect the bioavailability of the medication (e.g., the high rate of first-pass metabolism of oral propranolol causes the IV and oral dosing to be significantly different).
     - (2) Medication metabolites may cause a toxic response (e.g., cyanide liberation as a result of nitroprusside metabolism).
     - (3) Rapid metabolism and serum clearance may require continuous IV infusion (e.g., dopamine, dobutamine).
   - **d.** Excretion. Impaired renal function will markedly affect excretion of some medications (e.g., captopril, furosemide). This requires careful monitoring of the clinical response and serum medication levels.

Central Nervous System (CNS) Medications

A. Introduction.

1. In adult patients, these are the most widely used group of medications.
2. The value of pain control and mood alteration in the neonatal population has only recently been recognized.

3. Recent increased interest in the use of CNS medications in the neonatal population has caused a recognition that the body of knowledge about these medications is limited.
4. The use of these medications is increasing as neurobehavioral assessment skills increase among neonatal caregivers.

B. Definitions.

1. Analgesic medication: a medication (e.g., morphine, meperidine, acetaminophen) that provides diminished sensation of pain. These help to promote control of undesirable responses to a painful event.
2. Anesthetic medication: a medication that removes pain sensation either through peripheral nerve block (e.g., lidocaine) or through CNS effects (e.g., high-dose fentanyl). Not all anesthetic medications provide pain relief (e.g., inhalation gases, propofol, pentobarbital).
3. Sedative/hypnotic medications: medications that provide mood alteration in patients with anxiety. These are divided into two groups: barbiturates (e.g., phenobarbital) and nonbarbiturates (e.g., chloral hydrate, chlorpromazine, lorazepam). These medications do not provide relief from pain.
4. Addiction: a lifestyle change that occurs in a medication-dependent person. This lifestyle change involves a focus on medication use. This cannot occur in a neonate.
5. Tolerance: a condition that may occur with many types of medications. Tolerance exists when larger doses and higher serum concentrations of the medication are required to achieve the desired response, and commonly occurs in conjunction with physical dependence.
6. Dependence: a physiologic state in which the individual requires regular medication administration for continued physiologic well-being. Patients who develop dependence to a medication may need a dosage-tapering regimen rather than abruptly discontinuing the medication in order to prevent withdrawal symptoms.

C. Basic principles of CNS medication use.

1. Mechanism of action of most CNS medications is frequently not clearly understood.
2. Assessment of need for these medications must be carefully performed as an ongoing process.
   a. Close attention must be paid to differentiation of need for sedation, pain relief, or both.
   b. These medications may cause the development of medication tolerance and/or dependence.
3. Consideration must be made for the risks and benefits of the medication in relation to potential side effects or toxicities.
4. The science of the study of neonatal neurologic development is new, and much is yet to be learned. The effect that CNS medications may have on that development is largely unknown. Therefore nonpharmacologic methods to relieve pain should be exhausted before medications are administered (e.g., positioning, swaddling, sucrose pacifiers).

D. Specific considerations in the neonatal population.

1. Pharmacodynamics.
   a. Limited knowledge of CNS development in premature and term neonates mandates a special need for caution in the use of CNS-active medications.
   b. Specific physiologic characteristics in the neonatal population require careful observation for harmful side effects or toxicities (e.g., reduction in blood pressure with IV bolus doses of morphine).

c. Narcotic analgesics may cause respiratory depression and may precipitate respiratory failure in neonates.
d. Careful assessment of clinical response is necessary to determine the most safe and effective dose and interval.

2. Pharmacokinetics.
   a. Absorption.
      (1) Poor GI motility and high first-pass clearance may make oral administration highly unpredictable for many medications (e.g., morphine, meperidine).
      (2) Oral or rectal absorption of mild analgesics and sedatives is often adequate (e.g., acetaminophen).
   b. Distribution.
      (1) Because these agents work in the CNS, they must be lipid soluble in order to cross the blood-brain barrier.
      (2) As neonates increase their proportion of body fat, the doses required will increase.
      (3) Because these agents are stored in the body fat, patients must be monitored for the accumulation of these agents and hence prolonged effects.
   c. Metabolism.
      (1) Slower hepatic metabolism may cause a prolonged half-life.
      (2) Hepatic disease may markedly increase the risk of toxic effects (e.g., chloral hydrate).
      (3) Hepatic metabolism converts medications to either toxic metabolites (e.g., meperidine converts to normeperidine) or active metabolites (e.g., theophylline converts to caffeine).
   d. Excretion.
      (1) Limited renal function or failure may cause toxic effects as a result of accumulation of medication or metabolites (e.g., normeperidine).
      (2) Medication may have a direct effect on renal function.
         (a) Blood flow to kidney may be diminished (e.g., morphine).
         (b) Urinary output may be diminished (e.g., morphine-caused changes in smooth muscle tone; chlorpromazine effect on renal tubular function).

Diuretics

A. Introduction.

1. Commonly used in neonatal patients to promote the removal of excessive extracellular fluid.
2. Site of action of nearly all diuretic agents is the luminal surface of the renal tubular cell.

B. Basic principles of diuretic use.

1. Use must be based on a thorough understanding of function of the various segments of the nephron in the neonatal population.
2. Diuretic medications whose primary purpose is to cause the excretion of excess extracellular fluid commonly cause a secondary or side effect of loss of electrolytes, along with the desired water loss. The knowledge of the specific action for each diuretic medication will assist the clinician in monitoring electrolytes for undesirable losses.
3. The pharmacologic response is dependent on the existing level of renal function and the medication's ability to reach the target tissue in amounts adequate to produce the desired diuretic effect.

4. Any medication or therapy that increases glomerular filtration rate may have an indirect diuretic effect. Some medications that act on the cardiovascular system to increase cardiac output or increase renal blood flow through vasodilatation may cause diuresis (e.g., dopamine). Maximal water and electrolyte excretion usually occurs in the first days of use. Later, decreased GFR and hyperaldosteronism resulting from diuretic-induced hypovolemia limit these losses.

C. **Specific considerations in the neonatal population.**
1. Pharmacodynamics.
   a. Many diuretic medications are dependent on reaching the lumen of the proximal tubule to achieve diuresis.
   b. The renal tubular function is limited in all neonates and is more limited in less mature neonates.
   c. The clinical response to diuretic agents is commonly decreased because of existing poor renal tubular absorption. Therefore a larger dose is needed to achieve the response.
   d. Limited tubular function potentiates electrolyte loss with many diuretic agents (e.g., furosemide, hydrochlorothiazide).
2. Pharmacokinetics.
   a. Absorption. Oral absorption may be limited, requiring a larger per kilogram dose as compared with the IV dose to achieve the desired effect (e.g., furosemide). Other diuretics (e.g., hydrochlorothiazide, spironolactone) are well absorbed orally.
   b. Distribution. Some diuretic medications are strongly protein-bound. Some concern has been raised over displacement of bilirubin from albumin-binding sites (e.g., furosemide, spironolactone).
   c. Metabolism. Some diuretics are primarily metabolized by the liver (e.g., spironolactone).
   d. Excretion.
      (1) Low renal blood flow and low glomerular filtration rate, along with limited renal tubular function, may delay excretion and limit effectiveness of the medication (e.g., the plasma clearance of furosemide has been shown to be prolonged in extremely premature neonates and in neonates with renal failure) (John and Guignard, 1998).
      (2) Some diuretics are primarily eliminated unchanged in the urine (e.g., furosemide, hydrochlorothiazide).

Immunizations

A. **Introduction.**
1. Vaccines are commonly given to the hospitalized neonatal patient.
2. Each year in January, the Centers for Disease Control and Prevention (CDC)'s Advisory Committee on Immunization Practices publishes an updated version of the recommended immunization guidelines. Each nurse should be familiar with these guidelines.
3. The following documentation is required when vaccines are given:
   a. Name, title, and business address of person administering the vaccine.
   b. Vaccine administered.
   c. Manufacturer of the vaccine.
   d. Lot number of the vaccine.
   e. Expiration date of vaccine.
   f. Date of administration.

g. Site of administration.
h. Route of administration.
i. Documentation that the parents/guardians have been given an adequate explanation of the risks and benefits of the vaccination.

B. Basic principles of immunization use.

1. The goal of immunization is to prevent many viral and bacterial diseases and their sequelae.
2. For maximum effectiveness, the immunizations must be given at specific ages before the recipients have been exposed to the diseases.
3. Live vaccines (e.g., measles-mumps-rubella [MMR], varicella) should not be administered in the hospital setting.
4. All adverse events associated with immunization should be reported in detail in the patient's medical record and also on the vaccine adverse event reporting system (VAERS) form found on the U.S. Food and Drug Administration (FDA)'s website.

C. Types of immunizations.

1. Active immunization.
   a. Involves the administration of all or part of a microorganism or a modified product of that microorganism to evoke an immunologic response mimicking that of the natural infection. This usually presents little or no risk to the recipient.
   b. Some immunizing agents provide complete protection against disease for life, some provide partial protection, and some must be readministered at intervals (booster doses).
   c. Vaccines may be either live (attenuated) or killed (inactivated). Inactivated vaccines may not elicit the range of immunologic response provided by attenuated agents.
2. Passive immunization.
   a. Involves the administration of preformed antibody to a recipient.
   b. Most often utilized when a person exposed to a disease has a high likelihood of complications from that disease and time does not permit adequate protection by active immunization alone.
   c. Can be utilized when a disease is already present with the hope of reducing the reaction to the disease.
   d. Accomplished through the use of immune globulin preparations (e.g., hepatitis B immune globulin, varicella immune globulin, palivizumab).
   e. There are strict indications for the use of the products (American Academy of Pediatrics [AAP], 2000).

D. Specific considerations in the neonatal population.

1. Pharmacodynamics.
   a. Most immunizations are usually given starting at 2 months of age; the immune response to the vaccines may be limited if given before this age. Resistance to certain diseases before this time may be provided from the mother's antibodies that are transferred across the placenta.
   b. Premature infants should receive the vaccines at the same ages as term infants. The dose should NOT be decreased in this patient population.
   c. When a vaccine is given at birth to a preterm neonate (e.g., hepatitis B vaccine for neonates born to hepatitis B–positive mothers), this vaccine will not count in the total number of doses that are required (if given at birth, the preterm infant will receive a total of four doses of the hepatitis B vaccine instead of three doses).
   d. Antibody titers may be measured to prove adequate immune responses.

2. Pharmacokinetics.
   a. Absorption.
      (1) Injectable vaccines should be administered in sites that limit the risk of neural, vascular, or tissue injury.
      (2) The preferred sites for administration include the anterolateral aspect of the upper thigh.
      (3) The deltoid area of the upper arm can be used in older infants.
      (4) The upper, outer aspect of the buttocks should not be routinely used due to the possibility of damaging the sciatic nerve.
      (5) When necessary two vaccines can be given in the same limb but should be separated by 1 to 2 inches so that local reactions are not likely to overlap.
      (6) The recommended routes of administration are included in the package inserts of the vaccines (e.g., intramuscular [IM], subcutaneous [SC]).
   b. Distribution. Vaccines should be held when the neonate is on pressor agents because the blood flow to the muscle and subcutaneous tissues may be limited.
   c. Metabolism/excretion. Kidney and liver failure should not affect the administration of the vaccines.

E. **Misconceptions about vaccine contraindications.** Some health care professionals inappropriately consider certain conditions or circumstances to be contraindications to immunizations. The nurse should be familiar with the specific contraindications listed in the package inserts of the vaccine. The following are NOT contraindications to immunization:
   1. Mild acute illness with low-grade fever or mild diarrheal illness in an otherwise healthy child.
   2. Current antimicrobial therapy or the convalescent phase of illness.
   3. Reaction to a previous diphtheria and tetanus toxoids and acellular pertussis (DTaP) dose that involved temperature of less than 105° F.
   4. Prematurity.
   5. Pregnancy of mother or other household contact.
   6. Breast-feeding.
   7. Allergies to penicillin or any other antibiotic, except anaphylactic reactions to neomycin or streptomycin.
   8. Family history of convulsions in person considered for pertussis or measles vaccination.
   9. Allergies to duck meat or duck feathers.
   10. Family history of sudden death infant syndrome (AAP, 2000).

NURSING IMPLICATIONS FOR MEDICATION ADMINISTRATION IN THE NEONATE

A. **Nurses' responsibility** involves moral, legal, and ethical duties in patient care, which places the primary responsibility for providing safe medication administration on nurses in most cases.

B. **Specific in-depth knowledge** about the pharmacodynamics and pharmacokinetics of medications administered in the NICU is absolutely necessary in the assessment of the clinical response and potential for risk.

C. **Careful assessment of vital sign parameters and clinical responses** may assist in the evaluation of desirable or undesirable medication responses.

D. **Careful observation of the neonate for therapeutic and toxic medication effects** will allow medication administration to achieve the maximal desired response while minimizing toxic responses.
E. **Monitoring renal function through intake and output measurements** may alert the care team to potential changes in medication metabolism and/or excretion.
F. **Double check of medication doses** involves recalculating the weight-based doses and comparing written doses with current medication dosing reference books in order to prevent potential medication dosing errors.
G. **Meticulous medication dosing** involves giving the medication at the correct time and at the correct time interval, which is essential for the maximal desired effect by many medications, with minimal undesired effects.
H. **Facilitation of medication serum level monitoring with absolute accuracy** makes safe administration of medications, with a narrow margin between effective and toxic levels, possible.
I. **Cross-checking** on a regular basis is a nursing responsibility. Because of the very small volumes of medications commonly given to the NICU patient, a system for regular cross-checking of medication volume accuracy with medication concentration before administration should be established.
J. **Medications known to have specific recommendations for safe administration** should be given under a defined protocol for administration.
K. **Medication precautions** must be observed. Any medication or medication preparation known to have a high risk of adverse effects in the neonate should be removed from the patient care area or should be specifically labeled to avoid inadvertent administration.
L. **Precise documentation** of medication administration date, time, dose, route, and interval, or time medication levels are obtained are important in interpreting patient response to therapy.
M. **Facilitation of or participation in clinical trials** designed to evaluate a medication's efficacy does much to advance the body of knowledge related to neonatal pharmacology.
N. **Recognition of established clinical experience with individual medications in the neonatal population is essential.** Because some medications are introduced into the clinical area after only minimal study of specific medication response in the neonate, early observation of potential toxic effects may avert a later disaster.

REFERENCES

American Academy of Pediatrics. In L.K. Pickering (Ed.): *2000 Red Book: Report of the Committee on Infectious Diseases* (25th ed.). Elk Grove Village, IL, 2000, American Academy of Pediatrics, pp. 1-54.

Berry, D. D., Adcock, E. W., and Starbuck, A.: Fluid and electrolyte management. In G.B. Merenstein and S.L. Gardner (Eds.): *Handbook of neonatal intensive care* (5th ed.). St Louis, 2002, Mosby, pp. 283-297.

Chemtob, S.: Basic pharmacologic principles. In R.A. Polin and W.W. Fox (Eds.): *Fetal and neonatal physiology*. Philadelphia, 1998, W.B. Saunders, pp. 125-136.

John, E.G. and Guignard, J.P.: Development of renal excretion of drugs during ontogeny. In R.A. Polin and W.W. Fox (Eds.): *Fetal and neonatal physiology*. Philadelphia, 1998, W.B. Saunders, pp. 188-193.

Kraus, D.M. and Pham, J.T.: Neonatal therapy. In *Applied therapeutics: The clinical use of drugs*. Baltimore, 2001, Lippincott Williams & Wilkins, pp. 91-1–91-54.

Nagourney, B.A. and Aranda, J.V.: Physiologic differences of clinical significance. In R.A. Polin and W.W. Fox (Eds.): *Fetal and neonatal physiology*. Philadelphia, 1998, W.B. Saunders, pp. 239-249.

Nahata, M.C. and Taketomo, C.: Pediatrics. In J.T. Dipiro, R.L. Talbert, G.C. Yee, et al. (Eds.): *Pharmacotherapy: A pathophysiologic approach*. New York, 2002, McGraw-Hill, pp. 69-77.

Stewart, C.F. and Hampton, E.M.: Effect of maturation on drug disposition in pediatric patients. *Clinical Pharmacy*, 6(7): 548-564, 1987.

CHAPTER

13 Laboratory and Diagnostic Test Interpretation

DIANE M. SZLACHETKA

OBJECTIVES

1. Identify the types of laboratory testing in the neonatal intensive care unit (NICU).
2. Discuss the purpose of laboratory testing and diagnostics.
3. Review the process of specimen collection and the principles of test utilization.
4. Review the principles of laboratory interpretation.
5. Describe iatrogenic sequelae associated with laboratory testing and diagnostic procedures.
6. Discuss strategies to minimize iatrogenic sequelae associated with laboratory testing and diagnostic procedures.
7. Discuss the decision-making process of ordering and interpreting laboratory values—a decision tree.

Newborns delivered in the United States receive an average of one or two laboratory tests, typically in the form of screening for genetic disorders and birth defects. Additionally, all infants admitted to the NICU require laboratory testing to assess their clinical status. Given the U.S. birth rate of 4 million infants (Martin et al., 2002) and average NICU admission rate of 360,000 (Schwartz et al., 2000), this translates to a minimum of 8 million screening/laboratory tests per year.

It has been estimated that 10% to 15% of the U.S. national health budget is spent on laboratory testing constituting 15% to 20% of each patient's hospital bill (Sacher et al., 2000a). The impact of laboratory testing on the patient, health care, and its cost is significant.

Because all health care workers in the NICU are in some way involved in obtaining laboratory samples, understanding the principles of laboratory testing and the contribution of laboratory tests to patient care and cost is essential. Developing skills in laboratory interpretation at the NICU bedside provides a key element in comprehensive patient care.

This chapter features a review of the types and purposes of laboratory testing in the NICU, describes principles of laboratory testing and interpretation, and discusses potential iatrogenic sequelae. Included is a discussion of strategies to avoid sequelae, when to obtain laboratory testing, and a strategy to interpret results for patient care. A decision-making process for laboratory interpretation is presented.

LABORATORY TESTS IN THE NICU

A. Laboratory testing occurs daily in the NICU. Data obtained from laboratory analysis assist clinicians in determining diagnosis, measuring success of treatment, and monitoring trends in an infant's clinical course. The common laboratory tests performed in the NICU include (see Table 13-1):

1. **Chemistry analysis:** serum tests that measure the chemical activity or state of the body. Chemical substances reflect metabolic processes and disease states in the body. Measuring changes in chemical concentrations (chemical substances) is useful in diagnosis, planning care, monitoring of therapy, screening, and determining severity of disease and response to treatment.
   a. Four categories (Sacher et al., 2000b).
      (1) Chemical substances normally present with function in the circulation—laboratory examples: *electrolytes, calcium, magnesium, phosphorus, total proteins, albumin, hormones, and vitamins.*
      (2) Metabolites: nonfunctioning waste products in process of being cleared—laboratory examples: *bilirubin, ammonia, blood urea nitrogen (BUN), creatinine, and uric acid.*
      (3) Substances released from cells as a result of cell damage and abnormal permeability or abnormal cellular proliferation—laboratory examples: *alkaline phosphatase, alanine aminotransferase (ALT), aspartate aminotransferase (AST), and creatinine kinase.*
      (4) Drug and toxic substances—laboratory examples: *antibiotics, theophylline, caffeine, digoxin, phenobarbital, and substances of abuse.*
2. **Hematologic tests:** study of the blood and blood-forming tissues of the body such as the bone marrow and reticuloendothelial system (Sacher et al., 2000c). This area of testing also includes the study of hemoglobin structure, red cell membrane, and red cell enzyme activity. Whole blood is composed of blood cells suspended in plasma fluid (see also Chapter 30).
   a. Blood cells: erythrocytes (red blood cells), leukocytes (white blood cells), and thrombocytes (platelets)—laboratory examples: *hematocrit (Hct), reticulocyte (Retic) count, platelet (Plt) count, peripheral blood smear, complete blood count (CBC), Kleihauer-Betke test, white blood cell (WBC) count, and WBC differential count.*
   b. Plasma: plasma proteins, coagulation factors I through XIII, immunoglobulins—laboratory examples: *total protein, albumin, fibrinogen (factor I), prothrombin (factor II), partial thromboplastin time (factor III), factors IV through XIII assays, immunoglobulin G (IgG), A (IgA), and M (IgM).*
3. **Microbiology tests:** identification of infectious microorganisms causing disease. Tests include diagnostic bacteriology, mycology, virology, parasitology, and serology—laboratory examples: *culture of any body fluid, bacterial stain, and bacteria antigen detection.*
4. **Microscopy tests:** examination of body fluids and tissues under a microscope— laboratory examples: *cell counts, fecal blood, fecal fat, Apt test, and urinalysis.*
5. **Blood bank tests (transfusion medicine):** area of blood component preparation, blood donor screening and testing, blood compatibility testing, and blood and stem cell banking.
   a. Commonly used blood components in the NICU:
      (1) Whole blood: hematocrit (~35%) typically low for infants.
         (a) Used for large-volume replacement in surgery.
         (b) Used for extracorporeal membrane oxygenator (ECMO) pump.

TABLE 13-1
Common Laboratory Tests in the NICU by System

Fluids Electrolytes Nutrition	Respiratory	Cardiac	Gastro-intestinal	Renal	Endocrine/Metabolic	Neurologic	Hematology	Other
Electrolytes (serum)	Blood gas	Isoenzymes	Alkaline phosphatase	BUN (serum)	Thyroxine level	Phenobarbital level	CBC w/differential	Chromosome levels
Calcium (serum)	pH		Triglyceride levels	Creatinine (serum)	Thyroid-stimulating hormone	Dilantin level	Hct	Buccal smear
Magnesium (serum)	$Paco_2$		AST (SGOT)	Specific gravity	Cortisol level	Ammonia (serum)	Plt Plt antibody	CRP
Phosphorus (serum)	Pao_2		ALT (SGPT)	Urine sodium	Insulin level	Amino acid (serum)	Reticulocyte count	Drug levels (serum)
Alkaline phosphorus	Bicarbonate (HCO_3)		GGT (GGTP)	Urine potassium	Growth hormone	Amino acid (urine)	Direct Coombs'	Urine toxicology screen
Glucose (serum)	Base excess		Bilirubin (total and direct)	Urine osmolality	Testosterone levels	Organic acids (urine)	Blood type	Cultures (all sources)
Vitamin levels	Theophylline level		Ammonia (serum)	Drug levels	Aldosterone (serum and urine)	Glycine (serum and CSF)	G6PD	RPR
Serum osmolality	Caffeine level		α_1-antitrypsin	Uric acid (serum)	17-hydroxy-corticosteroids	Pyridoxine level	Sedimentation rate	Occult blood (fecal)
Albumin (serum)			Trypsin (stool)	Urinalysis	Parathyroid hormone	Lactic acid	Folic acid	PCR (serum)
Total protein			Pyridoxine level				Fibrinogen PT PTT Immunoglobulins Methemoglobin	

ALT, Alanine aminotransferase (SGPT); *AST,* aspartate aminotransferase (SGOT); *BUN,* blood urea nitrogen; *CBC,* complete blood count; *CRP,* C-reactive protein; *CSF,* cerebrospinal fluid; *GGT,* gamma-glutamyl transferase; *G6PD,* glucose-6-phosphate dehydrogenase; *Hct,* hematocrit; *PCR,* polymerase chain reaction; *Plt,* platelet; *PT,* prothrombin time; *PTT,* partial prothrombin time; *RPR,* rapid plasma reagin.

(2) Packed red blood cells: spun blood with supernatant removed to concentrate red blood cells ~ Hct 70%.
  (a) Reconstituted to an average Hct 50% and used for blood transfusions in treatment of anemia.
  (b) Used in exchange transfusions.

(3) Platelets: platelets separated from donor blood and stored suspended in plasma.
  (a) Often spun to concentrate platelets in smaller volume.
  (b) Used for platelet replacement in thrombocytopenia.

(4) Fresh frozen plasma: plasma separated from blood cells and stored frozen. Has some fibrinogen but cryoprecipitate is a better source.
  (a) Used for clotting factor replacement, rich in factors VIII and IX and contains other stable and labile coagulation factors.
  (b) Used in treatment of disseminated intravascular coagulopathy (DIC).

(5) Granulocytes: WBCs removed from fresh donor blood.
  (a) Used to replace WBCs in cases of severe neutropenia.

(6) Cryoprecipitate: a plasma preparation rich in factor VIII and XIII, and fibrinogen.
  (a) Used in treatment of hemophilia.
  (b) Used in treatment of DIC.

b. Common blood bank tests:
  (1) Blood typing and crossmatch.
  (2) Direct antiglobulin test (DAT).
  (3) Indirect antiglobulin test (IAT).
  (4) Erythrocyte Rosette test for fetomaternal hemorrhage.

6. **Immunoassays:** laboratory method based on antigen-antibody reactions employed in therapeutic drug monitoring, toxicology screening, detection of plasma proteins, and certain endocrine testing—laboratory examples: *urine and meconium toxicology test for "street drugs," latex agglutination test, and drug levels.*
7. **Cytogenetic tests:** testing used to determine genetic composition by chromosome analysis—laboratory examples: *simple karyotype (blood, amniotic fluid, tissue, bone marrow), chromosome-specific probes, and fluorescence in situ hybridization (FISH).*
8. **Immunology tests:** laboratory evaluation measuring immune system activity (Sacher et al., 2000d). This consists of complement activity and its cascade of activation, humoral, and cell-mediated immunity. Tests are used to diagnose immunodeficiency and autoimmune disorders—laboratory examples: *C-reactive protein, complement C3 and C4, IgG, IgM, IgA.*

PURPOSE OF LABORATORY TESTING

A. Laboratory testing in the NICU is multidimensional. The rationale for selecting, ordering, and interpreting laboratory tests needs to be scrutinized (considered) in order to maximize patient care, minimize patient risk, and contain health care costs. The purpose of laboratory testing is to:
  1. Determine the health state of the patient.
  2. Monitor the clinical status, trends, and disease severity.
  3. Assist in a differential diagnosis.
  4. Confirm a diagnosis or cure.
  5. Screen for common disorders and disease prevention.

6. Measure effect of therapy.
7. Assist in management of disease.
8. Establish a prognosis.
9. Assist in genetic counseling.
10. Evaluate specific events—example: *medication errors, sudden clinical decompensation, medical-legal problems, and postmortem tests.*

PROCESS OF LABORATORY COLLECTION

A. Collection of laboratory specimens requires meticulous technique to ensure the best possible results. Proper technique, source of laboratory sample, use of collection tubes, labeling, and laboratory processing combine to play a key role in patient treatment, in minimizing blood loss and painful stimuli, and in reducing cost of NICU care.
   1. **Types of laboratory collection** (see also Chapter 15).
      a. Capillary blood sampling: admixture of arterial, venous, and capillary blood and tissue fluid obtained from a warmed, well-perfused heel. Note: Finger-stick sampling is contraindicated in infants, because distance from skin surface to bone is less than 1.5 mm (Olsowka and Garg, 2001).
         (1) Most common route for obtaining small blood samples in the infant.
         (2) Heel stick no deeper than 2 mm (Garza and Becan-McBride, 2002a).
         (3) Avoid squeezing or milking site to obtain blood (Olsowka and Garg, 2001).
         (4) Cell counts such as WBC, Plt count, or blood gas Po_2 may not be accurate.
      b. Venipuncture: venous blood typically obtained from the hand, arm, foot, leg, or scalp. Venous blood can also be obtained from an umbilical vein catheter.
         (1) May need use of tourniquet to distend peripheral veins. *Tourniquet application ≥3 minutes may alter laboratory test results* (Garza and Becan-McBride, 2002b).
         (2) Venipuncture may be difficult to obtain in small infants.
         (3) May wish to ration available veins for future intravenous sites vs. use for laboratory drawing.
      c. Arterial puncture (see also Chapter 15): arterial blood typically obtained from an artery stick of the radial, tibial, or temporal arteries. Brachial artery stick is performed less often due to potential for arteriospasm of brachial artery supplying the lower arm. Femoral artery stick is rarely performed in the NICU population. Arterial blood can also be obtained from an umbilical artery catheter or percutaneous arterial line.
         (1) Allen test should be done prior to radial arterial stick (Henry et al., 2001; Olsowka and Garg, 2001).
         (2) Anticipatory pain management should be considered (see also Chapter 16).
      d. Point-of-care testing (POCT), alternate-site testing (AST), near-patient testing (NPT), patient-focused testing (PFT): tests done in the primary care setting, often at the bedside (Henry, et al., 2001).
         (1) Uses whole blood obtained from capillary stick, arterial, or venous sources.
         (2) Provides "real-time," rapid testing.
         (3) Utilizes small blood volumes, less than 0.5 ml.

(4) Common POCT assays obtained in the NICU include electrolytes, ionized calcium, BUN, creatinine, Hct, hemoglobin (Hgb), blood gas analysis, glucose.

e. Lumbar puncture (see also Chapter 15): procedure done to remove cerebrospinal fluid (CSF) from spinal canal.

(1) CSF evaluated in the laboratory for: (Henry, et al., 2001).

(a) Infection.

(b) Hemorrhage.

(c) Demyelinating diseases.

(d) Malignancy.

f. Urine sampling (see also Chapter 15): urine obtained for chemical analysis, bacterial cultures, or microscopic examination.

(1) Techniques for obtaining samples include:

(a) Bag collection.

(b) Straight catheterization.

(c) Bladder suprapubic tap.

g. Thoracentesis (see also Chapter 15): procedure using a needle tap or chest tube to remove abnormal collection of fluid (effusion) from thoracic cavity.

(1) Thoracic cavity fluid evaluated in laboratory for:

(a) Microorganisms: cultures, Gram stains.

(b) Chemistries: electrolytes, total protein, albumin, glucose, triglycerides.

(c) Hematology: WBC count and WBC differential count.

h. Peritoneal tap: procedure using a needle tap to remove an abnormal collection of fluid (ascites) from the abdomen.

(1) Peritoneal cavity fluid evaluated in laboratory for:

(a) Microorganisms: cultures, Gram stains.

(b) Chemistries: electrolytes, total protein, albumin, glucose, triglycerides.

(c) Hematology: WBC count and WBC differential count.

2. Process of laboratory collection.

a. Order request for test.

b. Check for appropriateness of order.

c. Cluster laboratory drawing as much as possible.

d. Prepare infant for laboratory test, for example:

(1) Wrap foot for capillary specimen—a wrapped foot arterializes specimen and helps promote blood flow (Garza and Becan-McBride, 2002c; Kaplan and Tange, 1998; Olsowka and Garg, 2001).

(2) Provide pain management.

e. Observe strict aseptic technique per institution guidelines.

f. Observe Standard Precautions per institution guidelines.

g. Obtain laboratory test using appropriate route, for example:

(1) *Capillary vs. arterial vs. venous.*

h. Obtain hematology specimens first to minimize platelet clumping, then chemistry and blood bank samples (Garza and Becan-McBride, 2002c)

i. Insert proper amount of specimen into proper specimen container.

j. Label specimen.

k. Place specimen in biohazard container or bag.

l. Promptly send specimen to laboratory.

3. Specimen tubes: color-coded containers indicating whether they contain whole blood, plasma (which contains fibrinogen), or serum. Tube colors in the NICU typically come in red, blue, green, lavender and yellow. Microtainers are the most common types of specimen collection tubes in the NICU. Microtainers allow for use of smaller blood volumes to obtain laboratory results. Blood culture tubes, sterile swabs, and glass slides are also used in the NICU for specimen collection. Tubes with anticoagulant coating should be gently inverted, end over end, 7 to 10 times for proper anticoagulant-blood mixing (Fischbach, 2002; Kee, 2002).

- **a.** Red tube (plain): no additives or anticoagulant. Clotted blood for serum testing. Hemolysis should be avoided—laboratory examples: *electrolytes, serology, blood bank, proteins, hormones, and drug monitoring.*
- **b.** Blue tube (light): contains sodium citrate, an anticoagulant that removes calcium to prevent clotting (Fischbach, 2002). Unclotted blood-plasma specimens—laboratory specimens: *prothrombin time (PT), partial prothrombin time (PTT), factor assays.*
- **c.** Green tube: contains anticoagulant heparin (sodium, lithium, ammonium) that inhibits thrombin activation to prevent clotting. Unclotted blood-plasma specimens—laboratory examples: *chromosome analysis (use sodium heparin tube*), ammonia levels, and hormone levels.
- **d.** Lavender tube: contains ethylenediaminetetraacetic acid (EDTA) that removes calcium to prevent clotting. Tube used for whole blood and plasma specimens—laboratory examples: *CBC, Retic count, Plt count, Hct.*
- **e.** Yellow tube/bottle cap—contains sodium polyethylene sulfonate (SPS) and used for blood cultures. These cultures should be processed quickly to minimize potential for decreased yield due to storage or prolonged exposure to SPS (Olsowka and Garg, 2001).

CONCEPTS OF LABORATORY TEST INTERPRETATION

A. It is important to be familiar with the limitations and applications of the laboratory data as they apply to patient care. A laboratory test has certain characteristics that influence how it is interpreted and used in the clinical setting. The following concepts are integral in the process of laboratory interpretation:

1. **Accuracy:** synonymous with "correctness," this term refers to how close a test result is to the true value (Oxley, et al., 2001).
    - **a.** Point-to-point variability in test results.
    - **b.** Variation in value may be more reflective of an analytic variation of automated chemistry systems than actual patient status.
2. **Precision:** synonymous with "reproducibility," this term describes the distribution of results when a sample is analyzed repeatedly.
    - **a.** Imprecision is known as random error.
    - **b.** Test precision is a more desirable test characteristic than accuracy in measuring treatment response or clinical changes.
3. **Sensitivity:** the ability of a test to correctly identify an individual with disease and not miss anyone by falsely testing "healthy." It refers to a test's ability to generate more true-positive results and fewer false-negative results.
    - **a.** Sensitive test has a low threshold for abnormality.
    - **b.** Sensitive test usually has a low specificity.
    - **c.** Certain testing requires sensitivity over specificity—example: blood bank donors screened for infectious diseases when it is better to err in

excluding donors who are falsely positive than include donors who are falsely negative.

4. **Specificity:** the ability of a test to identify *only* those individuals with disease as opposed to individuals testing positive when there is no disease. It refers to a test's ability to generate more true-negative results and fewer false-positive results.
   a. Specific test has a high threshold for "normal" or negative test results.
   b. Specific test usually has low sensitivity.
   c. Certain testing requires specificity over sensitivity—example: urine toxicology screen to detect presence of cocaine, cardiac isoenzymes to rule out a myocardial infarct.
5. **Reference range:** established upper and lower boundary levels of a laboratory value by which a patient's result will be measured for presence of disease. The range of normality (mathematical) is dependent on population subsets such as age, gender, pregnancy, and other patient attributes.
   a. Often referred to as "normal" range.
   b. Term "normal" is misleading—reference range determined based upon specific attributes of a population subset, not due to "normalcy" (Oxley et al., 2001).
   c. Approximately 5% of "healthy" laboratory results fall outside the reference range.
   d. Reference range can vary from laboratory to laboratory.

PRINCIPLES OF TEST UTILIZATION

A. Patient management depends upon good clinical skills, judicious use of laboratory testing, and careful interpretation of laboratory data. Once a laboratory value is determined and the patient's clinical status evaluated, the combined information is utilized to direct treatment. In an effort to optimize care, minimize patient discomfort, and contain health care costs, Wallach (2000) identifies key principles of test utilization:
   1. Under the best of circumstances, no test is perfect.
      a. Results can be misleading.
      b. Specificity or sensitivity of a test is never 100%.
   2. Choice of tests should be based on the prior probability of the diagnosis being sought, which affects the predictive value of the test.
      a. History, physical examination, and prevalence of a disease determine probability of diagnosis.
      b. Patient history and examination should precede choice of laboratory tests.
   3. The combination of short-term physiologic variation and analytical error is sufficient to render the interpretation of single determinations difficult when the concentrations are in the borderline range.
      a. Despite the high quality of the laboratory, any laboratory result may be incorrect.
      b. Laboratory test may need to be rechecked or redrawn, at times in another laboratory.
   4. Reference ranges vary from one laboratory to another.
      a. Age, gender, race, size, and physiologic status must be considered.
      b. 5% of test results will be outside reference range in absence of disease.
   5. Tables of reference values represent statistical data for 95% of the population; values outside these ranges do not necessarily represent disease.

a. Test results falling within the reference range may be abnormal from the patient's baseline range.
b. Certain conditions warrant serial testing.

6. Multiple test abnormalities are more likely to be significant than single test abnormalities.
   a. Two or more positive tests for a given disease reinforce diagnosis.
7. The greater the degree of abnormality of a test result, the more likely that a confirmed value is clinically significant or represents a real disorder.
8. Excessive repetition of tests is wasteful, and the excess burden increases the possibility of laboratory errors.
   a. Patient's acuity should dictate testing interval.
9. Tests should be performed only if they will alter the patient's diagnosis, prognosis, treatment, or management.
10. Clerical errors are far more likely than technical errors to cause incorrect results.
11. The effect of drugs on laboratory test values must never be overlooked.
    a. Certain drugs can produce false-negative and false-positive results-examples: *anticonvulsants, antihypertensives, and antiinfectives.*
12. The effect of artifacts can cause spurious values and factitious disorders *especially in the face of discrepant laboratory results.*
13. Negative laboratory (or any other type of tests) do not necessarily rule out a clinical disease.

IATROGENIC SEQUELAE OF LABORATORY TESTING—PREVENTIVE STRATEGIES

A. The goal of laboratory testing is to help diagnose and guide management of disease. Inadvertently, laboratory testing can complicate patient care by creating additional illness, stress, injury, and/or cost. An understanding of the potential sequelae associated with laboratory sampling and strategies that can be used to minimize sequelae is integral to patient care.

1. **Physiologic stress.**
   a. Adverse physical symptoms triggered by pain stimuli, sensory stimuli, and/or disease state.
   b. Laboratory sampling via skin puncture elicits a painful stimuli creating physiologic stress.
   c. Common physiologic stress symptoms include (see also Chapter 11):
      (1) Tachycardia or bradycardia.
      (2) Hypertension or hypotension.
      (3) Apnea or crying.
      (4) Cyanosis or respiratory distress.
      (5) Changes in skin color and temperature.
   d. An event creating physiologic stress can potentially alter a laboratory sample result—example:
      (1) *Change in P_{CO_2} and P_{O_2} reading when infant cries (Kaplan and Tange, 1998)*
      (2) *Altered blood pH if infant becomes hypothermic.*
   e. Strategies to minimize sampling-induced physiologic stress include:
      (1) Minimize skin punctures for laboratory sampling by minimizing or combining labwork.

(2) Utilize existing indwelling catheters (when available) to obtain laboratory samples.
(3) Employ noninvasive pain management techniques to assist infant in coping with painful stimuli (see also Chapter 16).
(4) Use of spring-loaded lancets for heel-stick sampling (Franck, 1998).
(5) Quick, efficient execution of laboratory sampling.
(6) Warm compress to the heel to promote blood flow and improve testing accuracy, avoiding repeat laboratory sampling.
(7) Venipuncture may be preferable to the heel-stick procedure in minimizing procedural-related pain in term neonates.

2. Pain (see also Chapter 16).

a. An unpleasant sensory and emotional experience associated with actual or potential tissue invasion (Franck, 1998).
b. Laboratory sampling by skin puncture evokes pain.
c. Pain causes adverse physiologic stress (see number 1, this section), including potential central nervous system (CNS) alterations.
d. It is difficult to differentiate between acute and chronic pain in the infant.
e. Strategies to minimize sampling-induced pain include:
(1) Strategies that minimize physiologic stress (see number 1, this section).
(2) Nonpharmacologic pain management strategies—examples: *swaddling, facilitated tucking, nonnutritive sucking, skin-to-skin contact*.
(3) Pharmacologic pain management strategies—examples: *sucrose, local anesthetic, and opioid and nonopioid analgesics*.
(4) Usefulness of topical local anesthesia for pain control in infants remains unclear (Franck, 1998).

3. Skin injury.

a. Alteration in normal barrier function of skin due to invasive procedures, adhesives to skin, reaction to skin antiseptics, and/or disease states (Kuller and Lund, 1998).
b. Arterial punctures, venipunctures, capillary heel-sticks used to obtain laboratory samples may potentially create skin injury. (LeFrak and Lund, 2001)
c. Potential skin injury from peripheral laboratory samples include:
(1) Bruising.
(2) Hematoma.
(3) Abrasion from antiseptic solutions, friction, or tape application.
(4) Dermal stripping from friction or tape application.
(5) Scarring from multiple punctures.
(6) Calcifications.
(7) Burns secondary to prewarming heel with a soak that is too hot; warm soak should not exceed 44° C.
d. Strategies to minimize sampling—induced skin injury from skin puncture include to:
(1) Minimize labwork.
(2) Avoid excessive "squeeze" when obtaining capillary bloodwork.
(3) Apply adequate pressure to puncture sites to minimize bleeding and formation of hematoma.
(4) Utilize nonadhering products to apply a dressing to puncture site—example:
(a) *Loose elastic wrap (Coban) around extremity holding gauze in place.*

(5) Thoroughly wash skin of antiseptic solutions.
(6) Use proper skin puncture devices when obtaining blood—example:
(a) *Spring-loaded lancet of proper length (no deeper than 2 mm) (Garza and Beacon-McBride, 2002a).*
(b) *Butterfly needle of proper gauge and length for site.*

4. Infection.

a. An important skin function is to provide a barrier to infection.
b. Any break in skin barrier creates potential for infection.
c. Common infections associated with altered skin barrier include:
(1) Bacterial/candidal skin surface infection.
(2) Cellulitis.
(3) Abscess formation at puncture site.
(4) Septicemia.
(5) Osteomyelitis.
(6) Urinary tract/bladder infection.
(7) Meningitis.
d. Strategies to minimize sampling-induced infection include:
(1) Minimize laboratory sampling.
(2) Avoid sampling in area of existing skin injury.
(3) Avoid repeated sampling from dedicated central lines—example: *routine laboratory sampling via percutaneous central line or Broviac catheter.*
(4) Meticulous aseptic technique when obtaining a laboratory sample.
(5) Use of nursing strategies to maintain optimal skin integrity (see Chapter 35).

5. Organ/nerve injury.

a. Needle puncture for laboratory sampling can potentially contribute to organ injury.
b. Potential organ injury associated with needle puncture includes:
(1) Damage to nerve and/or tissues in wrist or brachial area from arterial puncture.
(2) Damage to lung and/or breast tissue from thoracentesis.
(3) Damage to abdominal organs from peritoneal tap.
(4) Damage to bladder or nearby intestine from suprapubic bladder tap.
(5) Damage to nerves or tissue of spine from lumbar puncture.
(6) Damage to skin as mentioned in number 3, this section.
(7) Tissue ischemia from arterial vasospasm secondary to arterial puncture.
c. Strategies to minimize sampling-induced organ/nerve injury include:
(1) Prudent use of laboratory sampling.
(2) Proper technique for needlestick sampling (see also Chapter 15).
(3) Ultrasound guidance as needed for pleural and peritoneal aspiration.

6. Anemia.

a. Iatrogenic anemia due to blood loss from laboratory sampling (Kaplan and Tange, 1998; Shaw, 1998).
b. Iatrogenic anemia, along with physiologic anemia, constitutes the most common causes of chronic anemia in infants (Shaw, 1998).
c. Despite micro sampling and conservative laboratory sampling, sick infants can lose more than 5 cc of blood per day (Clapp, et al., 2001).
d. Removal of 1 cc of blood from a 1 kg infant equals removal of 70 cc of blood from an adult (Blackburn, 2003).
e. Iatrogenic blood loss correlates with degree of illness.

f. Laboratory sample overdraws (19% ± 1.8% more than needed) is common in the NICU (Blackburn, 2003).
g. Strategies to minimize sampling-induced anemia include:
   (1) Judicious use of laboratory sampling.
   (2) Micro sampling when possible.
   (3) Accurate documentation of blood loss.
   (4) Avoiding overdrawing of blood samples.

7. **False diagnosis.**
   a. Under the best circumstances, no test is perfect.
   b. Excess repetition of a test increases the possibility of laboratory error.
   c. The more laboratory samples drawn, the more likely one or more results will be outside the reference range.
   d. Clinical decision making should be based on trends or multiple laboratory values pointing to disease vs. spurious results.
   e. Strategies to minimize sampling-related false diagnosis include:
      (1) Obtain laboratory samples only when necessary to assist in diagnosis, prognosis, treatment, or management.
      (2) Verify spurious laboratory values.
8. **Cost factor.**
   a. 15% to 20% of a patient's hospital bill results from laboratory sampling.
   b. If the average ancillary cost of a NICU stay is $13,873, a patient spends $3308 for laboratory testing (Rogowski, 1999).
   c. Cost of hospitalization in the NICU is inversely related to gestational age.
   d. Rising cost of medical care is complicating delivery of care.
   e. Strategies to minimize sampling-related laboratory costs include:
      (1) Minimize laboratory sampling.
      (2) Prudent medical and nursing decision making regarding laboratory sampling.
      (3) Minimizing laboratory errors precipitating repeat sampling.

DECISION—QUESTIONS TO ASK PRIOR TO OBTAINING A LABORATORY TEST

A. Judicious use of laboratory testing is critical in any setting, particularly in the NICU, where acuity is high. Below are questions to consider *prior to* ordering and/or obtaining a laboratory sample. Asking oneself these questions will assist in refining critical thinking skills and aid in selective use of labwork (Box 13-1).
   1. **Does the patient require the laboratory test?**
      a. **Is the patient examination abnormal, whereby a laboratory test will help in diagnosis?**
         (1) Example:
            (a) Abnormal finding: model-jittery infant.
            (b) Possible laboratory tests: glucose, calcium, and urine toxicology screen.
      b. **Is the medical history helpful in directing which laboratory test to order?**
         (1) Example: model-jittery infant.
            (a) Infant of a gestational, class A1, diabetic mother (IDM-A1). Might choose to obtain a serum glucose and/or serum calcium vs. a urine toxicology screen.

BOX 13-1
QUESTIONS TO ASK *PRIOR TO* OBTAINING A LABORATORY TEST

- **Does the patient require the laboratory test?**
  Is the patient examination abnormal whereby a laboratory test will help in diagnosis?
  Is the medical history helpful in directing which laboratory test to order?
- **Will the laboratory test requested answer the "so what" question?**
  Is the laboratory result integral to the immediate clinical management of the infant?
  Is the laboratory result contributory to a patient's diagnosis?
- **Is the laboratory test requested still applicable to current clinical status?**
  Has the infant's clinical examination changed?
  Has the infant recovered?
- **Is the timing of the laboratory test appropriate?**
  When should the labwork be obtained?
- **Is the laboratory test ordered the "best" test to answer the clinical question?**
- **Does the laboratory test(s) require too much blood volume?**
- **Does the potential benefit of the laboratory test outweigh the risk of sequelae in the patient?**
- **If the laboratory sample is inadequate, faulty, or "lost," is it necessary to redraw?**
  Has the clinical status changed?
  Has the infant recovered?

(b) Infant with delayed drying of skin after birth and rectal temperature of 97° F? Might choose to place infant under heat source and not obtain labwork.

(c) Infant 1800 g, IDM-A1, and mother with minimal prenatal care? Might choose to obtain all possible laboratory tests.

2. Will the laboratory test requested answer the "so what" question?

a. Is the laboratory result integral to the immediate clinical management of the infant?

(1) Example: hypoglycemia in an IDM-A1 will mandate increasing the carbohydrate intake to treat the problem.

(2) Example: mild hypothermia in an otherwise healthy infant will not require a change in management directed by labwork.

b. Is the laboratory result contributory to a patient's diagnosis?

(1) Example: serum glucose result will help diagnose hypoglycemia as a cause of jitteriness.

(2) Example: serum glucose result will not help diagnose respiratory distress syndrome.

3. Is the laboratory test requested still applicable to current clinical status?

a. *Example: model-jittery infant.*

(1) Has the infant's clinical examination changed?

(a) 1-hour-old IDM-A1 whose jitteriness has changed to tonic-clonic movements of extremities in addition to serum glucose and calcium, will need to consider a urine toxicology screen and electrolytes.

(b) 3-hour-old IDM-A1 who breast-fed for 20 minutes and is no longer jittery may not require further testing, particularly if the original serum glucose was normal.

(c) Hypothermic infant who continues to remain hypothermic after 2 hours under heat source may need serum glucose, sepsis evaluation.

b. *Example: model-jittery infant.*
   (1) **Has the infant recovered?**
      (a) Infant with multiple normal glucose results: may no longer require frequent glucose testing.
      (b) Infant no longer jittery after acquiring a normal body temperature: may need to cancel labwork ordered to evaluate jitteriness.

4. **Is the timing of the laboratory test appropriate?**
   a. *Example: model-jittery infant.*
      (1) **When should the labwork be obtained?**
         (a) IDM-A1 at birth: might wait to check serum glucose at 30 minutes of age when result would reflect infant's status vs. maternal environment.
         (b) Jittery infant with normal serum glucose and calcium: might obtain *first* voided specimen for a urine toxicology screen.
5. **Is the laboratory test ordered the "best" test to answer the clinical question?**
   a. *Example: model-jittery infant.*
      (1) Should the jittery infant have a serum glucose sent to the laboratory or should a whole blood glucose be obtained at the bedside by POCT, NPT? A POCT glucose result is available in seconds, allowing for rapid clinical intervention.
      (2) Should the jittery infant with polycythemia have a POCT whole blood glucose or should a serum glucose be sent to the laboratory? A POCT glucose may not be accurate in the face of polycythemia.
6. **Does the laboratory test(s) require too much blood volume?**
   a. *Example: model-jittery infant.*
      (1) A 500-g infant with q2h serum glucose: POCT whole blood glucose testing requires average sample size of one drop to 0.1 ml of blood vs. serum glucose requiring average sample size of 0.5 ml.
      (2) A 5-ml sample of blood required for metabolic screening in a 500-g infant: 10% blood volume loss may not be tolerated; need to prioritize labwork and draw in stages based on most common to least common disorders.
7. **Does the potential benefit of the laboratory test outweigh the risk of sequelae in the patient?**
   a. *Example: model-jittery infant.*
      (1) A 500-g infant with hypoglycemia: frequent glucose testing needed to monitor treatment; benefit outweighs potential harm of blood loss. Also, using POCT can minimize blood loss.
      (2) A 5-ml blood sample for metabolic screening in a 500-g, symptomatic infant: potential harm of an acute 10% blood loss outweighs the need to simultaneously obtain all the ordered metabolic screening laboratories.
8. **If the laboratory sample is inadequate, faulty, or "lost," is it necessary to redraw?**
   a. *Example: model-jittery infant.*
      (1) **Has the clinical status changed?**
      (2) **Has the infant recovered?** (See number 3, of this section.) If status improves or infant recovers while waiting for sample, repeat sampling may not be indicated.

LABORATORY INTERPRETATION—DECISION TREE

A. Careful laboratory data interpretation is essential in providing accurate therapeutic interventions (Bishop, 1999). Asking focused questions will assist in refining critical thinking skills related to utilization of laboratory values in patient management. Below are questions to consider when utilizing laboratory results to *direct* patient care.

1. **Laboratory test result.** Is it reliable? Is it believable? (Box 13-2) A question tree ***if result too low:***
   a. **Is the sample diluted?** *Examples:*
      (1) A laboratory specimen can be contaminated with or diluted by fluids infusing through indwelling arterial and/or venous lines if the initial few drops of blood are incorporated into the sample.
      (2) A laboratory specimen can be diluted by interstitial fluid from the skin tissues if heel-stick puncture is not fresh, the puncture site is not prewarmed, or the infant is exceedingly edematous.
   b. **Was the sample handled correctly?** *Examples:*
      (1) A serum bilirubin can be falsely low if obtained while infant is under phototherapy or if exposed too long in the daylight unanalyzed.
      (2) A serum glucose can be falsely low if left in a microtainer and not processed and analyzed promptly.
      (3) An overfilled or underfilled hematology sample can precipitate clotting and falsely decrease platelet count.

BOX 13-2

LABORATORY INTERPRETATION. IS IT RELIABLE? IS IT BELIEVABLE?

Laboratory Test Result. Is it *reliable*? Is it *believable*?

Yes
- Implement appropriate clinical intervention, if needed.

No
- Consider repeating laboratory test when appropriate correction made.
- Consider repeating laboratory test if clinical status continues to warrant laboratory test.

Laboratory test result. Is it *reliable*? Is it *believable*?

If Result too Low
- Is the sample diluted?
- Was the sample handled correctly?
- Was the timing of the test an issue?
- Was medical therapy not implemented or inadequate?
- Was the specimen site condition a factor?
- Was the POCT device calibrated?
- Was there interference from past medical therapy?

If Result too High
- Was the laboratory specimen drawn too early?
- Was the sample handled correctly?
- Was medical therapy not implemented or inadequate?
- Was the source of the laboratory sample not appropriate?
- Was the POCT device calibrated?

POCT: Point-of-care testing.

c. **Was the timing of the test an issue?** *Examples:*
   (1) A serum gentamicin, vancomycin, or theophylline level will be too low if drawn too early in the drug treatment.
   (2) A serum glucose or POCT glucose obtained too soon after feeding the infant may remain falsely low due to lack of digestion time.
   (3) Electrolytes may remain falsely low if obtained too soon after electrolyte replacement.

d. **Was medical therapy not implemented or inadequate?** *Examples:*
   (1) A blood gas obtained prior to weaning the ventilator for a PCO_2 of 25.
   (2) A serum glucose or POCT glucose obtained prior to medical intervention for hypoglycemia.
   (3) A serum gentamicin, vancomycin, or theophylline level will be too low if the dose is inadequate or dose interval too long.
   (4) A theophylline level may be low due to intermittent doses being held due to tachycardia in the infant.

e. **Was the specimen site condition a factor?** *Examples:*
   (1) A capillary blood sample from an edematous infant can be falsely low due to excessive tissue fluids.
   (2) A nonwarmed heel can falsely lower a capillary blood gas pH, PO_2.

f. **Was the POCT device calibrated?** *Examples:*
   (1) Laboratory result may be unreliable if POCT device:
      (a) Not recently calibrated.
      (b) Calibrated by an untrained individual.
      (c) Reagent for calibration expired.
      (d) Sample cartridge expired or not room temperature.

g. **Was there interference from past medical therapy?** *Examples:*
   (1) An infant's blood culture may be falsely negative if a mother was treated with antibiotics during labor.
   (2) Phenobarbital use may decrease theophylline concentrations.

2. **Laboratory test result. Is it *reliable*? Is it *believable*?**A question tree ***if result too high*:.**

a. **Was the laboratory specimen drawn too early?** *Examples:*
   (1) A triglyceride level may be falsely elevated if drawn too soon after lipid infusion.
   (2) A serum calcium level may be falsely increased if drawn soon after a calcium gluconate bolus.
   (3) Electrolytes can remain elevated if drawn too soon after IV fluids increased.

b. **Was the sample handled correctly?** *Examples:*
   (1) A serum potassium may be falsely elevated due to hemolysis from squeezing the heel for capillary laboratory sampling.
   (2) A serum protein or potassium may be falsely elevated if a tourniquet is applied too tightly or too long (≥3 minutes).
   (3) A Hct can be falsely elevated if drawn from a poorly perfused heel.

c. **Was medical therapy not implemented or inadequate?** *Examples:*
   (1) A serum bilirubin can remain elevated if phototherapy not instituted long enough to measure change.
   (2) A PCO_2 can remain elevated if ventilator setting changes not sufficient to correct the respiratory ailment or the sample drawn too soon after corrective intervention.

d. **Was the source of the laboratory sample not appropriate?** *Examples*:
   (1) A Hct can be falsely elevated from a capillary sample vs. an arterial or venous sample.
   (2) An ammonia level can be falsely elevated if hemolyzed so needs to be drawn via artery or vein.
e. **Was the POCT device calibrated?** *Examples*:
   (1) Laboratory result may be unreliable if POCT device not recently calibrated, calibrated by an untrained individual, reagent for calibration expired, sample cartridge expired or not room temperature.

3. **Laboratory test result. Is it *reliable?* Is it *believable?* YES**
   a. **Implement appropriate clinical intervention, if needed.** *Examples*:
      (1) Alert physician or midlevel practitioner of laboratory result and implement appropriate medical or nursing corrective intervention as needed:
         (a) Medication dose change for inadequate drug level.
         (b) Ventilator setting change for under- or overventilation.
         (c) Blood product transfusion for anemia, thrombocytopenia.
         (d) Change in IV fluid concentration or rate for electrolyte imbalance or dehydration.
         (e) Change feeding interval for hypoglycemia.
4. **Laboratory test result. Is it *reliable?* Is it *believable?* NO**
   a. **Consider repeating laboratory test when appropriate correction made.** *Example:*
      (1) Repeat laboratory test at appropriate time for drug level measurement.
      (2) Warm heel prior to obtaining capillary sample.
      (3) Wait 2 to 3 hours after a milk feeding to obtain a postfeed serum glucose.
   b. **Consider repeating laboratory test if clinical status continues to warrant laboratory test.** *Examples:*
      (1) A clotted CBC sample after red blood cell transfusion or after antibiotic therapy: may not require a repeat sample or might wait for redraw until another blood sample needed.
      (2) A high Hct value taken from an acrocyanotic heel in a hypoglycemic infant would need a central Hct to determine if polycythemia is a cause of hypoglycemia.
5. **Laboratory test result. Is it *normal?* YES** (Box 13-3).
   a. **Consider a change in medical management.** *Examples*:
      (1) Normal electrolyte results in the face of electrolyte replacement may signal a need to decrease or stop the electrolyte supplementation.
      (2) A normal Hct may warrant cancellation of a projected red blood cell transfusion.
   b. **Consider implementing surveillance plans.** *Examples:*
      (1) Normal serum calcium, phosphorus, alkaline phosphatase may need weekly surveillance in very low birth weight infants to monitor for potential rickets.
      (2) Normal electrolytes may need frequent monitoring when initiating diuretic therapy.
6. **Laboratory test result. Is it *normal?* NO** (see Box 13-3).
   a. **Consider calling the laboratory to verify specimen.** *Examples:*
      (1) See numbers 1, 2, and 4 of this section.

BOX 13-3
LABORATORY INTERPRETATION: IS IT NORMAL?

Laboratory Test Result. Is it *normal?*

Yes	No
■ Consider a change in medical management. ■ Consider implementing surveillance plans.	■ Consider calling the laboratory to verify specimen. ■ Is the laboratory result in the appropriate reference range? ■ Review patient care practice at time of laboratory specimen sampling. ■ Consider medication interactions as etiology. ■ Institute corrective medical and/or nursing action.

(2) Call laboratory to verify that the result is indeed that of the patient in question.
(3) Ascertain that the abnormal laboratory value was taken from the patient in question.

b. **Is the laboratory result in the appropriate reference range?** *Examples:*
(1) A critical Hct value differs with age. A Hct of 55% in a newborn is normal as compared with an adult.
(2) Laboratory methods and equipment vary with different laboratories; need to confirm laboratory result with the laboratory used to analyze sample.

c. **Review patient care practice at time of laboratory specimen sampling.** *Examples:*
(1) See numbers 1, 2, and 4 of this section.

d. **Consider medication interactions as etiology.** *Examples:*
(1) Heparin in a blood sample will prolong PT, PTT.
(2) Narcotic sedation may depress respirations and increase Pco_2 level.
(3) Sulfonamides can increase serum bilirubin.
(4) Stool Hematest can be falsely positive when patient is on iron supplement, indomethacin, potassium preparations, or steroids.

e. **Institute corrective medical and/or nursing action.** *Example:*
(1) See number 3 of this section.

7. **Laboratory test *follow-up*—normal** test result (Box 13-4).

a. **Continue to watch for potential sequelae of treatment.** *Examples:*
(1) Periodic monitoring of electrolytes needed when patient on diuretic therapy.
(2) Periodic monitoring of renal function and electrolytes when patient on antifungal therapy.

b. **Consider a plan for implementing maintenance laboratory surveillance.** *Examples:*
(1) Routine weekly monitoring of electrolytes, liver function, and renal function when infant on prolonged hyperalimentation.
(2) Routine monitoring of skeletal integrity of the premature infant susceptible for rickets.

■ BOX 13-4
■ **LABORATORY INTERPRETATION: TEST FOLLOW-UP**

Laboratory Test *Follow-up*

Normal Test Result	**Abnormal Test Result**
■ Continue to watch for potential sequelae of treatment. ■ Consider a plan for implementing maintenance laboratory surveillance.	■ Consider a change in clinical practice. ■ Allow time for corrective action then repeat laboratory test to measure effective therapy.

8. **Laboratory test *follow-up*—abnormal** test result (see Box 13-4).
   a. **Consider a change in clinical practice.** *Examples:*
      (1) See number 3, of this section.
   b. **Allow time for corrective action, then repeat laboratory test to measure effective therapy.** *Examples:*
      (1) Weaning from ventilatory support may warrant blood gases every half hour to every 4 hours for an overventilated infant recovering from primary atelectasis.
      (2) Repeat serum glucose checks every half hour to every hour may be necessary after a hypoglycemic infant receives an IV glucose bolus.
      (3) Weekly or biweekly serum electrolytes may be necessary when adjusting oral electrolyte supplementation for borderline low serum electrolyte levels in infant on diuretics for chronic lung disease.

REFERENCES

Bishop, M.L.: Laboratory results in the newborn. In B.G. Davis, D. Mass, and M.L. Bishop (Eds.): *Principles of clinical laboratory utilization and consultation*, Philadelphia, 1999, Saunders, pp. 635-639.

Blackburn, S.T.: Hematologic and hemostatic systems. In S.T. Blackburn (Ed.): *Maternal, fetal and neonatal physiology: A clinical perspective* (2nd ed.). St Louis, 2003, Saunders, pp. 213-254.

Clapp, D.W., Shannon, K.M., and Phibbs, R.H.: Hematologic problems. In M.H. Klaus and A.A. Fanaroff (Eds.): *Care of the high-risk neonate* (5th ed.). Philadelphia, 2001, Saunders, pp. 447-479.

Fischbach, F.: Overview of the clinician's role: Responsibilities, standards, and requisite knowledge. In F. Fischbach (Ed.): *A manual of laboratory & diagnostic tests* (6th ed.). Philadelphia, 2002, Lippincott, pp. 2-33.

Franck, L.S.: Identification, management, and prevention of pain in the neonate. In C. Kenner, J.W. Lott, and A.A. Flandermeyer (Eds.): *Comprehensive neonatal nursing: A physiologic perspective* (2nd ed.). Philadelphia, 1998, Saunders, pp. 788-803.

Garza, D. and Becan-McBride, K.: Blood collection equipment. In D. Garza, and K. Becan-McBride (Eds.): *Phlebotomy handbook: Blood collection essentials*. New Jersey, 2002a, Prentice Hall, pp.181-230.

Garza, D. and Becan-McBride, K.: Complications in blood collection. In D. Garza, and Becan-McBride, K: *Phlebotomy handbook: Blood collection essentials*. New Jersey, 2002b, Prentice Hall, pp. 283-300.

Garza, D. and Becan-McBride, K.: Pediatric procedures. In D. Garza, and K: Becan-McBride, *Phlebotomy handbook: Blood collection essentials*. New Jersey, 2002c, Prentice Hall, pp. 307-333.

Henry, J.B., Kurec, A.S., and Derrwyler, M.T.: The clinical laboratory: Organization, purposes, and practice. In J.B. Henry (Ed.): *Clinical diagnosis and management by laboratory methods* (20th ed.). Philadelphia, 2001, Saunders, pp. 3-29.

Kaplan, L.A. and Tange, S.M. (Eds.): *Standards of laboratory practice.* Washington, DC, 1998, National Academy of Clinical Biochemistry (monograph).

Kee, J.L.: The importance of specimen collection. In J.L. Kee (Ed.): *Laboratory and diagnostic tests with nursing implication* (6th ed.). New Jersey, 2002, Prentice Hall.

Kuller, J.M. and Lund, C.H.: Assessment and management of integumentary dysfunction. In J. Kenner, J.W. Lott, and A.A. Flandermeyer (Eds.): *Comprehensive neonatal nursing: A physiologic perspective* (2nd ed.). Philadelphia, 1998, Saunders, pp. 648-681.

LeFrak, L. and Lund, C.H.: Nursing practice in the neonatal intensive care unit. In M.H. Klaus and A.A. Fanaroff (Eds.): *Care of the high-risk neonate* (5th ed.). Philadelphia, 2001, Saunders, pp. 223-242.

Martin, J.A., Hamilton, B.E., Ventura, S.J., et al.: Births: Final data for 2000. *National Vital Statistics Reports, 50*(5):February 12, 2002.

Olsowka, E.S. and Garg, U.: Specimen collection and point-of-care testing. In D.S. Jacobs, D.K. Oxley, and W.R. DeMott (Eds.): *Jacobs & DeMott laboratory test handbook* (5th ed.). 2001, Hudson, Ohio, Lexi-Comp, Inc, pp. 35-48.

Oxley, D.K., Garg, U., and Olsowka, E.S.: Maximizing the information from laboratory tests-The Ulysses syndrome. In D.S. Jacobs, D.K. Oxley, and W.R. DeMott (Eds.): *Jacobs & DeMott laboratory test handbook* (5th ed.). Hudson, Ohio, 2001, Lexi-Comp, Inc, pp.15-23.

Rogowski, J.: Section 2: Measuring the cost of neonatal and perinatal care. *Pediatrics, 103*(1):329-335, 1999.

Sacher, R.A., McPherson, R.A., and Campos, J.M.: Principles of interpretation of laboratory tests. In R.A. Sacher, R.A. McPherson, and J.M. Campos (Eds.): *Widmann's clinical interpretation of laboratory tests* (11th ed.). Philadelphia, 2000a, F.A. Davis, pp. 3-27.

Sacher, R.A., McPherson, R.A., and Campos, J.M.: General chemistry. In R.A., Sacher, R.A., McPherson, and J.M. Campos, (eds.): *Widmann's clinical interpretation of laboratory tests.* 11th ed. Philadelphia, 2000b, F.A. Davis, pp. 445-446.

Sacher, R.A., McPherson, R.A., and Campos, J.M.: Hematological methods. In R.A. Sacher, R.A. McPherson, and J.M. Campos (Eds.): *Widmann's clinical interpretation of laboratory tests* (11th ed.). Philadelphia, 2000c, F.A. Davis, pp. 31-32.

Sacher, R.A., McPherson, R.A., and Campos, J.M.: Principles of immunology and immunology testing. In R.A. Sacher, R.A. McPherson, and J.M. Campos (Eds.): *Widmann's clinical interpretation of laboratory tests* (11th ed.). Philadelphia, 2000d, F.A. Davis, p. 325.

Schwartz, R.M., Kellogg, R., and Muri, J.H.: Specialty newborn care: Trends and issues. *Journal of Perinatology, 20*(8 Pt 1):520-529, 2000.

Shaw, N.: Assessment and management of hematologic dysfunction. In C., Kenner, J.W., Lott, A.A Flandermeyer.: *Comprehensive neonatal nursing: A physiologic perspective,* 2nd ed. Philadelphia, 1998, W.B. Saunders, pp.520-563.

Wallach, J.: Introduction to normal values (reference ranges). In J. Wallach (Ed.): *Interpretation of diagnostic tests* (7th ed.). Philadelphia, 2000, Lippincott Williams & Wilkins, pp. 3-6.

CHAPTER

14 Radiologic Evaluation

LINDA K. BEAUMAN AND JANE DEACON

OBJECTIVES

1. Define common radiologic terms used to describe an x-ray.
2. Differentiate various densities that are evident on an x-ray.
3. Describe radiologic findings that are commonly seen in neonatal disease states.
4. Differentiate normal from abnormal findings on a chest x-ray.
5. Recognize findings on an x-ray that are consistent with congenital heart disease.
6. Describe an x-ray consistent with necrotizing enterocolitis.
7. Review correct line and endotracheal tube placement on an x-ray.

Radiographic interpretation of abnormalities in a sick newborn infant is an established part of diagnostic evaluation. This evaluation assists the clinician in determining a diagnosis or formulating a differential diagnosis for treatment of the patient. Rarely is a newborn infant admitted to the neonatal intensive care unit (NICU) without having at least one x-ray taken, and frequently several additional films are needed during the course of treatment. Nurses need to become familiar with common radiographic findings to add to the knowledge base on which patient care is founded. This chapter reviews essentials of radiologic interpretation, discusses pathologic findings, and presents x-rays with common findings.

BASIC CONCEPTS

A. **Radiographs are "composite shadowgrams" representing the sum of densities (white through black) interposed between the x-ray beam and the source (Kirks and Griscom, 1998).**
B. **From the shadow forms, densities, and shapes, information can be deduced or inferred regarding anatomy, pathology, and function.**

TERMINOLOGY

A. **Air bronchogram:** air in the bronchial tree visualized against a background of generalized alveolar atelectasis (Swischuk, 2003).
B. **Artifact:** an unnaturally occurring silhouette that is artificially reproduced on an x-ray and is not a part of the patient (e.g., electrocardiogram [ECG] leads, temperature probes).
C. **Cardiothoracic ratio:** computed by dividing the maximum cardiac width by the maximum thoracic width to determine the heart size (Kirks and Griscom, 1998).
D. **Carina:** bifurcation of the trachea, usually about the level of the third and fourth thoracic vertebrae (Kirks and Griscom, 1998). Used in determining location of endotracheal tube.

E. **Expiratory film:** obtained when the infant is in expiration; appears to increase cardiac size, accentuate lung markings, and decrease normal lung expansion.
F. **Exposure:** amount of radiation used, producing a film ranging from light to dark. An underpenetrated (underexposed) film causes images to appear light and hazy. Overpenetration (overexposure) causes the film to be dark and to lack contrast, in comparison with an appropriately penetrated and exposed film.
G. **Hyperexpanded lungs:** lungs expanded to greater than the ninth rib.
H. **Hypoexpanded lungs:** lungs expanded to less than the seventh rib.
I. **Inspiratory film:** obtained when infant is in full inspiration and the lungs project to the eighth rib above the right diaphragmatic dome, with the trachea shown in a straight projection. This is the most desirable for chest film interpretation.
J. **Interlobar fissure:** accumulation of fluid in the pleural space between the lung lobes. The fissure may be fluid filled and may appear as a distinctive line.
K. **Perihilar:** pertaining to radiographic area bordering mediastinal structures.
L. **Pleural effusion:** abnormal collection of fluid in the pleural space (Kirks and Griscom, 1998).
M. **Radiolucent:** pertaining to substances with varying degrees of transparency (Swischuck, 2003).
N. **Radiopaque:** pertaining to substances that are dense and nonpenetrable to x-rays (Swischuk, 2003).
O. **Rad:** fundamental unit of radiation measurement.
P. **Roentgen:** unit of exposure.
Q. **Rotation:** turned from the midline. Chest structures closest to the beam are magnified, making their shadows appear enlarged and distorted (Kirks and Griscom, 1998).
R. **Skinfold:** the most common artifact seen in the neonate. Manifests as a straight line of variable length that can travel across or outside the chest or across the diaphragm and into the abdomen. Results from folding of excessive skin; may mimic a pneumothorax. However, the obliquity of the line produced by a skinfold is opposite to that produced by the edge of the lung in pneumothorax (Swischuk, 2003).
S. **Proper technique:** signifies correct exposure, positioning, and timing in relation to inspiration and proper labeling of a film.
T. **X-ray:** radiant energy of very short wavelength that penetrates substances opaque to light differently according to wavelength (Kenner and Lott, 2003).

X-RAY VIEWS COMMONLY USED IN THE NEWBORN INFANT (Fig. 14-1)

A. **Anteroposterior view.** X-ray tube is positioned above the infant's chest, with the x-ray beam passing through from front to back. Most common view used in the neonate for general assessment.
B. **Cross-table lateral view.** X-ray beam passes horizontally through infant in the supine position. Used to verify line placement, for assessment of free air in the chest, and for general assessment.
C. **Lateral decubitus view.** X-ray beam passes horizontally through the patient, who is positioned with suspect side uppermost. The film is placed on the infant's back, and the patient is placed perpendicular to the bed, facing the x-ray tube. The patient is usually elevated on diapers or blankets, with the arm positioned above the head and out of the field of view. Free air will rise to the

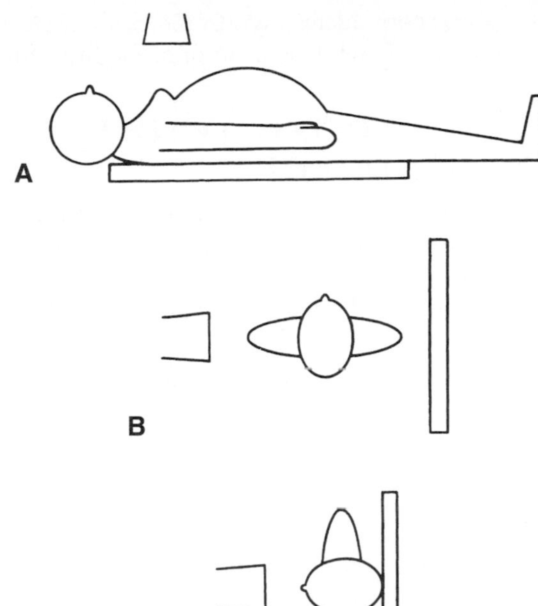

FIGURE 14-1 ■ X-ray views commonly used for the newborn infant. **A,** Anteroposterior view. **B,** Lateral view. **C,** Lateral decubitus view. (Courtesy Peter Honeyfield, M.D.)

highest portion of the thorax if a pneumothorax is present. If an abdominal perforation is present, free air will also rise above the liver when the patient is positioned with the left side down.

RADIOGRAPHIC DENSITIES

A. Radiodensities of various substances and tissues differ according to their composition (Kenner and Lott, 2003).

1. The least dense (radiolucent) substance will radiograph black or dark gray because the sparse molecules offer no obstacle to the rays.
2. A very dense (radiopaque) object such as lead will radiograph gray or white because no rays or few rays will penetrate it, so the film underneath will remain unchanged.
3. Subcutaneous fat is very radiolucent and produces a dark gray shadow on x-ray film.
4. Blood, muscle, and liver are of similar densities and will be seen as white and medium gray. Moist solid or fluid-filled organs and tissue masses have about the same radiodensity—greater than air but less than bone or metal.
5. Bone is composed of an organic matrix into which the complex bone mineral (primarily calcium) is precipitated. Organic substances will reduce the radiodensity of bone and will be seen as white with a tinge of gray.
6. Metal such as the surgical clip used for patent ductus arteriosus ligation is very dense and radiopaque. All the x-rays are absorbed by the metal, producing a white image on the film.

B. Differentiation of densities is the basis for interpretation of an x-ray film. For example, because of the contrast in densities between the fluid-filled heart, which radiographs white, and the air-filled lungs, which radiograph black, the heart can be seen against the lungs. Organs of the same density that are located side by side, such as the heart and the thymus, may be difficult to distinguish from each other. Changes in normal density can indicate a pathologic process, such as severe respiratory distress syndrome. Surfactant deficient lungs will appear on the film completely white instead of black, indicating areas of alveolar collapse.

RISKS ASSOCIATED WITH RADIOGRAPHIC EXAMINATION IN THE NEONATE

A. **Early radiation effects (Kenner and Lott, 2003).**
   1. Adverse effects of x-rays do not occur unless a threshold amount of radiation is delivered.
   2. Threshold amounts are far in excess of the radiation delivered during an x-ray examination.

B. **Delayed effects of x-rays.** The risk of radiation-induced childhood leukemia after abdominal radiography of the premature neonate would not be likely to exceed 0.02% unless 100 or more studies are performed.

C. **Risks to personnel.**
   1. Risks to personnel in the area where studies are properly done are too small to be of serious concern.
   2. At 2 m from the patient, the risk to personnel from an abdominal radiograph of the neonate is much less than the equivalent risk from 1 day of natural background radiation.

APPROACH TO INTERPRETING AN X-RAY

A. **Develop a systematic approach and a definite order for assessing a film to ensure that no pathology is missed.**

B. **Labeling.** Note name or identification of the patient, date and time of the film, and radiographic labeling on right or left side of the film.

C. **Assess for correct exposure of the film.**

D. **Note positioning.** Clavicles and ribs should be even on both sides of the chest. Rotation distorts structures.

E. **Individually assess all anatomic and pathologic changes on each film.**
   1. Lung fields.
      a. Normal lung expansion: Eight ribs projecting above the right diaphragmatic dome, with the trachea in a straight position.
      b. Lung volume, determined by noting the number of ribs expanded on an inspiratory film.
      c. Pulmonary vascularity: vessels branching from the lung root (hilum) and decreasing in size, with extension into the lung fields. Vascularity will be increased or diminished depending on pathologic state.
      d. Presence of free air: pneumothorax, pneumoperitoneum, pneumopericardium, and pneumomediastinum.
   2. Mediastinum.
      a. Heart.
         (1) Size.
         (2) Malposition: any inappropriate position of the heart—that is, any position other than the usual position in the hemithorax.
         (3) Contour: variable because of the influence of patient position and angulation of the x-ray beam.
         (4) Shape: may indicate pathologic change—for example, boot-shaped heart in tetralogy of Fallot and egg-shaped heart in transposition of the great vessels.
         (5) Pulmonary vascular markings: may be significantly diminished, as in pulmonary atresia, or increased, as in congestive heart failure (CHF).

b. Trachea.
   (1) Normally located within the mediastinum.
   (2) Assessment on x-ray film for presence and position of endotracheal tube.

c. Thymus.
   (1) Size.
   (2) Presence or absence.
   (3) Sail sign.

d. Diaphragm.
   (1) General pattern: two smooth, curved shadows on either side of the heart, taking off from the midline at the origin of the 10th and 11th ribs (Blickman, 1998; Swischuk, 2003).
   (2) Contour: possibly flattened with lung overdistention or elevated if there is abdominal distention.
   (3) Diaphragmatic hernia: abdominal contents passing through a hole in the diaphragm.
   (4) Eventration: herniation of bowel and liver against a weakened hemidiaphragm.

e. Gastrointestinal (GI) tract.
   (1) Esophagus. Distended, air-filled esophageal pouch may be visible in esophageal atresia.
   (2) Tracheoesophageal fistula. Fistula is present if an esophageal atresia exists and if air is visible in the stomach and intestine.
   (3) Passage of air through stomach and intestines.
   (4) Location of stomach bubble.
   (5) Bowel gas pattern.
   (6) Presence of pneumatosis intestinalis.
   (7) Presence of calcifications as a result of bowel perforation in utero.
   (8) Fluid, seen as a gasless abdomen. It is necessary to distinguish fluid from masses.
   (9) Pneumoperitoneum. Free air is seen within the peritoneal cavity.
   (10) Obstructions. Gaseous distention of the bowel is seen at various levels, depending on the location of the obstruction.

f. Skeletal system.
   (1) General skeletal assessment. Assess for symmetry, size, continuity, intactness, and abnormalities.
   (2) Fractures of long bones, clavicles, ribs, and skull. A dark line is seen along any portion of a fractured bone because of the air or tissue that settles between the bone fragments (Blickman, 1998; Kirks and Griscom, 1998).

g. Tubes and catheters.
   (1) Position of endotracheal tube, gastric tube, or chest tube.
   (2) Umbilical catheter placement.
   (3) Central venous line placement.

RESPIRATORY SYSTEM

A. The normal chest (Fig. 14-2).

1. Complete aeration of the chest occurs within a few breaths after onset of respirations at delivery (Blickman, 1998).
2. Residual fluid may be present in the alveoli after delivery. Early films (<6 hours after delivery) may show increased bronchovascular markings because of this fluid.

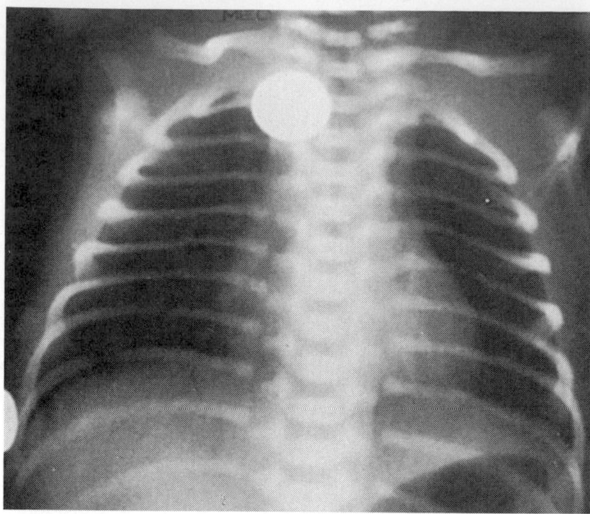

FIGURE 14-2 ■ Normal appearance of chest on x-ray film.

3. Normal lung pattern.
   a. Uniform radiolucent appearance.
   b. Hilar and perihilar regions show some increased density because of vascular, bronchial, and hilar structures, which produce some increase in density.
   c. Periphery shows few, if any, markings.
   d. Fluid in the various interlobar fissures represents a normal variation.

B. **Thymus.**
   1. Occupies the anterior part of the superior portion of the mediastinum and consists of right and left lobes (Hedlund et al., 1998).
   2. Appears as a smoothly rounded outline superior to the cardiac shadow and blending imperceptibly with the cardiac silhouette.
   3. Definite notch visible in some cases at the junction of the cardiac silhouette and the thymus.
   4. Generally more prominent on the right.
   5. Shape may alter markedly with degree of inspiration.
   6. Rapid involution during times of stress.
   7. Aplasia of the thymus (DiGeorge syndrome).
   8. Creation of "sail sign" when mediastinal air lifts the thymus upward.

C. **Trachea.**
   1. Trachea is normally displaced slightly to the right by the left aortic arch.
   2. Deviated trachea supports a mediastinal shift.
   3. On inspiration, the trachea dilates and lengthens.
   4. On expiration, the trachea constricts and shortens.
   5. On deep inspiration, the trachea and major bronchi are well distended and are easily identifiable.

PULMONARY PARENCHYMAL DISEASE

A. **Respiratory distress syndrome (hyaline membrane disease) (Fig. 14-3, *A*).**
   1. Pronounced under aeration. Fewer than eight ribs expand on inspiration on anteroposterior film with doming of the hemidiaphragms on lateral view.
   2. Bilateral diffuse alveolar infiltrates. Reticulogranular (ground-glass) appearance is due to microatelectasis of the alveoli (Hedlund et al., 1998).

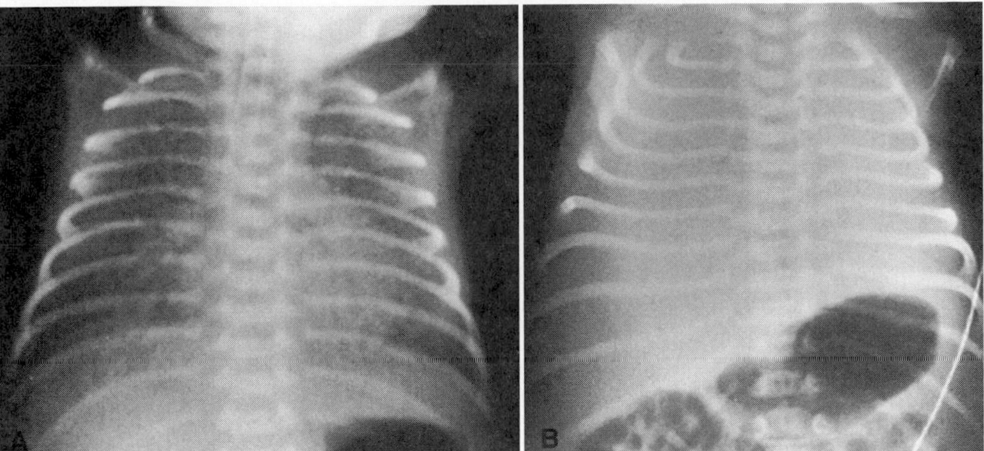

FIGURE 14-3 ■ **A,** *Hyaline* membrane disease. Note reticulogranular lung pattern and air bronchograms. **B,** Severe hyaline membrane disease. Note "white-out" appearance bilaterally with faint air bronchograms visible.

3. Homogeneous pattern throughout both lung fields.
4. Air bronchograms. Air-filled bronchi (black) are contrasted against the more radiopaque (whiter) lung fields (Blickman, 1998).
5. With severe disease a generalized opacity or frank "white-out" appearance (see Fig. 14-3, *B*).
6. Reticulogranular pattern and air bronchograms. May resemble those seen in group B streptococcal pneumonia and may be impossible to distinguish from respiratory distress syndrome.
7. X-ray findings after surfactant administration (Fig. 14-4).

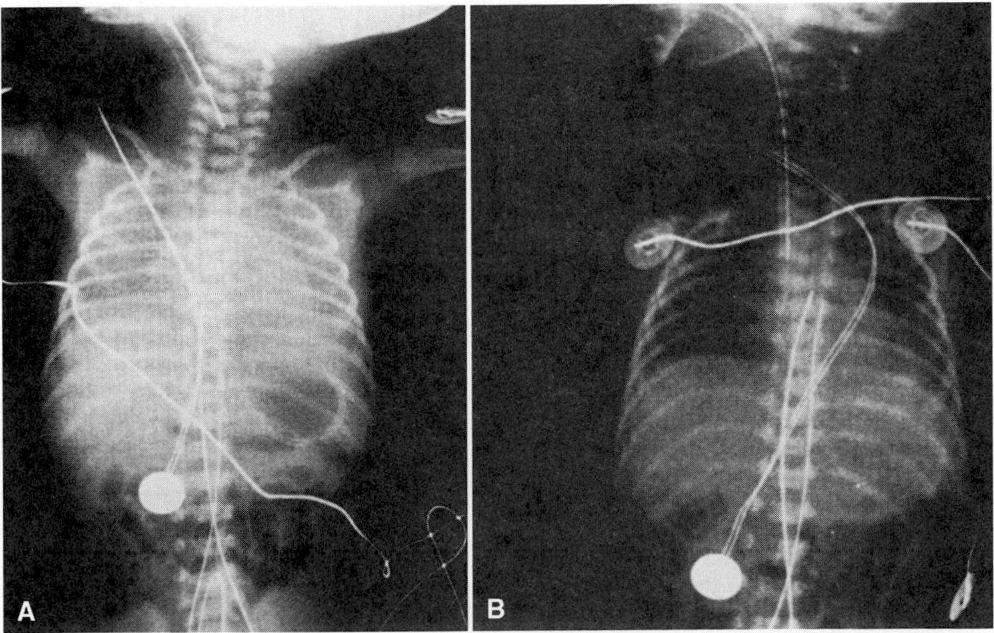

FIGURE 14-4 ■ Hyaline membrane disease before administration of surfactant (**A**) and significant clearing after administration (**B**).

a. Improvement in pulmonary aeration on x-ray.
b. Asymmetric distribution of surfactant, showing areas of improved lung alternating with areas of unchanged respiratory distress syndrome (RDS) (Blickman, 1998).
c. Poor prognosis with pulmonary interstitial emphysema after surfactant therapy (Blickman, 1998).

B. **Pulmonary interstitial emphysema (Fig. 14-5).**
1. Alveolar overdistention is due to assisted ventilation, visualized as multiple small, cystlike radiolucencies that are bilateral, unilateral, localized, or in a diffuse pattern (Fanaroff and Martin, 2002).
2. Condition may lead to a pneumothorax or other air leak.

C. **Bronchopulmonary dysplasia (BPD) (Fig. 14-6).**
1. Initial x-ray picture shows lung disease (e.g., respiratory distress syndrome, meconium aspiration syndrome) (Hedlund et al., 1998).
2. Radiologic appearance and course of BPD have changed since Northway and Rosan (1968) described four stages (Fanaroff and Martin, 2002).
   a. By the end of the first or second week, there is a persistent haziness of vessel margins progressing to linear densities that persist into the third or fourth week of life.
   b. Subsequently there is gradual development of a bubbly appearance of the lungs in association with hyperaeration, which is more pronounced at the lung bases. This persists after 1 month of age and represents a modified form of stage IV BPD.

D. **Transient tachypnea of the newborn (TTN) (retained fetal lung fluid, wet lung disease) (Fig. 14-7).**
1. Bilateral, symmetric perihilar streakiness due to increased interstitial and alveolar fluid (Fanaroff and Martin, 2002).
2. Mild to moderate overaeration of the lungs and occasionally pleural effusions (Swischuk, 2003).
3. Possible fluid in minor (or horizontal) fissure and major (or oblique) lobar fissure (Blickman, 1998).

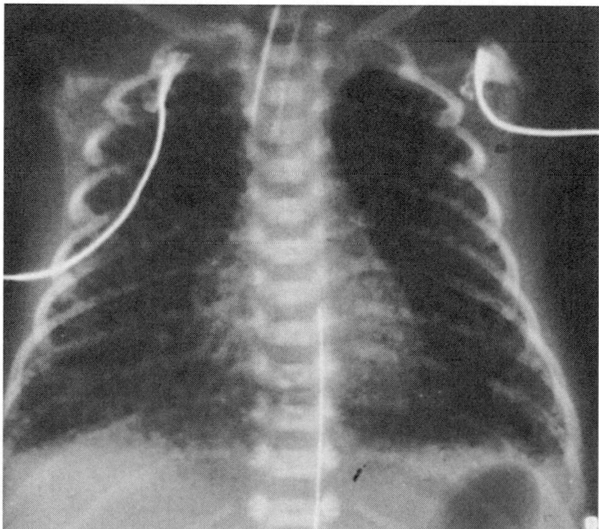

FIGURE 14-5 ■ Pulmonary interstitial emphysema. Note hyperexpansion bilaterally and pinpoint dark bubbles throughout both lung fields.

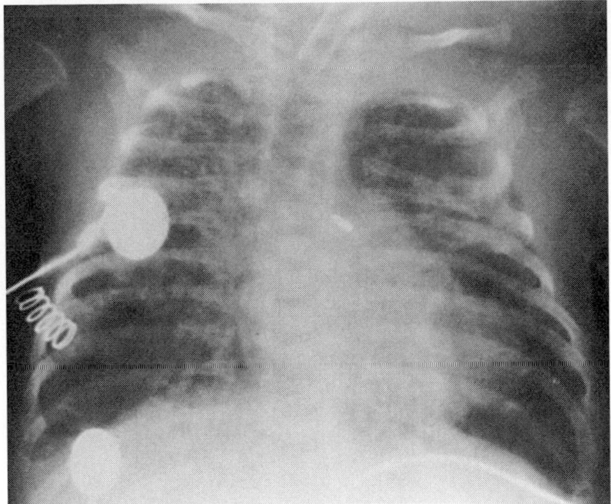

FIGURE 14-6 ■ Bronchopulmonary dysplasia. Note ill-defined densities bilaterally. Also note fractured rib in upper left portion of chest and pale-appearing ribs.

4. Mildly enlarged cardiothymic silhouette (Blickman, 1998).
5. Lung fields begin to clear in 24 to 48 hours (Swischuk, 2003).

E. **Meconium aspiration syndrome (Fig. 14-8).**
1. Mild cases may show a normal lung pattern to mild infiltrates with overexpanded lungs.
2. Bilateral asymmetric areas of atelectasis; hyperaeration with flattened hemidiaphragms (Blickman, 1998; Hedlund et al., 1998).
3. Hyperaeration of the lungs and flattened hemidiaphragms (Hedlund et al., 1998).
4. Possible atelectasis if airway is obstructed because of debris.
5. Possible air leaks (pneumothorax or pneumomediastinum) resulting from overdistention and rupture of the alveoli.

F. **Pneumonia.**
1. Patchy, occasionally asymmetric, radiating, bilateral interstitial infiltrate. A nodular pattern may predominate in hazy lungs, and an effusion is a common occurrence (Blickman, 1998).

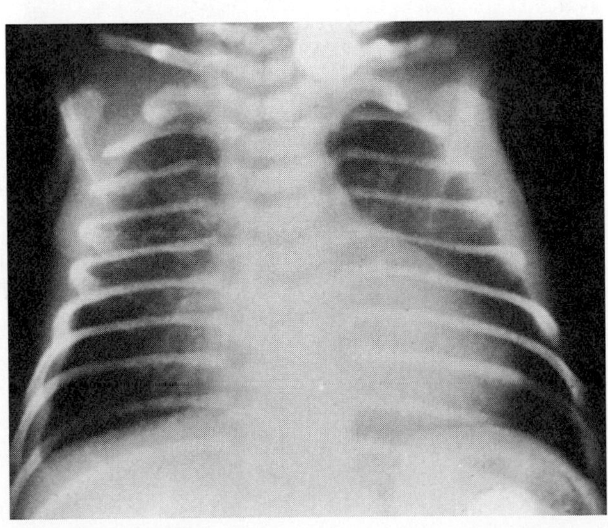

FIGURE 14-7 ■ Transient tachypnea of neonate. Note mild hyperexpansion and perihilar streakiness. A small pleural effusion is also present on right side.

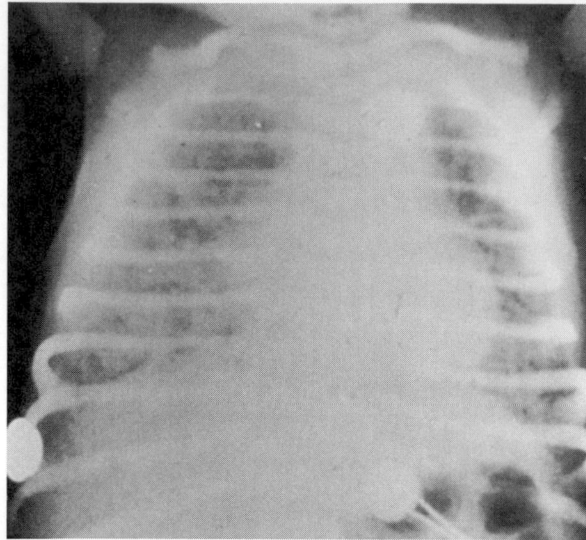

FIGURE 14-8 ■ Meconium aspiration syndrome. Note coarse, patchy infiltrates bilaterally.

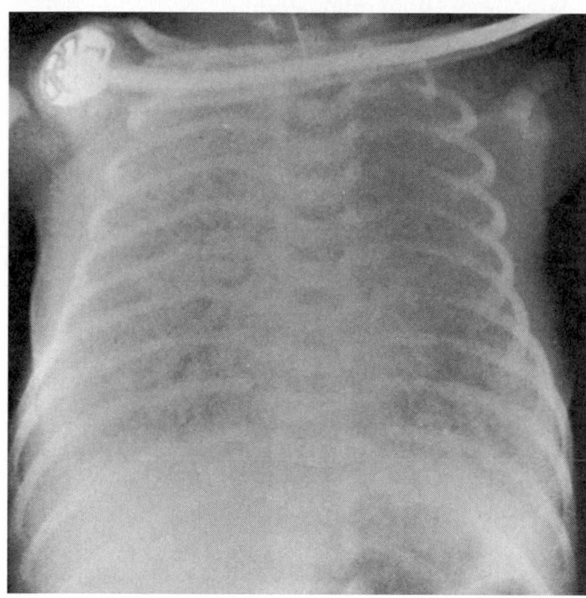

FIGURE 14-9 ■ Group B streptococcal pneumonia. Note reticulogranular appearance seen with hyaline membrane disease.

2. Reticulogranular pattern similar to that of respiratory distress syndrome. Some alveoli contain inflammatory exudate, which will appear more opaque and reticulogranular on x-ray than those filled with air (Hedlund et al., 1998; Swischuk, 2003).
3. Group B streptococcal pneumonia, often indistinguishable from RDS (Hedlund et al., 1998; Swischuk, 2003) (Fig. 14-9).

PULMONARY AIR LEAKS

A. Pneumothorax (Fig. 14-10, *A*).

1. Accumulation of air in the pleural space. Air can outline the lung circumferentially or can accumulate.
2. Mediastinal shift of structures away from the affected side as air accumulates (tension pneumothorax) (Swischuk, 2003).

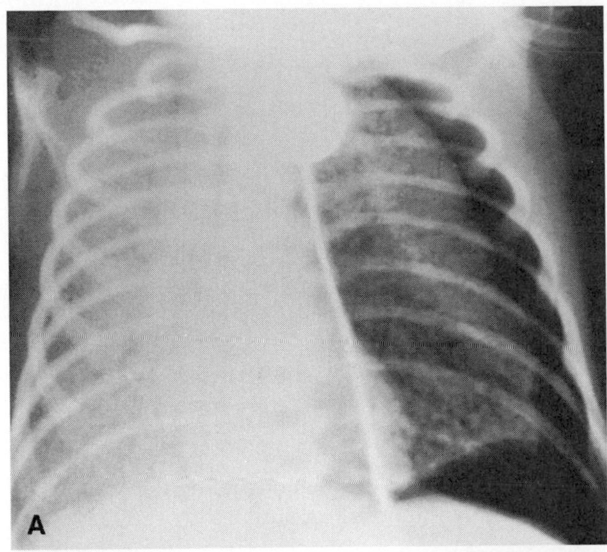

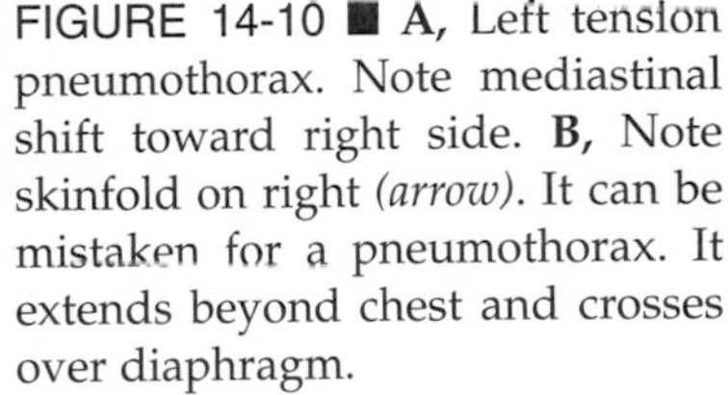
FIGURE 14-10 ■ **A,** Left tension pneumothorax. Note mediastinal shift toward right side. **B,** Note skinfold on right *(arrow)*. It can be mistaken for a pneumothorax. It extends beyond chest and crosses over diaphragm.

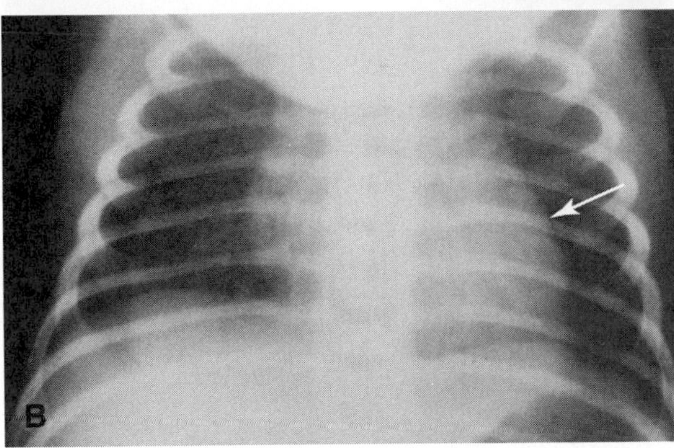

3. Outline of the collapsed lung, with a band of hyperlucency between the chest wall and the underlying lung (Swischuk, 2003).
4. Other findings related to pneumothorax.
   a. Pneumothorax not under tension may not exhibit a mediastinal shift.
   b. Diaphragm on affected side of a pneumothorax under tension will be flattened because of tension placed on it by air accumulation superior to it (Hedlund et al., 1998).
   c. Skinfold may mimic a pneumothorax (Swischuk, 2003) (see Fig. 14-10, *B*).

B. Pneumomediastinum (Fig. 14-11).
1. Mediastinal air collection, which produces irregular gas collections within the soft tissues of the superior mediastinum, with air frequently outlining the undersurface of the thymus gland and thus creating a "sail sign" (Swischuk, 2003).
2. Can accompany a pneumothorax.
3. On lateral film, a radiolucent area of hyperlucency in the superior retrosternal space.

C. Pneumopericardium (Fig. 14-12).
1. Radiolucent halo of free air surrounds the heart as air accumulates within the pericardial space (Hedlund et al., 1998).
2. Width of air around the heart is proportional to the amount of air present. Air is limited to the pericardium and cannot extend beyond the origins of the aorta and pulmonary artery (Hedlund et al., 1998).

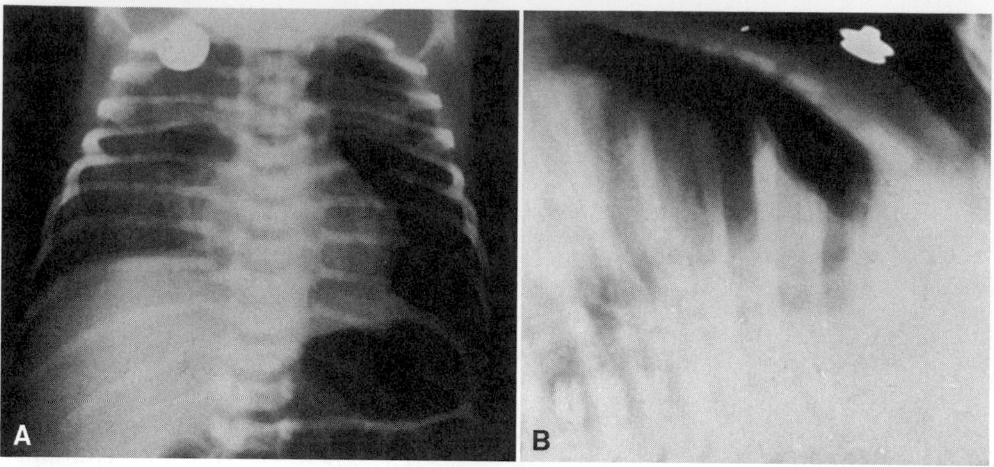

FIGURE 14-11 ■ **A,** Pneumomediastinum with thymus lifted, demonstrating the "sail sign." **B,** Pneumomediastinum on lateral view. Note air in anterior chest outlines thymus.

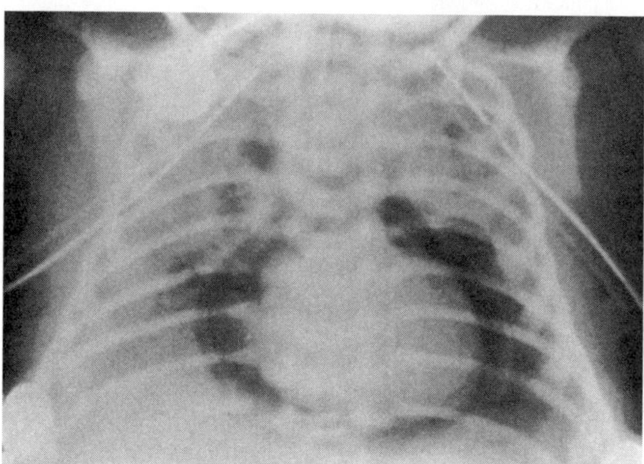

FIGURE 14-12 ■ Pneumopericardium. Note air completely encircles heart. Bilateral chest tubes are also in place.

3. Decreased cardiac size may indicate cardiac tamponade.
4. Other pulmonary air leaks and/or pulmonary interstitial emphysema are generally present.
5. Pneumopericardium is rare in the absence of assisted ventilation.

MISCELLANEOUS CAUSES OF RESPIRATORY DISTRESS

A. Diaphragmatic paralysis (phrenic nerve injury) (Fig. 14-13).

1. Elevation and fixation of a diaphragmatic leaflet (Swischuk, 2003).
2. More common on the right than the left side and usually unilateral.
3. Mediastinum may be shifted away from the affected side.
4. Most often results from obstetric injury to the brachial plexus (Swischuk, 2003).
5. Erb palsy an associated finding.

B. Eventration of the diaphragm (Fig. 14-14).

1. Weakness of the hemidiaphragm, with abdominal organs pushing up against it but not entering the chest because no opening exists.
2. Either partial or complete; usually right-sided (Hedlund et al., 1998).

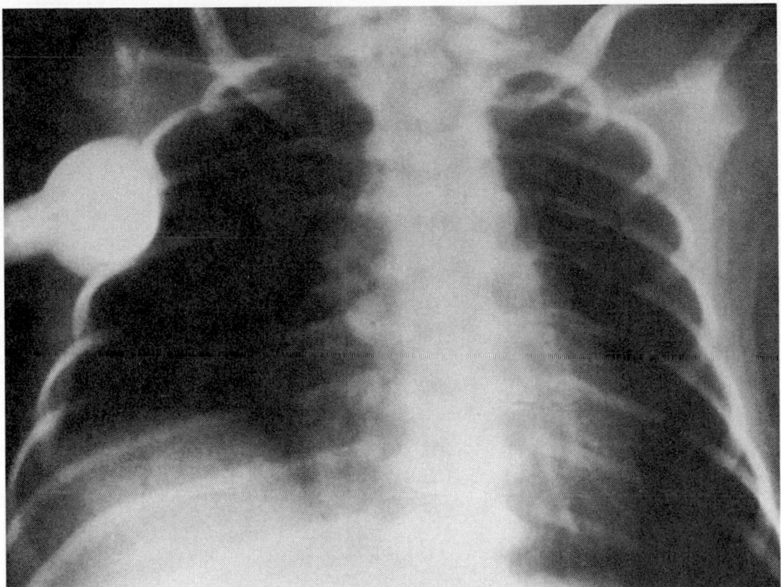

FIGURE 14-13 ■ Paralysis of right side of diaphragm. Note right side of diaphragm is markedly elevated in comparison with left side of diaphragm.

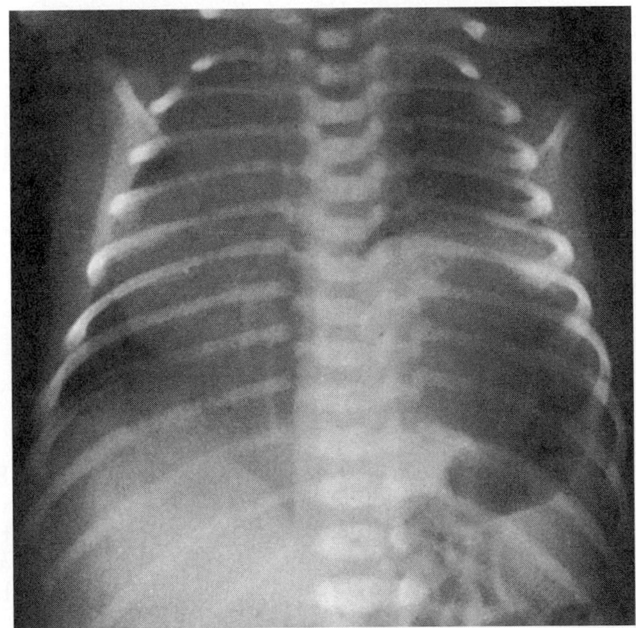

FIGURE 14-14 ■ Eventration of diaphragm. Note left side of diaphragm bulging upward, with stomach pushing upward against it.

C. **Pulmonary edema (Fig. 14-15).**

1. Increased pulmonary permeability is common in premature infants with lung injury that can manifest as diffuse haziness of the lungs to a white-out appearance (Swischuk, 2003).
2. Significant association between high fluid intake and subsequent occurrence of a clinically significant patent ductus arteriosus and BPD.
3. Also common with certain congenital heart defects due to increased pulmonary blood flow (coarctation of the aorta, hypoplastic left heart syndrome).

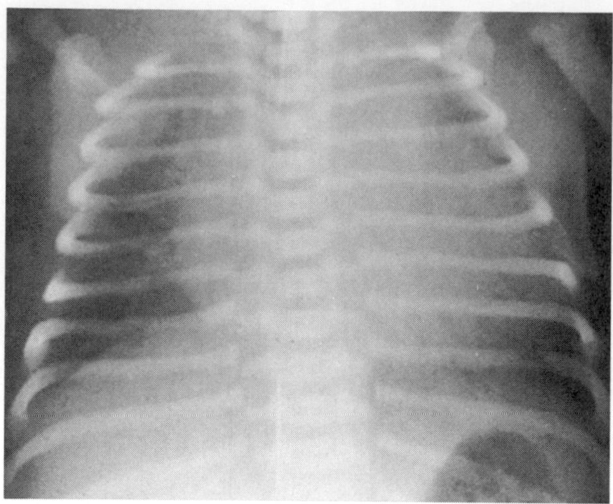

FIGURE 14-15 ■ Pulmonary edema. Note congested lung fields and cardiomegaly.

THORACIC SURGICAL PROBLEMS

A. Congenital diaphragmatic hernia (Fig. 14-16, *A*).

1. Herniation of abdominal contents through various portions of the diaphragm into the thoracic cavity, most commonly through the foramen of Bochdalek (Hedlund et al., 1998).
2. 75% occur on the left side (Swischuk, 2003).

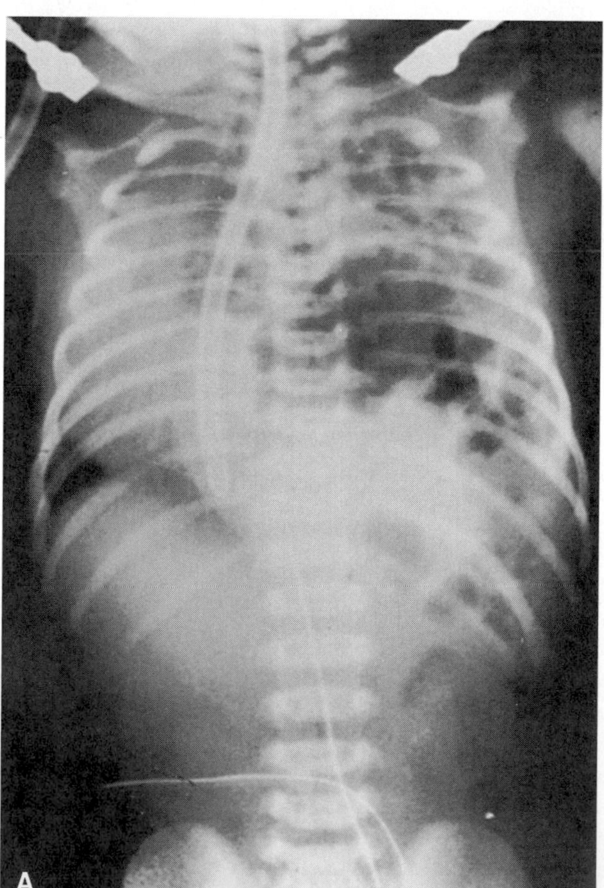

FIGURE 14-16 ■ **A,** Left diaphragmatic hernia. Note presence of bowel in left side of chest, a mediastinal shift to right, and lack of bowel in abdomen.

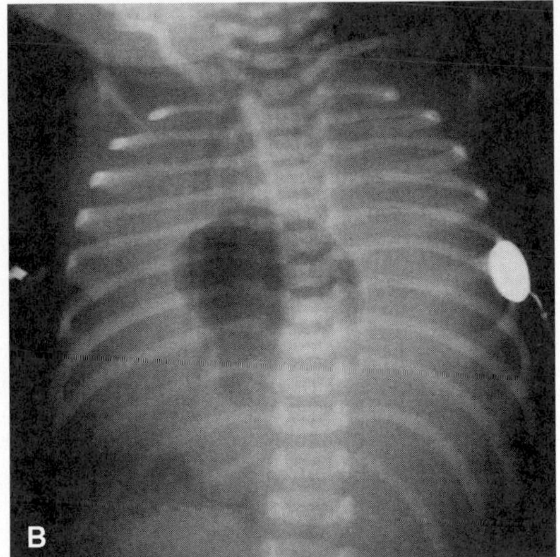

FIGURE 14-16, *cont'd* ■ **B,** Left diaphragmatic hernia before much air has expanded bowel. Note that trachea and heart have shifted to right.

3. Hemithorax filled with loops of bowel, stomach, and often liver; displaces the mediastinal structures away from the affected side (Swischuk, 2003).
4. Abdomen relatively gasless and may be scaphoid (Hedlund et al., 1998).
5. Contralateral pneumothorax possible with assisted ventilation or as a result of pulmonary hypoplasia on the unaffected side.
6. If the x-ray is obtained before the bowel is expanded with air, the affected hemithorax may appear entirely opacified with the mediastinal structures shifted to the opposite side (Swischuk, 2003) (see Fig. 14-16, *B*).

B. **Congenital lobar emphysema (Fig. 14-17).**
   1. Most common cause of cystic malformation of the lung.
   2. Air trapped within one or more lung lobes at birth, resulting in obstructive emphysema.
   3. Overdistended affected lobe, with mediastinum shifted to contralateral side.
   4. Possibly hyperlucent but may also be opaque because of fluid accumulation distal to the obstruction (Swischuk, 2003).
   5. Generally limited to the upper lobes.

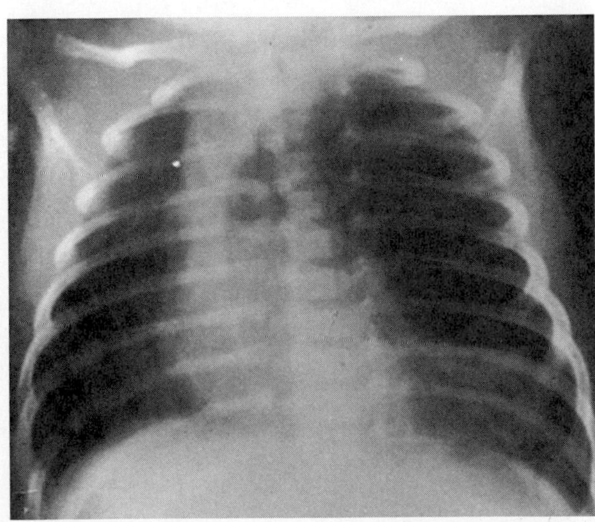

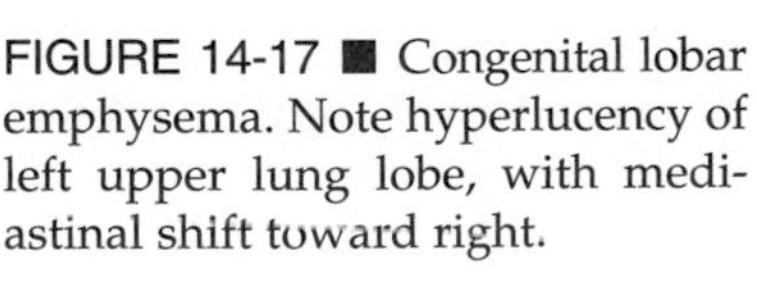
FIGURE 14-17 ■ Congenital lobar emphysema. Note hyperlucency of left upper lung lobe, with mediastinal shift toward right.

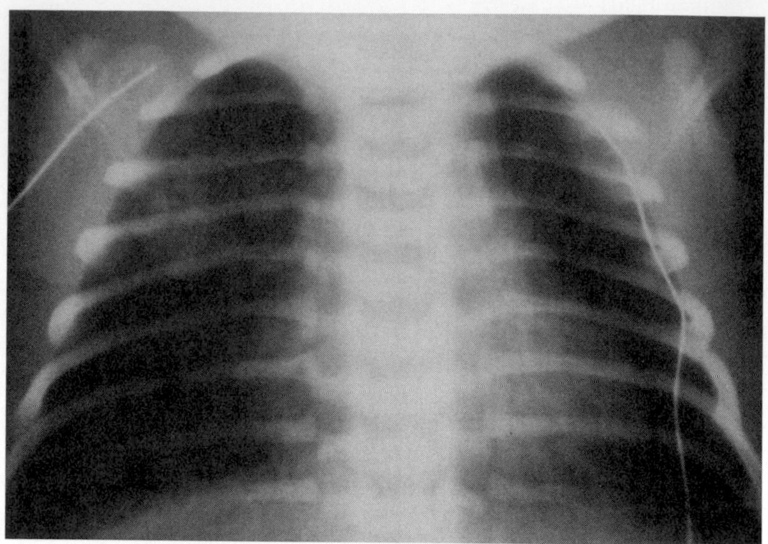

FIGURE 14-18 ■ Cystic adenomatoid malformation in right lung.

C. **Cystic adenomatoid malformation (Fig. 14-18).**
   1. Overdistention of affected lobe, with mediastinal shift to contralateral side.
   2. Lobar overdistention, caused by air and fluid.
   3. Upper lobes most frequently affected (Swischuk, 2003).
   4. X-ray findings: multiple air-filled cysts, mediastinal shift, and compression of opposite lung. Diaphragmatic hernia must be ruled out.

CARDIOVASCULAR SYSTEM

A. **Size of the heart.**
   1. Difficult to assess on anteroposterior film because of a large thymus. Lateral film assessing a specific chamber enlargement may be more useful (Swischuk, 2003).
   2. Enlargement suggested by cardiothoracic ratio greater than 65% (Strife et al., 1998) (Fig. 14-19).

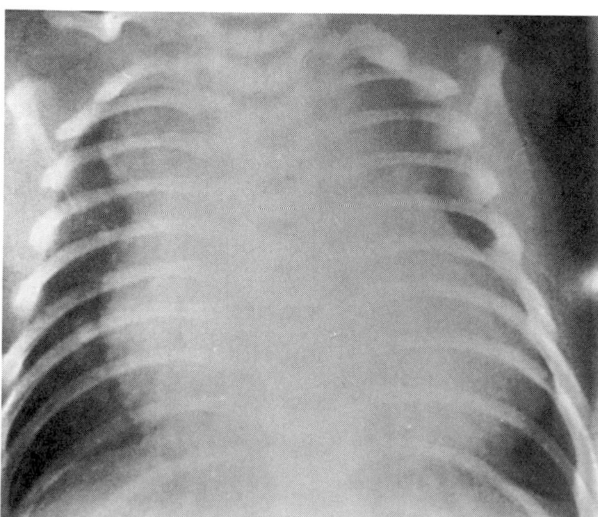

FIGURE 14-19 ■ Cardiomegaly. Note enlarged heart occupies majority of thorax.

3. Malpositioning: may represent cardiac displacement, developmentally abnormal cardiac position, or ambiguous rotation or site (Strife et al., 1998).
4. Possible transient enlargement as a result of polycythemia, perinatal anoxia, or normally increased fluid present at birth.

B. Pulmonary vascularity.

1. Normal vascular markings are seen in the middle one third of the lung fields (Fig. 14-20).
2. Decreased vascular markings occur with obstruction along the right ventricular outflow tract of the heart and are manifested as hyperlucency in both lung fields (Fig. 14-21).
3. Increased pulmonary vascularity occurs when excess blood flow causes congestion in the blood vessels and is manifested as increased streakiness, hazy lung fields, and increased densities as the condition worsens.

C. Positional anomalies of the heart.

1. Types of malposition are as follows:
   a. Dextrocardia: right-sided heart.
   b. Mesocardia: midline heart.
   c. Extrathoracic: ectopia cordis.
2. Position of other organs in relation to the heart is also incorporated into the definition of cardiac malposition. Positions of the abdominal organs are as follows:
   a. Situs solitus: normal abdominal organ position.
   b. Situs inversus: stomach and spleen on right, liver on left, and left atrium on right.
   c. Situs ambiguus: abdominal organs and atrial position are anatomically uncertain. The liver may be symmetric and at midline, and the stomach may be central. There may be duplication or absence of unilateral structures such as the spleen (asplenia or polysplenia).
3. "Mirror image" dextrocardia with situs inversus is the most common type of malposition; congenital heart disease is unlikely (Fanaroff and Martin, 2002) (Fig. 14-22).
4. Dextrocardia with situs solitus—dextrocardia is an isolated finding with all other organs in their normal position. Incidence of congenital heart disease is 95% to 98% (Strife et al., 1998).
5. Cardiac malposition caused by shift of the heart within the thorax must be differentiated from extracardiac causes, such as pneumothorax, hypoplastic lung, diaphragmatic hernia, decreased lung volume, and lung mass.

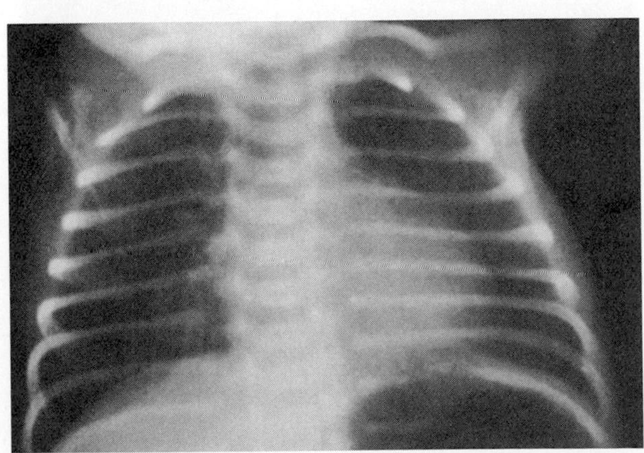

FIGURE 14-20 ■ Normal pulmonary vascularity. Note presence of vascularity radiating from perihilar region.

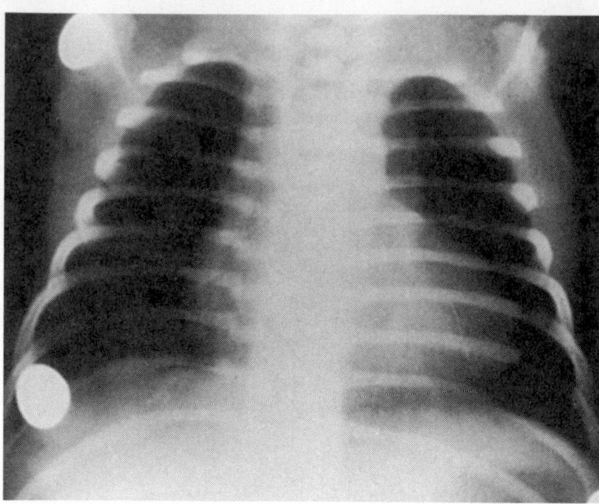

FIGURE 14-21 ■ Hyperlucent lung fields because of decreased blood flow to lungs.

D. Lesions with increased pulmonary vascularity.

1. Left-to-right shunt or intracardiac mixing.

a. Transposition of the great vessels. Plain film shows "egg on a string" appearance. Cardiac silhouette of normal size or mild cardiomegaly may be seen (Blickman, 1998). Pulmonary vascularity is variable, depending on the presence or absence of a ventricular septal defect or a patent ductus arteriosus.

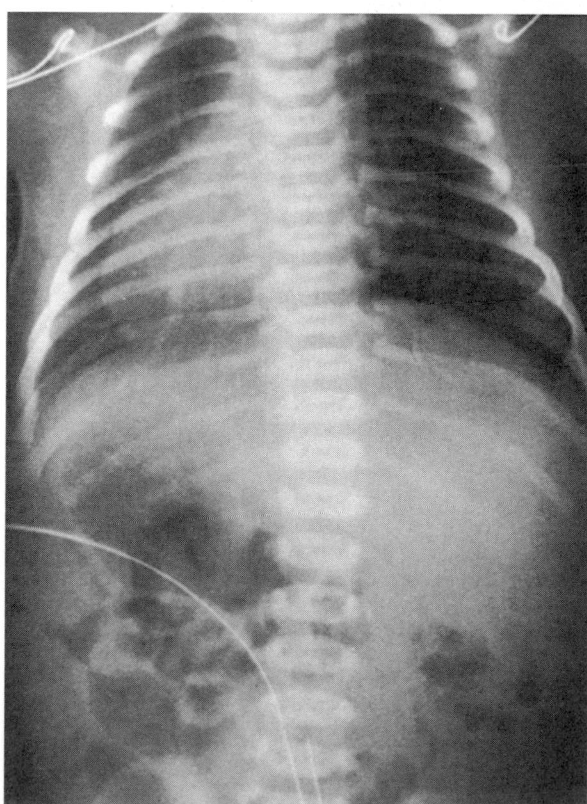

FIGURE 14-22 ■ "Mirror image" dextrocardia. Note apex of heart pointing to right, with stomach located on right and liver on left.

b. Total anomalous pulmonary venous return. X-ray film shows cardiomegaly; increased pulmonary vascularity; and enlargement of the right atrium, right ventricle, and pulmonary artery. The "snowman" appearance of the heart, caused by a characteristic widening of the superior mediastinum due to the connecting blood vessels, is rarely seen in the neonate because of the slow development of excessive pulmonary blood flow (Swischuk, 2003).

c. Atrioventricular canal defect (AV canal) (endocardial cushion defect). Pulmonary vascular resistance usually remains high enough to delay the onset of CHF until after the first 1 to 2 weeks, after which marked cardiomegaly and vascular congestion are evident.

d. Truncus arteriosus. Right and left ventricles are prominent, with left atrial dilation. As CHF develops, pulmonary vessels become indistinct and obscured by pulmonary edema.

e. Atrial septal defect. Chest x-ray may be normal, with small defects. With large left-to-right shunts, there are moderate cardiac enlargement and increased pulmonary vascularity. The right atrium and right ventricle are enlarged.

f. Ventricular septal defect. With small defects the heart size and vascularity may be normal. With moderate-sized defects, heart size may be enlarged, with increased pulmonary vascular markings. With large defects and increased blood flow, cardiomegaly is evident because of right and left ventricular enlargement. Pulmonary vascularity is markedly increased. CHF, interstitial edema, and alveolar fluid may be present.

g. Patent ductus arteriosus. Pulmonary vasculature and cardiac silhouette may be obscured by underlying lung disease of RDS. Lung fields may show pulmonary edema and increasing heart size compared with heart size on previous x-ray films.

2. Left-sided obstruction. Outflow of blood from the left side of the heart or return of blood from the lungs is obstructed, which will eventually cause CHF.

a. Hypoplastic left heart syndrome (aortic atresia, mitral atresia). Pulmonary vascularity may appear normal until significant cardiac decompensation is present, and then cardiomegaly and CHF become evident. Right atrial enlargement may also be seen (Swischuk, 2003). This is most common cause of CHF in the first few days of life.

b. Coarctation of the aorta. Heart size is normal, but left ventricular enlargement may subsequently be seen on lateral views (Swischuk, 2003). X-ray findings vary according to the degree of patency of the patent ductus arteriosus and the severity of the obstruction at the coarctation site. CHF occurs, with ductal closure resulting in cardiomegaly and pulmonary venous congestion.

c. Aortic stenosis. Normal cardiac size and vasculature may be seen, with mild stenosis of the aortic valve. Left ventricular enlargement occurs, with cardiac decompensation or associated aortic regurgitation resulting in cardiomegaly and venous congestion (Blickman, 1998).

3. Lesions with decreased pulmonary vascularity. All these lesions involve some form of obstruction to the normal flow of blood through the right outflow tract. They can be located anywhere from the tricuspid valve to the pulmonary artery.

a. Pulmonary valve atresia with intact ventricular septum. Pulmonary vascularity is reduced or normal, depending on alternative sources of pulmonary blood flow, such as a patent ductus arteriosus. A shallow or concave pulmonary artery is evident (Swischuk, 2003). Closure of the ductus arteriosus and obstruction of the right ventricular outflow tract cause decreased pulmonary blood flow. Pulmonary vessels are underfilled and appear small and thin, which results in dark, hyperlucent lung fields. Heart size is variable, but cardiomegaly is usually present because of right atrial and left ventricular enlargement (Swischuk, 2003).

b. Tricuspid atresia. Tricuspid valve has complete atresia, and the right ventricle and right outflow tract are underdeveloped. Chest x-ray shows a normal or small heart and diminished pulmonary blood flow (Strife et al., 1998).

c. Tetralogy of Fallot. Cardiac size and shape are frequently normal. Pulmonary vascular markings are decreased. A "boot-shaped" contour may occur from a small, concave pulmonary artery and a prominent cardiac apex as a result of right ventricular hypertrophy (Strife et al., 1998).

d. Pulmonary stenosis. Severe valvular obstruction is associated with hypoxemia because of a right-to-left shunt at the foramen ovale (Wechsler and Wernovsky, 1998). This is referred to as critical pulmonary stenosis. Neonate's chest x-ray is normal, but cardiomegaly with predominant right atrium and right ventricle, decreased pulmonary vascularity, and dilation of the pulmonary artery eventually occur.

GASTROINTESTINAL SYSTEM

A. Characteristics of the normal abdomen (Fig. 14-23).

1. Air is present in the stomach immediately after birth because of respiratory movement of the thorax and swallowing of air. By 24 hours of life, air should appear in the rectum (Blickman, 1998).

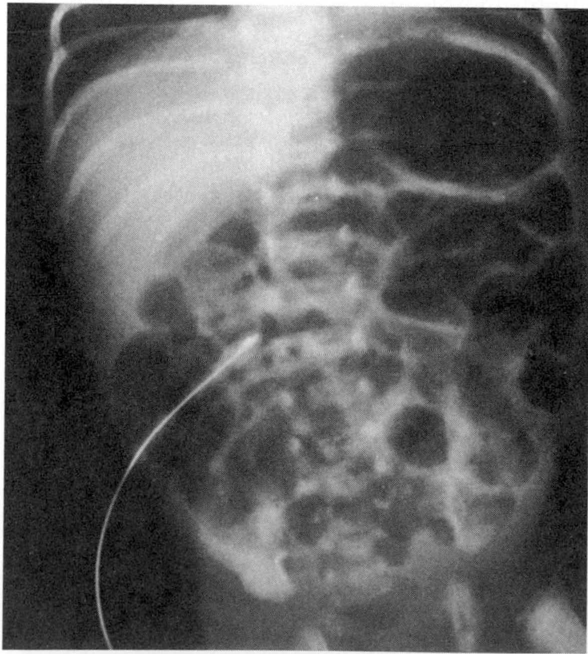

FIGURE 14-23 ■ Normal bowel gas pattern. Note presence of stomach bubble and air through entire abdomen to rectum.

2. A gasless abdomen may be seen in infants with decreased swallowing, decreased GI motility (i.e., with intubation or chemical paralysis), vomiting, or gastric decompression from suctioning.
3. Resuscitation may increase the amount of bowel gas seen on an x-ray.

B. **The esophagus.**
1. May show indentations near the aortic arch and left mainstem bronchus.
2. May assume peculiar configurations because of flexibility during the respiratory cycle.
3. Air in the esophagus a normal finding on regular chest films.

C. **Esophageal abnormalities.**
1. Esophageal atresia (Fig. 14-24, *A*). A portion of the esophagus is atretic, and both distal and proximal portions of the esophagus end in blind pouches.

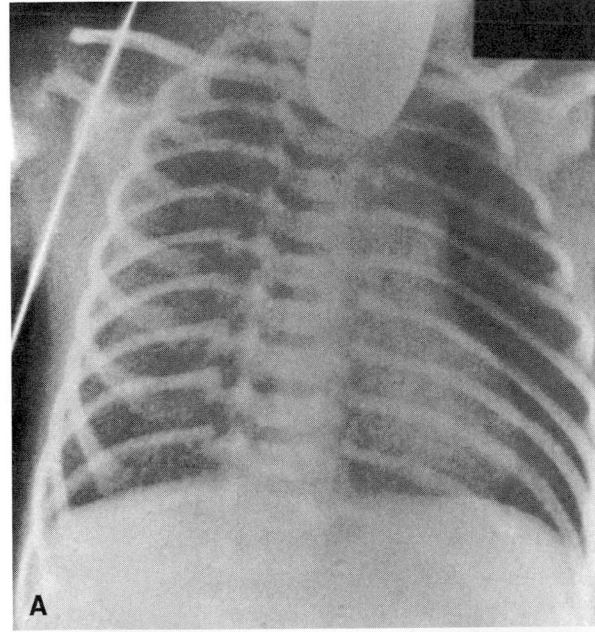

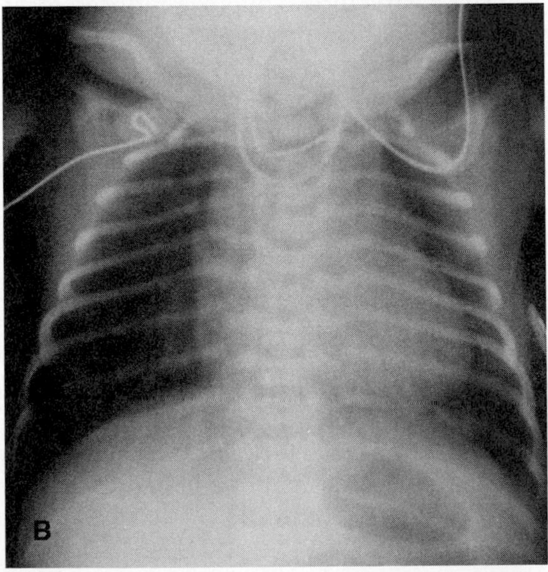

FIGURE 14-24 ■ **A,** Esophageal atresia. Contrast medium outlines esophagus, which ends in blind pouch. **B,** Esophageal atresia with tracheoesophageal fistula. Gastric tube cannot be advanced because of esophageal atresia. Air is in abdomen, confirming presence of tracheoesophageal fistula.

a. On x-ray a radiolucent, air-filled, distended proximal esophageal pouch is present. The abdomen is gasless because no air can enter (Swischuk, 2003). The proximal pouch can be identified by passing a radiopaque tube and obtaining a chest film. The tube will not advance beyond 9 to 11 cm (Blickman, 1998).
b. Aspiration pneumonitis of the upper lobes, especially the right upper lobe, is a common finding.

2. Esophageal atresia with tracheoesophageal fistula (see Fig. 14-24, *B*).
   a. Esophageal atresia with fistulous connection to the distal esophageal pouch is the most common esophageal anomaly.
   b. Excessive dilation of the stomach and/or small bowel, resulting from distal fistula communication between the lungs and the stomach, may occur (Blickman, 1998).
   c. Chest film should be obtained with a radiopaque tube in place. The tube will not advance into the stomach, and air will be present in the GI tract.
3. Tracheoesophageal fistula with no esophageal atresia (H type of fistula).
   a. Difficult to identify without a contrast study.
   b. Fistula characteristically assumes an upwardly oblique configuration on contrast study.
   c. Widespread pulmonary infiltrates are commonly present because of constant aspiration through the fistula into the lungs.

D. The stomach.

1. Visible directly beneath the left diaphragm.
2. Often appears large in the neonate as a result of dilation with air.
3. Mucosal folds are absent. Stomach wall appears smooth (Swischuk, 2003).
4. Begins to empty moments after being filled.

E. Abnormalities of the stomach.

1. Pyloric stenosis.
   a. Symptoms develop 2 to 8 weeks after birth (Swischuk, 2003).
   b. Plain films demonstrate a distended stomach and duodenum, with disproportionately less gas in the small bowel (Swischuk, 2003).
   c. Ultrasonography is the study of choice for the diagnosis.
2. Gastric perforation.
   a. Uncommon, but may result from gastric ulcers, hypoxia-induced focal necrosis, gastric tubes, or indomethacin therapy for closure of ductus arteriosus.
   b. Possible overinflation due to distal obstruction, as with mechanical ventilation.
   c. Common finding of free air (pneumoperitoneum) with absence of gastric gas.

F. Duodenal abnormalities (Fig. 14-25).

1. Duodenal atresia and stenosis.
   a. Infants with duodenal atresia present with vomiting in the first few hours of life. Those with stenosis present at variable times, depending on the degree of stenosis.
   b. Duodenal atresia and stenosis are present in approximately 33% of infants with Down syndrome (trisomy 21) (Blickman, 1998).
   c. X-ray demonstrates dilation of the stomach and proximal duodenum, producing the characteristic "double bubble" pattern. No air is present distal to the duodenum (Swischuk, 2003).

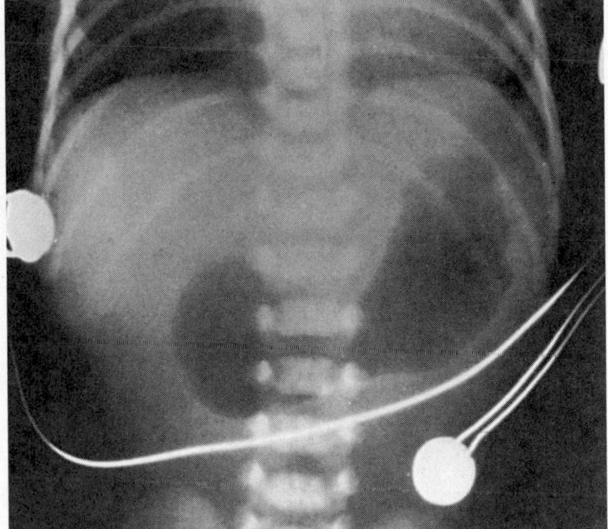

FIGURE 14-25 ■ Duodenal atresia with characteristic "double bubble" pattern.

2. Annular pancreas.
   a. Pancreas grows in the form of an encircling ring around the duodenum (Blickman, 1998).
   b. Presentation is similar to that of duodenal atresia or stenosis.
   c. X-ray findings are generally indistinguishable from duodenal atresia or stenosis (Swischuk, 2003). Identification is made with ultrasonography.

G. **Abnormalities of the small bowel.**
1. Small-bowel atresia and stenosis.
   a. Single or multiple areas of atresia or stenosis may exist.
   b. Clinically abdominal distention and bile-stained vomiting are apparent early on.
   c. Types of small-bowel atresia.
      (1) High jejunal obstruction. One or two loops of bowel are visible on x-ray.
      (2) Midjejunal obstruction. More dilated loops are visible on x-ray.
      (3) Distal ileal atresia. Many dilated loops are visible on x-ray.
2. Meconium ileus (Fig. 14-26).
   a. Approximately 20% of infants with cystic fibrosis present with meconium ileus at birth (Blickman, 1998).
   b. Obstruction results from impaction of thick, tenacious meconium in the distal portion of the small bowel. Ileal atresia or stenosis, ileal perforation, meconium peritonitis, and volvulus are common complications (Buonomo et al., 1998).
   c. Clinical presentation includes bile-stained vomiting, abdominal distention, and failure to pass meconium.
   d. X-ray shows a low small-bowel obstruction with numerous, variably sized air-filled loops of bowel (Blickman, 1998). There is a "soap bubble" appearance in the right lower quadrant as a result of trapping of air in meconium.
   e. A contrast-enema study will demonstrate a microcolon. A water-soluble contrast agent draws large amounts of fluid into the intestine and lubricates the meconium, allowing it to pass without surgical intervention. This technique is successful 30% to 50% of the time (Blickman, 1998).

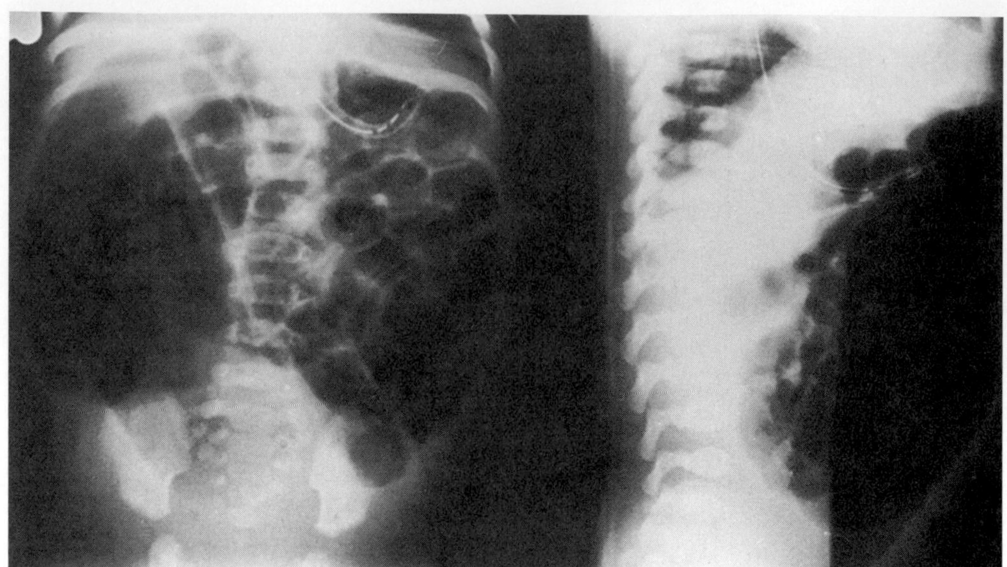

FIGURE 14-26 ■ Meconium ileus with perforation and free air visible on lateral film.

3. Midgut volvulus.
   a. Most common form of small-bowel volvulus.
   b. Twisting and spiraling of entire gut around the superior mesenteric artery, resulting in vascular compromise, necrosis, perforation, and gangrene.
   c. May present with bilious vomiting.
   d. May be difficult to determine on x-ray because findings are variable, from a normal abdomen to one suggesting a gastric outlet obstruction, partial obstruction of the duodenum, or small-bowel obstruction (Buonomo et al., 1998).
   e. Ultrasonography, barium enema, or x-ray of upper GI tract may be needed for diagnostic purposes or to demonstrate complete obstruction of third portion of duodenum (Buonomo et al., 1998).

H. **Abnormalities of the colon.**
1. Hirschsprung disease (aganglionosis of the colon) (Fig. 14-27).
   a. Typical presentation is vomiting, obstruction, and failure to pass meconium within the first 24 to 36 hours of life.
   b. Commonly involves the distal colonic segment—rectal and rectosigmoid areas.
   c. Plain films show some degree of low small-bowel or colonic obstruction, air-fluid levels, and distention of the bowel (Blickman, 1998). Rectal gas may be absent or sparse.
   d. Barium enema will support the findings, and a rectal biopsy will show absence of ganglion cells.
2. Meconium plug syndrome/small left colon syndrome.
   a. Normal meconium becomes impacted in the distal portion of the colon. In meconium plug syndrome, the obstruction is generally in the sigmoid colon. In small left colon, the site of obstruction is the splenic flexure.
   b. Functional immaturity of the colon, especially in infants of diabetic mothers, is thought to be the cause of the initial inability to pass meconium (Blickman, 1998).

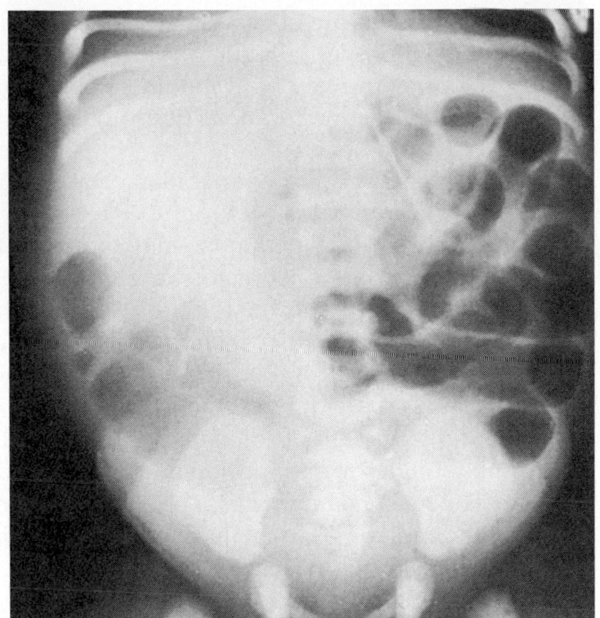

FIGURE 14-27 ■ Hirschsprung disease. Note abdominal distention with dilated loops of bowel and lack of air present in distal portion of bowel.

c. Condition is manifested within the first 23 to 36 hours of life with abdominal distention, bilious vomiting, and failure to pass meconium.
d. Diagnosis is by contrast-enema examination. The examination may also be therapeutic by dislodgment of the meconium (Swischuk, 2003).
e. Plain films are nonspecific and usually show a low small bowel with distention of the bowel obstruction.

3. Necrotizing enterocolitis (Fig. 14-28).
   a. X-ray findings include generalized distention caused by paralytic ileus, asymmetric distribution of bowel gas, and localized distention of bowel loops (Buonomo et al., 1998).

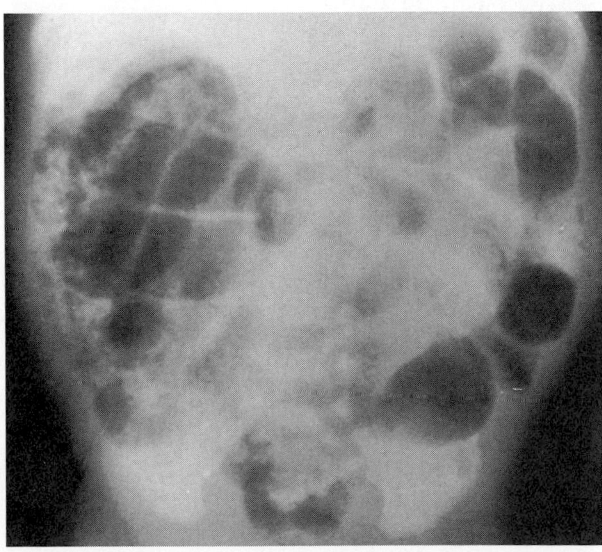

FIGURE 14-28 ■ Necrotizing enterocolitis. Note presence of distended bowel loops and pneumatosis intestinalis.

b. X-ray films are obtained every 6 to 8 hours to follow the progression of the disease in the acute phase (Swischuk, 2003). A cross-table lateral view, along with plain film, should be obtained to detect free air (Swischuk, 2003). Most perforations occur in the first 2 days of the diagnosis (Buonomo et al., 1998).
c. Subsequently, individual loops may become tubular, with thickened bowel walls.
d. Persistently dilated loops may be evident on consecutive films.
e. At any point, pneumatosis cystoides intestinalis can be seen. This represents gas formed in the intestinal wall by bacteria. The typical picture is linear or of a bubbly or foamy appearance. Air may be located in the submucosal or subserosal layer and can enter the GI tract or portal venous system (Blickman, 1998).
f. Right segment of colon and terminal ileum are most likely to be affected, although the entire colon may be affected.
g. The most common cause of intestinal perforation, is seen as free abdominal gas on plain film or in left lateral decubitus view.

I. Pneumoperitoneum (see Fig. 14-26).

1. Most commonly a result of perforation of the GI tract because of perinatal asphyxia, indomethacin therapy, gastric overdistention, iatrogenic perforation with a thermometer, and as a complication of necrotizing enterocolitis and GI obstruction (Swischuk, 2003).
2. Air may dissect from the neonate's chest during positive-pressure ventilation.
3. Presents with abdominal distention and respiratory distress, or abdominal wall erythema.
4. Supine x-ray may not reveal free air (Swischuk, 2003), necessitating lateral decubitus or cross-table view.

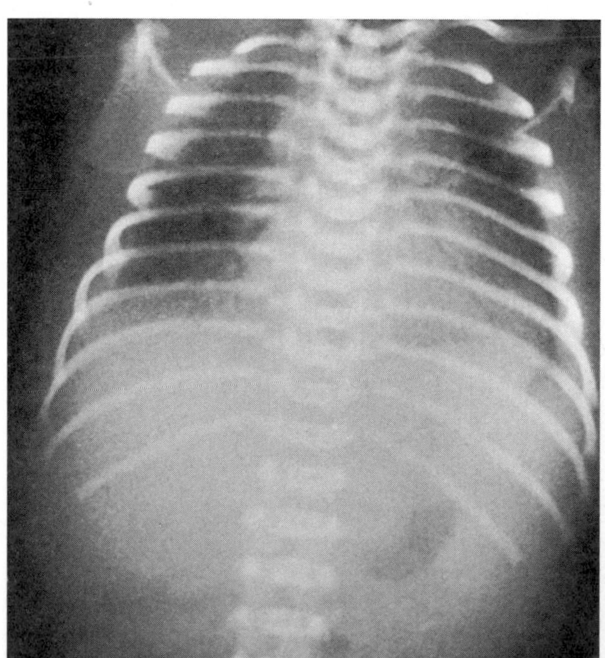

FIGURE 14-29 ■ Abdominal ascites with bilateral pleural effusions.

5. Abdomen is distended and radiolucent on x-ray (Swischuk, 2003). Individual loops of bowel are visible because of air inside and outside the bowel wall. Falciform ligament (an opaque stripe) may be visualized in the right upper quadrant or upper mid portion of the abdomen.

J. **Meconium peritonitis.**
1. Results from intrauterine GI perforation due to obstruction (atresia, stenosis, imperforate anus) and/or volvulus associated with meconium ileus (Swischuk, 2003).
2. Calcifications, which are easily identifiable on x-ray, assume a focal or diffuse, patchy, irregular pattern. Multiple white-speckled areas are seen in one area or throughout the abdomen and may be present in the scrotum (Swischuk, 2003).
3. Calcifications will slowly disappear.

K. **Abdominal ascites (Fig. 14-29).**
1. 25% of cases result from urinary tract obstruction. Other cases include infants with fetal hydrops, GI obstruction with perforation, and peritonitis (Buonomo et al., 1998).
2. Uniform density to the distended abdomen is noted with a gasless or centralized bowel gas pattern. Body wall edema may also be present in infants with fetal hydrops.

SKELETAL SYSTEM

A. **Fractures:** occur most often during delivery with an increased incidence during breech deliveries. In breech deliveries, fractures can occur in both upper and lower extremities.
1. Clavicle: fractured during delivery (Fig. 14-30). Fractures occur at the midclavicle most commonly. Fractured clavicle is common in large infants during difficult vaginal delivery (Swischuk, 2003).
2. Rib fractures: may occur at delivery and be asymptomatic (Swischuk, 2003). With multiple fractures the infant may show signs of respiratory distress and pain. Premature infants may have rib fractures as a result of osteopenia of prematurity 8 to 16 weeks after birth (Fig. 14-31) (Swischuk, 2003). These bones are fragile and will fracture with handling and chest physiotherapy. Fractures may be preceded by a thin, "washed out" appearance to the ribs or extremities.

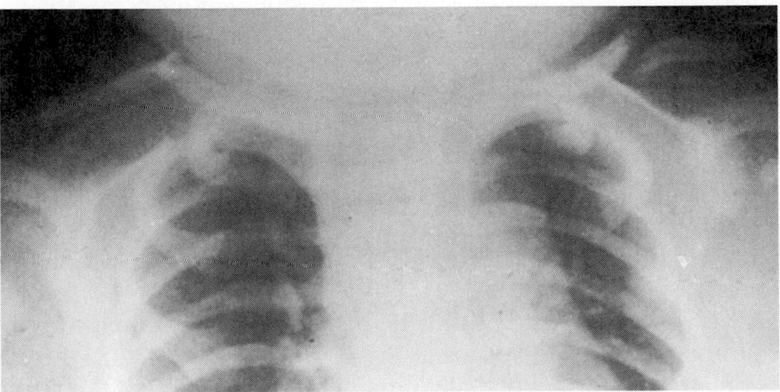

FIGURE 14-30 ■ Fractured left clavicle.

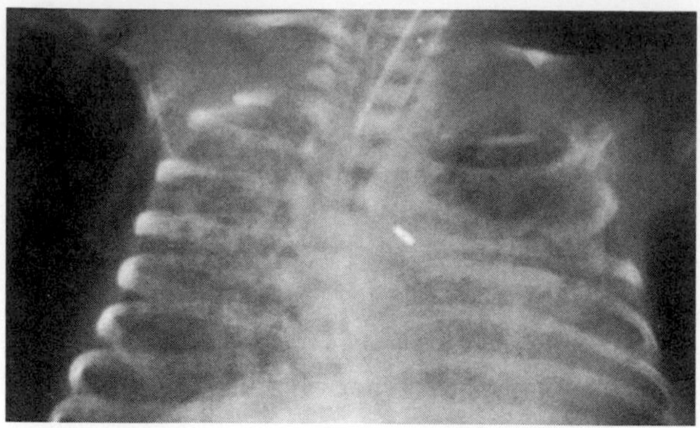

FIGURE 14-31 ■ Fractured rib on left, with pale, "washed out" ribs.

3. Skull fractures.
   a. Can be linear, buckled, or frankly depressed.
   b. Linear and buckling fractures most often occur in the parietal bone and may be suspected in the presence of cephalhematoma or other skull trauma.
   c. Computed tomography (CT) scan is more helpful than plain films for evaluation of skull fractures.

B. **Bony dysplasias.**
   1. Osteogenesis imperfecta (see Chapter 34).
   2. Dwarfism (common types) (Laor et al., 1998; Swischuk, 2003).
      a. Achondroplasia: short extremities and marked flaring of the metaphyses. Classic signs include spinal curvature and narrowed spinal canal; short, squared-off iliac wings; deep-set sacrum; flat acetabular roofs; and bulky proximal femurs.
      b. Thanatophoric dwarfism (type I) (Fig. 14-32): marked underdevelopment of the skeleton; extremely short, bent, or curved long bones; and flaring of the metaphyses. Vertebral bodies are very flat and underdeveloped. Thorax is small and narrow, with pulmonary hypoplasia. Condition is uniformly fatal in the perinatal period.

INDWELLING LINES AND TUBES

A. **Endotracheal tube.**
   1. Placement is 1.2 cm below the vocal cords and 2 cm above the carina, with the neonate's head in neutral position (Hedlund et al., 1998).
   2. Placement beyond the carina results in occlusion of a bronchus (usually the right mainstem bronchus), with subsequent atelectasis and clinical deterioration (Fig. 14-33).

B. **Umbilical artery catheter (Fig. 14-34, *A*).** Proceeds from the umbilicus down toward the pelvis, making an acute turn into the internal iliac artery and common iliac artery advancing into the aorta (Strife et al., 1998).
   1. Low placement: at third and fourth lumbar vertebrae.
   2. High placement: at sixth through tenth thoracic vertebrae.

C. **Umbilical venous catheter (see Fig. 14-34, *B*).** Passes cephalad to join the left portal vein.
   1. On lateral view the catheter is directly distal to the abdominal wall until it passes through the ductus venosus.
   2. Correct placement is above the diaphragm at the junction of the right atrium (Strife et al., 1998).

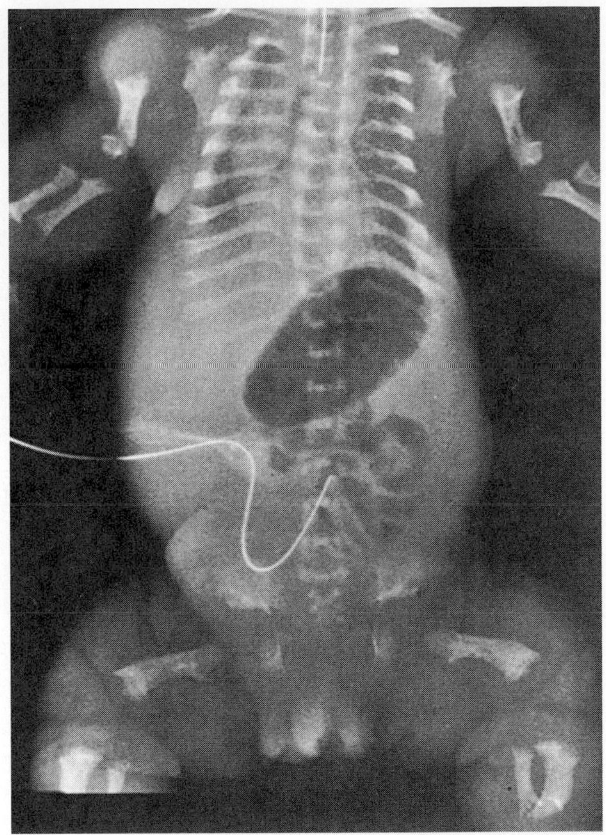

FIGURE 14-32 ■ Thanatophoric dwarf. Note small, narrow thorax and shortness of long bones.

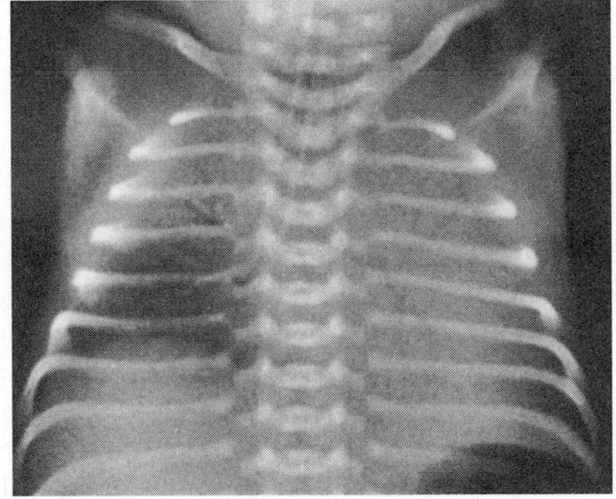

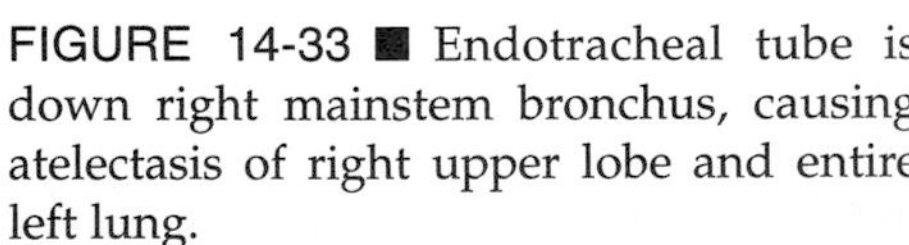

FIGURE 14-33 ■ Endotracheal tube is down right mainstem bronchus, causing atelectasis of right upper lobe and entire left lung.

D. **Chest tube.**
   1. X-rays are obtained to determine placement and effectiveness in reinflating the lung.
   2. Lateral chest x-ray film will determine anterior or posterior placement. For air evacuation, anterior placement is desirable. For fluid evacuation, posterior placement is most effective.
   3. Correct placement will show the tube in the midclavicular line with the distal chest tube hole inside the thoracic space.

E. **Central venous line.** Tip should be located in the superior vena cava or right atrium above the tricuspid valve.

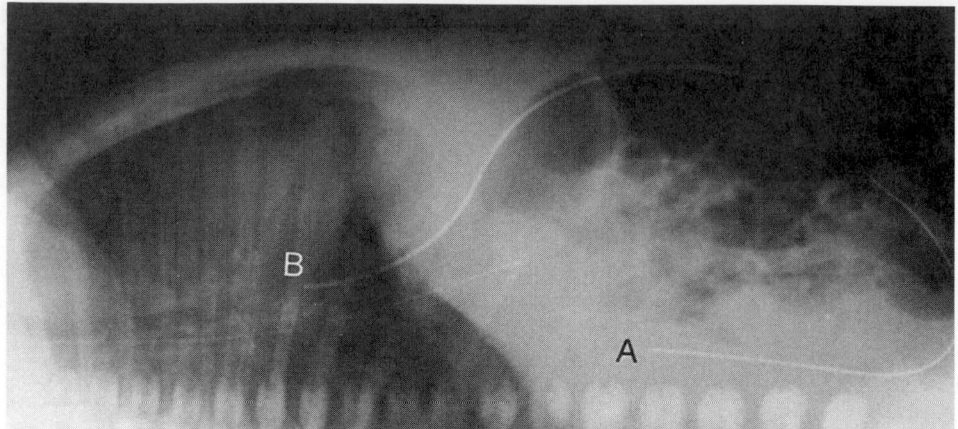

FIGURE 14-34 ■ Umbilical artery catheter (**A**) enters abdomen and proceeds distally as it enters aorta. Umbilical venous catheter (**B**) proceeds toward head, passes through ductus venosus, and lies in inferior vena cava.

F. **Percutaneous central venous line.** If placed in an upper extremity, the tip of the catheter should be located in the superior vena cava and is considered central once it crosses the midclavicular line. If placed in a lower extremity, the line should be positioned in the inferior vena cava and is considered central once it crosses to the pelvic cavity.
   1. A chest x-ray is obtained to confirm placement of a catheter placed in an upper extremity. Arm placement will affect the position of the line. The arm should be extended and at a 45-degree angle from the body to best represent normal arm position (Nadroo et al., 2002).
   2. An abdominal x-ray is obtained to confirm placement of a catheter placed in a lower extremity. Lower extremities should be extended and held in place for the abdominal x-ray.

DIAGNOSTIC IMAGING

A. **Ultrasound.**
   1. Uses sound waves to depict anatomic and functional motion of tissue. The sound waves evaluate varying density of tissues, the movement of tissue, and blood flow. The sound waves can be directed in a variety of planes and angles to enhance imaging (Kenner and Lott, 2003).
   2. Utilized to evaluate internal anatomic structures and some function. Unlike conventional radiography, ultrasound does not emit radiation. The images are typically recorded on videotape or magnetic disks (Kenner and Lott, 2003).
   3. Ultrasound is less expensive than CT or magnetic resonance imaging (MRI), is portable, and therefore more convenient for the evaluation of the unstable patient.
   4. Ultrasound is painless and generally does not require sedation. The procedure is performed at the bedside and the infant's environment is minimally disrupted. Peripheral IVs placed in the area of the anterior fontanelle may need to be relocated if brain imaging is required.
   5. Poor imaging technique, presence of bone and air in the imaging area, and patient position adversely affect quality of the exam. Infant should be supine with the head in midline position.

6. The nurse's role during an ultrasound exam is to correctly position infant, offer comfort measures if necessary, and monitor vital signs and infant's tolerance of the procedure.
7. Ultrasound is commonly used to evaluate brain parenchyma and ventricular size, myocardial function and structure, urinary tract anatomy and pathology, pelvic masses, liver anatomy, and blood flow in major vessels.

B. Computed Tomography (CT).

1. Obtains cross-sectional images of structures by emitting multiple x-ray beams through tissue. CT passes multiple fan x-ray beams through the same cross-sectional slice of tissue at different angles during different time intervals. The beams rotate about the infant, pass through the body, and the exit transmission of x-ray beam is monitored by a series of detectors (Alpen, 1998; Bushong, 2000).
2. CT provides a two-dimensional visualization of anatomy and can be further enhanced by the use of a radiographic contrast agent. Contrast enhancement can assist in the evaluation of blood flow and help define pathologic abnormalities (Bushong, 2000).
3. CT can distinguish changes in density in very small areas of tissue and allows identification of a variety of soft tissues. This allows for superior anatomic detail and precise clarity of tissue structure (Alpen, 1998; Bushong, 2000; Juhl. 1998).
4. CT requires the infant to be transported to the radiology department, so the infant's environment is disrupted. CT is painless but may require sedation depending on the infant's state.
5. Utilized to evaluate structure, function, malformation, and extent of disease process. Used commonly in the NICU to evaluate brain anatomy, intraventricular hemorrhage, and extent of parenchymal disease, subgaleal and subarachnoid and subdural bleeds.
6. The nurse's role in caring for an infant undergoing a CT examination is to swaddle the infant to decrease movement while in the scanner, thus diminishing artifacts from scan. The nurse must also provide comfort measures, evaluate the need for sedation, and monitor vital signs and infant's tolerance of procedure.

C. Magnetic Resonance Imaging (MRI).

1. Utilizes radio waves and magnetic fields to produce images. The image quality is excellent and the increased sensitivity allows for more precise imaging of even the smallest of structures.
2. Does not use ionizing radiation and has less artifact to obscure visualization.
3. Is costly and has limited availability. The magnetic field can interfere with monitoring devices and may restrict the availability to unstable infants.
4. Requires that the infant be transported to the MRI department, so the infant's environment is disrupted. MRI is painless but heavy sedation may be required for an optimal study, which may require mechanical ventilation.
5. May be useful in the early diagnosis of periventricular leukomalacia, or when more accurate definition of tissue structures is needed for evaluation and diagnosis (Kenner and Lott, 2003).
6. The nurse's role in MRI includes swaddling the infant and positioning in the scanner. The infant must be placed on a monitor designed to function within a magnetic field; specialty ventilators are also available for use with MRI. The nurse provides comfort measures and sedation as ordered, as well as monitors vital signs and infant's tolerance of procedure.

D. **Echocardiogram (ECHO).**
   1. Noninvasive diagnostic tool to evaluate cardiac structure and function.
   2. High-frequency sound waves send vibrations through the heart, which reflect energy, which is transmitted into a visual image (Patel et al., 2002).
   3. Poor imaging technique and infant movement adversely affect ECHO quality. It is portable and therefore available for even the unstable infant.

E. **Barium enema.**
   1. Used to evaluate the structure and function of the large intestine and diagnose disorders such as Hirschsprung disease, malrotation, and meconium plug syndrome (Kenner and Lott, 2003).
   2. A water-soluble contrast solution is instilled and a series of x-rays are taken under fluoroscopy. A series of follow-up x-rays may be taken at timed intervals to evaluate the evacuation of the solution from the bowel.

F. **Upper GI series with small bowel follow-through.**
   1. Used to evaluate the structure and function of the upper GI tract. The three main areas examined are (1) the esophagus (for size, patency, reflux, and presence of fistula or swallowing abnormalities), (2) stomach (abnormalities and motility), and (3) the small intestine (for strictures, patency, and function).
   2. A water-soluble contrast solution is swallowed and a series of x-rays are taken under fluoroscopy. A series of follow-up x-rays are obtained to evaluate emptying ability of the stomach, intestinal motility, and for potential obstruction (Kenner and Lott, 2003). Complications include reflux of the contrast solution, vomiting, and potential for aspiration.

G. **Voiding cystourethrogram (VCUG).**
   1. Used to evaluate the structure and function of the kidneys, bladder, and lower urinary tract.
   2. The infant's bladder is emptied by catheterization and then filled with a contrast solution. A series of x-rays are taken under fluoroscopy in a variety of positions during voiding. After voiding follow-up x-rays are taken to evaluate residuals in the bladder and any reflux into the kidneys (Kenner and Lott, 2003).
   3. The infant should be monitored for hematuria and signs of infection related to a contaminated catheterization (Kenner and Lott, 2003).

REFERENCES

Alpen, E.L.: *Radiation biophysics* (2nd ed.). Englewood Cliffs, NJ, 1998, Prentice Hall.

Blickman, H.: *Pediatric radiology: The requisites* (2nd ed.). St Louis, 1998, Mosby,.

Buonomo, C., Taylor, G.A., Share, J.C., and Kirks, D.R.: Gastrointestinal tract. In D.R. Kirks and N.T. Griscom (Eds.): *Practical pediatric imaging: Diagnostic radiology of infants and children.* Philadelphia, 1998, Lippincott-Raven, pp. 822-996.

Bushong, S.C.: *Essentials of imaging series: Computed tomography.* New York, 2000, McGraw-Hill.

Fanaroff, A.A. and Martin, R.J.: *Neonatal perinatal medicine: Diseases of the fetus and infant* (7th ed.). St Louis, 2002, Mosby.

Hedlund, G.L., Griscom, N.T., Cleveland, R.H., and Kirks, D.R.: Respiratory system. In D.R. Kirks and N.T. Griscom, (Eds.): *Practical pediatric imaging: Diagnostic radiology of infants and children.* Philadelphia, 1998, Lippincott-Raven, pp. 619-812.

Juhl, J.H., et al. (Eds.): *Paul and Juhl's essentials of radiologic imaging* (7th ed.). Philadelphia, 1998, Lippincott-Raven.

Kenner, C. and Lott, J.W.: *Comprehensive neonatal nursing: A physiologic perspective* (3rd ed.). Philadelphia, 2003, Saunders.

Kirks, D.R. and Griscom, N.T.: *Practical pediatric imaging: Diagnostic radiology of infants and children.* Philadelphia, 1998, Lippincott-Raven.

Laor, T., Jaramillo, D., and Oestreich, A.E.: Musculoskeletal system. In D.R. Kirks and N.T. Griscom (Eds.): *Practical pediatric imaging: Diagnostic radiology of infants and children.* Philadelphia, 1998, Lippincott-Raven, pp. 350-354.

Nadroo, A.M., Glass, R.B., Lin, J., et al.: Changes in upper extremity position cause migration of peripherally inserted central catheters in neonates. *Pediatrics, 110*(1):131-136, 2002.

Northway, W.H. Jr. and Rosan, R.C.: Radiographic features of pulmonary oxygen toxicity in the newborn: Bronchopulmonary dysplasia. *Radiology, 91*(1): 49-58, 1968.

Patel, C.R. et al.: Fetal cardiac physiology and fetal cardiovascular assessment. In A.A. Fanaroff and R.J. Martin (Eds.): *Neonatal-perinatal medicine: Diseases of the fetus and infant* (7th ed.). St Louis, 2002, Mosby.

Strife, J.L., Bissett, G.S., and Burrows, P.E.: Cardiovascular system. In D.R. Kirks and N.T. Griscom (Eds.): *Practical pediatric imaging: Diagnostic radiology of infants and children.* Philadelphia, 1998, Lippincott-Raven, pp. 512-613.

Swischuk, L.E.: *Imaging of the newborn, infant, and young child* (5th ed.). Philadelphia, 2003, Williams & Wilkins.

Wechsler, S.B. and Wernovsky, G.: Cardiac disorders. In J.P. Cloherty and A. Stark (Eds.): *Manual of neonatal care.* Philadelphia, 1998, Lippincott-Raven, p. 419.

CHAPTER

15 Common Invasive Procedures

GINA M. HEISS-HARRIS

OBJECTIVES

1. Understand the indications for endotracheal tube intubation, endotracheal tube suctioning, thoracentesis, peripheral intravenous (IV) line placement, peripherally inserted central venous catheter placement, peripherally inserted central venous catheter removal, umbilical vessel catheterization, capillary blood sampling, venipuncture, radial artery puncture, bladder catheterization, bladder aspiration, and lumbar puncture.
2. Know the equipment and supplies needed to perform common fundamental and advanced invasive procedures in the neonate.
3. Identify pertinent anatomic landmarks for commonly performed invasive procedures in the neonatal intensive care unit (NICU).
4. Describe the precautions and contraindications for each invasive procedure.
5. Describe complications related to selected invasive procedures.
6. Recognize the care, support, and sedation/pain management necessary for patients undergoing invasive procedures in the NICU.

Invasive procedures performed in neonatal intensive care were once the sole purview of physicians. However, qualified nursing personnel now commonly perform many of these same procedures. Whereas the ability to perform the procedure proficiently is a prerequisite, so is knowledge of the necessary precautions and complications associated with each procedure. Additionally, in recent years there has been much greater appreciation of the pain, discomfort, and adverse reactions possible when performing procedures on the neonatal patient. Awareness of these aspects is as essential as having the needed technical expertise.

The details pertaining to each of the covered procedures make up this chapter. Aspects that are common to each include the crucial issues listed below.

- Know your institution's protocols about the qualifications needed to perform any procedure.
- Know your institution's protocols about any specific ways in which procedures differ from the descriptions included here.
- Obtain informed consent whenever required for an invasive procedure. Discussion with family is key, even if signed informed consent is not required.
- Always use standard infection control precautions and implement aseptic technique whenever indicated.
- Provide for pain and comfort control before, during, and after the procedure.

Note: The author wishes to thank William H. Hyde, MD, for his assistance with this chapter.

- Monitor the patient's clinical status during the procedure. Minimally, monitoring will include oxygenation, ventilation, temperature, and reaction to the procedure.
- Make written documentation about pertinent aspects of the procedure and enter this into the medical record.

AIRWAY PROCEDURES

Endotracheal Tube Suctioning: Fundamental Procedure

A. Indications.
1. Facilitate oxygenation and ventilation.
2. Maintain patent airway.
3. Clearance of tracheobronchial secretions.
4. Obtain tracheal aspirate specimens.

B. Contraindications.
1. Recent surgical procedure to area.
2. Recent surfactant administration.
3. Pulmonary hemorrhage—suction only if needed to maintain tube patency.

C. Precautions.
1. Maintain aseptic technique.
2. Monitor vital signs and for adverse responses to procedure such as bradycardia and oxygen desaturations.
3. Loss of lung volume can occur with suctioning.
4. Suctioning should not be done by a routine schedule. Suctioning should be based on physical examination, blood gases, and character and amount of secretions.
5. Keep infant's head midline during suctioning to prevent jugular vein distention, which can increase intracranial pressure.
6. Pulmonary hemorrhage may be exacerbated by suctioning. However, suctioning may be needed to clear the blood from the airway or tube.
7. When feasible, use two caregivers to perform endotracheal suctioning. This may minimize adverse responses and shorten procedure time.

D. Equipment and supplies.
1. Sterile gloves.
2. Suction catheter (6F or 8F).
3. Resuscitation bag with 100% oxygen source and oxygen blender.
4. Suction source with vacuum control setting.
5. Manometer.
6. Stethoscope.
7. Specimen trap (if applicable).
8. Sterile normal saline (NS) solution or commercially prepared respiratory NS bullets (if necessary).

E. Procedure.
1. Determine the need to suction and suction only when indicated. The following situations *may* warrant suctioning:
   - **a.** Falling oxygen saturations.
   - **b.** Increasing oxygen requirements.
   - **c.** Diminished breath sounds.
   - **d.** Changes in vital signs.
   - **e.** Changes in blood gases.
   - **f.** Changes in respiratory rate and pattern.
   - **g.** Agitation.
   - **h.** Visible secretions in endotracheal tube (ETT).

2. Wash hands and ensure that equipment is in working order.
3. Determine suction catheter insertion distance by summing the length of the ETT and its adapter.
4. Gather supplies.
   a. Commercially prepared suction catheter kit or sterile suction catheter and sterile gloves. Closed-system suction catheter kits are available that remain attached to the ETT adapter and should be used per manufacturer's recommendations. This system allows for a closed-system suction technique that allows the infant to be suctioned without being removed from the ventilator and is recommended for those infants who require frequent suctioning.
   b. Appropriate sized suction catheter with measurement markings. Use an 8F suction catheter for ETTs 3 mm or larger. Use a 6F for ETTs smaller than 3 mm.
   c. If using a commercially prepared suction kit, open package and maintain sterility of contents. Remove and don sterile gloves, then remove catheter. If using separate gloves and catheter supplies, open suction catheter package, maintaining sterility of catheter then open and don gloves. Continue to maintain aseptic technique and remove catheter from package.
5. While maintaining aseptic technique attach suction catheter to suction tubing with nondominant hand (now considered contaminated). With sterile dominant hand hold suction catheter and maintain sterility of catheter.
6. Release suction tubing from nondominant hand and remove infant from ventilator. Provide oxygen and ventilation at necessary levels to maintain heart rate and provide adequate oxygen saturation. Infant may be ventilated by hand or by providing manual breaths from ventilator. If manual breaths are provided by the ventilator, use caution to allow adequate exhalation times.
7. Suction at 60 to 80 mm Hg or with just enough suction to extract secretions through catheter.
8. Advance catheter only to predetermined distance. If a cough reflex is initiated, catheter distance is too far. Advancing the catheter beyond the ETT can cause trauma to surrounding tissue, even perforation of the airway.
9. Apply suction only when withdrawing catheter and limit suction duration to 5 to 10 seconds. Ventilate patient between suction passes while monitoring vital signs, oxygen saturation, and chest wall movement.
10. Routine NS irrigation is not recommended.
11. Limit the number of suction passes. Suction until secretions are removed or infant shows signs of intolerance. Clear suction catheter with NS between suction passes. Most secretions can be cleared in one or two passes.
12. If obtaining tracheal specimen, attach sterile specimen trap to suction catheter and suction tubing prior to suctioning.
13. Return infant to previous oxygen requirement as tolerated.
14. Label and send tracheal specimen to laboratory, if applicable.
15. Document patient's tolerance, character of secretions (amount, color, and consistency), and breath sounds.

F. **Complications.**
   1. Hypoxia.
   2. Bradycardia.
   3. Apnea.

4. Accidental extubation or malpositioning of tube.
5. Trauma to trachea or bronchi.
6. Hemorrhage.
7. Atelectasis.
8. Infection.
9. Pneumothorax.
10. Increased intracranial pressure.

Endotracheal Intubation: Advanced Practice Procedure

A. Indications.

1. Bag-and-mask ventilation is ineffective or undesirable.
2. Need for mechanical ventilation.
3. Tracheal suctioning or lavage is required.
4. Obtain sterile tracheal aspirate specimen.
5. Protection of the airway is required.
6. Diaphragmatic hernia is present.
7. Administration of exogenous surfactant.

B. Precautions.

1. Patient's heart rate and oxygen saturation should be monitored continuously during the procedure.
2. Hypoxia during the procedure should be minimized.
3. Use free-flow oxygen held near the mouth and nose of any infant with respiratory effort, to maximize oxygenation during the procedure.
4. Limit intubation attempts to 20 seconds. The infant's condition should be stabilized with bag-and-mask ventilation between attempts.
5. Have all equipment necessary for intubation prepared and in working order prior to initiating procedure.
6. Consider sedation of infant prior to procedure for nonemergent intubation, using institutional protocol.
7. Maintain thermal homeostasis and developmental care.

C. Equipment and supplies.

1. Pediatric laryngoscope handle.
2. Laryngoscope blade with functioning secure bulb.
   - **a.** Size 00 blade for infants weighing less than 1000 g may be needed.
   - **b.** Size 0 blade for preterm infants or infants weighing 1000 to 3000 g.
   - **c.** Size 1 for term infants or infants weighing more than 3500 g.
3. ETT size:
   - **a.** Internal diameter (ID) 2.5 mm for infants weighing less than 1000 g or less than 28 weeks' gestation.
   - **b.** ID 3 mm for 1000-to 2000-g infant or infants with a gestational age of 28 to 34 weeks.
   - **c.** ID 3.5 mm for 2000- to 3000-g infant or infants with a gestational age of 34 to 38 weeks.
   - **d.** ID 3.5 mm to 4 mm ETT for infants weighing more than 3000 g or greater than 38 weeks' gestation.
4. Stylet (though use is optional, it should be available).
5. Suction catheters (size 6F to 10F) and suction source set at 60 to 80 mm Hg of negative pressure. For suctioning in the delivery room, it should be set at negative 100 mm Hg.
6. Resuscitation bag and mask of appropriate sizes. Alternatively, availability of infant ventilation device such as the NeoPuff.

7. 100% oxygen source set minimally at a flow rate of 5 to 10 L/minute with attached manometer.
8. Tape and other supplies to secure ETT according to hospital policy.
9. Cardiorespiratory monitor and oxygen saturation monitor.
10. Stethoscope.
11. Meconium aspirator, if applicable.
12. End-tidal CO_2 detector, colorimetric device.

D. Procedure.

1. Select ETT of the appropriate size.
2. Insert stylet (optional) and shape the ETT as desired. The stylet must be secured so that its tip does not extend below the tip of the ETT and also so the stylet cannot advance during the procedure. Keep the tube and stylet as clean as possible.
3. Prepare the resuscitation bag or ventilation device so that the infant may be given ventilation before and after the procedure.
4. Aspirate gastric contents and suction the oropharynx.
5. Position the patient supine on a flat surface, with the head midline and the neck slightly extended (optional: place a soft flat roll under neck). The person performing intubation must have easy access to the airway and equipment while positioned at the patient's head.
6. Hold the laryngoscope in the left hand between the thumb and first finger, with the blade pointing away.
7. Open the patient's mouth with the fingers of the right hand and gently slide the blade into the right side of the mouth.
8. Stabilize the left hand against the left side of the patient's face, advance the blade tip to the base of the tongue, and move the blade to the midline, pushing the tongue to the left.
9. Expose the pharynx by lifting the entire blade upward in the direction in which the handle is pointing. Do not rock the tip of the blade upward or use the upper gum as a fulcrum.
10. If unable to see the glottis, apply gentle pressure over the trachea with the fifth finger of the left hand and withdraw the blade slowly until the glottis is visible.
11. Remove any secretions that interfere with visualization by suctioning. Direct suctioning under laryngoscopy is ideal.
12. Identify anatomic landmarks (Fig. 15-1).
    a. Epiglottis is uppermost.
    b. Glottis is anterior, with vocal cords closing side to side.
    c. Esophagus is posterior.
13. After identifying the vocal cords, and with the cords in clear view, place the ETT into the right side of the patient's mouth with the right hand.

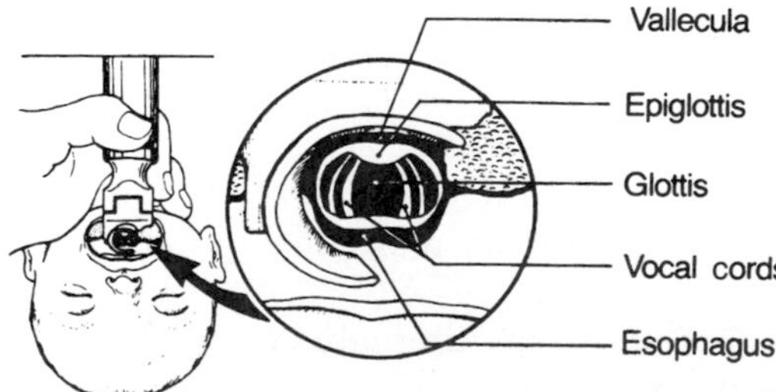

FIGURE 15-1 ■ Anatomic landmarks for endotracheal intubation. (From American Academy of Pediatrics/American Heart Association: *Textbook of neonatal resuscitation* [4th ed.]. Elk Grove Village, IL, 2000, the Associations.)

14. Keeping the cords in view, pass the ETT between the cords to the level of the vocal cord guide mark on the tube. This should position the tip of the tube approximately halfway between the vocal cords and the carina.
    a. If the vocal cords are closed or will not open, wait for spontaneous breath.
15. With the right hand, firmly grasp the ETT at the level of the patient's lip, stabilize the right hand against the patient's face, and carefully remove the laryngoscope with the left hand.
16. Carefully remove the stylet, if used, from the ETT.
17. Attach the resuscitation bag or alternative ventilating device (NeoPuff) to the ETT and deliver breaths.
18. Assess tube placement.
    a. Auscultate both sides of the chest for the presence and intensity of breath sounds.
    b. Assess chest movement with inflationary breaths.
    c. Auscultate over the epigastrium and visually assess for distention.
    d. Check for condensation in tube during exhalation.
    e. Check for color change on CO_2 detector, if available.
19. If the tube is in too far and placed in a right or left mainstem bronchus, auscultation may reveal unilateral or unequal breath sounds. The tube should be withdrawn 0.5 to 1 cm and placement reassessed.
20. If the tube is in the esophagus:
    a. Air may be heard entering the stomach with inflationary breaths.
    b. The stomach may become distended.
    c. No breath sounds will be heard on auscultation of the chest during inflationary breaths, though air movement may be heard, especially over the lower portion of the chest.
    d. Remove the ETT and discard it.
21. In very small infants, breath sounds may seem audible even with an ETT in the esophagus.
22. When the tube is assessed to be in good position, note the markings relative to the upper gum, or use the lip-to-tip rule (6 plus the weight in kilograms) and secure the tube according to hospital policy.
23. Position of the tube must be confirmed by chest radiograph. Its tip should lie approximately 1 cm above the carina (Fig. 15-2).
24. After confirming tube placement by chest radiograph, any length of tube that extends more than 4 cm beyond the lip should be cut off to limit dead space and to prevent kinking.
25. Document according to hospital policy: date, time, ETT size, centimeter marking at lip, chest radiograph, and patient's tolerance of procedure. Sedation interventions performed, if any, should also be documented.

E. Complications.

1. Hypoxia.
    a. During the procedure.
    b. Due to misplacement of tube.
2. Bradycardia.
    a. Due to hypoxia.
    b. Due to vagal stimulation from the laryngoscope, ETT, or suction catheter.
3. Infection.
4. Perforation of esophagus or trachea.
5. Trauma to oropharyngeal and laryngeal tissues.
6. Vocal cord injury.

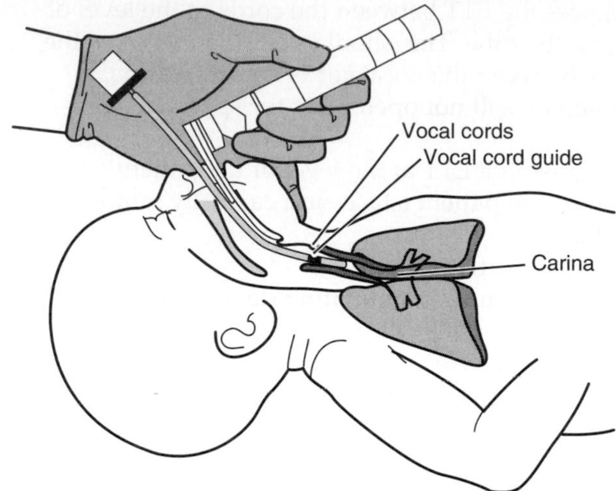

FIGURE 15-2 ■ Correct depth of insertion of endotracheal tube. (From American Academy of Pediatrics/American Heart Association: *Textbook of neonatal resuscitation* [4th ed.]. Elk Grove Village, IL, 2000, the Associations.)

7. Misplacement of tube into esophagus or bronchus.
8. Interference of oral development caused by oral ETT.
9. Tube obstruction or kinking.
10. Pain, agitation, or discomfort.

Thoracentesis: Advanced Practice Procedure

A. Indications.
1. Emergency evacuation of pneumothorax.
2. Emergency evacuation of pleural fluid.

B. Equipment and supplies.
1. Skin antiseptics according to hospital policy.
2. Large bore over-the-needle IV catheter (14 to 20 gauge). Use of a butterfly or hypodermic needle is discouraged due to potential injury to lung.
3. Three-way stopcock.
4. Syringe, 20 to 35 cc.
5. Local anesthetic, tuberculin (TB) syringe with small-bore needle, if medical condition permits.

C. Procedure.
1. Position the infant supine and restrain limbs if necessary.
2. Provide pharmacologic pain management if medical condition permits.
3. Identify entry site. Use second or third intercostal space along midclavicular line.
4. Prepare skin with antiseptic as per hospital policy.
5. Infiltrate the area with 1 cc of local anesthetic using a TB syringe and 25- to 27-gauge needle.
6. Puncture skin at 45-degree angle, angling over third or fourth rib, and advance needle/catheter at 90-degree angle. Inserting the catheter over the top of the rib will avoid blood vessels and nerves that run along the bottom of the rib. If thoracentesis is being done due to pleural fluid or effusion, the thorax should be punctured between the fifth and sixth intercostal spaces, midaxillae.
7. Remove needle from IV catheter while sliding the catheter into the pleural space.

8. Attach catheter hub to stopcock and syringe. The stopcock allows for aspiration of free air or fluid into the syringe and emptying of the syringe while maintaining a closed system.
9. When free air or fluid is obtained, stabilize the catheter and continue to aspirate until preparation for chest tube insertion is complete, or until the air leak or fluid accumulation is evacuated.
10. Document according to hospital policy: date, time, catheter size, location, amount of air/fluid evacuated, patient's tolerance of procedure. Pharmacologic interventions performed, if any, should also be documented.

D. Complications.
1. Hemorrhage.
2. Infection.
3. Needle injury to lung or adjacent structures.
4. Damage to breast tissue.
5. Pain.

CIRCULATORY ACCESS PROCEDURES

Peripheral Intravenous Line Placement: Fundamental Procedure

A. Indications.
1. Administration of medications.
2. Administration of fluids, volume expanders, or blood products.
3. Administration of parenteral nutrition.

B. Precautions.
1. Avoid areas of infection or loss of skin integrity near selected puncture site.
2. Use caution in infants with coagulation disorders, which may result in bleeding into surrounding tissues.
3. Padded armboard is to be used only if necessary to maintain line placement and must be of an appropriate size for gestational age.
4. Avoid sites that may be needed for possible central venous cannulation.
5. Differentiate between veins and arteries.

C. Equipment and supplies.
1. 22- to 27-gauge over-the-needle catheter device or a 23- to 27-gauge butterfly needle. Butterfly needles are discouraged due to damage to the vein caused by the metal against the vessel wall.
2. Tape and dressing supplies as per hospital policy.
3. Skin antiseptics as per hospital policy.
4. Tourniquet (a sanitized rubber band will suffice).
5. NS flush solution in a 3-ml syringe.
6. T-connector device, if applicable.
7. Transilluminator, if necessary.
8. Appropriately sized padded armboard, if necessary.
9. Nonsterile gloves.
10. Pain/developmental management: pacifier, sucrose pacifier, blankets for developmental swaddling, eye protection from bright lights.

D. Procedure.
1. Gather supplies, wash hands, and don gloves.
2. Determine vein for cannulation. Transilluminate to locate vein, if necessary (use caution to avoid skin burns from heated device).
3. Provide pain management such as pacifier for nonnutritive sucking, sucrose pacifier and/or developmental care with facilitated tucking or swaddling. Shield eyes from bright lights.

4. Flush T-connector device with NS flush solution. Flushing over-the-needle catheter is optional. Flush butterfly needle if utilizing this method.
5. Select vein (Fig. 15-3). Accomplish distention of the vessel by applying a gentle tourniquet proximal to the selected insertion site. Alternatively, an assistant may encircle the proximal extremity with hand/fingers and apply direct pressure for the same effect.
6. Position and stabilize puncture site to allow puncture in direction of blood flow.
7. Prepare skin at selected puncture site with antiseptic as per hospital policy.
8. Beginning a few millimeters distal to the anticipated site of the vessel puncture, insert the needle bevel up, at a 15- to 25-degree angle, depending on location of vein.
9. Advance needle until blood appears in the catheter or tubing.
10. If resistance is met or vein is not punctured, withdraw needle slowly to just below the level of the skin, relocate vein, and advance the needle again.
11. If a hematoma develops or bleeding occurs, occlude the vessel with pressure just proximal to the puncture site, remove tourniquet, withdraw the needle or catheter, and apply pressure until hemostasis has occurred.
12. If cannulation appears to be successful, remove the tourniquet and catheter needle (if using over-the-needle catheter), connect the T-connector to the catheter hub, and inject some of the flush solution gently to evaluate

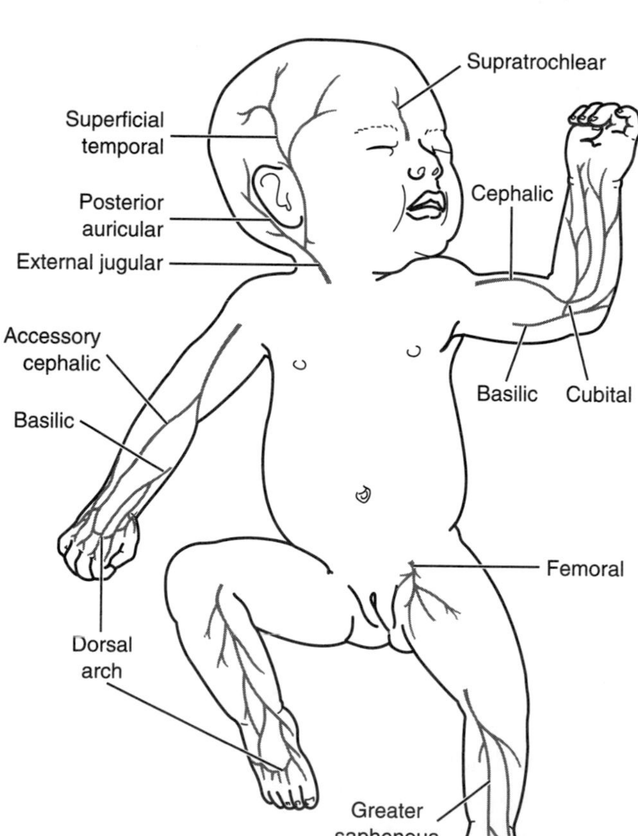

FIGURE 15-3 ■ Frequently used sites for venous access in the neonate. (From Gomella, T.L.: *Neonatology: Management, procedures, on-call problems, diseases, and drugs* (4th ed.). New York, 1999, Lange-Medical Books/McGraw-Hill.)

patency of the catheter. If flush solution infiltrates the tissues surrounding the catheter tip, occlude the vessel with pressure just proximal to the puncture site, withdraw the needle or catheter, and apply pressure until hemostasis has occurred.

13. If cannulation was successful and flush solution infuses without complications, connect T-connector and IV tubing with appropriate fluid to catheter, if applicable.
14. Tape catheter in position per hospital policy. Tape, dressing, and restraint must allow for easy inspection of insertion site, circulation of the distal extremity, and patency of the IV tubing. Avoid occlusion of the IV tubing with the tape or dressing.
15. Dispose of needle(s) in appropriate sharps container.
16. Document date, time, catheter size, site location, and patient's tolerance of procedure, according to hospital guidelines. Pain management interventions should also be documented.
17. Monitor for tissue infiltration or device dislodgment. Adverse signs may include the following:
    - **a.** Redness, blanching, or discoloration at or near IV insertion site.
    - **b.** Edema.
    - **c.** Pain with flushing.
    - **d.** Resistance with flushing.
18. Treatment for infiltration/extravasation:
    - **a.** Elevation of affected extremity.
    - **b.** Avoid cold or warm compresses.
    - **c.** Puncture site to express fluid (in extreme infiltrations).
    - **d.** Pharmacologic intervention:
        - (1) Hyaluronidase—indicated for the treatment of severe infiltration of intravenous solutions, especially hypertonic solutions or those containing calcium (examples: total parenteral nutrition [TPN], sodium bicarbonate, potassium chloride, and aminophylline). Do not use for infiltrations of vasoactive drugs such as dopamine, epinephrine, or norepinephrine. For best results use hyaluronidase within 1 hour of infiltration. Reconstitute product with NS to 15 mg/cc and inject five 0.2 cc injections subcutaneously around the periphery of the infiltration (do not inject directly into affected area), using a different 25- to 27-gauge needle for each injection. Not recommended for IV use. *Note:* Wydase is no longer available; however, hyaluronidase is available and can be compounded by hospital pharmacies.
        - (2) Phentolamine—indicated for treatment of infiltration of vasoactive drugs. For best results use within 12 hours of infiltration. Reconstitute product with NS to 0.5 mg/cc and inject 0.1 or 0.2 mg/kg (up to 5 mg maximum) subcutaneously into the area of infiltration using multiple small injections with a 25- to 27-gauge needle, changing the needle between each skin entry. Monitor patient for hypotension, tachycardia, and cardiac arrhythmias.

E. Complications.

1. Hematoma.
2. Infection.
3. Air, clot, or particle embolus.
4. Tissue injury (phlebitis, infiltration) and possible necrosis after infiltration of infused solutions and/or medications.

5. Injury to extremity from restraint.
   a. Compromised distal circulation.
   b. Pressure necrosis over bony areas.
   c. Limb deformity after prolonged immobilization.
   d. Pressure injury of peripheral nerves.
6. Inadvertent arterial line placement.
   a. Blood loss from inadvertent catheter or tubing dislodgment.
7. Pain from infiltration or ruptured blood vessel from unsuccessful cannulation.

Peripherally Inserted Central Catheter (PICC): Advanced Practice Procedure

A. Indications.
1. Intermediate or long-term intravenous therapy (>7 days).
   a. TPN.
   b. Antibiotic or other medicinal therapy.
2. Limited venous access.
3. Irritating drug therapy.
4. Very low birth weight (<1500 g).

B. Contraindications.
1. Active bacteremia or sepsis.
2. Inadequate vessel for cannulation.
3. Parental refusal.

C. Precautions.
1. Avoid areas of infection or loss of skin integrity near selected puncture site.
2. Avoid placement of PICC line in extremity with inadequate or poor circulation.
3. Obtain parental informed consent prior to the procedure.
4. Use caution in infants with coagulation disorders.
5. Use aseptic technique during insertion and care of PICC line.
6. Ensure attention to pain management, developmental care, and thermal homeostasis.
7. Infuse medication via medication infusion pump, avoid "pushes."
8. Use larger-bore syringes (>5 cc) that generate less pressure. Do not use a TB syringe.
9. Avoid tension on catheter and tubing.
10. Never pull catheter back through needle introducer because of the risk of damage or shearing of catheter.
11. Monitor for bradycardia and hypoxia during procedure.
12. Do not infuse blood products or obtain blood specimens from PICC lines.

D. Equipment and supplies. *Note:* Polyurethane catheters with a guidewire are available. However, due to the potential risk of perforation to vessels or organs, the discussion below will be limited to the more common Silastic catheters that do not utilize a guidewire.
1. Commercially prepared catheter insertion kit, *or* the following:
   a. Antiseptic per hospital policy or alcohol swabs (3) and povidone-iodine swabs (3).
   b. Forceps.
   c. Sterile measuring tape.
   d. Sterile gown and gloves, mask and surgical cap.
   e. Sterile NS or heparin flush solution.

f. Sterile gauze pads.
g. Sterile drapes and towels.
h. Sterile tourniquet (optional with preterm infants).
i. Transparent, semipermeable dressing.
j. Sterile adhesive strips.
k. Luer-Lock or T-connector device.

2. Neonatal percutaneous catheter of appropriate size.
   a. Silastic catheter without guidewire, with break-away needle or peel-away plastic cannula. Available commercially in 1.9F to 2.8F.
   b. If infant is less than 1000 g, the smallest catheter should be used.

E. Procedure.

1. Verify physician's order for PICC line.
2. Check to ensure informed consent obtained.
3. Gather equipment and supplies.
4. Provide sedation/analgesia.
5. Maintain thermoregulation and developmental positioning. Also provide environmental support by protecting infant's eyes from bright lights.
6. Select vein (see Fig. 15-3). Most common sites for neonates include the cephalic, basilic, and greater saphenous. A right-sided basilic or cephalic approach is preferred due to the shorter distance between the insertion site and the superior vena cava.
7. Position infant so selected vein is accessible. Restrain infant if necessary to prevent contamination of sterile field.
8. Measure length of catheter to be inserted. Optimal placement of catheter is with tip in a large-caliber central vein (i.e., superior or inferior vena cava). Measure from insertion site to the third or fourth intercostal space (upper extremity placement) or to xyphoid process (lower extremity placement).
9. Don mask and cap and perform 3- to 5-minute scrub.
10. Set up sterile field and open catheter kit, maintaining sterility of contents.
11. Don sterile gloves and prepare insertion site with povidone-iodine or antiseptic per hospital policy and allow to dry.
12. Discard first pair of sterile gloves and don gown and new pair of sterile gloves. Drape infant with sterile towels. Assemble equipment using aseptic technique. An alternate method is to have assistant don sterile gloves and elevate extremity while inserter prepares insertion site maintaining aseptic technique.
13. Trim the catheter to predetermined length.
    a. Catheter may be shortened by cutting catheter with sterile scissors, slightly longer than measured distance.
    b. Cut the tip of the catheter straight across to prevent the catheter from lying flush against the vessel wall and possibly obstructing the infusion flow.
14. Attach flush-syringe and prime catheter.
15. Apply sterile tourniquet (optional).
16. Puncture vessel at about 10- to 20-degree angle. Enter directly into the vein with catheter introducer. Entry into the vessel is signaled by blood leaking from puncture site or from the introducer needle/cannula (Fig. 15-4).
17. Two types of catheter introducers are available:
    a. Break-away needle—this technique utilizes a break-away introducer needle. The vessel is cannulated and the catheter advanced through the needle to the premeasured distance. The catheter needle is then retracted and pulled apart along its longitudinal axis and discarded.

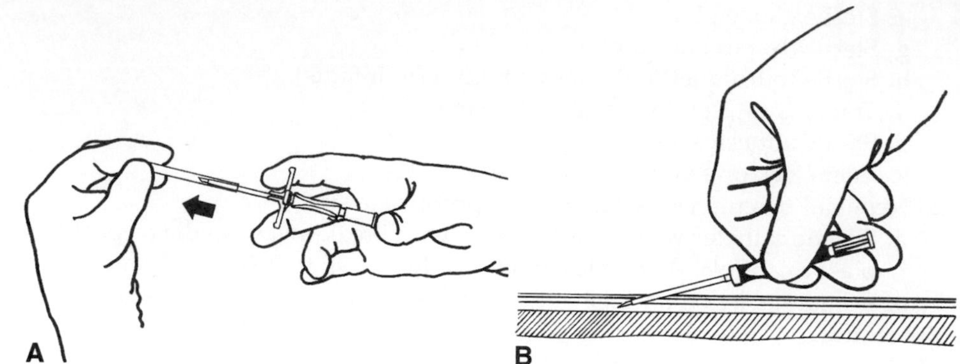

FIGURE 15-4 ■ *A* and *B*, Performing venipuncture for PICC insertion. (Courtesy NeoCare, a division of Arrow International, Inc., Reading, PA.)

   b. Peel-away plastic cannula—this technique utilizes a needle with a plastic cannula. The vessel is cannulated and the needle is removed, leaving the plastic cannula in the vessel for catheter insertion. Advance the catheter to the premeasured distance, then retract plastic cannula from vessel and pull the catheter apart along its longitudinal axis and discard.

18. Loosen tourniquet (if applicable) after venipuncture and before catheter advancement. Gentle pressure with finger distal to puncture site may reduce blood loss. Remove needle, leaving peel-away plastic cannula in place if utilizing this method (Fig. 15-5).

19. Advance flushed catheter to zero measure marking on catheter with forceps ⅛ to ¼ inch at a time. Catheter should advance smoothly, i.e., without resistance (Fig. 15-6).

20. Once catheter is advanced to predetermined distance, withdraw plastic cannula or break-away needle and pull apart (Figs. 15-7 and 15-8). Catheter may be pulled out slightly during splitting technique and may need to be advanced slightly when complete.

21. Aspirate on catheter to confirm blood return (Fig. 15-9).

22. Temporarily secure catheter with sterile adhesive strips and obtain chest radiograph for catheter placement while maintaining sterile field and aseptic technique.

23. Radiographically confirm placement in large-caliber vein prior to any infusions. Pull back or advance catheter, if necessary, to appropriate distance. Check for blood return and obtain another chest radiograph to confirm satisfactory position.

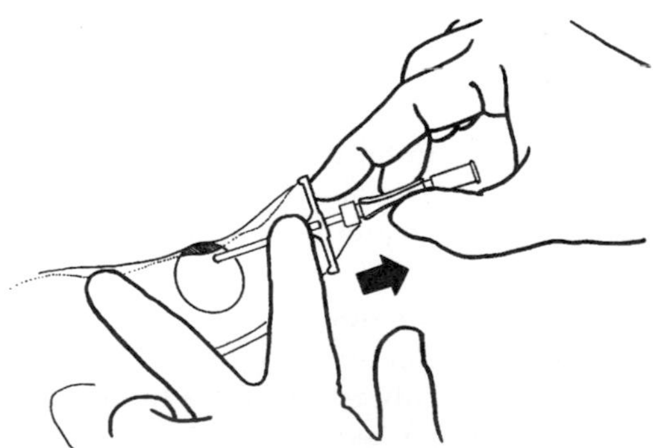

FIGURE 15-5 ■ Withdrawing introducer needle from introducer sheath. (Courtesy NeoCare, a division of Arrow International, Inc., Reading, PA.)

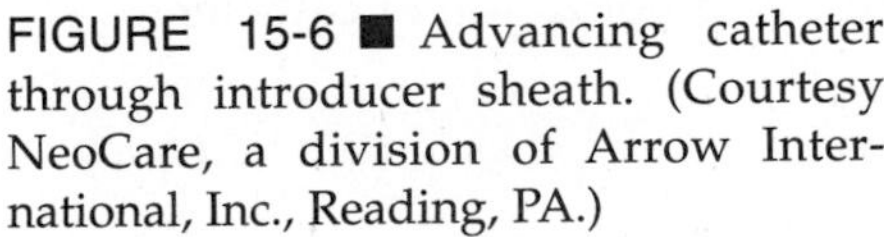

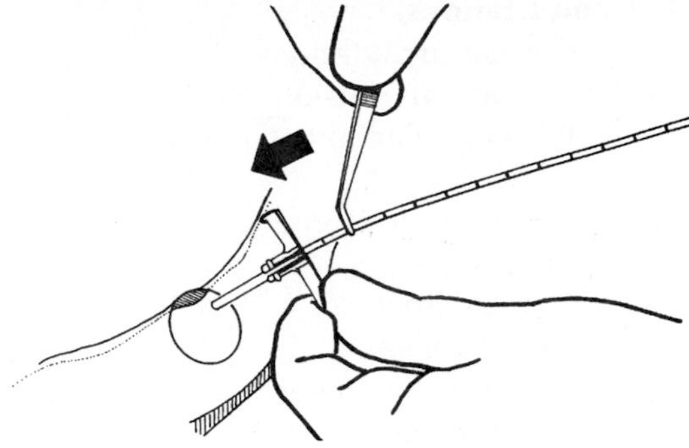

FIGURE 15-6 ■ Advancing catheter through introducer sheath. (Courtesy NeoCare, a division of Arrow International, Inc., Reading, PA.)

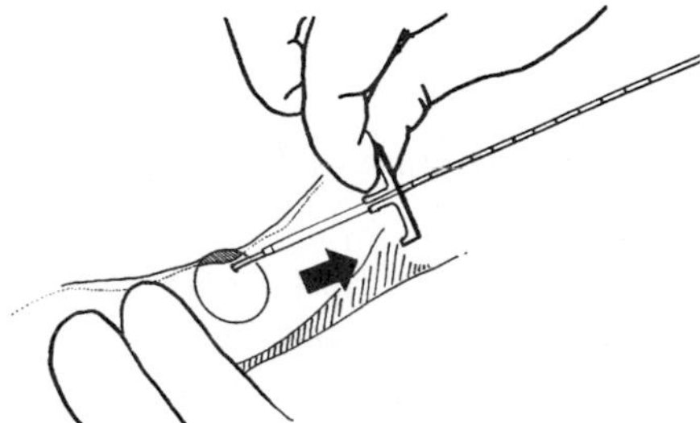

FIGURE 15-7 ■ Withdrawing introducer sheath. (Courtesy NeoCare, a division of Arrow International, Inc., Reading, PA.)

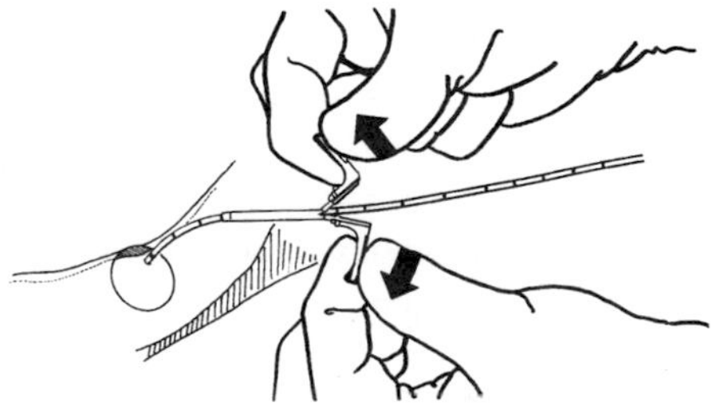

FIGURE 15-8 ■ Splitting and removing introducer sheath. (Courtesy NeoCare, a division of Arrow International, Inc., Reading, PA.)

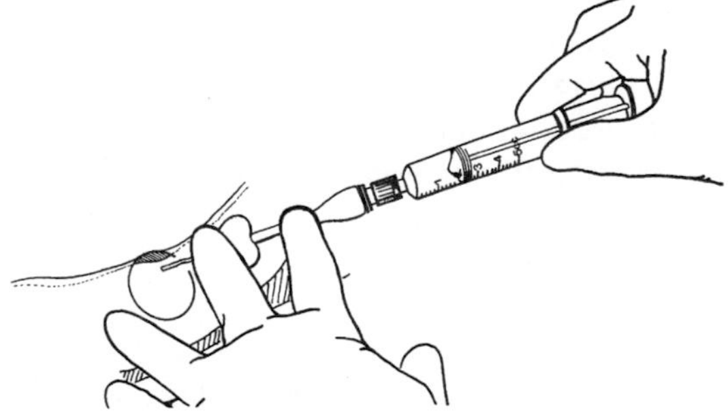

FIGURE 15-9 ■ Aspirating and flushing catheter. (Courtesy NeoCare, a division of Arrow International, Inc., Reading, PA.)

24. Remove antiseptic from surrounding skin with sterile water.
25. Secure and dress catheter per manufacturer's recommendations.
26. Document procedure including catheter lot number, catheter size, catheter type, location and insertion distance, location of catheter tip on radiograph, and sedation/analgesia provided.
27. Change dressing per manufacturer's recommendations.
28. Monitor for infiltration or extravasation:
    a. Redness.
    b. Edema.
    c. Difficulty with flushing or fluid infusion.

F. **Complications.**
1. Cardiac arrhythmias.
2. Pericardial effusion and tamponade.
3. Intravascular catheter shearing, followed by embolization of catheter fragment.
4. Thrombus formation.
5. Infection.
6. Nerve damage.
7. Air embolism.
8. Rupture of catheter (from using excessive infusion pressure, e.g., from using small-bore syringes).
9. Infiltration/extravasation.
10. Hemorrhage.

Umbilical Vessel Catheterization: Advanced Practice Procedure

A. **Indications.**
1. Arterial catheterization.
    a. Frequent arterial blood sampling.
    b. Continuous arterial blood gas monitoring.
    c. Continuous arterial blood pressure monitoring.
    d. Vascular access for intravenous fluids when other sites are not available or suitable.
    e. Exchange transfusion.
    f. Cardiac catheterization.
2. Venous catheterization.
    a. Emergency administration of drugs.
    b. Emergency measurement of P_{CO_2} and pH.
    c. Fluid administration (hypertonic solutions or inadequate peripheral access).
    d. Exchange transfusion.
    e. Central venous pressure monitoring.
    f. Blood sampling.

B. **Contraindications.**
1. Abdominal wall defects.
2. Necrotizing enterocolitis (controversial).
3. Vascular compromise below level of umbilicus.
4. Omphalitis.
5. Peritonitis.

C. **Precautions.**
1. Maintain thermal homeostasis.
2. Monitor heart rate and oxygen saturation throughout procedure.
3. Maintain aseptic technique.
4. Dilate artery before attempting vessel cannulation.
5. Do not force catheter past obstruction.

D. **Equipment and supplies.**
1. Commercially prepackaged sterile umbilical catheter tray or sterile instrument tray for umbilical catheterization to include the following:
    a. 4×4 gauze pads.
    b. Sterile drapes.
    c. Small container for antiseptic solution.
    d. Scissors.

e. Umbilical tape.
f. Measuring tape.
g. Syringes, 10 cc.
h. No. 11 scalpel with handle.
i. Mosquito hemostats (2).
j. Curved, nontoothed iris forceps (2).
k. Toothed iris forceps (1).
l. Needle holder.
m. Umbilical catheter of either argyle or silastic material. Silastic catheters may be more difficult to insert due to the lack of their rigidity.
n. Determine appropriate size catheter with either a single, double, or triple lumen, or as desired by your institution's medical staff.
   (1) Size 3.5F for infants weighing less than 1500 g.
   (2) Size 3.5, 4.0, or 5.0 F for infants weighing more than 1500 g
   (3) A 2.5 F argyle catheter is available for use in the extremely premature infant.
o. 3-0 silk suture.
p. 4-0 silk suture with curved needle.
q. Three-way Luer-Lock stopcock.
r. Dressings for securing (clear occlusive dressing and a hydrocolloid skin barrier).
s. Sterile heparin-flush solution (1 unit/cc).

2. Sterile antiseptic solution.
3. Mask, surgical cap, and sterile gown and gloves.
4. Standardized premeasurement graph (Fig. 15-10) *or* access to a formula to determine insertion depth.

E. Procedure.

Umbilical Artery Catheterization (UAC). *Note:* "Low position," catheter tip placed between the third and fourth lumbar vertebrae (L3-L4). "High position," catheter tip placed between the sixth and tenth thoracic vertebrae (T6-T10). Either position is accepted practice currently. Consult your institution's guidelines for desired positioning of UACs.

1. Inspect lower extremities for bruising and palpate pulses.
2. Assess umbilical cord to rule out umbilical anomaly such as a small omphalocele.
3. Place infant supine and restrain limbs.
4. Calculate insertion depth.
   a. Measure shoulder to umbilical distance (adding length of umbilicus stump) and multiply by 0.66 to arrive at insertion depth for a "low" placement (L3-L4), *or*
   b. 2.5 times body weight in kilograms plus 9.7 cm ($2.5 \times \text{weight} + 9.7$) for a "high" placement (T6-T10).
5. Don mask and cap and perform a 3- to 5-minute scrub.
6. Don sterile gown and gloves.
7. Have assistant hold heparin flush vial and draw up flush into sterile syringe.
8. Prepare catheter by attaching Luer-Lock stopcock to catheter and connect flush-filled syringe to stopcock and flush catheter.
9. Turn stopcock off to catheter.
10. Have assistant hold umbilical cord up and out of procedure area while you prepare cord with antiseptic solution. Scrub in a circular manner moving from the cord to approximately 5 cm in radius on surrounding abdomen.

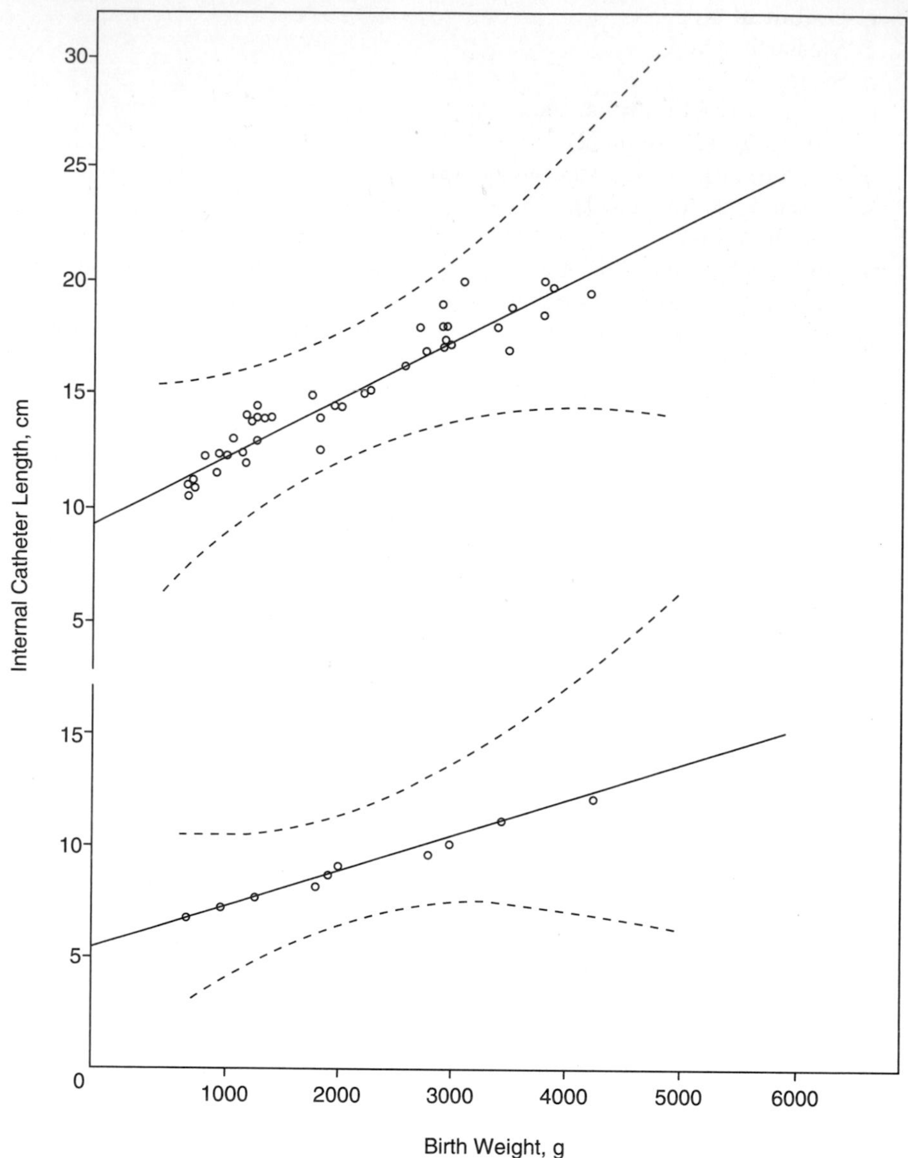

FIGURE 15-10 ■ Estimates of insertional length of umbilical catheters. (From Shukla, H. and Ferrara, A.: Rapid estimation of insertional length of umbilical catheters in newborns. *American Journal of Diseases of Children, 140*[8]:786-788, 1986.)

Do not let antiseptic drip down infant's side because this may cause burns, especially in extremely premature infants.

11. Drape procedure area with sterile towels.
12. Tie umbilical tape using a single hand knot tight enough to prevent bleeding at base of cord, not on the skin. Umbilical tape may have to be loosened to advance catheter or tightened to control bleeding.
13. Using a scalpel, cut through the umbilical cord 1 to 1.5 cm from skin.
14. Identify cord vessels.
    a. Arteries: two small, thick-walled, and white constricted vessels that may stick out slightly and typically located at the 4 and 8 o'clock positions.

   b. Vein: single, large, thin-walled vessel, often open and typically located at the 12 o'clock position.

15. Stabilize cord stump.
   a. Grasp portion of cut edge of cord with hemostat and apply gentle traction.
   b. Apply hemostats to opposite sides of the cord and roll them away from each other, causing the arteries to protrude from the cut surface of the cord.

16. Dilate artery.
   a. Insert one tip of curved iris forceps into selected artery and probe gently to a depth of about 0.5 cm.
   b. With tips of forceps together, gently probe artery to a depth of about 0.5 cm.
   c. Gently spread forceps apart, and then slowly withdraw forceps from artery, dilating lumen as forceps is withdrawn.
   d. Continue to dilate lumen (approximately 15-60 seconds) until forceps can easily be inserted to a depth of about 1 cm.

17. Insert catheter.
   a. Insert catheter into dilated artery.
   b. Thread catheter to predetermined depth.
   c. If resistance is met, *do not force catheter*. Apply gentle, steady pressure to catheter while applying gentle traction on cord.
   d. If catheter cannot be advanced to the desired distance, discontinue attempts and catheterize second artery.
   e. Observe for blanching of legs, toes, and/or buttocks.

18. Aspirate blood to ensure placement in vessel after catheter advanced approximately 5 cm. If blood obtained, clear catheter by injecting 0.5 ml flush solution. If blood cannot be aspirated, remove catheter and attempt catheterization of second artery.

19. Obtain radiograph to confirm catheter position.
   a. If catheter tip is too high, pull catheter back to proper position, and obtain another radiograph.
   b. If catheter tip is too low for "high position," pull back to "low position," if your institutional guidelines allow this.
   c. If catheter tip is too low for "low position," it should be adjusted to an acceptable position. Keep in mind that a catheter that is no longer sterile should not be advanced.

20. Suture catheter in place.
   a. Place pursestring suture around cord. Avoid piercing the vessels and catheters. Secure to umbilical skin or cord depending on your institution's guidelines.
   b. Knot suture securely in cord close to catheter per manufacturer's recommendations.
   c. If suture around catheter, it must be tight to prevent catheter from sliding, but not so tight that flow through catheter is obstructed.

21. Loosen umbilical tape.

22. Remove antiseptic as soon as possible from skin to prevent burns.

23. Secure catheter per hospital policy. The following are various securing techniques used to secure catheters:
   a. Commercially manufactured securing devices.
   b. "Bridge" or "goalpost" taping technique.
   c. Hydrocolloid skin barrier to umbilical area with clear occlusive dressing.

24. Document procedure according to hospital policy noting type of catheter, catheter size, distance catheter threaded, location of catheter tip on radiograph, adjustments made to catheter to correct malpositioned catheter, and assessment of color, pulses, and perfusion to lower extremities.

Umbilical Vein Catheterization. *Note:* Equipment for umbilical vein catheterization is the same as that for UAC insertion with the exception that an 8F catheter may occasionally be used for infants weighing greater than 3500 g.

1. Maintain aseptic technique.
2. Prepare cord as for umbilical artery catheter and identify the thin-walled vein.
3. Grasp the base of the cord with curved hemostats or toothed forceps, hold upright, and dilate vessel with the tip of iris forceps.
4. Insert the catheter to predetermined distance.
   a. Emergency placement (temporary catheter, low position): Insert 2 to 3 cm into vessel until blood is obtained. Once emergency medications and fluids have been administered and infant is stabilized, remove the catheter.
   b. Indwelling umbilical venous catheter (see Fig. 15-10):
      (1) Measure shoulder to umbilical distance and multiply by 0.75 to arrive at insertion depth, *or*
      (2) Calculate insertion depth with the formula 1.5 times body weight in kilograms plus 5.6 cm ($1.5 \times \text{weight} + 5.6$).
5. If resistance is met, withdraw the catheter 2 to 3 cm and attempt to reinsert. If cannulation remains unsuccessful, remove the catheter.
6. If cannulation is successful, connect and secure catheter and confirm position by radiograph. Correct radiographic position is 0.5 to 1 cm above the diaphragm.
7. Secure catheter per hospital policy.
8. Document procedure according to hospital policy, noting type of catheter, catheter size, distance catheter threaded, location of catheter tip on radiograph, and adjustments made to catheter to correct malpositioned catheter.

F. Complications of using umbilical catheters.

1. Vasospasm, embolism, thrombosis, distal ischemia:
   a. Blanching, cyanosis, and mottling of skin.
   b. Sloughing of skin.
   c. Necrosis of extremities.
   d. Paraplegia.
   e. Intestinal necrosis and perforation.
2. Infection.
3. Mechanical complications:
   a. Perforation of vessels.
   b. Perforation of peritoneum.
   c. False aneurysm.
   d. Knot in catheter or breaking of catheter.
4. Malpositioned catheter:
   a. Cardiac arrhythmias.
   b. Pericardial effusion.
   c. Hydrothorax.
5. Necrotizing enterocolitis (controversial).
6. Perforation of colon.
7. Hepatic necrosis.

8. Skin burns from antiseptics.
9. Hemorrhage; exsanguination.
10. Portal hypertension.
11. Death.

BLOOD SAMPLING PROCEDURES

Capillary Blood Sampling: Fundamental Procedure

A. **Indications**
  1. Small amount of blood collection is needed (<2.5 cc).
  2. Venous or arterial blood sample is not possible or necessary.
  3. Collection of blood specimen for blood gas sampling, routine laboratory sampling, state newborn metabolic screens.

B. **Contraindications.**
  1. Impaired circulation in selected limb or at puncture site.
  2. Infection near puncture site.

C. **Precautions.**
  1. Consider venipuncture if impaired skin integrity noted at selected puncture site (edema, bruising, multiple puncture marks).
  2. Hyperviscous blood may render sampling difficult. Consider venipuncture in infants with polycythemia.
  3. Use caution in infants with coagulation disorders.
  4. Avoid using the center of the heel.
  5. Avoid finger sticks.
  6. Avoid excessive squeezing that may cause hemolysis.

D. **Equipment and supplies.**
  1. Alcohol swabs or other site preparation material, as per institutional guideline.
  2. Spring-loaded lancet with tip not longer than 2.4 mm or manufactured lancets based on infant size.
  3. Sterile gauze pad.
  4. Warm compress. Caution: maximum temperature of 40° C.
  5. Nonsterile gloves.
  6. Pain management: pacifier, sucrose pacifier, and blankets for developmental swaddling.

E. **Procedure.**
  1. Select puncture site on lateral or medial aspect of the heel (Fig. 15-11). Avoid other areas due to the possibility of nerve damage or osteomyelitis.
  2. Warm heel with compress for 5 to 10 minutes to improve blood flow.
  3. Provide pain management: use spring-loaded lancets, consider venipuncture in term newborns, pacifier for nonnutritive sucking, sucrose pacifier, dim and quiet environment, skin-to-skin holding, and/or hand or blanket swaddling with selected extremity exposed.
  4. Gather supplies, wash hands, and don gloves.
  5. Prepare area selected for skin puncture with site prepping material or alcohol and allow to dry.
  6. Puncture heel perpendicular to the skin.
  7. Wipe away first drop of blood with sterile gauze pad.
  8. Collect specimen from free-flowing drops at puncture site.
     a. Blood flow is increased if the puncture site is dependent relative to the extremity.
     b. Gentle "pumping" of the extremity above the puncture site may encourage blood flow.

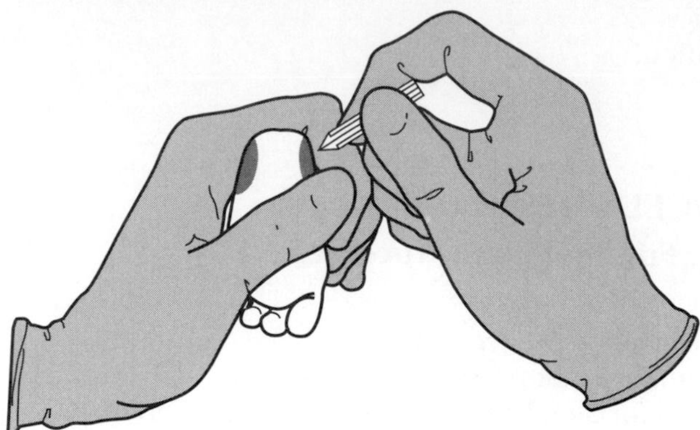

FIGURE 15-11 ■ Use shaded areas when performing heel stick in an infant. (From Gomella, T.L.: *Neonatology: Management, procedures, on-call problems, diseases, and drugs* (4th ed.). New York, 1999, Lange Medical Books/McGraw-Hill.)

9. After specimen is collected, elevate foot and apply pressure with sterile gauze pad until hemostasis has occurred.
10. Dispose of lancet in appropriate sharps container.
11. Document the heel-stick procedure, specimen obtained, date and time, nonpharmacologic interventions, and patient's tolerance.

F. Complications.

1. Bruising or loss of skin integrity.
2. Infection.
3. Scarring.
4. Calcified nodules.
5. Cellulitis.
6. Osteomyelitis.
7. Pain.
8. Erroneous laboratory values may result from the following:
   - **a.** Contamination of specimen with tissue fluid.
   - **b.** Contamination of specimen with alcohol.
   - **c.** Inadequate warming or poor circulation at puncture site.
   - **d.** Hemolysis of specimen.

Venipuncture (Phlebotomy): Fundamental Procedure

A. Indications.

1. Large quantity of blood required.
2. Arterial sample not possible or necessary.
3. Capillary sample not possible or sufficient.
4. Sterile collection for blood culture.
5. Specific laboratory tests requiring venous sampling.

B. Contraindications.

1. Inadequate or impaired circulation in selected limb.
2. Infection or loss of skin integrity near selected venipuncture site.

C. Precautions.

1. Use caution in infants with coagulation disorders.
2. Avoid sites that may be needed for possible central venous cannulation.
3. Differentiate between arteries and veins.

D. Equipment and supplies.

1. Antiseptic skin preparation per hospital policy.
2. 23- to 25-gauge butterfly needle or hypodermic needle attached to syringe.
3. Syringe(s) for specimen collection.
4. Appropriate specimen collection tubes.

5. Sterile gauze pad.
6. Tourniquet or rubber band.
7. Nonsterile gloves.
8. Pain management: pacifier, sucrose pacifier, blankets for swaddling leaving venipuncture site accessible, and/or cloth to protect eyes from bright lights.

E. **Procedure.**
1. Gather supplies, wash hands, and don gloves.
2. Choose vein to be used (see Fig. 15-3). Accomplish distention of the vessel by applying a gentle tourniquet proximal to the selected insertion site. Alternatively, an assistant may encircle the proximal extremity with his or her hand or fingers and apply direct pressure for the same effect.
3. Provide pain-relieving measures and developmentally position/swaddle with selected venipuncture site accessible.
4. Stabilize and position the selected puncture site to allow puncture in direction of blood flow.
5. Prepare skin at selected puncture site with antiseptic per hospital policy.
6. Puncture skin at a 15- to 45-degree angle, bevel up, just distal to anticipated vessel entry site, using shallow angle for smaller infants or superficial vessels.
7. Advance needle until blood appears in the tubing.
   a. If resistance is met or vessel is not punctured, withdraw needle slowly to just below level of the skin, relocate vessel, and advance the needle again.
   b. If a hematoma develops or bleeding occurs occlude the vessel with pressure just proximal to the puncture site, remove tourniquet, and withdraw needle. Apply pressure until hemostasis has occurred.
8. Upon entrance of blood into tubing, attach syringe and gently aspirate to obtain specimen. If a hypodermic needle with an intact hub was utilized, blood specimen may drip into laboratory collection container.
9. After specimen is obtained, using a gauze pad just proximal to puncture site, occlude vessel with pressure over entry site while removing tourniquet and withdrawing needle.
10. Apply pressure to site until hemostasis has occurred.
11. Dispose of needle in appropriate sharps container.
12. Document date, time, site location, specimen collected, amount of blood removed, nonpharmacologic interventions, patient's tolerance of procedure, and any complications according to hospital guidelines.

F. **Complications.**
1. Hematoma.
2. Infection.
3. Hemorrhage.
4. Needle injury to adjacent structures.
5. Pain.

Radial Artery Puncture: Advanced Practice Procedure

A. **Indications.**
1. Venous and/or capillary sites are not satisfactory.
2. Other arterial line is unavailable for sampling.
3. Arterial blood gas sampling.
4. Need to sample large quantities of blood.

B. Precautions.
1. Avoid area of infection or loss of skin integrity near selected puncture site.
2. Use caution in infants with coagulation defects.
3. Avoid puncture in extremity with inadequate or impaired circulation.
4. Consider need to preserve arterial site for possible cannulation.
5. Avoid extremity with inadequate collateral circulation distal to the selected puncture site.
6. Use of small-gauge needle reduces potential complications.

C. Equipment and supplies.
1. Antiseptic supplies to prepare for arterial puncture per hospital policy.
2. Butterfly needle 23- to 25-gauge or 23- to 25-gauge needle attached to a 3-cc syringe.
3. Extra syringes.
4. Sterile gauze pad.
5. Arterial blood gas (ABG) syringe, other applicable lab specimen containers.
6. Transilluminator (optional).

D. Procedure.
1. Determine puncture site.
   a. Transillumination may assist in vessel location.
   b. Extend wrist, do not hyperextend, which may occlude vessel (Fig. 15-12).
   c. Palpate artery at distal crease of wrist.
2. Perform modified Allen test to assess collateral circulation.
   a. Elevate hand.
   b. Massage the palm to blanch hand.
   c. Apply pressure to occlude both radial and ulnar arteries.
   d. Release pressure on ulnar artery.
   e. If color returns to hand in less than 10 seconds, adequate collateral circulation is suggested. If color returns in greater than 15 seconds, do not puncture artery due to poor collateral circulation.
   f. Doppler flow evaluation of ulnar, radial, and palmar circulation can also help determine adequacy of collateral flow.
3. Provide pain management such as pacifier for nonnutritive sucking, sucrose pacifier, and/or developmental care with facilitated tucking or blanket swaddling.
4. Position and stabilize extended wrist to allow puncture against direction of arterial flow.

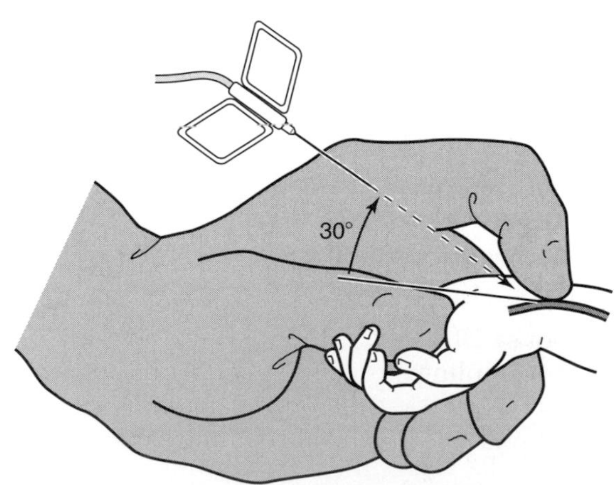

FIGURE 15-12 ■ Technique of arterial puncture in the neonate. (From Gomella, T.L.: *Neonatology: Management, procedures, on-call problems, diseases, and drugs* (4th ed.). New York, 1999, Lange Medical Books/McGraw-Hill.)

5. Prepare area with antiseptic for skin puncture (middle to outer third of wrist) per hospital policy.
6. Puncture skin with needle (bevel up) at 15- to 45-degree angle, using shallower angle for smaller infants or more superficial arteries.
7. Advance needle slowly to puncture artery.
   a. If resistance is met or blood is not obtained, withdraw needle slowly to just below skin level, palpate artery, and advance needle again in direction of artery.
   b. If hematoma or bleeding develops, occlude artery with gauze and pressure just proximal to the puncture site, withdraw needle, and apply pressure until hemostasis has occurred (approximately 5 minutes of direct pressure).
8. If arterial cannulation is successful, when blood enters the butterfly tubing, attach syringe and aspirate gently to obtain sample.
9. Apply firm, but not occlusive, pressure to artery with gauze just proximal to puncture site and withdraw needle. Apply pressure to site for 5 minutes or until hemostasis has occurred.
10. Ensure distal circulation after puncture.
    a. Evaluate color and temperature.
    b. Check capillary refill time.
    c. Palpate arterial pulse.
11. Document the following or according to hospital policy: Date, time, site location, Allen test result prior to procedure, pain management interventions, tolerance to procedure, specimen obtained, amount of blood drawn, hemostasis, distal circulation, and any complications if encountered.

E. Complications.
1. Hematoma.
2. Hemorrhage.
3. Infection.
4. Thrombosis, embolism.
5. Arteriospasm, tissue necrosis.
6. Needle injury to adjacent structures.
7. Pain.

MISCELLANEOUS PROCEDURES

Removal of Peripherally Inserted Central Catheter: Fundamental Procedure

A. Indications.
1. No longer needed or indicated.
2. Septicemia, especially fungal.
3. Malfunctioning.

B. Precautions.
1. Avoid catheter disruption.
2. Venospasm (if resistance is met, do not force catheter; apply warm compress for 20-30 minutes and reattempt).

C. Equipment and supplies.
1. Sterile gauze.
2. Measuring tape.
3. Transparent dressing.

D. Procedure.
1. Verify physician's order for removal.
2. Wash hands and don gloves.

3. Remove securing tape and dressing.
4. Gently withdraw catheter one centimeter at a time, grasping the catheter near insertion site.
5. Apply sterile gauze over insertion site as withdrawal is complete.
6. Continue to apply pressure with gauze until hemostasis is obtained. Once hemostasis is confirmed, cover site with transparent dressing.
7. Measure removed catheter and compare that distance with the recorded insertion depth.
8. Document date, time, site location, measurement of catheter removed in comparison to recorded insertion depth, patient's tolerance of procedure, and any complications according to hospital guidelines.

E. **Complications.**
1. Shearing of catheter inside patient, before complete removal.
2. Dislodgment of thrombus from tip.

Bladder Catheterization: Fundamental Procedure

A. **Indications.**
1. To obtain urine specimen/culture when suprapubic aspiration cannot be obtained.
2. To monitor urinary output.
3. To monitor bladder residuals.
4. To relieve urinary retention.
5. To accomplish genitourinary testing such as cystogram or voiding cystourethrogram.

B. **Contraindications.**
1. Anatomic malformations.

C. **Precautions.**
1. Use caution in infants with coagulation disorders.
2. Maintain aseptic technique.
3. Do not force catheter.
4. Remove catheter as soon as possible to minimize infection.
5. Use the smallest-diameter catheter to avoid trauma.
6. If using a urinary catheter with a stylet, remove stylet before insertion to minimize injury to urethra and/or bladder.
7. If Foley catheter is used, inflate the catheter per manufacturer's recommendation.

D. **Equipment and supplies**. *Note:* All equipment is sterile and is available in commercially prepared kits.
1. Urethral catheters.
   a. Size 3.5F umbilical artery catheter for infants weighing less than 1000 g may be used.
   b. Size 6F Foley catheter or 5F feeding tube for infants weighing 1000 to 1800 g.
   c. Size 8F feeding tube or Foley catheter for infants weighing greater than 1800 g.
2. Urinary catheter tray.
   a. Sterile gloves.
   b. Povidone-iodine solution swabs.
   c. Sterile drapes.
   d. Lubricant.
   e. Sterile specimen container or closed-urinary drainage system.

E. Procedure.

Male Catheterization.

1. Place infant supine and restrain legs or have assistant hold legs.
2. Don sterile gloves.
3. Clean penis:
   a. Hold the penis perpendicular to the body with the nondominant hand (which is now considered contaminated) and gently retract the foreskin (if not circumcised).
   b. Starting at the meatus and moving down the penis, clean with povidone-iodine solution swabs three times, using a new swab each time.
4. Drape sterile towels across infant's lower abdomen and across legs.
5. Apply sterile lubricant to appropriately sized catheter tip with the sterile dominant hand.
6. Place the catheter (held by the still sterile dominant hand) into the meatus while maintaining perpendicular position of the penis with the nondominant hand. Advance catheter along the urethra until urine appears. Slight resistance may be felt as the catheter passes through the external bladder sphincter. Steady, gentle pressure is usually needed to pass beyond this area; however, *never force the catheter* (Fig. 15-13).
7. Advance catheter slightly past the point where urine flow began. Inflate the balloon per hospital policy and manufacturer's recommendations, if applicable. Usually the catheter will function satisfactorily if simply taped in place. Balloon inflation may injure the urethra if the catheter is not properly positioned in the bladder.
8. If catheter is to remain indwelling, tape it to lower abdomen or to penile shaft.
9. Collect urine specimen in the sterile container and send to the laboratory or attach to a closed urinary drainage system.
10. Document procedure, catheter type and size, patient's tolerance, quantity, and characteristics of sample obtained, and any difficulties encountered.

Female Catheterization.

1. Place infant on back and secure legs in "frog-leg" position. You may secure with restraints or have an assistant hold the legs.
2. Don sterile gloves.
3. Separate the labia with nondominant hand (which is no longer sterile). With the sterile dominant hand, clean the area around the meatus with the povidone-iodine solution swabs, using front-to-back strokes, repeating with three separate swabs.

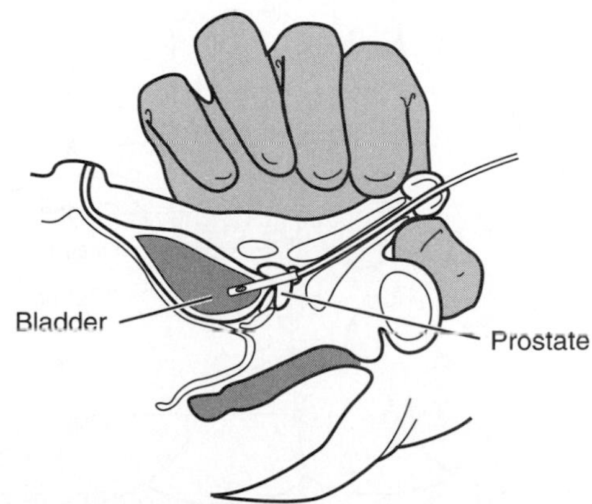

FIGURE 15-13 ■ Bladder catheterization in the male. (From Gomella, T.L.: *Neonatology: Management, procedures, on-call problems, diseases, and drugs* (4th ed.). New York, 1999, Lange Medical Books/McGraw-Hill.)

4. Drape sterile towels across infant's lower abdomen and across legs.
5. Spread the labia and identify the meatus and urethra (Fig. 15-14).
6. Apply sterile lubricant to an appropriately sized catheter tip using the sterile dominant hand.
7. Insert the catheter into the urethra and advance until urine appears.
8. Advance catheter slightly past the point where urine flow began. Inflate balloon per hospital policy and manufacturer's recommendations, if applicable. Usually the catheter will function satisfactorily if simply taped in place. Balloon inflation may injure the urethra if the catheter is not properly positioned in the bladder.
9. If catheter is to remain indwelling, secure to inner thigh.
10. Collect urine specimen in the sterile container and send to the laboratory or attach to a closed urinary drainage system.
11. Document procedure, catheter type and size, patient's tolerance, quantity, and characteristics of sample obtained, and any difficulties encountered.

F. Complications.

1. Infection.
2. Hematuria.
3. Trauma to urethra.
4. Stricture of urethra or at meatus.
5. Pain.

Bladder Aspiration: Advanced Practice Procedure

A. Indications.

1. To obtain sterile urine sample for culture.

B. Contraindications.

1. Recent void or dehydration.
2. No clinical evidence or ultrasound evidence of urine in bladder.
3. Infection or loss of skin integrity over puncture site.
4. Distention or enlargement of abdominal viscera.
5. Genitourinary anomaly or enlargement of pelvic structures.
6. Use caution in infants with coagulation disorders.
7. Acute enteropathy such as necrotizing enterocolitis (NEC).

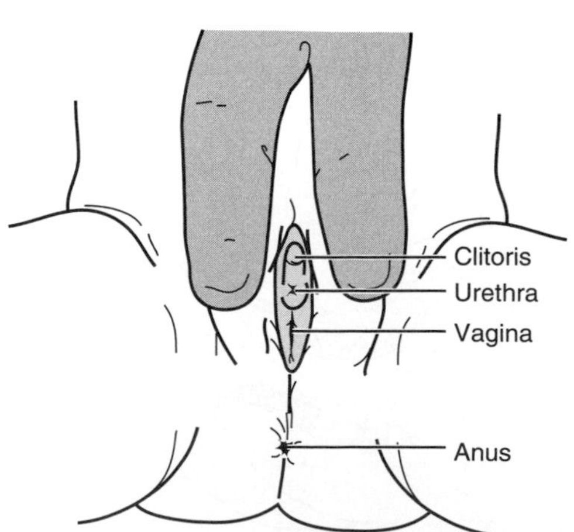

FIGURE 15-14 ■ Landmarks used in bladder catheterization in females. (From Gomella, T.L.: *Neonatology: Management, procedures, on-call problems, diseases, and drugs* (4th ed.). New York, 1999, Lange Medical Books/McGraw-Hill.)

C. Precautions.
1. Use aseptic technique.
2. Consider catheterization as an alternative for infants with coagulation defects or when previous needle aspirations were unsuccessful.
3. Avoid inserting the needle directly over the pubic bone or away from midline.
4. Aspirate using gentle suction. Too much suction can occlude the needle with the bladder mucosa preventing urine collection and increasing the risk of bladder injury.
5. Use latex precautions, if indicated (i.e., myelomeningocele, multiple surgeries).

D. Equipment and supplies. All equipment is sterile, except transillumination light or ultrasound equipment that may be covered with a sterile glove.
1. Gloves.
2. Povidone-iodine solution swabs or antiseptic per hospital policy.
3. 3-to 6-cc syringe.
4. 22- or 25-gauge with a 1- to 1½-inch needle.
5. Sterile specimen container.
6. Transillumination light or portable ultrasound (optional). Use of volumetric bladder ultrasound guidance will improve success rate.

E. Procedure.
1. Provide pain management such as pacifier for nonnutritive sucking, sucrose pacifier, and/or developmental positioning with blanket swaddling of upper extremities.
2. Determine the presence of urine in the bladder:
   a. Verify that the diaper has been dry for at least 1 hour.
   b. Transilluminate or use ultrasound guidance (optional).
   c. Consider prehydrating prior to procedure if medical condition permits.
3. Have the assistant restrain the infant in the supine frog-leg position.
4. Reflex urination may occur. Optimally, ask the assistant to pinch the base of the penis gently in a male infant.
5. Perform a 3-minute scrub and don gloves.
6. Prepare puncture site with hospital-approved antiseptic three times using separate swabs each time.
7. Locate puncture site:
   a. Palpate the symphysis pubis and locate puncture site that is approximately 1 cm above symphysis pubis.
8. Puncture bladder:
   a. Using the syringe with attached needle, maintain the needle at a 90-degree angle. Puncture skin and tissues over the bladder area and advance needle 2 to 3 cm and simultaneously aspirate with syringe. A slight decrease in resistance may be felt when the bladder is penetrated. Once urine has been obtained, do not advance the needle farther to avoid perforation of the posterior wall of the bladder.
9. Do not probe with the needle or attempt to redirect it to obtain urine.
10. Withdraw the needle if no urine is obtained and wait at least 1 hour before reattempting the procedure.
11. If urine is obtained, withdraw the needle and apply gentle pressure over the puncture site with sterile gauze.
12. Transfer urine to sterile specimen container. Send for culture and/or other diagnostic studies.

13. Dispose of needle in appropriate sharps container.
14. Document procedure, patient's tolerance, laboratory samples obtained, amount and characteristics of urine, and any pain/developmental interventions performed.

F. **Complications.**
1. Bleeding.
   a. Transient hematuria.
   b. Bladder wall hematoma.
   c. Abdominal wall hematoma.
   d. Pelvic hematoma.
2. Infection.
   a. Abdominal wall abscess.
   b. Sepsis.
   c. Osteomyelitis of pubic bone.
   d. Peritonitis.
3. Perforation of bowel or other pelvic organ.

Lumbar Puncture: Advanced Practice Procedure

A. **Indications.**
1. To obtain cerebrospinal fluid (CSF) to diagnose central nervous system (CNS) disorders such as infections or subarachnoid hemorrhage.
2. To monitor efficacy of antibiotic therapy in the presence of CNS infection (rare).
3. To drain CSF in communicating hydrocephalus associated with intracranial hemorrhage.
4. To administer medication.
5. To assist in the diagnosis of certain metabolic disorders.

B. **Contraindications.**
1. Evidence of increased intracranial pressure. Performance of the procedure could cause herniation.
2. Lumbosacral anomalies.

C. **Precautions.**
1. Avoid areas of infection or loss of skin integrity at puncture site.
2. Use caution in infants with coagulopathies.
3. Monitor for and be prepared to respond to cardiorespiratory instability.
4. Avoid flexion of the neck and ensure that a patent airway is maintained.
5. Obtain parental informed consent.
6. Always maintain aseptic technique.
7. Always use a needle with a stylet to avoid development of intraspinal epidermoid tumor.
8. To prevent traumatic tap caused by overpenetration, insert the needle slowly while removing the stylet at frequent intervals to detect CSF as soon as the subdural space is entered.
9. Never aspirate CSF with a syringe. Even a small amount of negative pressure can increase the risk of subdural hemorrhage or herniation.
10. Palpate landmarks accurately to prevent puncture above the L3 interspace.

D. **Equipment and supplies.** Prepackaged lumbar puncture kits are available, or obtain the following supplies:
1. Sterile gloves and gown, mask, and surgical cap.
2. Sterile cup with povidone-iodine or antiseptic per hospital policy.
3. Sterile gauze pads.

4. Sterile towels or transparent aperture drape.
5. Spinal needle with short bevel and stylet (20-or 22-gauge with 1-to 1½-inch needle).
6. Three or more sterile specimen tubes with caps.
7. Adhesive bandage.
8. Cardiorespiratory monitor and pulse oximeter and emergency equipment such as suction and oxygen source.
9. Analgesic agents and/or sedatives.
10. Pressure monitoring equipment, if planning to obtain CSF pressures.

E. Procedure.

1. Verify informed consent obtained.
2. Gather equipment and supplies.
3. Provide pain management such as pacifier for nonnutritive sucking or sucrose pacifier.
   a. Consider eutectic mixture of local anesthetics (EMLA) over puncture site if more than 37 weeks' gestation.
   b. Consider conscious sedation.
   c. Consider local anesthesia: 1% lidocaine drawn up in a 1-cc syringe with a 27- to 25-gauge needle for injection.
4. Examine and determine puncture site:
   a. Grasp both iliac crests at their highest points and following an imaginary line (that passes across the level of the fifth lumbar vertebra) palpate the interspace of the spinous process that falls immediately above or below the imaginary line drawn between the iliac crests.
   b. The preferred puncture site is between L3-4 and L4-5.
   c. The puncture site can be marked by making a small nail print impression, using a surgical marker, or applying a dab of iodine.
5. Don mask and cap and perform a 3-minute scrub and then don gown and sterile gloves.
6. Have an assistant open tray while maintaining the sterility of its contents.
7. Have assistant restrain the infant with hips flexed and back arched in the lateral decubitus (knee-chest) or sitting position, with spine flexed. An intubated infant must be positioned in the lateral decubitus position. Avoid flexion of the neck and ensure that a patent airway is maintained.
8. Clean the lumbar area three times with antiseptic using a new swab each time.
   a. Begin at the desired interspace, using a circular motion from puncture site outward to up and over the iliac crests.
   b. Allow antiseptic to dry.
9. If used, inject a wheal of local anesthetic at the puncture site. After several minutes, infiltrate the deeper tissues also.
10. Place one sterile drape under the infant and another that covers the patient with the exception of the puncture site and the infant's face. Transparent aperture drapes are available and recommended because they permit better observation of the infant.
11. Relocate the desired interspace and insert the needle in the midline.
    a. Angle slightly cephalad to avoid the vertebral bodies.
    b. If resistance is met, withdraw the needle slightly and redirect more cephalad.
    c. Hold a finger on the vertebral process above or below the interspace to aid in locating the puncture site if the infant moves.

12. Advance the needle slowly and in small increments (2-3 mm) to avoid puncture of posterior wall.
    a. Remove the stylet frequently to observe the needle hub for fluid. Always replace the stylet before readvancing the needle.
    b. A pop may be felt when the ligamentum flavum and dura are penetrated. Penetration of the dura may also be detected when a loss of resistance is met.
    c. Once fluid is noted in the needle hub, patiently wait for CSF, which may be slow.
13. Obtain pressure measurement reading, if desired.
    a. Opening pressure measurements are difficult and often unreliable, but possible in a quiet infant (though not in the seated position). If measuring pressure (only in the lateral decubitus position), attach the manometer and wait for the fluid oscillations to stabilize in the tube before recording the pressure. Normal values in the newborn are 7.5 to 12.5.
14. Allow CSF to collect dropwise into the collection tubes; never aspirate with a syringe.
15. If no fluid is obtained, try gently rotating the needle. If no fluid is obtained after repositioning needle, replace the stylet, remove the needle, and try one interspace above or below, using a new needle for each attempt.
16. Allow the CSF to drop from the needle hub to collect 0.5 to 1 cc aliquots of CSF in three or four of the specimen tubes for the following diagnostic studies:
    a. Tube 1: culture, Gram stain, and sensitivity studies.
    b. Tube 2: protein and glucose
    c. Tube 3: cell count and differential
    d. Tube 4: other diagnostic studies such as Venereal Disease Research Laboratory (VDRL) and/or viral studies.
    e. *Note:* If a traumatic (bloody) tap was performed, send the clearest specimen for cell count and differential. Bloody CSF can be differentiated from venous blood by dropping a sample onto filter paper. Bloody CSF will form a "water ring" around a central patch of erythrocytes.
17. Once specimens have been obtained replace stylet and remove needle/stylet unit in a single outward motion to prevent injury to the spinal cord and nerves.
18. Apply local pressure to the puncture site for 3 to 5 minutes to minimize the risk of CSF leakage. Then place an adhesive bandage over the puncture site.
19. Remove the surrounding antiseptic with sterile water to avoid skin injury.
20. Document procedure according to hospital policy noting position of the patient during procedure, needle size used, complications or difficulties encountered, CSF characteristics, pain management interventions, patient's tolerance, and specimens sent to laboratory for analysis.

F. Complications.

1. Infection from nonsterile conditions:
    a. Use of poor sterile technique.
    b. Bacteremia if blood vessel puncture during procedure, having passed through infected CSF.
2. Intraspinal epidermoid tumor from lack of stylet use.
3. Spinal cord and/or nerve damage if puncture performed above L3.
4. Cerebral herniation.
5. Apnea and/or bradycardia.

6. Hypoxia.
7. Spinal cord or epidural abscess.
8. Spinal fluid leakage into epidural space.
9. Vertebral body osteomyelitis.
10. Persistent bleeding, especially in patients with an underlying coagulopathy.
11. Pain.

REFERENCES

American Heart Association: *Textbook of neonatal resuscitation*. Dallas, TX, 2000.

American Society of Health-System Pharmacists (August, 2002): *Hyaluronidase Injection—discontinued*. Retrieved online on March 5, 2003 at www.ashp.org/shortage/hyaluronidase.cfm

Askin, D.F.: *Acute respiratory care of the neonate* (2nd ed.). Petaluma, CA, 1997, NICU Ink.

Blackwood, B.: Normal saline instillation with endotracheal suctioning: Primum non nocere (first do no harm). *Journal of Advanced Nursing, 29*(4):928-934, 1999.

Carbine, D., Finer, N.N., Knodel, E., and Rich, W.: Video recording as a means of evaluating neonatal resuscitation performance. *Pediatrics, 106*(4): 654-658, 2000.

Clark, C., Prieur, B., Ramirez, A., et al.: Reduction in the incidence of chronic lung disease following the implementation of a lung protective delivery room management strategy (July, 2003). *Respiratory Abstracts*. Retrieved online on September 13, 2003 at www.cardinal.com/mps/focus/respiratory/ab2002/of%202002%20group%207/of-02-053.asp.

Cloherty, J.P. and Stark, A.R.: *Manual of neonatal care* (4th ed.). Philadelphia, 1998, Lippincott-Raven.

Cordero, L., Sananes, M., and Ayers, L.: A comparison of two airway suctioning frequencies in mechanically ventilated, very low birth weight infants. *Respiratory Care, 46*(8):783-788, 2001.

Evans, M. and Lentsch, D.: Percutaneously inserted polyurethane central catheters in the NICU: One unit's experience. *Neonatal Network, 18*(6):37-44, 1999.

Finer, N.N. and Rich, W.: Neonatal resuscitation: Toward improved performance. *Resuscitation, 53*(1):47-51, 2002.

Finer, N.N., Rich, W., Craft, A., and Henderson, C.: Comparison of methods of bag and mask ventilation for neonatal resuscitation. *Resuscitation, 49*(3):299-305, 2001.

Fioravanti, J., Buzzard, C.J., and Harris, J.P.: Pericardial effusion and tamponade as a result of percutaneous Silastic catheter use. *Neonatal Network, 17*(5):39-42, 1998.

Gomella, T.L.: *Neonatology: Management, procedures, on-call problems, diseases, and drugs* (4th ed.). New York, 1999, Lange Medical Books/McGraw-Hill.

Green, C. and Yohannan, M.D: Umbilical arterial and venous catheters: Placement, use and complications. *Neonatal Network, 17*(6):23-27, 1998.

Hanrahan, K.S., Kleiber, C., and Berends, S.: Saline for peripheral intravenous locks in neontates: Evaluating a change in practice. *Neonatal Network, 19*(2):19-24, 2000.

Johnson, N., Deakins, K., Chatburn, R., and Myers, T.: Evaluation of manual ventilation using the Neopuff infant resuscitator during transport of the premature infant (July, 2003). *Respiratory Abstracts*. Retrieved online on September 13, 2003 at www.cardinal.com/mps/focus/respiratory/ab2001/a00000228.asp.

Kiechl-Kohlendorfer, U., Unsinn, K.M., Schlenck, B., et al.: Cerebrospinal fluid leakage after lumbar puncture in neonates: Incidence and sonographic appearance. *American Journal of Roentgenology, 181*(1):231-234, 2003.

Kinloch, D.: Instillation of normal saline during endotracheal suctioning: Effects on mixed venous saturation. *American Journal of Critical Care, 8*(4):231-239, 1999.

Klein C.: *The neonatal and pediatric workshop manual*. San Antonio, 1998, Klein Baker Medical.

MacDonald, M.G. and Ramasethu, J. (Eds.): *Atlas of procedures in neonatology* (3rd ed.). Philadelphia, 2002, Lippincott Williams & Wilkins.

Meehan, R.M.: Heelsticks in neonates for capillary blood sampling. *Neonatal Network, 17*(1):17-24, 1998.

Munir, V. Barnett, P., and South, M.: Does the use of volumetric bladder ultrasound improve the success rate of suprapubic aspiration of urine? *Pediatric Emergency Care, 18*(5):346-349, 2002.

Newborn Section Department of Pediatrics: *Guidelines for the acute care of the neonate.* Houston, TX, 2001, Baylor College of Medicine.

O'Brien Pharmacy (2001). *Hyaluronidase.* Retrieved online on March, 5, 2003, at www.obrienrx.com/o_brien_pharm/sterile/hyaluronidase/index.html

Page, N.E., Giehl, M., and Luḱe, S.: Intubation complications in the critically ill child. *AACN Clinical Issues, 9*(1):25-35, 1998.

Paisley, M.K., Stamper, M., and Brown, J.: The use of heparin and normal saline flushes in neonatal intravenous catheters. *Pediatric Nursing, 23*(5): 521-524, 1997.

Park, J.C., Chung, C.K., and Kim, H.J.: Iatrogenic spinal epidermoid tumor. A complication of spinal puncture in an adult. *Clinical Neurology and Neurosurgery, 105*(4):281-285, 2003.

Repetto, J.E., Donohue, P.K., Baker, S.F., et al.: Use of capnography in the delivery room for assessment of endotracheal tube placement. *Journal of Perinatology, 21*(5):284-287, 2001.

Roos, Ḱ.L.: Lumbar puncture. *Seminars in Neurology, 12*(1):105-114, 2003.

Roth, B. and Lundberg, D.: Disposable CO_2-detector: A reliable tool for determination of correct tracheal tube positioning during resuscitation of a neonate. *Resuscitation, 35*(2):149-150, 1997.

Smith, A.B. and Adams, L.L.: Insertion of indwelling urethral catheters in infants and children: A survey of current nursing practice. *Pediatric Nursing, 24*(3):229-234, 1998.

Squire, S.S., Harnung, T.L., and Kirchoff, K.T.: Comparing two methods of umbilical arterial catheter placement. *American Journal of Perinatology, 7*(1):8-12, 1990.

Trotter, C. and Carey, B.E. (Eds.): Tearing and embolization of percutaneous central venous catheters. *Neonatal Network, 17*(3):67-70, 1998.

Wrightson, D.D.: Suctioning smarter: Answers to eight common questions about endotracheal suctioning in neonates. *Neonatal Network, 18*(1):51-54, 1999.

Zenk, K.E., Sills, J.H., and Koeppel, R.M.: *Neonatal medications & nutrition* (2nd ed.). Santa Rosa, CA, 2000, NICU Ink.

CHAPTER

16 Pain Assessment and Management

MARLENE WALDEN

OBJECTIVES

1. Review the physiology of acute pain in preterm neonates.
2. Discuss current standards for assessing and managing pain in neonates.
3. Identify behavioral and physiologic responses that are indicative of pain in the neonate.
4. Select a valid and reliable composite measure for assessment of pain in neonates.
5. Discuss the evidence base for nonpharmacologic and pharmacologic approaches to the management of pain in neonates.

Since the mid-1980s, caregivers in neonatal intensive care have become more aware of the need to treat pain in neonates. Previously it was believed that infants did not experience pain because the level of myelinization prevented reception of pain. It was also believed that infants have no memory of painful procedures and that pharmacologic agents to control pain might be dangerous to the developing neonate, so that the risks would outweigh the benefits. Numerous researchers have since demonstrated that neonates are mature enough for pain perception and to have memory of painful procedures (Andrews and Fitzgerald, 1994; Craig et al., 1993; Franck, 1987; Stevens et al., 1994, 1995). Progress has been made in identifying pain in the neonate and interventions to alleviate neonatal pain. This chapter will review pain pathways, identification of pain, and interventions to alleviate pain in the neonate.

DEFINITION OF PAIN

The International Association for the Study of Pain (IASP) defines pain as "unpleasant sensory and emotional experience associated with actual or potential tissue damage, or described in terms of such damage" (1979, p. 250). The IASP definition implies that the meaning of pain must be learned through experience and articulated within the context of verbal language. This conceptualization of pain perpetuates the misconceptions that infants, who lack linguistic skills, do not experience pain (Anand and Craig, 1996). In neonates, physiologic, behavioral, and hormonal indicators provide objective and quantifiable information about the location, intensity, and duration of painful stimuli. These responses can be used in conjunction with other contextual indicators to infer the existence of pain.

NEONATAL INTENSIVE CARE UNIT (NICU) PROCEDURES THAT CAUSE PAIN

A. **Many activities and interventions in the NICU cause pain.** The most frequently occurring painful procedures include endotracheal suctioning and intubation, peripheral venous catheter insertion, and heel sticks (Barker and Rutter, 1995).

B. **Research evaluating invasive procedures in NICUs found frequency of invasive procedures was inversely related to gestational age and severity of illness** (Barker and Rutter, 1995; Porter et al., 1999; Stevens et al., 1999). Therefore, the smaller and sicker neonates are those subject to the greatest numbers of most painful procedures.
   1. In a study by Barker and Rutter (1995), one 23-week gestation, 560-g infant had 488 painful intrusive procedures performed during her hospital stay.
   2. Stevens and colleagues (1999) found that infants born between 27 and 31 weeks' gestation received on average a mean of 134 painful procedures within the first 2 weeks of life and approximately 10% of the youngest or sickest infants received more than 300 painful procedures.
   3. Porter and colleagues (1999) found that preterm infants experienced, on average, more than 700 painful procedures during their hospitalization. These procedures were characterized as mildly (insertion of gavage tube, umbilical arterial catheter insertion), moderately (heel sticks, venipunctures), or highly invasive (lumbar punctures, circumcision).

C. The International Evidence-Based Group for Neonatal Pain provides guidelines for preventing and treating neonatal procedural pain (Anand and International Evidence-Based Group for Neonatal Pain, 2001).

PHYSIOLOGY OF ACUTE PAIN IN PRETERM NEONATES

A. **An understanding of the physiology of acute pain in preterm neonates is essential to optimal pain management in the NICU.** Pain responses exhibited by neonates are the result of a concurrent set of reactions within the peripheral nervous system, spinal cord, and higher centers involved at the supraspinal/integrative level including the thalamus and cerebral cortex (Melzack, 1996).
   1. Peripheral nervous system (Evans, 2001).
      a. Fully mature and functional by 20 weeks' gestation
      b. Consists of two types of neuronal afferent fibers.
         (1) A-delta fibers: thinly myelinated, rapid-conducting fibers associated with sharp pain or "first pain" (e.g., sharp, localized, pricking).
         (2) C fibers: polymodal, unmyelinated, slow-conducting fibers associated with aching, burning, poorly localized, or "second pain."
      c. Density of nociceptors is equal to or greater than those in adult skin.
      d. Local tissue injury such as heel stick or venipuncture activates nociceptors of sensory afferent fibers to:
         (1) Transmit pain impulses to spinal cord and central nervous system (CNS).
         (2) Release biochemical mediators such as substance P and prostaglandins that results in *hyperalgesia* (increased sensitivity to painful stimuli) or *allodynia* (pain caused by a stimulus that ordinarily does not cause pain). This decreased pain threshold may persist for days or weeks.
         (3) Cause dendritic sprouting and hyperinnervation that results in hypersensitivity and lower pain threshold that may persist into adulthood.

2. Spinal cord (Evans, 2001).
   a. During the first postnatal week, weak linkages exist between peripheral nervous system and dorsal horn, resulting in either prolonged pain responses or no reaction to the painful stimuli.
   b. Receptive fields of the dorsal horn cells are larger than those of adults and begin to diminish 2 weeks after birth.
   c. Local spinal cord response to pain impulses from peripheral afferent fibers stimulate efferent somatomotor neurons in the anterior horn and produce reflex withdrawal.
   d. Afferent fiber neurotransmitters stimulate *N*-methyl-D-aspartate and tachykinin receptors in the dorsal horns, producing central sensitization (increased excitability of dorsal horn neurons that spreads to several adjacent segments of the spinal cord), "windup" (perceived increase in intensity or duration of painful stimuli), or secondary hyperalgesia (hypersensitivity elicited by both painful and nonpainful stimuli that extends to areas beyond the site of injury).
   e. Increases in autonomic responses such as heart rate and respiratory rate and facial responses such as brow bulge, eye squeeze, and nasolabial furrow in response to heel-stick procedures provide evidence of maturity of ascending pathways by 20 weeks of gestation.
   f. Preterm infants have a limited ability to modulate pain. Dopamine and norepinephrine are not available to modulate pain before 36 to 40 weeks of gestation. Serotonin is first released at approximately 6 to 8 weeks after birth.
3. Supraspinal/integrative level (Evans, 2001).
   a. Cerebral cortex has a full complement of neurons by 20 weeks of gestation.
   b. Cerebral cortex is functionally mature by 22 weeks of gestation and bilaterally synchronous by 27 weeks of gestation.
   c. Somatosensory-evoked potentials are slow and simple before 29 weeks of gestation, but short and complex by 40 weeks of gestation.
   d. Cortical cell migration is complete at approximately 24 weeks of gestation. However, the support structure of the germinal matrix remains highly vascular until 28 weeks. Therefore the neonate is vulnerable to intraventricular hemorrhage related to increases in blood pressure associated with pain.
   e. Maximum number of cortical neurons is reached at 28 weeks of gestation, and then approximately 70% cortical neurons are lost before birth through apoptosis.
   f. Neonates as early as 27 weeks' gestation can differentiate touch (sham heel stick from a noxious stimuli (heel stick) as evidenced by physiologic and facial response patterns.
   g. Neurologic connections are in place for the perception of, reaction to, and memory of pain on the cortical level as evidenced by mature visual and auditory response patterns on electroencephalogram in infants younger than 30 weeks' gestation and by measurements of in vivo cerebral glucose in the sensory areas of the brain.

B. Repetitive, unrelieved pain can lead to serious and adverse consequences for neonates (Anand and Hickey, 1987, 1992; Evans, 2001; Fitzgerald and Shortland, 1988).

1. Short-term physiologic consequences of painful procedures include decreased oxygen saturations and increased heart rates that can place

increased demands on the cardiorespiratory system (Craig et al., 1993; McIntosh et al., 1994; Stevens and Johnston, 1994; Stevens et al., 1993).

2. Pain can cause elevation in intracranial pressure, thereby increasing risk of intraventricular hemorrhage in preterm neonates (Anand et al., 1999; Evans, 2001; Stevens and Johnston, 1994; Stevens et al., 1993).
3. Pain and stress may also depress the immune system and contribute to increased susceptibility of neonates to infections (Evans, 2001).
4. Long-term consequences of repeated painful procedures include decreased sensitivity to the commonplace pain of childhood, higher incidence of somatic complaints and somatization of unspecified origin, and long-term structural changes in the brain and spinal cord (Evans, 2001; Fitzgerald and Shortland, 1988; Grunau et al., 1994).

STANDARDS OF PRACTICE

A. **Recognition of the widespread inadequacy of pain management promoted various professional and accrediting organizations to issue position statements and clinical recommendations in an effort to promote effective pain management in undertreated populations.** Organizations that support the importance of optimal pain assessment and management in hospitalized neonates include the National Association of Neonatal Nurses (Walden, 2001), the Association of Women's Health, Obstetric, and Neonatal Nurses (1995), the American Academy of Pediatrics/Canadian Paediatric Society (2000), and the Joint Commission on Accreditation of Healthcare Organizations (JCAHO, 1999). There is considerable consistency in the recommendations set by these various professional and accrediting organizations. Core principles contained within these guidelines and standards that are applicable to pain assessment and management in the NICU include:
   1. Education and competency assessment in pain assessment and management of new and current employees.
   2. Regular assessment and reassessment of pain using a valid and reliable multidimensional pain assessment instrument.
   3. Use both nonpharmacologic and pharmacologic approaches to prevent and/or manage pain.
   4. Health care team members should collaborate together and with the infant's family in developing an approach to pain assessment and management.
   5. Documentation should facilitate regular reassessment and follow-up intervention.
   6. Policies and procedures should be established to provide consistency and quality of pain assessment and management practices.
   7. Data should be collected to monitor the appropriateness and effectiveness of pain management practices.

B. The clinical challenge remains on how to implement these standards in various institutional settings based on patient types, frequently occurring clinical procedures performed, and current staffing patterns.

PAIN ASSESSMENT

A. **Pain assessment has been advocated as the "fifth vital sign" and should be assessed routinely (American Pain Society, 1995).**

B. **"The 'golden rule' of pain assessment must be:** What is painful to an adult is painful to an infant until proven otherwise" (Franck, 1989). This rule, along with the use of valid and reliable tools, must be used for the assessment and intervention of pain.
C. **Pain behaviors versus irritability/agitation behaviors.** Pain is often evaluated as irritability and agitation. These indicators are similar but can be distinguished from those of pain. Indicators that are similar and yet distinct are shown in Table 16-1.
D. **Because previous painful experiences may modify pain expression,** further research is needed to develop and test an instrument to assess chronic pain in the infant requiring prolonged hospitalization who has been subjected to multiple painful clinical procedures.
E. **Pain assessment is an essential prerequisite to optimal pain management.**
F. **Behavioral responses.**
   1. Facial activity offers the most specificity as an indicator of pain, namely brow bulge, eye squeeze, and nasolabial furrow (Grunau and Craig, 1987; Grunau et al., 1990; Stevens et al., 1993).

■ TABLE 16-1
■ ■ **Pain vs. Irritable Behaviors**

	Pain Behavior	Irritable Behavior
Cry	Sudden, high pitched	Whining
Facial expression	Grimace, lowered brows, eyes shut tight, furrowing of brow, open lips, quivering of chin	Frown, gaze aversion, worried faces
Motor response	Withdrawal, swiping, thrashing, increased tone, decreased tone	Rigid posture: arching, flailing of extremities, random head and body movement, tremulous
Complex response	Sleep/wake cycle changes: wakeful, increased irritability, listlessness, change in activity level, feeding difficulties, bonding interruption	Easily aroused, fuss/cry interchangeable, high level of persistence, ineffective in self-consoling, hyperalert
Physiologic	Increased HR up to 30%, increased RR up to 30%, increased BP up to 30%; shallow respiration, pallor, flushing, diaphoresis, palmar sweating, decreased transcutaneous Po_2, dilated pupils	Increased HR and BP with activity only, duskiness only after prolonged, transcutaneous Po_2 decreases after prolonged, no diaphoresis, increased respiratory rate and effort
Hormonal/metabolic	Decreased insulin secretion and thus hyperglycemia; increased catecholamines, cortisol levels, glucagon, aldosterone; decreased fat, protein, carbohydrate stores	

HR, Heart rate; *RR,* respiratory rate; *BP,* blood pressure.
Data from Agarwal R., Hagedorn, M.I., and Gardner, S.L.: Pain and pain relief. In G.B. Merenstein and S.L. Gardner (Eds.). *Handbook of neonatal intensive care* (4th ed.). St. Louis, 1998, Mosby, pp. 173-196: Shapiro, C.: Pain in the neonate: Assessment and intervention. *Neonatal Network, 8*(1):7-19, 1989; Broome, M.E., and Tanzillo, H.: Differentiating between pain and agitation in premature neonates. *Journal of Perinatal and Neonatal Nursing, 4*(1):53-62, 1990; and Craig, K.D., Whitfield, M.F., Grunau, R., et. al.: Pain in the preterm neonate: Behavioral and physiological indices. *Pain, 52*(3):287-299, 1993.

2. Acoustical and temporal characteristics of pain cries have been demonstrated to be different than other cry types in both preterm and full-term infants. Increases in peak fundamental frequency (pitch), peak spectral energy, cry duration, and intensity are reported features (Fuller, 1991; Grunau and Craig, 1987; Grunau et al., 1990; Levine and Gordon, 1982; Porter et al., 1986; Stevens et al., 1993; Stevens et al., 1994).
3. Many preterm infants do not cry in response to a noxious stimulus. The absence of response may only indicate the depletion of response capability and not lack of pain perception (Johnston et al., 1995; Johnston et al., 1999; Stevens et al., 1993; Stevens et al., 1994).
4. Healthy full-term newborns use swiping motions by the unaffected leg to the lanced foot, as if trying to push away the noxious stimulus (Franck, 1986).
5. Preterm infants demonstrate an increase in motor extension patterns, including finger play, saluting, and sitting on air during painful clinical procedures. These hyperextension motor patterns are quickly replaced with flaccidity in infants at younger postconceptional ages.

G. **Physiologic responses.**

1. Preterm infants respond to noxious stimuli in patterns similar to that of full-term neonates, including increases in heart rate (Craig et al., 1993; McIntosh et al., 1994; Stevens and Johnston, 1994; Stevens et al., 1993) and decreases in oxygen saturation (Craig et al., 1993; Stevens and Johnston, 1994; Stevens et al., 1993).
2. While physiologic measures provide greater objectivity in the assessment of pain, they also reflect the body's nonspecific response to stress and thus are not specific to pain (Barr, 1992; Gunnar et al., 1988). Therefore physiologic measures should be converged with behavioral measures that have been demonstrated to be more consistent and specific to pain in neonates (Craig et al., 1993; Grunau and Craig, 1987; Johnston et al., 1993; Walden, 2001).
3. Physiologic measures should be used to assess pain in infants who are paralyzed for mechanical ventilation or who are severely neurologically impaired (Walden, 2001).

H. **Contextual factors modifying pain responses.**

1. Developmental maturity, health status, and environmental factors may all contribute to an inconsistent, less robust pattern of pain responses between infants and even within the same infant over time and situations (Craig et al., 1993; Johnston et al., 1993; Shapiro, 1993). Therefore contextual factors that have been demonstrated to modify the pain experience must be considered when assessing for the presence of pain in neonates (Walden, 2001).
2. Infants in awake or alert states demonstrate a more robust reaction to painful stimuli than infants in sleep states (Grunau and Craig; 1987; Johnston et al., 1999; Stevens and Johnston, 1994; Stevens et al., 1996).
3. Research examining facial as well as bodily activity has demonstrated that the magnitude of infant response has been observed to be less vigorous and robust with decreasing postconceptional age (Craig et al., 1993; Johnston et al., 1995; Johnston et al., 1999). Craig and colleagues (1993) suggest that the less vigorous responses demonstrated by preterm infants "should be interpreted in the context of the energy resources available to respond and the relative immaturity of the musculoskeletal system" (p. 296).
4. Less mature behavioral responses to noxious stimuli are noted as the total number of invasive procedures that a preterm infant encounters increases with advancing postnatal age (Johnston and Stevens, 1996).

5. Postnatal age at time of study, postconceptional age at birth, time since last painful procedure, and behavioral state predict lack of response to a heel-stick procedure in preterm neonates (Johnston et al., 1999).
6. When pain stimuli or pain persists for hours or days without intervention, the infant exhibits a decompensatory response. The sympathetic nervous system, or the "fight or flight" mechanism, can no longer compensate. As a result, the physiologic parameters return to baseline (Shapiro, 1989). "Return to baseline" does not indicate that pain is no longer felt or is tolerated, but it does make the infant's pain more difficult to evaluate.

PAIN ASSESSMENT INSTRUMENTS

A. **Select a composite or multidimensional instrument that incorporates both physiologic and behavioral measures of pain.** Caregivers should select instruments with known reliability and validity. Aspects of clinical utility and feasibility should also be considered (Walden, 2001).

B. **CRIES:** a postoperative pain tool (Table 16-2) (Krechel and Bildner, 1995).
   1. Acronym for five behavioral and physiologic parameters: C = crying; R = requires oxygen to maintain saturation at greater than 95%; I = increased vital signs; E = expression; and S = sleeplessness.
   2. Demonstrates validity and interrater reliability for use in infants born at 32 weeks' gestation and later. Beginning establishment of clinical utility.
   3. Tool scoring system, 0 to 10, is structured in the same fashion as the Apgar score and was designed to make the tool easy to use and remember.
   4. Score is used postoperatively.
   5. Pain is assessed hourly for a period of not less than 24 hours. A score of 4 or above indicates pain, and any assessment of 4 or above should receive pain intervention. The neonate should then be reevaluated 15 to 30 minutes after analgesia to assess for pain relief.

C. **The Premature Infant Pain Profile (PIPP) (Stevens et al., 1996) (Table 16-3).**
   1. Seven-item, four-point scale for assessment of pain in premature infants through term gestation. The stimuli for the studies were handling, heel stick, and circumcision.
   2. Multidimensional: includes heart rate, oxygen saturation, brow bulge, eye squeeze, and nasolabial furrow.
   3. Unique in that it includes two contextual modifiers (e.g., gestational age and behavioral state).
   4. Good establishment of reliability and validity. Beginning establishment of clinical utility.
   5. Total pain score of 7 to 12 indicates mild pain and infant may benefit from use of nonpharmacologic comfort measures. Total pain score greater than 12 indicates moderate to severe pain and will most likely require pharmacologic intervention in conjunction with comfort measures.

D. **Neonatal Infant Pain Scale (NIPS) (Lawrence et al., 1993) (Fig. 16-1).**
   1. Six-item scale. Five behavioral items (facial expression, crying, arms, legs, and state of arousal) and one physiologic indicator (breathing pattern). Each behavior except cry has descriptors for the two possible scores of 0 and 1. Cry is scored on a three-point scale (0, 1, 2).
   2. Tested in preterm and full-term neonates who required capillary, venous, or arterial punctures.
   3. Total score can range from 0 to 7.

■ TABLE 16-2
■ ■ **CRIES: Neonatal Postoperative Pain Measurement Score**

	Score			
	0	**1**	**2**	**Tips for Scoring CRIES**
***C*rying**	No	High pitched	Inconsolable	Score 0: no cry or cry not high pitched Score 1: cry high pitched, but consolable Score 2: high-pitched cry, inconsolable
***R*equires O_2 for saturation >95%**	No	<30%	>30%	Score 0: no oxygen required from baseline Score 1: oxygen requirement <30% from baseline Score 2: oxygen requirement >30% from baseline
***I*ncreased vital signs**	HR and BP ≤ preoperative values	HR or BP ↑ <20% of preoperative values	HR or BP ↑ >20% of preoperative values	Score 0: HR and BP are both unchanged or at less than baseline Score 1: HR or BP is increased by <20% Score 2: HR or BP is increased by >20% *Note:* Measure BP last so as not to wake the infant.
***E*xpression**	None	Grimace	Grimace/grunt	Score 0: no grimace Score 1: grimace only is present Score 2: grimace and nonaudible grunt present *Note:* Grimace consists of lowered brow, eyes squeezed shut, deepening nasolabial furrow, and open lips and mouth.
***S*leepless**	No	Wakes at frequent intervals	Constantly awake	Score 0: continuously asleep Score 1: awakens at frequent intervals Score 2: awake constantly *Note:* Based on infant's state during previous hour.

BP, Blood pressure; *HR,* heart rate.
Neonatal pain assessment tool developed at the University of Missouri–Columbia.
From Krechel, S. and Bildner, J.: CRIES: A new neonatal post-operative pain measurement score: Initial testing of validity and reliability. *Paediatric Anaesthesia, 5*(1):53-61, 1995.

NURSING CARE OF THE INFANT IN PAIN

Skilled observation, assessments, and interventions are the responsibility of the care providers. Pain intervention may be provided by both nonpharmacologic and pharmacologic methods.

■ TABLE 16-3
■ ■ **Premature Infant Pain Profile**

Infant Study Number: ____________________
Date/time: ____________________
Event: ____________________

Process	Indicator	0	1	2	3	Score
Chart	Gestational age	36 weeks and more	32-35 weeks, 6 days	28-31 weeks, 6 days	Less than 28 weeks	
Observe infant 15 s	Behavioral state	Active/awake eyes open facial movements	Quiet/awake eyes open no facial movements	Active/sleep eyes closed facial movements	Quiet/sleep eyes closed no facial movements	
Observe baseline Heart rate _____	Heart rate Max _____	0-4 beats/min increase	5-14 beats/min increase	15-24 beats/min increase	25 beats/min or more increase	
Oxygen saturation _____	Oxygen saturation Min _____	0%-2.4% decrease	2.5%-4.9% decrease	5%-7.4% decrease	7.5% or more decrease	
Observe infant 30 s	Brow bulge	None 0%-9% of time	Minimum 10%-39% of time	Moderate 40%-69% of time	Maximum 70% of time or more	
	Eye squeeze	None 0%-9% of time	Minimum 10%-39% of time	Moderate 40%-69% of time	Maximum 70% of time or more	
	Nasolabial furrow	None 0%-9% of time	Minimum 10%-39% of time	Moderate 40%-69% of time	Maximum 70% of time or more	
					Total score _____	

From Stevens, B., Johnston, C., Petryshen, P., and Taddio, A.: Premature infant pain profile: Development and initial validation. *Clinical Journal of Pain, 12*(1):13-22, 1996.

A. Nonpharmacologic approaches to pain management.

1. Goals.
   a. To help minimize pain and stress while maximizing the infant's ability to cope with and recover from clinical procedures.
   b. To provide additive or synergistic benefits to pharmacologic therapy (Franck and Lawhon, 1998, 2000).
2. Preventive measures.
   a. Reduce the total number of painful procedures to which the infant is exposed by (Franck and Lawhon, 1998, 2000; Walden, 2001):
      (1) Evaluating all aspects of caregiving.
      (2) Evaluating the number and grouping of laboratory and diagnostic procedures.
      (3) Scheduling clinical procedures based on medical necessity versus a routine schedule.
   b. Use environmental interventions such as reduced lighting and noise levels to minimize infant stress (Anand and International Evidence-Based Group for Neonatal Pain, 2001; Franck and Lawhon, 2000; Walden, 2001).

	Before Time		During Time					After Time		
	1	2	1	2	3	4	5	1	2	3
Facial expression 0—Relaxed 1—Grimace										
Cry 0—No cry 1—Whimper 2—Vigorous										
Breathing patterns 0—Relaxed 1—Change in breathing										
Arms 0—Relaxed/restrained 1—Flexed/extended										
Legs 0—Relaxed/restrained 1—Flexed/extended										
State of arousal 0—Sleeping/awake 1—Fussy										
Total										

Note: Time is measured in 1-minute intervals.

FIGURE 16-1 ■ Neonatal Infant Pain Scale. (From Lawrence, J., Alcock, D., McGrath, P., et al.: The development of a tool to assess neonatal pain. *Neonatal Network, 12*[6]:59-66, 1993.)

3. Behavioral measures.
   a. Facilitated tucking (hand-swaddling technique that holds the infant's extremities flexed and contained close to the trunk). When implemented prior to the heel-stick procedure, this technique reduces pain responses in preterm neonates as young as 25 weeks' gestational age (Corff et al., 1995).
      (1) Preterm infants in the post–heel-stick recovery phase demonstrated significantly reduced heart rates and crying and more stability in sleep/wake cycles in the hand-swaddled position.
   b. Blanket swaddling following a painful procedure may help reduce infant physiologic and behavioral distress in the post–heel-stick recovery phase for older preterm infants (postconceptional age ≥31 weeks) (Fearon et al., 1997).
   c. Pacifiers ranked by NICU nurses as the first choice of pain intervention (Franck, 1987).
      (1) Nonnutritive sucking (NNS) is thought to modulate the transmission or processing of nociception through mediation by the endogenous nonopioid system (Blass et al., 1987; Gunnar et al., 1988).
      (2) The efficacy of NNS is immediate but appears to terminate almost immediately upon cessation of sucking.
      (3) NNS has been shown to reduce composite pain responses in preterm infants during heel sticks (Stevens et al., 1999).
      (4) Pain relief is greater in infants who receive both NNS and sucrose.

(5) NNS reduced the duration of cry and soothed infants more rapidly when compared with blanket swaddling (Campos, 1989) or rocking (Campos, 1994) during painful procedures.

d. Studies demonstrate that a single 2-ml dose of 0.24 to 0.50 g (12%-25%) sucrose given orally approximately 2 minutes before painful stimulus is associated with statistically and clinically significant reductions in crying after a painful stimulus (Stevens et al., 1997).

(1) Interval coincides with endogenous opioid release triggered by the sweet taste of sucrose (Stevens et al., 1999).

(2) Smaller doses of sucrose (as little as 0.05 ml) are shown effective in decreasing the percent of occurrence of facial expressions of pain when administered in either single or triple oral applications to preterm neonates between 25 and 34 weeks' gestation (Johnston et al., 1997; Stevens et al., 2000).

(3) Safety of implementing repeated doses of sucrose in very low birth weight infants has not been confirmed; therefore caution is advised before widespread use of repeated doses in preterm and critically ill neonates (Walden, 2001).

(4) In a recent study, no immediate adverse effects when administering a 24% sucrose-dipped pacifier during four random, consecutively administered routine heel-stick procedures were noted (Stevens et al., 1999).

B. Pharmacologic approaches to pain management.

1. Pharmacologic approaches to pain management should be used when moderate, severe, or prolonged pain is assessed or anticipated (U.S. Department of Health and Human Services, 1992).

2. Intravenous opioids remain the most common class of analgesics administered in the NICU, particularly that of morphine sulfate and fentanyl citrate (Franck and Miaskowski, 1998).

a. Systemic opioids induce analgesia by acting at various levels of the CNS (Deshpande and Anand, 1996).

(1) Spinal cord. Opioids impair or inhibit the transmission of nociceptive input from the periphery to the CNS.

(2) Basal ganglia. Opioids activate a descending inhibitory system.

(3) Limbic system. Opioids alter the emotional response to pain, making it more tolerable.

b. Special considerations in neonates are as follows:

(1) Longer dosing intervals are often required in neonates less than 1 month of age due to longer elimination half-lives and delayed clearance of opioids as compared with adults or children greater than 1 year of age (Franck and Miaskowski, 1998).

(2) Neonates should be monitored closely during opioid therapy and for several hours after opioids have been discontinued because enterohepatic recirculation in preterm and full-term neonates may result in higher plasma concentrations of opioids for longer periods as compared with older children (Franck and Miaskowski, 1998).

(3) Due to immature descending pain pathways, preterm infants may require significantly higher opioid concentrations to achieve adequate analgesia as compared with older children (Evans, 2001; Franck and Miaskowski, 1998).

(4) Efficacy of opioid therapy should be assessed using a valid and reliable neonatal pain scale (Walden, 2001).

(5) Opioid-induced cardiorespiratory side effects in neonates are uncommon (Farrington et al., 1993; Franck and Miaskowski, 1998; Koren et al., 1985; Purcell-Jones et al., 1987).

c. Fentanyl is used as follows (Young and Mangum, 2003):

(1) Bolus dose: 1 to 4 µg/kg/dose every 2 to 4 hours by slow IV push.

(2) Continuous infusion: 1 to 5 µg/kg/hour.

(3) Onset is almost immediately after IV administration.

(4) Adverse effects include respiratory depression, chest wall rigidity, tolerance and dependence, and urinary retention.

d. Morphine is used as follows (Young and Mangum, 2003):

(1) Bolus dose: 0.05 to 0.2 mg/kg/dose by IV slow push, intramuscularly, or subcutaneous route. Repeat as required, usually every 4 hours

(2) Continuous infusion: give loading dose of 100 to 150 µg/kg over 1 hour followed by a continuous infusion of 10 to 20 µg/kg/hour.

(3) Onset of action: beginning a few minutes after IV administration, with peak analgesia occurring at 20 minutes.

(4) Adverse effects: respiratory depression, hypotension, bradycardia, transient hypertonia, ileus, delayed gastric emptying, urinary retention, tolerance and dependence, and seizures.

e. Managing opioid tolerance and dependence (Franck and Vilardi, 1995; Suresh and Anand, 1998).

(1) Tolerance is decreasing pain relief with the same dosage over time and is exhibited by increased wakefulness and increased sympathetic responses such as high-pitched crying and tremors when handled or disturbed. Tolerance to opioids is usually managed by increasing the dose, although adjunctive analgesics or sedatives may also be clinically beneficial.

(2) Neonates who require opioid therapy for an extended time (>1 week) should be weaned slowly, usually by a dose reduction of 10% to 20% per day depending on duration of therapy and presence of clinical symptoms of withdrawal. Rapid weaning of opioids may lead to withdrawal symptoms such as signs of neurologic excitability, gastrointestinal dysfunction, autonomic signs, poor weight gain, and skin excoriation due to excessive rubbing. An opioid weaning scale such as the Finnegan Scoring System should be used to manage opioid withdrawal in neonates exposed to prolonged opioid therapy (Finnegan et al., 1975).

3. Nonopioid analgesics (Young and Mangum, 2003).

a. Acetaminophen is a nonsteroidal antiinflammatory drug commonly used for short-term use with mild to moderate pain in neonates.

(1) Oral dose: 20 to 25 mg/kg loading dose followed by 12 to 15 mg/kg/dose.

(2) Rectal dose: 30/mg/kg loading dose followed by 12 to 18 mg/kg/dose.

(3) Maintenance intervals are every 6 hours for term infants; every 8 hours for preterm infants older than 32 weeks; and every 12 hours for preterm infants younger than 32 weeks.

(4) Adverse effects: liver toxicity, rash, fever, thrombocytopenia, leukopenia, and neutropenia.

4. EMLA cream (eutectic mixture of local anesthetics, lidocaine and prilocaine).

a. Approved in children at birth with a gestational age of 37 weeks or greater.

b. EMLA cream reduces pain during venipuncture, circumcisions, arterial puncture, and percutaneous venous catheter placement but is not effective for management of pain associated with the heel-stick procedure (Taddio et al., 1998).
c. Local/topical dose: 1 to 2 g under occlusive dressing 60 to 90 minutes before procedure (Young and Mangum, 2003).
d. Adverse effects: methemoglobinemia, redness, and blanching.

5. Local pain control: lidocaine.
   a. Local anesthesia for procedures such as circumcision, chest tube insertion, and cutdown.
   b. Dose: 0.5% solution. Infiltration of less than 0.5 ml/kg/dose is recommended to prevent toxic effects (McClain and Anand, 1996).
6. Sedatives suppress the behavioral expression of pain and have no analgesic effects. Sedatives can even increase pain and should only be used when pain has been ruled out (Hartley et al., 1989). When administered with opioids, sedatives may allow more optimal weaning of opioids in critically ill, ventilator-dependent neonates who have developed tolerance from prolonged opioid therapy. The two most commonly used sedatives in neonates include midazolam and chloral hydrate. However, no research has been done to determine the safety or efficacy of combining sedatives and analgesics for the treatment of pain in infants (Walden and Carrier, 2003).
7. Neuromuscular blocking agents. Chemical paralysis is often used for severely ill neonates. Because the use of paralytic agents masks the behavior signs of pain, sedatives or analgesics should be used in conjunction with paralytics (Shapiro, 1989).

PAIN CONTROL USING REGIONAL ANESTHESIA

For regional anesthesia, an opioid and a local anesthetic are administered via the spinal or epidural (caudal) route. The opioids bind to the receptors in the dorsal horn of the spinal cord and can affect sensory neurons without affecting motor or sympathetic activities (Rasmussen, 1996). Morphine, because of its hydrophilic nature, tends to stay in the cerebrospinal fluid longer and to travel toward the brain (Rasmussen, 1996).

A. **Spinal route:** the space within the spinal canal.
B. **Epidural (caudal) route:** the space just outside the spinal canal where the nerve roots are located. Provides a route for anesthesia and analgesia during operative procedures and can be used for postoperative pain management and for operative procedures below the umbilicus, such as inguinal hernia repair, repair of low imperforate anus, and placement of central venous catheters (Valley, 1997). Spinal and epidural routes can be used with a one-time injection of an agent or a continuous infusion through a catheter.
   1. Agents used include morphine and fentanyl.
   2. Absolute and relative contraindications to regional anesthesia include:
      a. Systemic infection: septicemia, meningitis.
      b. Bleeding disorders: coagulopathy, thrombocytopenia.
      c. Allergy to local anesthetics.
      d. Parent/guardian refusal.
      e. Hypovolemia.
      f. Degenerative CNS diseases.
      g. Other: malformation of the spinal column, hydrocephalus with increased intracranial pressure, poorly controlled seizures.

3. Nursing care (Ochsenreither, 1997).
   a. Inspect catheter for kinking and ensure catheter connections are tight.
   b. Regularly inspect insertion site for leakage, drainage, hematoma, and erythema.
   c. Keep area clean and dry and reinforce with bio-occlusive dressing as necessary.
   d. Ensure correct infusate, dose, and rate of infusion.
   e. Regularly assess for catheter-related, anesthetic-related, and opioid-related side effects.

REFERENCES

American Academy of Pediatrics/Canadian Paediatric Society: Prevention and management of pain and stress in the neonate. *Pediatrics, 105*(2):454-461, 2000.

American Pain Society: Pain: The fifth vital sign [online]. Available: www.ampainsoc.org, 1995.

Anand K.J. and International Evidence-Based Group for Neonatal Pain: Consensus statement for the prevention and management of pain in the newborn. *Archives of Pediatrics and Adolescent Medicine, 155*(2):173-180, 2001.

Anand, K.J., Barton, B.A., McIntosh, N., et al.: Analgesia and sedation in preterm neonates who require ventilatory support: Results from the NOPAIN trial. *Archives of Pediatrics and Adolescent Medicine, 153*(4):331-338, 1999.

Anand, K.J. and Craig, K.D.: New perspectives on the definition of pain [editorial]. *Pain, 67*(1):3-6, 1996.

Anand, K.J. and Hickey, P.R.: Pain and its effects in the human neonate and fetus. *New England Journal of Medicine, 317*(21):1321-1329, 1987.

Anand, K.J.S. and Hickey, P.R.: Halothane-morphine compared with high-dose sufentanil for anesthesia and postoperative analgesia in neonatal cardiac surgery. *New England Journal of Medicine, 326*(1):1-9, 1992.

Andrews, K. and Fitzgerald, M.: The cutaneous withdrawal reflex in human neonates: Sensitization receptive fields, and the effects of contralateral stimulation. *Pain, 56*(1):95-102, 1994.

Association of Women's Health, Obstetric, and Neonatal Nurses: Position paper: *Pain in neonates*. Washington, DC, 1995, Author.

Barker, D.P. and Rutter, N.: Exposure to invasive procedures in neonatal intensive care unit admissions. *Archives of Disease in Childhood, Fetal and Neonatal Edition, 72*(1):F47-F48, 1995.

Barr, R.: Is this infant in pain? Caveats from the clinical setting. *American Pain Society Journal, 1*(3):187-190, 1992.

Blass, E., Fitzgerald, E., and Kehoe, P.: Interactions between sucrose, pain and isolation distress. *Pharmacology, Biochemistry, and Behavior, 26*(3):483-489, 1987.

Campos, R.G.: Soothing pain-elicited distress in infants with swaddling and pacifiers. *Child Development, 60*(4):781-792, 1989.

Campos, R.G.: Rocking and pacifiers: Two comforting interventions for heelstick pain. *Research in Nursing and Health, 17*(5):321-331, 1994.

Corff, K., Seideman, R., Venkataraman, P.S., et al.: Facilitated tucking: A nonpharmacologic comfort measure for pain in preterm neonates. *Journal of Obstetric, Gynecologic, and Neonatal Nursing, 24*(2):143-147, 1995.

Craig, K.D., Whitfield, M.F., Grunau, R., et al.: Pain in the preterm neonate: Behavioral and physiological indices. *Pain, 52*(3):287-299, 1993.

Deshpande, J.K. and Anand, J.S.: Basic aspects of acute pediatric pain sedation. In J.K. Deshpande and J.D. Tobias (Eds.): *The pediatric pain handbook.* St Louis, 1996, Mosby, pp. 1-48.

Evans, J.C.: Physiology of acute pain in preterm infants. *Newborn and Infant Nursing Reviews, 1*(2):75-84, 2001.

Farrington, E.A., McGuinness, G.A., Johnson, G.F., et al.: Continuous intravenous morphine infusion in postoperative newborn infants. *American Journal of Perinatology, 10*(1):84-87, 1993.

Fearon, I., Kisilevsky, B.S., Hains, S.M., et al.: Swaddling after heel lance: Age-specific effects on behavioral recovery in preterm infants. *Journal of Developmental and Behavioral Pediatrics, 18*(4):222-232, 1997.

Finnegan, L., Connaughton, J., and Kron, R.: A scoring system for evaluation and treatment of the neonatal abstinence syndrome: A new clinical and research tool. In P. Marselli, S. Garanttini, and F. Sereni (Eds.): *Basic and therapeutic aspects of perinatal pharmacology*. New York, 1975, Raven, pp. 139-152.

Fitzgerald, M. and Shortland, P.: The effect of neonatal peripheral nerve section on the somadendritic growth of sensory projection cells in the rat spinal cord. *Brain Research, 470*(1):129-136, 1988.

Franck L.S.: A new method to quantitatively describe pain behavior in infants. *Nursing Research, 35*(1):28-31, 1986.

Franck, L.S.: A national survey of the assessment and treatment of pain and agitation in the neonatal intensive care unit. *Journal of Obstetric, Gynecologic, and Neonatal Nursing, 16*(6):387-393, 1987.

Franck, L.S.: Pain in the nonverbal patient: Advocating for the critically ill neonate. *Pediatric Nursing, 15*(1):65-68, 90, 1989.

Franck, L.S. and Lawhon, G.: Environmental and behavioral strategies to prevent and manage neonatal pain. *Seminars in Perinatology, 22*(5):434-443, 1998.

Franck, L. and Lawhon, G.: Environmental and behavioral strategies to prevent and manage neonatal pain. In K. Anand, B. Stevens, and P. McGrath (Eds.): *Pain in neonates*. Amsterdam, 2000, Elsevier Science, pp. 203-216.

Franck, L.S. and Miaskowski, C.: The use of intravenous opioids to provide analgesia in critically ill, premature neonates: A research critique. *Journal of Pain and Symptom Management, 15*(1):41-69, 1998.

Franck, L. and Vilardi, J.: Assessment and management of opioid withdrawal in ill neonates. *Neonatal Network, 14(2)*:39-48, 1995.

Fuller, B.: Acoustic discrimination of three types of infant cries. *Nursing Research, 40*(3):156-160, 1991.

Grunau, R.V. and Craig, K.D.: Pain expression in neonates: Facial action and cry. *Pain, 28*(3):395-410, 1987.

Grunau, R.V., Johnston, C.C., and Craig, K.D.: Neonatal facial and cry responses to invasive and non-invasive procedures. *Pain, 42*(3):295-305, 1990.

Grunau, R.V., Whitfield, M.F., and Petrie, J.H.: Pain sensitivity and temperament in extremely low-birth-weight premature toddlers and preterm and full-term controls. *Pain, 58*(3):341-346, 1994.

Gunnar, M., Connors, J., Isensse, J., and Wall, L.: Adrenocortical activity and behavioral distress in human newborns. *Developmental Psychobiology, 21*(4):297-310, 1988.

Hartley, S., Franck, L.S., and Lundergan, F.: Maintenance sedation of agitated infants in the NICU with chloral hydrate: New concerns. *Journal of Perinatology, 9*(2):162-164, 1989.

International Association for the Study of Pain Subcommittee on Taxonomy: Pain terms: A list with definitions and notes on usage. *Pain, 6*(3):249-252, 1979.

Johnston, C., Stevens, B., Craig, K., and Grunau, R.: Developmental changes in pain expression in premature, full-term, two- and four-month-old infants. *Pain, 52*(2):201-208, 1993.

Johnston, C.C. and Stevens, B.J. Experience in a neonatal intensive care unit affects pain response *Pediatrics,* 98(5):925-930, 1996.

Johnston, C.C., Stevens, B.J., Franck, L.S., et al.: Factors explaining lack of response to heel stick in preterm newborns. *Journal of Obstetric, Gynecologic, and Neonatal Nursing, 28*(6):587-594, 1999.

Johnston, C.C., Stevens, B.J., Yang, F., and Horton, L.: Differential response to pain by very premature neonates. *Pain, 61*(3):471-479, 1995.

Johnston, C.C., Stremler, R.L., Stevens, B.J., and Horton, L.J.: Effectiveness of oral sucrose and simulated rocking on pain response in preterm neonates. *Pain, 72*(1-2):193-199, 1997.

Joint Commission on Accreditation of Healthcare Organizations: Pain management standards for 2001 [online]. Available: www.jcaho.org, 1999.

Koren, G., Butt, W., Chinyanga, H., et al.: Postoperative morphine infusion in newborn infants: Assessment of disposition characteristics and safety. *Journal of Pediatrics, 107*(6):963-967, 1985.

Krechel, S. and Bildner, J.: CRIES: A new neonatal post-operative pain measurement score: Initial testing of validity and reliability. *Paediatric Anaesthesia, 5*(1):53-61, 1995.

Lawrence, J., Alcock, D., McGrath, P., et al.: The development of a tool to assess neonatal pain. *Neonatal Network, 12*(6): 59-66, 1993.

Levine, J.D. and Gordon, N.C.: Pain in prelingual children and its evaluation by pain-induced vocalization. *Pain, 14*(2):85-93, 1982.

McClain, B.C. and Anand, K.J.S.: Neonatal pain management. In J. Deshpande and J. Tobias (Eds.): *The pediatric pain handbook.* St Louis, 1996, Mosby, pp. 197-234.

McIntosh, N., Van Veen, L., and Brameyer, H.: Alleviation of the pain of heel prick in preterm infants. *Archives of Disease in Childhood, 70*:F177-F181, 1994.

Melzack, R.: Gate control theory: On the evolution of pain concepts. *Pain Forum, 5*:128-138, 1996.

Ochsenreither, J.: Epidural analgesia in infants. *Neonatal Network, 16*:79-84, 1997.

Porter, F., Wolf, C., and Miller, P.: Procedural pain in newborn infants: The influence of intensity and development. *Pediatrics, 104*(1):e13-e16, 1999.

Porter, F.L., Miller, R.H., and Marshall, R.E.: Neonatal pain cries: Effect of circumcision on acoustic features and perceived urgency. *Child Development, 57*(3):790-802, 1986.

Purcell-Jones, G., Dormon, F., and Sumner, E.: The use of opioids in neonates: A retrospective study of 933 cases. *Anaesthesia, 42*(12):1316-1320, 1987.

Rasmussen, G.E.: Epidural and spinal anesthesia and analgesia. In J. Deshpande and J. Tobias (Eds.): *The pediatric pain handbook.* St Louis, 1996, Mosby, pp. 81-112.

Shapiro, C.: Pain in the neonate: Assessment and intervention. *Neonatal Network, 8*(1):7-19, 1989.

Shapiro, C.: Nurses' judgments of pain in term and preterm newborns. *Journal of Obstetric, Gynecologic, and Neonatal Nursing, 22*(1):41-47, 1993.

Stevens, B.J. and Johnston, C.C.: Physiological responses of premature infants to a painful stimulus. *Nursing Research, 43*(4):226-231, 1994.

Stevens B., Johnston C., Franck L., et al.: The efficacy of developmentally sensitive interventions and sucrose for relieving procedural pain in very low birth weight neonates. *Nursing Research, 48*(1):35-43, 1999.

Stevens, B.J., Johnston, C.C., and Grunau, R.V.: Issues of assessment of pain and discomfort in neonates. *Journal of Obstetric, Gynecologic, and Neonatal Nursing, 24*(9):849-855, 1995.

Stevens, B., Johnston, C., and Horton, L.: Multidimensional pain assessment in premature neonates: A pilot study. *Journal of Obstetric, Gynecologic, and Neonatal Nursing, 22*(6):531-541, 1993.

Stevens, B.J., Johnston, C.C., and Horton, L.: Factors that influence the behavioral responses of premature infants. *Pain, 5*(1)1:101-109, 1994.

Stevens, B., Johnston, C., Petryshen, P., and Taddio, A.: Premature infant pain profile: Development and initial validation. *Clinical Journal of Pain, 12*(1):13-22, 1996.

Stevens, B., Yamada, J., and Ohlsson, A.: Sucrose for analgesia in newborn infants undergoing painful procedures. *Cochrane Database of Systematic Reviews* 2000(2): CD001069.

Stevens, B., Taddio, A., Ohlsson, A., and Einarson, T.: The efficacy of sucrose for relieving procedural pain in neonates—A systematic review and meta-analysis. *Acta Paediatrica, 86*:837-842, 1997.

Suresh, S. and Anand, K.J.: Opioid tolerance in neonates: Mechanisms, diagnosis, assessment, and management. *Seminars in Perinatology, 22*(5):425-433, 1998.

Taddio, A., Ohlsson, A., Einarson, T.R., et al.: A systematic review of lidocaine-prilocaine cream (EMLA) in the treatment of acute pain in neonates. *Pediatrics, 101*(2):E1, 1998.

U.S. Department of Health and Human Services, Public Health Service, Agency for Health Care Policy and Research: Acute pain management in infants, children, and adolescents: Operative and medical procedures. In *Quick reference guide for clinicians* (DHHS publication No. [AHCPR] 92-0019.) Silver Springs, MD, 1992, AHCPR Clearinghouse, pp. 3-22.

Valley, R.D.: Anesthesia and postoperative pain management. In D.K. Nakayama,

C.L. Bose, N.C. Chesheir, and R.D. Valley (Eds.): *Critical care of the surgical newborn*. New York, 1997, Futura, pp. 148-157.

Walden, M.: *Pain assessment and management: Guideline for practice*. Glenview, IL, 2001, National Association of Neonatal Nurses.

Walden, M. and Carrier, C.T.: Sleeping beauties: The impact of sedation on neonatal development. *Journal of Obstetric, Gynecologic, and Neonatal Nursing, 32*(3): 393-401, 2003.

Young, T.E. and Mangum, B.: *Neofax: A manual of drugs used in neonatal care* (16th ed.). Raleigh, NC, 2003, Acorn Publishing.

CHAPTER

17 Families in Crisis

CAROLE KENNER

OBJECTIVES

1. Define the concept of crisis.
2. Recognize the psychologic tasks that the mother and family must accomplish to establish a healthy parent-child relationship after the crisis of the birth of a premature or sick infant.
3. Describe assessment strategies for identifying a family in crisis.
4. Identify the risks of teenage parenting on the adolescent and the infant.
5. Identify nursing interventions to support a family coping with stressful events surrounding the birth of their infant.
6. Evaluate maternal behaviors found to be predictive of specific parenting outcomes.
7. Recognize emotional characteristics related to grief.
8. Identify strategies for working with families experiencing perinatal or neonatal end-of-life (EOL) issues.
9. Identify specific behaviors to be assessed in determining parental attachment to their infant.
10. Describe the nursing strategies to promote parental attachment.
11. Identify cultural influences that impact on parenting a sick or dying neonate.

With the current technologic and genomic advances, even the most acutely ill or most premature infant has a good chance of going home. Neonates born as prematurely as 23 weeks' gestation are surviving. For parents, though these advances are increasing the odds of having a live neonate they also have brought on tremendous stress (Miles et al., 1998). The result may be a family that views the infant as medically fragile and vulnerable. This view changes the relationship between the family and child, especially the mother (Holditch-Davis et al., 2003c).

When an infant requires health care at birth because of prematurity, illness, or congenital malformations, or when an infant dies, the effects of these unexpected events on the parents can be overwhelming. The families of these infants may experience multiple crisis events during the infant's hospitalization (Kenner et al., 2003). Assessment skills are critical for the neonatal nurse who is caring for an infant and family at this period of crisis. The parents usually display signs of anxiety, fear, and powerlessness. It is the nurse who is viewed as the advocate for the family and who has the most continual interactions with them. Nursing care is generally concerned with both the physiologic and psychosocial needs of the patient and the family. However, the focus of this chapter is the psychosocial aspects of supporting parents who must cope with stressful events surrounding the birth of their infant. The chapter highlights various types of families who may experience a crisis when their infant requires a neonatal intensive care unit (NICU) stay or a perinatal/neonatal death. Many of the strategies or interventions are the same for all groups of parents because they represent parenting needs. Cultural influences must also be considered.

CRISIS AND THE BIRTH OF THE SICK OR PREMATURE INFANT

Pregnancy and transition to parenthood have been recognized as periods of stress and change during which mothers and fathers are attempting to master the normal developmental process of parenthood. These major life changes have been referred to as *developmental* or *maturational stressors*. In contrast, the birth of a premature or sick infant and the death of an infant are unexpected stressful life events for which a person or family is often psychologically unprepared. Such events are referred to as *situational* or *accidental stressors*. When such maturational and situational stressors occur simultaneously, the resulting pressure can overwhelm a person's usual coping resources and support systems. Rolland (1994) suggests there is a family life cycle that accompanies chronic illnesses. The five elements of psychosocial demands of this framework are onset, course, outcome, incapacitation, and uncertainty (Rolland, 1994; Street and Soldan, 1998). As health care professionals we need to recognize these stages of demands that families face. If they do not successfully work through these demands, ineffective coping may result. Ineffective coping causes personal and family psychologic disequilibrium or crisis, which continues until new ways of coping can be developed and maintained. Coping, however, is intimately tied to cultural values and beliefs, and in some instances, spirituality (Rivett and Street, 2001), so these must be taken into account.

A. **Several psychologic tasks** have been identified that the mother and family must accomplish to cope with the crisis of a premature birth or the birth of a sick infant and to establish a basis for a healthy parent-child relationship (Krebs, 1998). These must take into consideration the psychologic health of the mother and its impact on parent-infant interactions (Davis et al., 2003).
   1. *Preparation for the possible loss of the infant*. Parents must consider the possibility of disability or death of the infant while simultaneously hoping for the infant's survival.
   2. *Acknowledgment of failure to deliver a term infant*. The mother struggles with feelings of guilt and failure and searches for causes of the infant's condition. Family members may actually be, or be perceived as, blaming the mother for the premature infant.
   3. *Adaptation to the intensive care environment*. Parents must be helped to develop secure relationships in an unfamiliar and stress-provoking setting.
   4. *Resumption of interaction with the infant once the threat of loss has passed*. Parents must participate in the infant's care and gain confidence in their abilities. Parental interaction may be adversely affected due to effects of posttraumatic stress and fear that something might still happen to the infant. Taking part in their infant's care can ease the crisis, decrease guilt, and increase psychologic health (Mayes, 2003).
   5. *Preparation for taking the infant home*. Parents must understand the special needs and characteristics of the premature or sick infant and the necessary precautions that must be taken and yet maintain a positive relationship with the infant, realizing that these needs are only temporary. Failure to resolve these tasks can contribute to such maladaptive parenting as being overprotective, resulting in the "vulnerable child syndrome" and in other negative child outcomes such as failure to thrive, emotional deprivation, and battering (Docherty et al., 2002; Miles et al., 1998). Mothers and health care professionals may view the child as medically fragile when this may or may not be the case. The psychologic impact of having a sick infant can continue even after a successful discharge, resulting in maternal psychologic distress

(Davis et al., 2003). Whereas most of the current research focuses on the maternal role and their level of distress, fathers must be considered too. The father's perception of a crisis is just as important as the mother's, and interventions to ease their distress must be part of the preparation for taking an infant home (Pohlman, 2004).

B. **Definition of *crisis:*** a temporary disequilibrium that occurs when people face an important problem or transitional phase so stressful that they are unable to cope by using their customary problem-solving resources (Docherty et al., 2002; Wereszczak et al., 1997). It usually lasts from 4 to 6 weeks. This period is the optimal time for effective interventions with the family.

C. **Discussion.** During early stages of a crisis, parents are more receptive to overtures of help from other family members, friends, and the health care team. Nurses are in a key position because they work so directly with the parents to anticipate a family crisis and to promote positive coping and effective use of social supports (Mayes, 2003; Moore and Freda, 1998). A family in crisis cannot effectively interact with their newly born infant because all their energies are going toward the crisis. When interventions are put into place to promote effective coping and positive social support, the crisis will resolve and psychologic equilibrium, a necessary step toward the establishment of a healthy parent-child relationship, will be restored. Factors that influence a family's return to equilibrium include the following:
   1. Understanding of the infant's problem and the need for NICU care and understanding of their parental role.
   2. Resolving or at least lessening of the family's grief reaction to the need for NICU care.
   3. Viewing parents as partners in care and not visitors.
   4. Using positive coping and social supports (Kenner et al., 2003).

SPECIFIC POPULATION OF PARENTS: ADOLESCENTS

Parents who are adolescent have some unique needs. They undergo the crises of parenthood and of having an infant in the NICU. In addition, these parents are dealing with the normal developmental tasks of adolescence. Sometimes these tasks seem in conflict with their needs as new parents. The nurse must be aware of these conflicts and realize their unique blending needs of taking on a new role and being at their developmental stage.

Adolescence is a turning point, or change period. It moves a child from childhood toward the maturation of the adult. Many physiologic changes are occurring, first at puberty and then in the move toward adulthood. Physical appearance changes, and the adolescent is capable of childbearing. Maturation of the reproductive system now occurs much earlier than in the past. In the United States, girls are reaching menarche as young as 8 years of age. Adolescence is the time when childbearing becomes a potential reality for most individuals.

Development of the personality is tied to role attainment, much as for parents and the parenting role. Adolescents strive to have an identity unique from those of other family members. They are developing their self-concept and self-esteem. The peer group becomes important for validation of attitudes, values, and beliefs (Koshar et al., 1998). But adults can model this peer validation to enhance positive developmental outcomes for adolescent parents (Dishion et al., 2002). Adolescence is a time of constant change and usually turmoil—a period of maturational crisis.

A. **Some developmental tasks of this period are:**
   1. Independence from adults.

2. Preparation for financial security.
3. Gender identification.
4. A stable, realistic, positive sense of self.

B. **In addition, adolescence:**
1. Is characterized by high anxiety.
2. Can be anticipated; therefore preparation can be made.
3. Requires normal social support for a successful transition.
4. Is relatively easy to resolve because the individual's values usually do not conflict with societal expectations for the outcome, which is adult behavior.
5. Is a period of vulnerability to a crisis occurrence if a traumatic event is added to the transitional state.

While adolescents have unique needs they also are unique individuals. As health professionals we often make assumptions of what they need or what type parents they will be. The reality is they need to be assessed for their knowledge, level of crisis, and supports the same as any other individual or family. Perception is all there is—right or wrong—and we cannot or should not perceive that all adolescents will be bad parents, or immature in their actions, or be more concerned with peers than with their child. We must evaluate their needs certainly within the context of their developmental stage but also with consideration of their own personal, individualized needs.

THE FAMILY IN CRISIS

Assessment

A. **Determine parents' understanding of the situation** (i.e., realistic vs. distorted). The parents' ability to resolve the crisis depends on their realistic perception of their situation: they need to be fully informed about their infant's condition and expected progress. An inability to understand the crisis may be related to low socioeconomic status or cultural values and beliefs. Parents of a lower socioeconomic status may not fully understand what to expect of their infant or their role because they may lack good role models for themselves or the financial means to provide adequate, safe care for themselves or their infant. Cultural values and beliefs also may play a role because different cultures view the infant in relationship to parents in different ways and their view of health and death may be different from the typical U.S. views. In some countries, such as in India or China, only male offspring are valued and girl babies are dismissed as nonessential. Whereas we often crave control over the environment in Western culture, other cultures may view this as fate (Lynch and Hanson, 1998). Native Americans usually accept what is; blacks are more oriented to specific situations than time; Latinos value the inclusion of the extended family and view death as having rituals associated with it; touching an infant's head is threatening by some southeast Asians, Buddhists, and native Hawaiians; and Middle Eastern children make few independent decisions (consideration when working with adolescent parents if their extended family is not present) (Lynch and Hanson, 1998).

B. **Determine parents' grief response.** The extent to which they are experiencing a grief reaction must be determined. This grief may be in the form of anticipatory grief because they fear the infant might die, even though the physical condition does not appear to warrant this fear. Consider this within the cultural context of the family, because it may not be acceptable to express grief or worries to outsiders. If the child is dying then consider EOL issues such as advanced directives from the parents' perspectives and what they want or need from us as health professionals.

C. **Determine parents' adaptation to and coping** with the stressful event.
   1. Are the parents maintaining responsibilities related to activities of daily living (e.g., eating, personal grooming)?
   2. To what degree has the family's normal lifestyle been affected by the crisis? (Are they able to return to work? Keep house? Care for other children in the household?)
   3. Are the parents exhibiting positive coping skills within the context of their cultural values and beliefs?
   4. To what extent has the financial status of the family been affected?

D. **Determine what support systems exist** for the parents and whether they are being used. It is also important to determine whether these supports are positive. The parents may have several people in their support network, but if these people are critical of how the parents are conducting themselves, then they may not be viewed as positive supports.
   1. Who are the significant others in the lives of the parents? Consider biologic kinship (family) and/or emotional kinship (friends).
   2. What professional supports are available?
   3. Is a parent support group available?

E. **Understanding the origins of a crisis, and their links with the normal "ups and downs" of life, is crucial to successful assessment and intervention. Events that stimulate the occurrence of a crisis, such as those of the teenage parent in the NICU, can originate from:**
   1. Being in a transitional state, such as:
      a. Adolescence to adulthood.
      b. Childhood to parenthood.
   2. Being a part of a social-cultural structure and:
      a. Violating customs or cultural norms embedded in that structure, such as a teenager's becoming pregnant and having a newborn, *or*
      b. Behaving outside the accepted teenage social norms, as the role of parent would demand (although these examples are culture specific): for example, being tied down to taking care of a newborn or having to arrange for child care at a time when peers are freely going to sports games and dances and having fun.
      c. Being exposed to hazardous or disturbing situations, such as:
         (1) Birth of a first child. This is a disturbing situation because no one knows exactly what to expect of parenthood—a role never before experienced.
         (2) Lack of experience with parenthood.
         (3) Bearing of a sick newborn infant.

Problems Associated with Adolescent Pregnancy

When teens become pregnant, they often experience the following problems:

A. **Loss of peer group.** Adolescents' peers often disappear, leaving them without support and feeling socially isolated. Their self-concept changes as they approach parenthood because before the pregnancy the peer group helped shape their self-perception (Alpers, 1998; Dishion et al., 2002).

B. **Disruption of family ties.** The pregnant adolescent and her boyfriend often bring on direct conflict with their parents. The rationale for this conflict is that the parents of the adolescents often believe that adolescence is an inappropriate time to start a family and that the adolescents need to live by the parental house rules. At the same time, the adolescent parents may be trying to take on adult responsibilities while feeling that they are being treated as children. This conflict removes a possible positive social support. It also disrupts the effort to assume a parental role if the adolescents' parents try to make decisions regarding the coming infant.

C. **Maternal health problems.** The pregnant female adolescent often has engaged in risky behaviors besides being sexually active. She may smoke, drink, or use drugs. She is at risk of having human immunodeficiency virus (HIV) infection and other sexually transmitted infections (STIs). This risk is not unique to adolescents but is possible because of the feelings of invincibility that accompany this age. The pregnant adolescent may be emotionally immature and may have to interrupt her education to bear the child. She may be forced into a marriage she does not want or is not ready for at this time. She may lack knowledge about normal fetal and infant growth and development. She may have very unrealistic expectations of an infant and of herself as a parent. She may have sought pregnancy as a way to have someone need her. She may not seek prenatal care or may try to hide the pregnancy by limiting weight gain. These actions may put her health and her infant's health at risk. She also often lacks parenting skills.

D. **Paternal problems.** The adolescent father may have engaged in risky sexual behaviors. He may have been smoking or used alcohol or drugs. He also may be at risk of having HIV infection or other STIs. If he is infected, the pregnant adolescent and the fetus are also at risk because these infections can be passed on to the maternal-fetal unit. The male adolescent may be generally stable psychologically, but he may not be thinking about future consequences of his sexual behavior, such as his inability to fulfill his parenting role. For example, because of his risky behaviors, he may have contracted HIV, which will take him away from the pregnant adolescent and his future child. If his family, his significant other, or her family views his behaviors as irresponsible, he may be isolated from an active role in future parenting. He may feel excluded from decisions regarding the continuation of the pregnancy or the placement of the child after birth. He may interrupt his own education to provide financial support to his new "family." He may be forced into a marriage he neither wants nor is ready for at present.

E. **Risks to the infant.** The infant is at risk of having a faulty, or negative, parent-infant interaction, generally because of the parents' lack of understanding of the normal growth and development process. The parents also often have unrealistic expectations of the child, and their role as parents and may lack parenting skills. The infant may be small for gestational age or premature and may require an expensive hospitalization that the parents are not ready financially or cognitively to accept. The infant may be less responsive or organized in cues for care by the parents. He or she may be more at risk of having slowed or delayed growth because of the parents' lack of understanding of normal infant care and feeding practices. The infant may not receive the type and amount of stimulation necessary for positive cognitive or behavioral development. An infant who is premature tends to be more irritable, to feed poorly, to have poor self-regulatory behaviors, and to be difficult to console. This seeming lack of responsiveness to parenting efforts often reinforces the adolescent parents' poor self-esteem and poor self-concept, which often accompany adolescent pregnancy. The infant may also be at risk of experiencing abuse or neglect.

1. Prematurity, birth between 23 and 27 weeks' gestation, is more common among infants of adolescent mothers. The risk factors for delivering early are (Hall et al., 2003; Joffe and Wright, 2002):
   a. Low pregnancy weight.
   b. Lower socioeconomic status.
   c. Marital status: single.
   d. Tobacco use (smoking).
   e. Narcotic or other substance use.
   f. Anemia (hemoglobin concentration <11 g/dl).
   g. First child.
   h. Poor prenatal care.
2. Low birth weight (<2500 g) is also a risk factor for an adolescent's offspring. The risk can be as much as six times greater for 14-year-old and younger mothers (Hall et al., 2003; Joffe and Wright, 2002).

Intervention

A. **Be present with the physician or nurse practitioner** at the initial meeting with the parents.
B. **Talk with the mother and father** together whenever possible. Consider cultural values of each family. In some cultures the father must receive the information first (Kenner et al., 2003).
C. **Determine and address the parents' perceptions** of the infant's condition (Kenner et al., 2003).
D. **Be consistent with information** given to parents by the staff. If in an academic health care setting where the physicians or nurse practitioners rotate frequently, be sure that any changes in care that are reflective only of these staff changes are explained within that context. If parents do not understand the basis of these changes or are not told when their infant's condition really changes, then mistrust begins. Then the chance that the crisis will escalate is highly probable (Kenner et al., 2003; Miles et al., 1998).
E. **Do not overload parents with detailed information** about their infant during their initial visits to the NICU; provide basic facts and allow the parents some time to process the information.
F. **Assess the grief response.** Males and females express their grief in different ways. However, most, if not all, parents experience some form of grief by just having an infant who requires specialized care (Kenner et al., 2003). This reaction must be assessed throughout the hospital stay. Sometimes this response is directly tied to their understanding of the infant's condition. Other times it is related to cultural beliefs and values.
G. **Acknowledge any feeling of guilt that might be expressed** about the unexpected birth outcome. Let the parents know that these feelings are normal (Siegel et al., 2002).
H. **Facilitate adaptation of the parents' new role** by being a very good listener, by observing body language, and by helping them to verbalize their feelings (Siegel et al., 2002).
I. **Periodically assess the parents' understanding** of their infant's condition and their interpretation of the information that has been given to them. Information must be reinforced throughout the hospital stay. Whenever anyone is anxious, little information is actually heard or retained.
J. **Write notes from the infant to the parents** concerning current status (e.g., equipment, feedings, oxygen concentration) and take pictures of the infant

periodically. A notebook containing the notes and pictures can be kept at the infant's bedside for the parents. These can be memory books or scrapbooks that become especially important if the child dies. This intervention should be individualized because not all parents want this form of "communication." It is one strategy, however, for some parents that promotes positive attachment.

K. **Encourage the parents to keep a journal** concerning their experience of delivering a premature or sick infant. This action can assist families to work through their feelings as well as having memories to review what happened and reflect on issues that have been or are have not been resolved (Ullrich and Lutgendorf, 2002).
L. **Give parents the freedom to express negative ideas without being judged.** Fear and frustration over the inability to control their infant's circumstances are often the basis for parental anger displaced to staff. Remember that control is not acceptable in all cultures, so it is important to ask what is making them uncomfortable. Also a positive way to approach this and possibly decrease their anger is to ask them what would help them to feel more comfortable.
M. **Encourage parents to participate in the care as they desire.** Parents need to understand and develop their roles as parents. If professionals provide all the care, a clear message is conveyed to the parents that they are not capable of helping their infant. They must understand all the things they have to contribute to the team approach to care. Parents must be a part of the health care team and as such should have a say in health care decisions.
N. **Do not refer to parents as visitors.** Parents are not visitors. They are parents and are partners in the care of the infant. They are an integral part of the infant's care and should be a focus of nursing care.
O. **Promote a developmentally supportive environment for the family.** Use of individualized family-centered care is important if the family is to be helped through this crisis (Kenner and McGrath, 2004). For example, kangaroo care (skin-to-skin contact, done by placing the naked infant next to the parent's naked chest, with a blanket or gown draped over the parent and infant), dimmed lights or cycled lights, private areas for parent interaction with the infant, and swaddling or cuddling of the infant promote positive development of the infant and family (Davis et al., 2003; Gray et al., 1998; Gretebeck et al., 1998; Griffin, 1998).
P. **Determine parents' network of social support.** The social support network may include family, friends, clergy, and health professionals. Also determine whether the level of support is adequate from the parents' and the health professionals' standpoint.
Q. **Encourage parents to share their concerns and fears** with each other. Often it is not until the infant is discharged that parents share their feelings with each other. This is another area where culture plays a role. For some Asian cultures, expressions of concern are acceptable within the family unit but not with others. Health professionals may be viewed as authority figures and not ones to whom fears should be confided. It is important too to find out what this illness and hospitalization mean to the family and to what degree they are viewed as stress (Peebles-Kleiger, 2000).
R. **Assist parents in maintaining their relationship with one another.** Reinforce with them that they must take time for themselves as a couple. If the mother is alone, encourage her to maintain ties with other family members and her friends.
S. **Assist parents in maintaining their relationship with the infant's siblings** by helping them to recognize the needs of the other children and identify how the needs can be met.

T. **Assist the adolescent parents in defining their role with their own parents** by helping them to learn how to talk with their parents.

U. **Encourage parents to attend a parent support group if desirable.** Involvement in a parent support group has been demonstrated to facilitate parental grieving, reduce fears, and increase feelings of parental competence (Bracht et al., 1998; Geron et al., 2003; Levin, 1998; Raines, 1998). This intervention must be culture specific. In some cultures it is not acceptable to discuss family problems openly. It is also important to include the father's perspective. Some groups are for fathers only because this is a recognized growing need (Lurie, 1992).

V. **Assist families of dying infants to tell you what they need.** EOL issues are never easy but are especially difficult in this population when celebration of a birth is the expectation. Asking the family what they need from us as health care professionals is important. Understanding what this death means to them is critical to plan individualized care. Finding out if they want siblings and extended family involved, if clergy or spiritual healers are important, as well as what for them constitutes a good death are all important aspects of helping families cope (Kenner and Lott, 2004). Use of consistent information and the same message from all health care providers is important too. The use of a palliative care protocol is one method to ensure more consistency (Catlin and Carter, 2002; Glicken and Merenstein, 2002). Consideration of cultural differences once again is important (Lundqvist et al., 2003.)

Evaluation of Maternal Parenting Outcomes

A. **Predictors of good maternal parenting outcomes (Kenner et al., 2003).**
   1. Anxiety level is moderate to high: she worries about the infant's chances of surviving, the possibility of abnormality, and her competence as a mother.
   2. Seeks information about the infant.
   3. Demonstrates warmth toward infant and in other relationships.
   4. Has a support system (i.e., father of the infant, her mother, friends).
   5. Has had a previous successful experience with a premature infant (i.e., previous child, a sibling, other relative), which enables her to feel more experienced and confident.
   6. Recognizes positive attributes of the child (i.e., smiling) (Johnson-Crowley and Conrad, 2003).
   7. Views self positively.
   8. For an adolescent, has a centralized locus of behavioral control.
   9. Exhibits effective caregiving.
   10. Makes positive eye contact with the infant.

B. **Predictors of poor maternal parenting outcomes (Kenner et al., 2003).**
   1. Exhibits an inappropriately low anxiety level.
   2. Demonstrates passivity—does not actively seek out information related to infant's condition.
   3. Has limited verbal interaction.
   4. Visits infrequently and for short periods in the NICU. (Remember that sometimes infrequent visits are due to a lack of transportation and not true parenting problems.)
   5. Is unaware of the infant's needs.
   6. Has unrealistic expectations of the infant or the parenting role.
   7. Personalizes the infant's behavior as a failure of her ability to parent or that the infant is "bad."
   8. During pregnancy, expressed little desire to have a child.

9. Is more likely to express disappointment about the sex of the infant.
10. Has no support system.
11. Is an adolescent with little or no social supports.
12. Exhibits role confusion.

Grief and Loss

A. **Introduction.** Unfortunately, not all pregnancies result in a healthy term infant. When adverse neonatal events occur, often the parents are overwhelmed by grief. As the parents realize that their newborn is "less than perfect" and not the infant of their fantasies, acute grief reactions occur. One of the early tasks of parenting is to resolve the discrepancy between the idealized infant and the real infant. In the case of neonatal death, the parents also grieve for the lost opportunity to parent the child. To assist parents therapeutically in working through the feelings associated with loss, nurses working with high-risk infants must understand the grief process, recognize typical parental behaviors associated with grief, and provide appropriate nursing interventions.

B. **Definitions.**
   1. *Grief:* the response of sadness and sorrow to the loss of a valued object (Siegel et al., 2002).
   2. *Anticipatory grief:* grieving that occurs before an actual loss. If the outcome for the infant is healthy, then anticipatory grieving can lead to difficulties in attachment and problems in the parent-infant relationship.
   3. *Chronic grief:* unresolved or blocked grief; frequently seen in parents of a disabled child, who is a constant reminder of loss.

C. **Assessment.**
   1. Grief responses to death, premature birth, or the birth of an infant with a malformation are similar. These responses do not necessarily occur in the same sequence for all people. They are mediated by cultural beliefs and values as well as the parents' developmental stage. In addition, the responses may overlap and recur. Posttraumatic stress disorder (PTSD) often results from just having an infant in an NICU but is exacerbated if the child actually dies (Holditch-Davis et al., 2003a). Stages of grief (Siegel et al., 2002) are:
      a. Shock.
      b. Denial and/or panic: refusal to accept reality; intense anxiety.
      c. Anger, guilt, and shame; awareness of loss suffered becomes acute.
      d. Acceptance, adaptation, and reorganization; grief continues, but the individual is able to reestablish a state of equilibrium.
   2. One of the goals of the staff working with parents is to encourage the development of attachment, or an affectional tie, between the parent and infant. However, because the birth of a premature or a physically, psychologically, or neurologically challenged infant creates a sense of loss, the parents must first resolve their grief before attachment can be fully achieved (Nurses Association of the American College of Obstetricians and Gynecologists, 1991; Siegel et al., 2002).

Interventions for Facilitating Grief

A. **Listen:** parents need to be given the opportunity to express their feelings.

B. **Acknowledge the pain of their loss:** gives the parents permission to talk about their loss and provides support for acknowledging and working through their grief.

C. **Convey an attitude of acceptance, openness, and availability to the family:** grieving people need permission to experience their feelings, regardless of how uncomfortable or unpleasant (Siegel et al., 2002).

D. **Help the parents to understand the individuality of the grieving process.** Mothers and fathers usually have "incongruent grieving": they do not grieve at the same pace. This incongruence frequently leads to marital discord because of misconceptions about feelings and an inability to communicate (Kohner and Henley, 2001).

Interventions for Parents Experiencing a Perinatal Loss

A. **Encourage the family to see, hold, and spend time with the infant** before and after death (Catlin and Carter, 2002; Kenner and Lott, 2004).
   1. Be sensitive to individual and cultural differences in rituals of saying goodbye.
   2. Physically bring the family together and offer privacy. Some hospitals have a neonatal hospice program in which the family is involved with the infant's care (Catlin and Carter, 2002; Kavanaugh and Wheeler, 2003; Kenner and Lott, 2004; Sudia-Robinson, 2003).

B. **Provide the parents with the following mementos:** photograph of the infant, identification bracelet, footprints, completed crib card, blanket, wisp of hair, and birth certificate. Keep these mementos in a file in the nursery for future retrieval should parents choose not to take the items at the time of the infant's death. This intervention must be individualized according to the needs and desires of each family (Catlin and Carter, 2002; Kavanaugh and Wheeler, 2003; Kenner and Lott, 2004).

C. **Provide information about support groups and/or grief counseling.** Consideration for individual family wishes is important. Not all families want or would benefit from support groups. Family follow-up even if just a phone call from a NICU nurse or hospice nurse a few weeks after the loss is very helpful to many families.

D. **Encourage the parents to name the infant.**

E. **Provide a booklet about perinatal loss for the parents and siblings.** Pediatric hospice and palliative care programs have a number of resources for parents and the left-behind siblings. There are many books and videos that are age appropriate. A good resource is Children's Hospice International at www.chionline.org or 901 North Pitt Street, Suite, 230, Alexandria, VA 22314; phone 800-242-4453.

F. **Discuss options for autopsy, disposition of the body, and a memorial or funeral service.** It is important to ask what they need and what they would like. For some parents they wish to be an active participant in the plans. Other families want these arrangements to be done for them. Rituals surrounding death are culturally driven; for example, the taking of pictures after death is not acceptable to Native Americans, Eskimos, Amish, Hindus, and Muslims. It is the family's choice (Kavanaugh and Wheeler, 2003).

G. **Offer the option for the infant to be baptized.** This option is not acceptable in all cultures.

H. **Assist parents in understanding the importance of informing siblings about the death of the infant.** Suggest that they use simple statements based on the children's level of understanding (Siegel et al., 2002). Many times the siblings take the death much better than adults expect. Allowing them to see the infant after death may make the infant real to them. Of course parental wishes are always to be the guiding principle for how the siblings are informed of the death and what part they play in the rituals following the death.

I. **Talk with parents about possible responses** from family and friends, who often minimize the infant's death in an attempt to offer comfort. Encourage them to delegate or give tasks to those that call them. If they need the laundry done or groceries bought, then these are simple tasks that can be delegated to others that truly want to help and do not know what to do. More information on EOL issues can be obtained through the joint project of American Association of Colleges of Nursing (AACN) and the City of Hope (COH) End-of-Life Nursing Education Consortium (ELNEC) found at www.aacn.nche.edu/ELNEC/index.htm. A pediatric specific program is available.

Interventions for Parents with a Preterm or Physically, Developmentally, or Psychologically Challenged Infant

These interventions have been incorporated into the interventions listed in the previous section, The Family in Crisis, and in the following section, Family-Infant Bonding.

FAMILY-INFANT BONDING

Parents who have an infant who is born ill, prematurely, or physically or psychologically challenged are at risk of having parenting difficulties. These stressful events around the time of the infant's birth generate feelings of anxiety, disappointment, and grief in the parents. Moreover, early disruptions in the acquaintance and attachment process between parent and infant place these parents in a state of increased vulnerability for establishing a nurturing relationship with their infant. Opportunities for parents to learn to interpret their infant's unique needs and to develop reciprocal interaction through sensitivity to behavioral cues are also interrupted (Kenner et al., 2003; Krebs, 1998). The relationship between parent-infant attachment and later parenting behaviors has been well established. In addition, the parent-infant attachment is the basis for all the infant's subsequent attachments and is the relationship through which a sense of self is developed. Therefore an important component of nursing care of the high-risk infant is facilitation of parent-infant interaction and attachment.

A. Definitions.

1. *Bonding:* a gradual, reciprocal process that begins with acquaintance. It is a unique and specific relationship between two people and endures across time. Bonding occurs on a different timetable for mothers than for fathers. Although mothers experience a sharp increase in bonding around the fifth month of pregnancy and have intensifying feelings throughout the pregnancy, the father's feelings usually tend to develop more slowly than the mother's and become congruent after birth, when infant caretaking begins (Kenner et al., 2003; Krebs, 1998).
2. *Attachment:* the quality of the bond, or affectional tie, between parents and their infant, which begins early in the prenatal period, appears to increase when fetal movement is felt and is intensified with interaction between the parent and the infant after birth (Siegel et al., 2002).

B. Discussion. The development of a warm, nurturing, and reciprocal relationship between infant and parent is essential for a healthy psychologic outcome to the crisis of the birth of a premature, sick, or malformed infant (Kenner et al., 2003). "The parent 'at risk' cannot resolve a crisis surrounding birth of their infant and simultaneously establish warm attachment bonds while retaining his or her self-esteem without the support of others in the social system" (Mercer, 1977, p. 5). Neonatal nurses can provide this support by assessing the parents' responses to their infant and facilitating their acquaintance and attachment process with the infant.

C. Assessment.

1. Note pattern of parental visiting to the NICU, duration of visits, and frequency of phone calls. This pattern, if abnormal, is predictive of maternal

parenting difficulties. If parents are not visiting frequently, be careful to determine the reasons (i.e., cultural practices after childbirth, conflicting obligations between work and family roles, or lack of transportation to the hospital) before assuming that the parents are unconcerned or that parenting difficulties exist.

2. Identify the development of attachment behaviors. Mothers' activity with their infants has been found to be indicative of the initial adjustment to the infant, important past and present interpersonal relationships, and involvement in taking care of the infant (Siegel et al., 2002). Examples of attachment behaviors include:
   a. Touching: typical maternal progression of touching the premature infant is from fingertip touching of the infant's extremities to palmar stroking of the infant's trunk, to holding and embracing the infant. This progression of touch usually occurs during a period of several visits to the NICU.
   b. Looking *en face* : aligning head with infant's head in the same plane to make eye-to-eye contact with the infant.
   c. Talking to the infant, calling the infant by name.
   d. Bringing pictures, toys, and/or clothes to the hospital.
   e. Participating in caretaking activities, such as feeding, bathing, and clothing the infant.

Interventions to Encourage Family-Infant Bonding

A. **If at all possible, show the infant to the parents in the delivery room and allow them to touch the infant, if only for a few moments.** This helps to establish the reality of the infant for the parents (Kenner et al., 2003).

B. **Encourage the parents to visit** their infant in the intensive care nursery as soon as possible.
   1. Before the first visit to the nursery, prepare the parents for what to expect by giving them written information about the unit, describing the atmosphere of the nursery (i.e., noise, high activity level, infants attached to various kinds of equipment) and discussing the normal aspects of their infant as well as deviations.
   2. If the mother is unable to visit because of conditions such as ordered bed rest or transport of the infant to another hospital, the father can be given pictures of the infant for the mother. In addition, the mother should be given the phone number of the nursery and encouraged to call as often as desired.
   3. For the parents of an infant born with a malformation, encourage the parents to see the infant together as soon as possible, but do not force them to interact. Point out to the family the normal qualities of the infant as well as the abnormalities (Kenner et al., 2003; Krebs, 1998).

C. **Ensure that during the family's first visit the nurse assigned to the infant stays at the bedside** to explain equipment and the infant's condition, as well as to answer questions, provide emotional support, and encourage touching of the infant.

D. **Convey a positive, realistic attitude about the infant** rather than a negative or fatalistic viewpoint, which may alienate the parents and impair attachment (Kenner et al., 2003).

E. **Assist the parents with holding** and cuddling their infant as soon as possible, taking into consideration the infant's condition and the parents' readiness (e.g., assist in managing respiratory and monitoring equipment and intravenous [IV] lines). Some nurseries are implementing skin-to-skin care (also called kangaroo care) by parents as an alternative to the traditional modes of providing care to stable, hospitalized premature infants. This care consists of positioning the infant, dressed only in diapers, upright and prone between the mother's breasts. This vertical position in skin-to-skin contact provides tactile stimulation and warmth from the mother, as well as opportunities for eye-to-eye contact, auditory stimulation, and breast-feeding. Mothers usually wear their own front-opening blouses or dresses that are loosely fitted. Fathers can also be encouraged to engage in kangaroo care (Conde-Agudelo et al., 2003; Feldman et al., 2002; Holditch-Davis et al., 2003b; Ludington-Hoe et al., 1991.)

F. **Encourage the parents to participate in caretaking activities** as warranted by the infant's condition and tolerance for input. Explain to parents of very premature infants the relationship between neurologic maturity and the capacity for handling stimulation (Holditch-Davis et al., 2003b).

G. **Model nurturing parenting behavior** such as stroking, touching, and talking to the infant for parents who may need assistance in developing positive parenting behaviors.

H. **Give positive reinforcement** to parents as they interact with their infant. For example, say that "He seems to calm down when you talk with him," or "He really seems to sleep better after you have held him" (Kenner et al., 2003). Assisting parents to recognize positive changes in the infant in response to their caretaking has a strong impact on the parents and increases their feelings of success (Kenner et al., 2003).

I. **Use consistent caregivers for the premature or sick infant** to establish a rapport with the parents.

J. **Role-model caregiving techniques—one on one,** if possible, especially for adolescent parents.

K. **Avoid power struggles with parents by defining their role** and recognizing that they are the parents and that the infant is theirs, not the staff's.

L. **Suggest that the parents or siblings bring something** for the infant, such as a small toy, pictures of the family members to be taped on the infant's bed, and/or a tape recording of the parents' voices to be played for the infant. Share personalized information about the infant with the parents. This information can include statements such as "She really enjoys sucking on her pacifier" or "She was really active while I was giving her a bath," to assist the parents in individualizing and accepting the infant.

M. **Encourage sibling visitation** in the unit or window observation of the infant (Kenner et al., 2003; McGrath, 2003).

N. **Promote individualized family-centered developmental care that includes the family unit** in the plan of care and an environment that supports the parents. Provide a private area, or a transitional care area, to encourage parental stays within a more homelike environment, and encourage developmental care that includes parents as an integral part of the health care team (Kenner and McGrath, 2004).

O. **After the mother's discharge from the hospital, maintain communication** with the parents by providing them with the phone number of the unit. For parents of transported infants, sending pictures and cards from their infant to show current status, arranging for transportation assistance through social service agencies for parents who lack means of travel (Kenner et al., 2003), and maintaining frequent phone contact with parents can be helpful in promoting parent-infant attachment.

P. **Give the mother the opportunity to provide breast milk** for the infant should she so desire, and support her in this endeavor. However, be careful not to overemphasize the importance of breast-feeding. The rationale is that if she should be unsuccessful or decide to stop breast-feeding, feelings of guilt or disappointment may occur if breast-feeding has been touted as the ideal infant feeding method.

Q. **Identify situations in which there are difficulties in parent-infant interaction or problems in the family's functioning (Siegel et al., 2002).**
R. **Be sensitive to cultural practices** that may influence parent-infant behaviors while bonding and attachment remain strong.
S. **Identify infants who are at risk of having developmental difficulties (Siegel et al., 2002).**
T. **Identify the unique needs of the parent with lower socioeconomic status.** This parent may want to provide the best possible care to the infant but either may not know how to do so (poor role models) or may not have the means to provide for the infant's perceived needs.
U. **Assess the cultural needs of minority parents.** This means to be culturally sensitive to what the parenting role means in that culture and then gear the interventions toward these cultural values and beliefs.

Evaluation of Parent-Infant Bonding

Evaluation of parental behaviors should be based on ongoing patterns rather than on isolated incidents (Mercer, 1977).

A. **Positive attachment behaviors.** The parent:
   1. Visits frequently.
   2. Has named the infant.
   3. Makes positive comments when talking to or about the infant.
   4. Demonstrates increasing skill in holding the infant.
   5. Displays increasing eye and body contact between parent and infant (i.e., kissing, fondling, stroking, nuzzling).
B. **Behaviors of concern.** The parent:
   1. Is overly optimistic.
   2. Appears unconcerned about the infant's condition.
   3. Does not ask questions.
   4. Is passive or indifferent.
   5. Avoids close body contact by holding the infant at a distance; props the bottle whether or not the infant is held; positions the bottle in such a way that milk is unable to flow from the nipple.
   6. Is unable to describe any physical or behavioral features unique to the infant.
   7. Attributes inappropriate characteristics to the infant, such as "she's lazy and stubborn just like her father."
C. **Make sure these areas of concern are considered within the context of the culture of the parents. Different cultures approach parenthood and parent-infant interaction in different ways.**

SUMMARY OF PARENTAL NEEDS TO BE MET BY NICU STAFF

A. **Help mother reconceptualize image** of "ideal" infant to image of her premature, acutely ill, or malformed infant.
B. **Help mother deal with feelings of guilt.**
C. **Help parents develop affectionate ties** with infant through the infant's features (e.g., soft eyes; pretty, soft skin) and learn to read infant's behavioral cues.

D. **Assist parents in gaining confidence** in holding the infant by encouraging them to participate in caretaking tasks.
E. **Promote communication** between the parents.
F. **Be sensitive to the unique needs** of the individual families.
G. **Assist families in preparing for the transition** to home care after discharge (Kenner et al., 2003).
H. **Provide support for parents during the transition phase** after discharge of their infant from the NICU (Kenner et al., 2003).
I. **Assist parents in dealing with neonatal death** in a personally meaningful way.
J. **Assist the parents in describing their cultural values and beliefs,** if applicable, to understand their view of their infant and their role as parents.

REFERENCES

Alpers, R.R.: The changing self-concept of pregnant and parenting teens. *Journal of Professional Nursing, 14*(2):111-118, 1998.

Bracht, M., Ardal, F., Bot, A., and Cheng, C.M.: Initiation and maintenance of a hospital-based parent group for parents of premature infants: Key factors for success. *Neonatal Network, 17*(3):33-37, 1998.

Catlin, A. and Carter, B.: Creation of a neonatal end-of-life palliative care protocol. *Journal of Perinatology, 22*(3):184-195, 2002.

Conde-Agudelo, A., Diaz-Rossello, J.L., and Belizan, J.M.: Kangaroo mother care to reduce morbidity and mortality in low birthweight infants. *Cochrane Database of Systematic Reviews, 2003*(2):CD002771, 2003.

Davis, L., Edwards, H., Mohay, H., and Wolin, J.: The impact of very premature birth on the psychological health of mothers. *Early Human Development, 73*(1-2):61-70, 2003.

Davis, L., Mohay, H., and Edwards, H.: Mothers' involvement in caring for their premature infants: A historical overview. *Journal of Advanced Nursing, 42*(6):578-586, 2003.

Dishion, T.J., Bullock, B.M., and Granic, I.: Pragmatism in modeling peer influence: Dynamics, outcomes, and change processes. *Development and Psychopathology, 14*(4):969-981, 2002.

Docherty, S.L., Miles, M.S., and Holditch-Davis, D.: Worry about child health in mothers of hospitalized medically fragile infants. *Advances in Neonatal Care, 2*(2):84-92, 2002.

Feldman, R., Eidelman, A.I., Sirota, L., and Weller, A.: Comparison of skin-to-skin (kangaroo) and traditional care: Parenting outcomes and preterm infant development. *Pediatrics, 110*(1 Pt 1):16-26, 2002.

Geron, Y., Ginzburg, K., and Solomon, Z.: Predictors of bereaved parents' satisfaction with group support: An Israeli perspective. *Death Studies, 27*(5):405-426, 2003.

Glicken, A.D. and Merenstein, G.B.: A neonatal end-of-life palliative protocol—An evolving new standard of care? *Neonatal Network, 21*(4):35-36, 2002.

Gray, K., Dostal, S., Ternullo-Retta, C., and Armstrong, M.A.: Developmentally supportive care in a neonatal intensive care unit: A research utilization project. *Neonatal Network, 17*(2):33-38, 1998.

Gretebeck, R.J., Shaffer, D., and Bishop-Kurylo, D.B.: Clinical pathways for family-oriented developmental care in the intensive care nursery. *Journal of Perinatal and Neonatal Nursing, 12*(1):70-80, 1998.

Griffin, T.: The visitation policy. *Neonatal Network, 17*(2):75-76, 1998.

Hall, R.T., Santos, S.R., Cofield, F., et al.: Perinatal outcomes in a school-based program for pregnant teen-agers. *Missouri Medicine, 100*(2):148-152, 2003.

Holditch-Davis, D., Bartlett, T.R., Blickman, A.L., and Miles, M.S.: Posttraumatic stress symptoms in mothers of premature infants. *Journal of Obstetric, Gynecologic, and Neonatal Nursing, 32*(2):161-171, 2003a.

Holditch-Davis, D., Blackburn, S.T., and VandenBerg, K.: Newborn and infant neurobehavioral development. In C. Kenner and J.W. Lott (Eds): *Comprehensive neonatal nursing: A physiologic perspective* (3rd ed.). St Louis, 2003b, Saunders, pp. 236-284.

Holditch-Davis, D., Cox, M.F., Miles, M.S., and Belyea, M.: Mother-infant interactions of medically fragile infants and on-chronically ill premature infants. *Research in Nursing & Health, 26*(4):300-311, 2003c.

Joffe, G.M. and Wright, M.: Prenatal environment: Effect on neonatal outcome. In G.B. Merenstein and S.L. Gardner (Eds.): *Handbook of neonatal intensive care* (5th ed.). St Louis, 2002, Mosby, pp. 9-30.

Johnson-Crowley, N. and Conrad, L.: Systematic assessment and home follow-up: A basis for monitoring the neonate's integration into the family unit. In C. Kenner and J.W. Lott (Eds.): *Comprehensive neonatal nursing: A physiologic perspective* (3rd ed.). St Louis, 2003, Saunders, pp. 876-892.

Kavanaugh, K. and Wheeler, S.R.: When a baby dies: Caring for bereaved families. In C. Kenner and J.W. Lott (Eds.): *Comprehensive neonatal nursing: A physiologic perspective* (3rd ed.). St Louis, 2003, Saunders, pp. 108-126.

Kenner, C., Bagwell, G.A., and Spangler-Torok, L.: Assessment and management of the transition to home. In C. Kenner and J.W. Lott (Eds.): *Comprehensive neonatal nursing: A physiologic perspective* (3rd ed.). St Louis, 2003, Saunders, pp. 893-909.

Kenner, C. and Lott, J.W.: *Neonatal nursing handbook*. St Louis, 2004, Saunders.

Kenner, C. and McGrath, J.M.: *Developmental care of newborns and infants: A guide for health professionals*. St Louis, 2004, Mosby.

Kohner, N. and Henley, A.: *When a baby dies: The experience of late miscarriage, stillbirth, and neonatal death*. Routledge, NY, 2001, Routledge.

Koshar, J.H., Lee, K.A., Goss, G., et al.: The Hispanic teen mother's origin of birth, use of prenatal care, and maternal and neonatal complications. *Journal of Pediatric Nursing, 13*(3):151-157, 1998.

Krebs, T.L.: Clinical pathway for enhanced parent and preterm infant interaction through parent education. *Journal of Pediatric Nursing, 12*:38-49, 1998.

Levin, B.: Grief counseling. *American Journal of Nursing, 98*(5):69-72, 1998.

Ludington-Hoe, S.M., Hadeed, A.J., and Anderson, G.C.: Physiologic responses to skin-to-skin contact in hospitalized premature infants. *Journal of Perinatology, 11*(1):19-24, 1991.

Lundqvist, A., Nilstun, T., and Dykes, A.K.: Neonatal end-of-life care in Sweden: The views of Muslim women. *Journal of Perinatal and Neonatal Nursing, 17*(1):77-86, 2003.

Lurie, T.: Fathers and families: Forging ties that bind. *Ford Foundation Report, 23*(3):3-8, 1992.

Lynch, E.W. and Hanson, M.J.: *Developing cross-cultural competence* (2nd ed.). Baltimore, 1998, Paul Brooks Publishing.

Mayes, L.C.: Child mental health consultation with families of medically compromised infants. *Child and Adolescent Psychiatric Clinics of North America, 12*(3):401-421, 2003.

McGrath, J.M.: Family-centered care. In C. Kenner and J.W. Lott (Eds.): *Comprehensive neonatal nursing: A physiologic perspective* (3rd ed.). St Louis, 2003, Saunders, pp. 89-107.

Mercer, R.T.: *Nursing care for parents at risk*. Thorofare, NJ, 1977, Charles B. Slack.

Miles, M.S., Holditch-Davis, D., and Shepherd, H.: Maternal concerns about parenting prematurely born children. *MCN American Journal of Maternal Child Nursing, 23*(2):70-75, 1998.

Moore, M.L., and Freda, M.C.: Reducing preterm and low birthweight births: Still a nursing challenge. *MCN American Journal of Maternal Child Nursing, 23*(4):200-208, 1998.

Nurses Association of the American College of Obstetricians and Gynecologists: *NAACOG standards for the nursing care of women and newborns* (4th ed.). Washington, DC, 1991, Author.

Peebles-Kleiger, M.J.: Pediatric and neonatal intensive care hospitalization as traumatic stressor: Implications for intervention. *Bulletin of the Menninger Clinic, 64*(2):257-280, 2000.

Pohlman, S.: Father's role in NICU care: Evidence-based practice. In C. Kenner and J.M. McGrath (Eds): *Developmental care of newborns and infants: A guide for health professionals*. St Louis, 2004, Mosby.

Raines, D.A.: Values of mothers of low birth weight infants in the NICU. *Neonatal Network, 17*(6):41-64, 1998.

Rivett, M. and Street E.: Connections and themes of spirituality in family therapy. *Family Process, 40*(4):459-467, 2001.

Rolland, J.S.: Chronic illness and the life cycle: A conceptual framework. *Family Process, 26*(2):229-244, 1994.

Siegel, R., Gardner, S.L., and Merenstein, G.B.: Families in crisis: Theoretical and practical considerations. In G.B. Merenstein and S.L. Gardner (Eds.): *Handbook of neonatal intensive care* (5th ed.). St Louis, 2002, Mosby, pp. 725-753.

Street, E. and Soldan J.: A conceptual framework for the psychosocial issues faced by families with genetic conditions. *Families, Systems & Health, 16*(3):217-232, 1998.

Sudia-Robinson, T.: Hospice and palliative care. In C. Kenner and J.W. Lott (Eds.): *Comprehensive neonatal nursing: A physiologic perspective* (3rd ed.). St Louis, 2003, Saunders, pp. 127-131.

Ullrich, P.M. and Lutgendorf, S.K.: Journaling about stressful events: Effects of cognitive processing and emotional expression. *Annals of Behavioral Medicine, 24*(3):244-250, 2002.

Wereszczak, J., Miles, M.S., and Holditch-Davis, D.: Maternal recall of neonatal intensive care unit. *Neonatal Network, 16*(4):33-40, 1997.

CHAPTER

18 Patient Safety

DEBORA SIMMONS

OBJECTIVES

1. Define and discuss organizational approaches to error.
2. Describe types of health care errors.
3. Define safety-related terms.
4. Discuss human factors and the relation to common errors.
5. Describe special risks associated with neonatal intensive care units and the special vulnerabilities of neonates.
6. List Internet sites and organizations where reliable safety information can be found.

Nurses must recognize and understand the causes of errors in order to practice safely. The knowledge and skills associated with safety must become a routine part of nursing practice. Improving patient safety requires assimilation of knowledge from other disciplines and industries, and application of safety knowledge to health care.

Neonatal care is complex and with these complexities comes an increased chance of errors. Applying the principles of human factors, system complexities, and cognitive processes has increased safe practice in other complex and high-risk industries. Although the complexities of health care and especially neonatal care are a challenge, it is possible that nurses armed with basic knowledge of safety can decrease errors.

The following chapter offers an introduction of the basic principles and resources available for increasing safety in your nursing practice. At the end of the chapter is a list of Internet sites that may be used to increase your awareness and practice of safety.

A. **Organizational and professional approaches to errors in health care.**
   1. **Person-centered approach**—the response to error in health care has been the person-centered approach. The person-centered approach focuses on individual responsibility and does not recognize inevitable human fallibility. Under the person-centered approach errors are "solved" by blaming individuals for forgetfulness, inattention, or moral weakness (Reason, 2000).

      Reactions to errors under this approach include instituting increasingly complex or strict policy and procedures, hard rule disciplinary actions, retraining, and the infamous naming-blaming-and-shaming. Focusing on individual failure seldom addresses recurrent system failures and therefore does not decrease errors (Reason, 1997).
   2. **The systems approach**. A system is a set of interdependent and interacting parts that have a single goal (Kohn et al., 1999). Health and well-being are dependent upon the interaction and interdependence of cardiovascular, renal, and respiratory systems. Safety in health care is much like these

physiologic determinants. Changing one area may create a problem in another. Weaknesses or flaws in systems of the health care organization—whether they are in communication, teams, patient identification, drug dispensing, staffing, or policies—influence the ability to deliver consistently safe care.

By concentrating on the conditions in the workplace that influence the occurrence of errors, the systems approach builds defenses that will avert errors (Reason, 2000). The systems approach recognizes that human performance is not perfect and errors are to be expected. The focus is changed to analyzing the characteristics of the whole system and then making changes to decrease the likelihood of error occurring again (Leape et al., 1995). By moving the focus of responsibility for errors from individual practitioners to the system in which they work, the systems approach has achieved success in the aviation and nuclear industries, with safety practices that have intervened at the root cause of problems. Reviewing safety from the systems approach is an inclusive process and counts the relationships between providers, the exchange of information, environmental factors, and the practices of providers as influential.

The systems approach does not absolve individuals from the accountability of practice (Small and Barach, 2002) nor does it take away responsibility for quality work from individuals (Leape et al., 1995). A professional practicing under the systems approach recognizes a duty to report, pursue, and innovate new safe methods for delivering care in order to decrease errors (Small and Barach, 2002).

B. **Important milestones in patient safety.**

1. **"To Err Is Human: Building a Safer Health System."** The Institute of Medicine (Kohn et al., 1999) concluded that 44,000 to 98,000 patient deaths per year are attributable to preventable medical errors. The concept of failure in health care due to a lack of safety systems, even under the best intentions, was introduced for the first time. The report also promoted the concept of caring health care professionals who make honest mistakes owing to factors beyond their control. The culture of punishment of the health care practitioner is a barrier to safety because it forces providers to hide important safety information that can be learned from an analysis of errors. Included is a call for a national agenda for reducing medical errors through design of a safer health system and a decrease in medical errors by 50% in the next 5 years (the full report can be obtained free online at http://books.nap.edu).
2. **"Crossing the Quality Chasm."** This report (2001) followed the one above, and called for a massive redesign and sweeping changes in the health care delivery system in the United States with equitable patient-driven care delivered by teams of health care professionals (see online report at www.nap.edu).
3. **Council on Graduate Medical Education and the National Advisory Council on Nurse Education and Practice Meeting under the direction of the Health and Human Resources and Services Administration 2000).** The result of this meeting was a list of key recommendations including a call to reform the historical divide between medicine and nursing, and improve interdisciplinary training and practice.
4. **The Leapfrog Group** is an organization sponsored by the Business Roundtable to leverage purchasing power of large self-insured companies. The goal is to improve patient safety by directing their employees to health

care facilities that adhere to evidence-based practices that decrease errors and increase the quality of care (Small and Barach, 2002). This is the first consumer-driven initiative that includes reimbursement as a reward for safe and high-quality care.

5. **Denver, Colorado (October, 1996).** The death of a newborn is attributed to a medication error in this highly publicized case. The investigation revealed more than 50 systems factors that contributed to the error. The nurses were charged with criminally negligent homicide and later acquitted (Cohen, 1999) (see more analysis at www.ismp.org).

C. **Types of health care errors.**

1. **Medication errors.** Medication errors are the most commonly detected errors in health care and account for at least one third of adverse drug events (Bates et al., 1995). Medication errors happen throughout the stages of drug delivery and include preventable and nonpreventable adverse drug events (ADE).
2. **Common stages of medication ordering and delivery where errors occur.**
   a. **Prescribing.** In the general patient population, 71% percent of serious medication errors occur at the prescribing stage of the drug-ordering and delivery system (Senst et al., 2001). A high percentage of neonates, one of the most high-risk populations of patients due to their physiology, have been found to have medication errors that originate in the ordering stage (Kaushal et al., 2001). Weight-adjusted doses pose considerable risk for mathematical errors; the most frequent type of serious error being decimal point misplacement resulting in tenfold errors in prescriptions (Buck, 1999; Selbst et al., 1999).

   b. **Transcribing.** Poor handwriting and errors in transcription account for many errors in administration. Systems that rely on multiple transcriptions and "hand-offs" of written information increase the chance of an error in the transcription phase. Errors related to similarly spelled drug names and similarly sounding drug names are common. Equally problematic are ambiguous abbreviations (Cohen, 1999).

   c. **Dispensing.** Three primary types of dispensing errors are ambiguous names, mistaken abbreviations, and "look-alike" drugs that bear the same color and shape as other drugs (*Note:* the Institute for Safe Medication Practices has alerts with examples of "look-alike" packaging available at www.ISMP.org). Incorrect placement of computerized labels and poor storage techniques (for example, where lethal drugs are placed near others) also lead to dispensing errors (Cohen, 1999). In some cases, the order may be correct but the dose prepared is incorrect. Products available in multiple strengths such as digoxin and phenytoin may be confused with the more frequently used "adult" preparations by those unaccustomed to working with pediatric patients (Buck, 1999). Stock solutions require dilution routinely, increasing the risk of dilution errors (Kaushal et al., 2001).

   d. **Administration.** Errors are frequently detected at the point of administration although the error may have begun in an earlier stage. Although the errors are more easily detected at the point of administration, it is important to analyze the entire event and contributing factors in order to understand how to prevent the error in the future, i.e., perform a root cause analysis. Inadequate information at the point of care, incomplete medical orders, or mislabeled patient charts can cause administration errors (Buck, 1999). Infusion devices with poorly designed programming functions and high workloads can also contribute to errors in administration.

3. **Monitoring errors.** Failure to monitor a patient for a known or unknown complication may be due to lack of knowledge, inadequate resources, or human error in attention (for example, failure to reconnect a monitoring device, set alarm limits, or failure to recognize signs of adverse reactions) (Buchino et al., 2002). Complications may be due to new drug therapies or unknown interactions and may go unrecognized. Alarm limit functions that allow for suspension of alarms and do not revert after suspension may also cause a failure to monitor.
4. **Diagnostic errors.** Errors occur in all aspects of health care. Errors in diagnosis can be attributed to failed information sharing, failure to make an accurate diagnosis, or delays in diagnosis, as well as failure to perform appropriate tests to determine diagnosis (Leape, 1994). Diagnostic errors include decisions based on the wrong laboratory results or mislabeled test results.
5. **Errors in treatment** may be due to a lack of technical skills, errors made in administration, avoidable delays in treatment, and inappropriate care (Leape, 1994). Complex protocols, unfamiliar equipment, and new procedures also increase the risk for errors in treatment.
6. **Error of omission.** Omitting a procedure, treatment, or medication for a patient may have potential harmful results for the patient. Errors of omission may be the result of a wrong judgment by a skilled and knowledgeable practitioner (Wu et al., 1997).

D. **Terms related to safety.**

1. **Active failure**—an error that occurs at the level of the frontline operator and whose effects are felt almost immediately (Kohn et al., 1999). These are difficult to anticipate and have an immediate adverse impact on safety by breaching, bypassing, or disabling existing defenses (JCAHO, 2003a). They may be increased in overly strict policy and procedures that require breaches to complete tasks (Reason, 1997).
2. ADE—a response to a drug that is noxious, unintended, and occurs at doses normally used in adults for the prophylaxis, diagnosis, or therapy of disease, or for modification of physiologic function (Edwards and Aronson, 2000). This also includes an injury resulting from medical interventions related to administration of a drug (Leape et al., 1995).
3. **Adverse drug reaction (ADR)**—an undesirable response associated with use of a drug (JCAHO, 2003b).
4. **Blunt end**—describes the part of the error trajectory not apparent to the "sharp end" and indicates the beginnings of the error event. Decisions that seem harmless at the blunt end may create a sequence of events that lead to an error. Defenses against blunt-end errors include standardizing equipment and medications, including "frontline" providers in buying decisions and performing analysis of possible failures for new additions to the clinical area.
5. **Error**—an unintended act (whether of omission or commission) or an act that does not achieve its intended outcome (Leape, 1999).
6. **Failure mode and effects analysis (FMEA)**—a multidisciplinary exercise used to help proactively identify error prone circumstances. Use of FMEA allows for safety brainstorming before an error occurs. FMEA has been used as a quality process to identify weak system links and rank possible errors by severity and occurrence (Cohen, 1999).

7. **Five rights.** The "five rights" are rules traditionally thought to safeguard against errors. The five rights of medication administration (right patient, right drug, right dose, right route, and right frequency) are the basis of most education on drug administration and considered the "safe" way to administer medications. The five rights do not safeguard against major sources of error and may limit critical thinking (Mitchell, 2001).
8. **Forcing functions are** interventions that prevent error by "forcing" a safe action, such as removing concentrated potassium from the medication carts. Forcing functions are the strongest of interventions against human failure. A common example of a forcing function is designing oral syringes such that they cannot be connected to an intravenous port.
9. **Iatrogenic injury** is unintended injuries that result from therapeutic interactions. They can be a result of an act of omission or commission (Small and Barach, 2002).
10. **Latent failure.** Latent threats and errors come from faulty systems that have a delayed effect of causing an error (Reason, 1990). Latent failures pose the greatest danger to complex systems because they are difficult to track and defend (JCAHO, 2003a). Latent factors include aspects of the hospital, medical organization, or practice that are not always easily identifiable but that predispose the commission of errors or the emergence of overt threats (Helmreich, 2000). Examples of latent errors include workloads and schedules that increase fatigue and hasty decisions, shortsighted or exhausting staffing schedules, poor resource allocations, process and policies that impede workflow, and environmental or equipment designs that decrease the ability to remain attentive or accurate.
11. **Near miss or close call**—events that could have caused harm but were caught before they reached the patient (Cohen, 1997). Reports of close calls occur many more times than actual errors. They range from benign actions to near catastrophic events and are extremely valuable in preventing errors. Unfortunately, reporting of near miss or close calls can be blocked by the reporter's fear of retribution, being "blamed" or fear of being thought "not careful" (Reason, 1997) . Close call reporting systems that allow for anonymous reporting may increase reports and increase the creation of valuable safety practices. The University of Texas Close Call reporting system (www.UTCCRS.org) is one example of an anonymous reporting system to collect close call reports and share information with other hospitals.
12. **Negligence or negligent conduct**—a failure to use care and actions as a reasonably prudent and careful nurse would use under similar circumstances, or a failure to exercise the skill, care, and learning expected of a reasonably prudent health care provider, or a failure to recognize risk (JCAHO, 2003b). Errors attributed to individual negligence in the past have been shown to be due to a complex set of system circumstances. Fear of being labeled "negligent" may be one barrier to health care providers reporting unsafe conditions or circumstance.
13. **Nonpunitive approach**—a cultural change in health care that will increase learning about mistakes and errors, and reduce fear by focusing on the cause of an error and not the participants. This approach allows for learning and development of safety interventions (Cohen, 1999).
14. **Root cause and root cause analysis.** The root cause is the most fundamental reason for the failure or inefficiency of a process (JCAHO, 2003a). Root cause analysis is a process for identifying the basic or causal factor(s) such that learning can take place and errors avoided in the future.

15. **Sentinel event**—an unexpected occurrence that causes significant physical or psychologic harm or death, or has risk of causing significant harm (Cohen, 1997; JCAHO, 2003b). Such events are called sentinel because they signal the need for immediate investigation and response (JCAHO, 2003a). The root causes of sentinel events identified for 1995 through 2002 included deficits in communication, orientation and training, patient assessment, and availability of information (JCAHO, 2003a).
16. **Sharp end.** The frontline personnel at the human-system interface where the error becomes apparent are at the "sharp end." For example, the nurse who administers the wrong drug is at the sharp end as is the physician who removes the wrong leg in surgery. Research shows that the sharp end is greatly influenced by the decisions made "upstream" of the error (also called latent error or latent failure). Resources, constraints, incentives, and demands by the environment greatly influence the ability of the sharp end to operate safely (Reason, 1997).
17. **Threats** are factors that increase the likelihood of an error being committed. They may be environmental (such as lighting, colors, digital displays that look alike), person related (fatigue, stress, illness, fear), staff related (communication), or patient related (a difficult intubation, complicated comorbidities) (Helmreich, 2000).

E. **Human factors research and health care errors.** Human factors include the interrelationships between humans, the tools they use, and the environment in which they live and work. Human factors are at the root cause of many errors. The cognitive aspect of errors in health care makes use of "human factors" in the design of systems and equipment to safeguard against the inevitable faults in human performance. Human factor science evaluates how humans process information and is essential to design and safety in the health care system (Schneider, 2002). Equipment design failures often result from the failure to apply basic human factor principles to the design of equipment (Leape, 1999). Environmental factors such as poorly designed work areas can contribute to fatigue, poor teamwork, and ultimately errors (Cohen, 1999; Kaushal et al., 2001). The development of an understanding of the contributing human factors and modes of errors that result is the first step in decreasing errors.

F. **Error modes.**

1. **Automatic mode**—the state of mind in which familiar and/or scripted actions take place effortlessly. Tasks are often monotonous and frequent. We do not "think " about the task but are performing from our internal script. Errors that occur are often unconscious to the participant. Factors that increase automatic mode errors are fatigue, stress, and environmental stressors. There are two common types of automatic mode errors:
   a. **Slips**—errors made in familiar tasks; they are unconscious and often undetected by the person making the slip. Slips occur in familiar tasks that are usually done without effort and performed perfectly (for example, locking the keys in the car, forgetting to date/time an order, not latching the door on the IV pump) (Reason, 1990).
   b. **Lapses**—an error of not remembering what was done in automatic mode. Lapses are made in familiar tasks or task sequences and may also not be detected by the participant (for example, walking into the kitchen and forgetting to get what you came for, "forgetting" to chart an important fact or detail) (Reason, 1990).
2. **Nonautomatic mode**—types of errors that are made with the attention of the participant. They include errors in processing information and making

decisions. Nonautomatic mode errors are increased with fatigue and stressors. The participants may believe they are making the right choice but later wonder how they came to that conclusion. Nonautomatic mode errors are often called mistakes, and include errors in the thought process such as (Cohen, 1999; Reason, 1990):

a. Applying the wrong rule to a situation (rule based).
b. Similarity matching (this looks similar to that so it must be that).
c. Errors related to a lack of experience (failure of expertise).
d. Grabbing the first answer that comes to mind.
e. Misinterpretation of information.
f. Inadequate training.
g. Decisions made with incomplete information.
h. Wrong judgment or faulty knowledge.

G. **Special considerations for neonatal intensive care.** It has been suggested that neonates experience significantly higher rates of medication errors and adverse drug events (Kaushal et al., 2001). The most frequent medication errors were associated with bronchodilators, antiinfective agents, analgesics and sedatives, and electrolytes and fluids (Kaushal et al., 2001).

1. **Risks related to the neonate** include rapid changes in body weight, body water distribution, protein binding capacity, hepatic maturity or immaturity, variation in renal function, and being "therapeutic orphans" of drug testing considered routine in adults (Stokowski, 2001). There is an increased risk of errors related to dilution owing to the inavailability of medications that are appropriately diluted by the manufacturer for the patient's small size (Kaushal et al., 2001). In addition, critically ill neonates may not have the capacity to withstand errors because of fragile physiology.
2. **Risks related to the environment and equipment.** High-stress areas substantially increase the risk of human errors (Reason, 1990). Complex or poorly designed systems, poor teamwork, and environmental stressors also increase the frequency of errors (Kaushal et al., 2001). The need for precise dosing is hampered by the technology of the drug delivery system—small doses may get caught in the Y of intravenous connections, and diluting drugs in the same syringe does not allow for dead space that can increase the dose (Stokowski, 2001).There is also a lack of neonatal specific information and labeling information on many medications used in neonatal therapy (Levine et al., 2001).
3. **Risks related to medications.** Multiple factors in medication administration can contribute to errors. System improvements have been suggested to decrease risk and increase safety in neonatal care and include (Levine et al., 2001; Stokowski, 2001):
   a. Lack of published information related to dosing neonates, which may lead to problems in dosing and calculations.
   b. Poor labeling, which makes details hard to read and vital information easy to miss, is found in every area of the hospital.
   c. The use of unit stock medication and preparation of medication by nurses on the units without pharmacist assistance.
   d. Improper dilution techniques of very small doses (the needle hub dead space can contain enough of the substance for overdosage of a neonate).

H. **Recommendations for improvements.** Clearly the use of root cause analysis to reexamine the underlying system failures in errors have led to best practices that apply to every practice setting. The following list includes best practices from several sources and is by no means exhaustive. The absolute best practice is a commitment to safety that allows for learning and active participation of all persons in the health care continuum, from patient (and families) to provider. Please consult the reference list for more detail.

1. Instruction and practice in determining mathematical calculations related to neonatal populations. Independently checked calculations and calculations clearly stated on the medication order (Alert, 2002).
2. Standardized abbreviations (Cohen, 1999).
3. Standardized formulary.
4. Medication reference manual should include multiple dilutions of the same drug.
5. Storage of neonatal doses away from adult doses (Cohen, 1999).
6. Increased availability of dilute forms of drugs used in neonatal areas (Kaushal et al., 2001).
7. Use of technology that includes careful consideration of human factors (bar coding, computerized order entry) and the impact on the existing practice patterns. The use of failure mode and effects analysis before implementation of technology.
8. Regular use of failure mode and effects analysis and root cause analysis to identify and defend against risk.
9. Limits on verbal orders.
10. Read-back of new telephone orders after the order has been written on the chart (JCAHO, 2003a).
11. Use of at least two patient identifiers to increase accuracy of patient identification (JCAHO, 2003a).
12. Use of active communication to verify patient identity and call "time out" to verify identity prior to procedures (JCAHO, 2003a).
13. Removal of concentrated electrolytes from patient care units (JCAHO, 2003a).
14. Ensuring free-flow protection on all general-use intravenous pumps and implementation of limits on the amounts to be infused (JCAHO, 2003a).
15. Preferred use of "neonatal" intravenous pumps.
16. Implementation of regular preventive maintenance and testing of alarm systems. Ensure that alarms are activated with appropriate settings and are sufficiently audible with respect to distances and competing noise within the unit (JCAHO, 2003a).
17. Use of computer prescribing order entry (or CPOE) systems with features that integrate information between departments and verify correct dosages. Computerized "forcing functions" are functions that limit routes and frequencies of drugs that are ordered and are specific to neonates, such as weight in kilograms and age in days of life (Levine et al., 2001).
18. Staff education that builds and reinforces communication and recognition of unsafe circumstances (Levine, 2001).
19. Increased education, emphasis, and practice of teamwork skills. Teamwork in health care has been compared with other high-risk industries: nuclear power, aviation, and the chemical industry and lessons learned from their experience. The following team behaviors have been identified to increase risk of error (Helmreich, 2000; Sherwood et al., 2002):
    a. Poor communication between members.
    b. Failure to establish leadership.
    c. Interpersonal conflict.
    d. Hostility and frustration.
    e. Failure to plan for contingencies in treatment plan.
    f. Failure to support other team members.

I. Internet resources for patient safety.

1. Agency for Healthcare Research and Quality (AHRQ) Medical Errors Research Page. The contributions of Agency for Healthcare Research and Quality (formerly AHCPR) have resulted in a broader understanding of what the patient safety problems are and where they occur in the delivery of health care. AHRQ-supported research is leading to a rethinking of what does and does not work at the health care systems level. www.ahcpr.gov/qual/errorsix.htm
2. American Society of Health-System Pharmacists (ASHP) and its Research and Education Foundation have been helping pharmacists and others understand and prevent medication errors and adverse drug events for decades. This page includes a helpful section on "Medical Misadventures." www.ashp.org
3. American Society of Healthcare Risk Management (ASHRM) is a professional membership organization devoted to identification, evaluation, and control of risks that could cause injury to the patient and financial loss to the institutions they represent. www.ashrm.org/asp/home/home.asp.
4. Anesthesia Patient Safety Foundation (APSF). The mission of the APSF is to ensure that no patient shall be harmed by anesthesia. The purposes of the foundation are to foster investigations that will provide a better understanding of preventable anesthetic injuries, encourage programs that will reduce the number of anesthetic injuries, and promote national and international communication of information and ideas about the causes and prevention of anesthetic injuries. www.gasnet.org/societies/apsf.
5. "Crossing the Quality Chasm." This report (2001), following "To Err Is Human," called for a massive redesign of and sweeping changes in the health care delivery system in the United States with equitable patient-driven care delivered by teams of health care professionals (see online report at www.nap.edu).
6. ECRI (formerly Emergency Care Research Institute) is a nonprofit health services research agency. Its mission is to improve the safety, quality, and cost-effectiveness of health care. It is widely recognized as one of the world's leading independent organizations committed to advancing the quality of health care. www.ecri.org.
7. US Food and Drug Administration (FDA) MedWatch. MedWatch is an initiative designed to educate all health care professionals about the critical importance of being aware of, monitoring for, and reporting adverse events and problems, and to facilitate reporting to the agency. www.fda.gov/medwatch.
8. Institute for Healthcare Improvement (IHI) is an organization that hosts seminars and promotes a collaborative approach to reducing error in health care. One noted category of its program is the Breakthrough Series Collaborative on reducing adverse drug events and medical errors. www.ihi.org.
9. Institute for Safe Medication Practices (ISMP) is dedicated to making safety the highest performing function in its member organizations and to thereby ensure that facilities are as safe as possible for patients and staff. The organization has contributed countless alerts for health care professionals and patients. Links here include information to subscribe to *ISMP Medication Safety Alert!* and a special nursing newsletter. www.ismp.org.
10. Joint Commission on Accreditation of Healthcare Organizations (JCAHO) is a nationally recognized accreditation agency for hospitals, managed care entities, and other types of health care facilities. The website includes a

sentinel event alert, a glossary, a list of educational programs, and an annotated bibliography. In addition, information on how to perform a root-cause analysis is located here. www.jcaho.org.

11. The Leapfrog Group is an organization sponsored by the Business Roundtable to leverage purchasing power of large self-insured companies. The goal is to improve patient safety by directing their employees to health care facilities that adhere to evidence-based practices that decrease errors and increase quality of care (Small and Barach, 2002). This is the first consumer-driven initiative that includes reimbursement as a reward for safe and high-quality care. www.leapfroggroup.org.
12. Medical Device Safety Reports (MDSR) is a repository of medical device incident and hazard information independently examined by ECRI, a nonprofit health services research agency. MDSR is a collective look at the types of problems that have occurred with medical devices and lessons learned over the past three decades. www.mdsr.ecri.org/index.asp.
13. The National Patient Safety Foundation (NPSF) has many references for safety. The NPSF Clearinghouse Bibliography of patient safety literature is an extensive listing of references for medical error reduction research as well as an excellent online discussion group. www.NPSF.org.
14. Public Entity Risk Institute (PERI). The mission of the PERI is to serve public, private, and nonprofit organizations as a resource for the enhancement of risk management. www.riskinstitute.org.
15. The University of Texas Close Call Reporting System (UTCCRS) is a voluntary and anonymous tool designed to gather valuable information about close calls, which are situations that could have resulted in an accident, injury, or illness, but did not due to chance or a timely intervention. Information from narrow escape reports inform the development of targeted interventions and ultimately lead to the identification and implementation of best practices in quality improvement.
16. The Center for Patient Safety in Neonatal Intensive Care. The Vermont Oxford Network is a nonprofit voluntary collaboration of health care professionals dedicated to improving the quality and safety of medical care for newborn infants and their families. Established in 1988, the network is today composed of more than 400 neonatal intensive care units, predominantly in the United States. In support of its mission, the network maintains a database including information about the care and outcomes of high-risk newborn infants. The database provides unique, reliable, and confidential data to participating units for use in quality management, process improvement, internal audit, and peer review. www.vtoxford.org.
17. **"To Err Is Human: Building a Safer Health System."** This important work by the Institute of Medicine (Kohn et al., 1999) concluded that 44,000 to 98,000 patient deaths per year are attributable to preventable medical errors. The report introduced the concept of failure in health care even under the best intentions due to lack of safety systems. Also introduced was the concept of caring health care professionals who make honest mistakes owing to factors beyond their control. Included is a call for a national agenda for reducing medical errors through design of a safer health system and a decrease in medical errors by 50% in the next 5 years. (The full report can be obtained free online at http://books.nap.edu.)
18. Web morbity and mortality (M&M). AHRQ Web M&M is the nation's first web-based patient safety resource and journal. This site describes near misses in health care by population and performs a human factors and

systems analysis to identify strategies to prevent real harm in the future. www.webmm.ahrq.gov.

19. Talk About Prescriptions. This National Council on Patient Information and Education (NCPIE) website provides practical and educational resources, tips, and background articles for consumers and health care professionals concerned with ensuring safe, appropriate use of medications. www.talkaboutrx.org.
20. U.S. Food and Drug Administration Center for Devices and Radiological Health Evaluation and Research. The FDA provides educational programs and opportunities for information exchange to meet its regulatory and scientific needs using a variety of techniques. A cost-effective way of interacting with a large audience is with live satellite teleconferences. A satellite teleconference is a live program, broadcast to a satellite, that anyone interested can download and watch. www.fda.gov/cdrh/useerror/Index.html.
21. US Pharmacopoeia (USP) promotes public health by establishing and disseminating officially recognized standards of quality and authoritative information for the use of medicines and other health care technologies by health professionals, patients, and consumers. The page provides access to the USP Medication Errors Reporting (MEP) program, which facilitates the reporting of actual or potential medication errors. www.usp.org.
22. Veterans Administration Virtual Learning Center (VLC) was designed to provide a mechanism for individuals to post "lessons learned" and share knowledge. In particular, a section here is devoted to "Patient Safety" in which the sharing of lessons learned from adverse events, or from proactive actions aimed at preventing future occurrences, is encouraged. www.va.gov/med/osp/default.asp.

REFERENCES

Alert, I. M.S.: *ISMP medication safety alert.* 2002. www.ismp.org

Bates, D.W., Cullen, D.J., Laird, N., et al.: Incidence of adverse drug events and potential adverse drug events: Implications for prevention. *Journal of the American Medical Association, 274*(1):29-34, 1995.

Buchino J.J., Corey, T.S., and Montgomery V.: Sudden unexpected death in hospitalized children. *Journal of Pediatrics, 140*(4):461-465, 2002.

Buck, M. Preventing medication errors in children. A monthly review for health care professionals of the Children's Medical Center, 1999. Accessed 1/2/03.

Cohen, M.: *Medication errors.* Washington, DC, 1999, American Pharmaceutical Foundation.

Cohen, M.S.: Risk analysis and treatment. *Medication errors.* Sudbury, Mass, 20.1-20.34, 1997. Jones and Bartlett Publishers.

Council on Graduate Medical Education: National Advisory Council on Nurse Education and Practice and the Council on Graduate Medical Education. collaborative Education to Ensure Patient Safety. 2000. Health Resources and Services Administration, Washington, D.C.

Edwards, I.R., and Aronson, J.K.: Adverse drug reactions: Definitions, diagnosis, and management. *Lancet, 356*(9237): 1255-1259, 2000.

Helmreich, R.: On error management: Lessons from aviation. *British Medical Journal, 320*(7237):781-785, 2000.

The Institute of Medicine of National Academies, Crossing the Quality Chasm: The IOM Quality Initiative, 2001.

Joint Commission on Accreditation of Healthcare Organizations: *2003 National Patient Safety Goals.* Oakbrook Terrace, IL, 2003a, JCAHO.

Joint Commission on Accreditation of Healthcare Organizations: JCAHO Term Glossary. Oakbrook Terrace, IL, 2003b, JCAHO.

Kaushal, R., Bates, D.W., Landrigan, C., et al.: Medication errors and adverse drug events in pediatric patients. *Journal of the American Medical Association, 285*(16):2114-2120, 2001.

Kohn, L.T., Corrigan, J.M., and Donaldson, M.S.: *To err is human: Building a safer health system*. Washington DC, 1999, National Press.

Leape, L.: *The preventability of medical injury. Human error in medicine*. In MS Bogner (ed). Human Error in Medicine. Hillsdale, NJ, 1994, Lawrence Erlbaum Associates, pp.13-25.

Leape, L.: A system approach to medical error. In MR Cohen (Ed). *Medication errors*. Washington DC, 1999, American Pharmaceutical Association, p. 1-14.

Leape, L.L., Bates, D.W., Cullen, D.J., et al.: Systems analysis of adverse drug events. *Journal of the American Medical Association, 274*(1):35-43, 1995.

Levine S, C. M., et al.: Guidelines for preventing medication errors in pediatrics. *Journal of Pediatric Pharmacology and Therapeutics, 6*:426-242, 2001.

Mitchell, A.L.: *Challenges in pediatric pharmacotherapy: Minimizing medication errors*, 2001. http://www.medscape.com/viewarticle/421220.

Reason, J.: *Human error*. Cambridge, MA, 1990, Cambridge University Press.

Reason, J.: *Managing the risks of organizational accidents*. Burlington, VT, 1997, Ashgate Publishing Company.

Reason, J.: Human error: Models and management. *British Medical Journal, 320*(7237):768-770, 2000.

Schneider, P.J.: Applying human factors in improving medication-use safety. *American Society of Health-System Pharmacists, 59*(12):1155-1159, 2002.

Selbst, S.M., Fein, J.A., Osterhoudt, K., and Ho, W.: Medication errors in a pediatric emergency department. *Pediatric Emergency Care, 15*(1):1-4, 1999.

Senst, B.L., Achusim, L.E., Genest, R. P et, al.: Practical approach to determining costs and frequency of adverse drug events in health care network. *American Journal of Health-System Pharmacy, 58*(1): 1126-1132, 2001.

Sherwood, G., Thomas, E., Bennett, D.S., and Lewis, P.: A teamwork model to promote patient safety in critical care. *Critical Care Nursing Clinics of North America, 14*(4):333-340, 2002.

Small, S.D. and Barach, P.: Patient safety and health policy: A history and review. *Hematology/Oncology Clinics of North America, 16*(6):1463-1482, 2002.

Stokowski, L.: Using technology to improve medication safety in the newborn intensive care unit. *Advances in Neonatal Care, 1*(2):70-83, 2001.

Wu, A.W., Cavanaugh, T.A., McPhee, S.J., et al.: To tell the truth: Ethical and practical issues in disclosing medical mistakes to patients. *Journal of General Internal Medicine, 770*(12): 770-775, 1997.

CHAPTER

19 Discharge Planning and Transition to Home Care

KARIN GRACEY

OBJECTIVES

1. Describe the transition to home process for the high-risk neonate.
2. Identify individualized, clinical criteria for discharge.
3. Discuss the role of the family in the discharge of a high-risk infant.
4. Identify key components of infant and family care postdischarge.

INTRODUCTION

On an average day in the United States, 156 very low birth weight (VLBW) infants are born. The incidence of low birth weight (LBW) infants has risen steadily from 6.9% in 1988 to 7.6% in 1998, about 1 in 13 infants (March of Dimes, 2001). Survival of LBW infants, including the smallest of infants (less than 1000 g) continues to improve; 54% of infants weighing 510 to 750 g at birth survive to discharge. Survival increases as birth weight increases, with 86% of those born weighing 751 to 1000 g, 94% of those born weighing 1001 to 1250 g, and 97% of those weighing 1251 to 1500 g survive to discharge. Major morbidities tend to be highest in the smallest survivors (<600 g at birth) and can include problems such as bronchopulmonary dysplasia (BPD), necrotizing enterocolitis (NEC), and intraventricular hemorrhage (IVH) or periventricular leukomalacia (PVL), which have lasting effects well beyond hospital discharge. Also of particular concern is poor postnatal growth, which occurs in 99% of infants weighing less than 1000 g at birth (Lemons et al., 2001). Many infants are discharged from the neonatal intensive care unit (NICU) with chronic conditions and multiple, ongoing medical and social needs.

GENERAL PRINCIPLES

A. **Coordinated, comprehensive discharge planning and facilitating a smooth transition to home for the premature infant are critical for the health and well-being of both the infant and family.**
B. **Planning begins on admission to the NICU or special care nursery and continues throughout the hospital stay and into the home situation.**
C. **An interdisciplinary team made up of skilled individuals caring for the infant and family helps to ensure the successful transition to home** (Box 19-1).
D. **Parents are coping with a prolonged separation from their infant in addition to emotional, financial, and family stressors that impact the parent-child**

■ BOX 19-1
■ **MEMBERS OF THE INTERDISCIPLINARY DISCHARGE PLANNING/TRANSITION TO HOME TEAM**

Parents
Neonatologist/neonatal nurse practitioner (NNP)/resident
Primary pediatrician
Primary nurse
Social worker
Discharge planning coordinator/case manager
Developmental assessment and follow-up team member
Home care nurse
Infant specific support services as needed: occupational or physical therapist, nutritionist, lactation support, respiratory therapist, pharmacist
Durable medical equipment representative

relationship. Prolonged hospitalization has been shown to correlate with poor parent-infant relationships, failure to thrive, child abuse or abandonment, and grief (Raddish and Merritt, 1998). Unrecognized maternal depression may impact parent-child relationships (Beck, 2003).

E. **Recognition of parents as the constant in their child's life and individualizing care, based on the parents needs, will assist in the smooth transition to home.**

CURRENT HEALTH CARE TRENDS

A. **Trends in health care include early discharge from the NICU and transitioning the provision of care, many times complex, into the home.**
   1. The newborn period is a major source of uncompensated care and accounts for a high proportion of catastrophic cost cases (Zupancic et al., 2003).
   2. Economic pressures, including fair and equitable reimbursement for services, and the utilization of costly medical resources continue to be challenges many health care systems face when caring for the VLBW infant in the hospital setting.
   3. Advantages to early discharge of preterm infants include cost savings, improved outcomes, and improved emotional health of the family.

B. **Early discharge of the VLBW infant can be accomplished in a safe and positive manner, benefiting the infant and family when certain criteria are met.**
   1. Criteria include extensive predischarge parent preparation and extensive postdischarge home nursing by skilled neonatal nurses or nurse clinicians.
   2. Families need to demonstrate competency in caring for their infants prior to discharge (Raddish and Merritt, 1998).

C. **Current trends in discharge planning include utilizing the role of the case manager as a member of the multidisciplinary team.** Case managers assist in care coordination, utilization review, insurance reimbursement, and discharge preparation planning for the infant.

D. **Clinical pathways and care maps are examples of effective tools for tracking outcomes and planning for discharge during the transition to home.**

E. **Care provided in the NICU and home care setting, including discharge planning and the transition to home, should be continually evaluated from an evidence-based perspective.**

1. Several resources including the Cochrane Neonatal Reviews, the Vermont-Oxford Trial Group, and the National Institute of Child Health and Development (NICHD) Neonatal Research Group continually analyze the literature, publish care recommendations, and study groups of preterm infants during the discharge/convalescing phase of care. Guidance is provided for best practices in the NICU from these resources.
2. Additional organizations publish guidelines for transition of the preterm infant to home including the American Academy of Pediatrics (AAP), the National Association of Neonatal Nurses (NANN), Association of Women's Health, Obstetric and Neonatal Nurses (AWHONN), the March of Dimes, and the National Guideline Clearinghouse (see Resources).

DISCHARGE PLANNING AND SUCCESSFUL TRANSITION TO HOME

A. **Discharge planning begins at birth.** Active involvement in the care of the infant by the parents begins at the time of admission to the NICU. Continued parent education on disease process and outcomes, dealing with the hospitalization of a sick newborn, and stress and coping are educational topics that will benefit parents.

B. **Discharge teaching should begin weeks prior to the projected discharge date, with a comprehensive plan in place.**

C. **The discharge process and transition to home plan need to be clearly outlined with goals and objectives, including time frames to complete tasks for the parents and health care team members.** The Bronchopulmonary Dysplasia Interdisciplinary Discharge Planning Checklist (Gracey et al., 2003) is an example of a collaborative tool, utilized by staff and parents, to ensure all discharge criteria are met for a well-coordinated, comprehensive discharge (Fig. 19-1).

D. **Family members are active participants in the transition to home plan.** Parents should participate in infant care from birth and be intimately involved in the daily decisions for the care of their infant. Family educational, social, emotional, and financial needs must be assessed and individualized based on each discharge situation. Barriers to parental learning and participation in care need to be assessed, and resources identified to alleviate the barriers. Parents of infants in levels II and III units have similar concerns. Their concerns fall into five categories (Kenner et al., 2003):
   1. *Informational needs* including care of the newborn, both physical and behavioral. All care needs including equipment and an understanding of the prognosis and outcome need to be addressed.
   2. *Grief*—Recognition of the grief parents are experiencing and helping them with resolving any grief are important.
   3. *Parent-child development*—Expectations of parent and child roles need to be addressed during and after hospitalization. Helping parents to identify their role in the care and nurturing of their infant is important.
   4. *Stress and coping*—All parents experience a degree of stress with a sick, hospitalized infant. They need strategies to help cope with the daily stresses of life including dealing with a sick infant.
   5. *Social support*—Acknowledging parents' need for ongoing and meaningful support from staff, friends and family needs to be addressed.

Recognition of parental needs and addressing each area in the discharge plan will ease the transition to home.

Bronchopulmonary Dysplasia Interdisciplinary Discharge Planning Checklist
Nasal Cannula Home Oxygen

This checklist is intended to be used as a collaborative tool for staff and parents to prepare for discharge home. Supplemental teaching tools and methods should be selected to cover each area.

PROJECTED DISCHARGE DATE__________ **Beginning at least 2 to 3 weeks prior to anticipated discharge date**	Date Done	Initials	**At least 1 week prior to discharge** **Date teaching planned:**	Date Done	Initials
❑ Meet with parents to discuss upcoming discharge and teaching plan ○ Discuss medical criteria for discharge ○ Review basic infant care needs and ensure teaching is in progress ○ Discuss the anticipated course of recovery from illness, demands on family/caregiver time while transitioning to home ○ Clarify insurance coverage for durable medical equipment, supplies, and home nursing care ○ Identify insurance case manager or contact person for problem solving ❑ Health care provider selection ○ Parents to select health care provider, make contact prior to discharge, and provide name and number to staff ○ Follow-up appointment arranged for 3 to 5 days postdischarge ○ Discharge summary provided to parents and health care provider at the time of discharge ❑ Safe Sleep/Back to Sleep implementation ○ Literature reviewed with parents ○ Safe Sleep/Back to Sleep instituted in the hospital at least 2 to 3 weeks prior to discharge ❑ Cardiopulmonary resuscitation (CPR) training ○ CPR attended by family and caregivers and return demonstration completed ❑ Home evaluation done ○ Electricity, running water, plumbing, heating and cooling (esp. in summer months) in working condition ○ Check for availability and/or presence of ■ Fans/air conditioning ■ Space for infant and equipment ■ Electrical outlets ○ Phone in working order ❑ Safety planning ○ Emergency fire safety plan in place; carbon monoxide and smoke detectors installed and functioning ○ Home safety measures reviewed ○ Poison control phone number provided ○ Identification of nearest emergency department and preferred hospital for potential readmission ○ Notification of nearby fire, police, and ambulance service of technology-dependent infant home on oxygen ❑ Respite Care Plan is discussed and potential helpers identified ○ Social support network for parents identified ○ Church community (if appropriate) contacted for additional support ○ Specialized day care availability explored			❑ Overnight stay in care-by-parent area, with all home durable medical equipment arranged for family on Date:__________ ❑ Car seat selection and pulse oximetry testing ○ Car seat selection and safety review completed ○ Car seat pulse oximetry testing completed ❑ Circumcision ○ If desired, consent obtained and procedure performed if medically stable ❑ Immunizations • Initial doses given at 2 months of age • Record and upcoming schedule provided to parents and next scheduled doses reviewed • Flu vaccine recommended for family and siblings prior to discharge and at 6 months of age for this infant • Household contacts immunized ❑ Caregivers and equipment • Home care agency is __________ • Durable equipment supply company is __________ • Meeting with parents arranged • Home care nurse is __________ • Schedule for home care visits established **Care conference is scheduled with the team caring for the baby and parents, immediately prior to discharge, to review the baby's history, current problems, and follow-up care** Date and time:__________		

For legend see p. 427

Continued

Bronchopulmonary Dysplasia Interdisciplinary Discharge Planning Checklist
Nasal Cannula Home Oxygen

This checklist is intended to be used as a collaborative tool for staff and parents to prepare for discharge home. Supplemental teaching tools and methods should be selected to cover each area.

Special topics—To be completed prior to discharge	Date Done	Initials	Special topics—To be completed prior to discharge	Date Done	Initials

Home Oxygen Use
- ❑ Discuss the oxygen prescription
- ❑ Review reasons why baby is on oxygen, and reasons to keep baby on oxygen at prescribed times
- ❑ If prescribed, discuss the use of pulse oximetry, target saturation ranges, false alarms, and strategy for low saturations
- ❑ Review baby's normal breathing patterns (rate, effort, retractions, color) and signs of distress

Review of oxygen equipment:
- ❑ Company name and phone number:____________________
- ❑ Home safety issues
- ❑ Portable oxygen tank
- ❑ Stationary tank(s) at home
- ❑ Compressor
- ❑ Setting oxygen gauges/regulator
- ❑ Adjusting oxygen flow
- ❑ Plan to keep enough O_2 on hand/what to do if oxygen runs out
- ❑ Extra supplies (adaptors/tubing)

Oxygen cannula use
- ❑ Proper cannula position, securing techniques, skin protection, barrier use
- ❑ Changing cannula (frequency/technique)
- ❑ Obtaining additional supplies

Humidification use
- ❑ Importance of humidity
- ❑ Water sources, cleaning, infection risks

Chest physiotherapy (CPT) (if ordered)
- ❑ Signs infant displays when CPT is needed
- ❑ How often CPT is needed
- ❑ Technique and potential risks
- ❑ Equipment and supplies needed

Suctioning
- ❑ Signs baby shows when suctioning is needed
- ❑ How often suctioning is needed
- ❑ Technique to use
- ❑ Equipment and supplies needed

Traveling with oxygen
- ❑ Methods of securing oxygen tanks in vehicle
- ❑ Choosing a stroller or car seat to accommodate infant on oxygen
- ❑ Having extra supplies on hand
- ❑ Provide handicapped parking permit/access

Follow-up appointment with BPD or pulmonary clinic
- ❑ Schedule appointment prior to discharge and review with parents what to expect
  - ○ Expected length of time on oxygen, and how weaning decisions will be made

Respiratory Treatments

Respiratory medication(s) ordered:

Frequency:
- ❑ Recognition of signs of distress
- ❑ Assessing when treatments are needed
- ❑ Dealing with emergencies

Nebulizer use
- • Set-up and use of nebulizer
- • Cleaning and storage

Medications

Obtain corresponding medication teaching sheets for discharge medications

	Medication	Dose	Frequency
❑			
❑			
❑			
❑			

- ❑ Provide prescriptions, and request that parents bring the medications, from the home pharmacy, to perform a safety double-check on what was dispensed versus what was prescribed
- ❑ Provide parents with oral syringes appropriate for home use
- ❑ Adjust timing of doses for home use (avoid the middle of night)
- ❑ Review key points when administering medications (including signs of toxicity, storage)
- ❑ Discuss how to obtain medications and refills and the importance of using a consistent pharmacy

Anticipatory Guidance
- ❑ Review when to call the doctor/health care practitioner
- ❑ Share with parents current laboratory test findings (hematocrit [Hct], bone mineralization studies, others) and implications for baby
- ❑ State screen test and results discussed with parents
- ❑ Respiratory syncytial virus (RSV) and illness prevention
- ❑ Signs and symptoms of illness
- ❑ Synagis administration approved by parents and third-party payer
  - ○ Where to obtain
  - ○ First dose
  - ○ Subsequent doses
- ❑ Developmental milestone review
- ❑ Behavioral likes and dislikes reviewed
- ❑ Corrected age calculations
- ❑ Expectations in first weeks/months at home
  - ○ Transitioning from hospital to home ideas (lighting, noise, etc.)

Bronchopulmonary Dysplasia Interdisciplinary Discharge Planning Checklist
Nasal Cannula Home Oxygen

This checklist is intended to be used as a collaborative tool for staff and parents to prepare for discharge home. Supplemental teaching tools and methods should be selected to cover each area.

Special topics—To be completed prior to discharge	Date Done	Initials	Special topics—To be completed prior to discharge	Date Done	Initials
Nutrition ❑ Discharge formula and/or breastfeeding plan established ○ Review growth chart and discuss expected growth ○ Review normal stooling patterns and number of wet diapers per day ❑ Feeding amounts, frequency and duration ❑ Review feeding techniques ○ Breastfeeding ○ Bottle and nipple choices ○ Gavage, tube feeding, use of pump. Special equipment supplied by company:__________ phone:__________ ○ Occupational therapy, physical therapy, and/or nutritionist consultation made if appropriate ❑ Discuss formula preparation ○ Recipe for higher-calorie formula preparation reviewed ○ Written recipe given ○ Supplementation plan (amount, frequency, type) reviewed for medium chain triglycerides (MCT), polycose, powdered formula, or human milk fortifier ○ Vitamin and iron supplementation ❑ Discuss how to obtain formula and supplements ○ Obtaining formula ○ How to purchase supplements including breast milk fortifier ○ Women, Infants and Children (WIC) program; give parents completed forms/prescription for formula at least 1 week prior to discharge **Home Apnea Monitor Use** ❑ Company supplying equipment and phone number:__________ ❑ Why apnea monitor is needed ❑ When to use monitor ❑ Anticipated length of time on monitor ❑ Alarm limits, settings, application of leads, and false alarms ❑ Responding to alarms, keeping record of alarms ❑ Follow for apnea identified and appointment scheduled **Hearing** ❑ Screening completed and results reviewed ❑ Recommended rescreening at 6 months of age discussed with parents ❑ Appropriate referrals made for hearing screen failure			**Retinopathy of Prematurity** ❑ Eye examination findings and what they mean ❑ Visual developmental milestones expected ❑ Importance of eye examination follow-up visits ❑ Next eye examination date, time, and location:__________ **Specialty Follow-up** ❑ Coordinate all appointments so that conflicts do not occur, diagnostic studies are scheduled prior to seeing the specialist, and appointments are grouped together when possible ❑ Send discharge summaries to all specialists and make contact prior to discharge if necessary ❑ Obtain third-party approval for referrals if needed ❑ Ophthalmology ❑ Surgery ❑ Neurology ❑ Neurosurgery ❑ Genetics ❑ Audiology ❑ Cardiology ❑ Other: ❑ Other: ❑ Other: **Parent Resources/Advocacy (check all that apply)** ❑ Community resources identified ○ Volunteer agencies and local church ○ Easter Seals, March of Dimes ○ Public health department ○ Community mental health ❑ Local and national parent support groups and networks ❑ Parent resources in the community ❑ Internet resources ❑ Financial resources ❑ Other:		

FIGURE 19-1 ■ Bronchopulmonary Dysplasia Interdisciplinary Discharge Planning Checklist. (From Gracey, K., Talbot, D., Lankford, R., and Dodge, P.: The changing face of bronchopulmonary dysplasia: Part 2. Discharging an infant home on oxygen. *Advances in Neonatal Care, 3[2]*:88-98, 2003. With permission from National Association of Neonatal Nurses.)

E. **The transition to home process must include a multidisciplinary approach.** Consistency in care providers is critical, including identifying the primary care providers and key individuals caring for the infant and family. Include all individuals in the discharge process (see Box 19-1).

F. **Discharge criteria must be established and individualized to each infant and family.** Generic criteria serve as a model for assessing readiness for discharge and include evaluating infant readiness, family and home readiness, community readiness including home care resources and health care, and follow-up system readiness (Box 19-2).

G. **Intermittent care conferences throughout hospitalization ensure a smooth transition to home.**

H. **A comprehensive discharge-focused care conference should be completed several weeks prior to discharge.** All team members and family members should be present. It is at this time the criteria for discharge are discussed, the teaching plan is reviewed, the anticipated course of recovery and ongoing problems are outlined, and the home care/durable medical equipment needs are discussed.

I. **Included in the transition plan should be an opportunity for parents to care for their infant in an overnight/transition room prior to discharge.** This opportunity should be individualized based on the needs of the family and infant. This should be a strongly suggested component of the transition plan when the discharge is technologically complex or questions remain as far as the parental capabilities in coping with the complex needs of the infant.

J. **If the infant will have ongoing medical needs at discharge, selecting a primary health care practitioner and home care and durable medical equipment companies that will meet the needs of the infant and family is vital.**
   1. Choose a health care practitioner for the ongoing care needs before discharge, and establish a relationship. Preferably the individual or practice chosen for ongoing care will have experience caring for premature infants. A comprehensive discharge summary should be prepared for the physician, subspecialists, and home care agencies. Any issues of ongoing care must be discussed before discharge. Pertinent information should be given to parents for care providers at the time of discharge (Box 19-3).
   2. Home care personnel should be familiar with the type of condition(s) the infant is recovering from and should have skilled, experienced personnel on staff to make home visits. Examples of successful home care programs include personnel with experience caring for NICU infants (Swanson and Naber, 1997).
   3. Criteria for selecting a durable medical equipment agency to handle the home care should be considered including:
      a. Location of the agency.
      b. Availability of supplies and personnel.
      c. Ability to respond to emergencies.
      d. Availability of back-up equipment.
      e. Experience of care providers.
   4. All individuals caring for the infant in the community should be invited to participate in the discharge care conference prior to discharge.

K. **Discharge to alternative home settings may be necessary because of medical necessity, social problems, or family dynamics.** Alternatives vary widely from community to community but can include specialized foster care, pediatric rehabilitation hospitals, pediatric nursing homes, or inpatient hospice care (Cox and Zaccagnini, 1998).

BOX 19-2
READINESS CRITERIA FOR DISCHARGE

Is the infant medically stable with no acute illness? Is he/she physiologically stable with his/her chronic illness?

Does the infant meet the following general criteria?

- Ability to maintain temperature in an open crib for 24 to 48 hours prior to discharge
- Ability to take all feedings by bottle or breast without respiratory compromise or by gavage/tube feeding without difficulty
- Apnea and bradycardia free for 5 to 7 days prior to discharge
- Steady weight gain

Is the infant able to sit in a car seat without desaturations or respiratory distress for at least 60 minutes?

Are the hearing screen, newborn metabolic screen, and eye examinations completed and results reported to parents/medical professionals caring for the infant after discharge?

Family and Home

Is the family willing to assume responsibility for care? What have their previous experiences been caring for an infant (with ongoing medical issues)?

Has the discharge plan been tailored to simulate the home situation?

What is the family structure? Coping skills? Stress level? Social support and resources for respite care?

Any financial concerns? Are appropriate referrals made for financial assistance?

Are there language barriers or cultural beliefs that need to be addressed?

What is the home setting like? Is there electricity, running water, heating and cooling, plumb ing in working condition? If not, is it a safe environment for the infant? Is there space for the infant?

Do they have an emergency fire and emergency safety plan established?

Does the family have transportation available?

Is there a need for ongoing social work or mental health services postdischarge?

Community

Do the home care services and durable medical equipment agency provide specialized neonatal services?

Have the local emergency services (police, fire) and utility companies been notified of the discharge and need for ongoing medical services (oxygen, monitor, possible cardiopulmonary resuscitation, etc., if appropriate)?

Have referrals been made to community resources as appropriate?

Have support groups or networks been identified for the parents?

Health Care and Follow-up System

Is a primary care provider identified and willing to assume care for the infant and family? Does he/she have experience with caring for premature infants?

Are all subspecialty appointments coordinated for the family prior to discharge?

Are early intervention programs identified and contact made prior to discharge? Are all referrals made for services?

Is the developmental assessment program in the community contacted and appointment coordinated with other needs?

TRANSITION TO HOME PROCESS

Parental Needs and Role in the Transition Process

A. **The family is recognized as the constant in the infant's life from the beginning of the hospitalization and should be encouraged to be an active participant in care.** Parents learn about parenting by observing caregivers and

■ BOX 19-3

■ **PERTINENT INFORMATION FOR PARENTS AND CARE PROVIDERS AT TIME OF DISCHARGE**

Comprehensive discharge summary including resolved and ongoing problems
Recent test results including chest x-ray, head ultrasound, EEG, ECG, CT scan, MRI, Scintiscan, barium enema findings
Additional test results such as pneumograms, eye examination findings, hearing screen results, newborn metabolic/state screen
Pertinent laboratory values: recent complete blood count with hematocrit, hemoglobin and reticulocyte count, bone health, medication levels, blood gases
Immunizations given

CT, Computed tomography; *EEG,* electroencephalogram; *ECG,* electrocardiogram; *MRI,* magnetic resonance imaging.

actively participating in and/or demonstrating care on a daily basis. Caregivers should work with parents on an individual basis. Caregivers should assist parents in learning how to assess their infant's behaviors and provide individualized care based on their infant's responses (Lawhon, 2002).

B. **Assessment of parental knowledge base and previous infant care experience should be done and an individualized teaching plan established weeks prior to anticipated discharge.** Current caregiver knowledge level is assessed prior to teaching sessions and each session is individualized according to the needs of the infant and family. Experiences for learning can be offered through hands-on care, demonstration of specific care practices, and verbal reinforcement. Information can be obtained from a variety of sources including individual demonstration, group teaching sessions with other parents, published teaching tools, videos, written materials, and Internet resources.

C. **Parents are active participants in care conferences and involved in the discharge planning.** Overnight stays in a transition-to-home room can be beneficial in assessing for level of comfort in caring for the medically complex infant.

D. **Parents are encouraged to contact a health care provider in the community and make follow-up appointments prior to the infant discharge from the hospital.** The discharge coordinator, staff registered nurse, or advanced practice nurse can assist with the process.

E. **In addition to general infant care issues, infant care specifics related to prematurity need to be completed prior to discharge** including:

1. Cardiopulmonary resuscitation training.
2. Car seat selection and infant car seat fitted days prior to discharge.
3. Evaluation of home done. Safety planning reviewed. Emergency plan formulated.
4. Establishment of realistic plan for care at home including feeding schedules, medication schedules, and treatments needed.
5. Chronologic versus adjusted age calculations and developmental milestones.
6. Equipment and medication teaching completed (as needed).
7. Respite care explored including strategies to deal with stress.
8. Overnight stay in the transition room is successful.
9. Primary care practitioner chosen. Contact made with home care agency/nurse and durable medical equipment company, as appropriate.
10. Decision made for circumcision.
11. Safe sleep practices are reviewed.

NEONATAL TEACHING NEEDS

A. **Criteria for infant discharge need to be individualized and also established prior to discharge.** General criteria for discharge are listed in Box 19-2. Teaching topics needing to be completed prior to discharge include:
   1. Back to sleep/safe sleep practices implemented weeks prior to discharge.
   2. Car seat pulse oximetry testing completed and car seat fitted.
   3. Basic infant care practices such as bathing, feeding, nutrition, and growth, and diapering reviewed.
   4. Specialized teaching topics completed such as home oxygen use, tracheostomy care, suctioning, ostomy care, central line care, apnea monitor use, feeding alternatives, medications, and any special equipment needed for care.
   5. Anticipatory guidance. What to expect in weeks and months ahead explained to parents including expected growth and illness recovery guidelines.
   6. Infant temperament, developmental tasks, and milestones reviewed including sleep patterns, feeding patterns, and infant state regulation.
   7. Care issues such as vaccinations, traveling, and visitors are reviewed.
   8. Tips on adapting to home.

B. **Testing needs to be completed prior to discharge with all appropriate results and copies of examinations forwarded to health care practitioner(s) caring for the infant after discharge.** A comprehensive discharge summary including all resolved and ongoing problems must be forwarded with the family upon discharge to all appropriate individuals. Test results include:
   1. Recent test results including chest x-ray, head ultrasound, electroencephalogram (EEG), electrocardiogram (ECG), computed tomography (CT) scan, magnetic resonance imaging (MRI), Scintiscan, barium enema findings.
   2. Additional test results such as pneumograms, eye examination findings, hearing screen results, newborn metabolic/state screen.
   3. Pertinent laboratory values: recent complete blood count with hematocrit, hemoglobin, and reticulocyte count, bone health, medication levels.

FAMILY AND INFANT CARE POSTDISCHARGE

A. **The goal of a successful discharge plan and transition to home is facilitation of collaborative care postdischarge.** Encourage the parents to choose a pediatrician or health care provider that has experience with premature infants and their ongoing problems. Care has many aspects after NICU discharge and should be approached comprehensively and systematically.
   1. Primary health care provider and specialty follow-up appointments need to be coordinated and scheduled without conflicts, with the infant and family in mind. Often medically complex infants can have more than four specialist appointments in addition to a primary care provider.
   2. Ongoing assessment and assistance with family financial needs should occur (i.e., Social Security, state governmental assistance, private charities).
   3. Families should be made aware of community resources available to them such as early intervention services, case management services, counseling, and transportation assistance. Volunteer agencies, local and national parent support groups, and Internet resources should be recommended, as appropriate.
   4. Immunizations, including respiratory syncytial virus (RSV) prophylaxis arranged postdischarge.

BOX 19-4

PREMATURITY-RELATED PROBLEMS THAT PRESENT OR CONTINUE AFTER DISCHARGE

Respiratory
- Ongoing oxygen dependency
- Apnea
- Wheezing
- Infections

Cardiac
- ECG changes
- Right ventricular hypertrophy
- Cor pulmonale

Gastrointestinal Problems
- Oral and feeding aversions
- Regurgitation
- Gastroesophageal reflux
- Constipation
- Strictures and bowel obstruction
- Hernias (umbilical and inguinal)

Nutritional Problems
- Weight less than the 10th percentile
- Feeding fatigue
- Need for nutritional supplements or hypercaloric formula
- Need for adjunct feeding devices (e.g., tube feeding or gastrostomy)

Hematologic
- Anemia
- Thrombocytopenia

Dentition
- Delayed tooth eruption
- Altered oral and dental structures from prolonged intubation
- Enamel defects

Sensory
- Strabismus
- Retinopathy of prematurity (ROP)
- Hearing deficits

Speech and Language

Central Nervous System and Neurodevelopmental
- Differences in temperament and behavior
- Tone and movement abnormalities
- Posthemorrhagic hydrocephalus
- Periventricular leukomalacia
- Cerebral palsy
- IQ deficiencies
- Learning disabilities
- School problems

From Gracey, K., Talbot, D., Lankford, R., and Dodge, P.: The changing face of bronchopulmonary dysplasia: Part 2. Discharging an infant home on oxygen. *Advances in Neonatal Care,* 3(2):88-98, 2003. With permission from National Association of Neonatal Nurses.

B. **Problems related to prematurity often continue after discharge from the NICU** (Gracey et al., 2003) (Box 19-4). In addition, hospital readmissions can occur in close to half of the preterm infants discharged from the NICU in the first year of life (Elder et al., 1999). Parents need to be educated to recognize risk factors for readmission to the hospital and potential ongoing problems.

C. **Neurologic, developmental, neurosensory, and functional morbidities increase with decreasing birth weight.** Risk factors significantly associated with increased neurodevelopmental morbidity include BPD, grades III or IV IVH, PVL, steroids for chronic lung disease, NEC, and male gender (Vohr et al., 2000). Preterm infants have been shown to have a higher incidence of cerebral palsy and mental retardation than the general population. They also have a higher risk of disorders of cortical function, including language disorders, visual perception problems, attention deficits, and learning disabilities. In addition, virtually all infants born less than 1000 g at birth have weights at less than the 10th percentile at 36 weeks' postmenstrual age (Lemons et al., 2001). Particular attention needs to be focused on postnatal growth and developmental assessment postdischarge.

D. **An essential component of follow-up care for the VLBW or at-risk infant is referral to a developmental follow-up clinic**. Clinics often have criteria for referral. The goals of a clinic include early identification of developmental disability, parent counseling (anticipatory guidance), and identification and treatment of medical complications (Gomella, 1999). Clinics are staffed by a multidisciplinary team of specialists including neonatologists, pediatricians, and neurodevelopmental pediatricians. Other staff include occupational therapists, physical therapists, audiologists, psychologists, ophthalmologists, speech and language specialists, respiratory therapists, nutritionists, pediatric and orthopedic surgeons, and other subspecialists. The goals of a follow-up program are threefold (Cox and Zaccagnini, 1998):
   1. Management of the sequelae associated with the condition.
   2. Consultative assessment.
   3. Referral and monitoring of outcomes.
   4. The first visit usually occurs within weeks of discharge and continues for months to years, based on each infant's individualized needs.

RESOURCES

Cochrane Neonatal Reviews: www.cochrane.org/cochrane/revabstr/g030index.htm

Vermont-Oxford Trial Group: www.vtoxford.org/menu.htm

National Institute for Child Health and Development (NICHD): http://neonatal.rti.org

American Academy of Pediatrics (AAP): www.aap.org

National Association of Neonatal Nurses (NANN): www.nann.org

Association of Women's Health, Obstetric and Neonatal Nurses (AWHONN): www.awhonn.org

March of Dimes: www.modimes.org

National Guideline Clearinghouse: www.guideline.gov

REFERENCES

Beck, C.T.: Recognizing and screening for postpartum depression in mothers of NICU infants. *Advances in Neonatal Care, 3*(1):37-46, 2003.

Cox, K. and Zaccagnini, L.: Discharge planning. In J.P. Cloherty and A.N. Stark (Eds.): *Manual of neonatal care* (4th ed.). Philadelphia, 1998, Lippincott-Raven.

Elder, D., Hagan, R., Evans, et al.: Hospital readmission in the first year of life in very preterm infants. *Journal of Paediatrics and Child Health, 35*:145-150, 1999.

Gomella, T.L.: *Neonatology: Management, procedures on-call problems, diseases, drugs* (4th ed.). Stamford, CT, 1999, Appleton & Lange.

Gracey, K., Talbot, D., Lankford, R., and Dodge, P.: The changing face of bronchopulmonary dysplasia: Part 2. Discharging an infant home on oxygen. *Advances in Neonatal Care, 3*(2):88-98, 2003.

Kenner, C., Bagwell, G.A., and Torok, L.S.: Transition to home. In C. Kenner and J.W. Lott (Eds.): *Comprehensive neonatal nursing: A physiologic perspective* (3rd ed.). Philadelphia, 2003, Saunders.

Lawhon, G.: Facilitation of parenting the premature infant within the newborn intensive care unit. *Journal of Perinatal and Neonatal Nursing, 16*(1):71-82, 2002.

Lemons, J.A., Bauer, C.R., Oh, W., et al.: Very low birth weight outcomes of the National Institute of Child Health and Human Development Neonatal Research Network. *Pediatrics, 107*(1): 164-169, 2001.

March of Dimes: *March of Dimes data book for policy makers: Maternal, infant, and child health in the United States 2001*. Wilkes-Barre, PA, 2001, March of Dimes Fulfillment Center.

Raddish, M. and Merritt, T.A.: Early discharge of premature infants: A critical analysis. *Clinics in Perinatology, 25*(2): 499-520, 1998.

Swanson, S.C. and Naber, M.M.: Neonatal integrated home care: Nursing without walls. *Neonatal Network, 16*(7):33-38, 1997.

Vohr, B.R., Wright, L.L., Dusick, A.M., et al.: Neurodevelopmental and functional outcomes of extremely low birthweight infants in the National Institute of Child Health and Human Development Neonatal Research Network, 1993-1994. *Pediatrics, 105*(6):1216-1226, 2000.

Zupancic, J.A.F., Richardson, D.K., Lee, K., and McCormick, M.C.: Economics of prematurity in the era of managed care. *Clinics in Perinatology, 27*(2):483-497, 2003.

CHAPTER 20

Genetics: From Bench to Bedside

JULIEANNE SCHIEFELBEIN

OBJECTIVES

1. Define birth defects and possible causes.
2. Become familiar with genetic terminology.
3. Identify the number of chromosomes in a normal human cell.
4. Describe the characteristics and causes of structural and numeric chromosomal abnormalities, modes of inheritance of single-gene disorders, and multifactorial inheritance.
5. Describe what prenatal diagnostic tests are available and which anomalies they detect.
6. Describe the components and benefits of genetic counseling.
7. Identify three patient care management issues in genetic counseling.
8. Verbalize the systematic process used to evaluate the malformed infant.
9. List common congenital malformations and possible mechanisms of cause.

The neonate born with a genetic defect or fetal anomaly presents a challenge to the neonatal intensive care unit (NICU) team. A definitive diagnosis is essential for management and care of the neonate and the neonate's family.

Congenital malformations commonly have multiple causes. This chapter includes information on basic genetics, characteristics, and causes of some common fetal anomalies, and a systematic process for the evaluation of the malformed infant. Commonalities of patient care management issues are addressed, with the understanding that every family requires individualized care.

BASIC GENETICS

Terminology

A. **Birth defect:** an abnormality of structure, function, or metabolism, whether genetically determined or a result of environmental interference during embryonic or fetal life. A congenital defect may cause disease from the time of conception through birth or later in life (March of Dimes Foundation, 2003).

B. **Chromosome:** structural elements in a cell nucleus that carry the genes and convey genetic information.
   1. Each cell (except erythrocytes) in the body contains all the chromosomes received from both parents within its nucleus.
   2. There are 23 pairs of chromosomes, for a total of 46 chromosomes, with one maternal and one paternal chromosome creating each pair.

C. **Gene:** the smallest unit of inheritance of a single characteristic, responsible for a physical, biochemical, or physiologic trait and located with other genes in linear sequence along the chromosome.
D. **Genotype:** hereditary composition of an individual.
E. **Autosome:** one of 22 chromosomes that do not determine the sex of the individual.
F. **Sex chromosomes:** the X and Y chromosomes, which are responsible for sex determination—XX for female and XY for male.
G. **Diploid:** containing a set of maternal and a set of paternal chromosomes, for a total of 46 chromosomes.
H. **Gamete:** one of two cells, containing 23 chromosomes (haploid number), with the union of a male gamete and a female gamete required during sexual production to create a new individual (with the diploid number of chromosomes).
I. **Haploid:** having half the number of chromosomes found in the person's cells; characteristic of the gametes.
J. **Locus:** the position that the gene occupies on a chromosome.
K. **Karyotype:** pictorial representation of the chromosomal characteristics of an individual or species.
L. **Allele:** one of a series of alternate forms of a gene at the same locus on a chromosome (Gelehrter et al., 1998; Jones, 1997; Jorde et al., 2000).
M. **Penetrance:** The degree to which an inherited trait is manifested in the person who carries the affected gene (Nussbaum et al., 2001).

Dominance and Recessiveness

A. **Phenotype:** observable characteristics of an individual.
B. **Heterogeneous chromosomes:** differing pair of chromosomes, one from each parent, arraying differing genes for specific traits. When there are unlike genes on a locus, one gene dominates.
C. **Homologous chromosomes:** a matched pair of chromosomes, one from each parent, carrying the genes for the same traits.
D. **Dominant gene:** a gene that is expressed in the heterozygous state. In a dominant disorder, the mutant gene overshadows the normal gene. A dose of this gene is needed for expression.
E. **Recessive gene:** a gene whose effect is masked or hidden unless both genes of a set of homologous chromosomes at a given locus are abnormal, thus showing the disease. In a heterozygote (carrier) the normal gene overshadows the mutant gene.
F. **Possible combinations of chromosomes.**
   1. Both genes can be dominant—AA (homozygous).
   2. Both genes can be recessive—aa (homozygous).
   3. One gene can be dominant and one can be recessive—Aa (heterozygous).

Autosomal Disorders Total 13,807 (OMIM, 2003)

A. **Autosomal dominant disorders.**
   1. Characteristics of autosomal dominant disorders.
      a. Males and females are both affected equally; either parent can pass the gene on to sons or daughters.
      b. An affected offspring has an affected parent if the mutation is not new.
      c. Half the sons and half the daughters of an affected parent can be anticipated to have the disorder. There is a 50% chance with each pregnancy.

d. Unaffected offspring of an affected parent will have all normal offspring if the mate is an unaffected person (assuming complete penetrance).
e. If two affected people mate, three fourths of their offspring will be affected. A double dose of the mutant gene in any of the offspring will result in a lethal anomaly (except in the case of Huntington disease).
f. Family history of an anomaly indicates a vertical route of transmission through successive generations on one side of the family (if not a new mutation).

2. Examples of autosomal dominant disorders: myotonic dystrophy, neurofibromatosis, and coronary artery disease (Allanson and Cassidy, 2001; Jones, 1997).

B. Autosomal recessive disorders.

1. Characteristics of autosomal recessive disorders.
   a. Both males and females are affected equally.
   b. Parents of affected offspring are rarely affected and are usually heterozygous carriers.
   c. After the birth of an affected offspring, there is a 25% chance, with each pregnancy, of having another affected offspring and a 50% chance that the offspring will be a carrier.
   d. There may be a distant relative with the disorder.
   e. Affected people who mate with unaffected people will have offspring who will be heterozygous carriers.
   f. If two affected people mate, all offspring will be affected.
   g. No family history indicates a horizontal route of transmission in the same generation.
   h. There can be a difference in expression of the disorder: very mild in one member and extremely severe in another.
2. Examples of autosomal recessive disorders: cystic fibrosis, sickle cell anemia, Tay-Sachs disease, thalassemia major (Jones, 1997).

X-Linked Disorders: 819 Identified

A. X-linked dominant disorders.

1. Characteristics of X-linked dominant disorders.
   a. Both sexes can be affected; because females have a double chance of receiving the mutant X chromosome, they have twice the risk of being affected.
   b. Affected males will have all affected daughters and no affected sons.
   c. Affected females will transmit the disorders in the same manner as with autosomal dominant patterns.
   d. Two thirds of the time, affected females have an affected mother; one third of the time, they have an affected father.
   e. Family history shows no father-to-son transmissions.
2. Example: vitamin D-resistant rickets.

B. X-linked recessive disorders.

1. Characteristics of X-linked recessive disorders.
   a. Only male offspring are affected, with rare exceptions. A female offspring will be affected if she has both a carrier mother and an affected father.
   b. Carrier females transmit the disorder.
   c. All sons of affected males will be normal.
   d. All daughters of affected males will be carriers (with each pregnancy).

e. Heterozygous females transmit the gene to half their sons, who will be affected, and to half their daughters, who will be carriers.
f. Transmission is horizontal among males in the same generation; in addition, a generation will be skipped, and second-generation males will be affected.

2. Examples: Duchenne muscular dystrophy, hemophilia, color blindness, and glucose-6-phosphate dehydrogenase deficiency (Kingston, 2001).

CHROMOSOMAL DEFECTS

Abnormal Number

A. **Polyploidy:** more than two sets of homologous chromosomes, showing multiples of the haploid number.
B. **Nonmultiples** are designated by the suffix "-somy"; monosomy is one less than the diploid number (45), and trisomy is one more than the diploid (47).
C. **Causes.**
   1. Nondisjunction: failure of paired chromosomes to separate during cell division.
   2. Chromosome lag: failure of a chromosome to travel to the appropriate daughter cell.
   3. Anaphase lag: chromosome lag during third state of division of a cell nucleus in meiosis and mitosis.
D. **Mosaicism:** nondisjunction of an anaphase lag that occurs during mitosis after fertilization, resulting in two different cell lines in the same person (Jones, 1997).

Abnormal Structure

A. **Deletion:** loss of a chromosomal segment.
B. **Translocation:** occurrence of a chromosomal segment at an abnormal site, either on another chromosome or in the wrong position on the same chromosome (i.e., an inversion).
C. **Polygenic defects:** type of inheritance in which a trait is dependent on many different gene pairs with cumulative effects.
D. **Environmental influences.** Inadequate nutritional intake, certain drugs, irradiation, and viruses are examples that could alter the genetic makeup of an offspring while in vitro. Multifactorial: genes plus environment.
E. **Basic generalizations.**
   1. Loss of an entire autosome is usually incompatible with life.
   2. One X chromosome is necessary for life and development.
   3. If the male-determining Y chromosome is missing, life and development may continue but will follow female pathways.
   4. Extra entire chromosomes, the translocation of extra chromatin material, and the insertion of extra chromatin material are often compatible with life and development.
   5. Multiple congenital structural defects are present when gross aberrations are present (Gelehrter et al., 1998).
F. **Incidence.**
   1. Autosomal aberrations: 5:1000 births.
   2. Sex chromosome aberrations: 2:1000 births.
   3. Spontaneous abortions: 60% are associated with chromosomal aberration (Jorde et al., 2000).

PRENATAL DIAGNOSIS

Recent technologic advances and marked progress in the understanding of the etiology and pathogenesis of many common disorders have allowed many families a prenatal diagnosis.

Indications and Advantages of Prenatal Diagnosis

A. Indications.
1. Advanced maternal age.
2. Prior child with a chromosomal disorder.
3. Family history of neural tube defects.
4. Previous child with multiple malformations.
5. Carriers of X-linked diseases.
6. Carriers of chromosome translocation.
7. Couples at risk of having a child with a specific inborn error of metabolism (previous child or by carrier testing).
8. Ultrasonographic identification of major malformation, polyhydramnios, and/or intrauterine growth restriction (Jorde et al., 2000).

B. Advantages.
1. Knowledge that the fetus is unaffected.
2. Time to explore options and prepare for an affected newborn infant.
3. Opportunity electively to choose either to avoid starting a pregnancy or to abort an affected fetus.
4. Opportunity for the physician to plan delivery, management, and care of the infant when the disease is diagnosed in the fetus (Jorde et al., 2000).

Prenatal Tests

Maternal Serum Alpha-Fetoprotein (MSAFP) Test

A. **Screening test** done at 16 to 18 weeks' gestation to determine amount of protein produced by fetus and normally found in amniotic fluid. Smaller amounts normally cross the placenta and enter the mother's blood. This test is uninterpretable after 22 weeks' gestation.

B. **Preparation.** Explain to client that this is a screening test, *not* a diagnostic test. Explain that an abnormal result does not indicate an abnormality but will indicate the possible need for a diagnostic test to rule out abnormalities.

C. **Reasons for high MSAFP** (≥2 multiples of the median).
1. Greater gestational age than expected (incorrect due date).
2. Multiple gestation.
3. Risk of fetal complications, including spontaneous abortion, premature labor, or neonate who will not attain full birth weight.
4. Fetal structural defect: neural tube, abdominal wall, esophageal or intestinal obstruction, or renal anomalies.
5. Undetermined reason, with subsequent normal outcome of newborn infant.

D. **Reasons for low MSAFP** (≤ 0.5 multiple of the median).
1. Younger gestational age than expected (incorrect due date).
2. Chromosomal birth defect, Down syndrome being the most common.
3. Undetermined reason, with subsequent normal outcome of newborn infant.

E. **If abnormal MSAFP,** perform ultrasonography to confirm estimated gestational age and assess for anomalies.

F. **If overestimated or underestimated gestational age,** recalculate MSAFP on basis of corrected age; provide client with preliminary revised due date and recalculated MSAFP concentration. Reschedule follow-up ultrasonography in 2 to 3 weeks to confirm new due date.

G. **If confirmation of gestational age by ultrasonography subsequent to *high* MSAFP,** repeat MSAFP determination, schedule genetic counseling and offer amniocentesis for fetal chromosomes, amniotic fluid alpha$_1$-fetoprotein, and acetylcholinesterase.

H. **If confirmation of gestational age by ultrasonography subsequent to *low* MSAFP,** schedule genetic counseling and offer client amniocentesis for fetal chromosomes and alpha$_1$-fetoprotein. This ultrasonography should include Down syndrome screening for frontal lobe findings, mild ventriculomegaly, nuchal edema, cardiac defects, mild renal pelvis dilation, and abnormalities of the fetal hand.

Ultrasonography

A. **Preparation for ultrasonography.** Explain to the client that a transducer coated with ultrasonic gel will be placed on her abdomen, with high-frequency sound waves used to display sectional planes of the uterine contents on a monitor. Explain that ultrasonography cannot detect all anomalies and cannot guarantee fetal outcome.

B. **Initial assessment** recommended by 16 to 20 weeks for gestational age verification and evaluation.

C. **Ultrasonography:** to detect abnormalities of fetus, placenta, amniotic fluid, and uterus; to monitor changes in anatomy and growth with serial ultrasonography.

D. **Diagnostic capability:** only as good as the person's training—not just contingent on the equipment.

E. **No known harmful effects.**

F. **Critical to safety of amniocentesis:** chorionic villus sampling and percutaneous blood sampling.

G. **Anatomic landmarks commonly observed:** fetal spine, kidneys, bladder, stomach, three-vessel cord, cord insertion, four-chambered heart, face, upper lip, biparietal diameter, head circumference, abdominal circumference, femur length, transcerebellar diameter, placenta, amount of amniotic fluid, uterus, and adnexa.

H. **Detectable anomalies:** many, including those indicative of various syndromes. **Examples:** anencephaly, atrial septal defect, cardiac anomalies, choroid plexus cyst, cleft lip, craniosynostosis, cystic hygroma, cystic kidneys, encephalocele, gastroschisis, hydrocephalus, microcephaly, myelomeningocele, omphalocele, skeletal dysplasia (Gelehrter et al., 1998; Jorde et al., 2000).

Amniocentesis ("Amnio")

A. **Removal of 10 to 30 ml of amniotic fluid** through a needle placed into the woman's abdomen, for the purpose of chromosomal analysis and other biochemical tests as indicated.

B. **Preparation.** Review risks and benefits of the procedure, discuss options based on current information, and arrange to obtain results of amniocentesis. Explain that normal results of amniocentesis do not guarantee a good fetal outcome. Obtain written consent for this procedure. Obtain client's blood type before procedure. If she is Rh negative, obtain father's blood type.

C. **Usual timing of procedure:** 16 to 18 gestational weeks, but amniocentesis can be performed later in gestation and as early as 14 weeks.

D. **Indications.**
   1. Woman of advanced maternal age (>35 years at time of expected delivery).
   2. Previous fetus with Down syndrome.
   3. Previous fetus with neural tube defect.

4. Both parents known as heterozygous carriers of autosomal recessive chromosome.
5. Both parents known as carriers of sex-linked recessive disorder.
6. Client or partner with balanced chromosomal translocation of his or her chromosomes.
7. High or low MSAFP with accurate gestational age.

E. **Fluid analysis:** requires 2 to 3 weeks for cells to grow adequately for accurate analysis.

F. **Risks.** Overall risk to mother or fetus is 1%.
1. Spontaneous abortion: approximately 0.5% of cases.
2. Hemorrhage.
3. Infection.
4. Premature labor.
5. Rh sensitization from fetal bleeding into maternal circulation.
6. Trauma to fetus or placenta.

G. **Analysis.**
1. Fetal sex: determined through special staining techniques, karyotype, or amniotic fluid testosterone levels, providing risk information for X-linked disorder.
2. Alpha$_1$-fetoprotein: abnormally high or low levels raise concern (see earlier section on MSAFP test, under Prenatal Tests).
3. Biochemical: metabolism disorders, including Tay-Sachs disease (a lipid disorder) and amino acid, carbohydrate, and mucopolysaccharide metabolism disorders, can be discovered by 20 weeks' gestation.
4. Chromosomes: abnormalities, including Down syndrome, other trisomies, and other chromosomal abnormalities, can be detected at 16 weeks' gestation by karyotyping.

H. **Postamniocentesis care.**
1. Assess fetal heart activity.
2. Cleanse insertion site and apply protective cover.
3. Instruct client to rest for 24 hours, to lift no more than 10 pounds (approximately 4.5 kg), and to avoid straining.
4. Administer immune globulin (RhoGAM) if client is Rh negative and if father of fetus is either Rh positive or of unknown blood type. Do not give RhoGAM if Rh sensitization.
5. When results are available, explain their implications (Gelehrter et al., 1998).

Chorionic Villus Sampling

A. **Transvaginal or transabdominal sampling** of the chorionic villi. Obtain fetal cells for the purpose of chromosomal analysis and other biochemical tests. Chorionic villus sampling (CVS) cannot identify neural tube defects.

B. **Preparation.** Review risks and benefits of the procedure, discuss options, and arrange to obtain CVS results. Obtain written consent for this procedure.

C. **Timing of procedure:** usually 8 to 10 weeks of gestation.

D. **Indications.**
1. Client prefers to make decisions regarding pregnancy in first trimester.
2. Severe oligohydramnios.

E. **Contraindications.**
1. Multiple gestation.
2. Uterine bleeding during this pregnancy.
3. Active genital herpes infection or other cervical infection.
4. Uterine fibroids.

F. **Fetal cell analysis:** requires 24 to 28 hours for initial results.

G. **Risks:** overall, 2% to 3%.
   1. Infection.
   2. Bleeding.
   3. Cervical lacerations.
   4. Miscarriage: 1% to 5%.

H. **Techniques of CVS.**
   1. Vaginal CVS: Catheter is inserted through the vagina and cervix into the chorion outer tissue of the embryonic sac, and a tiny amount of the chorionic villi is aspirated by suction or cut with forceps.
   2. Abdominal CVS: Needle is inserted through the abdomen into the chorion to obtain a sample of the chorionic villi.

I. **Post-CVS care.**
   1. Same recommendations as for postamniocentesis care.
   2. Nothing in the vagina (tampon, douche, intercourse) for 24 hours.
   3. If transvaginal sample, instruct client to use sanitary napkins as needed for 24 to 48 hours.

Percutaneous Umbilical Blood Sampling (PUBS)

A. **Sampling:** removal of fetal blood through a needle placed into the woman's abdomen and into the umbilical vein.

B. **Preparation:** same as that recommended for CVS.

C. **Timing:** 18 weeks to term.

D. **Indications.**
   1. Client wants fast results to support her decision making regarding pregnancy.
   2. Abnormality is identified by ultrasonography late in pregnancy.
   3. Client has been exposed to infectious disease that could affect development of fetus.
   4. Blood incompatibility (Rh disease).
   5. Drug or chemical level in fetal blood needs to be assessed.

E. **Risks.**
   1. Same as amniocentesis: infection, bleeding, isoimmunization, miscarriage, trauma to the fetus—overall 1% to 5% risk factor.
   2. Perforation of uterine arteries, clotting in fetal cord.
   3. Premature delivery.

F. **Results:** fetal blood analysis takes 3 days.

G. **Postsampling care:** same as postamniocentesis care (Avery et al., 1999).

POSTNATAL TESTING

A. **Chromosome analysis/karyotype**—an ordered display of an individual's chromosomes. This can be done on amniotic fluid prenatally. Chromosomes are analyzed by staining techniques that result in visibility of dark and light bands that are designated in a standardized way from the centromere.

B. **High-resolution banding/prometaphase banding.** Some disorders cannot be seen reliably on standard chromosome analysis and require special handling during processing. Prometaphase banding is used because the cell growth during culturing is adjusted to maximize the number of cells in prometaphase, where the chromosomes are much less condensed and therefore longer, rather than in metaphase, where the cell growth is stopped in standard chromosome studies. High-resolution banding can have from 550 to 800 bands and allows a much more detailed analysis.

C. **Fluorescence in situ hybridization (FISH)** is a relatively new technique called molecular cytogenetics that combines chromosome analysis with the use of fluorescence-tagged molecular markers (probes) that are applied after the chromosome preparation is produced. This method relies on the phenomenon of hybridization of complementary pieces of deoxyribonucleic acid (DNA). FISH is a powerful tool useful not only in diagnosing relatively common microdeletion or microduplication disorders but also for identifying the origin of extra chromosome material (Allanson and Cassidy, 2001).

D. **Polymerase chain reaction (PCR)** is a powerful technique in amplifying many copies of a segment of DNA so that it can be analyzed. PCR is useful in disorders with recurring mutation, for example, achondroplasia.

HUMAN GENOME PROJECT

A. **What is the Human Genome Project?**
   1. The Human Genome Project is an international 13-year effort formally begun in October 1990 to discover all the estimated 30,000 to 35,000 human genes and make them accessible for further biologic study.
   2. The project started in the mid-1980s and is the single most important coordinated medical research initiative in the history of biomedical research. It culminated in the completion of the full human genome sequence in April 2000 (www.genome.gov).
   3. The goals of the project were to map genes on chromosomes and to determine the sequence of the nucleotides that make up human DNA, which is the basic genetic material. One of the top priorities was to generate complete sets of full-length chromosomal DNA (cDNA) clones and sequences for both human and model organism genes. It is expected that genome research will produce a ream of new information about the genes involved in inherited disorders, birth defects, and common conditions influenced by genetic factors.
   4. One insight already obvious is that even on a molecular level we are more than the sum of our 35,000 or so genes. However, surprisingly this new estimated number of genes is only one third of what was previously thought, although the numbers may be revised as more analyses are performed. This suggests to scientists that the genetic key to human complexity lies not in the number of genes but in how gene parts are used to build different products in a process called alternative splicing.
   5. In December 1999, the first human chromosome, chromosome 22, was sequenced. This is the location of defects that can cause DiGeorge syndrome, chronic myeloid leukemia, and neurofibromatosis. It is also the final autosome in the human sequence as outlined by the NIH Human Genome Report, 2003 (Collins et al., 2003).
   6. Though the outcome of the Human Genome Project itself is not ethically problematic, the use of the data generated presents major ethical questions that must be addressed. The future, then, presents the challenges of addressing the project's implications (Larsson, 2001).

B. **Ethical, legal, and social issues program.**
   1. Study is now under way on the ethical, legal, and social issues related to increasingly rapid progress in the field of human genetics. Four areas were identified for initial emphasis: privacy of genetic information, safe and effective introduction of genetic information in the clinical setting, fairness in the use of genetic information, and professional and public education.

2. The program also emphasizes the importance of understanding the cultural, ethnic, social, and psychologic influences that must inform policy development and service delivery issues.
3. With time these issues must be addressed to ensure that the maximal benefit is gained from the project (Gelehrter et al., 1998, Larsson, 2001).

GENETIC COUNSELING

A. **Definition:** a communication process that deals with the human problems associated with the occurrence, or the risk of occurrence, of genetic disorders in a family. This process involves collaboration of people from multiple disciplines (physician, sonographer, nurse, genetic counselor, social worker, neonatologist, and pediatric specialist, as indicated) and family support. Genetic counseling is a nondirective communication process that deals with the human problems associated with the occurrence, or the risk of occurrence, of a genetic disorder in a family.

B. **Principles of genetic counseling.**
   1. Based on correct diagnosis and pattern of inheritance.
   2. Nondirective.
   3. Reinforcement of information previously presented.
   4. Emphasis on communication with the primary care physician.

C. **Goal of genetic counseling** is to assist the family in comprehending:
   1. Diagnosis.
   2. Role of heredity.
   3. Recurrence risks and options.
   4. Possible courses of action.
   5. Methods of ongoing adjustment.

D. **Indications (Gelehrter et al., 1998).**
   1. Previously affected child, parent, grandparent.
      a. Congenital malformation.
      b. Sensory defect.
      c. Metabolic disorder.
      d. Mental retardation.
      e. Known or suspected chromosome abnormality.
      f. Neuromuscular disorder.
      g. Degenerative central nervous system (CNS) disease.
   2. Previously affected cousins.
      a. Muscular dystrophy.
      b. Hemophilia.
      c. Hydrocephalus.
   3. Consanguinity.
   4. Hazards of ionizing radiation.
   5. Recurrent miscarriages.
   6. Concern for teratogenic effect.
   7. Advanced maternal age.
   8. High or low MSAFP.

E. **Methods of obtaining information needed.**
   1. Questionnaire.
   2. Pedigree.
   3. Medical records.
   4. Physical examination.
   5. Laboratory tests.
   6. Carrier detection.

F. **Provision of medical facts.**
   1. Differential diagnosis.
   2. Risks to fetus and mother.
   3. Probable course of disorder.
   4. Recommended management for prenatal course.
   5. Type and timing of delivery.
   6. Neonatal, pediatric, and long-term care requirements.

G. **Explanation of hereditary factors** that contribute to the disorder.

H. **Discussion with parents** regarding all alternatives.
   1. Home care of newborn infant.
   2. Institutionalization.
   3. Adoption.
   4. Appropriate method of termination for gestational age.
   5. Objective information regarding fetus/neonate status. Provide statistical risk factors as they relate to this individual fetus.
   6. Identification of which normal characteristics can exist in the affected fetus. Point these out in pictures to promote awareness of total condition of fetus.
   7. Assistance to parents: understanding of causes, risks of recurrence, and limits of current treatments.
   8. Discussion of options available for dealing with risk of recurrence.
   9. Written information for parents and information regarding support groups.
   10. Explanation of recommended obstetric care, mode and timing of delivery, and neonatal care (Gelehrter et al., 1998; Jones, 1997).

NEWBORN CARE

Diagnosis

A. **Complete diagnosis:** important in planning care. Consideration for the infant's overall problems, in addition to the defect, is essential.

B. **Evaluation of infant with a birth defect.** A birth defect is a structural or functional abnormality of the body that is present from birth. The effects of a birth defect may be either immediate or delayed until later in life.

C. **Syndrome.**
   1. Definition: a constellation of anomalies that cannot be explained otherwise and that result in similar patterns of expression.
   2. Examples: fetal alcohol syndrome, trisomy 21.

D. **Sequence.**
   1. Definition: a primary event or anomaly that sets a pattern of other events (anomalies). Designates a series of anomalies resulting from a cascade of events initiated from a single malformation.
   2. Example: Pierre Robin sequence.

E. **Association.**
   1. Is a nonrandom occurrence in two or more individuals of multiple anomalies not known to represent a sequence or syndrome
   2. Example: Coloboma, Heart defect, Atresia choanae, Restricted Growth and/or Development, Genital anomalies and Ear Anomalies **(CHARGE)** Association

F. **Malformation.**
   1. Definition: an abnormality of morphogenesis due to intrinsic problems within the developing structures.
   2. Examples: neural tube defects, cleft lip and palate.

G. **Deformation.**
   1. Definition: an abnormality of morphogenesis due to intrinsic problems within the developing structures.
   2. Examples: Pierre Robin sequence, uterine position defects, oligohydramnios sequence.

H. **Disruption.**
   1. Definition: an abnormality of morphogenesis due to disruptive forces acting on the developing structure. Can be due to pressure on developing structures.
   2. Examples: amniotic bands, vascular accidents, infections.

I. **Genetic heterogeneity.**
   1. Definition: different causes may produce similar characteristics.
   2. Examples: hydrocephalus, cleft lip and palate.

History

A. **Family history.**
   1. History of three generations.
   2. Defects in the family history related to the problem in the child.
   3. Medical records and/or photos of similarly affected relatives.
   4. History of consanguinity.
   5. Reproductive history, such as frequent spontaneous abortions.
   6. Pattern of inheritance of the problems.

B. **Prenatal history.**
   1. Length of gestation.
   2. Fetal activity level.
   3. Maternal exposures: infections, illness, high fevers, medications, x-ray examinations, known teratogens, alcohol, smoking, and use of street and prescription drugs.
   4. Obstetric factors: uterine malformations, complications of labor, presenting fetal part.
   5. Neonatal factors: birth weight, length, head circumference, Apgar scores.

Examination and Care

A. **Physical examination.**
   1. General: asymmetry, problems of relationship, inappropriate size and strength.
   2. Face: configuration; centered features with normal spacing; round, triangular, flat, birdlike, elfin, coarse, or expressionless characteristics.
   3. Head: size of anterior fontanelle, prominence of frontal bone, flattened or prominent occiput, abnormalities in shape (proportionally large or small).
   4. Skin: intact, or presence of skin tags, open sinuses, tracts.
   5. Hair: texture, hairline, presence of whorls.
   6. Eyes: structure and color of iris, presence of colobomas, centering and spacing of epicanthal folds (hypotelorism or hypertelorism), ptosis, slanting, eyelash length.
   7. Ears: protruding or prominent shape, location, low set, unilateral or bilateral defect, presence and/or degree of rotation.
   8. Nose: beaked, bulbous, pinched, upturned, misshapen, two nares, flattened bridge, patency, centered on face.
   9. Oral: intact palate, presence of smooth philtrum, natal teeth; shape and size of tongue, mouth, jaw (micrognathia).

10. Neck: short and/or webbed, redundant folds.
11. Chest: symmetric; presence of accessory nipples.
12. Abdomen: number of cord vessels, presence of abdominal wall defects and abdominal musculature, prune belly.
13. Genitourinary system (male): hypospadias—four degrees, dependent on placement of meatus; chordee; ambiguous genitalia; testes descended.
14. Anus: position, patency.
15. Spine: intact, scoliosis, lordosis, kyphosis.
16. Extremities: length, shape, absence of bones.
17. Hands and feet: broad, square, or spadelike shape, polydactyly, clinodactyly, syndactyly, abnormal creases in the palm of the hand (simian or Sydney creases), contractures, abnormally large or small size, overriding fingers, proximally placed thumb, rocker-bottom feet.

B. Causation of defect.
1. Identify the primary abnormality.
2. Recognize etiologic heterogeneity (a defect having more than one cause).
3. Determine category of congenital malformation, according to etiology.
   a. Malformation.
   b. Deformation.
   c. Disruption.
   d. Syndrome.
   e. Association
   f. Sequence.
   g. Genetic heterogeneity.

C. Family care management for all genetic syndromes or disorders.
1. Provide grief counseling. Acknowledge short- and long-term grief; promote awareness that each of the parents may be in a different stage of the grief process, creating additional stress. Recommend that parents communicate their needs to each other and ask for support when needed.
2. Encourage genetic counseling.
3. Facilitate family use of support systems: social services; Aid to Families with Dependent Children; Women, Infants, and Children (WIC) program; March of Dimes; clergy; mental health services; support groups; Internet information.
4. Provide unconditional emotional support. Allow parents and siblings to verbalize feelings.
5. Identify normal aspects of neonate that can coexist with the syndrome or disorder.
6. Promote parent involvement in care; offer choices in care and interventions.
7. Discuss treatment options and their risks and benefits.
8. Provide literature.
9. Obtain legal and ethical counsel when parents prefer not to pursue medical interventions (Larsson, 2001).

Examples of Specific Disorders (for more specific disorders, see Chapter 34)

VATER Association

VATER is an acronym for *v*ertebral anomalies, *a*nal atresia, *t*racheo*e*sophageal fistula, and *r*adial and renal dysplasia.

A. Etiology and precipitating factors: unknown.

B. Incidence: 1.6:10,000.

C. **Clinical presentation.** Three or more of the following defects are present:
   1. Vertebral anomalies.
   2. Anal atresia with or without fistula.
   3. Tracheoesophageal fistula with esophageal atresia.
   4. Radial dysplasia, including thumb or radial hypoplasia, polydactyly, and syndactyly.
   5. Renal anomaly.
   6. Single umbilical artery.

D. **Complications and outcome.**
   1. Failure to thrive.
   2. Possibility of normal life after slow mental development during infancy.

E. **Care management.**
   1. Supportive: prognosis and management depend upon extent and severity of the anomalies.
   2. Surgery: surgical correction of anomalies.

VACTERL Association

VACTERL is an acronym for an association characterized by the sporadic, nonrandom association of specific abnormalities: *v*ertebral abnormalities, *a*nal atresia, *c*ardiac abnormalities, *t*racheo*e*sophageal fistula and/or esophageal atresia, *r*enal agenesis and dysplasia, and *l*imb defects.

A. **Etiology and precipitating factors.**
   1. Unknown.
   2. Injury between 4 and 6 weeks to a specific mesodermal area may produce simultaneous anomalies of the hindgut, lower vertebral column, lower urinary tract, and developing kidney.
   3. Abnormalities: average of 7 or 8 per patient.

B. **Incidence:** rare (about 250 reported cases worldwide).

C. **Clinical presentation** (Avery et al., 1999; Hooshang, 1998; Jones, 1997; Hockenberry, 2003).
   1. Vertebral anomalies.
   2. Anal atresia with or without fistula.
   3. Cardiac anomalies: commonly ventricular septal defects.
   4. Tracheoesophageal fistula with or without esophageal atresia.
   5. Radial dysplasia, including thumb or radial hypoplasia, polydactyly, and syndactyly.
   6. Renal anomaly.
   7. Single umbilical artery.

D. **Complications and outcome.**
   1. Failure to thrive.
   2. Normal life: minimal CNS anomalies with only occasional mental retardation.

E. **Care management** (Hockenberry, 2003).
   1. Supportive: prognosis and management depend on extent and severity of the anomalies.
   2. Surgery: surgical correction of anomalies.

RESOURCES

There are many resources available that cover the above disorders as well as many more. Information and explanation of diagnostic testing may be found in standard texts on genetics. A few resources that are particularly useful are listed on p. 449.

- Jones, K.: *Smith's recognizable patterns of human malformation* (5th ed.). Philadelphia, 1997, WB Saunders.
- Allanson, J.E. and Cassidy S.B. (Eds.): *Management of genetic syndromes*. New York, 2001, Wiley-Liss.

In addition, there are many online genetic resources available including:

- Online Mendelian Inheritance in Man (OMIM) (www.3ncbi.nlm.nih.gov/OMIM).
- GeneClinics (www.geneclinics.org).

Electronic databases can be purchased that aid in diagnosis and provide photographs and references for both common and rare genetic disorders.

POSSUM (Pictures of Standard Syndromes and Undiagnosed Malformations) (www.possum.net.au)

London Dysmorphology Database (www.hgmp.mrc.ac.uk/lddb) or (www.oup.com)

A resource for laboratories doing specialized diagnostic testing, both clinically and for research, for genetic syndromes and disorders is:

GeneTests (www.genetests.org).

Much more information for families and practitioners on individual syndromes is available on the Internet.

March of Dimes-Birth Defects Foundation. (www.modimes.org).

National Organization for Rare Diseases (NORD) (www.rarediseases.org).

REFERENCES

Allanson, J.E. and Cassidy S.B. (Eds.): *Management of genetic syndromes*. New York, 2001, Wiley-Liss.

Avery, G.B., Fletcher, M.A., and MacDonald, M.G.: *Neonatology: Pathophysiology and management of the newborn* (5th ed.). Philadelphia, 1999, JB Lippincott.

Collins, F.S., Green, E.D., Guttmacher, A.E., and Guyer, M.S.: A vision for the future of genomics research. *Nature*, 422(6934), pp. 835-848, 2003.

Gelehrter, T.D., Collins, F.S., and Ginsburg, D.: *Principles of medical genetics* (2nd ed.). Baltimore, 1998, Williams & Wilkins.

Hockenberry, M.J.: *Wong's nursing care of infants and children* (7th ed.). St Louis, 2003, Mosby.

Hooshang, T.: *Handbook of syndromes and metabolic disorders: Radiologic and clinical manifestations*. St Louis, 1998, Mosby.

Jones, K.: *Smith's recognizable patterns of human malformation* (5th ed.). Philadelphia, 1997, WB Saunders.

Jorde, L.B., Carey, J.C., Bamshed, M. J., and White, R.L.: *Medical genetics* (2nd ed.). St Louis, 2000, Mosby.

Kingston, H.M.: *ABC of clinical genetics* (4th ed.). London, 2001, BMJ Publishing.

Larsson, A.: Neonatal screening for metabolic, endocrine, infectious and genetic disorders: Current and future directions. *Clinics in Perinatology, 28*(2):449-461, 2001.

March of Dimes Foundation, White Plains, New York, 2003.

Nussbaum, R.L., McInnes, R.R., and Willard, H.F.: *Thompson and Thompson genetics in medicine* (6th ed.). Philadelphia, 2001, WB Saunders.

Online Mendelian Inheritance in Man (OMIM). www.3ncbi.nlm.nih.gov/OMIM.

CHAPTER 21

Intrafacility and Interfacility Neonatal Transport

S. LOUISE BOWEN

OBJECTIVES

1. Discuss planning for an intrafacility transport of a critically ill neonate.
2. Identify important considerations in the selection of transport vehicles.
3. Discuss the important factors to be considered selecting team composition.
4. Describe the process of neonatal transport from the referring call to transport of the patient to arrival at the receiving hospital.
5. List four methods to increase safety in the transport environment.
6. Discuss legal and ethical considerations relating to neonatal transport.

In the late 1950s and early 1960s, intensive care for newborn infants first became available. As the scope of care for critically ill infants expanded, so did the number of hospitals offering this service. Unfortunately because of the uneven distribution of these services, many areas remained without available resources. In the early 1970s the need to regionalize perinatal care was recognized by health care providers. In 1976 the National Foundation March of Dimes released the report "Toward Improving the Outcome of Pregnancy," which described regionalized care and identified criteria for level I, II, and III hospitals (Committee on Perinatal Health, 1976). The report also recommended the establishment of formal relationships between hospitals delivering different levels of care within a region so that every infant could receive appropriate care. The concept of regionalization led naturally to the need for the development of neonatal transport.

The United States Department of Health and Human Services reported that of the 4 million live births in the United States in 2001, 11.9% were premature (Martin et al., 2002). This percentage of preterm births was the highest level reported in 20 years. Advances in neonatology and technology have led to increased survival rates of these lower gestational age infants. These infants may be born outside a regional center and require transport to a neonatal intensive care unit. Infants with congenital anomalies or multisystem problems may also require transport to a regional neonatal intensive care center. The neonatal period is defined as the first 4 weeks of life and is the period of greatest mortality in childhood, with the highest risk occurring during the first 24 hours of life (March of Dimes, 2001). Intrafacility and interfacility transport of the critically ill neonate presents unique challenges. The goal is to transport these critically ill neonates in the most stable condition possible and to minimize adverse effects. The neonatal transport team must be knowledgeable about neonatal physiology and clinical requirements to provide optimal care and outcome. This chapter discusses various aspects of intrafacility and interfacility neonatal transport.

HISTORICAL ASPECTS

A. **1899:** When most infants were born at home, the first ambulance incubator was developed to transport premature infants from home to Chicago's Lying-In Hospital (Butterfield, 1993; Cone, 1985).

B. **1935:** The Chicago Board of Health operated a special ambulance with incubator, oxygen, and humidity and staffed with public health nurses (Chou and MacDonald, 1989).

C. **1948:** The New York City Department of Health, Maternity and Newborn Division, established a well-organized transport service staffed with ambulance drivers, nurses, a pediatrician, and a transport clerk (Losty et al., 1950; Wallace et al., 1952).

D. **1966:** Dr. Sydney Segal published guidelines for neonatal transport (Segal, 1966) that were expanded in 1972 into a comprehensive transport manual (Segal, 1972).

E. **1970s:** The number of organized transport programs increased due to regionalization of perinatal care (Bose, 1999).

PHILOSOPHY OF NEONATAL TRANSPORT

A. **The neonatal transport team is an extension of the neonatal intensive care unit (Bose, 1999).**

1. Interfacility neonatal transport is inherently different from typical emergency medical services (EMS) transport. Stabilization during interfacility transport is accomplished in the controlled setting of a medical facility, such as a hospital or medical clinic, in comparison with stabilization performed at the scene of an accident with limited support services. During interfacility transport, the patient is moved from a controlled setting, i.e., referring hospital, to the transport environment before arriving in the controlled setting of the receiving center. Scene-response systems move a patient from an uncontrolled setting to the controlled setting of a medical facility. The focus of EMS is on immediate short-term stabilization to sustain the patient until arrival at the medical facility. Interfacility transport systems focus on providing intensive care services from the referral facility and throughout the transport; thus more time is spent in stabilization at the point of origin. The level of care should remain the same or increase during neonatal interfacility transport.

B. **Crew and patient safety must be the highest priority of a transport program (American Academy of Pediatrics [AAP], 1999; Blumen, 2002; James, 2002).**

1. Crew and patient safety must be the highest priority for both ground and air neonatal transport programs. The focus of a transport safety program is accident prevention. However, when an accident does occur a systematic approach should be used to minimize the impact. Every team member is responsible for a safe program. Crew members' attitudes, participation, education, and judgment are variables that influence the safety program. Unsafe behaviors or practices are unacceptable in the transport environment.

C. **The neonate is a member of a family unit (Pillitteri, 2003).**
   1. Parents and family of a critically ill neonate experience a mixture of emotions. Reactions of the parents may vary based on the condition of their infant and on their perception of the situation, past experiences, support systems, and coping mechanisms. The transport team plays a pivotal role assisting the family to cope with the crisis.
   2. Intrafacility and interfacility neonatal transport should be planned and organized with appropriate transport staff and adequate equipment (Crain and Gershel, 2003).
   3. Intrafacility and interfacility preparation, stabilization, and transport should be performed as efficiently as possible using skilled staff and appropriate equipment. The continuum of care should not be interrupted during the transport process.

INTRAFACILITY NEONATAL TRANSPORT (Bowen, 2002)

A. **Preparation.**
   1. Neonates may require intrafacility transport for diagnostic and invasive procedures. The same concepts used for interfacility transport apply to intrafacility transport to avoid adverse outcomes.
   2. Level of care must be maintained or increased.

B. **Staffing.**
   1. Staff must be knowledgeable in neonatal physiology and pathophysiology and have excellent assessment skills. They must have the combined expertise and skills to provide safe transport.
   2. Number of personnel required is determined by patient acuity level and equipment.
   3. It is beneficial to have the bedside registered nurse as part of the staff because of patient knowledge. It may not be feasible with staffing shortages and patient care assignments.

C. **Effective communication** between staff of the neonatal intensive care unit, intrafacility transport team, and procedure department is critical.

D. **Equipment.**
   1. Type of equipment selected is based on patient acuity level.
   2. Anticipate potential complications.
   3. Maintenance of a neutral thermal environment during the procedure presents challenges. Prevention of hypothermia may require additional supplies.
      a. Radiant warming lights.
      b. Warm blankets.
      c. Hat.
      d. Crushable heat packs or thermal pad (do not place against fragile skin).
      e. Plastic wrap.
      f. A plastic bag may be used to reduce heat loss by placing the infant in the bag up to the neck.
   4. Monitoring devices should be compatible with the type of procedure performed.
   5. Equipment should have battery back-up capabilities. Plug in equipment to an electrical outlet to maintain the battery charge.

E. **Safety.**
   1. Use the most expeditious route between the unit and the procedure department.
   2. Anticipate and plan for potential problems, i.e., elevator not functioning.

3. Supplies and equipment should be packaged for safe transport.
4. Staff remaining with patient during the procedure should be provided with protective clothing and monitoring devices depending on type of procedure.
5. The neonate and monitoring equipment should be positioned for optimal visualization.
6. Staff may be required to stay with the neonate during the procedure given that other health care providers may not have the expertise to manage a neonate.
7. The neonate should be assessed frequently during the procedure.

INTERFACILITY NEONATAL TRANSPORT

Types of Transports (AAP, 1999)

A. One-way transports.
1. One-way transport uses services of personnel, equipment, and vehicles dispatched by the referral hospital to the receiving center.
2. Advantages of one-way transport.
   a. Time saving in patient arrival to the receiving center.
   b. Knowledge of the patient by referring staff.
3. Disadvantages of one-way transport.
   a. Justification of the expense of maintaining experienced staff and equipment is difficult because of the small number of transports.
   b. May deplete the resources of local EMS or the referring hospital for the duration of the transport.
   c. Referring hospital and local EMS staff may not have appropriate equipment or training for transport of neonates.

B. Two-way transport.
1. Two-way transport uses the services of personnel, equipment, and vehicles dispatched by the receiving center.
2. Advantages.
   a. More cost-effective use of expensive equipment.
   b. More experienced transport staff trained specifically in neonatal transport.
   c. Improved neonatal stabilization techniques.
   d. Provide equipment specifically for neonatal transport.
3. Disadvantages.
   a. Time delay in moving patient from referring facility.
   b. Expense of maintaining transport program.

C. Three-way transport.
1. The neonate is transported from the referring facility to the receiving facility by a transport team from a third facility or air medical company.

D. Back/return transport (Bose, 1999).
1. Neonates are transferred back to the local or birth hospital when they no longer require the resources of the regional neonatal intensive care center. The family should be involved in the decision of transferring the infant.
   a. Parents should visit the local or birth hospital prior to the transfer (Devane, 1999).
2. Advantages.
   a. More efficient use of beds at regional center.
   b. Improved relations between community hospitals and tertiary care center.
   c. Greater opportunity for parental involvement.
   d. Familiarity of primary physician with infant before discharge home.
   e. Decreased cost during convalescence.

3. Disadvantages.
   a. Financial analysis of cost to keep infant at the regional facility vs. cost of transport. Transfer of neonate back to referring hospital may depend on managed care or insurance contract.
   b. Potential need for transport back to higher-care facility if patient's condition deteriorates at community hospital.

E. Transfers out.

1. Neonates are transferred for a specialized procedure or treatment not available at the current facility, i.e., extracorporeal membrane oxygenation, surgical procedure.
2. Neonate may be transported by a team from the receiving, the referring hospital, or from a third facility or company.
3. Receiving facility should consider back transport after completion of the treatment or procedure.

SELECTION OF TRANSPORT VEHICLES

A. General considerations (AAP, 1999).

1. Appropriate vehicle selection may be dictated by diagnosis, clinical condition of the patient, available resources at the referring hospital, location of referring hospital, distance and duration of transport, geographic characteristics (road conditions, traffic conditions, construction detours), size of team, vehicle availability, weather, cost of the transport, and reimbursement.
2. Vehicles must be appropriately equipped, including power supplies, inverter, oxygen and air supply, suction, lighting, altitude pressurization where appropriate, means for securing incubators and all equipment, and room for adequate personnel.
3. An integrated system using multiple modes of transportation allows maximum flexibility to meet patient needs in a cost-effective manner.
4. Decisions regarding the appropriate vehicle for individual transport should be made by the medical control physician at the tertiary hospital, the transport team, and the referring physician in consideration of the impact on patient care and outcome, advantages and disadvantages of each vehicle, and cost.
5. Vehicle design and equipment placement must allow for continuation of patient care throughout the transport.
6. The vehicle must be equipped with appropriate locking devices and storage to secure the incubator and equipment.

B. Specific vehicle considerations.

1. Ambulance (AAP, 1999; Oakes, 2000).
   a. Advantages.
      (1) Lower transport costs.
      (2) Operate in weather conditions that restrict air transport.
      (3) Does not require a landing zone or runway.
      (4) Ability to carry equipment and personnel for two incubators in specially equipped ambulances.
      (5) Increased space and patient more accessible.
      (6) Ability to stop vehicle or divert to the closest hospital in an emergency.
   b. Disadvantages.
      (1) Long response times due to speed limitations, road conditions, traffic congestion, and geographic location.
      (2) Delay of admission to tertiary care center because of long-distance ground transport.

2. Helicopters (AAP, 1999; Arndt, 2003).
   a. Advantages.
      (1) Speed in response to calls and in returning patient to the receiving center for distances up to 200 miles.
      (2) Decreased response time to the referring facility.
      (3) Use of one-way helicopter transport to increase team's response time to referring hospital.
   b. Disadvantages.
      (1) Increased noise and vibration levels.
      (2) Difficult to identify problems when they occur because of noise and vibration (pneumothorax, extubation).
      (3) High operational costs.
      (4) Space and weight limitations.
      (5) Increased downtime due to weather.
      (6) May require ground transportation depending on landing zone location.
      (7) Securing the same incubator in a helicopter and ambulance may not be possible due to different mounts and stretcher configurations. This must be evaluated prior to the transport.
3. Fixed-wing aircraft (AAP, 1999).
   a. Advantages.
      (1) Primarily beneficial for long-distance transports, usually greater than 200 miles.
      (2) Although fixed-wing transportation is expensive, possible favorable cost comparison over long distances when staff time is taken into consideration.
   b. Disadvantages.
      (1) If no contractual agreements with aircraft vendors, possible inadequate equipment and unfamiliarity of team with the aircraft or with general vendor operation.
      (2) Requires coordination of ground transportation on both ends of the flight.
      (3) Space limitations.
      (4) Securing the same incubator in a fixed-wing aircraft and ambulance may not be possible due to different mounts and stretcher configurations. This must be evaluated prior to the transport.
      (5) Requires an airport for landing and takeoff.
      (6) Multiple patient movements from aircraft and ambulances.

TRANSPORT PERSONNEL

A. **Composition of a neonatal transport team varies with federal, state, and local regulations, budget, availability, professional standards, patient population, mission, referral area, expectations and available resources at referral hospital, skill and educational level of team, acuity, and volume of transports. The team must possess the combined expertise to assess, plan, implement, and evaluate actual and potential complications during transport of a critically ill neonate (Commission on Accreditation of Medical Transport Systems [CAMTS], 2001; James, 2002; Woodward et al., 2002).** The team may be staffed by using various combinations of personnel, with a minimum of two patient care providers trained in the management of critically ill neonates. These patient care providers are in addition to the ambulance drivers or pilots. At least one of the patient care providers should be a physician, registered nurse, or neonatal nurse practitioner. Team composition may remain constant or vary based on patient acuity (Woodward et al., 2002). When transporting two neonates in the same vehicle, specific patient care providers should be assigned to each infant. Cross-training staff within scope of practice and licensure increases efficiency of the team. Transport teams may be configured using a combination of the following personnel:

1. Physicians and neonatologists.
2. Fellows and residents.
3. Registered nurses.
4. Neonatal nurse practitioners.
5. Respiratory therapists.
6. Emergency medical technicians or paramedics.

B. Roles for transport personnel, including functions, responsibilities, qualifications, and competencies, must be clearly outlined in job descriptions.

1. Transport personnel should function as a team.
2. Cross-training personnel within scope of practice and licensure.
3. The program should have a written policy specific to job performance for physical requirements, and disqualifying mental conditions of team members.
   a. Weight and height requirements especially in air transport.
   b. General physical condition.
   c. Notification to transport administration of use of prescription and over-the-counter medications (certain medications may delay mental function and reflexes).
4. Staff should participate in neonatal transport with sufficient frequency to maintain expertise.

C. Team composition considerations (National Association of Neonatal Nurses [NANN], 1998).

1. Physicians.
   a. Neonatologists should be utilized when their additional expertise is required.
   b. May limit resources in a busy neonatal practice.
   c. Residents provide less consistency as a result of rotations and lack of educational experience in neonatal intensive care.
   d. Fellows provide more consistency and increasing levels of expertise as they advance through their fellowship.
2. Registered nurses.
   a. Requires advanced knowledge and experience in neonatal intensive care.
   b. May be the team leader.
   c. Educational requirements include in-service programs, national certifications and neonatal nurse practitioner programs, the American Academy of Pediatrics/American Heart Association Neonatal Resuscitation Program (NRP), and the American Academy of Pediatrics/American Heart Association Pediatric Advanced Life Support Course (PALS).
3. Neonatal nurse practitioners.
   a. Licensed in most states to perform diagnostic and therapeutic procedures.
   b. Highly skilled, in addition to their advanced knowledge of neonatal intensive care therapies.
   c. Increased cost in comparison to a registered nurse; however, this may obviate the need for resident/fellow/neonatologist presence.

4. Respiratory therapists.
   a. Frequent team members because of the majority of neonates transported have a respiratory problem.
   b. Require advanced knowledge in neonatal intensive care.
   c. May assist with nursing functions as licensed by the state.
   d. Responsible for respiratory equipment, airway maintenance, and maintaining adequate oxygenation and ventilation during transport.
5. Emergency medical technicians and paramedics.
   a. Role varies, depending on experience and education in neonatal care.
   b. Functions may include nursing or respiratory therapy responsibilities.
6. Expertise required within the transport team (Arndt, 2003; James, 2002; NANN, 1998).
   a. Assessment.
      (1) History taking.
      (2) Physical examination.
      (3) Interpretation of laboratory and radiologic findings.
   b. Knowledge of neonatal physiology and pathophysiology.
   c. Excellent communication and public relations skills.
   d. Clinical experience and expertise.
   e. Physical examination and fitness criteria (physical agility and stamina).
   f. Knowledge of aviation physiology.
   g. Transport safety.
   h. Knowledge of transport environment and vehicles.
   i. Independence and flexibility.
   j. Procedures (MacDonald and Ramasethu, 2002).
      (1) Bag-mask ventilation.
      (2) Endotracheal intubation.
      (3) Laryngeal mask airway (LMA) insertion (optional).
      (4) Arterial access (umbilical artery catheters, percutaneous artery catheters, arterial sampling).
      (5) Needle thoracostomy.
      (6) Thoracostomy tube insertion.
      (7) Venous access (umbilical venous catheters, peripheral intravenous [IV] lines).
      (8) Intraosseous insertion.
      (9) Administration of nitric oxide, nitrogen as applicable.
      (10) Mobile extracorporeal membrane oxygenation, as applicable.
      (11) Administration of surfactant.
7. Justification for a neonatal team.
   a. Staffing: dedicated, unit based, on call.
   b. Use of personnel when there are no transports.
   c. Volume of transports.
   d. Review of other systems that could transport neonates. These systems should demonstrate appropriate clinical expertise and possess equipment to transport a critically ill neonate.
   e. Cost and reimbursement.

D. **Medical director (AAP, 1999; Woodward et al., 2002).** The role of the neonatal transport team medical director, including qualifications, and responsibilities, must be clearly outlined in a job description.
1. A neonatologist or a physician with acute care expertise or subspecialty training in neonatology.
2. License to practice medicine in the transport program's state.

3. Knowledgeable in transport medicine.
4. Oversees medical aspects of the transport program.
5. Involved in the quality management program.
6. Involved in administrative aspects: selection of team members, orientation, education, program operation, public relations, and outreach education.

TRANSPORT EQUIPMENT (AAP, 1999; Oakes, 2000)

A. **Transport equipment and supplies must be checked regularly** to ensure that they are adequately stocked, functioning properly, and ready for immediate transport. Equipment should scheduled be for preventive maintenance program regularly.

B. **Recommended equipment must be operable on battery power.**
   1. Transport incubator.
   2. Cardiorespiratory monitor with pressure tracing and recorder.
   3. Pulse oximeter.
   4. Infant ventilator.
   5. End-tidal carbon dioxide monitor.
   6. Invasive and noninvasive blood pressure monitors.
   7. Intravenous infusion pumps.
   8. Transilluminator.
   9. Point-of-care testing including portable blood gas analyzer and glucometer (state regulations vary regarding use and quality control checks in mobile intensive care environments).
   10. Defibrillator/pacer (minimum capacity, 2 watt-seconds).
   11. Liquid oxygen, oxygen tank in vehicle, or portable oxygen cylinders.
   12. Air tank in vehicle, portable air cylinders or air compressor.
   13. Inverter in vehicle. Equipment should have battery back-up.
   14. Specialized equipment: nitric oxide, nitrogen, extracorporeal membrane oxygenation, and high-frequency ventilation during neonatal transport.

C. **Supplies for neonatal transport (Box 21-1).**

D. **Fixed-wing transports.**
   1. Ensure incubator fits through door of aircraft prior to the transport.

E. **Evaluate type and grounding of electrical outlets in vehicles prior to the transport.** Voltage and amp differences may affect equipment.

NEONATAL TRANSPORT PROCESS (AAP, 1999; Jaimovich and Vidyasagar, 2002; Salyer, 2003)

A. **Referral call.** The initial transport request call may be taken by a dispatch center, transport team, neonatologist, or neonatal intensive care staff. The referring physician is responsible for selection of an appropriate receiving facility and contacting the receiving physician to request patient transfer. During the initial call, at a minimum information should be obtained to activate the appropriate team, select the mode of transport, and anticipate any special supplies or equipment that may be required during the transport. A neonatologist may provide consultation to the referring hospital as needed until the transport team arrives. Management given via phone must be accurately documented. Transport computer data systems are available.

BOX 21-1
SUPPLIES FOR NEONATAL TRANSPORT

This supply list is designed for critical care interfacility neonatal transport.

Respiratory Equipment
Laryngoscope handle with blades, sizes Miller 00, 0, and 1
Spare laryngoscope bulbs and batteries
ET tube stylet
Anesthesia bag (not to exceed 750 ml) or self-inflating bag with oxygen reservoir
Manometer
Face mask (micropremie, premature, and term)
ET tubes, sizes 2.0, 2.5, 3.0, 3.5, and 4.0
Suction catheter and glove sets, sizes 5F, 6F, 8F, and 10F
Meconium aspirator
Blood gas kit
CPAP prongs
Nasal cannula (premature, infant)
Ventilator circuit
Thoracentesis setups:
  Syringe, 60 ml
  Three-way stopcock
  Angiocatheters, 20 and 22 gauge
  Tubing T-connector
Antiseptic solution
Heimlich valves
Chest tubes, sizes 8F, 10F, and 12F
Oxygen hood
Laryngeal mask airway
Bulb syringe
End-tidal carbon dioxide monitor

Intravenous Therapy Equipment
Bags of D_5W and $D_{10}W$
IV pump tubing
IV filters
Platelet and blood infusion sets
Umbilical catheters, sizes 3.5F and 5F
IV extension tubing
T-connectors, multiport connectors
Sterile drapes
Syringes, sizes 1 to 60 ml
Needles, assorted sizes, 18 to 25 gauge; or needleless system
Three-way stopcock and stopcock plugs
Antiseptic wipes
Scalp vein needles, 23 and 25 gauge
IV catheters, 22, 24, and 26 gauge
Disposable razors
Medication additive labels
Tape measure
Tongue blades
Armboards, sizes premature and infant
Intraosseous needles
Assorted tape
Umbilical tape

Continued

BOX 21-1
SUPPLIES FOR NEONATAL TRANSPORT—cont'd

Intravenous Therapy Equipment—cont'd
Antiseptic solution
Size 4-0 silk suture with curved needle
Umbilical catheter and thoracotomy set, including:
- Two sterile drapes
- Iris forceps
- Needle holders
- Scissors
- Curved forceps
- Tongue tissue forceps
- Sterile gauze pads, 2 × 2
- Scalpel and blade
- Blunt-end adapters, 17, 18, and 20 gauge

Thermoregulation and Monitoring Equipment
Hat
Plastic wrap, bubble wrap
Crushable heat packs and mattress
Space blankets
Thermometer
Chest electrodes; limb leads
Lead wires for heart monitor
Capillary tubes
Glucose monitoring device
Lancets
Arterial transducer tubing

Miscellaneous
Camera, film
Parent information
Blood culture bottles
Scissors and hemostat
Flashlight
Gauze pads, 2 × 2
Limb restraints
Rubber bands
Pacifiers (various sizes)
Cotton balls
Christmas tree adapters
Feeding tubes, sizes 5F and 8F
Salem sump tubes, sizes 10F and 12F
Dual-flow gastric tubes, sizes 10F and 12F
Sterile glove packs (assorted sizes)
Sphygmomanometer with blood pressure cuffs, sizes premature, neonate, and infant
Neonatal stethoscope
Trash bag; needle disposal system
Personal protective equipment (goggles, gowns, masks, gloves)
Visceral pack: normal saline solution, sterile gauze, sterile operating room drape, or sterile plastic bag

Medications
Epinephrine 1:10,000
Sodium bicarbonate, 4.2%
Atropine
Calcium gluconate 10%

BOX 21-1
SUPPLIES FOR NEONATAL TRANSPORT—cont'd

Medications—cont'd
Dopamine
Dobutamine
Isoproterenol (Isuprel)
Alprostadil (prostaglandin E_1)
Phenobarbital
Phenytoin (Dilantin)
Diazepam (Valium)
Paralytic agent; pancuronium bromide (Pavulon); vecuronium (Norcuron)
Analgesics
Concentrated sodium chloride and potassium acetate
Lidocaine (Xylocaine), 1%
Heparin (1000 U/ml)
Normal saline diluent, 0.9%
Sterile water diluent
Flush solution
Broad-spectrum antibiotics
Albumin 5% and/or normal saline solution
$D_{50}W$ (for making higher-glucose concentrated IV fluid)
Adenosine
Digoxin (Lanoxin)
Surfactant replacement therapy
Ophthalmic ointment
Vitamin K
Lorazepam (Ativan)
Sedative(s)
Milrinone
Reversals:
  Neostigmine (reverse neuromuscular blocking agents)
  Flumazenil (reverse benzodiazepine)
  Naloxone (reverse narcotic induced respiratory depression)

CPAP, Continuous positive airway pressure; *D_5W* and *$D_{10}W$*, 5% and 10% dextrose in water; *ET*, endotracheal; *IV*, intravenous.

Information to be obtained during the referral call includes the following:

1. Time and date of referral call.
2. Patient name and gender.
3. Parent's name and demographic information.
4. Referring physician.
5. Referring institution, including city, state, and phone number.
6. Maternal prenatal, labor, and delivery history.
7. Date and time of birth.
8. Gestational age, birth weight, and current weight.
9. Apgar scores.
10. Details of delivery room stabilization.
11. Subsequent neonatal course, including reason for transfer request.
    a. Significant findings of physical examination.
    b. Laboratory data.
    c. Radiographic findings.
    d. Vital signs.
    e. Respiratory support.

f. Fluid management. The infant should receive nothing by mouth before transport to prevent aspiration.
g. Other pertinent patient findings or medical management.

B. Selection and notification of team members.

C. Selection and dispatch of appropriate vehicle.

D. Selection of appropriate equipment and supplies.

E. Planning en route to referring hospital.

1. Team members will discuss provisional and differential diagnoses, proposed plan of care, and division of responsibilities.
2. Referring hospital should be notified of time of team's dispatch, mode of transport, and estimated time of arrival to referring hospital.
3. Emergency and anticipated medication dosages and intravenous fluid amounts are calculated on the basis of weight.
4. Potential complications are anticipated.
5. History and diagnostic study results to be obtained at referring hospital are identified.

F. Stabilization at referral hospital.

1. Introduce transport team members to referring physicians, staff, and family members. Check identification band on infant. All patients should be transported with identification band on. Parents' religious, cultural, and ethnic preferences should be incorporated into care.
2. Perform primary assessment of neonate to determine need for immediate interventions.
3. Obtain further details of history and current management.
4. Review previous radiographic images.
5. Obtain vital signs and glucose screening results. Determine blood gas values if clinical situation warrants.
6. Perform secondary assessment.
7. Pain assessment using a validated pain-scoring tool should be completed as part of the initial assessment and reassessed during the transport (Schechter et al., 2003).
   a. Recognition by the transport team that neonates feel pain.
   b. The neonate's response to pain becomes more defined with increased gestational age.
   c. Low birth weight and extremely low birth weight neonates display less organized and less vigorous response to pain.
   d. Transport team should observe for cues that the neonate is experiencing pain.
   e. The transport team should anticipate painful procedures to the neonate.
   f. The transport team should administer pain medication or sedation as ordered or by protocol.
   g. The neonate should be reassessed for effectiveness of therapy after treatment of pain.
8. Initiate monitoring systems as appropriate; may include cardiorespiratory, peripheral blood pressure, arterial blood pressure monitoring, end-tidal carbon dioxide, and pulse oximetry.
9. Consult with designated transport physician regarding management plan and anticipated complications en route, or follow transport protocols.
10. Attempt to achieve normal or optimal blood gas values, blood pressure, temperature, perfusion, serum glucose level, and acid-base balance according to the plan of care.

11. Begin switching to transport equipment, including ventilator and IV pumps, carefully monitoring changes in patient status.
12. Notify receiving unit of estimated time of arrival, current patient status, family's status, and equipment needs on admission.
13. Family support (Pillitteri, 2003). The transport team plays a pivotal role in recognizing the family in crisis, anticipating further crisis, intervening, and assisting the family through the transport process and admission to the receiving hospital.
    a. Identify members of the family unit, i.e., parenting dynamics and extended family members. The family unit is often diverse. The "family" should be viewed as the object of care.
    b. If possible, allow the parents to remain in the room as their newborn is prepared for the transport.
    c. Update current patient status; discuss anticipated complications during transport and treatment plans. The parents should be involved in the plan of care.
    d. Assess the parents' understanding of the infant's condition, plans for traveling to the receiving center, and their needs for physical and emotional support.
    e. Provide information about the receiving center, including location, phone numbers, directions, attending physician, primary/admitting nurse, and visiting policy.
    f. Obtain written transport consents.
    g. Take a picture of the infant or provide a set of hand or footprints of the infant to leave with the parents. Initiate the process for bedside video if available at the receiving hospital.
    h. The family may request that special objects, such as toys, pictures, or religious and cultural objects, be transported with their infant. The team should attempt to support the request if it does not interfere with safe transport and it is within the hospital policy.
    i. Leave a bonding agent (i.e., cloth) with a parent to keep against the skin that will be given to the infant during visitation.
    j. Discuss feeding options. If the mother is planning to breast-feed, discuss storage and transport of milk to receiving hospital.
    k. The parents should be allowed to touch the infant prior to departure. This is helpful in bonding and in making the birth seem more real.
    l. Depending on the team's policy and mode of transport, one parent may be allowed to accompany the infant.
14. Obtain copies of prenatal, maternal, and neonatal medical records. The records should be secured during the transport in accordance with the Health Insurance Portability and Accountability Act (HIPAA).
15. Distribute transport evaluation form to referring hospital staff and/or parents.

G. Planning en route to receiving hospital.

1. Infant should be secured in incubator with an approved restraint device. Loose equipment must never be placed inside the incubator.
2. Continuously monitor temperature, pulse, respirations, blood pressure, oxygenation/ventilation, and pain status as indicated.
3. Documentation at regular intervals, as indicated by infant's condition.
    a. Vital signs, blood pressure, color, pain level.
    b. Readings of oxygenation and ventilation monitors and of respiratory support settings (including altitude if appropriate).

c. Serum glucose screening.
d. Important documentation times for status of infant, including arrival at referring hospital, departure from referring hospital, and time of transfer of care to receiving hospital staff.

H. Arrival to receiving facility.
1. Transport team should notify the parents/family.
2. Follow-up may be provided to referring staff and physicians during the infant's hospitalization at the receiving center, maintaining patient confidentiality and following HIPAA regulations.

I. Neonates should be transported using individualized developmental care techniques (Bowen, 1999; Sweeney and Gutierrez, 2002; Symington and Pinelli, 2001).
1. The sick premature infant experiences significant physiologic stress when incoming stimuli resulting from high noise levels, increased vibration, lighting, and handling exceed the immature nervous system's ability to respond. The infant responds with autonomic instability, hypoxia, and increased oxygen requirements. Incorporating developmental care techniques may decrease these maladaptive responses.
2. Ear protection should be provided for the neonate especially on air transport.
3. Shield the neonate's eyes from light or glare by placing an eye shield on the infant or covering the incubator with a flame-retardant incubator cover. The infant's eyes should be covered prior to use of lights in the vehicle. Limit use of overhead fluorescent lighting. Install and use dimmer switches in the vehicle. Indirect lighting should be directed away from the neonate to facilitate staff needs.
4. The neonate should be positioned in the incubator to support posture and movement and promote a calm, regulated behavioral state. Nesting or boundaries support the infant's position and conserve energy by containing movement. Positioning aids may be purchased or blanket rolls may be used.
5. Incubator portholes and doors should be closed with care. Objects should not strike the incubator.
6. A gel mattress may be used to decrease vibration and aid in positioning.
7. Decrease noise levels inside the vehicle by reducing speech levels, excluding radio or television use, and responding promptly to monitor alarms. An intercom system may be used for staff communication.
8. On ground transport, request that the ambulance driver avoid rough areas in road.

J. Special transport stabilization considerations.
1. Very low birth weight infant (VLBW) (Polin et al., 2001; Thigpen, 2002).
   a. The VLBW infant presents unique challenges to the transport team.
   b. Ventilation.
      (1) Susceptibility to barotrauma with high peak inspiratory pressures.
      (2) Discuss oxygen saturation parameters with medical control.
      (3) Administration of surfactant replacement therapy by the transport team may be considered for infants meeting specific clinical criteria or for long-distance transports. Ventilatory status must be closely monitored to prevent pulmonary air leaks due to changes in lung compliance after surfactant administration. Transport from the referring hospital may be delayed to stabilize the infant and monitor lung compliance changes prior to departure in the vehicle.

(4) The VLBW infant may experience increased incidence of hypoxia and oxygen requirements due to the stresses of transport. Developmental care techniques should be incorporated into care. Sedation prior to transport may be required.

c. Hypothermia.

(1) May require supplemental warming devices in addition to the transport incubator. Due to the fragility of the skin, extreme care must be taken to not place warming devices in direct contact with skin.

(2) Transport incubator door and portholes should be kept closed as much as possible.

(3) Cover the outside of the incubator with a flame-retardant incubator cover.

(4) In cold weather preheat the vehicle prior to loading the incubator.

d. Skin fragility.

(1) Minimal to gentle handling.

(2) Use monitoring devices designed for the VLBW infant.

(3) Minimize invasive procedures and placement of monitoring devices on skin.

(4) Maintain appropriate level of hydration. Intravenous fluid administration is calculated on increased insensible water loss with decreased gestational age. Glucose should be closely monitored.

(5) Application of a semipermeable polyurethane membrane or specific products designed for the VLBW infant may be placed on the skin to maintain integrity and decrease insensible water loss.

2. Spinal immobilization (Jaimovich and Vidyasagar, 2002).

a. Traumatic injuries to the neonatal spinal cord are rare.

b. Injuries may occur due to a congenital defect, birth injury, fall, or nonaccidental trauma.

c. The spinal column in the neonate is more susceptible to hyperextension injury due to increased elasticity.

d. Spinal immobilization may be required. Immobilization device should fit into the incubator.

3. Inhaled nitric oxide (Griebel and Schmidt, 1999; Kinsella et al., 2002).

a. Inhaled nitric oxide (iNO) may be initiated at the referring hospital or by the transport team.

b. Requires continuous monitoring of all iNO delivery equipment.

c. Follow Federal Aviation Administration for rotor-wing and fixed-wing transports.

d. Ensure hand ventilation system is available.

4. High-frequency jet ventilation (HFV) (Jaimovich and Vidyasagar, 2002; Salyer, 2003).

a. May be initiated at the referring hospital or by the transport team.

b. Requires air and oxygen sources sufficient to support the HFV and the conventional ventilator.

c. Increased equipment weight.

DOCUMENTATION

A. Necessity of documentation. Patient status and the care provided must be documented throughout the transport.

B. Logistical documentation.

1. Time of transport call.

2. Time of departure en route to referring hospital.

3. Time of arrival at referring hospital.

4. Time of departure from referring hospital.
5. Time of arrival at receiving hospital.
6. Transport delays.
7. Names of transport staff.
8. Mode of transport.
9. Names of referring facility and physician.

C. **Patient care documentation.**
1. Significant maternal history, including medical history before pregnancy and prenatal, labor, and delivery history.
2. Date and time of birth.
3. Gestational age.
4. Birth weight.
5. Delivery room resuscitation, including Apgar scores.
6. Care provided before the team's arrival at the referring hospital, including laboratory and radiographic findings and medication administered.
7. Patient status on arrival of the transport team to the referring hospital, including physical assessment, vital signs, and current patient management.
8. Problem list, including current and resolved problems.
9. Ongoing documentation of patient assessment, management, and consultations with designated transport physician.
10. Patient status on arrival of the transport team to the receiving hospital, including assessment, vital signs, and monitor readings.

SAFETY (AAP, 1999; CAMTS, 2001; James, 2002)

A. **Safety must be the highest priority in any transport program.**
1. The transport program should develop a comprehensive safety program for team members and patients. Training should consist of orientation to the vehicle, emergency and evacuation procedures, survival training, crew resource management, and quality management.
2. During each transport the team should review evacuation procedures for the crew and the neonate.
3. Debriefing should be performed between crew members after each transport.
4. Critical incident stress management (CISM) should be available for each crew member.

B. **Uniforms.**
1. Team members should be appropriately attired when on transport.
   a. Flame- and heat-resistant uniforms.
   b. Garments such as jackets, gloves, socks, underclothing should be made from fire-retardant or natural fibers.
   c. Protective footwear.
   d. Helmets should be worn during helicopter transports. Visors should be available to protect the eyes and face from projectile objects. Helmets may also be worn during fixed-wing transport.
   e. Outer garments may be worn to protect against environmental conditions.
   f. Hearing protection should be worn by all crew who assist with patient loading and unloading while rotor blades are activated on the helicopter.

C. **Flotation vests should be worn by all crew members who fly over water.**

D. **Survival and first-aid kit should be located on each vehicle.**

E. **All equipment and articles in the ambulance or aircraft must be secured.**
1. The incubator may be mounted on a cart or stretcher.
2. The cart or stretcher must be locked into the vehicle.

3. Majority of vehicles use longitudinal placement of the incubator rather than horizontal placement.

F. **Restraint of all passengers, including the neonate, during transport.**
The neonate should be secured in the transport incubator with an approved restraint device. Due to different gestational ages, the restraint device must adjust to fit various sizes and weights. The restraint must not constrict the thoracic cavity. A cushioned head pad should be placed in the incubator to provide protection to the neonate's head.

G. **Establish a written policy on the use of lights and sirens.**
   1. Follow state and local regulations.
   2. Should only be used for life-threatening emergencies.

H. **Preaccident planning.**
   1. Ground and air transport programs must have a policy outlining the procedure to follow if the vehicle, staff, and patient are in an accident.
      a. Notification of transport and hospital administration, public relations.
      b. Provision for staff to receive care.
      c. Provision for patient care and completion of the transport. The patient may return to referring hospital for evaluation and treatment from the accident.
      d. Notification of transport team's emergency contact.
      e. Notification of the neonate's family.
      f. If appropriate, notification of other team members of the incident.
      g. If appropriate, lock-down of dispatch or transport office to limit amount of personnel in area.
      h. Assistance may be required to staff phones. Consider providing a separate phone number other than the team number to provide incident information and updates. A web site may also be used to disseminate information.
   2. Staff must complete an emergency contact form that is updated annually or when there is a change of information. The form should include:
      a. Name of employee.
      b. Home address.
      c. Name, address, phone, cell, and pager numbers of emergency contact.
      d. Alternate emergency contact information.
      e. Information on children.
      f. General directions to crew member's home.
      g. Current photograph in uniform.
      h. Fingerprints.
      i. Name, address, and phone number to obtain dental records.
   3. Contact local or state agencies for critical incident stress debriefing for the team. Immediate and long-term debriefing may be required.
   4. Staff should be aware of the benefits and services available prior to an incident.

I. **Infection control.**
Infection control and adherence to universal precautions should be planned due to the confined space of transport vehicle.

AIR TRANSPORT

A. **Altitude.**
   1. Anticipate increased oxygen requirement or ventilatory support at higher altitudes.
   2. Provide supplemental oxygen for staff above 10,000 feet if in a nonpressurized aircraft.

3. Neonates are at increased risk in developing hypoxia as the partial pressure of alveolar oxygen decreases during ascent.
4. Slow ascent and descent are recommended to prevent rapid reexpansion of gas, which increase the risk for pneumothorax and air embolism in the neonate.

B. **Dysbarism.**
1. Increased atmospheric pressure results in expansion of gases.
2. Anticipate expansion of "trapped" gases in body spaces (pulmonary air leaks, necrotizing enterocolitis, bowel obstruction).
   a. Gastrointestinal tract. Insert orogastric tube and empty stomach of air.
   b. Pulmonary air leaks. Consider needle thoracentesis or tube thoracotomy for decompression prior to the transport.
   c. Equalization of pressures in the eustachian tubes may be restricted in the neonate or in staff with upper respiratory or sinus problems. Providing a pacifier to the infant during descent, if appropriate, can maintain patency of the eustachian tubes.

C. **Effects of motion.**
1. Staff should recognize and understand the stresses of transport and flight.
2. Anticipate patient instability on ascent and descent.
3. Staff should be able to differentiate monitor artifact from actual recordings.

D. **Noise and vibration.**
1. Provide ear protection for staff and for the neonate (especially in rotor-wing aircraft).
2. Provide routine hearing screens for staff.
3. Minimize noise levels in patient compartment of vehicle.
4. Anticipate patient instability.
5. Use mattress and padding to minimize vibration in incubator.

E. **Evaluation for extubation and pulmonary air leaks: possibly difficult during transport, especially in rotor-wing aircraft.** Anticipate problems during transport on the basis of diagnosis and clinical presentation.

F. **Out-of-state and international transport.**
1. The team should be knowledgeable regarding out-of-state and international transport regulations and issues.
   a. Language barriers.
   b. Time change issues.
   c. Landing permits and fees.
   d. Airport hours of operation.
   e. Fueling.
   f. Ground ambulance: availability, type, fees.
   g. Customs/immigration.
   h. Communication with regional neonatal intensive care center.

G. Plan for crew hydration and nutrition on long-distance transports.

H. Transport configuration and on-loading/off-loading procedures should be predetermined, documented, and practiced prior to an actual patient transport.

LEGAL AND ETHICAL CONSIDERATIONS

A. **Legal issues (AAP, 1999; Bose, 1999).**
1. Determination of the level of responsibility of the receiving and referring staffs and institutions during the transport process has not been clearly defined and is open to legal interpretations.

a. Referring institution's level of responsibility gradually decreases as the receiving physician and transport team assume increasing responsibility for the management and care of the infant.
b. Transport team should be aware of national and state regulations regarding transport and professional standards: Federal Aviation Administration; National Health, Transportation and Safety Administration; Department of Transportation; Federal Communications Commission; Health Care Financing Agency; Joint Commission on Accreditation of Healthcare Organizations; the Clinical Laboratories Improvement Act; Health Insurance Portability and Accountability Act; and the Consolidated Omnibus Budget Reconciliation Act.
c. Receiving institution acquires increasing responsibility from the time of the transport call and the initial consultation, until the time of admission to the receiving hospital.

2. Parents or legal guardian must receive information regarding the infant's status, treatment options, the risks and benefits of transport, and risk of not transferring.
   a. The transport program should have a policy on transporting a neonate in an emergency situation and the parent(s) are not able to provide consent.
3. Responsibilities of transport team members should be clearly outlined in their job functions and should be compatible with practice acts.
4. The transport program may not be able to perform neonatal transport for a specific period due to external and internal factors.
   a. The program may not be able to perform transports due to:
      1. Weather, i.e., hurricanes, tornadoes, snowstorms.
      2. Transport accident.
      3. Neonatal intensive care bed status.
   b. Develop plan on how to communicate this information to referral centers.
   c. If team operational, develop plan for performing three-point transports. Team and facility will maintain relationship with referring hospital.
   d. If team is not operational, develop plan for contacting another neonatal transport service.

B. **Ethical issues.** Dilemmas regarding the transport of neonates should be addressed by administrative, medical, and transport staff and should include information on the following:
   1. Infants with expected poor outcomes, including those with genetic disorders, severely asphyxiated infants, extremely low birth weight infants, and those with lethal anomalies.
   2. Debriefing of the team may be required.

TOTAL QUALITY MANAGEMENT

The transport program should develop a quality management program to monitor, evaluate, and improve the service.

A. **Quality indicators may include the following:**
   1. Transport statistics (number of transports, referral hospitals, referral physicians).
   2. Equipment malfunction, failure, or supply.
   3. Transport delays.
   4. Stabilization times.
   5. Crew and patient safety issues.
   6. Number of transports per team member.

7. Procedures performed by crew on transport.
8. Documentation of patient care and medications.
9. Vehicle out-of-service time.
10. Patient outcome.
11. Family and referring hospital customer satisfaction.
12. Staff education and skills.

B. **Quality improvement may be attained through a number of mechanisms.** A combination of these mechanisms is probably most effective (NANN, 1998).
1. Case review by the team, medical director, and transport director.
2. Use of peer review.
3. Regular staff meetings.
4. Case review with team members, which can be effectively accomplished by review of selected cases, including the following:
   a. Initial referral call.
   b. Transport logistics.
   c. Stabilization of the infant by the referring hospital as well as the transport team.
   d. Care provided during transport.
   e. Patient outcome.

C. **Peer review may be used to provide feedback to individuals.**
1. Appropriateness of care provided.
2. Clarity of treatment plan.
3. Treatment plan rationale and outcome.
4. Documentation.

D. **Issues identified through any of these mechanisms should be addressed with recommendations and plans for follow-up.**

REFERENCES

American Academy of Pediatrics: *Guidelines for air and ground transport of neonatal and pediatric patients* (2nd ed.). Elk Grove Village, IL, 1999, Author.

Arndt, K.: *Standards for critical care and specialty rotor-wing transport.* Lexington, KY, 2003, Transport Nurses Association.

Blumen, I.: *A safety review and risk assessment in air medical transport.* Salt Lake City, 2002, Air Medical Physician Association.

Bose, C.: Neonatal transport. In G. Avery, M.A. Fletcher, and M.G. MacDonald (Eds.): *Neonatology pathophysiology and management of the newborn* (5th ed.). Philadelphia, 1999, Lippincott Williams & Wilkins, pp. 35-47.

Bowen, S.L.: *The effects of individualized developmental care on oxygenation and oxygen requirements in the premature infant during transport* [master's thesis]. Tampa, FL, 1999, The University of Tampa.

Bowen, S.L.: Transport of the mechanically ventilated neonate. *Respiratory Care Clinics, 8*:67-82, 2002.

Butterfield, L.J.: Historical perspectives of neonatal transport. *Pediatric Clinics of North America, 40*(2):221-239, 1993.

Chou, M. and MacDonald, M.G.: Landmarks in the development of patient transport systems. In M.G. MacDonald and M.K. Miller (Eds.): *Emergency transport of the perinatal patient.* Boston, 1989, Little, Brown.

Commission on Accreditation of Medical Transport Systems: *Best practices.* Anderson, SC, 2001, Author.

Committee on Perinatal Health: *Toward improving the outcome of pregnancy.* White Plains, NY, 1976, National Foundation of March of Dimes.

Cone, T.E.: *History of the care and feeding of the premature infant.* Boston, 1985, Little, Brown.

Crain, E.F. and Gershel, J.C.: *Clinical manual of emergency pediatrics*. New York, 2003, McGraw-Hill.

Devane, S.P.: Transport of ill infants. In J.M. Rennie and N.R.C. Roberton (Eds.): *Textbook of neonatology*. New York, 1999, Churchill Livingstone, pp. 1424-1428.

Griebel, J. and Schmidt, J.: Transporting infants on inhaled nitric oxide. *Advance for Managers of Respiratory Care, 64*:69, November, 1999.

Jaimovich, D.G. and Vidyasagar, D.: *Handbook of pediatric and neonatal transport medicine* (2nd ed.). Philadelphia, 2002, Hanley & Belfus.

James, S.E.: *Standards for critical care and specialty ground transport*. Lexington, KY, 2002, Transport Nurses Association.

Kinsella, J.P., Griebel, J., Schmidt, J.M., and Abman, S.H.: Use of inhaled nitric oxide during interhospital transport of newborns with hypoxemic respiratory failure. *Pediatrics, 109*(1):158-161, 2002.

Losty, M.S., Orlofsky, I., and Boles, T.: A transport service for premature babies. *American Journal of Nursing, 50*:10-12, 1950.

MacDonald, M.G. and Ramasethu, J.: *Atlas of procedures in neonatology* (3rd ed.). Philadelphia, 2002, Lippincott Williams & Wilkins.

March of Dimes. *Health library, infant health statistics*. Retrieved May 14, 2001, from www.modimes.org.

Martin, J., Hamilton, B.E., Ventura, S., et al.: Birth: Final data for 2001. *National Vital Statistics Reports, 51*(2):1-103, 2002.

National Association of Neonatal Nurses: *Neonatal nursing transport guidelines*. Petaluma, CA, 1998, Author.

Oakes, D.: *Neonatal/pediatric respiratory care: A critical care pocket guide* (4th ed.). Orono, ME, 2000, Health Educator Publications, Inc.

Pillitteri, A.: *Maternal and child health nursing: Care of the childbearing and childrearing family* (4th ed.). Philadelphia, 2003, Lippincott Williams & Wilkins.

Polin, R.A., Yoder, M.C., and Burg, F.D.: *Workbook in practical neonatology* (3rd ed.). Philadelphia, 2001, Saunders.

Salyer, J.W.: Transport of infants and children. In M. Czervinske and S. Barnhart (Eds.): *Perinatal and pediatric respiratory care* (2nd ed.). Philadelphia, 2003, Saunders, pp. 693-707.

Schechter, N.L., Berde, C.B., and Yaster, M.: *Pain in infants, children and adolescents* (2nd ed.). Philadelphia, 2003, Lippincott Williams & Wilkins.

Segal, S.: Transfer of a premature or other high-risk newborn infant to a referral hospital. *Pediatric Clinics of North America, 13*(4):1195-1205, 1966.

Segal, S. (Ed.): *Manual for the transport of high-risk newborn infants*. Sherbrooke, Quebec, 1972, Canadian Pediatric Society.

Sweeney, J.K. and Gutierrez, T.: Musculoskeletal implications of preterm infant positioning in the NICU. *Journal of Perinatal and Neonatal Nursing, 16*(1):58-70, 2002.

Symington, A. and Pinelli, J.: Developmental care for promoting development and preventing morbidity in preterm infants. *Cochrane Database of Systematic Reviews, 4*:CD001814, 2001.

Thigpen, J.: Developmental considerations for resuscitation of the VLBW infant. *Neonatal Network, 21*(4):21-26, 2002.

Wallace, H.M., Losty, M.A., and Baumgartner, L.: Report of two years' experience in the transportation of premature infants in New York City. *Pediatrics, 22*:439-447, 1952.

Woodward, G.A., Insoft, R.M., Pearson-Shaver, A.L., et al.: The state of pediatric interfacility transport: Consensus of the second national pediatric and neonatal interfacility transport medicine leadership conference. *Pediatric Emergency Care, 18*(1):38-43, 2002.

CHAPTER

22 Care of the Extremely Low Birth Weight Infant

DENISE POIRIER MAGUIRE

OBJECTIVES

1. Discuss atraumatic care techniques for the extremely low birth weight (ELBW) infant that eliminate or minimize the psychologic and physical distress experienced by infants and their families.
2. Identify principles of nursing management specific to the ELBW infant population and their families.

The ELBW infant challenges all assessment and management strategies and exemplifies the importance of holistic nursing care in the neonatal intensive care unit (NICU). Nursing skills must be finely honed and fully developed before assignment to care for the ELBW infant. The overriding approach must be one of extreme gentleness, with constant appreciation of the fragility before us. Every cell of the ELBW infant is immature and delicate, and demands special consideration. The purpose of this chapter is to describe a developmentally appropriate approach to nursing care of ELBW infants that emphasizes the special physiologic considerations pertinent to their care and management. Recent authors define extremely low birth weight infants as birth weight less than 1000 g, the definition adopted for this chapter (Blickstein et al., 2002; Msall and Tremont, 2002; Tommiska et al., 2003).

PRENATAL CONSIDERATIONS

A. **Whenever possible, ELBW infants should be delivered in a tertiary care facility with a NICU.** The best method of transportation for the infant is within the mother's womb, unless the mother is in danger herself. The safety of maternal transport must be weighed against the risks of infant transport (Ringer, 1998).
   1. Neonatology consultation. Women who threaten to deliver an infant on the brink of viability should have a neonatal consultation. Consultations should be requested and performed as soon as possible to minimize the stress for parents. Consultations that occur when delivery is imminent are of little value. The goal of the consultation is to initiate a relationship with the mother and father that will build trust and facilitate decision making. Consultations are typically performed by neonatologists, as well as neonatal nurse practitioners (NNP).
   2. Parent participation in decision making. Understanding the parents' thoughts, wishes, and concerns will guide discussion and enable the family to participate in decision making. Collaborating with families on decision

making ensures a family-centered approach that minimizes opportunities for paternalism. Parents must learn about the challenges and unknowns of ELBW infant delivery and resuscitation. Information should be provided in a nonbiased and factual manner. In the best situation, parents should be given time to reflect and talk with family, friends, and clergy. They should be encouraged to ask as many questions as they need to. Finally, they must feel supported by the care team in the decisions they make.

DELIVERY ROOM MANAGEMENT

A. **Whenever possible, the neonatal team should prepare for the birth of an ELBW infant in advance.**
   1. A neonatologist or NNP should attend the delivery, as well as a NICU nurse. Both should be skilled in the American Academy of Pediatrics/American Heart Association's Neonatal Resuscitation Program (NRP), and at least one should be skilled in intubation (NRP Steering Committee, 2000). Before the infant is born, the neonatal team should clearly define their roles with each other to avoid confusion in a stressful situation. If twins or other multiples are expected, one team should be assigned to each infant.
   2. The usual resuscitation equipment must be available and its function verified. The warming table should be prewarmed, and warmed blankets available. The delivery room itself should be warm, at least so the clinicians do not need gowns to stay warm.

B. **At the time of delivery:**
   1. As the infant is gently placed on the warming table, the clinician responsible for intubation should evaluate the infant's breathing, heart rate, and color. The NRP guidelines should be used to resuscitate if necessary (NRP Steering Committee, 2000). This clinician should also determine Apgar score at the appropriate times.
   2. The second clinician should be responsible for thermoregulation by gently drying the infant and removing wet blankets. Care should be taken to avoid shearing the skin from excessive or vigorous rubbing. The wet blankets should be removed so the infant can lie on a dry blanket for any intervention that is necessary. There is some evidence that placing the ELBW infant in a polyurethane bag (i.e., sterile bowel bag) immediately following delivery and before any intervention may be beneficial in reducing hypothermia (Knobel et al., 2003; Vohra et al., 1999).
   3. As soon as possible, the infant's arms and legs should be gently flexed and supported with blanket rolls. If a small diaper is to be used, it should be slid under the buttocks rather than lifting the legs to avoid a rapid shift in cerebral blood flow.
   4. Transfer the infant to the NICU as soon as possible in a warmed incubator equipped with the necessary gases and equipment. If the infant is intubated, the ventilator should be used rather than hand-bagging to minimize risk of pneumothorax. The infant should be secured to the mattress with a blanket tucked under side to side to minimize bouncing and provide a sense of security. Care should be taken when moving the incubator over breaks in the floor, such as entry into an elevator or the change from tile to carpeting.
      a. Hospital transfer. Increased precautions must be taken to protect the ELBW infants transported in an ambulance or fixed- or rotor-wing aircraft. Ensuring as smooth a ride as possible, minimizing bright lights,

and avoiding loud talking or noises will contribute to a developmentally supportive environment.

ADMISSION TO THE NICU

A. Monitoring.

1. Cardiac leads placed on the infant for transport should be used if they are functional. If they are not functional, replace them with water-based gelled leads.
2. Umbilical arterial catheters should be transduced with alarms.
3. Skin temperature must also be monitored, whether the infant is admitted to a warming table or incubator.
4. Oxygen saturation.
5. End-tidal CO_2 (if the infant is mechanically ventilated).
6. Ventilator alarms (if the infant is mechanically ventilated).

B. Thermoregulation. ELBW infants are unable to thermoregulate themselves, and require diligent attention to their temperature. Although research has not yet established an appropriate neutral thermal environment (NTE) for infants less than 1000 g, caregivers must provide an adequate amount of heat to keep the ELBW infant warm. The NTE is achieved by providing the appropriate amount of warmth so the infant does not need to expend energy. ELBW infants lose a tremendous amount of heat and water through their thin skin, so interventions focused on their skin will contribute to maintaining an NTE.

1. A temperature probe should be placed on a fleshy part of the abdomen, avoiding bony prominences, and extremities. Apply a heat reflector if radiant heat or phototherapy is in use. Placing the probe on the left lateral side of the abdomen enables the infant to be repositioned on the back, front, and right side without moving the probe.
   a. Incubators and radiant warmers should be prewarmed with the linens.
   b. The temperature mode should be set to servocontrol, and the desired temperature set manually (36.2°C-36.5° C).
2. Other interventions reported in the literature to maintain NTE include
   a. Addition of humidity to the microenvironment.
   b. Application of a semitransparent membrane on large skin surface areas.
   c. Application of plastic wrap across a radiant warmer.
   d. Application of a preservative-free topical ointment on the skin (Nopper et al., 1996).

C. Skin care. The importance of excellent skin care in the ELBW infant population cannot be overstated. Their integumentary system does not provide a significant barrier against pathogens, infections, topical teratogens, and insensible water loss. Skin tears and shears easily because there is a minimal bond between the epidermis and dermis. Depending upon gestational age, the stratum corneum may be as little as 1 or 2 cells thick (Rutter, 1996). The *Neonatal Skin Care Guidelines for Practice* (National Association of Neonatal Nurses [NANN], 1997) provides an evidenced-based approach to skin care. The guidelines were tested in a multicenter research utilization project that demonstrated improved skin conditions after guidelines were implemented (Lund et al., 2001).

1. Vernix caseosa appears to provide a measure of antimicrobial activity (Yoshio et al., 2003), yet only the "larger" ELBW infants will have any.
2. ELBW infants may need as many as 8 weeks for the stratum corneum to provide an effective barrier, and it may take 3 weeks for the skin pH to fall from 6.0 to 5.0 (Fox et al., 1998).
3. Protect the skin with a piece of a pectin-based skin barrier that has a keyhole the size of the probe cut into it. Tape the probe to the skin barrier.

These products should also be used to protect the skin when taping endotracheal tubes and umbilical lines (NANN, 1997).

4. Never use skin adhesives or solvents on the skin. Adhesives will create a stronger bond than that between the dermis and epidermis. Solvents will be absorbed into the skin, and are associated with liver and kidney toxicity (NANN, 1997).
5. Minimize the use of tape on the skin. In most cases, gel-based adhesives are available to avoid skin trauma (NANN, 1997).
6. Clean the skin with sterile water. Soap is not necessary, and may be drying (NANN, 1997).
7. Remove antimicrobials (such as povidone-iodine and chlorhexidine) as soon as possible to minimize absorption (NANN, 1997).
8. Application of a preservative-free topical ointment on the skin every 6 to 8 hours may help to protect the skin (NANN, 1997).
9. Cover wounds and cracks on skin with transparent adhesive dressings (Donahue et al., 1996; Lund et al, 2001; NANN, 1997), hydrocolloid or pectin-based barrier, or nonadherent hydrogel dressing (NANN, 1997).
   a. Cover up dry wounds to keep them moist: do not let wounds dry out. Use transparent adhesive dressings, hydrocolloid or pectin-based barrier, or nonadherent hydrogel dressing.
   b. Soak up wet wounds with a gel dressing.
   c. Fill up deep wounds with a sterile petroleum-based gauze dressing.
   d. Cover up shallow wounds to keep them moist: do not let wounds dry out. Use transparent adhesive dressings, hydrocolloid or pectin-based barrier, or nonadherent hydrogel dressing.
10. Avoid using isopropyl alcohol on the skin (NANN, 1997), including the umbilical cord (Dore et al., 1998). Alcohol is drying to the skin, and is absorbed through the umbilical cord. It can also be absorbed through the skin if evaporation is decreased, as occurs under a sterile drape. The cord should be kept dry to enable it to fall off naturally.

PARAMETERS OF CLINICAL ASSESSMENT AND NURSING MANAGEMENT

A. **Respiratory support.**
   1. It is the rare ELBW infant who does not require ventilatory support. Although some may require only blow-by oxygen or Oxyhood shortly after birth, ELBW infants may quickly tire breathing, and should be assessed closely for signs of respiratory failure.
   2. Continuous positive airway pressure (CPAP) provides alveolar distention, which decreases the work of breathing in ELBW infants with respiratory distress syndrome. The least traumatic method should be chosen to reduce stress. Care should be taken to ensure the correct device size because ELBW infants are quite small. Both mask and nasal prongs have the potential to cause pressure ulcers, but the nasopharyngeal (NP) and endotracheal (ET) methods are more invasive.
   3. Mechanical ventilation. Mechanical ventilation is indicated when the ELBW infant is not exchanging gases sufficiently, is acidotic, apneic, or bradycardic. Several different modes of mechanical ventilation are available (see Chapter 25.)
      a. Barotrauma associated with mechanical ventilation is responsible for the development of chronic lung disease.

B. **Nursing management.** Vigilant attention to all details is constantly necessary. Consistent nursing caregivers enable subtle changes to be recognized early.

1. Minimize oxygen consumption.
   a. Conserve heat.
   b. Maintain blood pressure and hematocrit.
   c. Buffer metabolic acidosis as ordered.
   d. Handle minimally, and provide cue-based, individualized care.
   e. Sedate with extreme caution. Midazolam is associated with adverse neurologic events such as death, grades III through IV intraventricular hemorrhage (IVH), and periventricular leukomalacia (PVL) (Anand et al.,1999; Ng et al., 2003).
   f. Monitor for complications such as patent ductus arteriosus (PDA), pneumothorax, heart failure, and disseminated intravascular coagulation (DIC).
2. Use supportive measures to decrease metabolic demands.
   a. Provide adequate fluid and caloric support.
   b. Accurately assess intake, output, and daily weights.
   c. Monitor glucose.
   d. Monitor serum electrolytes.
   e. Monitor blood and urine cultures.
   f. Review differential and platelet counts.
   g. Provide antibiotic therapy when indicated.
3. Maintain ventilatory support and supplemental oxygen.
   a. Maintain and protect patent airway.
   b. Monitor vital signs continuously.
   c. Monitor oxygen saturations.
   d. Sample and monitor blood gases frequently or as clinically indicated.
   e. Maintain PaO_2 50 to 70 mm Hg.
   f. Wean oxygen and ventilator settings as tolerated.
   g. Obtain x-rays, as clinically indicated.
   h. Administer surfactant replacement.
4. Assess airway patency, breathing patterns, and work of breathing. High risk of pulmonary hemorrhage and air leak.
5. Assess changes in breathing following interventions (pulse oximetry, grunting, flaring, retracting).
6. Assess changes in oxygenation and ventilation following interventions (pulse oximetry, blood gases, end-tidal CO_2).
7. Ensure continuous and excellent fit of mechanical devices. All have a tendency to move or dislodge with patient movement.
8. Maintain developmentally appropriate body positioning. Support rounded shoulders and hips; flexed extremities; tucked head; hand to mouth.
9. Regularly assess and reassess comfort and pain level with a standardized tool. Although sucrose appears to be safe in most preterm infants, it may be detrimental in the ELBW population (Johnston et al., 2002). Johnston and colleagues reported increased risk of poor neurobehavioral development and physiologic outcomes related to repeated use of sucrose in infants less than 31 weeks' gestation. However, opioids should be considered for moderate and severely painful procedures (i.e., chest tube placement) (Anand, 2001).

C. **Cardiovascular support.** ELBW infants have approximately 90 to 105 ml/kg of circulating blood.
   1. Blood pressure. Blood pressures tend to be lower in ELBW infants, but should rise in the first 24 hours of life.
      a. Persistent low mean arterial pressure (MAP) has been associated with an increased risk of cerebral hemorrhage and ischemic lesions (Watkins et al., 1989; Bada et al, 1990).

b. Blood pressures correlate directly with birth weights above 750 g.
c. Mean arterial pressures less than or equal to 28 torr at 3 hours have been identified as a reasonable but not absolute predictor of the need for treatment (Cordero et al., 2002).

2. PDA is the fourth most common congenital heart lesion. As pulmonary vascular resistance (PVR) decreases and systemic vascular resistance (SVR) increases, blood is shunted left to right through the PDA, which increases pulmonary blood flow.
   a. The incidence of PDA is inversely related to gestational age; as high as 80% in infants with birth weight less than 1200 g.
   b. Incidence of PDA in the ELBW infant is increased because the lack of smooth muscle in the ductus prolongs patency.
   c. PDA often manifests at 3 to 7 days when respiratory distress improves and the PVR resistance decreases. Classic signs (which may be subtle) include increased pulmonary vasculature, increased oxygen requirements, cardiomegaly, bounding peripheral pulses, widening pulse pressure, hyperactive precordium, and murmur.
   d. Patients are typically managed with conservative measures (fluid restrictions, diuretics, and positive end-expiratory pressure (PEEP), indomethacin (many contraindications), or surgical management. Little and colleagues (2003) reported that birth weight less than 1000 g was highly predictive of indomethacin failure.
   e. Increased pulmonary blood flow demands that systemic blood flow will decrease. ELBW infants with a PDA may be at increased risk for necrotizing enterocolitis and renal failure.
3. Blood transfusions. Blood removed for laboratory analysis far exceeds the ability of the ELBW infant to replace volume lost.
   a. Low hematocrit triggers bone marrow to increase red blood cell production, but this is a weak stimulus in the ELBW infant.
   b. Packed red blood cell transfusions may be needed occasionally to raise the hematocrit and improve oxygen-carrying capacity. Benefits must be weighed against known risks.
   c. Erythropoietin has been shown to reduce the need for transfusion in ELBW infants, if started on days 3 to 5 of life (Maier et al., 2002).
4. Nursing management. Vigilant attention to all details is constantly necessary. Consistent nursing caregivers enable subtle changes to be recognized early so that interventions can be made to decrease or minimize severity of symptoms. Nursing care includes diligent accounting for all blood removed, including estimates of bleeding episodes if necessary.

D. Fluid and electrolyte balance.

1. The principles of nursing assessment and management include:
   a. Knowledge of daily requirements.
   b. Assessment of any unusual losses or gains.
   c. Prediction and measurement of ongoing losses or gains.
2. Basic elements of fluid and electrolyte balance.
   a. Body water is the major constituent of body tissue, approximately 85% in ELBW infants. Any large change in weight reflects water balance. A 20% weight loss in ELBW infants is expected, and beneficial. Most losses occur in the extracellular fluid (ECF) compartment.
   b. Electrolytes. In solution, they dissociate into ions (charged particles).
      (1) The chief cations are sodium (Na^{++}, extracellular) and potassium (K^{+}, intracellular). Hydrogen (H^{+}) is also a cation.

(2) The chief anions are chloride (Cl^-) and bicarbonate (HCO_3^-).

c. pH. An alteration in pH always alters electrolyte balance. For example, hyperventilation increases the pH, and the kidneys respond by wasting bicarbonate to compensate for the elevated pH, and serum potassium is driven into the cells.

3. Body water is contained in two large compartments. The intracellular (55%) and extracellular (interstitial 40%, intravascular 5%) compartments freely exchange water.
   a. ELBW infants have severely decreased glomerular filtration rate (GFR), increased basal metabolic rate (BMR), and increased surface area in relation to body weight.
   b. Indicators of body water are weight, urine output, electrolyte balance, blood urea nitrogen (BUN), skin turgor, fontanelles, and cranial sutures.
4. Fluid and electrolyte imbalances common in ELBW infants.
   a. Hypernatremia due to excessive water losses from immature kidney function. This diagnosis should be suspected when there is increased urine output (>2 cc/kg/hour), and increasing serum sodium levels. Hypernatremia is treated by increasing fluid intake and considering decreasing sodium intake.
   b. Hyponatremia due to syndrome of inappropriate antidiuretic hormone (SIADH), in which a normal or excess ECF volume exists. The diagnosis should be suspected when there is sudden weight gain, no edema, increased urine osmolality, and decreased urine output. ELBW infants at risk of SIADH are those having intraventricular hemorrhage, pain, birth asphyxia, pneumothorax, positive pressure ventilation, or opiates. Treatment of SIADH is to restrict fluids if serum sodium is less than 120, and replace urinary sodium.
   c. Nonoliguric hyperkalemia is a common problem in the ELBW infant population, resulting from movement of potassium from the intracellular space to the extracellular space. Although little research exists on the best treatment methods, Mildenberger and Versmold (2002) advocate administration of calcium, infusion of insulin and glucose, and correction of acidosis based on the best evidence available.
5. Transepidermal water loss (TEWL) is a measurable parameter, but is usually estimated.
   a. The Evaporimeter (ServoMed, Stockholm, Sweden) has been used in research (Vernon et al., 1990), as well as the Nova 9003 Dermal Phase Meter (DPM) (NovaTech Corp, Portsmouth, NH) (Okah et al., 1995). Although expensive, the DPM 9003 is easy to use and not affected by changes in the microenvironment.
   b. High humidity decreases TEWL and heat loss. Humidity also decreases fluid requirements, improves electrolyte balance, and increases urine output (Gaylord et al., 2001).
   c. ELBW infants can lose up to 200 cc/kg/day in combined TEWL and urine output (Simmons, 1998). The sum of evaporation and radiant water loss is inversely proportional to weight.
   d. 85% to 90% humidity in the first week of life is needed to effect a difference (Kuller and Lund, 1993).
   e. The use of double-walled incubators decreases TEWL (NANN, 1997).
   f. The use of emollients or plastic wrap blankets may be used to decrease TEWL (Siegfried, 1998).

E. **Sepsis.** Early-onset sepsis is eight times more common in ELBW infants than in infants greater than 2000 g (Guerina, 1998). Infants with early-onset sepsis are more likely to die than uninfected infants (Stoll et al., 2002).
 1. Increased susceptibility to sepsis is due to:
  a. Decreased antibody levels.
  b. Poor response to antigenic stimuli.
  c. Limited production of type-specific antibodies.
  d. Impaired circulating antibody.
  e. Depressed complement pathways.
  f. Decrease in neutrophil storage pool.
  g. Failure to increase stem cell proliferation during infection.
  h. Altered neutrophil functions.
 2. Environmental risk factors include:
  a. Prolonged length of stay.
  b. Multiple invasive procedures.
  c. Frequent use of antibiotics.
 3. Reduce the risk of nosocomial bloodstream infections.
  a. Practice excellent handwashing skills.
  b. Use waterless hand disinfectants between patients after good handwashing.
  c. Use sterile technique when inserting invasive (venous or arterial) catheters.
  d. Use skin antimicrobials according to directions.
  e. Institute quality improvement measures to decrease the number of intravenous and central line days and improve nutrition.
  f. Prevent catheter hub contamination.
  g. Consider trophic feeds, preferably with breast milk (Edwards, 2002; Furman et al., 2003).

F. **Nutrition.** Nutritional management of ELBW infants is inconsistent among NICU settings. General uncertainty exists regarding when to begin parenteral nutrition, feeding, what type of feeding is most easily tolerated, and how quickly to advance feedings.
 1. The goal of feeding is to provide nutrition that supports "postnatal growth that approximates the in utero growth of a normal fetus" (AAP, 1998).
  a. Nutrition must support the tremendous amount of physiologic growth that occurs toward the end of the second trimester. Growth and development are vulnerable to nutritional deprivation.
  b. The ELBW infant gut is incapable of performing digestion and absorption successfully at birth, and is at high risk of developing necrotizing enterocolitis.
  c. Parenteral nutrition (PN) should be initiated as soon as possible, at least within the first 24 hours of life (Evans and Thureen, 2001; Ziegler et al., 2002).
   (1) Early administration of amino acids at 3 g/kg/day appears to be efficacious and safe (Paisley et al., 2000).
   (2) Serum blood glucose must be followed closely for evidence of hyperglycemia. Titrating infusion rates down and/or decreasing dextrose content in the infusate may be necessary to prevent hyperglycemia.
   (3) Continuous insulin infusion enables control of plasma glucose while increasing increased energy intake to promote growth. Although not fully studied, insulin administration to promote ELBW infant growth is used with caution in many centers.

(4) Lipids provide essential fatty acids and long-chain polyunsaturated fatty acids. Ziegler and colleagues (2002) recommend starting 10% lipids within 24 hours of birth at 1 g/kg/day, and increased gradually to 3 g/kg/day. They change to 20% emulsion when 2 g/kg/day is reached, and the rate of infusion never exceeds 150 mg/kg/hour.

d. Enteral nutrition.

(1) ELBW infants have random, irregular motility, which causes gastric residuals. It often leads to a misdiagnosis of "feeding intolerance" when in fact it is a benign finding. The pattern reverts back to normal when feedings are started early (Berseth and Nordyke, 1993).

(2) Withholding feedings for prolonged periods leads to atrophy of the gut. Initiation of feedings that have been withheld for a prolonged period may actually be more unsafe in a gut that has atrophied due to starvation.

(3) Although the etiology of necrotizing enterocolitis (NEC) is unclear, it does not seem related to gastric residuals. Berseth, Bisquera and Paje (2003) reported that NEC may be related to the rate at which feedings are incrementally increased. The incidence of NEC increased so drastically in their study group whose feeds were advanced from 20 to 140 ml/kg/day, that they closed the study early.

(4) The preferred first feed is breast milk. Ziegler and colleagues (2002) recommend 1 to 2 ml per feed every 3 to 6 hours. Then advance slowly when gastric residuals are less than 0.5 ml.

(5) The transition from gavage to oral feedings must be attempted cautiously. Breathing compromise, oxygen desaturation, and bradycardia are likely to occur during oral feeds with a nasogastric (NG) tube in place (Shiao et al., 1995). Apnea appears to be an important factor that increases the length of time it takes a preterm infant to reach full oral feedings (Mandich et al., 1996).

G. Developmentally appropriate care. There is no more important subgroup of high-risk infants to integrate developmentally appropriate care into nursing than the ELBW infant. Ideally, developmentally appropriate care should be more of a philosophic approach to care than specific interventions. Developmentally appropriate care should be so well integrated into neonatal nursing that it becomes invisible and cannot be discerned from "regular" nursing care. Evidence exists that measures taken to minimize pain and stress may reduce the incidence of intraventricular hemorrhage and periventricular leukomalacia (McLendon et al., 2003).

1. Stress. The most common sign of stress in the ELBW infant population is decreased activity and lack of "fight." They may become floppy and nonreactive.

a. Protect from stress.

(1) Use gentle touch when handling the infant.

(2) Avoid swift changes in cerebral blood flow by gentle repositioning.

(3) Create a stress-free, womblike environment. Consider alternating a heavy cover over the incubator with a light cover to alternate light levels. Some evidence exists that the circadian system is responsive to light, and that low-intensity lighting can help regulate the developing clock (Rivkees and Hao, 2000).

(4) Create a quiet environment.

(5) Provide long periods of restful sleep.

(6) Use an incubator or warming table that converts to incubator from the time of admission.

b. Minimize stress.
   (1) Provide comfort measures after stressful events, continuing until the ELBW infant has recovered.
   (2) Use "facilitated tucking," a technique that brings flexed arms and legs to midline. Facilitated tucking mimics the fetal position, which is a universally comforting position. It is particularly useful following a stressful event, or one in which the infant is in an extended position.
   (3) Avoid clustering many stressful procedures together. Give the ELBW infant time and support to recover.
   (4) Enable hand-to-mouth positioning by flexing the arms and bringing the hands up to the mouth. This position also mimics the fetal position. In order to promote hand-to-mouth activities, avoid using hands as an intravenous (IV) site.
   (5) Support position so shoulders and hips are rounded, and chin is tucked toward neck. Avoid supine positioning. Side-lying or prone is preferable.
   (6) Use ventral support.
   (7) Use close boundaries, as in a nest (see Chapter 11).
   (8) Provide nonnutritive sucking and handholding.
   (9) Locate ELBW infant beds in quiet areas, away from telephones, sinks, and other noise producers.

c. Learn ELBW infant cues.
   (1) Notice the emerging patterns of response from ELBW infants to caregiver's interventions.
   (2) Structure and time nursing interventions based on individual ELBW infant response.

d. Involve family.
   (1) Teach family how ELBW infant cues are interpreted.
   (2) Consider skin-to-skin holding (kangaroo care) when appropriate.

H. **Pain management**. Untreated or inappropriately treated pain can have devastating effects on the ELBW infant. Unfortunately we do not yet know all that causes pain in this population. Clinicians should proceed with caution, closely assessing ELBW infant response—and nonresponse—to all procedures and interventions.

1. Procedures known to cause moderate or severe pain (such as chest tube insertion) should be treated with an opioid such as morphine or fentanyl.
2. Procedures known to cause mild pain (i.e., heel stick) and those suspected of causing mild pain (i.e., endotracheal tube suctioning) should be treated using nonpharmacologic measures.
3. Sucrose has been reported to be effective in decreasing pain responses when administered in single oral applications to preterm infants between 26 and 34 weeks' gestation (Stevens et al., 2001). Not enough evidence exists regarding the safety of implementing sucrose interventions in ELBW infants to recommend its widespread use for repeated painful procedures in the NICU (Walden, 2001).
4. Eutectic mixture of local anesthetic (EMLA) is not approved for use in infants less than 37 weeks gestation.
5. ELBW infants treated with continuous opioid infusions for management of postoperative pain should be assessed at least every 3 to 4 hours for pain, using a valid and reliable pain scale developed specifically for preterm infants. The Premature Infant Pain Profile (PIPP) is such a pain scale (Ballantyne et al., 1999; Stevens et al., 1996).

a. Infants on continuous opioid infusions may be oversedated, even at a low starting dose. All continuous doses must be titrated to achieve the desired effect. Titration occurs when the dose is decreased periodically throughout the 24-hour day when little or no pain is assessed to enable achievement of the right amount of opioid without oversedating the ELBW infant.
b. The safety of sedatives in the ELBW infant population is not established, and should be avoided. Sedatives also blunt the infant's behavioral responses to pain without providing pain relief (Walden and Carrier, 2003).
c. Continuous infusions of opioids beyond 7 days will cause physical dependence. Depending upon the dose and length of treatment, the dose should be reduced (weaned) on a regular schedule, while signs of withdrawal are closely assessed and treated if necessary.
d. Withdrawal symptoms should be treated with opioids rather than sedatives or anticonvulsants, which mask rather than treat the symptoms.

I. **Palliative care** provides an integrated interdisciplinary approach by caregivers to support both the ELBW infant and the family through a difficult period (Carter and Bhatia, 2001). Palliative care is not limited to infants who are terminally ill or actively dying. Rather, it is a family-centered approach to care that should be offered to any family whose infant is admitted to the NICU. A program of palliative care may have several "levels" in which interventions change or escalate.
1. A supportive family-centered environment in which parents are encouraged to discuss concerns with health care providers is the first level of palliative care. Parents are active participants in their infant's plan of care. Clinicians spend time educating parents about their infant and condition.
2. Helping parents make decisions about resuscitation or withdrawing life support is another level of palliative care. When a model of palliative care is used as described above, decisions about life and death occur in a trusting relationship.
3. Infants with a lethal condition such as trisomy 13 who survive the initial neonatal period will require a higher level of palliative care. Parents may take home such an infant, but need help from community sources and respite care.
4. Infants who are actively dying require their care to be "redirected" to comfort care rather than treatment in the final level of palliative care. Clinicians caring for these patients and families must be sensitive to parents' wishes and cultural beliefs. They are intimately involved in creating the memory that parents and families will always have with them.

REFERENCES

American Academy of Pediatrics Committee on Nutrition: *Pediatric nutrition handbook* (4th ed.). Elk Grove Village, IL, 1998, The Academy.

Anand, K.J.: Consensus statement for the prevention and management of pain in the newborn. *Archives of Pediatric and Adolescent Medicine, 155*(2):173-180, 2001.

Anand, K.J., Barton, B.A., McIntosh, N., et al.: Analgesia and sedation in preterm neonates who require ventilatory support: Results from the NOPAIN trial. *Archives of Pediatric and Adolescent Medicine, 153*(4):331-338, 1999.

Bada, H.S., Korones, S.B., Perry, E.H., et al.: Mean arterial blood pressure changes in premature infants and those at risk for intraventricular hemorrhage. *Journal of Pediatrics, 117*(4):607-614, 1990.

Ballantyne, M., Stevens, B., McAllister, M., et al.: Validation of the premature infant pain profile in the clinical setting. *Clinical Journal of Pain, 15*(4):297-303, 1999.

Berserth, C.L., Bisquera, J.A., and Page, V.U.: Prolonging small feeding volumes early in life decreases the incidence of necrotizing enterocolitis in very low birthweight infants. *Pediatrics, 111*(3):529-534: 2003.

Berseth, C.L. and Nordyke, C.: Enteral nutrients promote postnatal maturation of intestinal motor activity in preterm infants. *American Journal of Physiology, 264*(6 Pt 1):G1046-G1051, 1993.

Blickstein, I., Jacques, D.L., and Keith, L.G.: The odds of delivering one, two or three extremely low birth weight (<1000 g) triplet infants: A study of 3288 sets. *Journal of Perinatal Medicine, 30*(5):359-363, 2002.

Carter, B.S. and Bhatia, J.: Comfort/palliative care guidelines for neonatal practice: Development and implementation in an academic medical center. *Journal of Perinatology, 2*(5):279-283, 2001.

Cordero, L., Timan, C.J., Waters, H.H., and Sachs, L.A.: Mean arterial pressures during the first 24 hours of life in < or = 600-gram birth weight infants. *Journal of Perinatology, 22*(5):348-353, 2002.

Donahue, M.L., Phelps, D.L., Richter, S.E., and Davis, J.M.: A semipermeable skin dressing for extremely low birth weight infants. *Journal of Perinatology, 16*(1):20-24, 1996.

Dore, S., Buchan, D., Coulas, S., et al.: Alcohol versus natural drying for newborn cord care. *Journal of Obstetric, Gynecologic, and Neonatal Nursing,* 27(6):621-627, 1998.

Edwards, W.H.: Preventing nosocomial bloodstream infection in very low birth weight infants. *Seminars in Neonatology,* 7(4):325-333, 2002.

Evans, R.A. and Thureen, P.: Early feeding strategies in preterm and critically ill neonates. *Neonatal Network, 20*(7):7-18, 2001.

Fox, C., Nelson, D., and Wareham, J.: The timing of skin acidification in very low birth weight infants. *Journal of Perinatology, 18*(4):272-275, 1998.

Furman, L., Taylor, G., Minich, N., et al.: The effect of maternal milk on neonatal morbidity of very low birth weight infants. *Archives of Pediatric and Adolescent Medicine, 15*(1):66-71, 2003.

Gaylord, M.S., Wright, K., Lorch, K., et al.: Improved fluid management utilizing humidified incubators in extremely low birth weight infants. *Journal of Perinatology, 21*(7):438-443, 2001.

Guerina, N.G.: Bacterial and fungal infections. In J.P. Cloherty and A.R. Stark (Eds.): *Manual of neonatal care.* Philadelphia, 1998, Lippincott-Raven, pp. 271-300.

Johnston, C.C., Filion, F., Snider, L., et al.: Routine sucrose analgesia during the first week of life in neonates younger than 31 weeks' postconceptual age. *Pediatrics, 110*(3):523-527, 2002.

Knobel, R.B., Wimmer, J.E., Ahearn, C.J., et al.: *Placing infants <29 weeks' gestation in polyurethane bags after birth to reduce hypothermia.* Abstract, Southern Nursing Research Society, 17th Annual Conference, Orlando, FL, Conference Proceedings, February 13-15, 2003.

Kuller, J.M. and Lund, C.H.: Assessment and management of integumentary dysfunction. In C. Kenner, A. Brueggemeyer, and L.P. Gunderson (Eds.): *Comprehensive neonatal nursing: A physiologic perspective.* Philadelphia, 1993, Saunders, pp. 742-781.

Little, D.C., Pratt, T.C., Blalock, S.E., et al.: Patent ductus arteriosus in micropreemies and full-term infants: The relative merits of surgical ligation versus indomethacin treatment. *Journal of Pediatric Surgery, 38*(3):492-496, 2003.

Lund, C.H., Osborne, J.W., Kuller, J., et al.: Neonatal skin care: Clinical outcomes of the AWHONN/NANN evidence-based clinical practice guideline. *Journal of Obstetric, Gynecologic, and Neonatal Nursing, 30*(1):41-51, 2001.

Maier, R.F., Obladen, M., Müller-Hansen, I., et al.: Early treatment with erythropoietin beta ameliorates anemia and reduces transfusion requirements in infants with birth weights below 1000 g. *Journal of Pediatrics, 141*(1):8-15, 2002.

Mandich, M.B., Ritchie, S.K., and Mullett, M.: Transition times to oral feeding in premature infants with and without apnea. *Journal of Obstetric, Gynecologic, and Neonatal Nursing, 25*(9):771-776, 1996.

McLendon, D., Check, J., Carteaux, P., et al.: Implementation of potentially better practices for the prevention of brain hemorrhage and ischemic brain injury in very low birth weight infants. *Pediatrics, 111*(4 Part 2):e497-e503, 2003.

Mildenberger, E. and Versmold, H.T.: Pathogenesis and therapy of non-oliguric hyperkalemia of the premature infant.

European Journal of Pediatrics, 161(8): 415-422, 2002.

Msall, M.E. and Tremont, M.R.: Measuring functional outcomes after prematurity: Developmental impact of very low birth weight and extremely low birth weight status on childhood disability. *Mental Retardation and Developmental Disabilities Research Reviews 8*(4):258-272, 2002.

National Association of Neonatal Nurses (NANN): *Neonatal skin care: Guidelines for practice.* Petaluma, CA, 1997, NANN.

Ng, E., Taddio, A., and Ohlsson, A.: Intravenous midazolam infusion for sedation of infants in the neonatal intensive care unit. *Cochrane Database of Systematic Reviews* (1):CD002052, 2003.

Nopper, A.J., Horii, K.A., Sookdeo-Drost, S., et al.: Topical ointment therapy benefits premature infants. *Journal of Pediatrics 128*(5 Part 1):660-669, 1996.

NRP Steering Committee: *Textbook of neonatal resuscitation*, Elk Grove Village, IL, 2000, American Academy of Pediatrics and American Heart Association.

Okah, F.A., Wickett, R.R., Pickens, W.L., et al.: Surface electrical capacitance as a noninvasive bedside measure of epidermal barrier maturation in the newborn infant. *Pediatrics, 96*(4 Part 1):688-692, 1995.

Paisley, J.E., Thureen, P.J., Baron, K.A., et al.: Safety and efficacy of low versus high parenteral amino acid intakes in extremely-LBW (ELBW) neonates immediately after birth. *Pediatric Research, 47*:293A, 2000.

Ringer, S.: Care of the extremely low-birth-weight infant. In J.P. Cloherty and A.R. Stark (Eds.): *Manual of neonatal care.* Philadelphia, 1998, Lippincott-Raven, pp. 73-76.

Rivkees, S.A. and Hao, H.: Developing circadian rhythmicity. *Seminars in Perinatology, 24*(4):232-242, 2000.

Rutter, N.: The immature skin. *European Journal of Pediatrics, 155* (Suppl 2):S18-S20, 1996.

Shiao, S.Y., Youngblut, J.M., Anderson, G.C., et al.: Nasogastric tube placement: Effects on breathing and sucking in very-low-birth-weight infants. *Nursing Research, 44*(2):82-88, 1995.

Siegfried, E.C.: Neonatal skin and skin care. *Dermatologic Clinics, 16*(3):437-446, 1998.

Simmons, C.F.: Fluid and electrolyte management. In J.P. Cloherty and A.R. Stark (Eds.): *Manual of neonatal care.* Philadelphia, 1998, Lippincott-Raven, pp. 87-100.

Stevens, B., Johnston, C., Petryshen, P., and Taddio, A.: Premature infant pain profile: Development and initial validation. *Clinical Journal of Pain, 12*(1):13-22, 1996.

Stevens, B., Yamada, J., and Ohlsson, A.: Sucrose for analgesia in newborn infants undergoing painful procedures. *Cochrane Database of Systematic Review* (4):CD001069, 2001.

Stoll, B., Hansen, N., Fanaroff, A.A., et al.: Changes in pathogens causing early-onset sepsis in very-low-birth-weight infants. *New England Journal of Medicine, 347*(4):280-281, 2002.

Tommiska, V., Heinonen, K., Kero, P., et al.: A national two year follow up study of extremely low birthweight infants born in 1996-1997. *Archives of Disease in Childhood, Fetal Neonatal Edition, 88*(1):F29-F35, 2003.

Vernon, H.J., Lane, A.T., Wischerath, L.J., et al.: Semipermeable dressing and transepidermal water loss in premature infants. *Pediatrics, 86*(3):357-362, 1990.

Vohra. S., Frent, G., Campbell, V., et al.: Effect of polyethylene occlusive skin wrapping on heat loss in very low birth weight infants at delivery: A randomized trial. *Journal of Pediatrics, 134*(5):547-551, 1999.

Walden, M.: *Pain assessment and management: Guidelines for practice.* Glenview, IL, 2001, National Association of Neonatal Nurses.

Walden, M. and Carrier, C.T.: Sleeping beauties: The impact of sedation on neonatal development. *Journal of Obstetric, Gynecologic, and Neonatal Nursing, 32*(3):393-401, 2003.

Watkins, A.M.C., West, C.R., and Cooke, R.W.: Blood pressure and cerebral haemorrhage and ischaemia in very low birthweight infants. *Early Human Development, 19*(2):103-110, 1989.

Yoshio, H., Tollin, M., Gudmundsson, G.H., et al.: Antimicrobial polypeptides of human vernix caseosa and amniotic fluid: Implications for newborn innate defense. *Pediatric Research, 53*(2):211-216, 2003.

Ziegler, E.E., Thureen, P.J., and Carlson, S.J.: Aggressive nutrition of the very low birthweight infant. *Clinics in Perinatology, 29*(2):225-244, 2002.

SECTION THREE

Pathophysiology: Management and Treatment of Common Disorders

CHAPTER

23 Respiratory Distress

KSENIA ZUKOWSKY

OBJECTIVES

1. Describe the anatomic and biochemical events associated with lung development.
2. Discuss the physiology of respiration.
3. Describe common respiratory disorders seen in the newborn infant.
4. Discuss common findings in respiratory distress syndrome (RDS), meconium aspiration syndrome, pneumonia, pulmonary hypertension, and bronchopulmonary dysplasia.
5. Describe nonpulmonary causes of respiratory distress.
6. Identify treatment strategies for common respiratory problems.
7. Formulate a plan of care for infants with respiratory disorders.

The most common group of life-threatening diseases in newborns is respiratory in origin. This is evidenced by the number of infants admitted to the neonatal intensive care unit (NICU) in respiratory distress. Respiratory distress syndrome, retained lung fluid syndromes, aspiration syndromes, air leaks, and congenital pneumonia account for approximately 90% of all respiratory distress in newborns. Pulmonary disease, however, is not the cause of all respiratory distress in newborn infants. Congenital malformations, metabolic abnormalities, central nervous system (CNS) disorders, and congenital heart disease may also present with respiratory distress. This chapter discusses common respiratory problems of the newborn infant, along with pathophysiology, clinical presentation, differential diagnosis, and management.

LUNG DEVELOPMENT

A. **Anatomic events.** Five stages of lung development have been identified and are described as follows (Larsen, 2001; Moore and Persaud, 2003):
   1. Embryonic development (weeks 1-5). The endoderm-derived embryonic foregut provides a single lung bud that begins to divide ventrocaudally through the mesenchyme surrounding the foregut. The pulmonary vein develops and extends to join the lung bud. The trachea develops at the end of the embryonic period. There are three divisions on the right side and two on the left side that will eventually become the lobes of the lungs.
   2. Pseudoglandular period (weeks 5-17). All conducting airways are formed. Cartilage appears; main bronchi are formed; demarcation of major lobes occurs; formation of new bronchi are complete; capillary bed is formed with connecting bronchial blood supply; no connection made with terminal air sacs. The lung at this time undergoes 14 more generations of branching and the formation of the terminal bronchioles. The lung resembles an exocrine organ because of surrounding loose mesenchymal tissues, hence the name, pseudoglandular.

3. Canalicular period (weeks 17-24). Formation of gas-exchanging acinar units (i.e., respiratory units). The appearance of glycogen-rich cuboidal cells and inclusions for surface-active material storage are seen; capillaries invade terminal airway walls; type II alveolar epithelial cells appear. Airway changes from glandular to tubular and increases in length and diameter. Vascular system proliferates and the capillaries are now closer to the epithelium-conducting airways. Respiratory bronchioles that will participate in gas exchange can be differentiated.
4. Terminal sac period (weeks 24-37). Between weeks 24 and 26 alveolar sacs are formed; air-blood surface area is limited for gas exchange; and type II cells are unable to release surfactant in sufficient quantity to maintain air breathing. Capillary loops increase; type II cells cluster at alveolar ducts, become numerous and mature; more budding occurs from alveolar ducts; and lung size increases rapidly because there is an exponential increase in surface area for gas exchange.
5. Alveolar period (week 37 to 8-10 years). This phase is characterized by continued alveolar proliferation and development.

B. Biochemical events.

1. Surface-active phospholipids line terminal air spaces and maintain alveolar stability by reducing surface tension.
2. Surfactant is a mixture of at least six phospholipids and four apoproteins.
   a. Dipalmitoylphosphatidylcholine (DPPC) is the major surface-active lipid component of surfactant. DPPC reduces the surface tension at the air–water interface in the alveolus almost to zero (Jobe and Ikegami, 2001).
   b. Surfactant includes cholesterol and cholesterol esters, proteins, complex carbohydrates, and glycolipids.
   c. Phospholipids are responsible for the surface-active properties of surfactant. Surfactant proteins have recently been found to have important properties.
   d. The two groups of surfactant proteins: the hydrophilic surfactant proteins A and D (SP-A and SP-D) and the hydrophobic surfactant proteins B and C (SP-B and SP-C). Group SP-B and SP-C is known to enhance the surface tension–lowering properties of surfactant and facilitate its absorption and spread.
      (1) SP-A binds phospholipids, requires calcium ions, and with SP-B, forms the tubular myelin lattice network. SP-A holds the corners of the lattice network together and probably has a role in the recycling of surfactant. SP-A activates alveolar macrophages and thus has a role in host defenses. SP-A is the most abundant of the surfactant proteins.
      (2) SP-B is important in the formation of tubular myelin, enhances the uptake of phospholipids by the type II cell, and is also important in the recycling of surfactant.
      (3) SP-C may have a role in surfactant dispersement and recycling, enhancing the rate of absorption and spreading of surfactant. It is a hydrophobic protein that constitutes roughly 0.4% of the surfactant by weight.
      (4) SP-D is calcium dependent and also may have a role in host defense mechanisms (Jobe and Ikegami, 2001; Moise and Hansen, 2003).
   e. Surfactant reduces surface-tension forces in the alveoli that are capable of producing collapse at expiration (Jobe and Ikegami, 2001).
      (1) Surfactant is produced in the type II pneumocyte beginning at 24 to 28 weeks' gestation and continuing to term (Shapiro, 1988). Type II

pneumocytes synthesize, store, secrete, and recycle surfactant (Moise and Hansen, 2003; Notter, 1988).
   (2) When the lungs are inflated, receptors in type II cells mobilize intracellular calcium, which causes the release of the contents of lamellar bodies into the air space. After secretion, surfactant may be taken back into type II cells and converted back into lamellar bodies for resecretion, with a turnover time of 10 hours (Moise and Hansen, 2003).

3. The changing pattern of phospholipids in amniotic fluid can be used to assess surfactant production and maturation of pathways.
   a. Material from the fetal lung contributes to amniotic fluid.
   b. Concentrations of various phospholipids can be measured and will assist in determining lung maturity.
4. Sphingomyelin concentration remains stable, with a small peak at 28 to 30 weeks.
5. Lecithin and phosphatidylinositol concentrations remain low until 26 to 30 weeks, when an increase begins. A peak occurs at 36 weeks.
6. Phosphatidylglycerol (PG) appears at 30 weeks, peaks at 35 to 36 weeks, and increases as the phosophatidylinositol level falls.
   a. When PG is present, the risk that RDS will develop in the infant is less than 1%.
   b. PG is measured as absent or present.
   c. Blood and meconium do not affect test results.
7. The lecithin/sphingomyelin ratio (L/S) has been used to assess fetal lung maturity.
   a. An L/S ratio greater than 2:1 is considered to indicate fetal lung maturity.
   b. An infant of a diabetic mother may develop RDS even with a mature L/S ratio (presence of PG ensures lung maturity).
   c. Chronic fetal stress (e.g., maternal hypertension, retroplacental bleeding, maternal drug use, smoking) will tend to accelerate surfactant production, resulting in a mature L/S ratio in premature infants.
8. Fetal lung maturity (FLM).
   a. Measures ratio of surfactant to albumin.
   b. Sample should be free of blood and meconium.
   c. Less than 50 = immaturity; 50 to 70 = borderline maturity; greater than 70 = mature lungs.

C. Role of antenatal steroids.

1. Antenatal corticosteroids and glucocorticoids (e.g., betamethasone or dexamethasone) affect lung maturation and present a strategy for preventing RDS. Betamethasone appears to significantly decrease neonatal death and morbidity (Maher et al., 1994; NIH Consensus, 2000). Steroids accelerate the normal pattern of lung growth by increasing the rate of glycogen depletion and glycerophospholipid biosynthesis. This leads to thinning of the intraalveolar septa and increases the size of the alveoli. The number of surfactant-producing type II pneumocytes increases as do the number of lamellar bodies inside the cells. This leads to increased synthesis of surfactant phospholipids. Steroids may also increase the amount of fibroblast pneumocyte factor, which increases surfactant production (Blackburn, 2003).
   a. Treatment with steroids is recommended for:
      (1) Maternal risk of preterm delivery between 24 and 34 weeks.
      (2) Premature rupture of the membranes at less than 30 to 32 weeks, without chorioamnionitis, because of the risk of intraventricular hemorrhage (IVH).

(3) Treatment with corticosteroids less than 24 hours prior to delivery is still associated with a decrease in mortality, RDS, and IVH. It should be given unless immediate delivery expected.
(4) Complicated pregnancies in which expected delivery is at less than 34 weeks' gestation, unless adverse effect on mother is anticipated (Moise and Hansen, 2003).

b. Repeated administration of corticosteroids in premature rupture of the membranes is not associated with a higher risk of chorioamnionitis (Ghidini et al., 1997). The recommendation from the National Institutes of Health (NIH) consensus statement is the use and efficacy of a single course of antenatal corticosteroid (NIH Consensus 2000).

c. Glucocorticoids are given concurrently with tocolytic agents (e.g., terbutaline, ritodrine, magnesium sulfate) for premature labor.

d. Two doses of betamethasone 12 mg. should be given intramuscularly (IM) 24 hours apart or four doses of dexamethasone 6 mg should be given IM every 12 hours in patients at risk for preterm delivery between 24 and 34 weeks of gestation with intact membranes or between 24 and 32 weeks of gestation for patients with ruptured membranes. Repeated courses of glucocortioids should not be routinely used (American Academy of Pediatrics and American College of Obstetricians and Gynecologists [AAP/ACOG, 2002]).

2. Infants exposed to chronic stress in utero are usually small for gestational age and have more mature lungs (they also have small thymuses and large adrenal glands, suggesting high glucocorticoid levels in utero).

PHYSIOLOGY OF RESPIRATION

Refer to Chapters 4 and 25.

RESPIRATORY DISORDERS

Respiratory Distress Syndrome

A. Definition.

1. Developmental disorder starting at or soon after birth and occurring most frequently in infants with immature lungs.
2. Increasing respiratory difficulty in first 3 to 6 hours, leading to hypoxia and hypoventilation.
3. Progressive atelectasis.

B. Incidence.

1. Approximately 20,000 to 30,000 infants per year affected in the United States (Whitsett et al., 1999). The American Lung Association (ALA) (2003) estimated that 24,764 infants were born alive in the United States with RDS in 2001.
2. The incidence of RDS is inversely related to gestational age: 60% of infants born at less than 28 weeks; 30% of those born at 28 to 34 weeks gestation, and less than 5% of those born after 34 weeks are affected (ALA, 2003).

C. Etiology.

1. Surfactant deficiency.
2. Pulmonary hypoperfusion.
3. Anatomic immaturity.
4. Precipitating factors associated with incidence and/or severity of RDS.
   - **a.** Prematurity.
   - **b.** Cesarean delivery without labor.

c. Maternal diabetes, especially if infant was born at less than 38 weeks' gestation.
d. Acute antepartum hemorrhage.
e. Second twin.
(1) May be due to greater risk of asphyxia.
(2) First twin usually smaller, suggesting chronic stress leading to early lung maturation.
f. Asphyxia at birth.
g. Male/female ratio of 2:1.

D. **Pathophysiology.**
1. Production of surfactant is inadequate, occurring when the utilization of surfactant exceeds the rate of production. This leads to diffuse alveolar atelectasis, pulmonary edema, and cell injury (Liley and Stark, 1998). Progressive worsening of these three factors will contribute to a loss of functional residual capacity, alteration in ventilation perfusion ratio, and uneven distribution of ventilation (Whitsett et al., 1999).
2. Serum proteins, which inhibit surfactant function, leak into the alveoli. The increased water content, immature mechanisms for clearance of lung liquid, lack of alveolar-capillary apposition, and decreased surface area for gas exchange, typical of the immature lung, also contribute to the disease (Liley and Stark, 1998).
3. Histologic findings are the presence of hyaline membranes and an eosinophilic material derived from injury to epithelial cells. The alveolar spaces are generally collapsed, with pulmonary edema, hemorrhage, and hemorrhagic edema noted (Whitsett et al., 1999).

E. **Clinical presentation.**
1. Almost exclusively in premature infants.
a. May appear to be a normally grown, healthy premature infant with good Apgar scores at birth.
b. Distress begins at or soon after birth.
2. Increasing respiratory difficulty related to progressive atelectasis. Symptoms are progressive.
a. Tachypnea (>60 breaths per minute) is usually the first sign; color is maintained.
b. Audible expiratory grunt.
(1) Heard during first few hours.
(2) Caused by forcing of air past a partially closed glottis.
(3) Used to maintain positive end-expiratory pressure (PEEP) at alveolar level in an attempt to prevent alveolar collapse.
(4) More pronounced with severe disease.
c. The chest wall in an infant is very compliant. When an infant breathes spontaneously, pleural pressure decreases during inspiration. When there is parenchymal disease, the chest wall produces greater negative pressure and the more compliant chest wall caves inward with a moderate decrease in pleural pressure, which results in retractions. Retractions are seen at the xiphoid and intercostal markings of the infant's chest (Guillory and Cabrera-Meza, 2003).
d. Nasal flaring.
e. Cyanosis due to increasing hypoxemia.
3. Oxygen requirements increase to maintain arterial Po_2 at 50 to 70 mm Hg due to decreased lung compliance secondary to decreased surfactant. Additional physical effort is needed to keep terminal airways open, resulting in increased work of breathing.

4. Paradoxic seesaw respirations may be seen.
5. If signs and symptoms are unattended, infant becomes obtunded and flaccid.
   a. Pale gray color obscures severe central cyanosis.
   b. Poor capillary filling time (>3-4 seconds).
   c. Progressive edema, usually seen in the face, palms, and soles.
6. Oliguria is common in the first 48 hours.
7. Breath sounds diminish and lung auscultation is usually described as "poor air entry" despite vigorous effort on the infant's part.
8. Rales occur as the disease progresses.
9. Cardiac murmurs are generally not heard until after 24 hours of age.
10. Tachycardia (heart rate >160 beats per minute [bpm]) is common and even more prevalent if acidosis and hypoxemia are present.

F. **Diagnosis.**
1. Signs and symptoms as previously described.
2. Hypoxemia (defined as arterial Po_2 level <50 mm Hg in room air) as a result of ventilation-perfusion mismatch and right-to-left intrapulmonary shunting, responding to supplemental inspired oxygen; respiratory failure secondary to alveolar hypoventilation (Pco_2 >50; pH ≤ 7.25).
3. Chest x-ray reveals low lung volumes, hazy lung fields, and a fine reticulogranular pattern of density with air bronchograms. Occasionally the disease may appear worse in one lung than the other (Moise and Hansen, 2003).
4. Diagnostic studies.
   a. Chest x-ray examination.
   b. Arterial blood gas (ABG) measurements.
   c. Blood cultures, complete blood cell count. Pneumonia caused by group B streptococcus has similar radiographic features; therefore infection must be considered.
   d. Other blood studies as needed (e.g., electrolytes, calcium and blood glucose levels).

G. **Differential diagnosis.**
1. Pneumonia. Similar signs, symptoms, and radiologic features can be found in neonates with pneumonia and those with RDS.
2. Transient tachypnea of the newborn (TTN) can present with the same signs and symptoms, but these infants usually require ≤ 40% Fio_2, improve quicker, and have larger lung volumes on chest x-ray (CXR).
3. Pulmonary edema. A primary cardiac disorder with pulmonary edema (caused by patent ductus arteriosus [PDA]) can mimic RDS.

H. **Complications.**
1. Pulmonary.
   a. Air leaks.
   b. Pulmonary edema.
   c. Bronchopulmonary dysplasia (BPD).
2. Cardiovascular.
   a. PDA.
   b. Systemic hypotension.
3. Renal.
   a. Oliguria.
      (1) Most likely to follow hypoxia, hypotension, or shock ("prerenal" renal failure).
   b. Immature renal function with decreased glomerular filtration in very low birth weight infants.

c. Natural diuresis will occur at approximately 48 to 72 hours of age, as infant's condition improves.

4. Metabolic.
   a. Acidosis. Atelectasis with increased work of breathing will lead to hypoxemia and acidemia, resulting in vasoconstriction of the pulmonary vasculature. This then limits alveolar capillary blood flow, which further impedes the production of surfactant and compounds the problem (Hagedorn et al., 2002).
   b. Hyponatremia or hypernatremia.
   c. Hypocalcemia.
   d. Hypoglycemia.
5. Hematologic.
   a. Anemia—may be iatrogenic due to blood loss required for diagnostic testing. Hematocrit should be near normal to ensure adequate oxygen carrying capacity.
6. Neurologic.
   a. Seizures: may result from hypoglycemia or an IVH.
   b. Ventilator manipulations, rapid fluid infusions, shock, and acidosis are all factors causing changes in cerebral blood flow that may precipitate an IVH (Paige and Carney, 2002).
7. Other.
   a. Secondary nosocomial infections.
   b. Retinopathy of prematurity (ROP).
   c. Dislodged endotracheal tubes.
   d. Thrombus formation. Complication of umbilical catheters needed to monitor respiratory status.

I. **Management.** RDS is a disease that is self-limited and transient. Adequate surfactant can be produced by the premature infant within 48 to 72 hours.

1. Goal of treatment is supportive until disease resolves and to prevent further lung injury (Moise and Hansen, 2003).
2. Surfactant replacement therapy.
   a. Benefits include (Kattwinkel, 1998; Moise and Hansen, 2003):
      (1) Reduced morbidity and mortality rates.
      (2) Improved compliance and decreased resistance in surfactant-poor acini, thereby reducing the pressure needed to inflate the lungs and decreasing work of breathing.
      (3) Improved ventilation in low-volume lung units, which increases the $Pa{O_2}$, decreases the right-to-left intrapulmonary shunt, and improves overall oxygenation of the infant.
   b. Surfactants approved by U.S. Food and Drug Administration (FDA) for treatment of RDS:
      (1) Natural surfactants: Beractant (Survanta), Poractant alfa (Curosurf), and Calfactant (Infasurf.) Composed of minced bovine, porcine, or calf lung with added lipids.
      (2) Synthetic surfactants: (Exosurf).
   c. Two treatment methods are related to timing.
      (1) Prophylaxis. Treatment soon after birth: infants born at less than 27 to 30 weeks' gestation; dose given via endotracheal tube after initial resuscitation. Additional doses may be given if necessary.
      (2) Rescue. Treatment of infants with progressive oxygen requirements (usually $\geq$ 40% $Fi{O_2}$) in the first day of life; multiple doses can be given. Studies have shown that surfactant response is improved when

it is given early. The goal of intervention is to avoid progressive alveolar atelectasis leading to respiratory failure requiring intermittent positive pressure ventilation (IPPV) (Egberts et al., 1993; Kattwinkel et al., 1993; Kendig et al., 1991).

(3) Beractant (Survanta): Dose is 4 ml/kg given in four quarter-doses as the infant is repositioned. Inject each quarter-dose gently into a 5 F. Orogastric catheter threaded through the endotracheal tube over 2 or 3 seconds, ventilating the infant after each quarter-dose until stable. Repeated doses can be given every 6 hours during the first 48 hours of life (Zenk et al., 2000).

(4) Poractant alfa (Curosurf): Initial dose is 2.5 ml/kg given in 2 aliquots via a 5 F. orogastric catheter threaded through the endotracheal tube, ventilating the infant after each half-dose for at least 30 seconds until stable. Two subsequent doses of 1.25 ml/kg can be administered at 12-hour intervals if needed (Young and Mangum, 2003).

(5) Calfactant (Infrasurf): Dose is 3 ml/kg divided in 2 aliquots, every 12 hours for a total of three doses. Ventilation is continued during administration over 20 to 30 breaths for each aliquot. After each aliquot, the infant is repositioned in either the right or left side dependent positions to enhance distribution in the lungs (Young and Mangum, 2003).

(6) Synthetic surfactant (Exosurf): Dose is 5 ml/kg administered in 2 half doses via the side port of a special adapter that is provided. Do not interrupt mechanical ventilation. Instill each dose slowly over 1 to 2 minutes in small bursts timed with inspiration. Administer with the infant in midline position. After the first half of the dose, turn the infant 45 degrees to the right for 30 seconds. Then turn the infant 45 degrees to the left, and after 30 seconds, return the infant to midline position (Young and Mangum, 2003).

3. Provide warm, humidified oxygen to maintain normal PaO_2.
4. Provide continuous positive airway pressure via nasal prongs or endotracheal tube if indicated.
5. Use assisted ventilation for profound hypoxemia (PaO_2 <50 mm Hg) and/or hypercapnia ($PaCO_2$ >60 mm Hg).
6. Monitor oxygenation by pulse oximetry and/or transcutaneous monitoring.
7. Monitor pulmonary status with chest x-ray examination, as clinically indicated.
8. Other measures.
   a. Stabilize temperature.
   b. Provide adequate fluid and electrolyte intake. Monitor intake and output, serum BUN, and creatinine.
   c. Restore acid-base balance by administration of sodium acetate and/or sodium bicarbonate ($NaHCO_3$) for metabolic acidosis.
   d. Monitor arterial/capillary blood gases, electrolytes, calcium, bilirubin, and glucose.
   e. Monitor blood pressure for hypotension. Give volume replacement and pharmacotherapeutic agents (e.g., dopamine or dobutamine) as indicated.
   f. Maintain hematocrit.
   g. Administer antibiotics for associated pneumonia/rule out sepsis.

J. Prevention of RDS.

1. Maternal glucocorticoid administration prenatally.
2. Use of L/S ratio, fetal lung maturity, and PG determination for timing labor induction or elective cesarean delivery.

3. Perinatal management to avoid situations leading to pulmonary circulation compromise in the fetus or newborn infant.
   a. Obstetric.
      (1) Maternal hypotension.
      (2) Oversedation.
      (3) Maternal hypoxia.
      (4) Fetal distress without prompt delivery.
   b. Neonatal.
      (1) Delayed resuscitation.
      (2) Uncorrected hypoxia or acidosis.
      (3) Hypothermia, hypoglycemia, and hypovolemia.

K. Outcome.

1. Infants with chronic lung disease improve slowly and progressively if they can be kept infection free. May have episodes of bronchiolitis and pneumonia (especially pneumonia caused by respiratory syncytial virus [RSV]); long-term sequelae are related to specific complications (e.g., BPD, IVH, ROP).
2. Infants who weigh greater than 1500 g who have mild to moderate RDS have the same developmental outcome as infants of the same gestational age without RDS. The infants with the most severe developmental outcomes are those who weigh less than 1500 g and who have had an IVH (Hagedorn et al., 2002).
3. Cerebral palsy (CP)—the most prevalent major impairment encountered in premature infants. Premature infants less than 3.3 pounds are 30 times more likely to develop CP than term infants (March of Dimes, 2003). Respiratory distress has only a modest association with CP with an odds ratio ranging from 1.3 to 2.1. Infants with pneumothorax and respiratory distress increase their incidence of CP. Infants who develop chronic lung disease have an increased incidence of CP with an odds ratio of 2.4 to 5.8. Infants who have been treated with dexamethasone to decrease the risk of chronic lung disease (CLD), increase their risk of CP (Stark et al., 2001).
4. The sickest infants with RDS have a 10% to 20% chance of a major neurologic deficit: CP, hydrocephalus, seizures, and mental retardation diagnosed within the first 2 years of life (Hagedorn et al., 2002).

Pneumonia

A. Definition. Infection of the fetal or newborn lung; may be intrauterine or neonatal.

1. Intrauterine infection.
   a. Passage of infecting agent by infection of fetal membranes.
   b. Transplacental transmission.
   c. Aspiration of meconium or infected amniotic fluid during delivery.
2. Neonatal infection.
   a. Acquired during nursery stay.
   b. Pathogens are generally different from those acquired in utero.
   c. Results by passage from other infants, equipment, or caretakers.

B. Incidence.

1. Neonatal pneumonia occurs 1% in the term infant and 10% in the preterm infant (Carey and Trotter, 2000). The incidence varies by institution and according to causative agent.
2. Bacterial pneumonia incidence is comparable with that of sepsis.

C. **Etiology.**
   1. Risk of infection greatest in premature infants because of immature immune system and lack of protective maternal antibodies. Pneumonia can occur by several routes: transplacental, amniotic fluid, at delivery, and nosocomially (Moise and Hansen, 2003).
   2. Immature ciliary system in the tracheobronchial tree, leading to suboptimal removal of inflammatory debris, mucus, and pathogens. The number of pulmonary macrophages are insufficient for bacterial clearance (Orlando, 1997).
   3. Multiple agents cause neonatal pneumonia (Box 23-1).

D. **Pathophysiology.**
   1. Congenital pneumonia.
      a. Infant may be born critically ill or stillborn to a mother with a history of chorioamnionitis. Evidence of pulmonary inflammation is found in 15% to 38% of stillborn infants at autopsy (Speer and Weisman, 2003). Other factors linked to congenital pneumonia include excessive obstetric manipulation, prolonged labor with intact membranes, and maternal urinary tract infection (Orlando, 1997).
      b. Prolonged rupture of membranes (>24 hours); ascending organisms may infect amniotic fluid. If mother is in active labor, contamination occurs more rapidly.
      c. Infective organisms may cross the placenta and enter the fetal circulation, causing septicemia that may present as pneumonia.

BOX 23-1
COMMON ORGANISMS ASSOCIATED WITH NEONATAL PNEUMONIA

Transplacental
- Rubella
- Cytomegalovirus
- Herpes simplex virus
- Adenovirus
- Mumps virus
- *Toxoplasma gondii*
- *Listeria monocytogenes*
- *Mycobacterium tuberculosis*
- *Treponema pallidum*

Amniotic Fluid
- Cytomegalovirus
- Herpes simplex virus
- Enteroviruses
- Genital mycoplasma
- *L. monocytogenes*
- *Chlamydia trachomatis*
- *M. tuberculosis*
- Group B streptococcus (GBS)
- *Escherichia coli*
- *Haemophilus influenzae* (nontypeable)
- Ureaplasma urealyticum

At Delivery
- GBS
- *E. coli*
- *Staphylococcus aureus*
- *Klebsiella* sp.
- Other streptococci
- *H. influenzae* (nontypeable)
- *Candida* sp.
- *C. trachomatis*
- Ureaplasma urealyticum

Nosocomial
- *S. aureus*
- *S. epidermidis*
- GBS
- *Klebsiella* sp.
- *Enterobacter*
- *Pseudomonas*
- Influenza viruses
- Respiratory syncytial virus
- Enteroviruses

From Weisman, L.E. and Hansen, T.N.(Eds.): *Contemporary diagnosis and management of neonatal respiratory diseases* (3rd ed.). Newtown, PA, 2003, Handbooks in Health Care (division of AMM Co.), p. 142.

d. Infants usually show signs of generalized illness from birth, but signs of illness may be delayed hours to days if the infective fluid is aspirated during delivery.

2. Neonatal pneumonia.
   a. Infection occurs days to weeks after birth.
   b. Pathogenic organism is acquired from hospital personnel, parents, or other infected infants. Poor handwashing, contaminated blood products, infected human milk, and open skin lesions are common ways of transmitting infection to the neonate (Orlando, 1997).
   c. Both bacterial and viral pathogens are associated with neonatal pneumonia. The most common bacterial organisms include Group B streptococcus, *Escherichia coli*, *Klebsiella*, *Pseudomonas*, *Serratia marcescens*, *Staphylococcus epidermidis*, group A streptococci, *Listeria*, *Enterobacter*, *Treponema pallidum*, and *Staphylococcus aureus*. Viral infections such as herpes, cytomegalovirus (CMV), varicella zoster, respiratory syncytial virus, enterovirus, adenovirus, and parainfluenza virus are also seen (Carey and Trotter, 2000; Whitsett et al., 1999).

E. Clinical presentation.

1. Labor greater than 24 hours.
   a. Prolonged rupture of membranes (>24 hours).
   b. Maternal fever/chorioamnionitis.
   c. Foul-smelling or purulent amniotic fluid.
   d. Fetal tachycardia.
   e. Decreased fetal heart rate variability.
2. Signs and symptoms.
   a. Often indistinguishable from those of other forms of respiratory distress and sepsis.
   b. Tachypnea, grunting, retractions, cyanosis, hypoxemia, hypercapnia, and hypoglycemia.
   c. With severe involvement, shock-like syndrome, usually in the first 24 hours of life, with recurrent apnea followed by cardiovascular collapse, profound hypoxemia, and persistent pulmonary hypertension. These signs represent a poor prognosis.
3. Physical examination.
   a. Physical signs are variable.
   b. Diminished breath sounds may be present over one or more areas.
   c. In addition, localized dullness, harshness, or rales may be audible.
   d. Radiologic findings can mimic those seen with RDS. In addition, pleural effusions may be seen on chest x-ray with Group B Streptococci (GBS) pneumonia.

F. Diagnostic evaluation.

1. History of any previously mentioned contributing factors is suggestive.
2. Infant may require resuscitation in the delivery room.
3. Chest x-ray findings are variable.
   a. Unilateral or bilateral alveolar infiltrates.
   b. Diffuse interstitial pattern.
   c. Pleural effusions.
4. Samples for blood and viral cultures (including RSV) should be obtained, although results are rarely positive unless there is generalized bacterial sepsis.
5. A complete blood cell count may show neutropenia/leukopenia or may have an abnormal ratio of immature to total neutrophils.

6. Urine collection for latex particle agglutination (LPA) and counterimmunoelectrophoresis (CIE) to detect GBS may be helpful because the results can be obtained faster than culture results.
7. Polymerase chain reaction (PCR) can be used to detect herpes viruses.
8. ABG values should be obtained because metabolic acidosis may be severe.
9. Tracheal aspirate culture should be obtained, especially if the infant has an endotracheal tube in place.
10. Cerebrospinal cultures should be obtained when infant is stable, because meningitis often accompanies pneumonia.

G. **Differential diagnosis.**
1. RDS.
2. Sepsis/meningitis.
3. TTN.
4. Meconium aspiration.
5. Lung hypoplasia.
6. Pulmonary hemorrhage.
7. Congenital heart disease.

H. **Complications.**
1. Gram-negative pneumonia; cardiopulmonary complications similar to those of RDS.
2. Septic shock.
3. Disseminated intravascular coagulation (DIC).
4. Persistent pulmonary hypertension.
5. Meningitis.

I. **Management.**
1. Antibiotic therapy (see Chapter 31).
2. Maintain normal temperature.
3. Monitor glucose levels.
4. Monitor blood pressure and treat hypotension.
5. Use oxygen with or without assisted ventilation to maintain normal ABG values.
6. Correct respiratory and metabolic acidosis.
7. Provide adequate fluid and electrolyte intake.
8. Monitor for evidence of DIC.
9. High-frequency ventilation, nitric oxide, and extracorporeal membrane oxygenation have been used for patients who are critically ill with pneumonia, with variable outcomes.
10. Provide support for the family.

Retained Lung Fluid Syndromes

A. **Definition:** delayed clearance of the fetal lung fluid—TTN.

B. **Clinical presentation.**
1. Term and near-term infants.
2. In first few hours, tachypnea results in respiratory rates of 60 to 120 breaths per minute; grunting and retractions may also be present.
3. Minimal cyanosis may require fractional inspired oxygen of 0.30 to 0.40; ABGs may show mild respiratory alkalemia, with P_{CO_2} values often less than 30 mm Hg.
4. Duration may be 1 to 5 days.

C. **Etiology.**
1. Delay in removal of lung fluid.
2. Excessive amount of lung fluid.

D. Pathophysiology.

1. Fetal lung fluid has a higher chloride concentration than plasma, interstitial fluid, or amniotic fluid. During labor, active transport of chloride stops and the fluid is reabsorbed via a protein gradient and removed by the lymphatic system. Two thirds of the lung fluid are removed before birth. Infants born without labor or prematurely may not have the time to reabsorb the fetal lung fluid (Speer and Hansen, 2003).
2. Infants at highest risk for retained fetal lung fluid include:
   a. Birth near or at term.
   b. Cesarean delivery without labor.
   c. Breech delivery.
   d. Second twin.
   e. Intrauterine growth restriction.
   f. Precipitous delivery.
   g. Delayed cord clamping (results in a transfusion of blood, which may transiently elevate the central venous pressure).
   h. Macrosomia.
   i. Male sex.
   j. Maternal sedation.
3. TTN may originate from reduced lung compliance because of delayed reabsorption of lung fluid at the time of birth and/or the distention of interstitial spaces by fluid, leading to alveolar air trapping and decreased lung compliance. (Whitsett et al., 1999).
4. Delayed clearance of lung fluid by pulmonary lymphatic system. The retained fetal lung fluid accumulates in the peribronchiolar lymphatics and bronchovascular spaces and interferes with forces promoting bronchiolar patency, and results in bronchiolar collapse with air trapping or hyperinflation. Hypoxemia results from continued perfusion of poorly ventilated alveoli and hypercarbia results from mechanical interference with alveolar ventilation. Decreased lung compliance results in tachypnea and increased work of breathing (Lawson, 1998).
5. Promotion of interstitial fluid results in:
   a. Hypoalbuminemia.
   b. Increased interstitial oncotic pressure.

E. Diagnosis.

1. Early signs and symptoms may be difficult to distinguish from those of other respiratory problems; however, they are usually milder.
2. Chest x-ray examination reveals diffuse haziness and streakiness in both lung fields, with clearing at the periphery. Fluid may be present in the interlobar fissures, and mild hyperinflation may be present.
3. Diagnosis is frequently one of exclusion.

F. Differential diagnosis.

1. RDS.
2. Pneumonia/sepsis.

G. Management.

1. Because diagnosis is not conclusive, other disorders should be ruled out.
2. Supportive management.
   a. Oxygen.
   b. Temperature regulation.
   c. Adequate fluid intake.
   d. Maintain ABGs within normal levels.
   e. Maintain blood glucose at normal levels.

3. If respiratory rate is greater than 60 breaths per minute, delay feedings to avoid possible aspiration.
4. If history indicates risk of infection, broad-spectrum antibiotics (e.g., ampicillin and gentamicin) should be administered until culture results are negative.

H. Outcome.

1. Self-limited.
2. Oxygen requirement and tachypnea decrease steadily over several days. Infant may remain mildly tachypneic beyond the need for oxygen.
3. Some infants with TTN have high pulmonary artery pressures documented by echocardiography. If hypoxemia and tachypnea persist, a further complication may be persistent pulmonary hypertension of the newborn.

Persistent Pulmonary Hypertension of the Newborn

A. Definition. Persistent pulmonary hypertension of the newborn (PPHN) is caused by right-to-left shunting through the fetal shunts at the atrial and ductal levels. It is secondary to persistent elevation of pulmonary vascular resistance (PVR) and pulmonary artery pressure (Harris and Wood, 1996). Seventy-seven percent of infants are diagnosed in the first 24 hours of life; 93% diagnosed by 48 hours of life; and 97% of the infants by 72 hours of life. Incidence is 1.9 per 1000 live births (Hagedorn et al., 2002; Walsh-Sukys et al., 2000).

B. Pathophysiology.

1. After delivery, adequate oxygenation depends on lung inflation, closure of fetal shunts, decreased PVR, and increased pulmonary blood flow.
2. Over the first 12 to 24 hours of life, PVR falls by 80% of its total decline.
3. When PVR remains high, adaptation from fetal to neonatal circulation is impaired.
4. Neonatal pulmonary vessels have greater vasoactive properties than adult pulmonary vessels and respond to hypoxia and acidosis with vasoconstriction. Numerous factors increase and decrease PVR (Box 23-2).
5. Development of increased vascular smooth muscle contributes to vasospasm. Development of pulmonary artery musculature occurs late in gestation, making PPHN generally a condition of the term and postterm infant.
6. High PVR and pulmonary hypertension impede pulmonary blood flow, which promotes hypoxemia, acidemia, and lactic acidosis.
7. Once vasoconstriction is induced, it can persist even when the precipitating cause is removed (Kinsella and Abman, 1995; Morin and Stenmark, 1995; Steinhorn et al., 1995).
8. Studies have described low plasma arginine and nitric oxide metabolites in infants with PPHN, suggesting a genetic link of the urea cycle may contribute to this process of PPHN (Pearson et al., 2001).

C. Etiology.

1. Maladaptation. The pulmonary vascular bed is structurally normal, but PVR remains high. Maladaptation generally results from active vasoconstriction, which may be transient or persistent.
   a. Hypoxia/asphyxia. This is the most common precipitating factor in PPHN. It is correlated with abnormal muscularization and remodeling of small pulmonary arteries. Acute asphyxia may induce persistent pulmonary vasospasm.
   b. Pulmonary parenchymal disease (RDS, meconium aspiration, pneumonia, other aspiration syndromes) can cause pulmonary vasospasm and may be associated with vascular remodeling.

■ BOX 23-2

FACTORS THAT MODULATE PULMONARY VASCULAR RESISTANCE IN THE NEAR-TERM AND TERM TRANSITIONAL AND NEONATAL PULMONARY CIRCULATION

Lowers PVR	**Increases PVR**
Endogenous mediators and mechanisms	Endogenous mediators and mechanisms
Oxygen	Hypoxia
Nitric oxide	Acidosis
PGI_2, E_2, D_2	Endothelin-1
Adenosine, ATP, magnesium	Leukotrienes
Bradykinin	Thromboxanes
Atrial natriuretic factor	Platelet activating factor
Alkalosis	Ca^+ channel activation
K^+ channel activation	α-adrenergic stimulation
Histamine	$PGF_{2\alpha}$
Vagal nerve stimulation	Mechanical factors
Acetylcholine	Overinflation or underinflation
β-adrenergic stimulation	Excessive muscularization, vascular remodeling
Mechanical factors	Altered mechanical properties of smooth muscle
Lung inflation	Pulmonary hypoplasia
Vascular cell structural changes	Alveolar capillary dysplasia
Interstitial fluid and pressure changes	Pulmonary thromboemboli
Shear stress	Main pulmonary artery distention
	Ventricular dysfunction, venous hypertension

ATP, Adenosine triphosphate; *PGI_2,* E_2, D_2, prostaglandins I_2, E_2, and D_2; *$PGF_{2\alpha}$,* prostaglandin $F_{2\alpha}$; *PVR,* pulmonary vascular resistance. From Kinsella, J.P. and Abman, S.H.: Recent developments in the pathophysiology and treatment of persistent pulmonary hypertension of the newborn. *Journal of Pediatrics 126*(6):853-864, 1995.

c. Bacterial sepsis. The underlying mechanism may be endotoxin-mediated myocardial depression or pulmonary vasospasm associated with high levels of thromboxanes and leukotrienes.

d. Prenatal pulmonary hypertension.
  (1) Fetal systemic hypertension.
  (2) Premature closure of ductus arteriosus (associated with maternal use of aspirin, prostaglandin inhibitors, phenytoin [Dilantin], lithium, or indomethacin).

e. Any condition preventing normal circulatory transition at delivery (CNS depression, delayed resuscitation, hypothermia).

f. Hypothermia and hypoglycemia contributing to acidosis, which will potentiate pulmonary vasoconstriction.

g. Hyperviscosity/polycythemia. This may lead to a functional obstruction of the pulmonary vascular bed.

2. Maldevelopment: abnormal pulmonary vessels. Musculature is hypertrophied and extends into normally nonmuscularized arteries. The excessive muscularization impacts lumen size, which increases vascular resistance. Causes of maldevelopment include:

a. Intrauterine asphyxia. Increases systemic arterial blood pressure in the fetus and diverts more blood to the lung, resulting in pulmonary vessel development.

b. Intrauterine aspiration of meconium. Contributes to intrauterine hypoxia.

c. Fetal ductal closure. Forces cardiac output from the right ventricle through the lungs, resulting in maldevelopment.
d. Congenital heart disease. Abnormal pulmonary vessels resulting from various defects.
3. Underdevelopment: decreased number of pulmonary vessels. Blood is shunted because there are too few vessels for blood to flow through the lungs. There is a decreased cross-sectional area available for gas exchange. Severity depends on the timing of the interruption of lung development in utero: reduced numbers of bronchial generations if early (<16 weeks) and decreased number of alveoli if later in gestation. Contributing conditions include:
a. Pulmonary hypoplasia (i.e., Potter sequence).
b. Space-occupying lesions or lung masses (e.g., diaphragmatic hernia, cystic adenomatoid malformation) that prevent normal development of lung tissue and the capillary bed.
c. Congenital heart disease. Pulmonary atresia or tricuspid atresia may lead to decreased blood flow and vascular underdevelopment (Van Marter, 1998; Wearden and Hansen, 2003).

D. Clinical presentation.
1. Near-term, term, or postterm infants.
2. History of hypoxia or asphyxia at birth.
a. Low Apgar scores.
b. Infant usually slow to breathe or difficult to ventilate.
c. Meconium-stained fluid, nuchal cord, abruptio placentae or any acute blood loss, and maternal sedation.
3. Respiratory abnormalities.
a. Symptoms seen before 12 hours of age.
b. Tachypnea/TTN.
c. Retractions if airway is obstructed (e.g., because of aspiration).
d. Cyanosis out of proportion to degree of distress (may not see cyanosis with PaO_2 <50 mm Hg); cyanosis of sudden onset that often is intractable.
e. Low PaO_2 despite high oxygen concentration administration because of right-to-left shunting. Differences are seen between pre- and postductal oxygenation.
f. Chest x-ray may be normal unless aspiration or pneumonia present (will see infiltrates in these cases).
4. Cardiovascular abnormalities.
a. Blood pressure is usually lower than normal.
b. Electrocardiogram will show a right axis deviation.
c. Systolic murmur is frequently heard, usually from a PDA, foramen ovale, or tricuspid insufficiency. Single loud second heart sound (S_2), resulting from high pulmonary pressures may be heard.
d. Echocardiogram shows dilated right side of the heart and evidence of pulmonary hypertension.
e. Congestive heart failure has been reported occasionally.
5. Metabolic abnormalities.
a. Hypoglycemia.
b. Hypocalcemia.
c. Metabolic acidosis.
d. Decreased urine output or coagulopathy caused by kidney and liver damage from asphyxia may occur.

E. **Diagnosis.**
1. PPHN will be suspected on the basis of history and clinical course.
2. Shunt study. Because of the right-to-left shunting at the level of the ductus arteriosus, there will be a preductal and a postductal $Pa{O_2}$ difference. Difference in $Pa{O_2}$ of 10 mm Hg or greater documents ductal shunting.
3. Hyperoxia test. A right-to-left shunt is demonstrated if $P{O_2}$ does not increase in 100% oxygen. Cause may be either PPHN or congenital heart disease.
4. An echocardiogram will rule out structural heart disease, evaluate myocardial function, measure pulmonary artery pressures, and diagnose right-to-left shunting at the level of the PDA or foramen ovale.
5. Chest x-ray may or may not be helpful, but should be taken to rule out other lung pathology.
6. Electrolytes, calcium and glucose levels, and complete blood cell count should be obtained.

F. **Differential diagnosis.**
1. Congenital heart disease.
2. Pulmonary disease.
   a. Severe disease may mimic PPHN.
   b. Disease may coexist with PPHN.

G. **Complications.**
1. Pulmonary.
   a. Air leaks. Related to high mean airway pressures used in ventilator management.
   b. BPD.
2. Cardiovascular.
   a. Systemic hypotension.
   b. Congestive heart failure.
3. Renal.
   a. Decreased urine output related to asphyxia and hypotension.
   b. Acute tubular necrosis caused by asphyxia.
   c. Hematuria, proteinuria.
4. Metabolic.
   a. Hypoglycemia, hypocalcemia.
   b. Metabolic acidosis.
5. Hematologic.
   a. Thrombocytopenia.
   b. DIC: depends on precipitating cause of PPHN.
   c. Hemorrhage (e.g., gastrointestinal, pulmonary).
6. Neurologic.
   a. CNS irritability.
   b. Seizures.
7. Iatrogenic.
   a. Thrombus formation or complications of invasive monitoring equipment.
   b. Dislodged endotracheal tube.
8. Other.
   a. Edema due to third spacing.
   b. Side effects of pharmacologic agents used for treatment.

H. **Management.**
1. Main goal is to correct hypoxia and acidosis (major contributing factors) and promote pulmonary vascular dilation, as well as support extrapulmonary systems.
2. Management will depend on the cause of PPHN.

3. Supportive care.
   a. Monitor vital signs.
   b. Temperature stabilization.
   c. Adequate IV fluid infusion.
   d. Monitor electrolytes, glucose, calcium, complete blood cell count, ABGs.
   e. Correction of metabolic abnormalities.
   f. Blood cultures and antibiotics.
4. Specialized monitoring.
   a. Umbilical catheters.
      (1) Arterial: blood gas access, arterial pressure monitoring.
      (2) Venous: central pressure monitoring, infusion of vasopressors.
   b. Right radial arterial line.
   c. Transcutaneous monitoring and pulse oximetry. Preductal and postductal applications can be helpful.
5. Oxygen. Most potent pulmonary vasodilator.
6. Ventilation.
   a. Conventional mechanical ventilation (CMV).
   b. High-frequency ventilation (HFV); high-frequency oscillatory ventilation (HFOV). Used when CMV fails or when excessive barotrauma is a concern.
   c. While many NICUs may use hyperventilation and/or buffers (e.g., sodium bicarbonate, tromethamine) to promote alkalization (e.g., pH between 7.45 and 7.55), data supporting the benefits of alkalization for treatment of PPHN is sparse.
      (1) Hyperoxygenation.
         (a) Goal is to keep $Pa{O_2}$ at greater than 90 mm Hg.
         (b) Danger of retinopathy of prematurity is minimal because most infants are born at or near term.
      (2) Hyperventilation to keep $Pa{CO_2}$ values in low normal range. Hyperventilation may aid in reducing acidosis and pulmonary artery pressure caused by the vasodilatory effect of alkalosis.
   d. Inhaled nitric oxide (iNO).
      (1) iNO is a selective pulmonary vasodilator.
         (a) Potent and short acting, with half-life of 3 to 5 seconds.
         (b) Combines with hemoglobin and becomes inactivated.
         (c) Inactivation results in formation of methemoglobin; levels need to be monitored during treatment.
      (2) Exact dosage has not been determined. Current evidence supports using starting doses of 20 ppm in term newborn infants with PPHN (Kinsella and Abman, 1995; 1998; Moise and Gomez, 2003).
      (3) iNO withdrawal (weaning) needs to be systematic; abrupt discontinuation may result in rebound increased PVR (Kinsella and Abman, 1998).
      (4) Infants with severe parenchymal lung disease/underinflation and PPHN respond better to iNO when it is combined with HFOV.
   e. Surfactant replacement: especially if etiology based on significant parenchymal disease (Kattwinkel, 1998).
   f. Extracorporeal membrane oxygenation (ECMO) may be used when conventional therapies are unsuccessful.
7. Minimal stimulation and handling.
   a. Infants will show marked fluctuation (generally decreases) in their $Pa{O_2}$ if handled or manipulated.

b. The pulmonary arteries are very reactive to changes in Pa_{O_2}; therefore any action that causes a decrease in Pa_{O_2} (e.g., suctioning, blood sampling, vital signs, ventilator changes) will cause further vasoconstriction.
c. Suction only as needed to maintain a patent airway.
d. Sedatives and analgesics are used for procedures and treatments.
e. The bedside nurse must be a strong advocate for these patients and keep noise and environmental stimuli to a minimum.

8. Pharmacologic support.
   a. Muscle relaxants.
      (1) Used when infant's own respirations interfere with assisted ventilation.
      (2) Paralysis prevents resisting the ventilator, reduces pulmonary vascular resistance, and reduces the risk of air leaks and BPD.
      (3) Pancuronium bromide (Pavulon). Dosage: 0.04 to 0.15 mg/kg every 1 to 2 hours, or as needed for paralysis (Young and Mangum, 2003; Zenk et al., 2000).
      (4) Vecuronium. Dosage: 0.1 mg/kg IV every 1 to 2 hours or as needed (Young and Mangum, 2003; Zenk et al., 2000)
   b. Vasopressors.
      (1) Goal is to keep the systemic pressure above pulmonary pressure to decrease right-to-left shunting.
      (2) Dopamine is the drug of choice. Dopamine is an endogenous catecholamine with a short half-life and must be given by constant infusion. Dosage: 2 to 20 μg/kg/min of continuous IV infusion. Begin at lowest dose and titrate by monitoring effects (i.e., blood pressure, urine output, capillary refill, perfusion, and heart rate (Hagedorn et al., 2002; Young and Mangum, 2003; Zenk et al., 2000).
      (3) Dobutamine is a synthetic catecholamine with primary β_1 effects to support blood pressure in patients with shock and hypotension related to myocardial ischemia, pulmonary hypertension, and cardiomyopathy. Dosage: 2 to 25 μg/kg/min by continuous infusion; titrate by monitoring effects (i.e., blood pressure, urine output, capillary refill, perfusion, and heart rate (Hagedorn et al., 2002; Young and Mangum, 2003; Zenk et al., 2000).
      (4) Nitroprusside increases cardiac output by decreasing left ventricular preload and afterload, acting on the arterial and venous smooth muscle. Dose 0.3 to 6 μg/kg/min. Closely follow thiocyanate and cyanide levels (Hagedorn et al., 2002; Zenk et al., 2000).
      (5) Amrinone is a bipyridine derivative that increases the sensitivity of contractile proteins in the heart to calcium, thus enhancing the heart's contractility. Amrinone also causes decreases in systemic vascular resistance and pulmonary vascular resistance. Dosage: a loading dose of 3 to 4.5 mg/kg is given, followed by a constant infusion of 3 to 5 μg/kg/min (Zenk et al., 2000).
   c. Pulmonary vasodilators.
      (1) iNO (previously described).
      (2) Isoproterenol (Isuprel). Dilates the pulmonary arteries and airways, and increases cardiac output. Tachycardia and systemic hypotension may be seen. Dosage: 0.05 to 0.5 μg/kg/min continuous IV infusion (Young and Mangum, 2003; Zenk et al., 2000).
   d. Analgesics and sedatives.
      (1) Fentanyl citrate. In addition to analgesic effect, fentanyl produces a sedative effect. Dosage: 1 to 4 μg/kg per dose by IV slow push. Repeat

as required (usually every 2-4 hours). Frequently used as a constant infusion at 1 to 5 μg/kg/hour. Tolerance may develop rapidly requiring weaning to prevent significant withdrawal symptoms (Young and Mangum, 2003: Zenk et al., 2000).

(2) Morphine sulfate. Dosage: 0.05 to 0.2 mg/kg per dose IV. Repeat as required, usually every 4 hours. For continuous infusion, usual dose is 10 to 20 μg/kg/hr. Tolerance may develop with prolonged use requiring slow weaning to prevent significant withdrawal symptoms (Young and Mangum, 2003; Zenk et al., 2000).

I. Outcome.

1. PPHN mortality rate and need for ECMO are 20% to 40%.
2. Residual chronic lung disease is common, though recently low-dose iNO has reduced the need for ECMO and has reduced the occurrence of chronic lung disease in neonates with hypoxemic respiratory failure (Clark et al., 2000).
3. Sensorineural hearing loss is higher among children treated for PPHN.
4. Incidence of abnormal neurologic outcome is 12% to 25% (Wearden and Hansen, 2003).

Meconium Aspiration Syndrome

A. Definition and etiology of meconium aspiration syndrome (MAS).

1. Meconium is a mixture of epithelial cells and bile salts found in the fetal intestinal tract.
2. With intrauterine stress or asphyxia, peristalsis is stimulated and relaxation of the anal sphincter occurs, releasing meconium into the amniotic fluid.
3. Aspiration may occur whenever meconium passes into the amniotic fluid, but the risk increases when repeated episodes of severe asphyxia lead to gasping respirations in utero.

B. Incidence. Meconium-stained amniotic fluid (MSAF) is present in approximately 13% of all newborns delivered. Of these, 5% to 12% develop MAS (Wiswell, 2001).

C. Pathophysiology.

1. Complete or partial airway obstruction can occur.
2. Atelectasis or ball-valve air trapping leads to hyperinflation.
3. A chemical pneumonitis develops (probably caused by bile salts). Hemorrhagic pulmonary edema in the alveoli interferes with surfactant production and increases surface tension (Wiswell, 2001).
4. Meconium decreases the levels of surfactant proteins, SP-A and SP-B, and large number of phospholipids (Cleary et al., 1997).

D. Clinical presentation/diagnosis.

1. MAS is a disease of term or postterm infants. MAS is rarely seen in infants born at less than 36 weeks' gestation.
2. Asphyxia and the results of chronic hypoxia may predispose these infants to PPHN.
3. Vigorous resuscitation is frequently needed in the delivery room because of central depression.
4. Respiratory distress signs are nonspecific and may include tachypnea, nasal flaring, and retractions.
5. Respiratory distress may range from mild and transient to severe and prolonged.

6. If there has been prolonged placental insufficiency, infants may appear to be wasted, with hanging skinfolds (usually around knees, buttocks, and axillae).
7. Nailbeds and skin are usually stained a yellow-green.
8. The chest may appear to be hyperinflated or barrel shaped.
9. Chest x-ray shows hyperexpanded lucent areas mixed with areas of atelectasis throughout lung fields.
10. Expiration phase of respirations may be prolonged.
11. Rales and rhonchi are common on auscultation.
12. No specific laboratory data are useful for diagnosis of MAS.
13. ABGs will show the following:
    a. Respiratory and metabolic acidosis in severe cases.
    b. Low Pao_2 even with 100% oxygen administration.

E. Complications.

1. Pulmonary.
   a. Air leaks (pneumothorax and pneumomediastinum) due to ball-valve phenomenon leading to overinflation and air trapping and high ventilator pressures.
   b. Pneumonia.
   c. PPHN.
   d. BPD.
2. Metabolic.
   a. Acidosis.
   b. Hypoglycemia.
   c. Hypocalcemia.
3. Neurologic: will depend on degree of asphyxia.

F. Management and prevention.

1. Delivery room management.
   a. Suction nasopharynx, oropharynx, and hypopharynx with delivery of head to remove any meconium before first breath is taken.
   b. If the infant is depressed with no respiratory effort, muscle tone and/or has a heart rate less than 100, direct suctioning of the trachea soon after delivery is indicated, before respirations are established. While administering free-flow oxygen, clear the mouth and posterior pharynx with a suction catheter to facilitate visualization of the glottis. Tracheal suctioning with an endotracheal tube is recommended. Using a meconium aspirator, suction as you slowly withdraw the endotracheal tube. This procedure should be repeated, if necessary (American Academy of Pediatrics [AAP], 2001).
2. Respiratory care.
   a. ABGs to determine degree of respiratory compromise and type of therapy needed.
   b. Oxygen and/or assisted ventilation.
      (1) Use same parameters for therapy as with RDS. May want to use a lower PEEP (to avoid inadvertent PEEP) and a higher respiratory rate to induce alkalosis and prevent PPHN.
      (2) May choose HFV.
      (3) iNO if PPHN develops.
   c. Improved oxygenation and reduced pulmonary morbidity has been demonstrated in infants given surfactant within 6 hours after birth (Johnson et al., 2003). The use of surfactant in infants with MAS has also decreased the need for ECMO (Lotze et al., 1998; Wiswell, 2001). Although

surfactant therapy seems to be effective in the management of MAS, this treatment strategy has not been approved by any regulatory agencies (Wiswell, 2001).
   - **d.** For infants with MAS requiring ventilation, the use of sedatives and paralytics may be necessary.

G. Outcome.
1. The prognosis for infants with mild cases of MAS is generally excellent unless complications such as seizures, PPHN, or severe asphyxia occur during the course of the disease.
2. In more severe cases, neurologic sequelae are common and death may occur despite vigorous, maximal support.

Bronchopulmonary Dysplasia

A. Definition.
1. In 1967 Northway, Rosan, and Porter originally described the four stages of BPD based on the time that the change occurred (from birth to 30 days of life) and on the type of alveolar and bronchial damage and repair that occurred.
2. A more clinically useful definition now is a 36-week postconceptional age infant with an O_2 requirement, an abnormal Chest x-ray, and abnormal physical examination findings (Barrington and Finer, 1998; Farrell and Fiascone, 1997).
3. A new proposed definition is an infant less than 32 weeks' gestation who has reached 36 weeks' postmenstrual age, was treated with oxygen greater than 28 days, and requires oxygen at 36 weeks' postmenstrual age or positive pressure. Extensive validation of this definition still needs to be determined (Jobe and Bancalari, 2001).

B. Incidence.
1. Statistics vary because of the difference in diagnostic criteria.
2. Overall, BPD seems to be increasing, but the population of infants receiving assisted ventilation has changed since first described (Farrell and Fiascone, 1997).
3. BPD estimates.
   - **a.** Less than 700 g: 85% affected.
   - **b.** Greater than 1500 g: 5% affected.

C. Etiology.
1. Oxygen toxicity can be a cause of BPD.
   - **a.** High inspired oxygen concentrations cause the production of reactive oxygen species and the release of chemotactic factors that attract neutrophils to the lung, initiating the inflammatory cycle. An ongoing inflammatory process in the lung ensues that causes and continues parenchymal damage (Barrington and Finer, 1998; Farrell and Fiascone, 1997).
   - **b.** Inflammatory mediators and proteolytic enzymes are released. The preterm infant has lower levels of antiproteases such as α_1-protease (α_1-antitrypsin) and the antioxidant enzymes dismutase and glutathione. Oxidative damage causes the α-protease to become inactive. These together make the premature pulmonary system especially vulnerable to oxygen toxicity (Barrington and Finer, 1998).
   - **c.** Oxygen radicals appear in the lung as a result of cellular metabolism and are supplementally provided with treatment for the ongoing pulmonary process (Farrell and Fiascone, 1997).

2. There are three pathways of injury that occur in the clinical evolution of BPD.
   a. Structural injury to the airway and alveoli in conjunction with inhibition of maturational processes.
   b. Stimulation of elastic tissue production and the accelerated fibrosis.
   c. Activation of an intense inflammatory response, which contributes to ongoing airway damage (Adams and Cooper, 2003).
3. Assisted ventilation with positive pressure and barotrauma contributes to BPD development.
   a. Intubation interrupts normal pulmonary function (mucociliary function is damaged; dead space is increased, leading to increased pressure needs).
   b. Correlation exists between the severity of the initial pulmonary process and BPD (Barrington and Finer, 1998).
   c. Barotrauma is related to the intensity and amount of time exposed to elements of positive-pressure ventilation (peak inspiratory pressure [PIP], inspiratory time, and PEEP). Repeated distention of distal airways during mechanical ventilation of infants with poor alveolar compliance results in ischemia. Because of the immaturity of the pulmonary system, the alveolar capillary unit is further disrupted by mechanical ventilation, leading to pulmonary edema (Farrell and Fiascone, 1997). Many factors contribute to barotrauma such as the structure of the tracheobronchial tree and the physiologic effects of surfactant deficiency. Changes in the method of ventilation are being evaluated in order to prevent barotrauma (Davis and Rosenfeld, 1999).
4. Increased shunting (left to right) via a PDA has been described as a possible cause of BPD. Improved lung compliance may follow PDA ligation in infants with RDS.
5. Excessive fluid intake in the first 4 days of life contributes to the development of BPD (Barrington and Finer, 1998).
6. Colonization by *Ureaplasma urealyticum, Chlamydia or CMV* has been associated with higher incidence of BPD (Adams and Cooper, 2003; Barrington and Finer, 1998; Davis and Rosenfeld, 1999; Jobe and Bancalari, 2001).
7. Gestational age plays an important role in the development of BPD.
   a. Damage to the developing lung is more likely in infants weighing less than 1500 g.
   b. Damage may occur with less exposure to the previously noted factors in the infant < 1250 g.

D. **Pathophysiology.** All levels of the tracheobronchial tree are involved.
1. Large airways.
   a. Submucosal glandular hypertrophy.
   b. Increased bronchial smooth muscle.
   c. Bronchial mucosa replaced by metaplastic squamous epithelium.
   d. Submucosal fibrosis.
   e. Inflammatory infiltrates.
   f. Granulation tissue.
   g. Loss of cilia.
   h. Tracheomalacia or bronchiomalacia frequently develops.
2. Small airways.
   a. Bronchiolar smooth muscle hypertrophy.
   b. Focal mucosal squamous metaplasia.
   c. Chronic inflammation.
   d. Peribronchial edema.

- **e.** Peribronchiolar fibrosis.
- **f.** Necrosis with intraluminal debris.
- **g.** Luminal narrowing.
- **h.** Excessive production of mucus.

3. Alveoli.
   - **a.** Decreased number of alveoli.
   - **b.** Enlarged alveoli.
   - **c.** Alveolar septal destruction, which leads to emphysematous blebs.
4. Pulmonary vascular bed.
   - **a.** Muscular hypertrophy of the medial layer of pulmonary arterioles leads to increased pulmonary pressures.
   - **b.** Fibrosis.
   - **c.** Endothelial cell hyperplasia, which leads to a decreased cross-sectional area.
5. Reactive airway disease (Farrell and Fiascone, 1997).

E. Clinical presentation.

1. Predisposing risk factors.
   - **a.** Oxygen, intubation, and assisted ventilation.
   - **b.** Gestational age<32 weeks.
   - **c.** Nutritional deficiencies.
   - **d.** Underlying lung disease.
   - **e.** Air leaks.
   - **f.** Infection.
2. Increase in ventilatory requirements or inability to be weaned from ventilator.
3. Hypoxia, hypercapnia, and respiratory acidosis.
4. Audible rales, rhonchi, and wheezing.
5. Retractions.
6. Increased secretions.
7. Bronchospasm.
8. Electrocardiogram showing right ventricular hypertrophy and right axis deviation.
9. Chest x-ray showing hyperinflation, infiltrates, blebs, and cardiomegaly.
10. Fluid intolerance, evidenced by increase in weight, edema, and decrease in urine output, despite no change in fluid intake.

F. Diagnosis.

1. Diagnosis of exclusion.
2. Chest x-ray findings (see Chapter 14).
3. Clinical signs (e.g., tachypnea, hypercapnia, hypoxia, rales) help make diagnosis.

G. Complications.

1. Intermittent bronchospasm.
2. Inability to be weaned from ventilator and/or oxygen supplementation.
3. Recurrent infections.
   - **a.** Pneumonia.
   - **b.** Upper respiratory tract infections.
   - **c.** Otitis media.
4. Congestive heart failure from cor pulmonale.
5. BPD "spells."
   - **a.** Infant becomes irritable, agitated, and dusky; has increased respiratory effort, hypoxia, and hypercapnia.
   - **b.** Cause is unknown but may be bronchospasm or increased pulmonary vascular resistance.

6. Gastroesophageal reflux.
7. Developmental delays.
8. Sudden death reported; cause not completely understood (Farrell and Fiascone, 1997).

H. Prevention.

1. Administration of antenatal steroids reduces the incidence of RDS and the need for mechanical ventilation.
2. Surfactant rescue therapy decreases mortality rates, and prophylaxis may decrease the incidence of BPD slightly.
3. Routine use of steroids (e.g., dexamethasone) for prevention of treatment of chronic lung disease in preterm infants is not recommended (AAP Committee on Fetus and Newborn, 2002).
4. Gentle ventilation, permissive hypercapnia, and early extubation have all been suggested as ways to decrease BPD but have not yet been confirmed by randomized, controlled trials.
5. Synchronized intermittent mandatory ventilation (SIMV) is associated with less severe BPD because the incidence of pulmonary air leaks decreases.
6. HFOV: A recent trial of HFOV after surfactant therapy demonstrated a decrease in the incidence of BPD (Barrington and Finer, 1998; Farrell and Fiascone, 1997).
7. Aggressive nutrition is needed to promote lung growth, maturation, and repair, and protect the damaged lung from infection (Davis and Rosenfeld, 1999; Jobe and Bancalari, 2001).

I. Management.

1. Continued respiratory support.
   a. Continue assisted ventilation.
      (1) Weaning should be *slow*, to allow time for the infant to compensate.
      (2) Decrease the rate because of the need for high PIP to deliver adequate tidal volume, but always assess each infant individually.
   b. After extubation, oxygen is needed to prevent hypoxia and avoid cor pulmonale.
      (1) Oxygen inhalation alleviates airway constriction seen in infants with BPD.
      (2) Maintain PaO_2 at greater than 55 mm Hg and pH at greater than 7.25.
      (3) Supplemental oxygen may enhance overall growth of the infant.
   c. Weaning can usually be accomplished by use of pulse oximetry and occasional monitoring of blood gas and/or serum bicarbonate levels (to assess compensation).
2. Diuretics are used to control fluid retention leading to pulmonary edema. Furosemide (Lasix) is used most often. Benefits include decreased airway resistance, increased airway compliance, and a decrease in total body water, extracellular water, and interstitial water. Metabolic alkalosis may result in compensatory hypoventilation. Calcium wasting may lead to nephrocalcinosis, cholelithiasis, and osteopenia (Zenk et al., 2000). Chlorothiazide (Diuril) has been used with results similar to those seen with furosemide. Follow serum electrolyte values to monitor for hyponatremia, hypokalemia, and metabolic alkalosis (Zenk et al., 2000).
3. Bronchodilators.
   a. Commonly used inhaled bronchodilators include albuterol, metaproterenol, ipratropium, and cromolyn sodium. The inhaled dose is extremely variable. Long-term outcome data on prolonged treatment with bronchodilators are lacking in this population (Barrington and Finer, 1998; Zenk et al., 2000).

   b. Systemic bronchodilator: theophylline (aminophylline). Use varies with individual centers; levels must be monitored. Can cause tachycardia and gastrointestinal (GI) irritation.

4. Fluid restriction may help reduce pulmonary edema and right-sided heart failure.
5. Cardiac evaluation for complications.
   a. Cor pulmonale (right ventricular hypertrophy) due to prolonged pulmonary hypertension.
   b. Electrocardiography and echocardiography should be performed periodically to evaluate the progression/development of right ventricular hypertrophy.
6. Optimal nutrition. Provide increased calories to compensate for increased work of breathing and fluid restriction. Infant may need 150 to 180 kcal/kg/day. Growth failure is common.
7. Monitor for osteopenia beginning at 6 weeks and follow every 2 to 3 weeks (Rusk, 1998). BPD infants are at high risk due to their gestational age, often protracted respiratory course, and medications (e.g., diuretics).
8. Chest physiotherapy and suctioning may be helpful in loosening and removing bronchial secretions. Caregivers must use caution so as not to precipitate a BPD "spell" or cause a rib fracture.
9. Evaluate infant for tracheostomy after 6 to 8 weeks of assisted ventilation and inability to wean off the ventilator. Reduces risk of airway complications (e.g., tracheomalacia, bronchomalacia).
10. Use of steroids.
    a. Early administration of systemic dexamethasone in preterm neonates who are mechanically ventilated may reduce the incidence of chronic lung disease and extubation failure, but can cause complications (Stark et al., 2001; AAP Committee on Fetus and Newborn, 2002).
    b. Complications include impairment of growth, possible increase in neurodevelopmental abnormalities, hypertension, myocardial hypertrophy, gastrointestinal hemorrhage and perforation, gastric ulcerations, nosocomial sepsis, hyperglycemia, and transient adrenal suppression (AAP/ACOG, 2002; Parad and Berger, 1998; Stark et al., 2001).
    c. Have not been found to have a substantial impact on long-term outcomes such as duration of supplemental oxygen requirement, length of hospital stay, or mortality (Parad and Berger, 1998).
    d. Early treatment of inhaled corticosteroids to very low birth weight infants has no discernible benefits in the prevention and treatment of chronic lung disease (AAP Committee on Fetus and Newborn, 2002).
11. RSV: BPD infants are at high risk for RSV outbreaks and account for many readmissions, with 25% of BPD infants needing assisted ventilation. Treament modalities include:
    a. Benefits of RSV Prophylaxis:
       (1) RespiGam (RSV IGIV). Decreases the severity of RSV infection, decreases hospitalizations, and reduces the incidence of concurrent otitis media (Impact-RSV Study Group, 1998; Welliver, 1998).
       (2) Palivizumab (Synagis). Humanized monoclonal antibody against RSV. Unlike RSV-IGIV, Palivizumab is not a human blood product and therefore is not associated with the risk of bloodborne pathogens (AAP/ACOG, 2002). Impact-RSV Study Group (1998) found 55%

decrease in hospitalizations caused by RSV infection, fewer hospital days, and a lower rate of intensive care unit admissions compared with the control group.

b. AAP recommendations include:

(1) Prophylaxis to infants who are less than 2 years of age with chronic lung disease requiring medical management within the preceding 6 months, infants born 29 to 32 weeks' gestation (prophylaxis up to 6 months of age), and infants born 28 weeks' gestation and younger (prophylaxis until 12 months of age)

(2) Prophylaxis is contraindicated for infants with cyanotic congenital heart disease (AAP/ACOG, 2002). However, patients with symptomatic acyanotic heart disease who were born preterm or have chronic lung disease may benefit from RSV prophylaxis.

c. RSV IGIV dose is 750 ml/kg per dose IV, repeated monthly during RSV season (Young and Mangum, 2003). Dosing should resume after recovery if RSV infection develops (AAP, 1997, 1998; Farrell and Fiascone, 1997). Immunizations with measles-mumps-rubella and varicella vaccines should be deferred for 9 months after the last dose (AAP/ACOG, 2002).

d. Palivizumab-dose is 15 mg/kg, intramuscular route, given monthly during RSV season, with the first dose to be given before the start of the season (AAP, 1997, 1998; Impact RSV-Study Group, 1998; Young and Mangum, 2003).

J. Outcome.

1. Mortality rate:

a. Approximately 10% to 15% by 1 year of age (Davis and Rosenfeld, 1999). May vary with the increased use of surfactant and the decreased use of steroids.

b. After discharge, mortality rate is less than 10%.

(1) Death is usually not caused by respiratory failure.

(2) Complications such as cor pulmonale or infection are the usual causes of death.

2. Some infants will be discharged home with oxygen supplementation.

3. Recurrent pulmonary infections and growth restriction are seen commonly among survivors. The pattern of growth is usually between the 10th and 25th percentiles (Farrell and Fiascone, 1997).

4. Pulmonary function:

a. Little improvement occurs before 6 months of age.

b. By three years of age, pulmonary compliance is near normal, however, airway resistance may be 30% higher than that of controls (Adams and Cooper, 2003).

5. Neurologic and developmental sequelae.

a. Cerebral palsy. The most common major neurologic disorder in the first 2 years of life in very low birth weight infants (Vohr and Msall, 1997). Recent studies have revealed that there is a higher incidence of CP with chronic lung disease. Prolonged treatment with dexamethasone decreases the risk of CLD, but infants are noted to have a higher incidence of CP and poorer neurodevelopmental outcome (Stark et al., 2001).

b. Sensorineural hearing loss. Incidence of 0.7% to 2% in very low birth weight infants. Conductive hearing loss has an incidence of 14% to 42%. Retinopathy of prematurity is reported at 23% to 57%, with myopia common (Dusick, 1997).

CHRONIC LUNG DISEASE IN PREMATURE INFANTS (Pulmonary Insufficiency of Prematurity, Chronic Pulmonary Insufficiency of Prematurity, Wilson-Mikity Syndrome)

A. **Definition.**
   1. Changes in pulmonary structure and function occur without underlying disease.
   2. Majority of cases are seen in infants weighing less than 1500 g.

B. **Incidence.** Incidence is unknown. Wide variation in population, clinical practice, and definition account for variation in incidence.

C. **Etiology/pathophysiology.**
   1. Abnormal distribution of air (overexpansion and atelectasis) due to characteristics of the premature lung.
   2. At the end of the first week, the functional residual capacity (FRC) decreases, resulting in hypoxia and hypercapnia, which lead to apnea and atelectasis.
   3. Chest x-ray reveals poorly defined, diffuse, hazy lung parenchyma (Cooper, 2003).

D. **Clinical presentation and diagnosis.**
   1. Can be seen in premature infants with minimal exposure to increased oxygen.
   2. Symptoms appear at 7 to 10 days of life and include transient cyanosis, hyperpnea, and retractions.
   3. Symptoms increase in severity for 2 to 6 weeks.
   4. Increasing oxygen dependency and retention of carbon dioxide.

E. **Management.** Provide supportive care.
   1. Oxygen to maintain normal PaO_2.
   2. Chest physiotherapy.
   3. IV fluids.
   4. Caffeine for apnea.
   5. Nasal continuous positive airway pressure (CPAP) until about 30 weeks' postconceptional age (Cooper, 2003).

F. **Outcome.**
   1. Mortality rates of 10% to 30% have been reported with these forms of chronic lung disease.
   2. Generally there is complete clearing of symptoms by 2 to 6 months.
   3. Condition often resolves with growth.

PULMONARY AIR LEAKS (Pneumomediastinum, Pneumothorax, Pneumopericardium, Pulmonary Interstitial Emphysema [PIE])

A. **Definition.** Alveolar overdistention and rupture. May occur spontaneously or as a secondary cause, usually when assisted ventilation is used.

B. **Incidence.** In infants receiving assisted ventilation, the incidence ranges from 2% to 8% but among low birth weight infants may be as high as 20% (Hagedorn et al., 2002).

C. **Pathophysiology.**
   1. Generally iatrogenic, resulting from the use of excessive airway pressure during resuscitation or with assisted ventilation.
   2. Can occur spontaneously if there is uneven air distribution at birth.
      a. Some areas are expanded, while others remain collapsed.
      b. Infant will generate pressure to expand unopened areas, leading to greater pressure in already expanded areas, which results in the air leak.

3. Frequently, underlying lung disease is present.
   a. Obstructive: such as ball-valve trapping of air, seen with MAS.
   b. Poor lung compliance: such as seen with RDS.
4. Overdistention of alveoli leads to rupture, with gas moving into nonventilated tissues. Air travels via vascular sheaths to the lining of the lung. Interstitial air can dissect around blood vessels or along lymphatics becoming PIE. Air can move from the lining to the mediastinum, resulting in pneumomediastinum, through to the thoracic cavity and visceral pleura, resulting in a pneumothorax. When the air moves along the great vessels to the pericardium, a pneumopericardium results. If air dissects down from the mediastinum through the sheaths of the great vessels, pneumoperitoneum results.

D. Clinical presentation and diagnosis (see Chapter 14 for x-ray findings).

1. Pneumothorax.
   a. Sudden deterioration.
   b. Decreased breath sounds on the affected side, hypotension, skin mottling, and shift of the mediastinum (detected by shift of the point of maximal cardiac impulse on auscultation) to the unaffected side.
   c. Obtain chest x-ray.
   d. Transillumination (translucent glow when fiberoptic light is placed against the skin) of the chest wall may confirm presence of pneumothorax, without having to wait for a chest x-ray.
   e. If the air leak is small, may be asymptomatic.
2. Pneumomediastinum.
   a. Should be anticipated with MAS.
   b. Signs include increased anteroposterior diameter of chest and indistinct heart sounds.
   c. Chest x-ray may show "sail sign," indicating elevation of the thymus surrounded by air.
3. Pneumopericardium.
   a. Immediate presentation with hypotension, muffled heart sound, and bradycardia from cardiac tamponade.
   b. Life threatening.
   c. Chest x-ray will show air encircling the heart, halo appearance.
4. PIE.
   a. Difficult to interpret.
   b. Limited to infants with poor lung compliance receiving CPAP or positive-pressure ventilation.
   c. Chest x-ray shows microcystic areas throughout one or both lungs; may show hyperinflated lungs and flattened diaphragm.
   d. May progress to pneumomediastinum and/or pneumothorax.
   e. Hypoxia and hypercapnia commonly present.

E. Management.

1. Pneumothorax.
   a. If asymptomatic, will often resolve without treatment.
   b. Symptomatic (tension) pneumothorax requires emergency removal of air. Associated with hypoxia, hypotension, and cardiopulmonary arrest.
      (1) Thoracentesis (needle aspiration to remove air) may be necessary, until a chest tube can be placed, if infant's condition has acutely deteriorated or until adequate pain pharmacologic support can be administered.
      (2) Thoracostomy tube is placed in the anterior chest and connected to underwater seal drainage system, with continuous negative pressure

of 10 to 15 cm H_2O, and left in place until air ceases to bubble from the chest tube for at least 24 hours and pneumothorax is resolved by chest x-ray examination. The chest tube is then placed to the water seal for 24 hours, and the infant is observed for reaccumulation of air. The chest tube is removed 12 to 24 hours after the tube has been placed to water drainage if the infant remains free of symptoms.

(3) In asymptomatic infants or nonventilated infants, administration of 100% oxygen may aid the absorption of the air in the pneumothorax by the pleural capillaries. Due to the toxic effects of oxygen, this treatment is not recommended for preterm infants.

2. Pneumomediastinum.
   a. Usually not treated.
   b. If associated with pneumothorax (common occurrence), high oxygen concentration may help resolve condition, as described previously.
3. Pneumopericardium. Emergency treatment is required by placement of a long catheter or chest tube into the pericardial sac with constant application of gentle negative pressure.
4. PIE.
   a. If unilateral and persistent, intubation of mainstem bronchus supplying opposite lung may show improvement in condition.
   b. If bilateral, supportive treatment is given (e.g., oxygen, ventilation, fluids).
   c. Minimize positive inspiratory pressure and shorten inspiratory time.
   d. High-frequency ventilation.
   e. Place affected side in dependent position.

F. Outcome.

1. Outcome depends on underlying lung pathology.
2. Mortality rate is high with pneumopericardium, bilateral pneumothoraces, and bilateral PIE.
3. In survivors of bilateral PIE, the risk of chronic lung disease is high.

PULMONARY HYPOPLASIA

A. Definition. Defective or inhibited growth of the lungs, either unilateral or bilateral. Developmental disorder that results in decreased numbers of alveoli, bronchioles, and arterioles.

B. Pathophysiology.

1. Conditions that compress the lungs or limit lung growth (e.g., diaphragmatic hernia, cystic adenomatoid malformation) are one cause of pulmonary hypoplasia.
2. Conditions that result in oligohydramnios (e.g., renal disorders, amniotic fluid leakage) are associated with pulmonary hypoplasia caused by thoracic compression.
3. Associated congenital malformations, such as renal dysgenesis (Potter syndrome), phrenic nerve absence, and vertebral and chromosomal anomalies, should be considered.

C. Diagnosis.

1. Often very difficult to diagnose.
2. Any of the above conditions are suggestive of pulmonary hypoplasia.
3. Usually present with severe respiratory distress.
4. Higher than usual pressures needed for ventilation; pneumothorax common.
5. Hypercapnia difficult or impossible to treat early in disease course.
6. Chest x-ray will usually show decreased volume of the thorax.
7. Symptoms of PPHN possible.

D. **Management.** Treatment is supportive and directed at respiratory failure.
   1. Assisted ventilation/HFV.
   2. Treatment of PPHN.
   3. iNO (nitric oxide).
   4. ECMO.

E. **Outcome.**
   1. Degree and etiology of hypoplasia determines outcome.
   2. Mortality rate is high.
   3. Management is difficult, but infant can function adequately if treatment and support can be continued until lung growth occurs, although this outcome is rare.

PULMONARY HEMORRHAGE

A. **Definition.**
   1. Localized areas of bleeding into alveoli (generally found at autopsy); also known as hemorrhagic pulmonary edema.
   2. Can be a massive generalized bleeding event.

B. **Etiology and pathophysiology.**
   1. Usually occurs as a complication of other disorders such as prematurity, erythroblastosis, intracranial hemorrhage, asphyxia, aspiration, heart disease, sepsis, hypothermia, PDA, and surfactant replacement.
   2. May be due to trauma from improper suctioning technique.
   3. Usually due to large increase in capillary hydrostatic pressure; results in capillary rupture and fluid transudation from other capillaries (Welty and Hansen, 2003).

C. **Clinical presentation.**
   1. May present with sudden, severe respiratory distress.
   2. Bright red blood may be suctioned from the trachea.

D. **Management.**
   1. Use of assisted ventilation is necessary to maintain gas exchange and PEEP.
   2. Transfusion of packed red blood cells if large hemorrhage with decreased hematocrit/hemoglobin.
   3. Identify any clotting abnormalities and treat.
   4. Treat underlying disease.

E. **Outcome.**
   1. If bleeding is massive, death will occur quickly despite vigorous management.
   2. If hemorrhage is small or isolated, infant will recover and outcome will be dependent on underlying disease.

OTHER CAUSES OF RESPIRATORY DISTRESS

A. **Upper airway disorders.**
   1. Choanal atresia:
      a. Incidence is 2 to 4 in 10,000 births with female/male ratio of 2:1.
      b. Bone or membrane protrudes into nasal passages, causing blockage or narrowing.
      c. If condition is bilateral, gasping respirations and cyanosis occur immediately after birth because neonates are obligate nose breathers. Many infants have associated anomalies (Treacher Collins syndrome, tracheoesophageal fistula, palatal abnormalities, CHARGE association [*c*oloboma, *h*eart disease, *a*tresia choanal, *r*estricted growth and

development, *g*enital hypoplasia, and *e*ar anomalies]), congenital heart disease.

d. Signs of distress are intermittent when condition is unilateral.
e. Failure to pass a catheter through the nasal passages to the posterior oropharynx will make the diagnosis.
f. Initially treat by placing infant in prone position with a large oral airway taped securely in place (an endotracheal tube can be used if placement of an oral airway is difficult).
g. Surgical correction of the problem is necessary and consists of perforation of the obstruction and serial dilation by use of obturators.

2. Micrognathia.
   a. Defined as mandibular undergrowth.
   b. Occurs with certain syndromes and sequences such as Pierre Robin syndrome, trisomy 18, trisomy 22, and cri-du-chat syndrome (deletion of the short arm of chromosome 5).
   c. Airway distress may be alleviated by prone positioning with the infant's head placed downward.
   d. Use of an oral airway or endotracheal tube will provide an open airway.
   e. If an endotracheal tube is in place, humidification will be needed to prevent the drying of secretions.
   f. Tracheostomy may be necessary.
   g. Generally mandibular growth "catches up" by 6 to 12 months of age.
3. Cystic hygroma.
   a. Form of cystic lymphangioma, with benign water cysts occurring most frequently in the neck (80%); can also be found in the groin, axilla, and mediastinum.
   b. Usually seen at birth.
   c. Mass will occupy the submandibular region and may compromise the airway in 25% of cases.
   d. Symptoms depend on the size and location.
   e. Treatment is related to complications.
      (1) If infant is free of symptoms, surgical excision is performed between 4 and 12 months of age.
      (2) Excision must be performed at an earlier age if the airway is compromised or if infections are recurrent.
      (3) Multiple excisions are usually performed to prevent damage to nerves and vascular structures.
4. Obstruction of larynx or trachea.
   a. Stridor is a major symptom and usually requires no specific treatment, but mechanical causes must be ruled out.
   b. Direct laryngoscopy will reveal structural abnormalities such as polyps, webs, and granulomas.
   c. Hemangiomas of the larynx or trachea may cause obstruction.
   d. Extrinsic compression of the upper airway occurs with thyroglossal duct cyst, cervical neuroblastoma, vascular ring, and double aortic arch.
   e. Laryngotracheomalacia results from collapse of the larynx and cervical trachea, which produces stridor; condition is usually self-limiting and resolves by 6 to 12 months of age, when the tracheal diameter increases and the cartilage matures.
5. Tracheoesophageal fistula (refer to Chapter 28.)

B. Thoracic disorders.
1. Cystic adenomatoid malformation (CAM).
   a. Primary pulmonary tissue dysplasia with failure of terminal bronchioles to canalize, which leads to intrapulmonary mass consisting of multiple small cysts.
   b. Three types.
      (1) Type I CAM is the most common, occurring in 70% of cases. It presents as a single or multiple large (3 to 10 cm) cysts that communicate with the bronchi; 11% are associated with anomalies; 90% survival rate.
      (2) Type II CAM is found in 18% of cases. It is composed of multiple medium size, evenly distributed cysts that resemble terminal bronchioles (0.5 cm to 2.0 cm); 50% of these infants have other anomalies, and only 56% survive. Most common anomalies associated are sirenomelia, renal agenesis, and extralobar pulmonary sequestration.
      (3) Type III CAM is found in 10% of cases. It is a large bulky lesion, composed of evenly distributed small (<0.2 cm in size) cysts. This type resembles the early canalicular stage of fetal lung development and may be the result of an insult at the time of lung bud branching. Only 60% of these infants survive (Johnson and Cooper, 2003).
   c. Respiratory distress may be seen at birth, or the malformation may cause no symptoms.
   d. May be confused with diaphragmatic hernia or pulmonary sequestration on x-ray.
   e. Treatment of choice is surgical excision of the involved lobe.
2. Bronchogenic cyst.
   a. Mucus-producing cyst.
   b. May cause tracheal, bronchial, or esophageal obstruction.
   c. Distress usually not severe.
   d. Treatment is surgical excision.
3. Congenital lobar emphysema.
   a. Overdistention of one or more lobes of the lung (upper lobes generally affected; 10% in right middle lobe).
   b. Inability of the lung to deflate properly, possibly because of a defect in bronchial cartilage.
   c. Possibility of severe respiratory distress within hours of birth but usually delayed for weeks or months.
   d. Chest x-ray examination is diagnostic (refer to Chapter 14).
   e. Treatment of choice: surgical resection.
4. Chondrodystrophies.
   a. Group of disorders of bone growth, resulting in short stature.
   b. Possible respiratory distress because of small thoracic cavities.
   c. Treatment: based on degree of distress.
5. Neuromuscular disorders.
   a. Conditions resulting in hypotonia, such as spinal muscular atrophy and myotonic dystrophy, result in varying degrees of respiratory distress.
   b. Management will depend on degree of distress.

C. CNS disorders.
1. Seizures.
2. Hypoxic-ischemic injury.
3. Intracranial hemorrhages.

4. Drugs.
5. Meningitis.

D. **Cardiovascular and hematologic disorders.**
1. Congenital heart disease.
2. Anemia.
3. Polycythemia.
4. Shock.
5. Sepsis.
6. Respiratory distress, varying from mild to severe.
7. Treatment in relation to underlying cause.

E. **Diaphragmatic disorders (see also Chapter 14).**
1. Diaphragmatic hernia.
2. Diaphragmatic paralysis.
3. Diaphragmatic eventration.

F. **Renal disorders.**
1. Pulmonary hypoplasia results from renal agenesis or renal dysgenesis.
2. Conditions are usually untreatable, and death will occur within hours or days.

REFERENCES

Adams, J.M. and Cooper, T.R.: Bronchopulmonary dysplasia. In L.E. Weisman and T.N. Hansen (Eds.): *Contemporary diagnosis and management of neonatal respiratory diseases* (3rd ed.). Newtown, PA, 2003, Handbooks in Health Care, pp. 163-178.

American Academy of Pediatrics Committee on Infectious Diseases: Respiratory syncytial virus immune globulin intravenous: Indications for use. *Pediatrics, 99*(4):645-650, 1997.

American Academy of Pediatrics and Canadian Paediatric Society: Postnatal corticosteroids to treat or prevent chronic lung disease in preterm infants. *Pediatrics, 109*(2):330-338, 2002.

American Academy Pediatrics Policy Statement: Prevention of respiratory syncytial virus infections: Indications for the use of Palivizumab and update on the use of RSV-IGIV. *Pediatrics, 102*(5):1211-1216, 1998.

American Academy of Pediatrics: Initial Steps in Resuscitation. In J. Kattwinkel (Ed.): *Textbook of neonatal resuscitation* (4th ed.). Elk Grove Village, IL, 2001, American Academy of Pediatrics, pp. 2-1 to 2-25.

American Academy of Pediatrics and The American College of Obstetricians and Gynecologists: *Guidelines for perinatal care* (5th ed.). Elk Grove Village, IL, 2002, AAP/ACOG, pp. 125-306.

American Lung Association: *American Lung Association Fact Sheet: Respiratory distress syndrome of the newborn*. American Lung Association State of the Art. New York, 2003, American Lung Association.

Barrington, K.J. and Finer, N.N.: Treatment of bronchopulmonary dysplasia: A review. *Clinics in Perinatology, 25*(1):177-202, 1998.

Blackburn, S.T.: *Maternal, fetal, and neonatal physiology: A clinical perspective* (2nd ed). St Louis, 2003, Saunders, pp. 282-321.

Carey, B.E. and Trotter, C.: Neonatal pneumonia. *Neonatal Network, 19*(4):44-50, 2000.

Clark, R.H., Kueser, T.J., Walker, M.W., et al.: Low-dose nitric oxide therapy for persistent pulmonary hypertension of the newborn: Clinical Inhaled Nitric Oxide Research Group. *New England Journal of Medicine, 342*(7):469-474, 2000.

Cleary, G.M., Antunes, M.J., Ciesielka, D.A., et al.: Exudative lung injury is associated with decreased levels of surfactant proteins in a rat model of meconium aspiration. *Pediatrics, 100*(6):998-1003, 1997.

Cooper, T.R.: Chronic pulmonary insufficiency of prematurity. In L.E. Weisman and T.N. Hansen (Eds.): *Contemporary diagnosis and management of neonatal respiratory diseases*. (3rd ed.), Newtown, PA, 2003, Handbooks in Health Care, pp. 162-163.

Davis, J.M. and Rosenfeld, W.: Chronic lung disease. In G.B. Avery, M.A. Fletcher, and M.G. MacDonald (Eds.): *Neonatology: Pathophysiology and management of the newborn* (5th ed.). Philadelphia, 1999, J.B. Lippincott, pp. 509-532.

Dusick, A.M.: Medical outcomes in preterm infants. *Seminars in Perinatology, 21*(3): 164-177, 1997.

Egberts, J., de Winter, J.P., Sedin, G., et al.: Comparison of prophylaxis and rescue treatment with Curosurf in neonates less than 30 weeks' gestation: A randomized trial. *Pediatrics, 92*(6):768-774, 1993.

Farrell, P.A., and Fiascone, J.M.: Bronchopulmonary dysplasia in the 1990s: A review for the pediatrician. *Pediatrics, 27*:129-172, 1997.

Ghidini, A., Salafia, C.M., Miniar, V.K., et al.: Repeated courses of steroids in preterm membrane rupture do not increase the risk of histologic chorioamnionitis. *American Journal of Perinatology, 14*(6): 309-313, 1997.

Guillory, C. and Cabrera-Meza, G.: Approaches to the patient with respiratory disease. In L.E. Weisman and T.N. Hansen (Eds.): *Contemporary diagnosis and management of neonatal respiratory diseases*. (3rd ed.). Newtown, PA, 2003, Handbooks in Health Care, pp. 54-62.

Hagedorn, M.I.E., Gardner, S.L., and Abman, S.H.: Respiratory diseases. In G.B. Merenstein and S.L. Gardner (Eds.): *Handbook of neonatal intensive care* (5th ed.). St Louis, 2002, Mosby, pp. 485-575.

Harris, T.R. and Wood, B.R.: Physiologic principles. In J.P. Goldsmith and E.H. Karotkin (Eds.): *Assisted ventilation of the neonate*. Philadelphia, 1996, Saunders, p. 53.

Impact-RSV Study Group: Palivizumab, a humanized respiratory syncytial virus monoclonal antibody, reduces hospitalization from respiratory syncytial virus infection in high-risk infants. *Pediatrics, 102*(3 Part 1):531-537, 1998.

Jobe, A.H.: Surfactant treatment. In R.A. Polin and W.W. Fox (Eds.): *Fetal and neonatal physiology* (2nd ed.). Philadelphia, 1998, Saunders, pp. 1321-1335.

Jobe, A.H. and Bancalari, E.: Bronchopulmonary dysplasia. *American Journal of Respiratory Care Medicine, 163*(7):1723-1729, 2001.

Jobe, A.H. and Ikegami, M.: Biology of surfactant. *Clinics in Perinatology, 28*(3): 655-669, 2001.

Johnson, K.E. and Cooper, T.R.: Congenital diseases affecting the lung parenchyma. In L.E. Weisman and T.N. Hansen (Eds.): *Contemporary diagnosis and management of neonatal respiratory diseases*. (3rd ed.), Newton, PA, 2003, Handbooks in Health Care, pp. 186-200.

Johnson, K.E., Cooper, T.R., and Hansen, T.N.: Meconium aspiration syndrome. In L.E. Weisman and T.N. Hansen (Eds.): *Contemporary diagnosis and management of neonatal respiratory diseases (3rd ed.)*. Newtown, PA, 2003, Handbooks in Health Care, pp. 135-141.

Kattwinkel, J.: Surfactant: Evolving issues. *Clinics in Perinatology, 25*(1):17-32, 1998.

Kattwinkel, J., Bloom, B.T., Delmore, P., et al.: Prophylactic administration of calf lung surfactant is more effective than early treatment of respiratory distress syndrome in neonates 29 through 32 weeks' gestation. *Pediatrics, 9*(1)2:90-98, 1993.

Kendig, J.W., Notter, R.N., Cox, C., et al.: A comparison of surfactant as immediate prophylaxis and as rescue therapy in newborns of less than 30 weeks' gestation. *New England Journal of Medicine, 324*(13):865-871, 1991.

Kinsella, J.P. and Abman, S.H.: Recent developments in the pathophysiology and treatment of persistent pulmonary hypertension of the newborn. *Journal of Pediatrics, 12*(6)6:853-864, 1995.

Kinsella, J.P. and Abman, S.H.: Controversies in the use of inhaled nitric oxide therapy in the newborn. *Clinics in Perinatology, 25*(2):203-218, 1998.

Larsen, W.J. Embryonic foldings. In *Human Embryology* (3rd ed.), New York, 2001, Churchill Livingstone, pp. 134-155.

Lawson, M.E.: Respiratory disorders: Transient tachypnea of the newborn. In J.P. Cloherty, and A.R. Stark (Eds.): *Manual of neonatal care*. Philadelphia, 1998, Lippincott-Raven, pp. 369-371.

Liley, H.G. and Stark, A.R.: Respiratory distress syndrome: Hyaline membrane disease. J.P. Cloherty, and A.R. Stark (Eds.): *Manual of neonatal care*. Philadelphia, 1998, Lippincott-Raven, pp. 329-335.

Lotze, A., Mitchell, B.R., Bulas, D.I., et al.: Multicenter study of surfactant (beractant) use in the treatment of term infants with severe respiratory failure. *Journal of Pediatrics, 132*(1):40-47, 1998.

Maher, J.E., Cliver, S.P., Goldenberg, R.E., et al.: The effect of corticosteroid therapy in the very premature infant. *American Journal of Obstetrics and Gynecology, 170*(3):869-873, 1994.

March of Dimes: Cerebral palsy. In *Professional and researchers: Quick reference and fact sheet*. Birth Defect and Genetics, www.march of dimes.com/professionals/681-1208.asp, 2003.

Moise, A.A., and Gomez, M.R.: Nonventilatory management of respiratory failure. In L.E. Weisman and T.N. Hansen (Eds.): *Contemporary diagnosis and management of neonatal respiratory diseases*. Newtown, PA, 2003, Handbooks in Health Care, pp. 286-291.

Moise, A.A. and Hansen, T.N.: Acute, acquired parenchymal lung disease. In L.E. Weisman and T.N. Hansen (Eds.): *Contemporary diagnosis and management of neonatal respiratory diseases*. (3rd ed.). Newtown, PA, 2003, Handbooks in Health Care, pp. 90-107.

Moore, K.L. and Persaud, T.V.N.: The respiratory system. In *Before we are born: Essentials of embryology and birth defects* (6th ed.). Philadelphia, 2003, Saunders, pp. 190-199.

Morin, F.C., III and Stenmark, K.R.: Persistent pulmonary hypertension of the newborn. *American Journal of Respiratory and Critical Care Medicine, 151*(6):2010-2032, 1995.

National Institutes of Health Consensus Development Panel: Antenatal corticosteroids revisited: Repeat course. *NIH Consensus Statement, 17*(2):1-18, 2000.

Northway, W.H., Rosan, R.C., and Porter, D.Y.: Pulmonary disease following respiratory therapy of hyaline membrane disease. *New England Journal of Medicine, 276*(7):357-368, 1967.

Notter, R.H.: Biophysical behavior of lung surfactant: Implications for respiratory physiology and pathophysiology. *Seminars in Perinatology, 12*(3):180-212, 1988.

Orlando, S.: Pathophysiology of acute respiratory distress. In D.F. Askin (Ed.): *Acute respiratory care of the neonate*. Petaluma, CA, 1997, NICU Ink Books, pp. 37-41.

Paige, P.L. and Carney, P.R.: Neurologic disorders. In G.B. Merenstein and S.L. Gardner (Eds.): *Handbook of neonatal intensive care* (5th ed.). St Louis, 2002, Mosby, pp. 644-678.

Parad, R.B. and Berger, T.M.: Chronic lung disease. In J.P. Cloherty and A.R. Stark (Eds.): *Manual of neonatal care*. Philadelphia, 1998, Lippincott-Raven, pp. 378-387.

Pearson, D.L., Dawling, S., Walsh, W.F., et al.: Neonatal pulmonary hypertension: Urea-cycle intermediates, nitric oxide production, and carbamoyl-phosphate synthetase function. *New England Journal of Medicine, 344*(24):1832-1838, 2001.

Rusk, C.: Rickets screening in the preterm infant. *Neonatal Network, 17*(1):55-57, 1998.

Shapiro, D.L.: The development of surfactant therapy and the various types of replacement surfactants. *Seminars in Perinatology, 12*(3):174-179, 1988.

Speer, M.E. and Hansen, T.N.: Transient tachypnea of the newborn. In L.E. Weisman and T.N. Hansen (Eds.): *Contemporary diagnosis and management of neonatal respiratory diseases*. Newtown, (3rd ed.). PA, 2003, Handbooks in Health Care, pp. 108-113.

Speer, M.E. and Weisman, L.E.: Pneumonia. In L.E. Weisman and T.N. Hansen (Eds.): *Contemporary diagnosis and management of neonatal respiratory diseases*. (3rd ed.). Newtown, PA, 2003, Handbooks in Health Care, pp. 140-144.

Stark, A.R., Carlo, W.A., Tyson, J.E., et al.: Adverse effects of early dexamethasone treatment in extremely-low-birth-weight-infants: National Institute of Child Health and Human Development Neonatal Research Network. *New England Journal of Medicine*, 344(2):95-101, 2001.

Steinhorn, R.H., Millard, S.L., and Morin, F.C.: Persistent pulmonary hypertension of the newborn. *Clinics in Perinatology, 22*(2):405-428, 1995.

Van Marter, L.J.: Persistent pulmonary hypertension of the newborn. In J.P. Cloherty and A.R. Stark (Eds.): *Manual of neonatal care*. Philadelphia, 1998, Lippincott-Raven, pp. 364-369.

Vohr, B.R. and Msall, M.E.: Neuropsychological and functional outcomes of low birth weight infants. *Seminars in Perinatology, 21*(3):202-220, 1997.

Walsh-Sukys, M.C., Tyson, J.E., Wright, L.L., et al.: Persistent pulmonary hypertension of the newborn in the era before nitric oxide: Practice variation and outcomes. *Pediatrics, 105*(1):14-20, 2000.

Wearden, M.E. and Hansen, T.N.: Persistent pulmonary hypertension of the newborn. In L.E. Weisman and T.N. Hansen (Eds.): *Contemporary diagnosis and management of neonatal respiratory diseases.* (3rd ed.). Newtown, PA, 2003, Handbooks in Health Care, pp. 113-124.

Welliver, R.C.: Respiratory syncytial virus immunoglobulin and monoclonal antibodies in the prevention and treatment of respiratory syncytial virus infection. *Seminars in Perinatology, 22*(1):87-95, 1998.

Welty, S.E. and Hansen, T.N.: Pulmonary hemorrhage. In L.E. Weisman and T.N. Hansen (Eds.): *Contemporary diagnosis and management of neonatal respiratory diseases.* (3rd ed.). Newtown, PA, 2003, Handbooks in Health Care, pp. 130-135.

Whitsett, J.A.: Composition and structure of pulmonary surfactant. In B.R. Boynton, W.A. Carlo, and A.H. Jobe (Eds.): *New therapies for neonatal respiratory failure.* New York, 1994, Cambridge University Press, pp. 3-15.

Whitsett, J.A., Pryhuber, G.S, Rice, W.R. and Warner, B.B.: Acute respiratory disorders. In G.B. Avery, M.A. Fletcher, and M.G. MacDonald (Eds.): *Neonatology: Pathophysiology and management of the newborn* (5th ed.). Philadelphia, 1999, J.B. Lippincott, pp. 485-508.

Wiswell, T.E.: Expanded uses of surfactant therapy. *Clinics in Perinatology, 28*(3): 695-711, 2001.

Young, T.E. and Mangum, O.B.: *Neofax: A manual of drugs used in neonatal care.* Raleigh, NC, 2003, Acorn Publishing.

Zenk, K., Sills, J., and Koeppel, R.: *Neonatal medications and nutrition.* Santa Rosa, CA, 2000, NICU Ink.

CHAPTER

24 Apnea

MARTHA GOODWIN

OBJECTIVES

1. Define types of apnea seen in the newborn infant.
2. Identify three causes of apnea.
3. Describe the pathogenesis of apnea in the premature infant.
4. Describe the evaluation process for the infant with apnea.
5. Discuss management techniques for controlling apnea.
6. Discuss the current status of home monitoring.

Apnea represents one of the most frequently encountered respiratory problems in the premature infant. It is not known why some infants are affected and others are not, although certain factors have a good predictive value. Apnea in the term infant is not ever a normal finding and must always be investigated. In the preterm infant, apnea that presents in the first 24 hours has historically been perceived as pathologic, whereas that occurring later has most often been attributed to immaturity. The mechanism of action is not fully understood but can be characterized as an immature respiratory system faced with demands it is ill equipped to handle. This chapter will provide a comprehensive review of apnea of the premature infant, including causes, evaluation, treatment, and long-term home follow-up.

DEFINITIONS OF APNEA

A. Periodic breathing.

1. Definition: recurrent sequences of pauses in respiration lasting 5 to 10 seconds followed by 10 to 15 seconds of rapid respiration (Miller et al., 2002).
2. Seen in less than 2% of well term infants and in 30% to 95% of healthy preterm infants more than 24 hours of age.
3. Not accompanied by cyanosis or changes in heart rate.
4. Episodes of periodic breathing in the preterm infant decrease significantly by 39 to 41 weeks' postconception age (Razi et al., 2002).
5. Controversy exists as to whether periodic breathing is associated with significant apnea or sudden infant death syndrome (SIDS). Recent studies suggest that periodic breathing is not associated with these two entities (Miller and Martin, 1998).

B. Apnea.

1. Definition: cessation of respiration for at least 10 to 15 seconds, frequently complicated by cyanosis, pallor, hypotonia, or bradycardia (Miller et al., 2002).
2. Most apnea occurs in the healthy preterm infant without organic disease. Up to 80% of infants weighing less than 1000 g and 25% weighing less than 2500 g at birth will have apnea during their neonatal course (Miller and Martin, 1998).

TYPES OF APNEA

A. **Primary apnea.**
   1. Definition: initial cessation of respiratory movements after a period of rapid respiratory effort as a result of asphyxia during the delivery process.
   2. Exposure to stimulation and/or oxygen will usually induce spontaneous respiratory effort.

B. **Secondary apnea.**
   1. Definition: apnea occurring after a period of deep, gasping respirations, and fall in blood pressure and heart rate, brought about by prolonged asphyxia during the delivery process. The gasping becomes slower and weaker and then ceases.
   2. Infant will not respond to stimulation and will require more vigorous resuscitation.
   3. For each minute in secondary apnea before resuscitation, there is a 2-minute delay before gasping is reestablished and another 2 minutes before the onset of regular respirations.
   4. It is not usually possible to distinguish primary from secondary apnea at birth (Kattwinkel, 2000).

C. **Central apnea.**
   1. Definition: absence of airflow and respiratory effort.
   2. Cause of central apnea in the preterm infant is not fully understood.
   3. Contributing factors are thought to include (Miller and Martin, 1998):
      a. Chest wall afferent neuromuscular signals and chest wall instability.
      b. Diaphragmatic fatigue.
      c. Immature, paradoxic response of neonate to hypoxia and hypercapnia.
      d. Altered levels of local neurotransmitters in brain stem region of the central nervous system (CNS).
   4. Fifteen percent of apnea episodes are central in origin.
   5. Closure of upper airway occurs in about half of cases of central apnea.

D. **Obstructive apnea.**
   1. Definition: absence of airflow with continued respiratory effort, associated with blockage of airway at level of pharynx and/or larynx (Miller and Martin, 1998).
   2. Hyperextension or flexion of the neck may induce obstruction of the airway.
   3. May be caused by obstruction of airflow at the mouth or nose as a result of anatomic abnormalities such as macroglossia (Beckwith-Wiedemann syndrome, congenital hypothyroidism) or micrognathia (Pierre Robin syndrome).
   4. Up to 30% of apnea episodes are obstructive in origin.

E. **Mixed apnea.**
   1. Definition: a combination of central and obstructive apnea, obstruction usually at the level of the pharynx.
   2. Fifty to sixty percent of neonatal apnea episodes are mixed.

F. **Idiopathic apnea, or *apnea of prematurity*.**
   1. Diagnosis after exclusion of pathologic processes in the premature infant.
   2. Not necessarily associated with the presence of periodic breathing.
   3. Recurrent apnea seen in preterm infants who show no other abnormalities.
   4. Onset within the first week of life, usually at 24 to 48 hours. If not present within the first week of life, will usually not appear unless later illness develops.
   5. More likely to be obstructive than central in the first 2 days of life.
   6. Episodes of apnea cease by term in 95% of infants: may persist longer in infants born at less than 28 weeks' gestational age (Eichenwald et al., 1997).

PATHOGENESIS OF APNEA IN THE PREMATURE INFANT

A. Immature central respiratory center.

1. Decreased afferent traffic occurs as a result of:
   a. Poor CNS myelinization.
   b. Decreased number of synapses.
   c. Decreased dendritic arborization (Miller and Martin, 1998).
2. Decreased amounts of neurotransmitters have been measured in infants with apnea and may play an important role in respiratory control (Kattwinkel, 1977).
3. Fluctuating respiratory center output has been implicated.

B. Chemoreceptors.

1. Located in the medulla (central) and the carotid and aortic bodies (peripheral), chemoreceptors relay information to the respiratory center in the brain regarding pH, Po_2, and Pco_2 via the vagus and glossopharyngeal nerves.
   a. Hypoxemia is sensed in the carotid and aortic bodies and results in an increase in alveolar ventilation. Premature infants with apnea do not respond to hypoxemia as effectively as infants who do not have apnea (Miller et al., 2002).
   b. Hypercapnia is sensed centrally. The normal response to an increased arterial Pco_2 is an increase in minute ventilation. Neonates can increase ventilation by only three or four times the baseline values, in comparison with the 10- to 20-fold increase that adults can obtain. Premature infants exhibit a blunted response to elevated Pco_2, resulting in ongoing hypoventilation and hypercapnia. This diminished response predisposes them to apnea (Forster et al., 2000).
2. Biphasic response of the premature infant to hypoxia.
   a. During the first minute of hypoxia, a brief increase in respiratory effort occurs. It is followed in the next 2 to 3 minutes by a decrease in respiratory rate and by periodic breathing, respiratory depression, and apnea. Initial stimulation of the peripheral chemoreceptors is followed by overriding depression of the respiratory centers as a result of hypoxia (Martin et al., 1998).
   b. At 7 to 18 days of postnatal age, an infant can maintain the adult response to hypoxia of sustained hyperventilation.
3. Depressed response to hypercapnia. The premature infant exhibits decreased sensitivity to increased levels of carbon dioxide, requiring higher levels of carbon dioxide to stimulate respirations (Miller and Martin, 1998).

C. Thermal afferents.

1. Apnea is increased in an environment that may be too warm for the infant (Bader et al., 1998).
2. Thermal receptors in the trigeminal area of the face produce an apneic response to stimulation by a cold gas mixture.

D. Mechanoreceptors.

1. Stretch receptors alter the timing of respiration at various lung volumes.
   a. Head's paradoxic reflex: a gasp followed by apnea after abrupt lung inflation.
   b. Hering-Breuer reflex.
      (1) Vagally mediated, it acts to inhibit inspiration and/or prolong expiration.
      (2) Lung inflation initiates inhibitory impulses that terminate inspiration and prolong expiratory time.
      (3) Mechanoreceptors are very active in the neonate but rarely seen in the adult (Weintraub et al., 2001).
2. Pharyngeal collapse and airway obstruction are produced by negative pharyngeal pressure generated during inspiration.

3. Intercostal phrenic inhibitory reflex, an inward movement of the ribcage during inspiration, prematurely ends inspiration (Miller and Martin, 1998).

E. **Protective reflexes.**
1. Stimulation of the posterior portion of the pharynx with suctioning, endotracheal or gavage tube placement, or gastroesophageal reflux can stimulate apnea.
2. Pulmonary irritant receptors can produce an apneic response to direct bronchial stimulation.
3. Laryngeal taste receptors can produce an apneic response to various chemical stimuli (Kattwinkel, 1977).

F. **Sleep state.**
1. Eighty percent of the neonate's day is spent in sleep.
2. Respiratory depression occurs predominantly in rapid eye movement (REM) or transitional sleep (Miller et al., 2002).
   a. May be influenced by central mechanisms at the level of the brainstem.
      (1) May be due to a defect in a sleep-related feedback loop or respiratory command.
      (2) Variability of respiratory rhythmicity is seen in active sleep (Miller and Martin, 1998).
   b. May be related to paradoxic respirations in which chest wall movements are out of phase, resulting in ribcage collapse with abdominal expansion during inspiration. This would lead to a decrease in lung volume and functional residual capacity.
   c. May be related to decreased skeletal muscle tone of the tongue and pharynx during sleep, which could lead to increased resistance and obstruction in the upper airway (Miller and Martin, 1998).

CAUSES OF APNEA

A. **Prematurity.**

B. **Hypoxia.**

C. **Respiratory disorders.**
1. Respiratory distress syndrome.
2. Pneumonia.
3. Aspiration.
4. Acidosis.
5. Airway obstruction.
6. Pneumothorax.
7. Atelectasis.
8. Pulmonary hemorrhage.
9. Postextubation status.
10. Congenital anomalies of the upper airway.

D. **Cardiovascular disorders.**
1. Hypotension.
2. Arrhythmias.
3. Congestive heart failure.
4. Patent ductus arteriosus.

E. **Infection.**
1. Sepsis.
2. Pneumonia.
3. Meningitis.
4. Viral infections.
5. Necrotizing enterocolitis.

F. **CNS disorders.**
  1. Congenital malformations.
  2. Seizures.
  3. Asphyxia.
  4. Intracranial hemorrhage.
  5. Kernicterus.
  6. Tumors.

G. **Drugs.**
  1. Maternal drugs.
    a. Narcotics.
    b. Analgesics.
    c. Anesthesia.
    d. β-blocker antihypertensive agents.
    e. Magnesium sulfate.
  2. Neonatal drugs.
    a. Anticonvulsants: phenobarbital, pentobarbital.
    b. Cardiovascular drugs: prostaglandin E_1.
    c. Narcotics/analgesics.
      (1) Fentanyl (Sublimaze).
      (2) Morphine.
      (3) Midazolam hydrochloride (Versed).
      (4) Lorazepam (Ativan).

H. **Metabolic disorders.**
  1. Hypocalcemia.
  2. Hypoglycemia.
  3. Hypomagnesemia.
  4. Hyponatremia.
  5. Acidosis.
  6. Hyperammonemia.

I. **Hematopoietic disorders.**
  1. Polycythemia.
  2. Anemia.

J. **Reflex stimulation.**
  1. Posterior pharyngeal stimulation.
  2. Gastroesophageal reflux.

K. **Environmental factors.**
  1. Rapid warming.
  2. Hypothermia.
  3. Hyperthermia.
  4. Elevated environmental temperature.
  5. Feeding.
  6. Stooling.
  7. Painful stimuli.

EVALUATION FOR APNEA

A. **History.**
  1. Perinatal risk factors.
    a. Maternal bleeding, drugs, fever, hypertension, prolonged rupture of membranes, polyhydramnios, chorioamnionitis, decreased fetal movements, abnormal fetal presentation.
    b. Fetal hypoxia, trauma.

2. Neonatal risk factors.
   a. Prematurity.
   b. Cardiorespiratory disease.
   c. Metabolic abnormalities.
   d. Temperature instability.
   e. Infection.
   f. Environmental causes.
   g. CNS disorders.

B. **Physical examination.** A complete physical and neurologic examination should be performed. Observe for congenital malformations, especially those involving the airway. Observe for signs of respiratory distress and heart disease. Abnormal behavior, tone, or posturing may be associated with a neurologic focus. An abdominal examination should be performed, which may reveal symptoms related to obstruction, infection, necrotizing enterocolitis, or congestive heart failure.

C. **Documentation of apnea episodes.** A record of apnea episodes should be maintained as part of the infant's record. This allows the caregiver to determine a pattern, if any, to the apnea. It may also provide information about precipitating events or specific events associated with the apnea. Information documented should include the following:
   1. Duration of apnea episode.
   2. Time of apnea episode and any relation to feeding, activity, stooling, sleep, or procedures.
   3. Infant's position: prone or supine, with head of bed elevated or flat.
   4. Associated bradycardia.
   5. Associated color change and/or oxygen desaturation.
   6. Type of stimulation required to resolve the episode:
      a. None, self-resolved.
      b. Gentle tactile stimulation.
      c. Vigorous tactile stimulation.
      d. Oxygen.
      e. Bag-mask ventilation.

D. **Laboratory evaluation.**
   1. Basic evaluation to look for infection, respiratory deterioration, and metabolic problems.
      a. Complete blood cell count, with differential cell and platelet counts.
      b. Blood gas.
      c. Serum glucose, electrolytes, calcium.
      d. Blood culture, lumbar puncture for evaluation of cerebrospinal fluid, urine culture.
   2. Extensive laboratory evaluation for less common causes of apnea.
      a. Toxicology screen.
      b. Urine collection for detection of amino acids and organic acids (metabolic screen).
      c. Serum ammonia.

E. **Other.**
   1. Echocardiogram or electrocardiogram: may detect cardiac abnormality or conduction disorders.
   2. Electroencephalogram: may confirm suspected seizures.
   3. Chest x-ray film: may demonstrate respiratory or cardiac abnormalities.
   4. Cranial ultrasound/computed tomography: may demonstrate structural abnormalities or hemorrhages.

5. Barium swallow and pH study: to evaluate pharyngeal function or gastroesophageal reflux.
6. Polysomnogram: examines eye movements, muscle activity, end-tidal CO_2, transcutaneous O_2 levels, oral or nasal airway, chest and abdominal wall movements, and cardiorespiratory patterns to detect type of apnea and relate it to sleep state. (Very rarely used.)
7. Pneumogram.
   a. Measures chest wall movement, heart rate, oxygen saturation, and nasal airflow by thermistor or carbon dioxide probe; measures esophageal pH.
   b. No predictive value for SIDS; newer recording monitors are as effective at detecting apnea over a prolonged period (Gibson et al., 1996; National Institutes of Health [NIH], 1986).

MANAGEMENT TECHNIQUES

A. **Treat underlying cause if determined.**
B. **Provide needed medical or surgical intervention.**
C. **Maintain environmental temperature at the low end of the neutral thermal zone.**
D. **Avoid triggering reflexes:**
   1. Vigorous catheter suctioning.
   2. Hot or cold to the face.
   3. Sudden gastric distention.
E. **Maintain infant in the prone position whenever possible.** Prone positioning is associated with higher oxygen saturation, shorter gastric emptying time, and decreased incidence of regurgitation and aspiration. Supine positioning has been associated with an increase in apnea and severity of apneic episode. Elevation of the head of the bed by 15 degrees reduces hypoxemic events in preterm infants (Jenni et al., 1997).
F. **Maintain the neck in a neutral position,** not flexed or hyperextended. Use of a neck roll is recommended.
G. **Avoid vigorous manual ventilation** to prevent intermittent hyperoxia, hypocapnia, and blunting of the CO_2 response.
H. **Attempt to control apnea by avoiding painful stimuli, loud noises, extremely vigorous tactile stimulation, or potent odors.** No evidence supports effectiveness of kinesthetic stimulation in reduction of apnea (Henderson-Smart and Osborn, 2002).
I. **Consider providing continuous positive airway pressure.**
   1. Increases end-expiratory lung volumes and splints the upper airway and weak chest wall, thereby improving compliance and oxygenation and decreasing respiratory muscle work so that diaphragmatic movements are less tiring and more effective (Barrington et al., 2001).
   2. Complicates gavage feedings and may increase risk of aspiration. Increases risk of air leak.
   3. Nasal intermittent positive-pressure ventilation (IPPV) may be helpful in infants whose apnea is severe and not well controlled on nasal continuous positive airway pressure (CPAP) alone (Lemyre et al., 2002).
J. **Pharmacologic therapy.**
   1. Methylxanthine (aminophylline/theophylline, caffeine), administered orally or intravenously. Used to treat apnea of prematurity after pathologic causes have been eliminated.
      a. Mechanisms of action include:
         (1) Stimulation of central respiratory chemoreceptors.
         (2) Increased ventilatory response to carbon dioxide.

(3) Increased oxygenation.
(4) Increased minute ventilation (theophylline).
(5) Stabilization of oscillations in breathing (theophylline).
(6) Improved diaphragmatic contractility.
(7) Relaxation of bronchial smooth muscle (theophylline).
(8) CNS excitation.
(9) Increased respiratory drive.
(10) Increased respiratory muscle activity.
(11) Increased skeletal muscle activity.

b. Pharmacokinetics.
(1) Half-life of aminophylline/theophylline is approximately 30 hours.
(2) Half-life of caffeine is approximately 100 hours.
(3) Both theophylline and caffeine are rapidly absorbed intravenously. Oral absorption of caffeine is rapid, and oral absorption of theophylline is variable.
(4) Metabolism of caffeine and theophylline takes place in the liver. This is slower in the neonate than in the adult.
(5) Theophylline is metabolized to caffeine by a metabolic pathway unique to the preterm infant.
(6) Serum concentrations must be checked to avoid toxic levels.

c. Dosage:
(1) Aminophylline.
(a) Route: intravenous (IV).
(b) Loading dose: 5 mg/kg.
(c) Maintenance dose: 1 to 2 mg/kg every 8 to 12 hours.
(d) Therapeutic level: 5 to 15 μg/ml.
(2) Theophylline.
(a) Route: by mouth.
(b) Loading dose: 5 mg/kg.
(c) Maintenance dose: 1 to 2 mg/kg every 8 to 12 hours.
(d) Therapeutic level: 5 to 15 μg/ml.
(3) Caffeine.
(a) Route: IV or by mouth.
(b) Loading dose: 10 mg/kg, caffeine base; 20 mg/kg, caffeine citrate.
(c) Maintenance dose: 2.5 mg/kg, caffeine base; 5 mg/kg, caffeine citrate; every 24 hours.
(d) Avoid use of caffeine benzoate preparation, which can displace bilirubin from albumin binding sites (Ahlfors, 2001).
(e) Therapeutic level: 5 to 20 μg/ml.
(f) Higher doses and therapeutic levels have been studied, with no reported adverse effects, but not in common use (Lee et al., 1997).

d. Side effects.
(1) Caffeine: tachycardia, cardiac dysrhythmias, increased wakefulness, increased active sleep, gastrointestinal distention, gastrointestinal bleeding, and diuresis with sodium loss.
(2) Theophylline: tachycardia, cardiac dysrhythmias, seizures, jitteriness, feeding intolerance, gastroesophageal reflux, dehydration, hyperglycemia, hypotension, increased cerebrovascular resistance (Hochwald et al., 2002).

e. Caffeine versus theophylline.
(1) Theophylline is a more potent vasodilator.
(2) Theophylline causes a more rapid and sustained tachycardia.
(3) Caffeine diffuses more rapidly in the CNS.

(4) Caffeine is given only once a day.
(5) Caffeine has a wider therapeutic index.
(6) Caffeine may be effective in apnea not responsive to theophylline and vice versa.
(7) Caffeine has a longer half-life, resulting in smaller changes in its plasma concentration.
(8) Based on higher therapeutic ratio, more reliable enteral absorption and longer half-life caffeine is recommended over theophylline for treatment of apnea of prematurity. Effectiveness over placebo demonstrated in multicenter, randomized controlled study (Comer et al., 2001; Erenberg et al., 2000).

2. Doxapram.
a. Potent respiratory stimulant for apnea refractory to methylxanthine therapy.
b. Mechanism of action thought to be stimulation of the peripheral chemoreceptors at low doses (0.5 mg/kg/hour) and of the CNS at higher doses (Blanchard and Aranda, 1986; Brion et al., 1991).
c. Increases minute ventilation, tidal volume, and mean inspiratory flow and decreases PCO_2.
d. Pharmacokinetics.
(1) Half-life is approximately 10 hours in the first few days of life and 8 hours at 10 days of age.
(2) Steady-state levels are reached within 24 hours.
e. Dosage.
(1) Route: IV.
(2) Dosage range: 0.25 to 2.5 mg/kg/hour, administered by continuous infusion (Yamazaki et al., 2001).
(3) Controversy exists over therapeutic and toxic plasma levels. Guidelines include the following:
(a) Therapeutic level: less than 5 mg/L.
(b) Toxic level: 5 mg/L. Levels greater than 3.5 mg/L may produce side effects (Yamazaki et al., 2001).
f. Side effects.
(1) Jitteriness, irritability, vomiting, seizures, abdominal distention, increased gastric residuals, hyperglycemia, and glycosuria.
(2) Hypertension, tachycardia, and increased cardiac output.
(3) Increased work of breathing resulting from respiratory stimulation; consequent increased oxygen consumption and carbon dioxide production; increased tidal volume and respiratory rate.
(4) Increased risk of intraventricular hemorrhage if used in first few days of life.
g. Contraindication: use in newborn infant not recommended because preparation contains benzyl alcohol.
(1) Benzyl alcohol is associated with "gasping syndrome," characterized by metabolic acidosis, renal failure, liver failure, and cardiovascular collapse (Ahlfors, 2001).
(2) Cumulative doses might be toxic for the liver, kidney, or brain (Miller and Martin, 1998; Sreenan et al., 2001).
(3) Insufficient data exist on clinical benefit and long-term effects, therefore is infrequently used.

K. Assisted ventilation. Used for apnea resistant to other methods of therapy.

HOME MONITORING

A. **Effectiveness of home monitoring.** The Consensus Development Conference Statement on Infant Apnea and Home Monitoring (NIH, 1986) states that cardiorespiratory monitoring is effective in preventing death from apnea for certain selected infants but is clearly inappropriate for others, with the primary objective being to serve the best interest of the infant based on the infant's history.

B. **Indications for home monitoring.**
   1. Premature infant with symptoms of idiopathic apnea of prematurity who is otherwise ready for hospital discharge.
   2. A survivor of an apparent life-threatening event (ALTE) defined as apnea, cyanosis, altered muscle tone, choking, or gagging.
   3. Having two or more siblings with SIDS.
   4. Tracheostomy.
   5. A sleep apnea syndrome caused by a neurologic disorder, periodic breathing, upper airway abnormality, or idiopathic syndromes.
   6. Other conditions of ill or high-risk infants, as determined on an individual basis.

C. **Home monitoring is not indicated in** prevention of SIDS in symptom-free, healthy infants (American Academy of Pediatrics [AAP], 2000).

D. **Monitoring technology.**
   1. Transthoracic impedance combined with electrocardiography is current standard.
      a. Electrodes are placed on infant's chest or inside an adjustable belt worn around the chest.
      b. A small electric current passes between the electrodes. The impedance to this current is measured as the chest wall diameter changes. Monitor senses this change, which is equated with respiration.
      c. Electrocardiograph reads cardiac activity.
      d. High and low limits for respirations and heart rate are set by the clinician.
      e. Monitor is compact and portable, weighing less than 5 pounds. A battery pack is available for use outside the home.
   2. Technical problems include artifact from signal interference, false alarms caused by shallow breathing, and the monitor's inability to detect obstructive apnea. Incorrect placement of leads can result in false alarms as well.
   3. Recent advances in technology allow recording of home monitor events for evaluation by the clinician.
      a. Recording of events allows monitoring of compliance.
      b. True events can be distinguished from false alarms.
      c. Fewer rehospitalizations are needed.
      d. Recording is as sensitive as a pneumogram for evaluating whether monitoring can be discontinued.
      e. Fewer monitor days are needed for infants without events.

E. **Follow-up care.**
   1. Multidisciplinary team includes physician, nurse, social worker, and equipment company representatives.
   2. Family and other caretakers of the infant are trained in cardiopulmonary resuscitation before hospital discharge. Thorough education in use of the monitor is also provided before discharge.

3. Care includes close telephone contact—within 24 hours after discharge and every week to 2 weeks afterward as needed.
4. Visiting nurse makes home visit within the first week and then as needed.
5. A team member is available 24 hours a day for answering questions and solving problems. Equipment company representative is available as needed for problems and information.
6. Home follow-up does not replace clinic visits.
7. In 80% of infants apnea of prematurity will cease between 40 and 44 weeks' postconceptual age; in asymptomatic infants home monitoring can be stopped at 45 weeks' postconceptual age (Tauman and Sivan, 2000).

REFERENCES

Ahlfors, C.E.: Benzyl alcohol, kernicterus, and unbound bilirubin. *Journal of Pediatrics, 139*(2):317-319, 2001.

American Academy of Pediatrics: Policy Statement: Changing Concepts of Sudden Infant Death Syndrome: Implications for Infant Sleeping Environment and Sleep Position (RE9946). *Pediatrics, 105*(3): 650-656, 2000.

Bader, D., Tirosh, E., Hodgins, H., et al.: Effect of increased environmental temperature on breathing patterns in preterm and term infants. *Journal of Perinatology, 18*(1):5-8, 1998.

Barrington, K., Bull, D., and Finer, N.: Randomized trial of nasal synchronized intermittent mandatory ventilation compared with continuous positive airway pressure after extubation of very low birth weight infants. *Pediatrics, 107*(4):638-641, 2001.

Blanchard, P.W. and Aranda, J.V.: Drug treatment of neonatal apnea. *Perinatology-Neonatology, 10*(2):21-28, 1986.

Brion, L.P., Vega-Rich, C., Reinersman, G., and Roth, P.: Low-dose doxapram for apnea unresponsive to aminophylline in very low birth weight infants. *Journal of Perinatology, 11*(4):359-364, 1991.

Comer, A.M., Perry, C.M., and Figgitt, D.P.: Caffeine citrate: A review of its use in apnoea of prematurity. *Paediatric Drugs, 3*(1):61-79, 2001.

Eichenwald, E.C., Aina, A., and Stark, A.R.: Apnea frequently persists beyond term gestation in infants delivered at 24-28 weeks. *Pediatrics, 100*(3 Part 1):354-359, 1997.

Erenberg, A., Leff, R.D., Haack, D.G., et al.: Caffeine citrate for the treatment of apnea of prematurity: A double blind, placebo-controlled study. *Pharmacotherapy, 20*(6):644-652, 2000.

Forster, H.V., Pan, L.G., Lowry, T.F, et al.: Important role of carotid chemoreceptor afferents in control of breathing of adult and neonatal mammals. *Respiration Physiology, 119*(2-3):199-208, 2000.

Gibson, E., Spinner, S., Cullen, J.A., et al.: Documented home apnea monitoring: Effect of compliance, duration of monitoring, and validation of alarm reporting. *Clinical Pediatrics, 35*(10):505-513, 1996.

Henderson-Smart, D.J. and Osborn, D.A.: Kinesthetic stimulation for preventing apnea in preterm infants. *Cochrane Database of Systematic Reviews, 92*(2): CD000373, 2002.

Hochwald, C., Kennedy, K., Chang, J., and Moya, F.: A randomized, controlled, double-blind trial comparing two loading doses of aminophylline. *Journal of Perinatology, 22*(4):275-278, 2002.

Jenni, O.G., von Siebenthal, K., Wolf, M., et al.: Effect of nursing in the head-elevated tilt position (15 degrees) on the incidence of bradycardic and hypoxemic episodes in preterm infants. *Pediatrics, 100*(4):622-625, 1997.

Kattwinkel, J.: Neonatal apnea: Pathogenesis and therapy. *Journal of Pediatrics, 90*(3): 342-347, 1977.

Kattwinkel, J.: *Textbook of neonatal resuscitation* (4th ed.). Elk Grove Village, IL, 2000, American Academy of Pediatrics and American Heart Association.

Lee, T.C., Charles, B., Steer, P., et al.: Population pharmacokinetics of intravenous caffeine in neonates with apnea of prematurity. *Clinical Pharmacology and Therapeutics, 61*(6):628-640, 1997.

Lemyre, B., Davis, P.G., dePaoli, A.G.: Nasal intermittent positive pressure ventilation (NIPPV) versus nasal continuous positive airway pressure (NCPAP) for apnea of prematurity. *Cochrane Database of Systematic Reviews*, (1), CD002272, 2002.

Martin, R.J., DiFiore, J.M., Jana, L., et al.: Persistence of the biphasic ventilatory response to hypoxia in preterm infants. *Journal of Pediatrics, 132*(6):960-964, 1998.

Miller, M. and Martin, R.: Pathophysiology of apnea of prematurity. In R. Polin and W. Fox (Eds.): *Fetal and neonatal physiology* (2nd ed.). Philadelphia, 1998, Saunders, pp. 1129-1140.

Miller, M.J., Fanaroff, A.A., and Martin, R.: Respiratory disorders in preterm and term infants. In A. Fanaroff and R. Martin (Eds.): *Neonatal-perinatal medicine: Diseases of the fetus and infant* (7th ed.). St Louis, 2002, Mosby, pp. 1038-1043.

National Institutes of Health: Consensus Development Conference Statement on Infant Apnea and Home Monitoring. *NIH Consensus Statement*, *6*(6):1-10, 1986.

Razi, N., M., DeLauter, M., and Pandit, P. B.: Periodic breathing and oxygen saturation in preterm infants at discharge. *Journal of Perinatology*, *22*(6):442-444, 2002.

Sreenan, C., Etches, P.C., Demianczuk, N., and Robertson, CM.: Isolated mental developmental delay in very low birth weight infants: Association with prolonged doxapram therapy for apnea. *Journal of Pediatrics, 139*(6):832-837, 2001.

Tauman, R. and Sivan, Y.: Duration of home 1991 monitoring for infants discharged with apnea of prematurity. *Biology of the Neonate, 78*(3):168-173, 2000.

Weintraub, Z., Cates, D., Kwiatkowski, K., et al.: The morphology of periodic breathing in infants and adults. *Respiration Physiology, 127*(2-3):173-184, 2001.

Yamazaki, T., Kajiwara, M., Itahashi, K., and Fujumura, M.: Low dose doxapram therapy for idiopathic apnea of prematurity. *Pediatrics International, 43*(2):124-127, 2001.

CHAPTER

25 Assisted Ventilation

DEBBIE FRASER ASKIN AND WILLIAM DIEHL-JONES

OBJECTIVES

1. Identify the concepts of FRC, VT, VC, and TLC and describe their importance in the physiology of ventilation.
2. Describe the concepts of elastic recoil, compliance, resistance, and gas trapping and their importance in ventilating the lungs of the newborn infant.
3. Explain the relationship of fetal hemoglobin, pH, and temperature to the oxyhemoglobin dissociation curve.
4. List potential causes of respiratory and metabolic acid-base disturbance in the newborn infant. Identify ranges of pH, Pao_2, $Paco_2$, HCO_3^-, and base excess/deficit in various respiratory disease states in the newborn infant.
5. Identify treatment modalities for neonates in respiratory distress.
6. Describe various types of mechanical ventilation devices available for the neonate.
7. List nursing interventions required to care for ventilated infants, based on the theories of mechanical ventilation.
8. Differentiate among the three types of high-frequency ventilation: jet, oscillatory, and high-frequency positive-pressure ventilation.
9. Identify the nursing interventions required for high-frequency ventilation that differ from those required for conventional ventilation.
10. Identify changes in patient status that indicate potential complications with assisted ventilation.
11. Describe various medications used to enhance lung status in the ventilated patient.

Caring for an infant requiring assisted ventilation is a challenge. It is necessary for the nurse to understand the normal pulmonary physiology as well as the pathophysiology of pulmonary diseases in the neonate. An understanding of the basic mechanical principles of various ventilators is important to providing optimal care for a neonate. New ventilation techniques are being developed rapidly, and the choices for ventilating the neonate are greater now than ever before. The focus of this chapter is to provide the basic knowledge needed to care for the infant requiring oxygen therapy or mechanical ventilation.

PHYSIOLOGY

A. Definitions (Blackburn, 2003).

1. Tidal volume (VT): the amount of air that moves into or out of the lungs with each single breath at rest (6 ml/kg).
2. Vital capacity (VC): the volume of air maximally inspired and maximally expired (40 ml/kg).
3. Functional residual capacity (FRC): the volume of gas that remains in the lungs after a normal expiration (30 ml/kg).

4. Total lung capacity (TLC): the amount of air contained in the lung after a maximal inspiration (63 ml/kg).
5. Physiologic dead space: anatomic plus alveolar dead space (Loper, 1997).
   a. Anatomic dead space: the volume of gas within the area of the pulmonary conducting airways that cannot engage in gas exchange.
   b. Alveolar dead space: the volume of inspired gas that reaches the alveoli but does not participate in gas exchange because of inadequate perfusion to those alveoli.
6. Mechanical dead space: gas that fills the ventilator circuit for availability in inspiration, as well as exhaled gas. Minimal dead space is desirable. Excessive dead space can cause increased retention of carbon dioxide.

B. Concepts.

1. Elastic recoil: the natural tendency for a stretched object to return to the original resting volume. With inhalation, alveoli stretch to a certain point, and during exhalation the alveoli return to their original size in an infant with normal lungs.
2. Lung compliance: the change in volume that occurs with a change in pressure (elasticity of the lung). It also refers to the relationship between a given change in volume and the pressure required to produce that change. An infant with severe hyaline membrane disease will have decreased compliance (because of lack of surfactant) requiring increased pressure to overcome the resistance generated by the surface tension in the alveoli. The major force contributing to elastic recoil of the lung is surface tension at the air-liquid interface in distal bronchioles and alveoli. The amount of distal airway pressure needed to counteract the tendency of the alveoli and bronchioles to collapse is demonstrated by the Laplace relationship: the relationship between pressure, surface tension, and the radius of a structure. The pressure needed to stabilize an alveolus is directly proportional to twice the surface tension and inversely proportional to the radius of that alveolus.
3. Lung resistance: the result of friction between moving parts. It refers to the relationship between a given change in pressure and a given change in flow. An increase in airway resistance increases the time needed for air to reach the alveoli (Hodson and Truog, 1999). High rates of airflow increase airway resistance by creating turbulence. Resistance to gas in a 2.5-mm endotracheal tube (ETT) is higher than in a 3.5-mm ETT because of the narrow lumen of the smaller tube. It takes greater pressure to force air through a small tube. Anatomic sources of resistance in the newborn infant include nasal passages, the glottis, the trachea, and the main bronchi. During intubation the ETT is also a source of resistance.
4. Gas trapping: more gas entering the lung than leaving the lung. A partially occluded ETT can cause gas trapping. Debris from meconium can allow gas into the lung but may occlude the airway during exhalation (known as a ball-valve effect).
5. Inadvertent positive end-expiratory pressure (PEEP): a result of gas trapping in which volume and pressure increase in the distal airways through end expiration. Providing oxygen by nasal cannula can result in inadvertent PEEP in the small premature infant.
6. Ventilation-perfusion ratio ($\dot{V}A/\dot{Q}C$) (Fig. 25-1). Matching pulmonary ventilation and perfusion is necessary for efficient gas exchange. The relationship between ventilation and perfusion is expressed as a ratio and describes the relationship between alveolar ventilation and capillary perfusion of the lungs. A 1:1 ratio indicates that the alveoli are in perfect

contact with the pulmonary capillaries, allowing exchange of O_2 and CO_2. A $\dot{V}_A/\dot{Q}_C$ ratio of zero indicates a shunt whereby no ventilation occurs during passage of blood through the lungs. Abnormalities of the $\dot{V}_A/\dot{Q}_C$ ratio may be due to:

a. Too little ventilation with normal blood flow.
b. Too little blood flow with normal ventilation.
c. Combination of the above.

7. Mean airway pressure (MAP): mean or average pressure transmitted to the airways throughout an entire respiratory cycle (Hagedorn et al., 2002).

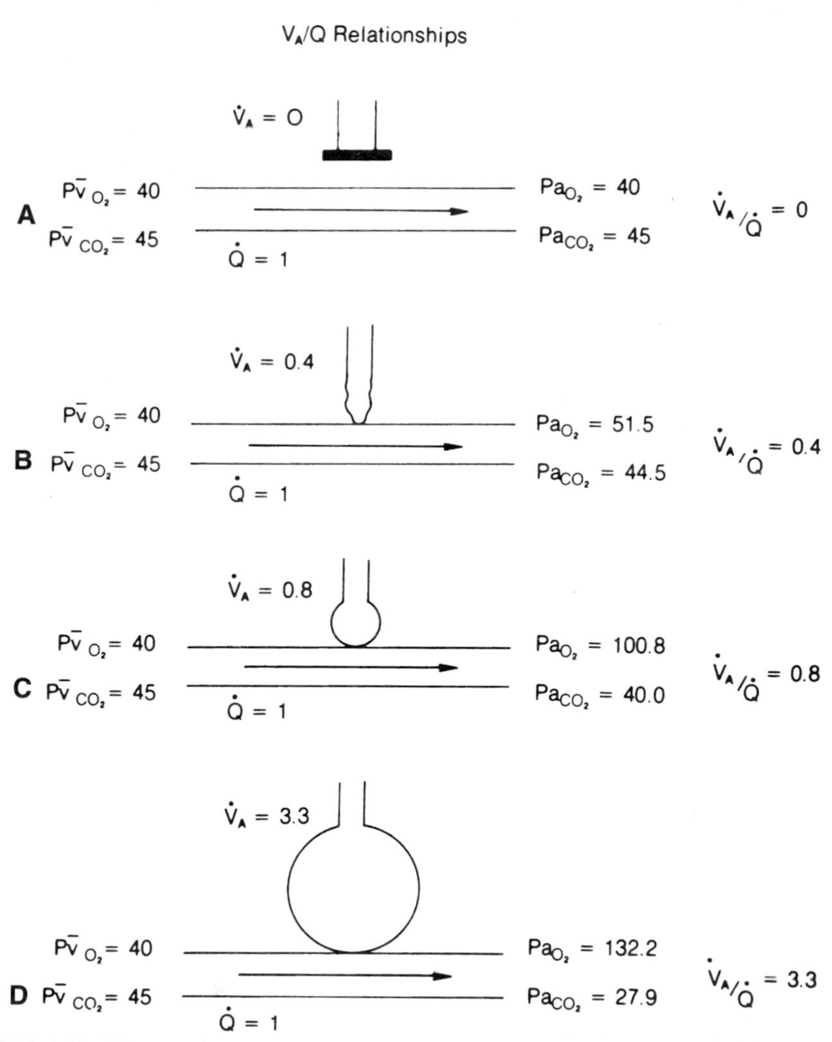

FIGURE 25-1 ■ Effects of various ventilation-perfusion ratios on blood gas tensions. **A,** Direct venoarterial shunting ($\dot{V}_A/\dot{Q} = 0$). Venous gas tensions are unaltered, and arterial blood has the same tension as venous blood. **B,** Alveolus with a low $\dot{V}_A/\dot{Q}$ ratio. Only partial oxygenation and CO_2 removal take place in this alveolus because of underventilation in relation to perfusion. **C,** Normal alveolus. **D,** Underperfused alveolus with high $\dot{V}_A/\dot{Q}$ ratio. Note that although the oxygen tension is 32 mm greater than alveolus (C), this results in only a slightly higher saturation and O_2 content. (From Thibeault, D.W. and Gregory, G.A.: *Neonatal pulmonary care.* Norwalk, CT, 1986, Appleton-Century-Crofts.)

MAP is dependent on the ventilator rate, gas flow through the ventilator circuit, peak inspiratory pressure (PIP), PEEP, and inspiratory time. Increasing MAP can greatly influence the management of respiratory distress in decreasing atelectasis and true intrapulmonary shunting and is a useful tool in determining oxygenation.

8. Permissive hypercapnia: ventilation strategy that allows carbon dioxide levels to remain elevated providing the pH does not fall below 7.25. This strategy is designed to minimize barotrauma by avoiding the use of mechanical ventilation or by using minimal ventilatory rates and pressures.

C. **Oxygen transport.**
1. The amount of oxygen that can be delivered to the tissues is dependent on cardiac output and the oxygen content of the blood.
2. Oxygen is transported to tissue cells bound reversibly to hemoglobin and dissolved in plasma O_2. The amount of O_2 that is dissolved in the plasma is small (0.3 ml of O_2 dissolved in 100 ml of plasma per 100 mm Hg of O_2) compared with the amount that is bound to hemoglobin (1.34 ml of O_2 per gram of 100% saturated hemoglobin).
3. The amount of oxygen carried in the blood by hemoglobin depends on the hemoglobin concentration and the percent saturation of the hemoglobin. Adequate saturation is affected by the amount of hemoglobin available. Hemoglobin is almost fully saturated at a PO_2 of 80 to 100 mm Hg.
4. The binding of oxygen to hemoglobin varies with the PaO_2. The relationship is nonlinear and gives rise to an S-shaped curve—the oxyhemoglobin dissociation curve. The amount of oxygen that combines with hemoglobin at a given PO_2 depends on the position of the hemoglobin-oxygen dissociation curve (Fig. 25-2). Factors that determine the position of the dissociation curve are:
   a. Concentration of 2,3-diphosphoglycerate and the proportion of hemoglobin A (adult) to hemoglobin F (fetal).
   b. Temperature.
   c. PCO_2.
   d. pH.
5. With decreased affinity (shift to the right), hemoglobin releases O_2 more easily to the tissues.
6. With increased affinity (shift to the left), oxygen is unloaded less rapidly and efficiently in the peripheral tissues.

D. **Control of breathing (Hagedorn et al., 2002).** Control of ventilation (Box 25-1) is affected by both neurologic and chemical factors. The neurologic factors include central nervous system (CNS) maturity, sleep state, and reflexes. The chemoreflexes include responses to hypoxemia, hyperoxia, and hypercapnia.

E. **Hypoxia.** Delivery of O_2 to tissues is inadequate. Causes include:
1. Heart failure.
2. Anemia. Hemoglobin available to transport oxygen is reduced although completely saturated. PaO_2 levels are usually normal.
3. Abnormal hemoglobin. O_2 is not released to the tissues.
   a. Methemoglobin.
   b. Bart hemoglobin.
4. Cardiogenic or hypovolemic shock.

F. **Hypoxemia.** O_2 content of arterial blood is low because of extrapulmonary or intrapulmonary shunts. The blood has bypassed adequately ventilated alveoli.
1. Intrapulmonary shunt.
   a. Ventilation-perfusion mismatch caused by lung diseases such as atelectasis, hyaline membrane disease, and pneumonia.

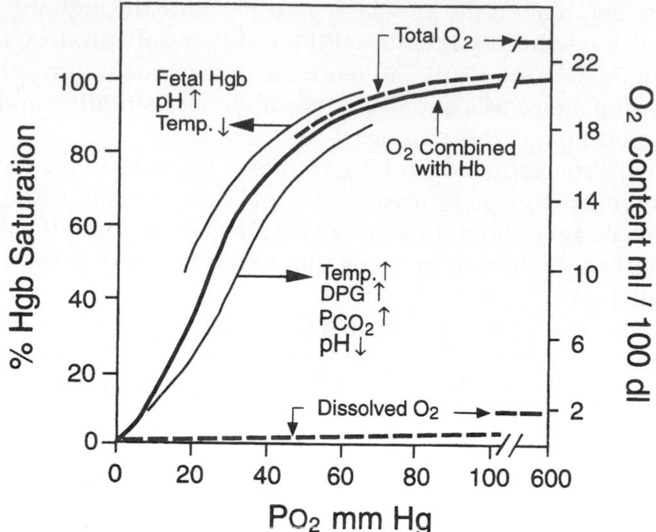

FIGURE 25-2 ■ Hemoglobin-oxygen dissociation curve. Nonlinear or S-shaped oxyhemoglobin curve and the linear or straight-line dissolved O_2 relationships between the O_2 saturation ($Sa{O_2}$) and the $P{O_2}$. Total blood O_2 content is shown with division into a portion combined with hemoglobin and a portion physically dissolved at various levels of $P{O_2}$. Also shown are the major factors that change the O_2 affinity for hemoglobin and thus shift the oxyhemoglobin dissociation curve either to the left or to the right. DPG, 2, 3-diphosphoglycerate. (Modified from West, J.B.: *Respiratory physiology: The essentials* (2nd ed.). Baltimore, 1979, Williams & Wilkins, pp. 71, 73.)

   b. Can occur whenever alveoli are inadequately ventilated (hypoventilation).
2. Extrapulmonary shunt.
   a. Cyanotic congenital heart disease. Abnormal heart structure causes blood to bypass the lungs for oxygenation.
   b. Pulmonary artery hypertension. Blood shunts from the right side of the heart to the left side via a patent foramen ovale or ductus arteriosus, or both, causing blood to bypass the lungs.
      (1) Comparison of the $Pa{O_2}$ or O_2 saturation of preductal and postductal blood can help determine whether a right-to-left shunt is present.
      (2) In the presence of shunting, preductal blood obtained from the right radial artery has a greater than 5% difference in saturation from postductal blood obtained from the umbilical artery or posterior tibial artery.

TREATMENT MODALITIES

A. **Blow-by oxygen.** Free flow of O_2 from a bag and mask or flow of O_2 through O_2 tubing near the infant's face may be useful for short-term O_2 delivery to an infant who is breathing but needs an O_2-enriched atmosphere for oxygenation (i.e., in the delivery room, during caregiving activities, during placement of an intravenous (IV) line into the scalp, during weighing). There is no way to determine the exact content of O_2 delivered to the infant. O_2 content depends on O_2 concentration, flow rate, the distance of the O_2 source from the infant, and the ventilatory efforts of the infant.

BOX 25-1

FACTORS AFFECTING CONTROL OF VENTILATION IN THE SPONTANEOUSLY BREATHING NEONATE

A. Neurologic Factors

1. "Maturity" of the CNS.
   a. Degree of *myelination,* which largely determines speed of impulse transmission and response time to stimuli affecting ventilation.
   b. Degree of *arborization,* or dendritic interconnections (synapses) between neurons, allowing summation of excitatory potentials coming in from other parts of the CNS, and largely setting the neuronal depolarization threshold and response level of the respiratory center.
2. Sleep state (i.e., REM sleep vs. quiet or non-REM sleep).
   a. *REM sleep* is generally associated with irregular respirations (both in depth and frequency), distortion, and paradoxic motion of the ribcage during inspiration, inhibition of Hering-Breuer and glottic closure reflexes, and blunted response to CO_2 changes.
   b. *Quiet sleep* is generally associated with regular respirations, a more stable ribcage, and a directly proportional relationship between Pco_2 and degree of ventilation.
3. Reflex responses.
   a. *Hering-Breuer reflex,* whereby inspiratory duration is limited in response to lung inflation sensed by stretch receptors located in major airways. Not present in adult humans, this reflex is very active during quiet sleep of newborn babies but absent or very weak during REM sleep.
   b. *Head reflex,* whereby inspiratory effort is further increased in response to rapid lung inflation. Thought to produce the frequently observed "biphasic sighs" of newborn infants that may be crucial for promoting and maintaining lung inflation (and therefore breathing regularity) after birth.
   c. *Intercostal-phrenic reflex,* whereby inspiration is inhibited by proprioception (position-sensing) receptors in intercostal muscles responding to distortion of the lower ribcage during REM sleep.
   d. *Trigeminal-cutaneous reflex,* whereby tidal volume increases and respiratory rate decreases in response to facial stimulation.
   e. *Glottic closure reflex,* whereby the glottis is narrowed through reflex contraction of the laryngeal adductor muscles during respiration, "breaking" exhalation and increasing subglottic pressure (as with expiratory "grunting").

B. Chemical Drive Factors (Chemoreflexes)

1. *Response to hypoxemia (falling Pao_2) or to decrease in O_2 concentration breathed* (mediated by peripheral chemoreceptors in carotid and aortic bodies):
   a. Initially there is increase in depth of breathing (tidal volume), but subsequently (if hypoxia persists or worsens), there is depression of respiratory drive, reduction in depth and rate of respiration, and eventual failure of arousal.
   b. For the first week of life, at least, these responses are dependent on environmental temperature (i.e., keeping the baby warm).
   c. Hypoxia is associated with an increase in periodic breathing and apnea.
2. *Response to hyperoxia* (increase in $Fio_{2)}$ breathing causes a transient respiratory depression, stronger in term than in preterm infants.
3. *Response to hypercapnia* (rising $Paco_2$ or $[H^+]$) *or to increase in CO_2 concentration breathed* (mediated by central chemoreceptors in the medulla):
   a. Increase in ventilation is directly proportional to inspired CO_2 concentration (or, more accurately stated, to alveolar CO_2 tension), as is the case in adults.
   b. Response to CO_2 is in large part dependent on sleep state: in quiet sleep, a rising $Paco_2$ causes increase in depth and rate of breathing, whereas during REM sleep the response is irregular and reduced in depth and rate. The degree of reduction closely parallels the amount of ribcage deformity occurring during REM sleep.
   c. Ventilatory response to CO_2 in newborn infants is markedly depressed during behavioral activity such as feeding, and easily depressed by sedatives and anesthesia.

CNS, Central nervous system; *REM,* rapid eye movement.

From Goldsmith, J.P. and Karotkin, E.H.: *Assisted ventilation of the neonate* (3rd ed.). Philadelphia, 1996, W.B. Saunders, p. 26.

B. **Oxygen hood.** Warm, humidified oxygen is provided at a measured concentration via a plastic hood placed over the infant's head.
   1. Indications are respiratory distress, hypoxemia, and cyanosis.
   2. Disadvantages are the necessity of restraining the infant's movements, temperature instability, loss of O_2 when hood is removed, and the possibility that the oxygen tubing will become disconnected from the hood.
   3. O_2 concentration must be measured with an appropriately calibrated oxygen analyzer.
   4. Pulse oximeter should be used to monitor O_2 saturation.
   5. Adequate gas flow is required to avoid CO_2 accumulation within the hood.
   6. Hood size should be appropriate to the size of the infant.
   7. A blender system should be used to provide a fixed oxygen concentration to the hood.

C. **Nasal cannula.** Humidified O_2 is delivered at a set flow rate via a cannula, with the flow directed into the nares. The exact concentration of oxygen delivered by nasal cannula cannot be measured.
   1. Conventional nasal cannula. O_2 is delivered at 100% through the cannula and is regulated by the flow (measured in liters). Low-flow meters are capable of delivering amounts as small as 0.02 L/minute.
   2. High-flow nasal cannula. Flow is 0.5 to 2 L/minute, with oxygen blended to a known concentration. High flow rates may result in the delivery of inadvertent continuous positive airway pressure (PEEP) similar to that of nasal CPAP (Sreenan et al., 2001).
   3. A blender can be used to adjust the concentration of oxygen being delivered by cannula although the amount of oxygen entering the infant's lungs cannot be accurately determined because of the entrainment of room air around the cannula.
   4. Indications. A nasal cannula is used when there is a need for prolonged oxygen therapy as in chronic lung disease, transfer or transport, and increased mobility of the infant for feedings or for other developmental activities.
   5. Complications. Pressure-related tissue damage may occur because of improper or infrequent changing, O_2 concentration may vary, hypoxemia may result from a displaced cannula, and the cannula may be occluded by nasal secretions (may cause significant respiratory distress). Flow through the cannula may result in drying of the nasal mucosa, predisposing the infant to tissue damage and thickened nasal secretions.

D. **CPAP.**
   1. Mask CPAP: delivery of positive pressure (2-8 cm H_2O pressure) with variable amounts of O_2 via face mask. Requires appropriate-sized mask and tight seal around the nose and mouth.
      a. Indications: atelectasis, apnea, respiratory distress, and pulmonary edema.
      b. Advantages: short-term use to assist with alveolar expansion and to inhibit alveolar collapse (atelectasis); intubation not required.
      c. Complications: pulmonary hyperexpansion potentially leading to air leaks (i.e., pneumothorax, pneumomediastinum), aspiration of stomach contents, and ineffective ventilation leading to increasing respiratory difficulty.
   2. Nasal CPAP: generally 5 to 8 cm H_2O pressure (Polin and Sahni, 2002) delivered by prongs that fit into the nares, in addition to a measured concentration of oxygen.

a. Indications: atelectasis, apnea, mild to moderate respiratory distress, and pulmonary edema.
b. Advantage: intubation not required.
c. Complications: ineffective ventilation, pneumothorax, variable pressure delivery when infant's mouth is open, molding of the head from securing straps, erosion of the septum from poorly fitting prongs, nasal obstruction as a result of increased secretions, agitation, dislodging of prongs by an active infant, and gastric distention and perforation.

3. Nasopharyngeal CPAP: delivered by ETT, which is passed through one of the nares and positioned with the tip of the tube in the oropharynx.
   a. Indications: atelectasis, apnea, respiratory distress, pulmonary edema, and to assist in weaning from mechanical ventilation.
   b. Advantage: stable placement of tube, which an infant is less likely to dislodge than with nasal CPAP.
   c. Disadvantages: need for a skilled provider to place the tube, possible damage to the nasal septum and oropharynx, more invasive than other forms of CPAP, variable pressure delivery when infant's mouth is open, and gastric distention.
4. Endotracheal CPAP: delivered via an ETT placed orally or nasally into the trachea.
   a. Indications: atelectasis, apnea, respiratory distress, pulmonary edema, improved pulmonary suctioning, upper airway obstruction, and CNS disorders.
   b. Advantage: constant delivery of O_2 and pressure.
   c. Disadvantage: skilled provider required for intubation. Intubation is an invasive procedure exposing the neonate to potential infection, tissue damage during intubation, and as a result of the presence of a tube in the trachea. Breathing through an ETT increases airway resistance and may result in increased work of breathing.
   d. Complications: malpositioned or dislodged tube, trauma resulting from intubation, port of entry for pathogens, hypoventilation, mucous plugging, possible airway injury (subglottic stenosis, laryngomalacia, tracheomalacia) with prolonged use, and increased risk of pulmonary air leaks.
5. Mechanical ventilation: respiratory support of infant using mechanical assistance.
   a. Gas exchange mechanisms in spontaneous and conventional mechanical ventilation.
      (1) Convection (bulk flow) in large airways goes to approximately the eighth bronchial generation. Gas moves along a negative pressure gradient from the upper airways to the alveoli.
      (2) Molecular diffusion occurs in terminal airways and alveoli. This is the exchange of gases in adjacent spaces.
      (3) The status of alveolar ventilation is determined as follows: Alveolar ventilation = Respiratory rate × (Tidal volume delivered – Anatomic dead-space volume).
   b. Indications: respiratory failure (hypoxemia, hypercapnia, and/or acidemia), pulmonary insufficiency, need for surfactant administration, severe apnea and bradycardia episodes, cardiovascular support, CNS disease, and surgery.
   c. Advantages: consistent delivery of assisted ventilation and oxygen therapy; decreases the work of breathing; stabilizes the airway.

d. Disadvantages: intubation by skilled provider, x-ray examination to confirm placement, possible intermittent x-ray examinations to verify placement or lung status, continuous monitoring of vital signs and oxygen saturation. Exposes the neonate to potential volutrauma/barotrauma of the lung tissue.
e. Complications: tube malposition or dislodgment, underventilation or overventilation, tracheobronchial injury, pulmonary air leaks, infection, intracranial hemorrhage, bronchopulmonary dysplasia, and retinopathy of prematurity.

Types of Assisted Ventilation

A. **Negative-pressure ventilator (derivative of "iron lung").** Provides ventilation by chest wall movement and eliminates the need for intubation. It requires a sealed chamber to provide negative pressure to the chest, which limits access to the infant for providing routine care. It was used in ventilating newborn infants in the early 1970s. With its limitations and the advent of the pressure-limited time-cycled ventilator, it is seldom used today.

B. **Positive-pressure devices.**
1. Bag-and-mask ventilation. Positive pressure and O_2 are delivered via face mask applied with an adequate seal around the mouth and nose. Maximal pressure relief valves should be present to prevent administration of excessive pressure. A manometer can measure pressure delivered to the patient. Device does not require intubation and can be very effective for short-term use including initial resuscitation.
2. Pressure-cycled ventilator. Inspiratory phase ends when a preset pressure is reached within the ventilator circuit, regardless of the volume of gas delivered during inspiration.
3. Time-cycled, pressure-limited, continuous-flow ventilator. A predetermined pressure of gas is administered; the duration of inspiration and expiration can be adjusted. Ventilator also allows for the infant's spontaneous respiratory efforts, facilitating a gradual reduction of support. The operator determines the rate, PIP, PEEP, inspiratory time, and flow. This is the most commonly used ventilator in neonatal care.
4. Volume-cycled ventilator. Inspiration ends when a preset volume of gas is delivered, regardless of the pressure reached within the ventilator circuit. The pressure used to deliver the breath will vary inversely with the infant's lung compliance and respiratory effort. An increase in ventilation is achieved by increasing V_T or rate; oxygenation is improved by increasing PEEP, FiO_2 or V_T (Schwartz, 2003).
5. Pressure-support ventilator (PSV): PSV supports breaths initiated by the infant by delivering a mechanical breath to a preset volume. PSV uses a variable inspiratory time to allow the infant greater control and synchrony with the ventilator. PSV is flow cycled such that when inspiratory flow decreases by a certain percentage, inspiration ends. PSV ventilators usually have a maximum **inspiratory time (T_i)** that is preset. PSV is mainly used as a weaning mode of ventilation (McGettigan et al., 1998).

Ventilator Modes

A. **Intermittent mandatory ventilation.** "Breaths" are delivered at a predetermined rate, regardless of where the patient is in the respiratory cycle.

The ventilator continues to deliver fresh gas, which allows spontaneous respirations as well. It is possible to stack a ventilator breath on top of a spontaneous breath during either inspiration or expiration. This may lead to air trapping, air leaks, CNS dysfunction, and irregularity of blood pressure and cerebral blood flow.

B. Patient-triggered ventilation (PTV). Mechanical breaths are delivered in response to a signal derived from the patient and detected as a spontaneous respiratory effort. The signal may be derived from a sensor that detects airflow, airway pressure, chest wall movement, or esophageal pressure (Schwartz, 2003). Some very immature infants may not generate a significant enough inspiratory effort to trigger the ventilator (Carlo and Ambalavanan, 1999). The goal of PTV is to avoid asynchrony of breathing by the patient and breaths given by the ventilator. Asynchrony may lead to air trapping, air leaks, CNS dysfunction, and irregularity of blood pressure and cerebral blood flow. Patient-triggered ventilation has been shown to improve gas exchange, decrease the need and duration of ventilation, reduce the incidence of air leaks and provide ventilation that better matches the infant's own efforts (Baumer, 2000; Beresford et al., 2000; Cole and Fiascone, 2000; Greenough et al., 2001; Lockridge, 1999; Schulze, 2000).

1. Synchronized intermittent mandatory ventilation.
   - **a.** Preset number of ventilator breaths is synchronized with the onset of spontaneous breaths. When the infant initiates a breath, the ventilator supports that breath according to the preset PIP and inspiratory time.
   - **b.** Unassisted breaths occur between ventilator breaths, with continuous flow of gas from the ventilatory circuit.
   - **c.** Partial asynchrony may occur if inspiratory times are different, in that the patient may attempt to terminate the inspiratory effort while the ventilator continues to be in the inspiratory phase.
2. Assist/control mode of ventilation.
   - **a.** A synchronized breath is delivered each time a spontaneous patient breath meeting the threshold criteria is detected, or mechanical breaths are delivered at a preset regular rate if the patient does not exhibit spontaneous respiratory effort (i.e., if the patient has apnea).
   - **b.** A detection system signals the start of inspiratory effort, which allows for synchronous initiation of inspiration.
   - **c.** Asynchronous expiratory-phase breaths may still occur.
3. Volume-targeted ventilation.
   - **a. Volume-targeted ventilation (VG)** can be used in conjunction with synchronized intermittent mandatory ventilation (SIMV) or Assist/Control modes in patient-triggered ventilation.
   - **b.** A VT is set by the operator based on the infant's weight and disease condition.
   - **c.** The benefits of VG include lower peak inspiratory pressures; enhanced spontaneous respiratory effort (Herrera et al., 2002).

NURSING CARE OF THE PATIENT REQUIRING RESPIRATORY SUPPORT OR CONVENTIONAL MECHANICAL VENTILATION

A. Care of O_2 delivery devices.

1. Oxygen hood. Warm, humidified (to prevent heat loss) O_2, delivered via head hood, is usually blended to select the appropriate amount needed. The percentage of O_2 in the hood must be monitored by a properly calibrated O_2 analyzer placed in the hood near the infant's nose. Ensure a hood of correct

size for each infant. To prevent buildup of CO_2, do not block openings in the hood and ensure an adequate flow of 5 to 7 L/minute. Clean and change per unit protocol.

2. Nasal cannula. Remove and clean secretions every 4 to 6 hours as needed. Inspect surrounding tissue for pressure-related injury. If sudden onset of respiratory distress occurs, inspect cannula for secretions and suction nasopharynx for mucus. Change cannula according to unit protocol. Some infants receiving oxygen by nasal cannula benefit from the administration of saline drops to moisten the mucosa. These should be administered according to unit protocol.
3. Nasopharyngeal or nasal prong CPAP. Ensure that CPAP device is of the correct size to decrease the incidence of pressure necrosis of the nares. Nasal CPAP units come in a variety of sizes and should be short and wide, with thin walls to allow for maximal airflow. They should be soft and flexible and should be easy to secure and maintain. Humidification of 90% to 100% should be provided in the CPAP system to prevent drying out of the mucous membranes and subsequent formation of thick secretions. Evaluate the need for suctioning every 2 to 4 hours. Inspect surrounding tissue for pressure-related injury. Secure the device to a stockinette cap or with soft straps provided by some manufacturers. Lightweight tubing is helpful for ease in securing the device and in keeping the unit in the nose. The infant can be positioned supine, on either side, or prone, generally with the head of the bed at approximately a 30-degree angle. Observe for abdominal distention resulting from excessive air entering the stomach from the CPAP device. Consider aspirating every few hours with an orogastric tube or leaving it in place continuously to vent gas in the stomach. Feeding is not contraindicated during delivery of CPAP. The clinical condition must be evaluated before institution of feedings. During CPAP delivery, feedings must be administered via orogastric tube either intermittently or by continuous drip. Change prongs according to unit protocol, generally every 2 or 3 days.
4. ETT. After correct placement has been determined, note the depth of the tube at the gum or lip and post at the bedside. This is important for future reference in case the tube slips, reintubation is needed, or to determine suction catheter length. Secure the ETT with tape or other method. Each institution generally develops a method that works well for the staff and patients. Observe for evidence of slipping or tape loosening and secure again when necessary to prevent accidental extubation. Position the infant supine, on either side, or in the prone position, with the head in a neutral position. Be aware that the tube moves with the chin and can move several centimeters with flexion or extension of the head. Signs of extubation include sudden deterioration in clinical status, abdominal distention, crying, decreased chest wall movement, breath sounds in the abdomen, agitation, cyanosis, or bradycardia. Notify the physician or neonatal nurse practitioner if extubation is a concern and prepare for reintubation as soon as possible. Intubation equipment should be readily available. A bag and mask with pressure manometer should also be available at each bedside and should be tested during each shift. Suction the ETT when necessary. Complications of an ETT include palatal grooves (consider a palate protector, which can be made by a pediatric dentist or is commercially available), nasal erosion, subglottic stenosis, tracheoesophageal perforation during insertion of the tube, aspiration, infection, and tracheal granuloma.

5. Tracheostomy tube. Daily changing of the dressing and weekly changing of the tube are usually adequate. Inspect the site for signs of tissue pressure and/or necrosis. Suctioning is necessary to keep the airway clear of secretions. Family members need to be included in this procedure, thus facilitating discharge.

B. Suctioning the airway.

1. Nontracheal tubes.
   a. Suctioning of the mouth, nose, and tubes should be performed on an as-needed basis. The presence of a foreign body in the mouth or nose will cause an increase in secretions.
   b. Suctioning can coincide with the cleaning or changing of the tubes or with routine caregiving.
2. Endotracheal tubes.
   a. The amount of secretions will be disease related. Infants with resolving respiratory distress syndrome, patent ductus arteriosus (PDA), bronchopulmonary dysplasia, and pneumonia are more likely to require suctioning because of an increased production of mucus. Patients with early-stage respiratory distress syndrome and those with most types of congenital heart disease will not have much mucus and will require less suctioning. Suctioning is done on an as-needed basis, never on a routine schedule (Hagedorn et al., 2002). Criteria for suctioning include evidence of secretions (audible or visible); changes in vital signs; agitation or restlessness; and changes in oxygenation or ventilation.
   b. Protocols for suctioning vary from one institution to another. Administering manual breaths with the ventilator or hand ventilating for 30 to 60 seconds (with an increase in fraction of inspired oxygen [FIO_2]) before and after suctioning may be necessary to maintain oxygenation during the procedure.
   c. In-line suction devices allow suctioning while ventilation continues and are associated with a decreased risk of infection, smaller changes in cerebral blood flow, and other hemodynamic changes (Ruof and Fahwenstich, 2000).
   d. Do not advance the suction catheter farther than the distance of the ETT, and do not suction too vigorously.
   e. Vacuum pressure range should be 60 to 100 mm Hg (Hagedorn et al., 2002). A 5F or 6F suction catheter for a 2.5 to 3.5 ETT, or an 8F suction catheter for a 4 to 4.5 ETT, is usually appropriate.
   f. Complications of suctioning include hypoxemia, bradycardia, barotrauma, changes in blood pressure, alterations in cerebral blood flow, intraventricular hemorrhage, tracheal damage, atelectasis, infection, and pneumothorax.

C. Initiating mechanical ventilation. The goal of mechanical ventilation is to assist in providing adequate tissue oxygenation and eliminating CO_2.

1. Establish an airway. Endotracheal intubation should be performed by a skilled provider (see Chapter 15).
2. Ventilator selection. The ventilator selected for use is based on the patient's condition and disease process, the patient's response to previous ventilatory support, and staff experience and comfort with the device. The most common ventilator used in the neonatal intensive care unit (NICU) is a synchronous time-cycled, volume- or pressure-limited continuous-flow device. This type of ventilator allows the operator to adjust peak pressure or volume, PEEP, inspiratory time, flow rate, rate of intermittent mandatory ventilation, and FIO_2.

3. Parameters to be set and/or monitored during mechanical ventilation.
   a. Rate of intermittent mandatory ventilation. Infants without respiratory failure have a resting respiratory rate of approximately 40/minute, whereas infants with respiratory failure may have a respiratory rate of zero to more than 100/minute. A beginning ventilator rate of 30 to 40/minute for an infant with respiratory failure should be adequate. For infants without respiratory failure, a rate of 20 to 30/minute should be adequate. The ventilator rate will affect the ability to blow off CO_2. The rate is adjusted to maintain the arterial tension of CO_2 in the range of 40 to 50 mm Hg and to avoid excessive respiratory effort, which would exhaust the infant. A rate greater than 40/min may shorten the expiratory phase of ventilation and cause air trapping.
   b. PIP. PIP is the primary factor used for determining tidal volume and affecting PaO_2. Determining the appropriate PIP requires careful and skilled assessment. The complications of excessive PIP include air leaks, decreased venous return, and decreased cardiac output. Factors such as weight, gestational age, disease process, lung compliance, and airway resistance must be considered. Auscultation of breath sounds to assess aeration and compliance is necessary. Experimenting with an anesthesia bag to find the best rate and pressure may be useful and allows the clinician to determine the infant's ventilation needs. Visual inspection of chest wall movement, in conjunction with the use of a pressure gauge connected to the anesthesia bag, may guide your assessment. A beginning PIP of 20 cm H_2O is appropriate for most preterm infants. The lowest PIP that will provide adequate ventilation is ideal, with the goals of preventing barotrauma and volutrauma, and decreasing the incidence of air leaks and chronic lung disease (Clark et al., 2000; Cole and Fiascone, 2000). Certain conditions may warrant use of high PIP, including poor compliance, atelectasis, or pulmonary hypertension. Before connecting the patient to the ventilator, ensure that the inspiratory pressure is correct. Recheck after the connection has been made, and adjust as necessary.
   c. VT: VT is the primary factor affecting both oxygenation and ventilation. When using volume-targeted ventilation, the operator determines the desired volume to be delivered with each breath rather than setting the PIP. Based on averaging a series of breaths, the ventilator determines the PIP needed to deliver the desired volume of gas. An upper limit for the PIP can be set by the operator to prevent the delivery of excessive pressure.

      An increase in ventilation is achieved by increasing the volume of gas to be delivered (VT) or the rate. Increased oxygenation is achieved by increasing the FiO_2, the PEEP, or the VT (Schwartz, 2003). Determination of tidal volume is based on the infant's weight, with a beginning VT of 4 to 5 ml/kg being most common.
   d. PEEP. This measure aids in maintaining functional residual capacity, stabilizing and recruiting atelectatic areas for gas exchange, improving compliance, and improving ventilation-perfusion matching in the lung (Hagedorn et al., 2002). PEEP is important in assisted ventilation for infants with surfactant deficiency because of the likelihood of alveolar collapse. Physiologic PEEP is estimated at 2 cm H_2O. Levels lower than 2 cm H_2O are not generally recommended. In most instances, medium levels, about 4 to 7 cm H_2O, are recommended. Levels greater than 8 cm H_2O are associated with pulmonary air leaks and reduction of cardiac output.

e. Inspiratory/expiratory (I/E) ratio: ratio of time spent in inspiration and time spent in expiration. Determining this time should be based on the underlying reason for ventilation. A physiologic I/E ratio in a nondisease state is equal to 1:2 or 1:3, meaning a short inspiratory time with a longer expiratory time. Prolonged expiratory time is useful during weaning, when oxygenation is not as problematic. The I/E ratio will affect the PaO_2 and $PaCO_2$. Changes affect mean airway pressure and oxygenation.
f. Flow rate: flow of gas (measured in liters per minute) through the patient's circuit. The flow rate determines the ability of the ventilator to deliver the desired amount of PIP, waveform, I/E ratio, and respiratory rate. A flow rate of at least twice the infant's minute ventilation ensures that the ventilator can reach the desired pressure. Flow rates of 8 to 10 L/minute are common (Gomez et al., 1998). With low flow rates (<3 L/min), inspiratory pressure gradually builds to a peak just before expiration, closely resembling a sine waveform (normal breaths are shaped like a sine waveform). There may be less barotrauma to the airways with a sine waveform. High flows of 4 to 10 L/minute or higher are necessary with square waveform ventilation or when high rates are used. A square waveform pattern moves the ventilator breath rapidly from the resting or expiratory pressure level to the PIP. Because the PIP is reached sooner than with a sine waveform, the PIP is held for a longer period (Fig. 25-3). This may be advantageous with atelectatic areas of the lung. It may also contribute to barotrauma.
g. MAP: average distending pressure throughout a complete respiratory cycle. It is the major determinant of oxygenation. MAP, most affected by changes in PEEP, PIP, and I/E ratio, is digitally displayed on newer ventilators. Separate devices can be attached to older ventilators to display MAP. Increases in oxygenation are directly related to increases in MAP, and increased barotrauma to the lungs can result with high MAP. Close attention to the MAP during ventilation is essential, especially once the underlying disease begins to resolve.

4. For effects of different ventilator changes, see Box 25-2.

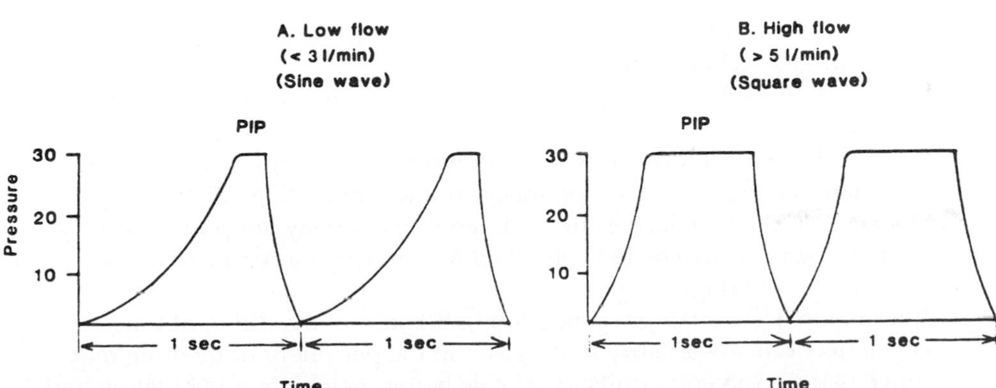

FIGURE 25-3 ■ Comparison of ventilator waveforms. *A,* Relative sine wave. *B,* Relative square wave. (From Goldsmith, J.P. and Karotkin, E.H. (Eds.): *Assisted ventilation of the neonate* (3rd ed.). Philadelphia, 1996, Saunders, p. 169.)

■ BOX 25-2
■ **SPECIFIC EFFECTS OF DIFFERENT VENTILATOR CHANGES**

Increasing PIP
1. Increases V_T and Ve
2. Adds little to MAP unless combined with a reversal of I/E ratio or prolongation of IT
3. Affects maximum dilation of alveoli already open, contributing to barotrauma
4. Opens alveoli with high critical opening pressures

Reversing I/E Ratio (for lengthening IT while respiratory rate is kept constant)
1. Has little effect on V_T or Ve beyond the minimum IT needed to deliver V_T or reach desired PIP level (or both)
2. Can contribute on more than one-to-one basis to MAP, depending on original PIP and degree of reversal of I/E ratio
3. Allows expansion of atelectatic alveoli at lower PIP
4. May cause inadvertent PEEP, overinflation of alveoli, and reduction of pulmonary blood flow

Increasing Background CPAP or PEEP
1. Decreases V_T and Ve unless significant atelectasis is overcome
2. Adds to MAP on a one-to-one basis
3. Holds open alveoli and terminal airways on end-expiration, thus raising closing volume and aiding in equal distribution of ventilation
4. Reduces likelihood of inadvertent PEEP

CPAP, Continuous positive airway pressure; *I/E,* inspiratory/expiratory; *IT,* inspiratory time; *MAP,* mean airway pressure; *PEEP,* positive end-expiratory pressure; *PIP,* peak inspiratory pressure; *V_T,* tidal volume; *Ve,* expired volume per unit time.

From Goldsmith, J.P. and Karotkin, E.H. (Eds.): *Assisted ventilation of the neonate* (3rd ed.). Philadelphia, 1996, W.B. Saunders, p. 62.

HIGH-FREQUENCY VENTILATION

High-frequency ventilation (HFV) is any of several forms of mechanical ventilation that use small tidal volumes and rapid ventilator rates to ventilate patients with severe respiratory failure. The advantage of HFV over conventional mechanical ventilation is the ability to deliver adequate minute volumes with lower proximal airway pressures.

A. **Gas-exchange mechanisms in HFV.** The tidal volumes used may be less than or equal to anatomic dead-space volume. According to gas-exchange theories for conventional ventilation, alveolar ventilation during HFV should be zero.

B. **Theories of gas exchange during HFV.**
   1. Augmented (facilitated) diffusion. Gas molecules diffuse higher in the airways.
   2. Coaxial diffusion. Fresh gases travel down the center of the airway, and CO_2 elimination occurs along the periphery of the airway (Fig. 25-4).
   3. Entrainment. Gas molecules from higher in the airway are pulled into the area of low pressure created behind a high-velocity gas entry point, such as a jet cannula port (Fig. 25-5).
   4. Interregional gas mixing ("pendelluft"). Because of the different time constants of the respiratory units, gases in the periphery of the lung may move between alveolar units to provide better matching of ventilation and perfusion.

C. **Effectiveness of gas exchange.** All forms of HFV produce gas exchange with lower PIPs, theoretically reducing the risk of barotrauma.

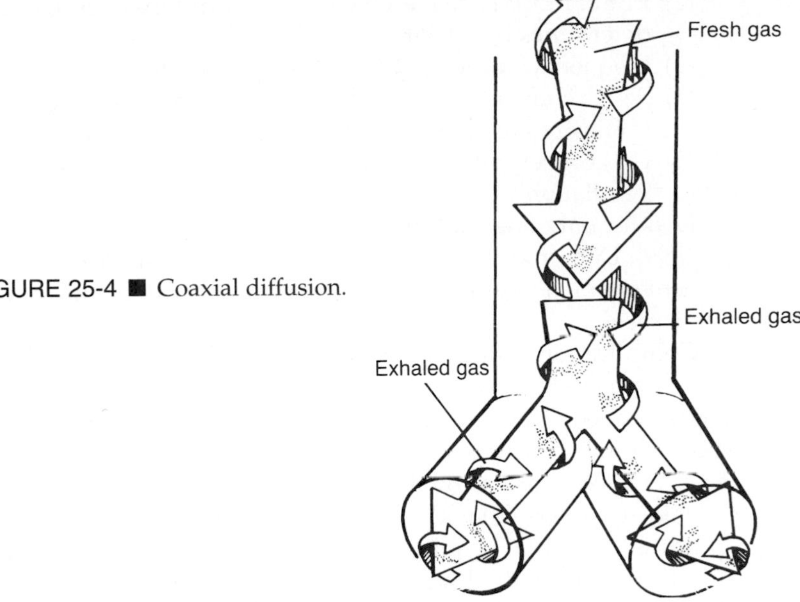

FIGURE 25-4 ■ Coaxial diffusion.

D. Types of high-frequency ventilators.

1. High-frequency flow interrupter (HFFI):
   - **a.** These ventilators have both high-frequency and conventional options.
   - **b.** Flow interrupters are neither oscillators nor jet ventilators. They operate with a microprocessor-controlled pneumatic valve to interrupt the gas flow to achieve a pulsatile flow.
   - **c.** Sigh breaths can be given with the conventional ventilator.
   - **d.** Inhalation: active; exhalation: passive.
   - **e.** Indications for use:
     - (1) Severe pulmonary air leaks.
     - (2) Lung diseases unresponsive to conventional mechanical ventilation.
   - **f.** Parameters to be set and/or monitored during HFFI:
     - (1) PIP: CO_2 elimination is dependent on the difference between the PIP and PEEP in this mode.

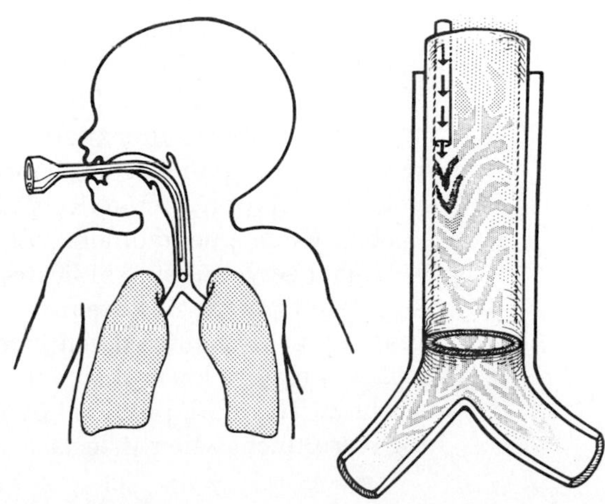

FIGURE 25-5 ■ Entrainment during high-frequency jet ventilation. Gas molecules near the jet orifice are "entrained," or dragged along with the jet pulse, whereby additional volume is delivered to the patient without substantially increasing static airway pressure. (From Harris, T.R.: Physiologic principles. In J.P. Goldsmith and E.H. Karotkin (Eds.): *Assisted ventilation of the neonate* (2nd ed.). Philadelphia, 1988, Saunders.)

(2) PEEP: PEEP is delivered by the conventional ventilator and determines oxygenation.
(3) Frequency: number of "breaths per minute."
(4) Sighs: conventional breaths given periodically to recruit alveoli and minimize atelectasis. (Sighs are optional with this mode.)
(5) FiO_2 concentration: set on the ventilator as with conventional ventilation.

g. Results: only one clinical trial using HFFI has been reported (Thome et al., 1999). Data from this study demonstrated no difference between HFFI and conventional ventilation with respect to the development of chronic lung disease.

h. Complications: inadequate gas delivery during inspiration and incomplete lung emptying during expiration.

2. High-frequency jet ventilation (HFJV): Bunnell Life Pulse Jet Ventilator (Bunnell Inc., Salt Lake City, Utah).

a. A jet injector or narrow-bore cannula that delivers short, rapid, high-velocity pulses from a pressurized gas source directly into the trachea via a small cannula. Requires the use of a triple-lumen ETT (Hi-Lo Jet Tube), which is specially designed for use during HFJV (requires reintubation) or a triple-lumen ETT adapter ("jet nozzle") that attaches to a standard ETT. The tube has a standard ETT lumen, a pressure-monitoring port located at the distal tip, and a jet injector port located within the tube wall.

b. Servocontrolled driving pressure: continuously adjusts the pressure of the gas supply to the jet cannula to maintain desired peak airway pressure.

c. Solenoid valve: opens and closes gas supply to the jet cannula.

d. Humidification system: built in-line.

e. Proximal airway pressures: monitored and continuously displayed; used in servocontrol of pressure delivery.

f. Conventional ventilator: used in tandem to provide gas for entrainment, PEEP, and background ventilation (sighs).

g. Exhalation: passive.

h. Indications for use: effective with disorders in which CO_2 elimination is the major problem. CO_2 elimination is achieved at lower peak and mean airway pressures than with high-frequency positive pressure ventilation (HFPPV) or high-frequency oscillatory ventilation (HFOV).

i. Parameters to be set and/or monitored:

(1) PIP: set on both the jet and the conventional ventilator.
   (a) Jet PIP is usually initially set at the same PIP required during conventional ventilation, and the conventional ventilator PIP is lowered by 2 to 5 cm H_2O.
   (b) A higher conventional PIP may cause interruption of the jet.

(2) Servocontrolled pressure: internal adjustment of driving pressure by the ventilator as patient compliance and pressure settings change.
   (a) Lower servopressure reflects worsening lung disease, airway obstruction, pneumothorax, or kinked ventilator tubing.
   (b) Higher servopressure indicates improved lung compliance or a leak in the patient/system.

(3) PEEP: set on conventional ventilator; displayed on jet ventilator. Value displayed may be lower than value set, because of where and how it is measured. The PEEP provided by the conventional ventilator assists in lung recruitment when atelectasis is a problem.

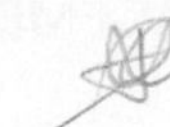

(4) Jet valve on time: percentage of time that the jet valve is open; similar to inspiratory time, usually 0.02 second.

(5) Rate set on jet and conventional ventilators:

(a) The jet rate is usually 400 to 500 breaths per minute; Bunnell default setting of 420/minute appears to be most effective for that ventilator.

(b) The rate for conventional intermittent mandatory ventilation is usually set between 5 and 20 breaths per minute to provide background ventilation (sigh breaths), which helps to prevent atelectasis.

(6) FiO_2: set on jet and conventional ventilators.

j. Weaning from HFJV is usually accomplished by 7 to 14 days. Air leaks should be resolved for 1 or 2 days before switching back to conventional mechanical ventilation. Weaning is accomplished by decreasing the PIP and reducing the HFJV rate to 250 to 350 breaths per minute. Support from conventional mechanical ventilation is increased using small tidal volume breaths.

k. Patient care assessment.

(1) Patient may undergo reintubation with special ETT that has a jet port and a pressure-monitoring port built in (Fig. 25-6), or an ETT adapter may be attached to the standard ETT.

(2) Suctioning may be performed with HFJV on or off.

(a) Placing jet ventilator on stand-by mode during suctioning may prevent airway damage caused by the shearing force of opposing positive and negative pressures.

(b) Suctioning with the jet ventilator on may help decrease respiratory decompensation during the procedure in some patients.

(c) If suctioning is performed with the jet ventilator running, suction must be applied as the catheter is inserted, as well as when withdrawn, to prevent overpressurization of the circuit and alveolar rupture.

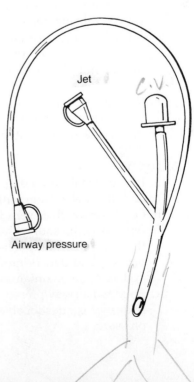

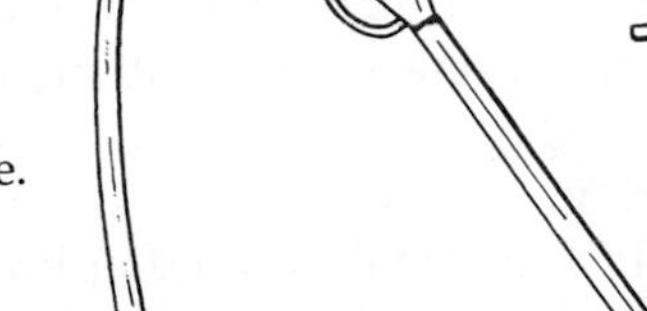

FIGURE 25-6 ■ Triple-lumen endotracheal tube.

(3) Humidification of gases is important with HFJV in preventing obstruction of the ETT.
   (a) Jet port should be irrigated with 0.5 ml normal saline solution or air every 3 to 4 hours.
   (b) Main port of ETT is suctioned as usual.

(4) Tubing to the conventional ventilator must never be kinked because overpressurization of the circuit and alveolar rupture may occur if expiratory gas cannot escape.

(5) Vibration of the chest wall is an indicator of lung compliance, airway patency, and effectiveness of ventilator settings.
   (a) Chest wall vibration must be assessed after head position changes to ensure that the jet port of the ETT has not been occluded by the tracheal wall.
   (b) Sudden decrease in chest wall vibration may indicate a plugged ETT or a pneumothorax.

(6) Vibration may interfere with electrical monitoring of heart rate and respiratory rate.
   (a) Use pulse from arterial line or pulse oximeter to monitor heart rate if necessary.
   (b) Respiratory rate cannot be monitored.

(7) Jet ventilation is more efficient at CO_2 elimination than at oxygenation.
   (a) Increasing the background ventilation rate may improve oxygenation.
   (b) Pressure difference between PIP and PEEP is the major determinant of ventilation.
   (c) MAP is the major determinant of oxygenation.

(8) Patients are generally weaned to a low PIP and then switched back to conventional ventilation before extubation.

l. Complications and problems:
   (1) Airway obstruction, which may be indicated by decreased chest wall vibration, increased P_{CO_2}, and decreased servopressure.
   (2) Necrotizing tracheobronchitis (inflammatory injury to tracheal mucosa).
   (3) Microatelectasis and poor oxygenation, possible after prolonged HFJV; necessitates return to conventional ventilation.
   (4) Air trapping occurs at very high rates or with excessive jet valve on-times.

m. Results: A Cochrane Review of jet ventilation in newborns has demonstrated a reduction in chronic lung disease at 36 weeks' gestation in infants electively ventilated with the jet (Bhuta and Henderson-Smart, 2003).

3. HFOV.
   a. Piston, or vibrating diaphragm, that moves a small volume of gas toward and then away from patient.
   b. Oscillators deliver very little bulk gas. A continuous flow of fresh gas flows past the source that powers the oscillations, producing bias gas flow in a resulting push-pull fashion and thereby eliminating CO_2 buildup and delivering O_2. A low-pass filter allows gas to exit the system while maintaining vibration of gas in the airway (Schwartz, 2003).
   c. Proximal airway pressure is monitored by the ventilator, but clinical relevance is questionable because it probably does not reflect alveolar pressure.

d. HFOV allows for the use of higher MAP with less barotrauma, in comparison with conventional-mechanical ventilation and ventilation with small tidal volumes.

e. Exhalation is active, assisted by the oscillating device.

f. Indications for use are:

(1) Severe lung disease that is unresponsive to conventional ventilation.

(2) Pulmonary air leaks, pulmonary interstitial emphysema, pneumothorax, and bronchopleural fistula.

(3) Pulmonary hypoplasia and diaphragmatic hernia: treated with limited success. HFV can be used to stabilize the condition of these patients.

(4) Persistent pulmonary hypertension and meconium aspiration syndrome: treated with mixed results. The improved CO_2 exchange may provide a respiratory alkalosis that would result in dilation of the pulmonary vascular bed.

(5) Failure of conventional mechanical ventilation.

g. Parameters to be set or monitored:

(1) MAP: affects oxygenation.

(2) Amplitude: size of pressure wave produced by oscillator (another way to describe volume delivered).

(3) Sighs: conventional breaths given periodically to recruit alveoli and minimize atelectasis.

(4) FiO_2: set on the ventilator as with conventional ventilation.

(5) Frequency: 180 to 900 "breaths" per minute (3-5 Hz).

h. Patient care and assessment:

(1) No special ETT is required.

(2) Suctioning procedure is performed as usual. Infants on high-frequency ventilation often benefit from the use of an in-line suctioning device to minimize postsuctioning atelectasis.

(3) Chest wall vibration is assessed, rather than breath sounds, to determine effectiveness of ventilator settings and lung compliance changes. Breath sounds are not audible during HFOV.

(4) Vibration may interfere with electrical monitoring of heart rate and respiratory rate.

(a) Use pulse from arterial line or pulse oximeter for heart rate monitoring if necessary.

(b) Respiratory rate cannot be monitored.

(c) Sighs help to reduce microatelectasis and improve oxygenation.

(5) Complications and problems are:

(a) Microatelectasis, poor oxygenation.

(b) Increased incidence of intraventricular hemorrhage in collaborative trial of HFV using oscillators for treatment of respiratory distress syndrome in preterm infants (HIFI Study Group, 1989; Moriette et al., 2001). Other recent studies have failed to demonstrate an increased risk (Thome et al., 1999).

i. Results: Studies evaluating the use of HFO ventilation have demonstrated mixed results depending on the volume strategy used. Bhuta and colleagues (2003) completed a Cochrane Review of HFOV for term or near-term infants and found no data to support the routine use of HFOV. A Cochrane Review comparing HFOV to conventional ventilation for preterm infants found that elective HFOV resulted in a reduction in chronic lung disease at term. Results were inconsistent across studies and some short-term neurologic morbidity was found, but this did not reach statistical significance (Henderson-Smart et al., 2003). Other benefits include decreased need for surfactant replacement (Moriette et al, 2001) and decreased days on oxygen and ventilation (Rimensberger et al., 2000).

4. Liquid ventilation: currently experimental but thought to be a powerful addition to pulmonary care for the future.
   a. Elimination of the air-liquid interface in the alveolus decreases surface tension, which results in a high degree of solubility for respiratory gases. Perfluorocarbon liquids are being studied as the basis for liquid ventilation.
   b. Indications for use include: rescue therapy for extremely low birth weight (ELBW) infants failing to respond to surfactant therapy; infants with pulmonary hypoplasia; term infants approaching the need for extracorporeal membrane oxygenation (ECMO) (Hodson and Truog, 1999), respiratory distress syndrome, and secondary surfactant deficiency.
   c. Monitoring is dependent on the delivery system. The circuit, similar to that used in extracorporeal membrane oxygenation, requires constant monitoring to ensure that there is no loss of tidal volume or any impairment of gas exchange. The circuit allows the fluid to flow into and out of the pulmonary airways, either by gravity or with a pump. Chest wall movement indicates patency and position of the ETT and V_T. Change of position is necessary to allow for even distribution of the lung liquid.
   d. Perfluorocarbons provide decreased alveolar surface tension, recruit lung volume, allow ventilation with decreased pressures, improve ventilation-perfusion matching, and clean debris from the lungs.
   e. Research and clinical trials are ongoing.

NURSING CARE DURING THERAPY

A. Physical assessment.

1. Observation. One of the most valuable tools in assessing an infant's respiratory status is observation. Does the infant appear to be comfortable while breathing, or does the infant show signs and symptoms of distress by grunting, flaring, and retracting? The Silverman-Andersen score is a screening tool that uses five signs or symptoms to assess respiratory distress in the newborn infant (Fig. 25-7). Assess the skin color of the infant. It should be uniformly pink. Skin color that is blue, dusky, or pale needs to be evaluated further. A dramatic change in skin color needs to be investigated immediately to rule out a pneumothorax versus a mechanical obstruction. Observe the infant's respiratory rate. Is it within the normal range (40-60 breaths per minute)? When observing the respiratory rate, consider variables such as environment, temperature, and the infant's state of activity or inactivity, which can increase or decrease the respiratory rate. Observe whether the chest rises symmetrically; if asymmetric, suspect a possible pneumothorax, diaphragmatic hernia, or phrenic nerve palsy. With accidental extubation, chest movement may not be observable or may be decreased from previous observations.
2. Auscultation. Listen to the breath sounds carefully to determine differences in the upper and lower lung fields and differences in the left and right lung fields. Is aeration equal bilaterally? Are fine coarse crackles evident? Are other abnormal sounds audible? A finding in a ventilated infant may be louder breath sounds on the right; if so, suspect that the ETT may have slipped into the right bronchus or that a pneumothorax may have occurred,

SILVERMAN-ANDERSEN RETRACTION SCORE

	UPPER CHEST	LOWER CHEST	XIPHOID RETRACT.	NARES DILAT.	EXPIR. GRUNT
GRADE 0	SYNCHRONIZED	NO RETRACT.	NONE	NONE	NONE
GRADE 1	LAG ON INSP.	JUST VISIBLE	JUST VISIBLE	MINIMAL	STETHOS. ONLY
GRADE 2	SEE-SAW	MARKED	MARKED	MARKED	NAKED EAR

FIGURE 25-7 ■ Silverman-Andersen scale to assess respiratory distress in the newborn infant. (Adapted from Silverman, W.A. and Andersen D. H.: A controlled clinical trial of effects of water mist on obstructive respiratory signs, death rate, and necropsy findings among premature infants. *Pediatrics, 17*(1):1-10, 1956.)

necessitating evaluation. Rule out other noises and their points of origin. Bowel sounds heard in the chest are an indication of a diaphragmatic hernia. In the patient receiving HFV, chest wall vibration is an indicator of lung compliance, airway patency, and effectiveness of ventilator settings. Chest wall vibration must be assessed after repositioning. Sudden decrease in chest wall vibration may indicate a plugged ETT or a pneumothorax.

3. ETT observation. Fogging or condensation in the ETT is a sign that the infant is intubated. The condensation occurs on exhalation and is visible in the ETT. Observation of the tube position more than 1 cm from its desired location may indicate extubation or placement in the right mainstem bronchus.
4. Signs of extubation:
   a. Audible crying.
   b. Absent or decreased breath sounds.
   c. Cyanosis.
   d. Bradycardia.
   e. Hypoxemia.
   f. Agitation, restlessness.
   g. Increased abdominal distention.

B. **Equipment function.** All ventilators used for conventional mechanical ventilation should have been approved by the U.S. Food and Drug Administration and should display rate (intermittent mandatory ventilation), peak inspiratory pressure, PEEP, tidal volume (where applicable), inspiratory time, I/E ratio, mean airway pressure, and O_2 concentration. Ventilators must be plugged into an electrical outlet that provides emergency power in the event of a power failure.

1. All mechanical ventilators should have:
   a. Alarms activated to alert caregivers to ventilator malfunction or disconnection.
   b. Preset pressure relief valves to ensure against administration of excessive PIP and PEEP.

c. Frequently scheduled inspections by licensed respiratory therapists.
d. Ventilator tubing changed routinely per unit policy.
e. O_2 concentration analyzed routinely and documented in the patient record.
f. Routine cleaning between patient use.

2. The following equipment, to be located in the immediate area of all infants requiring mechanical ventilation, should be checked for proper functioning and replaced as needed:
   a. Laryngoscope with blade.
      (1) Size 0 for infants weighing less than 3 kg.
      (2) Size 1 for infants weighing more than 3 kg.
   b. Sterile ETTs.
      (1) Size 2.5 for infants weighing less than 1000 g.
      (2) Size 3 for infants weighing 1000 to 2000 g.
      (3) Size 3.5 for infants weighing 2000 to 3000 g.
      (4) Size 3.5 or 4 for infants weighing more than 3000 g.
   c. Sterile stylet (plastic coated).
   d. Magill forceps (nasal intubation).
   e. Suction tubing and catheters (suction control gauge set at 60-100 mm Hg).
   f. Sterile orogastric tubes.
      (1) Size 5F for infants weighing less than 1 kg.
      (2) Size 8F for infants weighing more than 1 kg.
   g. Anesthesia bag with manometer and mask: capable of delivering blended O_2, and O_2 source.
   h. Tape, scissors.

C. **Noninvasive monitoring.**

1. All infants receiving O_2 therapy should be considered as potential candidates for mechanical ventilation and should be monitored with the following:
   a. Heart rate monitor: audible beat-to-beat capability and alarm device for bradycardia (<100 beats per minute [bpm]) or tachycardia (>180 bpm); should provide visual display of electrocardiogram and actual heart rate.
   b. Respiratory monitor: visual display of respiratory wave pattern and actual respiratory rate; should include alarm device for apnea and tachypnea. Respiratory rate trend mode is preferred.
   c. Blood pressure monitoring: peripheral (cuff) blood pressure or arterial blood pressure monitoring, performed on a scheduled interval and documented on the permanent record.
   d. O_2 analyzer: continuous monitoring of O_2 content of the gas delivered to the patient, with mandatory alarm device for O_2 concentration greater than or less than desired range.
   e. Pulse oximetry: continuous monitoring for critically ill infants; intermittent checks with documentation of peripheral O_2 saturations indicated for infants not critically ill.
   f. Additional requirements for all infants requiring mechanical ventilation, based on clinical condition:
      (1) Arterial access (usually via umbilical artery catheter) for:
         (a) Blood gas sampling.
         (b) Blood pressure monitoring.
      (2) Transcutaneous Po_2 and Pco_2 monitoring as indicated by clinical status.

2. Pulse oximetry.
   a. Pulse oximetry is a noninvasive and continuous method of measuring hemoglobin O_2 saturation. With the use of red and infrared light, the saturation of hemoglobin bound to O_2 is determined by a digital readout displayed by the monitoring device. The main advantage of pulse oximetry is the short response time in determining O_2 saturation in a neonate. It also reduces the number of invasive blood gas measurements necessary for a particular infant. It can be used in various settings outside the NICU (e.g., in neonatal transport, delivery room care, and surgery). The alarm device will alert attendants if O_2 saturations are at less than or greater than the desired range.
   b. An accurate reading is dependent on several factors, a primary factor being the perfusion status of the infant. The accuracy of pulse oximetry decreases with low-perfusion states. Phototherapy, motion artifact, dyes (ink from footprints), and vasoconstricting drugs (dopamine) can affect saturation readouts. Pulse oximetry does not eliminate the need for blood gas analysis because clinical signs of ventilation and acid-base balance must still be evaluated. Continuous saturations greater than 96% may indicate that an infant is ready to be weaned from O_2 therapy, depending on the acute or chronic nature of the infant's disease. Cifuentes and associates (2003) suggested that saturations between 92% and 97% are associated with a safe range of PaO_2. Table 25-1 gives percentage parameters for O_2 saturation monitoring.
3. Transcutaneous oxygen monitoring.
   a. Transcutaneous oxygen monitoring (TCOM) is the measurement of skin O_2 tension rather than arterial tension. The correlation between skin O_2 tension and arterial O_2 tension is excellent. A heated electrode measures the O_2 flow across the skin (skin PO_2) by making the skin more permeable to O_2, which occurs when the lipid layer under the skin is altered and the O_2 dissociation curve is shifted to the right. Thus O_2 is not bound as tightly to the hemoglobin molecule and is more readily released to the

■ TABLE 25-1
■ ■ **Practical Hints for O_2 Saturation Monitoring**

	Acute	Chronic
Acceptable Limits	**87%-95%**	**90%-95%**
Oxygen management parameters	Wean from O_2 when infant stable and SaO_2 readings are consistently >95% every 15-30 minutes	Wean from O_2 when infant stable and SaO_2 readings are consistently >95% every 12-24 hours
Blood gas requirements	When SaO_2 <85% or >97% consistently >15-30 minutes Monitoring and electrocardiographic heart rate not correlating and perfusion status poor	When SaO_2 <87% or >95% consistently >1 hour

From Dziedzic, K., and Vidyasagar, P.: Pulse oximetry in neonatal intensive care. *Clinics in Perinatology, 16*(1): 177-197, 1989.

tissues. The correlation between skin and arterial O_2 tension is best with normal perfusion, body temperature, and blood pressure. The advantage of TCOM is the same as for the pulse oximeter. TCOM reduces the number of invasive blood gas measurements and also can be used in various settings outside the NICU. The TCOM also has several disadvantages. The readout on the TCOM is not immediate—a warming period is required (10-20 minutes), and after about 4 to 6 hours the TCOM begins to lose its measurement reliability, requiring change of the probe. The TCOM requires frequent calibration during use. The electrode has been reported to cause burns in premature infants, and the probe adhesive may cause skin breakdown in the VLBW preterm infant. Further, the readout time of the transcutaneous PO_2 values lags 5 to 10 seconds behind the PaO_2 value. The accuracy of transcutaneous monitoring can change if the infant has poor perfusion or hypotension, with transcutaneous PO_2 values much lower (Cifuentes et al., 2003). TCM should be used for trending measurements. The TCOM does not replace the need for monitoring arterial blood gases.

b. Transcutaneous PCO_2 monitoring can be beneficial in caring for infants with respiratory problems characterized by hypercapnia. It is also beneficial in determining complications of pneumothorax or mechanical obstruction before they are clinically evident in the infant. Correlation with transcutaneous PCO_2 is fairly accurate, but transcutaneous PCO_2 values can be overestimated because of skin production of CO_2 (Cifuentes et al., 2003).

4. End-tidal CO_2 monitoring.

a. Measures CO_2 tension through gas analysis during respiration.

b. Most accurate when infants have normal lung function and a normal ventilation to perfusion ($\dot{V}_A/\dot{Q}_A$) ratio.

c. Markedly less accurate in infants with severe lung disease (large alveolar-arterial gradient) and cannot be relied on for accuracy.

d. May be useful in premature infants with mild to moderate lung disease and in infants with normal lung function.

e. Transcutaneous CO_2 monitoring is more accurate in the infant with severe lung disease.

D. Blood gas measurement. Blood gas measurement is the standard method for monitoring oxygenation, ventilation, and acid-base balance in the ill neonate. Different methods are available for obtaining the blood sample, with umbilical arterial catheterization being the most common. Other methods for sampling include the use of indwelling peripheral arterial catheters, intermittent arterial puncture, and capillary sampling. Arterial samples are preferred over capillary samples (heel stick or finger stick) because arterial samples are more reliable in obtaining an accurate PaO_2 value. Capillary samples are useful for measuring PCO_2 and pH in infants with chronic lung disease. All these methods are invasive, with the potential for complications (see Chapter 15).

MEDICATIONS USED DURING VENTILATION THERAPY

A. Surfactant: A deficiency of surfactant in the lungs of premature infants results in impaired gas exchange and increased work of breathing. Administration of exogenous surfactants is routinely carried out in preterm infants with evidence of respiratory distress syndrome (RDS). Surfactant therapy may also be indicated for more mature infants with meconium aspiration or pulmonary hypertension (American Academy of Pediatrics, 1999). Exogenous surfactant may be in a natural form taken from the lungs of pigs or calves (Beractant [Survanta], Bovine Lung Exogenous Surfactant [BLES], Curosurf, Infasurf) or manufactured artificially (Exosurf). Exogenous surfactant is a liquid preparation administered directly into the endotracheal tube.

1. Dose: depends on the product used; approximately 4 or 5 ml/kg/dose.
2. Administration: suction the infant 10 to 15 minutes prior to surfactant administration. Ensure that the endotracheal tube is in proper position prior to beginning surfactant administration. Follow the manufacturer's recommendations regarding positioning for administration.
3. Monitor: continuous cardiac, respiratory, and oxygen saturation monitoring during and after administration, frequent vital signs and blood pressure, ongoing assessment of air entry and chest excursion.
4. Considerations: infants may become hypoxic, bradycardic, or distressed during surfactant administration. Rapid changes in lung compliance may occur during and immediately following dosing. Changes in lung compliance increase the risk of pulmonary hemorrhage in infants with a PDA.
5. Endotracheal suctioning is delayed for at least one to two hours after dosing to avoid removing the drug.
6. Results: Cochrane Review of natural surfactant use in preterm infants found an improvement in respiratory status, a decreased risk of pneumothorax, a decrease in pulmonary interstitial emphysema, a decreased risk of bronchopulmonary dysplasia, and a decreased mortality (Soll, 2003).

B. Bronchodilators.

1. Methylxanthines: two drugs, theophylline and caffeine citrate, are routinely used to stimulate respirations in preterm neonates (see Chapter 24). In addition to improving respiratory drive, methylxanthines also increase the contractility of the diaphragm and enhance chemoreceptor sensitivity to carbon dioxide. Both drugs improve renal and pulmonary blood flow, causing mild diuresis and bronchodilation, and increased heart rate and cardiac output (Gannon, 2000).
   a. Theophylline (aminophylline).
      (1) Dose: loading dose, 5 to 6 mg/kg; maintenance dose, 2 to 3 mg/kg/dose every 8 to 12 hours; by continuous IV infusion, IV, or by mouth (Zenk, 2003).
      (2) Monitor: trough level obtained 30 minutes before dose, 72 hours after therapy is initiated; therapeutic range: apnea: 5 to 15 μg/ml (Zenk, 2003).
      (3) Aminophylline is approximately 80% theophylline.
      (4) Considerations: holding dose if heart rate exceeds 180 bpm.
      (5) Adverse effects: gastrointestinal upset, tachycardia, diuresis, poor weight gain, hyperreflexia, jitteriness, and reduced sleep.
   b. Caffeine: preferred by many clinicians over theophylline because it is given once daily and has fewer adverse effects. Caffeine does not have as great a bronchodilator or diuretic effect as theophylline.
      (1) Dose: loading dose, 10 mg/kg of caffeine base; maintenance 2.5 mg/kg caffeine base every 24 hours beginning 24 hours after loading dose (Zenk, 2003).
      (2) Write orders in terms of caffeine base. Caffeine citrate is 50% caffeine base.
      (3) Serum drug concentrations are not routinely monitored.
      (4) Adverse effects: usually well tolerated. Tachycardia, jitteriness, and mild glycosuria may occur at higher serum concentrations.

2. Albuterol: achieves bronchodilator effect similar to aminophylline but with less cardiac stimulation; enhances clearance of mucociliary secretions.
   a. Dose: aerosol, 0.5 to 1 mg/kg per dose every 4 hours via nebulized solution; metered dose inhaler: 1 or 2 puffs every 6 hours (Zenk, 2003).
   b. Monitor: serum concentration not determined; heart rate and respiratory effect monitored.
   c. Considerations: dilution of aerosol preparation with normal saline solution before use; signs of toxicity: tachycardia, arrhythmia, tremors, and irritability.

C. **Diuretics.**

1. Furosemide (Lasix): affects chloride transport in the loop of Henle, causes loss of chloride, sodium, potassium, and calcium. Diuresis may decrease pulmonary blood flow, decrease vascular resistance, and increase pulmonary compliance.
   a. Dose: 1 to 2 mg/kg/dose IV or by mouth (Zenk, 2003); a higher oral dose may be required because of reduced bioavailability. Interval: premature infant, every 24 hours; term, every 12 hours; full-term greater than 1 month, every 6 to 8 hours. Long-term therapy: consider a dose every other day.
   b. Monitor: accurate intake and output; specific gravity to evaluate response; frequent electrolyte values to monitor losses and replacement.
   c. Considerations: ototoxic, with transient and permanent hearing losses reported; renal calculi reported with long-term use.
2. Spironolactone (Aldactone): exerts inhibitory effect of aldosterone on the tubules, with resultant increase in sodium losses and sparing of potassium.
   a. Dose: 1 to 3 mg/kg/dose by mouth every 24 hours (Zenk, 2003).
   b. Monitor: accurate intake and output; specific gravity to evaluate response; electrolyte values after 48 to 72 hours to detect hyperkalemia.
   c. Considerations: may cause rash, vomiting, and diarrhea. Use with caution in infant with impaired renal function.
3. Chlorothiazide (Diuril): inhibits sodium reabsorption in the distal renal tubule; has potentiating effect on furosemide; calcium sparing.
   a. Dose: 10 to 30 mg/kg/dose by mouth every 12 hours (Zenk, 2003).
   b. Monitor: accurate intake and output; specific gravity to measure response; electrolyte, sodium, potassium, chloride, calcium, phosphorus, magnesium, and bicarbonate concentrations to evaluate losses and replacement.
   c. Considerations: optimal response when used with furosemide or spironolactone; may cause electrolyte disturbances and hyperglycemia; avoid with significant renal or hepatic dysfunction.
4. Hydrochlorothiazide with spironolactone (Aldactazide): Thiazides inhibit sodium reabsorption in the distal nephron, resulting in increased excretion of sodium chloride. The spironolactone is an aldosterone antagonist that helps to prevent potassium excretion and hypokalemia.
   a. Dose: 1 to 3 mg/kg/day given as a single daily dose or divided every 12 hours (Zenk, 2003).
   b. Monitor: accurate intake and output when first starting spironolactone; signs of dehydration; serum electrolytes.
   c. Considerations: may cause hyperglycemia or altered glucose tolerance; hypokalemia may result despite the potassium sparing effect of spironolactone.

D. **Corticosteroids.**

1. Dexamethasone (Decadron): a long-acting antiinflammatory medication used in the treatment of chronic lung disease and tracheal edema before and after extubation. Recent studies have documented an increased risk of adverse neurodevelopmental outcomes in infants receiving systemic steroid therapy.

These findings have resulted in the following recommendations developed by the American Academy of Pediatrics and the Canadian Paediatric Society (AAP and CPS, 2002):

a. Routine use of corticosteroids for the prevention or treatment of chronic lung disease in low birth weight (LBW) infants is not recommended.
b. The use of corticosteroids outside of randomized control trials should be limited to exceptional clinical circumstances.
c. Monitoring of long-term neurodevelopmental outcomes of infants in systemic steroid clinical trials is strongly encouraged.
d. Clinical trials investigating alternative antiinflammatory corticosteroids are needed before further recommendations can be made.
e. Further recommendations suggest that dexamethasone use be restricted to ventilator-dependent infants unlikely to survive without corticosteroids (Halliday, 2001); that informed parental consent be obtained (Halliday, 2000); and that the lowest dose and shortest course possible be prescribed (Halliday, 2001).

2. Monitor serum and urine glucose; blood pressure; gastric aspirates for blood. Echocardiogram is indicated if treatment continues longer than 7 days.
3. Considerations: adverse effects—hyperglycemia, glycosuria, hypertension, cardiac effects, sodium and water retention, poor weight gain, hypokalemia, hypocalcemia, and increased risk of sepsis.

E. **Paralytic agents.**

1. Pancuronium (Pavulon): pharmacologic relaxation/paralysis of the skeletal muscle to promote improved mechanical ventilation with improved oxygenation/ventilation; decreased barotrauma; decreased fluctuations in cerebral blood flow.
   a. Dose: 0.1 mg/kg/dose (0.02-0.15 mg/kg/dose) IV push. Interval: every 1 to 4 hours as needed for paralysis (Zenk, 2003).
   b. Monitor: vital signs frequently; blood pressure continuously.
   c. Considerations: mandatory availability of mechanical ventilation before use; adequate pulmonary toilet mandatory because no swallow or gag reflex is present; eye lubricant necessary. Signs of toxicity: tachycardia, hypertension, or hypotension.
2. Vecuronium: similar to pancuronium, but shorter acting. Dose: 0.1 mg/kg/dose IV push every 1 to 2 hours as needed for paralysis (Zenk, 2003).

F. **Pain control/sedation (see Chapter 16).**

G. **Inhaled nitric oxide (iNO):** endogenous nitric oxide is released from the endothelium and is responsible for vascular smooth muscle relaxation. iNO is used to promote relaxation of the pulmonary smooth muscle to facilitate perfusion of the lung and gas exchange. iNO has been approved by the FDA for the treatment of near-term and term infants with persistent pulmonary hypertension of the newborn (PPHN) (Hagedorn et al., 2002). Use of iNO in preterm infants remains experimental.

1. Dose: initial 20 parts per million (ppm); after 4 hours reduce dose to 6 ppm. iNO is then weaned by 20% in a stepwise fashion to a dose of 1 ppm before discontinuation (Zenk, 2003).
2. Duration of therapy: usually less than 5 days.
3. Monitor: vital signs frequently, blood pressure continuously, complete blood count (CBC), methemoglobin levels, environmental levels of NO.
4. Considerations: may cause methemoglobinemia, a decrease in platelet aggregation.
5. Results: term and near-term infants: significant reduction in the need for ECMO (Field, 2002; Finer, 2000). Cochrane Review concluded that enough

evidence exists to recommend iNO for this population of infants with hypoxic respiratory failure who do not have diaphragmatic hernia (Finer and Barrington, 2002). A randomized controlled trial of iNO in preterm infants found a decreased need for mechanical ventilation, improved survival without intraventricular hemorrhage (IVH), and a trend toward a decrease in chronic lung disease (Kinsella et al., 1999). A metaanalysis of iNO in preterm infants failed to demonstrate a decrease in mortality or incidence of chronic lung disease (Barrington and Finer, 2002; Hoehn et al., 2000).

WEANING FROM CONVENTIONAL VENTILATION

A. **Indications.**
   1. Clinical status of infant consistent with beginning resolution of pulmonary condition.
   2. Ventilation becomes easier with less support and may result in hypocapnia.
   3. Less inspiratory pressure is required to achieve desired VT.

B. **Techniques.**
   1. Physical assessment of respiratory status: breath sounds, aeration, chest wall excursion, and spontaneous respiratory rate. Physical assessment of cardiovascular status: color, perfusion, heart rate, pulses, blood pressure, and presence or absence of murmur. Physical assessment of neurologic status: presence of spontaneous respirations, tone, irritability, and reflexes.
   2. Radiographic evaluation: useful in documenting improved lung status and absence of pathologic changes.
   3. Laboratory analysis: fluid, electrolyte, and hematologic stability.
   4. Blood gas analysis: primary information for weaning an infant from conventional mechanical ventilation. If all other assessments indicate improvement, blood gas analysis provides information about the appropriate ventilator settings to adjust. To decrease the PaO_2, alter the MAP: reduce PIP, FiO_2, inspiratory/expiratory time (I/t) ratio, or PEEP. To increase $PaCO_2$, decrease ventilation: decrease rate or tidal volume. During weaning it is important to try to decrease the most injurious parameters first. O_2 toxic effects from free O_2 radicals damage lung tissue, and O_2 is associated with retinopathy of prematurity. Therefore it is important to keep O_2 use at a minimum. PIP, PEEP, I/t ratio, and rate are all associated with barotrauma, so weaning should be achieved as soon as possible.

C. **Extubation from mechanical ventilation.** When low ventilator parameters have been achieved (intermittent mandatory ventilation, 10-20/min; PIP, 14-18; VT 3.5-5 ml/kg; FiO_2, 0.21-0.30), the infant should be evaluated for extubation. Is the infant capable of maintaining respiration without ventilator support? Some infants may need a transition to nasal CPAP, nasal prong, cannula, or O_2 hood.

Nursing Care During Weaning Process

A. **Airway management, equipment function, and monitoring of the infant do not change during the weaning process.**

B. **Frequent assessment of the infant's vital signs, blood pressure, O_2 saturation, and neurologic status is essential.** Documentation of this assessment will facilitate appropriate changes in ventilator support.

C. **Be alert for decompensation of respiratory or cardiovascular status during this time, and notify the appropriate personnel when necessary.**

D. **Preparation for extubation.**

1. Equipment for reintubation available at the bedside.
2. Suction of ETT and oropharynx.
3. Postextubation equipment ready for use.
4. Blood gas determination after extubation.
5. X-ray examination of chest to rule out atelectasis if decompensation occurs.
6. Frequent physical assessment every 1 to 2 hours after extubation for 24 hours.
7. Frequent position changes; suctioning as needed.
8. Explanation of the plan and process to the family before extubation.

INTERPRETATION OF BLOOD GAS VALUES

The purpose of obtaining blood gas values in the neonate is to determine whether the patient has adequate ventilation and perfusion. Blood gas values also facilitate analysis of oxygenation and acid-base status. Oxygenation is determined by the Pao_2. The Pao_2 is the amount of O_2 dissolved in the serum—3% of the total O_2 content. The remainder of the body's O_2 is bound to hemoglobin. Acceptable arterial blood gas values are illustrated in Table 25-2. Capillary Pao_2 reliability is uncertain. The value is lower than with an arterial specimen. Acid-base balance is indicated by the pH and the base deficit or excess. Ventilation is measured by Pco_2.

A. **Acidosis and alkalosis.** Changes in the pH from the normal range indicate a change in the acid-base status of the infant. An elevated pH, greater than 7.45, is alkalosis, which is caused by excess base or decreased acid in the blood. A decreased pH, less than 7.35, is acidosis, which is caused by decreased base or increased acid in the blood.
   1. Respiratory acidosis ($Paco_2$ >45; pH <7.35), caused by the accumulation of CO_2, the respiratory acid, results from hypoventilation.
   2. Respiratory alkalosis ($Paco_2$ <35; pH >7.45), caused by the decrease of CO_2, results from hyperventilation.
   3. Metabolic alkalosis (HCO_3^- >26, base excess > +2; pH > 7.45) is caused by a failure to excrete HCO_3^-, which is controlled by kidney function.
   4. Metabolic acidosis (HCO_3^- <22, base deficit > −2 and <7.35) is caused by failure to retain HCO_3^- or by an increase in blood acid, which is controlled by the kidney.
   5. For causes of acidosis and alkalosis, see Table 25-3.

B. **Disorders of acid-base balance (see Chapter 8).**

C. **Interpreting a blood gas value.**
   1. Evaluate the pH. Is there an acidosis or an alkalosis?
   2. Evaluate the $Paco_2$. If it is not normal, does it contribute to the acid-base status? Or is it a compensating factor?
   3. Evaluate the HCO_3^- and the base excess or deficit. If they are not normal, do they contribute to the acid-base status? Or are they compensating factors?

TABLE 25-2
Normal Arterial Blood Gas Values

pH	7.35-7.45
$Paco_2$	35-45 mm Hg
Pao_2	50-80 mm Hg
HCO_3^-	22-26 mEq/L
Base excess	−2 to +2

■ TABLE 25-3
■ ■ **Causes of Acidosis and Alkalosis**

Cause	Mechanism
Respiratory Acidosis (↑$Paco_2$, ↓pH)	
CNS depression	Maternal narcotics during labor, asphyxia, intracranial hemorrhage, neuromuscular disorder, CNS dysmaturity (apnea of prematurity)
Decreased ventilation-perfusion ratio	Obstructed airway, meconium aspiration, choanal atresia
Decreased lung compliance	Hyaline membrane disease, pulmonary insufficiency, diaphragmatic hernia
Injury to the thorax	Phrenic nerve paralysis, pneumothorax
Metabolic Acidosis (↓HCO_3^-, pH, and base excess [negative value])	
Decreased tissue perfusion	Increased lactic acid production
Sepsis, congestive heart failure	
Renal failure	Increased organic acids
Renal tubular acidosis	Renal loss of base
Diarrhea	Gastrointestinal loss of base
Respiratory Alkalosis (↓$Paco_2$, ↑pH)	
Iatrogenic	Excessive mechanical ventilation
Hypoxemia	Increase in alveolar ventilation
CNS irritation (pain)	
Metabolic Alkalosis (↑HCO_3^-, pH and base excess [positive value])	
Gastric suction	Loss of acid
Vomiting	Loss of acid
Diuretic therapy	Renal losses of H^+ ion
Iatrogenic	Administration of HCO_3^- (base added)

CNS, Central nervous system.

4. Evaluate the Pao_2. Is there hypoxia or hyperoxia?
5. From this information, you can attempt to identify the specific cause of the abnormal acid-base status and treat as indicated.

REFERENCES

American Academy of Pediatrics and Canadian Paediatric Society: Postnatal corticosteroids to treat or prevent chronic lung disease in preterm infants. *Pediatrics, 109*(2): 330-338, 2002.

American Academy of Pediatrics Committee on Fetus and Newborn: Surfactant replacement therapy for respiratory distress syndrome. *Pediatrics, 103*(3):684-685, 1999.

Barrington, K.J. and Finer, N.N.: Inhaled nitric oxide for respiratory failure in preterm infants (Cochrane Review). In *Cochrane Library,* Issue 3, Oxford, UK, 2002, Update Software.

Baumer, J.H.: International randomized controlled trial of patient triggered ventilation in neonatal respiratory distress syndrome. *Archives of Disease in Childhood, 82*:F5-F10, 2000.

Beresford, M.W., Shaw, N.J., and Manning, D.: Randomized controlled trial of patient triggered and conventional fast rate ventilation in neonatal respiratory distress syndrome. *Archives of Disease in Childhood, 82*:F14-F18, 2000.

Bhuta, T., Clark, R.H., and Henderson-Smart, D.J.: Rescue high frequency oscillatory ventilation vs conventional mechanical ventilation for infants with severe pulmonary dysfunction born at or near term (Cochrane Review). In *The Cochrane Library,* Issue 3, Oxford, UK, 2003, Update Software.

Bhuta, T. and Henderson-Smart, D.J.: Elective high frequency jet ventilation versus conventional ventilation for respiratory distress syndrome in preterm infants (Cochrane Review). In *The Cochrane Library,* Issue 1, Oxford, UK, 2003, Update Software.

Blackburn, S.T.: *Maternal, fetal, and neonatal physiology: A clinical perspective* (2nd ed.). Philadelphia, 2003, Saunders.

Carlo, W.A. and Ambalavanan, N.: Conventional mechanical ventilation: traditional and new strategies. *Pediatrics in Review, 20*(12):e117-e126, 1999.

Cifuentes, J., Segars, A.H., and Carlo, W.A.: Respiratory system management and complications. In C. Kenner and J. Lott (Eds.): *Comprehensive neonatal nursing: A physiologic approach* (3rd ed.). Philadelphia, 2003, Saunders, pp. 348-362.

Clark, R., Slutsky, A., and Gerstmann, D.: Lung protective strategies of ventilation in the neonate. What are they? *Pediatrics, 105*(1 Pt 1):112-114, 2000.

Cole, C. and Fiascone, J.: Strategies for prevention of neonatal chronic lung disease. *Seminars in Perinatology, 24*(6): 445-462, 2000.

Field, D.: Alternative strategies for the management of respiratory failure in the newborn-clinical realities. *Seminars in Neonatology, 7(5)*:429-436, 2002.

Finer, N.N.: Inhaled nitric oxide in term and near-term infants: Neurodevelopmental follow-up of the neonatal inhaled nitric oxide study group (NINOS). *Journal of Pediatrics, 136*(5):611-617, 2000.

Finer, N.N. and Barrington, K.J.: Nitric oxide for respiratory failure in infants born at or near term (Cochrane Review). In *Cochrane Library,* Issue 3, Oxford, UK, 2002, Update Software.

Gannon, B.A.: Theophylline or caffeine: Which is better for apnea of prematurity? *Neonatal Network, 19*(8):33-36, 2000.

Gomez, M., Hansen, T., and Corbet, A.: Principles of respiratory monitoring and therapy. In H.W. Taeusch and R.A. Ballard (Eds.): *Avery's diseases of the newborn* (7th ed.). Philadelphia, 1998, Saunders, pp. 576-594.

Greenough, A., Milner, A.D. and Dimitriou, G.: Synchronized mechanical ventilation for respiratory support in newborn infants (Cochrane Review). In *The Cochrane Library,* Issue 1, Oxford, UK, 2001, CD000456. Update Software.

Hagedorn, M.I., Gardener, S.L., and Abman, S.H.: Respiratory diseases. In G.B. Merenstein and S.L. Gardener (Eds.): *Handbook of neonatal intensive care* (5th ed.). St Louis, 2002, Mosby, pp. 485-575.

Halliday, H.L.: Perinatal corticosteroid treatment-helpful or harmful. *Archives of Perinatal Medicine, 6*:7-9, 2000.

Halliday, H.L.: Postnatal steroids: A dilemma for the neonatologist. *Acta Paediatrica, 90*:116-118, 2001.

Henderson-Smart, D.J., Bhuta, T., Cools, F., and Offringe, M.: Elective high frequency oscillatory ventilation vs conventional ventilation for acute pulmonary dysfunction in preterm infants (Cochrane Review). In *Cochrane Library,* Issue 1, Oxford, UK, 2003, Update Software.

Herrera, C.M., Gerhardt, T., Claure, N., et al.: Effects of volume-guaranteed synchronized intermittent mandatory ventilation in preterm infants recovering from respiratory failure. *Pediatrics, 110*(3):529-533, 2002.

HIFI Study Group: High-frequency oscillatory ventilation compared with conventional mechanical ventilation in the treatment of respiratory failure in preterm infants. *New England Journal of Medicine, 320*(2):88-93, 1989.

Hodson, W.A. and Truog, W.E.: Principles of management of respiratory problems. In G.B. Avery, M.A. Fletcher, and M.G. MacDonald (Eds.): *Neonatology: Pathophysiology and management of the newborn.* Philadelphia, 1999, Lippincott Williams & Wilkins, pp. 533-555.

Hoehn, T., Krause, M.F., and Buhrer, C.: Inhaled nitric oxide in preterm infants: A meta-analysis. *Journal of Perinatal Medicine, 28*(1):7-13, 2000.

Kinsella, J.P., Walsh, W.F., Bose, C.L., et al.: Inhaled nitric oxide in premature neonates with severe hypoxaemic respiratory failure: A randomized controlled trial. *Lancet, 354*(9184):1061-1065, 1999.

Lockridge, T.: Following the learning curve: The evolution of kinder, gentler neonatal respiratory technology. *Journal of Obstetric, Gynecologic, and Neonatal Nursing, 28*(4):443-455, 1999.

Loper, D.L.: Physiologic principles of the respiratory system. In D.F. Askin (Ed.): *Acute respiratory care of the neonate.* Petaluma, CA, 1997, NICU Ink, p. 21.

McGettigan, M.C., Adolph, V.R., Ginsberg, H.G., and Goldsmith, J.P.: New ways to ventilate newborns in acute respiratory failure. *Pediatric Clinics of North America, 45*(3):475-509, 1998.

Moriette, G., Paris-Llado, J., Walti, H., et al.: Prospective randomized multi-center comparison of high-frequency oscillatory ventilation and conventional ventilation in preterm infants of less than 30 weeks with RDS. *Pediatrics, 107*(2):363-372, 2001.

Polin, R.A. and Sahni, R.: Newborn experience with CPAP. *Seminars in Neonatology, 7*(5):379-389, 2002.

Rimensberger, P., Beghetti, M., Hanquinet, S., et al.: First intention high-frequency oscillation with early lung volume optimization improves pulmonary outcome in VLBW infants with RDS. *Pediatrics, 105*(6):1202-1208, 2000.

Ruof, H. and Fahwenstich, H.: Closed versus open ET suctioning in ventilated preterm infants. *Pediatric Research, 47*:430A, 2000.

Schulze, A.: Enhancement of mechanical ventilation of neonates by computer technology. *Seminars in Perinatology, 24*(6):429-444, 2000.

Schwartz, J.E.: New technologies applied to the management of the respiratory system. In C. Kenner and J. Lott (Eds.): *Comprehensive neonatal nursing: A physiologic perspective* (3rd ed.). Philadelphia, 2003, Saunders, pp. 363-375.

Soll, R.F.: Prophylactic natural surfactant extract for preventing morbidity and mortality in preterm infants (Cochrane Review). In *Cochrane Library,* Issue 1, Oxford, UK, 2003, Update Software.

Sreenan, C., Lemke, R., Hudson-Mason, A., et al.: High-flow nasal cannulae in the management of apnea of prematurity: A comparison with conventional nasal continuous positive airway pressure. *Pediatrics, 107*(5):1081-1083, 2001.

Thome, U., Kossel H., Lipowsky G., et al. Randomized comparison of high frequency ventilation with high-rate intermittent positive pressure ventilation in preterm infants with respiratory failure. *Journal of Pediatrics, 135*(1):9-11, 1999.

Zenk, K.: *Neonatal medications and nutrition: A comprehensive guide* (3rd ed.). Santa Rosa, CA, 2003, NICU Ink.

ADDITIONAL READINGS

Askin, D.F.: Interpretation of neonatal blood gases. Part I. Physiology and acid-base homeostasis. *Neonatal Network, 16*(5):17-21, 1997.

Askin, D.F.: Interpretation of neonatal blood gases. Part II. Disorders of acid-base balance. *Neonatal Network, 16*(6):23-29, 1997.

Clark, R.H. and Gerstmann, D.R.: Controversies in high-frequency ventilation. *Clinics in Perinatology, 25*(1):113-122, 1998.

Donn, S.M. and Sinha, S.K.: Controversies in patient triggered ventilation. *Clinics in Perinatology, 25*(1):49-61, 1998.

Donn, S.M. and Sinha, S.K.: Newer techniques of mechanical ventilation: An overview. *Seminars in Neonatology, 7*(5):401-407, 2002.

Grier, D.G. and Halliday, H.L.: Corticosteroids in the prevention and management of bronchopulmonary dysplasia. *Seminars in Neonatology, 8*(1):83-91, 2003.

Hansen, T.N., Cooper, T.R., and Weisman, L.E.: *Contemporary diagnosis and management of neonatal respiratory diseases* (2nd ed.). Newtown, PA, 1998, Handbooks in Health Care.

Ho, J.J., Subramaniam, P., and Henderson-Smart, D.J.: Continuous distending pressure for respiratory distress syndrome in preterm infants (Cochrane Review). In *Cochrane Library,* Issue 1, Oxford, UK, 2003, Update Software.

Kattwinkel, J. (Ed.): *Textbook of neonatal resuscitation* (4th ed.). Elk Grove Village, IL, 2000, American Heart Association–American Academy of Pediatrics.

Mariani, G.L. and Carlo, W.A.: Ventilatory management in neonates: Science or art. *Clinics in Perinatology, 25*(1):33-48, 1998.

McGettigan, M.C., Adolph, V.R., Ginsberg, H.G., and Goldsmith, J.P.: New ways to ventilate newborns in acute respiratory failure. *Pediatric Clinics of North America, 45*(3):475-509, 1998.

Sinha, S.K. and Donn, S.M.: Weaning newborns from mechanical ventilation. *Seminars in Neonatology, 7*(5):421-428, 2002.

Zenk, K.: *Neonatal medications and nutrition.* Santa Rosa, CA, 2003, NICU Ink, p. 429.

CHAPTER

26 Extracorporeal Membrane Oxygenation

CAROLYN HOUSKA LUND

OBJECTIVES

1. Discuss the history of neonatal extracorporeal membrane oxygenation (ECMO) and related survival statistics.
2. Discuss indications and contraindications for ECMO.
3. Discuss the criteria used to determine an infant's need for ECMO.
4. Review the technical and mechanical aspects of the ECMO procedure.
5. Review the physiology of extracorporeal circulation.
6. Discuss the general care given to infants undergoing the ECMO procedure and the support provided to their families.
7. Review follow-up and outcome of ECMO survivors.

ECMO is the use of a modified heart-lung machine for days or weeks to support life and allow treatment and recovery during severe cardiac or pulmonary failure (Bartlett et al., 2000). Despite recent advances in ventilatory management, respiratory failure remains the most frequent cause of neonatal death. ECMO is used as a "rescue" therapy for the 2% to 5% of critically ill infants who do not respond to maximal ventilatory, pharmacologic, and surgical treatments.

ECMO: A HISTORICAL PERSPECTIVE

A. **John Gibbon (1937) invented the first heart-lung machine** and was the first physician to use the technology to perform cardiac surgery successfully. This prototype required direct exposure of the blood to oxygen and a roller pump.
B. **Development of a membrane lung by Clowes (1956)** allowed for separation of the blood and gas phases and dramatically reduced complications (thrombocytopenia, hemolysis, organ failure) of the direct exposure of blood to oxygen.
C. **Development of silicone rubber by Kammermeyer (1957)** made the membrane lung feasible for long-term support.
D. **Kolobow (1969-1970) demonstrated the safe use of extracorporeal support for up to 7 days in lambs,** using a coiled silicone membrane lung.
E. **Prolonged ECMO support for moribund neonates in respiratory failure was attempted from 1965 to 1971.** Bartlett began extensive clinical studies and

reported improvements in survival and morbidity rates (Bartlett, 1986; Bartlett and Gazzaniga, 1978; Bartlett et al., 1982, 1985).

F. **First survivor was successfully treated in 1975.**
   1. Survival rate of 55% in 1981 (Bartlett et al., 1982).
   2. Survival rate of 100% in 1985 (Bartlett et al., 1985).

G. **Bartlett's success prompted randomized, prospective clinical trials at ECMO centers.**
   1. O'Rourke and colleagues (1989), in a prospective clinical trial, demonstrated that the overall survival rate of ECMO-treated infants was 99%, in comparison with 60% of infants treated with conventional mechanical therapy.
   2. The UK Neonatal ECMO Trial Group (1996) found the mortality in infants who were randomized to ECMO support was 29%, compared with 61% for the control infants who received maximal conventional therapy.

H. **Extracorporeal Life Support Organization (ELSO) International Registry Report (January 2003) lists a total of 17,878 infants treated since 1975, with an overall survival rate of 78%.** A total of 120 ECMO centers reported. Survival by diagnosis was as follows: meconium aspiration syndrome 94%, persistent pulmonary hypertension of the newborn/persistent fetal circulation 79%, respiratory distress syndrome/hyaline membrane disease 84%, pneumonia/sepsis 76%, air-leak syndrome 69%, congenital diaphragmatic hemia 53%, sepsis 75%, pneumonia 58%, and other diagnoses 66%.

CRITERIA FOR USE OF ECMO

A. **Neonatal ECMO patient criteria (Finer, 2000).**
   1. Gestational age greater than 34 weeks.
   2. Birth weight greater than 2000 g.
   3. No significant coagulopathy or uncontrollable bleeding.
   4. No major intracranial hemorrhage.
   5. Mechanical ventilation for fewer than 10 to 14 days.
   6. Reversible lung injury.
   7. No lethal malformations.
   8. No major cardiac malformations (except in infants requiring stabilization and life support before or after surgery).

B. **Acute and reversible respiratory or cardiac pathology.**
   1. Respiratory distress syndrome.
   2. Meconium aspiration syndrome.
   3. Persistent pulmonary hypertension of the newborn.
   4. Congenital diaphragmatic hernia.
   5. Sepsis.
   6. Life support before or after cardiac surgery.
   7. Acute respiratory distress syndrome.

C. **Cranial and cardiac ultrasonography findings** ruling out severe intracranial hemorrhage and cyanotic congenital heart disease.

D. **Objective criteria for final selection predictive of greater than 80% mortality rate** (Box 26-1). To achieve specificity, each ECMO center must determine its own mortality indicators and criteria. Criteria may differ in different disease states, such as septic shock, congenital diaphragmatic hernia (CDH), or severe air leak caused by barotrauma.

E. **Pre-ECMO stabilization, including optimal ventilatory management and trial of high-frequency ventilation, volume support, vasopressors, vasodilator medications, surfactant, and nitric oxide if indicated.** These should be used at

■ BOX 26-1
■ **NEONATAL ECMO PATIENT QUALIFYING CRITERIA**

Alveolar-Arterial Difference in Partial Pressure of Oxygen: 600 to 624 mm Hg for 4 to 12 Hours at Sea Level

$$AaDo_2 = \frac{\text{Atmospheric pressure} - 47 - (Paco_2 + Pao_2)}{Fio_2}$$

Note: 47 is the partial pressure of water vapor.

Oxygenation Index: 25 to 60 for 30 Minutes to 6 Hours

$$OI = \frac{MAP \times Fio_2 \times 100}{Pao_2}$$

where MAP is mean airway pressure.

Pao_2: 35 to 50 mm Hg for 2 to 12 Hours

Acute Deterioration

Pao_2 ≤30-40 mm Hg
pH ≤7.25 for 2 hours
Intractable hypotension

From Rosenberg, E. and Seguin, J.: Selection criteria for use of ECLS in neonates. In J. Zwischenberger and R.H. Bartlett (Eds.): *ECMO: Extracorporeal Cardiopulmonary Support in Critical Care.* Ann Arbor, 1995, Extracorporeal Life Support Organization.

a center where ECMO can be initiated quickly if the infant does not respond adequately.

VENOARTERIAL PERFUSION

A. Technique for venoarterial perfusion (VA).

1. Deoxygenated blood is drained from the right side of the heart through a cannula placed in the right atrium via the right internal jugular vein.
2. Venous cannula must be a size that is capable of delivering total cardiac output (120-150 ml/kg/min) to the membrane lung; cannulas of largest possible internal diameter (8F-14F) are inserted.
3. Oxygenated blood is returned through a cannula placed into the ascending aorta via the right common carotid artery (Peek and Firmin, 2000).

B. Advantages.

1. Technique provides both respiratory and cardiac support by decompressing pulmonary circulation, decreases pulmonary artery and pulmonary capillary filtration pressure, and supports circulation by augmenting the pumping action of the heart.
2. Positive-pressure ventilation can be reduced to minimal parameters: peak inspiratory pressure, 15 to 20 cm H_2O; positive end-expiratory pressure, 5 to 10 cm H_2O; ventilator rate, 10 to 20/minute; and fractional concentration of oxygen in inspired gas (Fio_2), 21%.

C. Disadvantages.

1. Emboli (air or particulate) could be infused directly into the arterial circulation.
2. Ligation of carotid artery may affect cerebral perfusion.

VENOVENOUS PERFUSION

A. Technique for venovenous (VV) perfusion.

1. Double-lumen cannula is used (size 12F, 14F, or 15F). Deoxygenated blood is drained from the venous limb, positioned in the right atrium.

2. Blood is returned through the arterial limb, also located in the right atrium, with side holes positioned at the tricuspid valve.
3. Blood flow is directed across the valve, into the right ventricle, and through the pulmonary circulation. It returns to the left atrium before entering the systemic circulation via the aorta.

B. **Advantages (Pettignano et al., 2000).**
1. No ligation of the carotid artery is necessary.
2. Oxygenated blood flows through pulmonary circulation, which may help to reverse pulmonary hypertension.
3. Oxygenated blood is provided to the coronary arteries.
4. Emboli (air or particulate) are less likely to result in severe compromise to the infant because blood is not returned directly to the arterial circulation.

C. **Disadvantages (Pettignano et al., 2000).**
1. VV perfusion can be used only with adequate cardiac function because systemic flow is dependent on cardiac output. In the event of cardiac "stun," or decreased function, emergent conversion to VA ECMO may be needed.
2. Recirculation of oxygenated blood can occur. Oxygenated blood returned to the right atrium may be emptied again into the venous side of the double-lumen cannula, rather than across the tricuspid valve.
3. Use of somewhat higher ventilatory support may be required because lower flow rates are achieved with the smaller lumens of the double-lumen cannula.
4. Vasopressor therapy may need to be continued to support blood pressure and ECMO flow.

CIRCUIT COMPONENTS AND ADDITIONAL DEVICES

A. **Cannulas (Fig. 26-1).**
1. Cannulas remove deoxygenated venous blood and return oxygenated blood to the circulation.

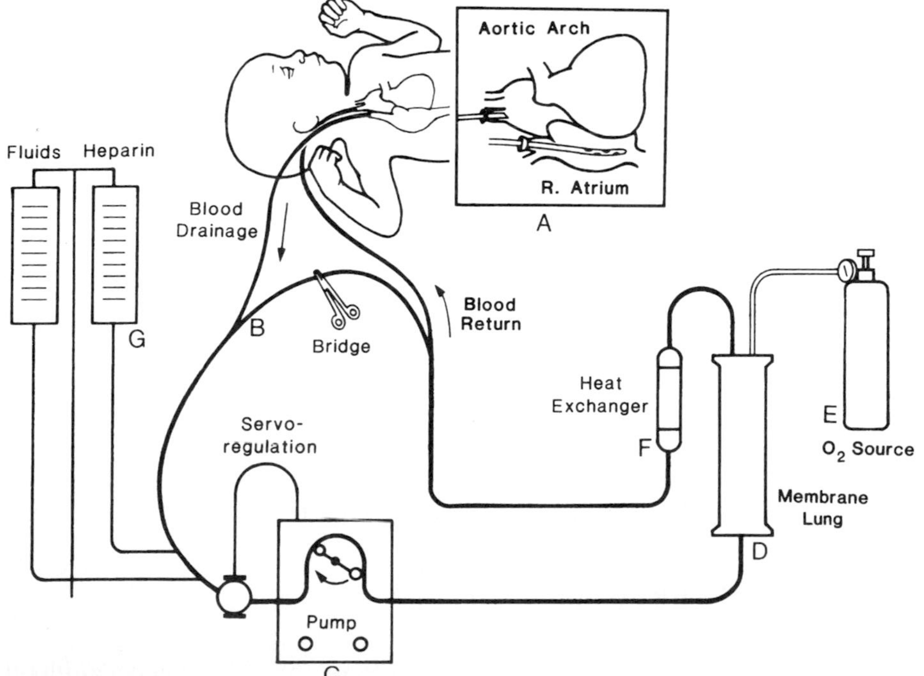

FIGURE 26-1 ■ Components of ECMO circuit: cannulas, polyvinyl chloride tubing, roller head pump, membrane oxygenator (lung), gas source, heat exchanger, and infusion pumps.

2. Before insertion of the cannulas, the infant is paralyzed and given opiates to prevent respiratory movement and air embolism, and systemic heparin is given to prevent clotting of the cannulas and the circuit (Nugent and Matranga, 1997).
3. In VA ECMO the venous cannula tip is positioned in the right atrium to drain blood flow from the inferior vena cava and the superior vena cava. The arterial cannula tip reaches just to the aortic arch.
4. In VV ECMO the double-lumen cannula is positioned in the right atrium, with the arterial side directed toward the tricuspid valve.

B. Polyvinyl chloride (PVC) tubing.

1. Tubing consists of Luer-Lok connectors, stopcocks, infusion sites, and silicone bladder.
2. Blood circulates throughout all components of the ECMO circuit; parenteral fluids, medications, and blood products are administered into the venous side of circuit (before the membrane oxygenator).
3. Only platelets are infused on the arterial side of circuit, or into the patient directly, to prevent adherence to the membrane oxygenator.
4. Precautions and guidelines for placing medications and blood products into the circuit are the same as those for safely administering medications and blood products directly to patients.

C. Silicone bladder for venous pressure monitoring.

1. Collapsible silicone bladder distends with returning venous blood.
2. Inadequate flow (decreased venous return) into the ECMO circuit causes the bladder to collapse, which triggers a microswitch and an audible alarm and stops the roller head pump.
3. When the bladder reexpands, the microswitch reengages the pump and normal pump operation continues.
4. Adequate venous return is critical for maintaining cardiorespiratory support; therefore, the cause of decreased return must be recognized and corrected immediately.
5. Servomechanism regulation of ECMO flow can also be achieved by transducers placed in the circuits. Premembrane (venous) pressure and postmembrane (arterial) pressure may be monitored continuously to signal extracorporeal flow problems before collapse of the silicone bladder. This allows for early detection and timely intervention.
   a. Fall in premembrane pressure indicates decreased venous return.
   b. Rise in postmembrane pressure indicates malfunction of membrane oxygenator or heat exchanger.

D. Pumps.

1. Roller head pumps are the most commonly used. They compress and displace the blood in the PVC tubing placed in the pump raceway.
2. Blood is pushed forward, creating gentle suction in the venous cannula and assisting left ventricular function when VA bypass is used.
3. Digital display indicates circuit flow in cubic centimeters per minute.
4. Electrically powered; must be hand cranked or attached to battery pack if power failure occurs.
5. Centrifugal pumps generate flow by means of a spinning motor; commonly used for bypass during cardiovascular surgery and, at some centers, for ECMO bypass.
6. Recently developed "M-pump" is a passively filled, nonocclusive roller pump that does not generate negative pressure.

E. **Membrane oxygenator.**
 1. Solid silicone polymer membrane envelope with plastic space screen is wrapped spirally around a spool; encased in a silicone rubber sleeve.
 2. Oxygenator of choice because it eliminates the damaging blood gas interface, ensures constant blood volume, and is relatively easy to operate (Hirschl, 2000).

F. **Heat exchanger.**
 1. Located downstream from the oxygenator.
 2. Rewarms blood to 37.2° C (normothermia) before returning it to the infant's circulation.
 3. Heat loss occurs from cooling effect of ventilating gases inside the oxygenator and circuit exposure to ambient air temperature.

G. **Bubble detector.**
 1. Placed distal (patient side) to heat exchanger to detect air in blood flowing through arterial side of pump as the blood is returned to the patient.
 2. In some systems, when air is detected, the roller head pump is shut off and flow to the patient ceases.

H. **Activated clotting time (ACT) monitoring.**
 1. Intermittent (every 30-60 minutes) monitor of the infant's ACT (Nugent and Matranga, 1997).
 2. Infusion pump for continuous infusion of heparin solution (25-60 units/kg/ml) into ECMO circuit (Nugent and Matranga, 1997).
 3. Titration of heparin solution to keep ACT within the desired range (180-220 seconds) (Pettignano and Cornish, 2000).
 4. For control of heparin administration, no heparin added to any other medications or fluids (an exception may be the fluids being infused into umbilical or peripheral arterial lines).
 5. Factors that influence heparin requirements: thrombocytopenia, abnormal clotting studies, urinary output, and infusions of blood products that contain clotting factors.

I. **Blood gas monitoring.**
 1. Mixed venous oxygen saturation ($S\bar{v}O_2$), monitored continuously, is the optimal parameter to assess tissue oxygen delivery. It can be measured through fiberoptic catheters or by using optical reflectance technology. Correlation with cooximeter values measured by a blood gas machine is required.
 2. Arterial blood gas measurements obtained beyond the membrane oxygenator in the ECMO circuit reflect the function of the membrane lung.
 3. Patient blood gas values and noninvasive oxygen saturation monitoring are used to assess the recovery of lung function and the infant's acid-base balance.

PHYSIOLOGY OF EXTRACORPOREAL CIRCULATION

The physiology of extracorporeal circulation has been discussed by Bartlett (2000), Nugent and Matranga (1997), and Torosian and coworkers (1996).

A. **Blood flow.**
 1. VA bypass is instituted by draining venous blood into the ECMO circuit; a like amount of oxygenated blood is returned to the arterial circulation.
 2. As bypass flow increases, flow through the pulmonary artery decreases faster than bypass flow and reduces total flow in the systemic circulation, causing peripheral and pulmonary hypotension.

3. Blood volume replacement is required for optimal tissue perfusion.
4. ECMO perfusion is nonpulsatile (pulse contour decreases as flow rate increases); kidneys interpret this as inadequate flow and promote the release of renin and aldosterone, which causes sodium retention, extracellular fluid expansion, and a decreased total body potassium concentration.
5. Total patient flow is the sum of ECMO flow and pulmonary blood flow; adequate flow is reached when oxygen delivery and tissue perfusion result in normoxia, normal pH, normal $S\bar{v}O_2$, and normal organ function.
6. Total gas exchange and support are achieved at a flow rate of 120 to 150 ml/kg/minute.

B. Gas exchange.

1. The membrane lung has two compartments divided by a semipermeable membrane: ventilating gas is on one side, and blood is on the other.
2. Oxygen diffuses into the blood because of a pressure gradient between the elevated oxygen pressure in the gas compartment and the low oxygen pressure in the venous blood.
3. Carbon dioxide diffuses from the blood compartment to the gas compartment as a result of a pressure gradient between venous carbon dioxide pressure and the ventilating gas. The carbon dioxide transfer rate is six times greater than oxygen transfer. The ventilating gas mixture is usually enriched with carbon dioxide to prevent hypocapnia.

C. Blood-surface interface.

1. During ECMO up to 80% of the cardiac output is exposed to a large artificial surface each minute.
2. Clot formation is prevented by systemic heparinization; platelet destruction is minimized by preexposure of the circuit to albumin.
3. Platelets show the greatest effect of exposure to a foreign surface, as evidenced by decreased platelet count (thrombocytopenia) and function.
4. Hemolysis is monitored regularly by measuring plasma free hemoglobin levels. It is usually not significantly altered by ECMO flow, although increases may indicate problems with red blood cell destruction in the membrane oxygenator or small-lumen cannula.
5. All types of white blood cells decrease in concentration, and phagocytic activity is significantly decreased.
6. After cessation of ECMO, platelets and white blood cell counts return to normal.

CARE OF THE INFANT DURING ECMO

Nugent and Matranga (1997), Sheehan (1999), and Torosian and coworkers (1996) have discussed the responsibilities of the ECMO specialist and the bedside nurse in the care of the infant during ECMO.

A. Cannulation.

1. Cannulation requires the initiation of systemic anesthesia and analgesia; the operating room staff is in attendance.
2. See Table 26-1 for nursing responsibilities and interventions.
3. ECMO specialist responsibilities:
   a. Maintain and monitor ECMO circuit.
   b. Assess physiologic stability.
   c. Maintain physiologic parameters such as blood gas values, blood pressure, platelet count, $S\bar{v}O_2$ and arterial oxygen saturation (SaO_2) and ACT.

TABLE 26-1
Nursing Responsibilities and Interventions for ECMO

Responsibility	Intervention
BEFORE CANNULATION	
Obtain and document baseline physiologic data.	Record weight, length, head circumference. Draw blood samples for CBC, electrolytes, calcium, glucose, BUN, creatinine, PT/PTT, platelet count and function, arterial blood gas values. Record vital signs: heart rate; respiratory rate; systolic, diastolic, and mean blood pressure; and temperature.
Ensure adequate supply of blood products for replacement.	Draw, type, and cross-match samples for two units of packed red blood cells and fresh frozen plasma. Keep one unit of packed cells and fresh frozen plasma always available in the blood bank.
Maintain prescribed pulmonary support.	Maintain ventilator parameters. Administer muscle relaxants if indicated.
Assemble and prepare equipment.	Prepare infusion pumps to maintain arterial lines and infusion of parenteral fluids and medications into the ECMO circuit. Place the infant on a radiant warmer with the head positioned at the foot of the bed to provide thermoregulation and access for cannulation. Attach infant to physiologic monitoring devices to monitor heart rate, intraarterial blood pressure, transcutaneous oxygen, and other parameters. Insert urinary catheter and nasogastric tube; place to gravity drainage. Remove IV lines just prior to heparinization (optional). Prepare loading dose of heparin (50-100 units/kg). Prepare heparin solution for continuous infusion (100 units/ml 5% dextrose in water). Prepare paralyzing drug (pancuronium bromide, 0.1 mg/kg, or succinylcholine, 1-4 mg/kg). Assist in insertion of arterial line (umbilical or peripheral). Administer prophylactic antibiotics.
DURING CANNULATION	
Monitor cardiopulmonary status during procedure.	Monitor heart rate and intraarterial blood pressure continuously. Obtain blood gas values after paralysis and during cannulation, as indicated by the infant's response to the procedure.
Be prepared to administer cardiopulmonary support.	Have medications and blood products available to correct hypovolemia, bradycardia, acidosis, and cardiac arrest.
Administer medications.	Give loading dose of heparin systemically when vessels are dissected free and are ready to be cannulated. Give paralyzing drug systemically just before cannulation of internal jugular vein if infant has not been previously paralyzed. Give analgesia for anesthetic effect.
Reduce ventilator parameters to minimal settings.	Once adequate bypass is achieved, reduce PIP to 16-20 cm H_2O, PEEP to 4 cm H_2O, ventilator rate to 10 to 20 breaths per minute, and Fio_2 to 21% to 30%. Patients undergoing VV bypass may require greater respiratory support.

■ TABLE 26-1
■ ■ **Nursing Responsibilities and Interventions for ECMO—cont'd**

Responsibility	Intervention
DURING ECMO RUN	
Monitor and document physiologic parameters.	Record hourly: heart rate, blood pressure (systolic, diastolic, mean), respirations, temperature, oxygen saturation, ACT, ECMO flow. Measure hourly accurate intake and output of all body fluids (urine, gastric contents, blood); test all stools for occult blood. Assess hourly: color, breath sounds, heart tones, murmurs, cardiac rhythm, arterial pressure waveform, peripheral perfusion. Assess hourly: level of consciousness, reflexes, tone, and movement of extremities; assess neurologic exam including fontanelle tension, pupil size and reaction every 8 to 12 hours. Record ventilator parameters hourly. Assess weight and head circumference daily.
Monitor and document biochemical parameters.	Draw samples for arterial blood gas values from umbilical or peripheral line as indicated. All other blood specimens are drawn from ECMO circuit by ECMO specialist: electrolytes, calcium, platelets, Chemstrip blood tests, hematocrit every 4 to 8 hours, CBC, PT/PTT, BUN, creatinine, total and direct bilirubin, plasma hemoglobin, fibrinogen, fibrin split products, and blood culture as indicated.
Administer medications.	Remove air bubbles and double-check dosages before infusion. Administer no medications intramuscularly or by venipuncture. Place all medications and fluids into the venous side of the ECMO circuit. Prepare and administer the arterial line (umbilical or peripheral) infusion. Administer parenteral alimentation.
Provide pulmonary support.	Perform endotracheal suctioning according to individual assessment and need. Maintain patent airway; be alert to extubation or plugging. Obtain daily chest films and tracheal aspirate cultures as indicated. Maintain ventilator parameters.
Prevent bleeding.	Avoid all of the following: rectal probes, injections, venipunctures, heel sticks. Avoid invasive procedures. Do not change nasogastric tube, urinary catheters, or endotracheal tube unless absolutely necessary; use premeasured endotracheal tube suction technique. Observe for blood in urine, stools, and endotracheal or nasogastric tubes.
Maintain excellent infection control.	Change all fluids and tubing daily. Change dressings daily and as needed. Maintain closed system for urinary catheter drainage. Maintain strict aseptic and handwashing techniques. Use universal barrier precautions.

Continued

TABLE 26-1
Nursing Responsibilities and Interventions for ECMO—cont'd

Responsibility	Intervention
DURING ECMO RUN—cont'd	
Provide physical care.	Keep skin dry, clean, and free of pressure points. Give mouth care as needed. Provide range of motion as indicated. Turn side to side every 1 to 2 hours.
Provide pain management, sedation, stress reduction.	Minimize noise level. Cluster patient care to maximize sleep period. Administer analgesia: fentanyl or morphine as continuous IV drip. Manage iatrogenic physical dependency by following dose reduction regimen.
Be alert to complications and emergencies.	See text.

ACT, Activated clotting time; *BUN*, blood urea nitrogen; *CBC*, complete blood cell count; *Fio_2*, fractional concentration of oxygen in inspired gas; *PEEP*, positive end-expiratory pressure; *PIP*, peak inspiratory pressure; *PT/PTT*, prothrombin time/partial thromboplastin time; *VV*, venovenous.

Adapted from Nugent, J. and Matranga, G.: Extracorporeal membrane oxygenation. In D.F. Askin (Ed.): *Acute respiratory care of the newborn* (2nd ed.). Petaluma, CA, 1997, NICU Ink, pp. 341-368.

d. Assist nurse in general care of infant.
e. Be prepared for circuit emergencies.

B. During ECMO "run."

1. Bypass is gradually instituted until approximately 80% (120-150 ml/kg/min) of cardiac output is diverted through the ECMO circuit.
2. At maximal flow, blood gas values should normalize and $S\bar{v}O_2$ is maintained at greater than 70%.
3. $S\bar{v}O_2$ is an excellent indicator of adequate flow during VA ECMO because it is a measure of tissue perfusion and efficiency of extracorporeal circulation in meeting metabolic demands.
4. Oxygenation during VV ECMO is assessed by infant's arterial blood gas values and continuous oxygen saturation monitoring via pulse oximetry. $S\bar{v}O_2$ is not an accurate reflection of deoxygenated blood because of recirculation; $S\bar{v}O_2$ is used as a trending parameter during VV ECMO.
5. Ventilator settings are reduced to a minimum; vasopressor therapy and chemical paralysis are usually discontinued; enteral feedings are generally withheld because of concern about hypoxic injury to the gastrointestinal tract, which has never been exposed to nutrients; and blood loss is quantified and replaced.
6. Emergencies during ECMO (Chung and Zwischenberger, 2000).
   a. Circuit emergencies.
      (1) Air embolism.
      (2) Tubing rupture.
      (3) Oxygenator malfunction.
      (4) Accidental decannulation.
      (5) Power failure.
      (6) Gas source failure.
   b. Responsibilities of the nurse during a circuit emergency.
      (1) Notification of physician.
      (2) Ventilation.

(3) Anticoagulation.
(4) Chemical resuscitation.
(5) Blood loss replacement.

c. Responsibilities of the ECMO specialist during a circuit emergency.
(1) Clamp catheters.
(2) Open bridge.
(3) Remove gas source.
(4) Repair circuit.

C. ECMO patient complications (Chung and Zwischenberger, 2000; Nugent and Matranga, 1997).

1. Electrolyte/glucose/fluid imbalance. Sodium requirements decrease; potassium requirements increase because of the action of aldosterone. Calcium replacement may be needed if citrate-phosphate-dextrose anticoagulated blood is used. Hyperglycemia may necessitate a decrease in the glucose concentration of IV fluids.
2. Central nervous system (CNS) deterioration: cerebral edema, intracranial hemorrhage, and seizures. Deterioration results from initial hypoxia, acidosis, hypercapnia, or vessel ligation.
3. Generalized edema. The extracellular space is enlarged by the distribution of crystalloid solution and the action of aldosterone and antidiuretic hormone. The use of diuretics or hemofiltration may be necessary if edema causes brain or lung dysfunction.
4. Renal failure. Acute tubular necrosis results from pre-ECMO hypotension and hypoxia. Indicators of renal failure are abnormal blood urea nitrogen and creatinine values. Low-dose dopamine therapy and/or hemodialysis may be necessary.
5. Hemorrhage due to thrombocytopenia, coagulopathy.
6. Decreased venous return and/or hypovolemia due to inadequate circulating blood volume, pneumothorax, and/or partial venous catheter occlusion or malposition.
7. Hypertension due to overinfusion of blood products, renal ischemia, and excretion of renin-angiotensin.
8. Patent ductus arteriosus. Left-to-right shunting may cause increased blood flow to the lung, necessitating high pump flows without the expected increase in PaO_2. Ligation may be necessary.
9. Cardiac "stun." Transient loss of ventricular contractility (1-3 days) is manifested by hypotension, decrease in aortic pulse pressure, poor peripheral perfusion, and decreased PaO_2. It is possibly due to mismatch between afterload and ventricular contractility during ECMO.
10. Mechanical complications. These include incorrect catheter placement, oxygenator failure, power failure, and accidental decannulation.

D. Weaning/decannulation.

1. Signs of improvement and indicators that the infant is ready to be weaned are as follows:
   a. Improvement of lung fields on chest x-ray examination.
   b. Clinical findings: improved breath sounds, rising PaO_2 on fixed ECMO flow, improvement in lung compliance.
2. Once improvement has been ascertained, flow rate is decreased slowly in 10 to 20 ml increments until ECMO support is no longer needed to maintain adequate gas exchange at low ventilator settings (Nugent and Matranga, 1997).
3. When flow rate is 50 to 100 ml/kg/minute, a state of "idling" is achieved; the infant remains at this lowest possible flow rate for 4 to 8 hours.

4. If improvement in lung function remains stable, cannulas are clamped, heparin is infused directly into the infant, and the circuit is recirculated via a bridge. If blood gas values deteriorate, the cannulas are unclamped and ECMO support is resumed.
5. During VV ECMO the cannulas are not clamped during the "trial off" procedure; gas flow to the membrane oxygenator is discontinued. Low flow rates are maintained, and patient response is assessed by measurement of blood gases.
6. Decannulation proceeds if blood gas values remain satisfactory.
7. Before decannulation, the infant undergoes chemical paralysis and ventilator parameters are increased to compensate for loss of spontaneous respiratory function.
8. After adequate anesthesia and analgesia has been administered, the cannulas are removed. Both the internal jugular vein and the carotid artery are ligated. In some ECMO centers, carotid reconstruction is attempted (Cheung et al., 1997; Levy et al., 1995). The efficacy of this procedure is still debated because of clot formation at the site of reconstruction.
9. After decannulation, the infant is weaned as tolerated from the ventilator and routine NICU care is resumed.

POST-ECMO CARE

A. **Lung recovery is achieved through weaning of the infant from assisted ventilation.** Occasionally the use of steroids and/or diuretics is necessary to improve recovery.

B. **Assessment of neurologic recovery involves clinical evaluation and computed tomography (CT) scan.** It may be difficult to assess neurologic status during opiate use or while the infant is recovering from significant illness, so assessment may be deferred until the infant is ready for discharge.

C. **Weaning from opiate analgesics and sedatives involves a gradual reduction of doses and careful monitoring for withdrawal symptoms.** Infants receiving ECMO therapy require opiate infusions or scheduled dosing of opiates and sedatives throughout their course of ECMO to prevent excessive movement, which can dislodge the cannulas (Arnold et al., 1990; Caron and Maguire, 1990; Franck and Vilardi, 1995).

D. **Establishing oral feedings may be difficult.** Prolonged respiratory compromise, the effect of opiates on state control, alterations in swallowing caused by neck dissection during cannula placement, and gastroesophageal reflux, particularly in infants with CDH, are some of the causes of feeding problems in the post-ECMO infant. Feeding difficulties are generally more common in infants with CDH than in those with other diagnoses such as meconium aspiration syndrome or persistent pulmonary hypertension of the newborn.

PARENTAL SUPPORT

A. **The ECMO candidate's parents are in crisis.** They are aware that ECMO is a method of last resort with no guarantee of positive result, and the technology is overwhelming.

B. **Parents need concise, accurate information** about their child's condition and the required procedures.

C. **Parent-to-parent support, using parents of "ECMO graduates,"** is efficacious and a positive experience.

D. **Parents should have access to their infant.** The ECMO candidates have an increasingly bright outcome, and every effort should be made to encourage involvement and bonding.

FOLLOW-UP AND OUTCOME

The follow-up and outcome of ECMO have been discussed by Bernbaum and associates (1995), Boggs and LaPrade-Wolf (1992); Glass and associates (1989, 1995, 2000), Hofkosh and colleagues (1991), and Kanto (1994).

A. **Critical scrutiny of survivors is essential to assess the value and safety of ECMO.** Survivors should be evaluated at 4 to 6 months, and then yearly until school age. The following are assessed:
   1. Growth and development.
   2. Cardiorespiratory development.
   3. Cerebrovascular status.
   4. Neurologic and psychologic functioning.

B. **Medical morbidity includes poor somatic growth, feeding problems, chronic lung disease, and rehospitalizations.** Predictors include diagnosis of CDH, lower birth weight, and age at initiation of ECMO.

C. **The incidence of auditory deficits among ECMO survivors is approximately 10% (range, 4%-21%). The incidence of significant sensorineural handicap including neurocognitive disability, neuromotor disability, and seizure disorder is 15% (Glass et al., 2000).** Predictors include cardiopulmonary resuscitation before ECMO, neuroimaging abnormalities, and seizures.

D. **School-age ECMO survivors are twice as likely as other children to have neuropsychologic deficits and are at risk of having academic problems.** Predictors include lower birth weight, abnormal findings on neurologic imaging, chronic lung disease, and failure to thrive. However, even children who do not have these risk factors can have neuropsychologic testing to predict the need for special education services.

E. **Psychologic morbidity, including behavioral problems, is also reported and may be due to altered parenting styles and family stress.** Early trauma from severe illness may set the stage for problems in parent-child interactions.

REFERENCES

Arnold, J., Truog, R., Orav, E.J., et al.: Tolerance and dependence in neonates sedated with fentanyl during extracorporeal membrane oxygenation. *Anesthesiology, 73*(6):1136-1140, 1990.

Bartlett, R.: Respiratory support: Extracorporeal membrane oxygenation in newborn respiratory failure. In K. Welch et al. (Eds.): *Pediatric surgery*. Chicago, 1986, Year Book Medical Publishers, pp. 74-77.

Bartlett, R.: Physiology of extracorporeal life support. In J. Zwischenberger, R.H. Steinhorn, and R. Bartlett (Eds.): *ECMO: Extracorporeal cardiopulmonary support in critical care* (2nd ed.). Ann Arbor, 2000, Extracorporeal Life Support Organization, pp. 41-66.

Bartlett, R., Andrews, A.F., Toomasian, J.M., et al.: Extra-corporeal membrane oxygenation for newborn respiratory failure: Forty-five cases. *Surgery, 92*(2):425-433, 1982.

Bartlett, R. and Gazzaniga, A.: Extracorporeal circulation for cardiopulmonary failure. *Current Problems in Surgery, 12*(5):1-96, 1978.

Bartlett, R., Roloff, D.W., Cornell, R.G., et al.: Extracorporeal circulation in neonatal respiratory failure: A prospective randomized study. *Pediatrics, 76*(2):479-487, 1985.

Bartlett, R., Roloff, D.W., Custer, J.R., et al.: Extracorporeal life support: The University of Michigan experience. *Journal of the American Medical Association, 283*(7):904-908, 2000.

Bernbaum, J., Schwartz, I.P., Gerdes, M., et al.: Survivors of extracorporeal membrane oxygenation at 1 year of age: The relationship of primary diagnosis with health and neurodevelopmental sequelae. *Pediatrics, 96*(5 Pt 1):907-913, 1995.

Boggs, K. and LaPrade-Wolf, P.: Beyond survival: Strategies for establishing a follow-up program for infants with extracorporeal membrane oxygenation. *Neonatal Network, 11*(1):7-13, 1992.

Caron, E. and Maguire, D.: Current management of pain, sedation and narcotic physical dependency of the infant on ECMO. *Journal of Perinatal and Neonatal Nursing, 4*(10):63-74, 1990.

Cheung, P.Y., Vickar D.B. Hallgren R.A., et al.: Carotid artery reconstruction in neonates receiving extracorporeal membrane oxygenation: A 4-year follow-up study. Western Canadian ECMO Follow-up Group. *Journal of Pediatric Surgery, 32*(4):560-564, 1997.

Chung, D.H. and Zwischenberger, J.B.: Emergencies during extracorporeal membrane oxygenation and their management. In J. Zwischenberger, R.H. Steinhorn, and R. Bartlett (Eds.): *ECMO: Extracorporeal cardiopulmonary support in critical care* (2nd ed.). Ann Arbor, 2000, Extracorporeal Life Support Organization, pp. 269-294.

Finer, N.: Neonatal selection criteria for ECMO. In J. Zwischenberger, R.H. Steinhorn, and R. Bartlett (Eds.): *ECMO: Extracorporeal cardiopulmonary support in critical care* (2nd ed.). Ann Arbor, 2000, Extracorporeal Life Support Organization, pp. 357-362.

Franck, L. and Vilardi, J.: Assessment and management of opioid withdrawal in ill neonates. *Neonatal Network, 14*(2):39-48, 1995.

Glass, P., Miller, M., and Short, B.: Morbidity for survivors of extracorporeal membrane oxygenation: Neurodevelopmental outcome at 1 year of age. *Pediatrics, 83*(1)3:72-78, 1989.

Glass, P., Wagner, A., and Coffman, C.: Outcome and follow-up of neonates treated with ECMO. In J. Zwischenberger, R.H. Steinhorn, and R. Bartlett (Eds.): *ECMO: Extracorporeal cardiopulmonary support in critical care* (2nd ed.). Ann Arbor, 2000, Extracorporeal Life Support Organization, pp. 409-420.

Glass, P., Wagner, A.E., Papero, P.H., et al.: Neurodevelopmental status at age five years of neonates treated with extracorporeal membrane oxygenation. *Journal of Pediatrics, 127*(3):447-457, 1995.

Hirschl, R.B.: Devices. In J. Zwischenberger, R.H. Steinhorn, and R. Bartlett (Eds.): *ECMO: Extracorporeal cardiopulmonary support in critical care* (2nd ed.). Ann Arbor, 2000, Extracorporeal Life Support Organization, pp. 199-232.

Hofkosh, D., Thompson, A., Nozza, R., et al.: Ten years of extracorporeal membrane oxygenation: Neurodevelopmental outcome. *Pediatrics, 87*(4):549-555, 1991.

Kanto, W.P.: A decade of experience with neonatal extracorporeal membrane oxygenation. *Journal of Pediatrics, 124*(3): 335-347, 1994.

Levy, M.S., Share, J.C., Fauza, D.O. et al.: Fate of the reconstructed carotid artery after extracorporeal membrane oxygenation. *Journal of Pediatric Surgery, 30*(7):1046-1049, 1995.

Neonatal ECMO Registry Report, January. Ann Arbor, 2003, Extracorporeal Life Support Organization.

Nugent, J. and Matranga, G.: Extracorporeal membrane oxygenation. In D.F. Askin (Ed.): *Acute respiratory care of the newborn* (2nd ed.). Petaluma, CA, 1997, NICU Ink, pp. 341-368.

O'Rourke, P. Crone, R.K., Vacanti J.P., et al.: Extracorporeal membrane oxygenation and conventional medical therapy in neonates with persistent pulmonary hypertension of the newborn: A prospective randomized study. *Pediatrics, 84*(6):957-963, 1989.

Peek, G.J. and Firmin, R.K.: Vascular access for extracorporeal organ support. In J. Zwischenberger, R.H. Steinhorn, and R. Bartlett (Eds.): *ECMO: Extracorporeal cardiopulmonary support in critical care* (2nd ed.). Ann Arbor, 2000, Extracorporeal Life Support Organization, pp. 253-268.

Pettignano, R., Clark, R.H., and Cornish, J.D.: Principles and practice of venovenous extracorporeal membrane oxygenation. In J. Zwischenberger, R.H. Steinhorn, and R. Bartlett (Eds.): *ECMO:*

Extracorporeal cardiopulmonary support in critical care (2nd ed.). Ann Arbor, 2000, Extracorporeal Life Support Organization, pp. 113-131.

Pettignano, R. and Cornish, J.D.: Clinical management of neonates on venoarterial ECMO. In J. Zwischenberger, R.H. Steinhorn, and R. Bartlett (Eds.): *ECMO: Extracorporeal cardiopulmonary support in critical care* (2nd ed.). Ann Arbor, 2000, Extracorporeal Life Support Organization, pp. 363-382.

Sheehan, A.: Bedside nursing care and ECMO specialist responsibilities. In Van Meurs, K. (Ed.): *ECMO specialist training manual* (2nd ed.), Ann Arbor, 1999, Extracorporeal Life Support Organization, pp. 199-206.

Torosian, M.B., Statter, M.B., and Arensman, R.M.: Extracorporeal membrane oxygenation. In J.P. Goldsmith and E.H. Karotkin (Eds.): *Assisted ventilation of the neonate* (3rd ed.). Philadelphia, 1996, Saunders, pp. 242-243.

UK Neonatal ECMO Trial Group: UK collaborative randomised trial of neonatal extracorporeal membrane oxygenation. *Lancet, 348*(9020):75-82, 1996.

ADDITIONAL READINGS

American Academy of Pediatrics Committee on Fetus and Newborn. Recommendations on extracorporeal membrane oxygenation. *Pediatrics, 85*(4):618-619, 1990.

Anderson, H.L., Snedecor, S.M., Otsu, T., and Bartlett, R.H.: Multicenter comparison of conventional venoarterial access versus venovenous double-lumen catheter access in newborn infants undergoing entracorporeal membrane oxygenation. *Journal of Pediatric Surgery, 28*(4):530-535, 1993.

Faulkner, S.: Mobile extracorporeal membrane oxygenation. *Critical Care Nursing Clinics of North America, 7*(2):259-266, 1995.

Krause, K. and Youngner, V.: Nursing diagnoses as guidelines in the care of the neonatal ECMO patient. *Journal of Obstetric, Gynecologic, and Neonatal Nursing, 21*(3):169-176, 1992.

Stolar, C., Crisafi, M., and Driscoll, Y.: Neurocognitive outcome for neonates treated with extracorporeal membrane oxygenation: Are infants with congenital diaphragmatic hernia different? *Journal of Pediatric Surgery, 30*(2):366-371, 1995.

CHAPTER

27 Cardiovascular Disorders

SHARYL L. SADOWSKI

OBJECTIVES

1. Describe how to differentiate between cyanosis that is cardiac in origin and that which is pulmonary in origin.
2. Name the major classifications of congenital heart disease; list two anomalies in each.
3. Define and describe the anatomy, clinical manifestations, and the possible medical and/or surgical treatment of tetralogy of Fallot, coarctation of the aorta, patent ductus arteriosus (PDA), ventricular septal defect (VSD), atrial septal defect (ASD), and hypoplastic left heart syndrome (HLHS).
4. Describe the basic medical rationale for care of the newborn infant with a suspected or identified cardiac defect.
5. Describe basic surgical rationale for treatment of major cardiovascular defects.
6. List signs and symptoms of congenital heart abnormalities in the newborn infant.
7. Describe a cardiac catheterization and list the major postoperative nursing concerns.
8. List the signs and symptoms of PDA and the current medical, transcatheter, and surgical interventions.
9. Discuss the treatment modalities employed in congestive heart failure, including the risks and benefits to the neonate.
10. Define the three classifications of shock and list one cause under each category.
11. Discuss the major complications and sequelae of open-heart surgery and list two factors that contribute to the sequelae.

Until the twentieth century, there was limited clinical interest in congenital heart disease. In the majority of cases, the cardiac anomaly was incompatible with life; in the others, no treatment existed either to remedy the condition or to relieve its symptoms. Today, with advances in treatment of congenital heart defects, the survival and quality of life of infants with congenital heart disease have markedly improved.

Advances in fetal echocardiography have resulted in the prenatal diagnosis of many congenital heart defects, allowing parents time to make decisions about treatment prior to birth (Cuneo, 2002). In addition, advancements have been made in echocardiography, angiography, and interventional catheterization, which coupled with a more complete understanding of newborn physiology, have led to improvements in diagnostic capabilities with decreased risk. Additionally, the advent of deep hypothermia with circulatory arrest permits the total correction of many forms of congenital heart disease in the neonatal period. In some cases, early intervention is essential to prevent long-term morbidity or early death.

Whereas these advances have allowed for correction of many congenital heart defects, one would be remiss not to mention the long-term data, now available, that address neurodevelopmental complications following neonatal heart surgery. del

Nido (2002) identified seizures and motor and sensory deficits as late neurodevelopmental complications in infants following arterial switch procedures. In addition, Limperopoulos and colleagues (2001) assessed 134 infants undergoing their first cardiac surgery prior to and 12 to 18 months after surgery and found that 37% had moderate disability and another 6% showed severe disability. The disabilities were identified as motor and cognitive impairments, including 41% with neurologic abnormalities, 42% with gross and fine motor deficiencies, and 35% with behavioral problems.

Many studies have linked these outcomes with the deep hypothermic cardiac arrest and cardiopulmonary bypass that is used during open-heart surgery. In the past few years, pediatric heart surgeons have begun to perform some of these procedures on "beating" hearts, circumventing the need for circulatory arrest. It remains to be seen if this approach will improve the adverse neurodevelopmental outcomes presently linked to open-heart surgery in the neonatal period.

CARDIOVASCULAR EMBRYOLOGY AND ANATOMY

Cardiac Development

Fetal cardiac development occurs rapidly from day 18 to the 12th week of fetal life (Table 27-1) (Collins-Nakai and McLaughlin, 2002).

A. Cardiac tube.

1. Heart development is first identified at 18 to 19 days of fetal life. At the cephalic end of the embryo, splanchnic mesenchyme form the heart cords that then canalize to become primitive heart tubes. According to Collins-Nakai and McLaughlin (2002), fusion of the paired heart tubes is complete by 21 days of embryonic life (Fig. 27-1, *A*).
2. The heart tube elongates and develops dilatations and contractions that will later form the ventricles, bulbus cordis, and outflow tracts. This segmentation of the primitive heart begins at 21 days (Fig. 27-1, *B*).

■ TABLE 27-1
■ ■ **Timeline for Fetal Heart Development**

Age (Days)	Cardiovascular Morphogenesis
18	Angiogenic tissue appears
19-20	Endothelial heart tubes appear
21	Fusion of endothelial heart tubes
23-25	Differentiation of atria, ventricle, and bulbus cordis; heart begins to beat
25	Fusion of atria, dorsal mesocardium regresses, formation of bulboventricular loop
26-27	Circulation is established
32	Appearance of septum primum
33	Intraventricular septum begins to form
35	Foramen secundum present
36-37	Fusion of atrial endocardial cushions
43	Ridges form in the bulbus cordis
46	Closure of ventricular septum, formation of coronary arteries
47	Septum secundum appears

Data from Collins-Nakai, R. and McLaughlin, P.: How congenital heart disease originates in life. *Cardiology Clinics, 20*(3):367-383, 2002; Park, M.K.: *Pediatric cardiology for practitioners* (4th ed.). St Louis, 2002, Mosby; Theorell, C.: Cardiovascular assessment of the newborn. *Newborn and Infant Nursing Reviews*, 2(2):111-127, 2002.

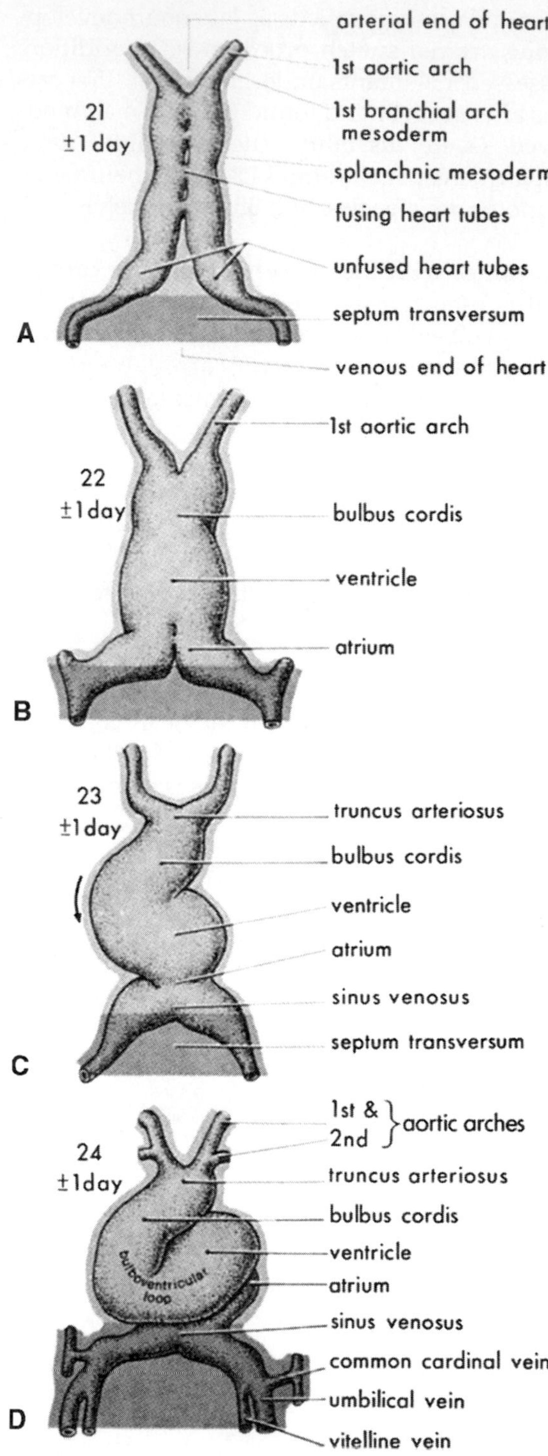

FIGURE 27-1 ■ Sketches of ventral views of developing heart (at 20-25 days), showing fusion of endocardial heart tubes to form a single heart tube. Bending of heart tube to form a bulboventricular loop is also illustrated. (Adapted from Moore, K.L. and Persaud, T.V.N.: *The developing human: Clinically oriented embryology* [7th ed.]. Philadelphia, 2003, Saunders, p. 336.)

3. The pairs of aortic arches develop from the cephalic, extracardial portion of the heart tube. The caudal end will form the early ventricle. The bulbus cordis and ventricle grow faster than other regions of the heart, resulting in the heart tube bending upon itself, thus forming a U shape (Fig. 27-1, *C, D*).
4. As the looping continues, the S-shaped heart becomes apparent (Fig. 27-2).

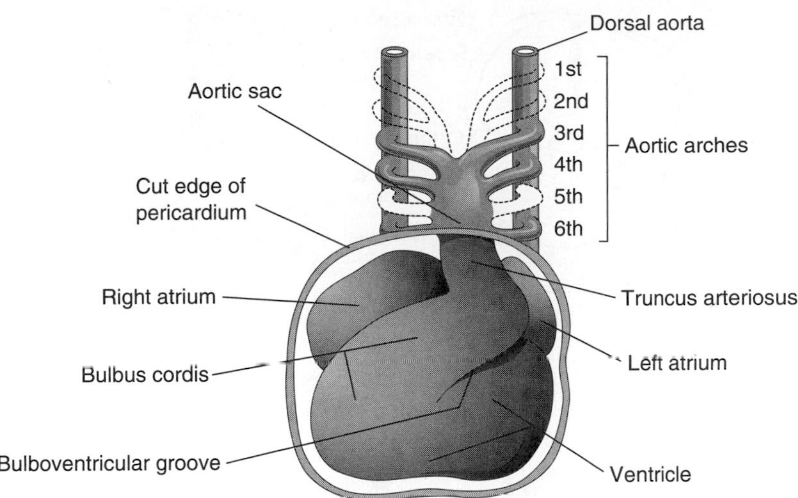

FIGURE 27-2 ■ Ventral view of heart and aortic arches (about 35 days). Ventral wall of pericardial sac has been removed to show heart in pericardial cavity. (From Moore, K.L. and Persaud, T.V.N.: *The developing human: Clinically oriented embryology* [7th ed.]. Philadelphia, 2003, Saunders, p. 339.)

5. Abnormal development during formation of the bulboventricular loop include corrected transposition and dextrocardia (Collins-Nakai and McLaughlin, 2002).

B. Cardiac septation: begins in the middle of the fourth week and is complete by the end of the fifth week of fetal life.

1. Atrial septum and foramen ovale are formed from two septa and endocardial cushions.
   a. Atrial septum primum is formed by unidirectional growth from the top of the atrium toward the endocardial cushions, resulting in formation of the septum. A septum formed in this manner can never be complete; there is always an opening, which in this case is the ostium primum.
   b. Perforation occurs high in the septum primum to form the ostium secundum; growth of the endocardial cushions eliminates the ostium primum.
   c. A second septum (septum secundum) appears to the right of the septum primum and grows to overlap the ostium secundum. Thus the flapped opening, the foramen ovale, is created (Fig. 27-3).
2. Ventricular septation results from fusion of the endocardial cushions (forming the membranous portion of the ventricular septum) and dilation and fusion of the ventricles (creating the muscular ventricular septum) (Fig. 27-4).
3. Tissue of endocardial cushion forms the atrioventricular valves (Fig. 27-5).
   a. Tricuspid valve: between right atrium and ventricle.
   b. Mitral valve: between left atrium and ventricle.
4. Abnormal development during cardiac septation can lead to the following:
   a. VSD, ASD, and endocardial cushion defect (atrioventricular canal).
   b. Absence, deformation, stenosis, or atresia of the tricuspid and/or mitral valves.

Great Vessel Development

A. Single vessel (truncus arteriosus) extends from the ventricles until the fourth week of fetal life.

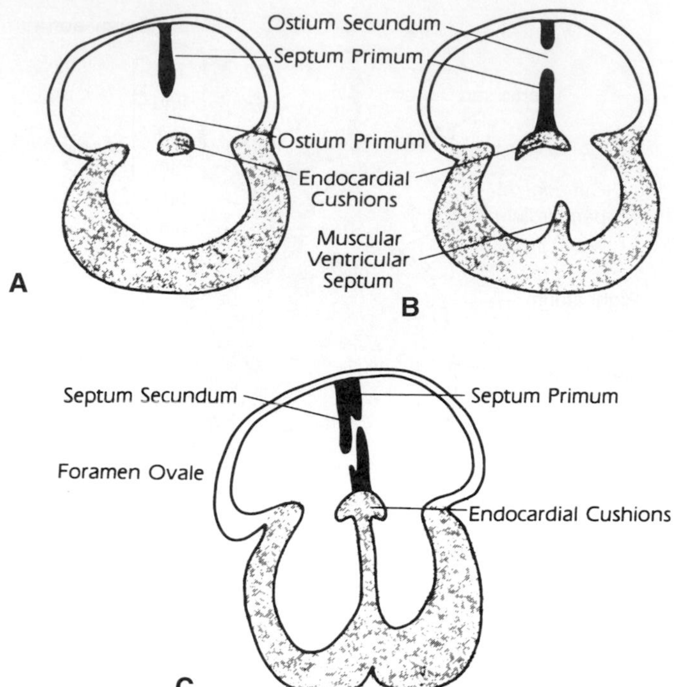

FIGURE 27-3 ■ Atrial septation. **A,** Septum primum begins to form, extending toward endocardial cushion (note ostium primum). **B,** Ostium primum is closed and perforation (called ostium secundum) forms in septum primum. **C,** Septum secundum forms, creating foramen ovale. (From Hazinski, M.F.: Congenital heart disease in the neonate. *Neonatal Network, 21*[3]:31-42, 1983.)

B. **Fifth week:** Ridges appear within the truncus arteriosus and the bulbus cordis. These ridges extend and spiral, separating the truncus arteriosus into the aorta and the pulmonary artery (Fig. 27-6).
   1. Swellings at the base of the truncus appear and fuse to form the right and left ventricular outflow tracks.
   2. Neural crest cells migrate to the outflow tract, where they help form the septum. The septation occurs distal to proximal, resulting in elongation of the aorticopulmonary septum. In the proximal one third, the crest cells form

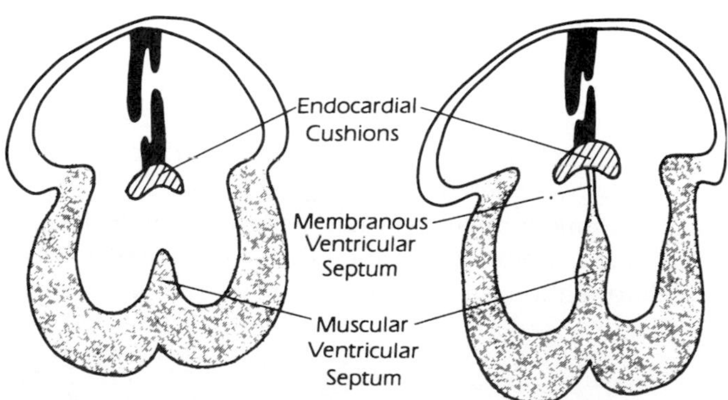

FIGURE 27-4 ■ Ventricular septation (with muscular and membranous septum). (From Hazinski, M.F.: Congenital heart disease in the neonate. *Neonatal Network 21*[3]:31-42, 1983.)

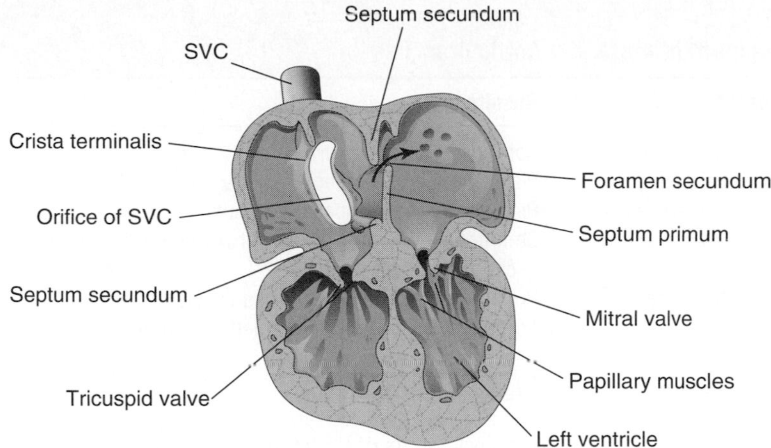

FIGURE 27-5 ■ The developing heart about 8 weeks, showing heart after it is partitioned into four chambers. Arrow indicates flow of well-oxygenated blood from right to left atrium. (From Moore, K.L. and Persaud, T.V.N.: *The developing human: Clinically oriented embryology* (7th ed.). Philadelphia, 2003, Saunders, p. 342.)

truncal and conal ridges that extend to separate the truncus arteriosus into the aorta and pulmonary artery.

3. The semilunar valves (aortic and pulmonic valves) develop from three ridges of tissue at the opening to the aorta and pulmonary trunk.

C. Development of aorta and aortic branches (Table 27-2). The truncus arteriosus connects with the aortic sac, which in turn connects with the paired aortic branches. A series of six paired aortic arches then form in succession (Fig. 27-7).
   1. First and second arches are the first to form and the first to disappear.
   2. The third arches become part of the common carotid arteries.
   3. The right fourth arch becomes the proximal portion of the right subclavian artery.
   4. The left fourth arch becomes the aortic arch segment between the left common carotid artery and left subclavian artery.
   5. The fifth arch regresses.
   6. The left sixth arch becomes part of the left pulmonary artery and the ductus arteriosus.

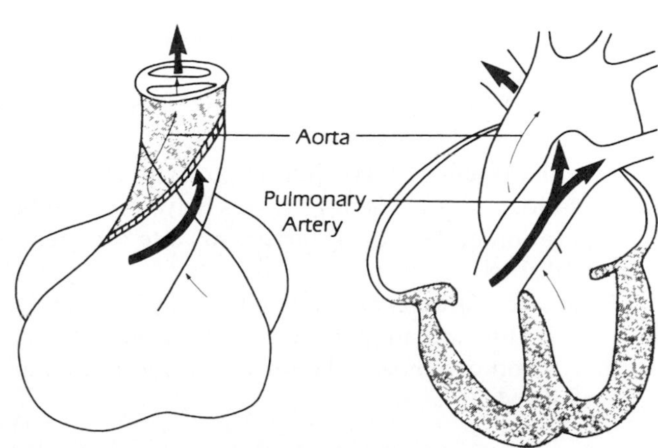

FIGURE 27-6 ■ Closing of truncus arteriosus and division into pulmonary artery and aorta. (From Hazinski, M.F.: Congenital heart disease in the neonate. *Neonatal Network, 21*[3]:31-42, 1983.)

TABLE 27-2
Development of Aorta and Aortic Branches

Embryonic Vessel	Results In
Truncus arteriosus	Aorta and pulmonary artery
First pair of aortic arches	Pieces remain as stapedial arteries
Second pair of aortic arches	Pieces remain as stapedial arteries
Third pair of aortic arches	Common carotid arteries and proximal portion of internal carotid arteries
Fourth pair of aortic arches	Proximal portion of the right subclavian artery
Right	Aortic arch segment between left common carotid and left subclavian artery
Left	
Fifth pair of aortic arches	Regresses totally
Sixth pair of aortic arches	
Left	Proximal portion of the left pulmonary artery and ductus arteriosus
Right	Proximal portion of the right pulmonary artery

Data from Collins-Nakai, R. and McLaughlin, P.: How congenital heart disease originates in life. *Cardiology Clinics, 20*(3):367-383, 2002; Park, M.K.: *Pediatric cardiology for practitioners* (4th ed.). St Louis, 2002, Mosby; Theorell, C.: Cardiovascular assessment of the newborn. *Newborn and Infant Nursing Reviews, 2*(2):111-127, 2002.

7. The right sixth arch forms the right pulmonary artery
8. Abnormalities include interrupted aortic arch and coarctation of the aorta.

D. Developmental abnormalities of truncal septation include (Collins-Nakai and McLaughlin, 2002):
1. Truncus arteriosus.
2. Tetralogy of Fallot.
3. Pulmonary and/or aortic valve atresia or stenosis.
4. Transposition of the great vessels (dextroposition).
5. Double outlet right ventricle.

Circulatory Development

A. **Heart contractions begin around 21 days;** the atrium and ventricle muscle layers are continuous. Contractions result in a rhythmic peristalsis. The initial circulation is an ebb-and-flow type.

B. **Coordinated contractions** established by the fourth week of gestation provide a unidirectional flow.

C. **Electrical conduction system** is functional around 10 weeks, with normal sinus rhythm seen by 16 weeks (Witt, 1997).

D. **Establishment of fetal circulation.** With completion of atrial and ventricular septation, development of valves between chambers and outflow tracks, and separation of the truncus arteriosus into the great vessels, fetal circulation is established.

E. **Fetal circulation is anatomically and physiologically different from adult circulation, and adaptation after birth is necessary** (Park, 2002). For a full discussion of fetal circulation and cardiopulmonary adaptation at birth, see **Chapter 4.**

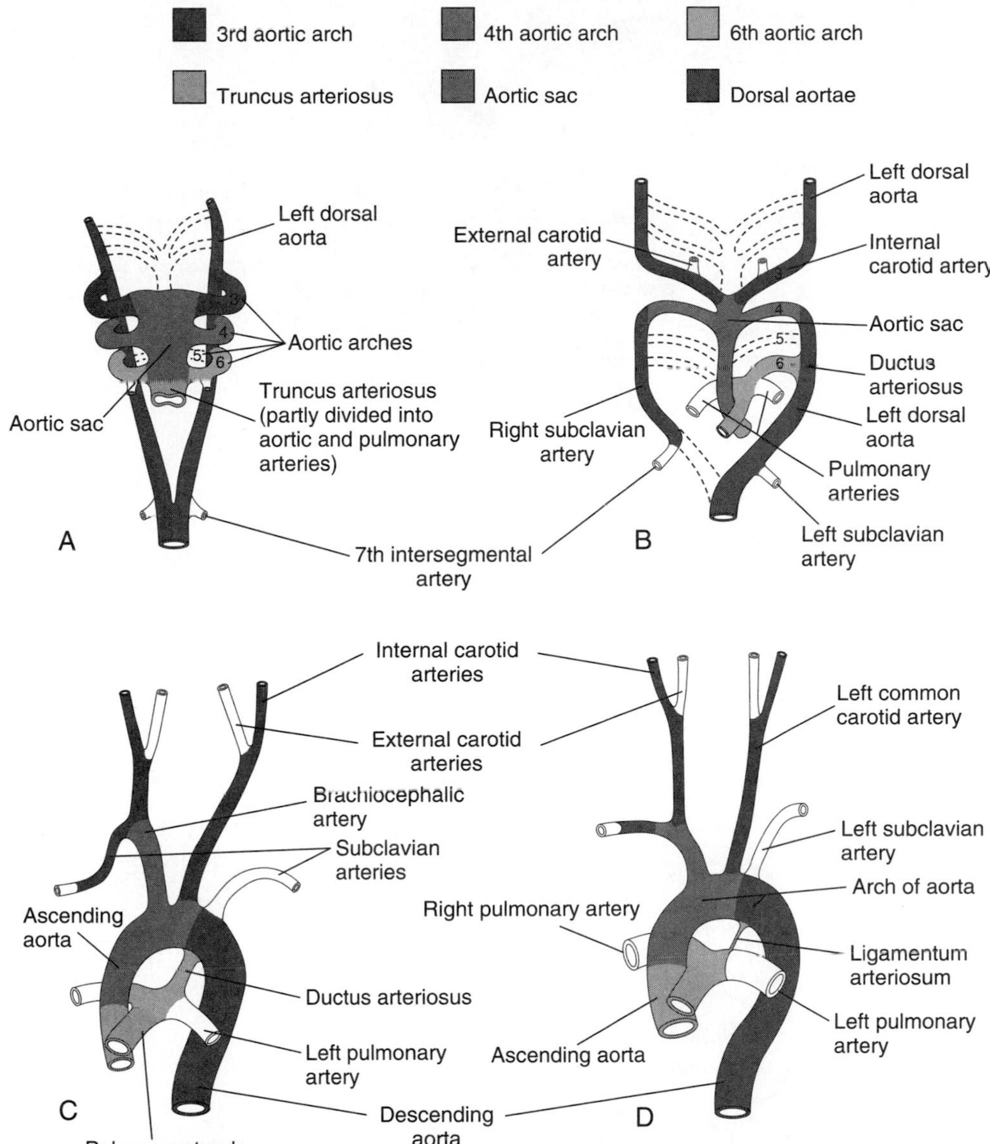

FIGURE 27-7 ■ Schematic drawings illustrating arterial changes that result during transformation of truncus arteriosus, aortic sac, aortic arches, and dorsal aortas into adult arterial pattern. **A,** Aortic arches at 6 weeks. **B,** Aortic arches at 7 weeks. **C,** Arterial arrangement at 8 weeks. **D,** Sketch of arterial vessels of 6-month-old infant. (From Moore, K.L. and Persaud, T.V.N.: *The developing human: Clinically oriented embryology* [7th ed.]. Philadelphia, 2003, Saunders, p. 364.)

Cardiovascular Physiology

A. Normal circulation (Fig. 27-8).

1. Oxygen-poor blood enters the right atrium and passes through the tricuspid valve into the right ventricle, where it is pumped through the pulmonary artery to the lungs.
2. As the blood flows through the lungs, it gives up carbon dioxide and gains oxygen.

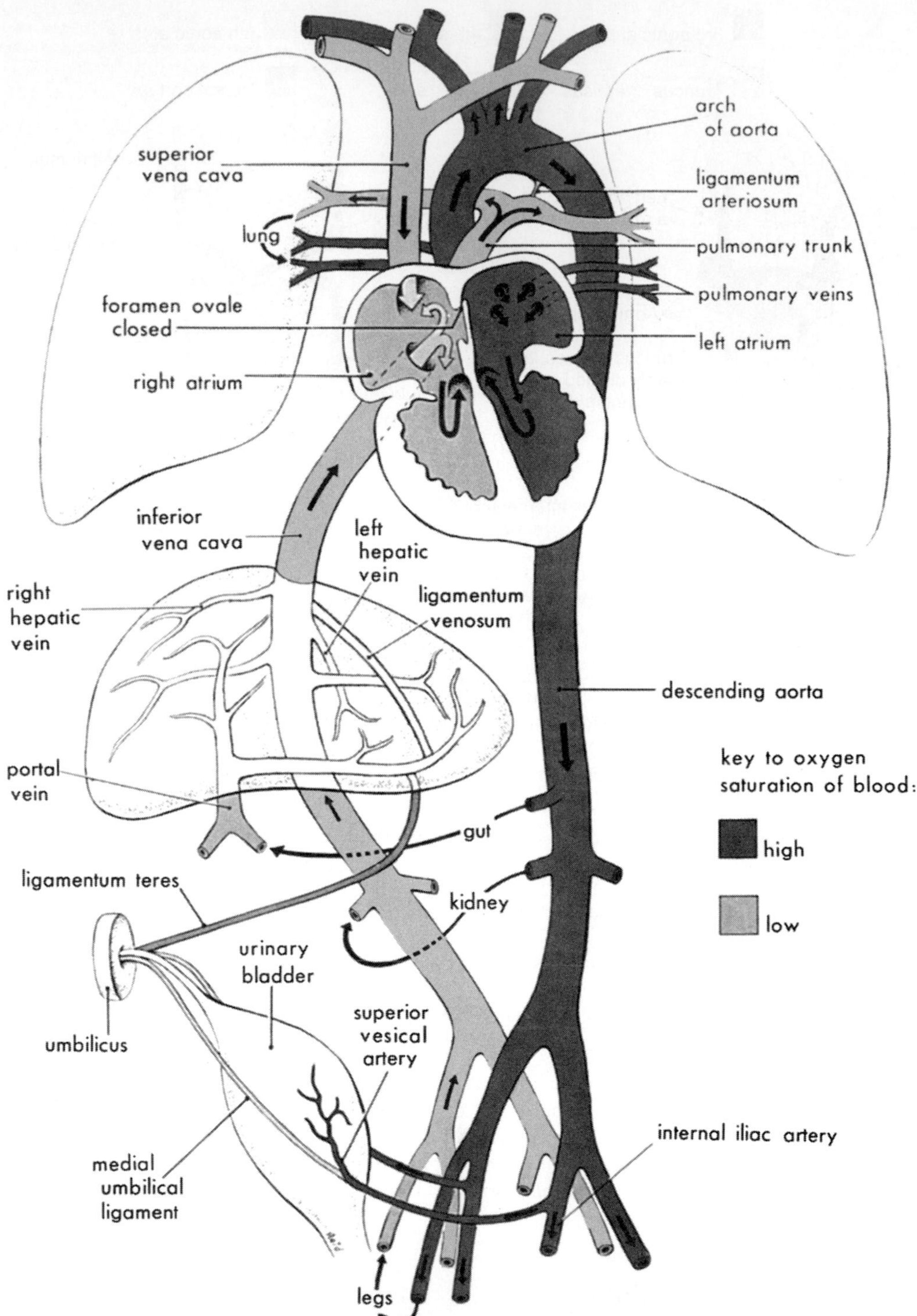

FIGURE 27-8 ■ Neonatal circulation. Adult derivatives of fetal vessels and structures that become nonfunctional at birth are shown. Arrows indicate course of neonatal circulation. (Organs not drawn to scale.) After birth, three shunts that short-circuited the blood during fetal life cease to function, and pulmonary and systemic circulations become separated. (From Moore, K.L. and Persaud, T.V.N.: *The developing human: Clinically oriented embryology* [7th ed.]. Philadelphia, 2003, Saunders, p. 373.)

3. Oxygen-rich blood returns from the lungs through the pulmonary veins. It enters the left atrium and then passes through the mitral valve into the left ventricle, which pumps it through the aortic valve and into the aorta.
4. The aorta then delivers oxygenated blood to all body organs and tissues.

B. Cardiac depolarization (Guyton and Hall, 1996).

1. Cardiac depolarization, which results from the electrical discharge across the myocardial cell (total net movement of ions across the cell wall), is measured by the electrocardiograph (ECG).
2. Shortening of muscle fibers (contraction) usually follows cardiac depolarization. Strength of cardiac (ventricular) contraction is measured by blood pressure or arterial pulse palpation.
3. Cardiac electrical activity does not ensure adequate cardiac function.
   a. Congenital defects or surgical injury to the conduction system may result in arrhythmias or heart block.
   b. Electrolyte disturbance (i.e., altered fluid composition surrounding the cells) can affect electrical activity.
      (1) Hypokalemia and hyperkalemia.
      (2) Hypocalcemia and hypercalcemia.
      (3) Hypoxia.
      (4) Acidosis.

C. Cardiac output.

1. Cardiac output is the volume of blood ejected by the heart in 1 minute. Approximations vary from 120 to 200 ml/kg/minute.
2. Cardiac output = stroke volume × heart rate (in liters per minute).
   a. As heart rate fluctuates, so will cardiac output.
      (1) Normal term newborn heart rate is 110 to 160 beats per minute (bpm), although it may range from 70 to 180 bpm on an individual basis (Park, 2002).
      (2) Significant or persistent bradycardia will result in a drop in the neonate's cardiac output.
   b. Tachycardia seems to be an effective mechanism for improving cardiac output as long as the tachycardia does not compromise diastolic filling time and decrease coronary artery perfusion.
3. Stroke volume is relatively fixed at 1.5 ml/kg and is affected by three factors: preload, contractility, and afterload.
   a. Preload: the volume of blood in the ventricles before contraction.
      (1) Clinically, preload is a measurement of pressure, rather than volume, in the ventricles before contraction.
      (2) Increasing the volume in the ventricles, consequently lengthening the myocardial fibers before contraction, should result in improved stroke volume (Frank-Starling law) (Patterson and Starling, 1914). The newborn infant is capable of increasing stroke volume provided there is no increase in systemic vascular resistance or rapid rise in aortic pressure. Given the neonate's smaller contractile mass, less compliant myocardium, and normal maximization of myocardial fiber length, volume infusions are likely to increase aortic pressure and afterload, resulting in a decline in stroke volume (Bell, 1998).
   b. Contractility: speed of ventricular contraction.
      (1) Cardiac cycle consists of ventricular contraction (systole), followed by ventricular relaxation (diastole). As contraction time decreases,

relaxation time (diastole) increases, with an increase in ventricular filling volume (preload) before contraction.
(2) Ventricular contractility cannot be directly measured. Measurements of cardiac shortening fractions and ejection fraction provide an indirect assessment of contractility.
(3) Contractility in neonates is influenced by the following:
(a) Exogenous catecholamine (dopamine/dobutamine) use, which increases blood pressure and cardiac output (Bell, 1998).
(b) Factors that decrease contractility.
(i) Acidosis, which impairs myocardial response to catecholamines.
(ii) Hypoxia.
(iii) Electrolyte disturbances.
(iv) Hypoglycemia.

c. Afterload: the resistance to blood leaving the ventricle.
(1) Dependent on systemic vascular resistance (SVR) and pulmonary vascular resistance (PVR); if SVR or PVR increases, afterload increases.
(2) The neonate's myocardium is very sensitive to increased afterload; with small increases in afterload, stroke volume can fall significantly.
(3) Afterload can be reduced by intravenous (IV) infusion of vasodilators (e.g., nitroglycerin and nitroprusside). Dobutamine can be used to decrease PVR (Bell, 1998).

4. Concepts of blood flow.
a. Flow is directly proportional to pressure/resistance.
b. Blood flow will always take the path of least resistance.
c. If heart action (pressure) remains unchanged but vasoconstriction or dilation or obstruction to flow (resistance) changes, flow will change (i.e., cardiac output will vary).
d. PVR starts to fall after delivery and declines to levels less than 50% of systemic arterial pressure (Ivy et al., 1998). This normal decline is influenced by prematurity, low birth weight, and hypoxia episodes.

CONGENITAL HEART DISEASE

Occurrence

A. Incidence: congenital heart disease (CHD) occurrence varies from 3.7 to 8:1000 live births (<1%) according to Carey (2002).
1. 90% of cases due to multifactorial causes.
2. 8% are from chromosomal/genetic factors.
3. 2% come from exposure to environmental teratogens (Strife and Sze, 1999).

B. Genetic factors. Chromosomal abnormalities: overall incidence of CHD in patients with a chromosome aberration is 30%.
1. Incidence of CHD varies with chromosomal abnormality.
a. Trisomy 21: 50%.
b. Trisomy 18: 90% to 100%.
c. Trisomy 13: 90%.
d. Chromosome deletion syndromes 18, 13, 5, and 4: 25% to 50%
e. DiGeorge deletion 22q: 50%.
2. Single-mutant-gene syndromes: 1% to 2% of all cardiovascular abnormalities in newborn infants. Both autosomal dominant and recessive syndromes have been associated with CHD.

3. Multifactorial: approximately 90% most likely due to genetic predisposition coupled with a causative factor.
   a. Cornelia de Lange: approximately 30%.
   b. VACTERL (**V**ertebral anomalies, **A**nal atresia/stenosis, **C**ardiac defects, **T**racheo-**E**sophageal fistula, **R**adial defects, **L**imb anomalies) (Baraitser and Winter, 1996).
   c. CHARGE (**C**oloboma, **H**eart defects, choanal **A**tresia, **R**estriction of growth and development, **G**enital anomalies, **E**ar anomalies) (Baraitser and Winter, 1996).

C. **Environmental factors and teratogens can include fetal exposure to drug, chemical, infectious, or physical agents; maternal disease or altered metabolic state with the period of greatest risk at 14 to 50 days of fetal life** (Carey, 2002).
1. Cardiac teratogenesis is associated with maternal ingestion of:
   a. Thalidomide: dramatically illustrates the extraordinarily deleterious effects of prescribed drug on a developing fetus.
   b. Anticonvulsants: 2% to 3% of infants exposed to anticonvulsants will have associated congenital cardiac defects such as pulmonary stenosis, coarctation of the aorta, PDA.
      (1) Phenytoin.
      (2) Carbamazepine (Tegretol).
      (3) Valproate.
      (4) Trimethadione: increased incidence of transposition of the great vessels, tetralogy of Fallot, and hypoplastic left heart syndrome.
      (5) Pentobarbital: no confirmed specific embryopathy but may potentiate the effects of other drugs taken concurrently.
   c. Anticoagulants.
      (1) Warfarin (Coumadin) causes abortion or fetal embryopathic development in weeks 6 to 9 of gestation. Cardiac malformations have been identified, but no consistent cardiac defect has been noted.
      (2) Heparin, because of its larger molecular weight, does not cross the placenta.
   d. Antineoplastic medications.
      (1) Aminopterin: cardiac manifestations include dextroposition but are not as prominent as other defects resulting from drug ingestion.
      (2) In general, the disorders for which antineoplastic agents are used are serious enough to preclude pregnancy.
   e. Lithium: approximately 10% of infants exposed will have defects such as Ebstein anomaly, ASD, and tricuspid atresia.
   f. Retinoic acid: aortic arch abnormalities, other congenital heart malformations (Brent, 2001).
   g. Isotretinoin.
   h. Alcohol. Fetal alcohol syndrome (FAS) is accompanied by a variety of cardiac lesions (e.g., VSD with or without subpulmonic and subaortic stenosis, coarctation of the aorta, aortic regurgitation, and ASD).
   i. Amphetamine: 5% to 10% will have congenital cardiac defects such as VSD, PDA, ASD, and transposition of the great arteries (Montoya and Washington, 2002).
2. Exposure to environmental hazards such as radiation, heat, and gases may produce teratogenic effects, but there are no specific associated cardiac malformations.

D. Maternal disease and viral infections (Box 27-1).

1. Women with diabetes mellitus, especially insulin-dependent, have a five times greater risk of their children being born with cardiac anomalies than the general population of pregnant women have. Disorders include hypertrophy of the septum and myocardium, VSD, double-outlet right ventricle, transposition of the great vessels, truncus arteriosus, and coarctation of the aorta.
2. Maternal lupus erythematosus may be linked to neonatal heart block.
3. Rubella is the only viral illness that produces clinically significant heart disease (Ayres, 1998). Disorders seen are PDA, pulmonary stenosis and branch pulmonary artery stenosis, VSD, and ASD.

Sex Preferences Associated with Cardiac Lesions

A. Males.

1. Coarctation of the aorta.
2. Aortic stenosis.
3. Transposition of the great vessels (TGV).

BOX 27-1

CLASSIFICATION OF MATERNAL DISEASES AFFECTING THE FETAL CARDIOVASCULAR SYSTEM

Category I: Maternal Diseases That Directly Affect the Fetal Cardiovascular System (Excluding Teratogenic Effects)

Pheochromocytoma
Hyperthyroidism
Diabetes mellitus
Collagen vascular disease (e.g., Ro antibody)
Smoking
Rubella
Cytomegalovirus
Enterovirus infection
Toxoplasmosis
Listeriosis
Maternal group B streptococcal colonization with fetal invasion
Syphilis
Inherited metabolic diseases

Category II: Maternal Diseases That May Indirectly Affect the Fetal Cardiovascular System as a Result of Abnormalities of Uteroplacental Function

Neoplastic diseases
Diabetes mellitus
Maternal cardiac disease
Anemia (including the hemoglobinopathies)
Hypertensive disorders
Collagen vascular disease (e.g., lupus anticoagulant and systemic lupus erythematosus)
Renal disease (associated with hypertension)
Smoking
Asthma
Cholestatic jaundice of pregnancy
Cytomegalovirus
Bacterial infections

From Katz, V. and Bowes, W.: Maternal diseases affecting the fetal cardiovascular system. In W. Long, (Ed.): *Fetal and neonatal cardiology.* Philadelphia, 1990, W.B. Saunders, p. 135.

B. Females.
1. ASD.
2. PDA.

APPROACH TO DIAGNOSIS OF CARDIAC DISEASE

History (Theorell, 2002)

A. Gestational age.
1. Preterm. Infants born prematurely are much more likely to have pulmonary problems resulting in cyanosis than to have congestive heart disease (CHD), but they do have a higher incidence of:
   a. PDA.
   b. Left-to-right shunts (e.g., VSD or atrioventricular canal).
2. Term. The majority of infants with CHD are term infants.

B. Maternal history (see Box 27-1).
1. Infants of mothers with uncontrolled diabetes have an increased risk of:
   a. TGV.
   b. VSD.
   c. Cardiomyopathy.
   d. Complex congenital heart disease.
2. Lupus may cause congenital heart block.
3. Viral and bacterial illnesses may directly and indirectly affect the fetal cardiovascular system.
4. Seizures or coagulation disorders can be linked to congenital heart defects because the medications used may be teratogens.
5. Maternal congenital heart disease can lead to an increased risk of same defect in infant.
6. Maternal age older than 35 years increases risk.
7. Alcohol consumption: increase in cardiac defects seen with FAS.

C. Familial.

Incidence of congenital heart defects increases by three- to fourfold when a first-order relative (parent or sibling) has congenital heart disease (Park, 2002). Risk increases by tenfold if two first-order relatives have congenital heart disease (Table 27-3).

D. Congenital diseases or syndromes may have associated cardiac anomalies.
The following associations have been noted:
1. Trisomy 13: PDA and/or VSD.
2. Trisomy 18: VSD, PDA.
3. Trisomy 21: ASD, VSD, atrioventricular canal, PDA.
4. Turner syndrome: coarctation of the aorta.
5. DiGeorge syndrome: PDA, peripheral pulmonary stenosis.
6. Rubella syndrome: PDA, peripheral pulmonary stenosis.
7. FAS: VSD, ASD, tetralogy of Fallot.

E. Perinatal history.
1. Intrauterine growth pattern and birth weight.
2. Prenatal diagnosis with ultrasound.
3. Mode of delivery.
   a. Vaginal delivery most common for CHD, and initial Apgar scores are usually good.
   b. History of cesarean section and poor Apgar scores more indicative of asphyxia and respiratory distress.

TABLE 27-3
Familial Recurrence Risks

Cardiac Anomaly	Family Member with Congenital Heart Defect	Risk (%)
PDA—patent ductus arteriosus	Mother	3.5-4
	Father	2.5
	Sibling	3
VSD—ventricular septal defect	Mother	6
	Father	2
	Sibling	3
ASD—atrial septal defect	Mother	4-4.5
	Father	1.5
	Sibling	2.5
AVC—atrioventricular canal	Mother	14
	Father	1
	Sibling	2
Tetralogy of Fallot	Mother	6-10
	Father	1.5
	Sibling	2.5
Aortic stenosis	Mother	13-18
	Father	3
	Sibling	2
Pulmonary stenosis	Mother	4-6.5
	Father	2
	Sibling	2
Coarctation of the aorta	Mother	4
	Father	2
	Sibling	2
Other defects (TGA, tricuspid atresia, truncus arteriosus, HLHS)	Sibling	1.4 (average)

Data from Park, M.K.: *Pediatric cardiology for practitioners* (4th ed.). St Louis, 2002, Mosby; Theorell, C.: Cardiovascular assessment of the newborn. *Newborn and Infant Nursing Reviews, 2*(2):111-127, 2002.
HLHS, Hypoplastic left heart syndrome; *TGA,* transposition of the great arteries.

Clinical Presentation

A. **Cyanosis** (in the first week may be sole evidence of a heart lesion).
   1. With cardiovascular problems, cyanosis is unexpected or gradual in onset.
   2. Cyanosis observation.
      a. Dependent on hemoglobin levels; at least 5 g of desaturated hemoglobin/dl is necessary before cyanosis becomes apparent.
      b. Will be influenced by presence of anemia or polycythemia and the levels of 2,3-diphosphoglycerate.
   3. Differentiation between central and peripheral cyanosis.
      a. Peripheral cyanosis results from sluggish movement of blood through the extremities and increased tissue oxygen extraction.
         (1) Persists from birth and can last several days.
         (2) Does not involve mucous membranes.
         (3) May be caused by peripheral vasomotor instability.
      b. Central cyanosis results from desaturated blood leaving the heart.
         (1) Seen as bluish discoloration of tongue and mucous membranes, reflecting arterial desaturation.

(2) Central cyanosis may present difficulties in making a differential diagnosis between respiratory and cardiac origin.

B. Respiratory pattern.

1. Useful in the differentiation of cyanosis.
2. Tachypnea (respiratory rate >60) without dyspnea is an important if subtle clue to cardiac anomalies. In the absence of cyanosis, may indicate a left-to-right shunt lesion. Tachypnea is significant if coupled with feeding difficulty and infant must stop feeding to catch its breath is suggestive of congestive heart failure.
3. Hyperpnea (increased respiratory depth) is observed in congenital heart lesions resulting in diminished pulmonary blood flow.
4. Crying may exacerbate cyanosis in neonates with CHD because of increased oxygen consumption by the tissues.

C. Heart sounds.

1. First heart sound (S_1) represents closure of the mitral and tricuspid valves at the onset of ventricular systole.
   a. Best heard at fourth intercostal space in left midclavicular line (mitral) and at fourth intercostal space at sternal borders (tricuspid).
   b. S_1 is accentuated with the following:
      (1) Increased cardiac output.
      (2) Increased flow across atrioventricular valves.
      (3) Specific conditions such as:
         (a) PDA.
         (b) VSD with increased mitral flow.
         (c) Total anomalous pulmonary venous return (TAPVR).
         (d) Arteriovenous malformation.
         (e) Tetralogy of Fallot.
         (f) Anemia.
         (g) Fever.
   c. Conditions decreasing S_1 include the following:
      (1) Decreased atrioventricular conduction.
      (2) Congestive heart failure (CHF).
      (3) Myocarditis.
2. Second heart sound (S_2) occurs at the end of ventricular systole from closure of aortic and pulmonic valves.
   a. Heard best at upper left sternal border.
   b. Split S_2 is a normal occurrence, reflecting closure of aortic valve before the pulmonic valve.
      (1) Increases on inspiration.
      (2) Single S_2 is often heard in the first 2 days of life because of increased PVR.
      (3) Splitting of S_2 is influenced by:
         (a) Abnormalities of aortic or pulmonic valves.
         (b) Conditions altering PVR or SVR.
   c. Conditions widening the S_2 are influenced by:
      (1) ASD.
      (2) TAPVR.
      (3) Tetralogy of Fallot.
      (4) Pulmonary stenosis.
      (5) Ebstein anomaly.
   d. Absent S_2 splits occur in the following:
      (1) Pulmonary atresia and severe pulmonary stenosis.
      (2) Aortic stenosis/atresia.

(3) Persistent pulmonary hypertension.
(4) L-TGV.
(5) Truncus arteriosus.

3. Third heart sound (S_3) comes from increased flow across the atrioventricular (AV) valves from rapid, passive ventricular filling from the atria.
   a. Follows S_2 and is a low-pitched, broad sound.
   b. Prominent in situations of increased atrioventricular flow and increased ventricular filling (Duff and McNamara, 1998).
      (1) Left-to-right shunts (e.g., ASD, VSD, PDA).
      (2) Anemia.
      (3) Mitral valve insufficiency.
4. Fourth heart sound (S_4) occurs at the final phase of ventricular filling and active atrial contraction during late diastole.
   a. Occurs just before S_1 and is low pitched.
   b. Rarely heard in the newborn infant.
   c. Always pathologic and indicates decreased ventricular compliance.
5. Ejection clicks are heard as snapping sound just after the first heart sound in the first 24 hours of life.
   a. Abnormal (except during first 24 hours of life) and indicate cardiac disease.
   b. Audible for short duration after S_1.
   c. Associated with dilation of the great vessels or deformity of aortic or pulmonic valve.
   d. Other conditions associated with ejection clicks include the following:
      (1) Aortic valve stenosis.
      (2) Truncus arteriosus.
      (3) Tetralogy of Fallot (severe).
      (4) Pulmonary valve stenosis.
      (5) Hypoplastic left heart syndrome.
      (6) Coarctation of the aorta.
6. Murmurs.
   a. Murmurs are audible vibrations resulting from turbulence of blood flow and may be due to:
      (1) Abnormal valves.
      (2) Septal defects.
      (3) Regurgitated flow through incompetent valves.
      (4) High blood flow across normal structures.
   b. Physiologic murmurs have been noted in 50% of neonates in the first 48 hours of life (Theorell, 2002). Generally, these murmurs are due to:
      (1) Transient left-to-right flow via the ductus arteriosus.
      (2) Increased flow over pulmonary valve associated with fall in PVR.
      (3) Mild bilateral peripheral pulmonary arterial stenosis because of size and pressure differences between the main pulmonary trunk and the left and right pulmonary arterial branches.
   c. Absence of murmur does not indicate absence of significant cardiac disease.
   d. Evaluation of murmurs includes the following:
      (1) Intensity of sound.
         (a) Murmurs are graded I through VI. Grade III or less generally present no hemodynamic problems (Duff and McNamara, 1998).
            (i) Grade I: barely audible, only after careful auscultation.
            (ii) Grade II: soft, easily audible on auscultation.

(iii) Grade III: moderately loud, not associated with a thrill.
(iv) Grade IV: loud murmur associated with a thrill.
(v) Grade V: very loud, with a thrill. May be heard with stethoscope just touching the chest wall.
(vi) Grade VI: extremely loud, with a thrill. Can be heard with stethoscope off the chest wall.

(b) Presence of a thrill on palpation is associated with a loud murmur of at least grade 4.

(2) Timing within cardiac cycle.

(a) Systolic: heard during ventricular systole (i.e., between S_1 and S_2) or if feeling the pulse during auscultation, at the upstroke of the pulse.
(i) Identified as early, mid-, or late systolic.
(ii) Pansystolic (holosystolic): heard throughout systole. Heard in mitral or tricuspid insufficiency and VSD.
(iii) Ejection murmurs: turbulence of blood flow leaving the heart; noted in aortic or pulmonic valve stenosis, tetralogy of Fallot, ASD, and TAPVR. The majority of innocent murmurs are systolic ejection murmurs (Pelech, 1999).

(b) Diastolic: heard during period of ventricular filling (i.e., between S_2 and S_1).
(i) Early: results from aortic or pulmonic valve insufficiency.
(ii) Mid: increased blood flow across normal mitral or tricuspid valve.
(iii) Late: associated with stenotic mitral or tricuspid valve.

(c) Continuous: audible throughout cardiac cycle but can be louder in systole or diastole (e.g., PDA).

(3) Quality and pitch.

(a) Pitch: reflects frequency of vibrations.
(i) High-pitched sound from turbulent blood flow from a high-pressure area to a low-pressure area. Generally reflects valve insufficiency on left side of heart, whereas a low-pitched sound reflects right-sided valve insufficiency.
(ii) Low-pitched sound is from a low-pressure difference in turbulent blood flow reflecting right-sided valve insufficiency.

(b) Quality is described as:
(i) Harsh.
(ii) Blowing.
(iii) Musical.

(4) Location: in terms of maximal intensity described by anatomic location on chest wall.

(5) Radiation if present.

D. Peripheral pulses (Theorell, 2002).

1. Pulses should be synchronous with equal intensity.
2. Upper and lower extremity pulses should be palpated simultaneously and differences documented.
3. Discrepancies (e.g., pulses that are greater in upper than in lower extremities) raise the possibility of an abnormal aortic arch.
4. Right brachial artery pulse should be compared with pulses in lower extremities because the right subclavian is always preductal.
5. Pulse volume graded from 0 to 4+.
   a. 0 = absent.

   b. 1+ = weak.
   c. 2+ = weak to average.
   d. 3+ = strong.
   e. 4+ = bounding.
6. Weak pulses indicate low cardiac output as seen in:
   a. Left heart outflow obstructive lesions.
   b. Myocardial failure.
   c. Shock.
7. Bounding pulses indicate aortic runoff.
   a. PDA.
   b. Aortic insufficiency.
   c. Systemic to pulmonary shunts.
8. Visible precordial impulse persisting after the first 12 hours of life occurs in defects with volume overload.

E. Blood pressure.

1. Normal values are dependent on birth weight and gestational age. The mean arterial pressure (MAP) is reported as being the same as the gestational age of the infant (Seri and Evans, 2001). In 1996, Hegyi and associates reported that blood pressure increases steadily in the first week of life for all infants.
   a. Healthy term infant: average systolic pressure is 56 to 77 mm Hg; average diastolic pressure is 33 to 50 mm Hg. Mean arterial pressure (MAP) is 42 to 60 mm Hg (Sansoucie and Cavaliere, 2003).
   b. Premature infant's blood pressure varies with size and gestational age, but the lower limit of the MAP is similar numerically to the gestational age for those infants 26 to 32 weeks' gestation. For neonates weighing less than 800 g, the MAP may be lower than the gestational age (Lee et al., 1999).
2. Blood pressure values may also be affected by postnatal age, body temperature, infant's behavioral state, and cuff size.
3. Cuff width should be 25% greater than the width of the extremity. If the width is too narrow, the blood pressure will have a false high reading. If the cuff width is too wide, the blood pressure will have a false low reading (Theorell, 2002).
4. Compare upper- and lower-extremity pressures. Systolic blood pressure of the upper extremities 20 mm Hg above that of lower extremities is suggestive of:
   a. Coarctation of the aorta. PDA may mask these pressure differences.
   b. Aortic arch abnormalities.
      (1) Additionally, blood pressure differences between the upper extremities are seen with aortic arch abnormalities.
      (2) To evaluate, simultaneously measure blood pressure in both arms and one leg. Either leg can be evaluated because the blood supply to both legs comes from the descending aorta below the level of the defect.
5. In a term infant, neonatal hypertension is defined as a systolic blood pressure greater than 90 mm Hg and a diastolic pressure greater than 60 mm Hg.
   a. In a premature infant, systolic pressure greater than 80 mm Hg and diastolic pressure greater than 50 mm Hg indicates hypertension.
   b. Structural and/or functional renal abnormalities are most common causes of hypertension.

F. Congestive heart failure (CHF).

1. CHF is defined as inadequate delivery of oxygen by the heart (O'Laughlin, 1999) and is typically associated with congenital heart lesions. The

timing of CHF appearance may assist in diagnosis of the lesion (Park, 2002).

2. Structural heart defects leading to a presentation of CHF symptoms:
   a. At birth:
      (1) Hypoplastic left heart syndrome.
      (2) Severe tricuspid or pulmonary regurgitation.
      (3) Large systemic arteriovenous fistula.
   b. First week of life:
      (1) Transposition of the great arteries.
      (2) Premature infant with large PDA.
      (3) Total anomalous pulmonary venous return below the diaphragm.
   c. 1 to 4 weeks of life:
      (1) Critical aortic or pulmonary stenosis.
      (2) Coarctation of the aorta.
3. Noncardiac causes.
   a. Birth asphyxia resulting in transient myocardial ischemia.
   b. Metabolic, including hypoglycemia and hypocalcemia.
   c. Severe anemia.
   d. Overhydration.
   e. Neonatal sepsis.
4. Primary myocardial disease.
   a. Myocarditis.
   b. Transient myocardial ischemia.
   c. Cardiomyopathy (seen in infants of diabetic mothers).
5. Disturbances in heart rate.
   a. Supraventricular tachycardia.
   b. Atrial flutter or fibrillation.
   c. Congenital heart block.
6. Late-onset CHF may result from bronchopulmonary dysplasia or other pulmonary stressors (see Chapter 23).
7. Clinical Presentation
   a. Depends on the cause of the CHF and the age of the patient.
      (1) Newborns. The CHF interferes with the breathing and feeding, crying or stooling. Poor perfusion is the hallmark sign, with pale, cyanotic, or gray coloring, poor capillary refill, and diaphoresis. These newborns may take as long as 45 to 60 minutes to finish a feeding that should only take 10 to 15 minutes.
   b. Physical examination (Montoya and Washington, 2002).
      (1) Respiratory rate greater than 60, tachypnea from interstitial pulmonary edema.
      (2) Heart rate. Tachycardia from compensation for decreased cardiac output, may have a gallop rhythm.
      (3) Four-limb blood pressure may yield a higher blood pressure in right arm than in either leg, indicating an aortic obstruction.
      (4) Central or peripheral cyanosis may be a clue to poor perfusion.
      (5) Decreased peripheral pulses and mottling of extremities from redistribution of blood flow to vital tissues.
      (6) Precordium may be hyperactive.

Diagnostic Adjuncts

A. **Arterial blood gas values** are used primarily to help differentiate lung disease vs. heart disease as the cause of cyanosis.

1. $PaCO_2$: generally normal in CHD and elevated in pulmonary parenchymal disease.
2. Hyperoxygen test.
   a. Sample arterial PO_2, with infant breathing 100% oxygen for at least 10 minutes vs. room air.
      (1) Umbilical artery sample may detect right-to-left shunts via PDA. The lowered PaO_2 is usually a reflection of lung disease and not of primary heart disease.
      (2) Administration of oxygen to infants with cardiac disease resulting in high pulmonary blood flow and CHF will improve oxygen levels (i.e., increased PaO_2) through decreased PVR and increased pulmonary blood flow.
      (3) Most accurate assessment of cardiac vs. pulmonary disease can be made if the right radial or temporal (preductal) and umbilical artery samples (postductal) are taken simultaneously.
      (4) Monitoring of preductal and postductal transcutaneous oxygen pressure or pulse oximetry provides a noninvasive evaluation for cardiac versus pulmonary disease.
   b. Preductal PaO_2 will rise to greater than 100 mm Hg with pulmonary disease; whereas an increase to less than 100 mm Hg is consistent with cardiac disease. However, the response of arterial PO_2 in the hyperoxitest should be interpreted in view of the clinical picture (Park, 2002).

B. Chest x-ray examination is used to:

1. Rule out pulmonary parenchymal disease (Penny and Shekerdemian, 2001).
2. Identify increased pulmonary vascular markings, as seen in lesions with left-to-right shunting.
3. Evaluate aortic arch (Strife and Sze, 1999).
4. Evaluate cardiac size, shape, and position.
   a. Cardiomegaly: defined as cardiac/thoracic ratio greater than 0.6.
   b. See Chapter 14 for chest x-ray findings in heart disease.

C. Electrocardiography (ECG).

1. Reflects abnormal hemodynamic burdens placed on the heart.
2. Used to determine severity of disease by assessing the degree of atrial or ventricular hypertrophy. Right ventricular predominance is normal shortly after birth. (In utero the right ventricle does most of the cardiac work.)
3. Changes in ST segments or T waves may suggest myocardial ischemia.
   a. Tall, peaked P waves are common in right-sided heart failure.
   b. Wide, notched P waves are seen with left-sided heart failure.
4. ECG is the major diagnostic tool for evaluating arrhythmias and the impact of electrolyte imbalances (e.g., potassium and calcium) on electrical conductivity.
5. Normal ECG values in term neonates:
   a. Heart rate: 110 to 160 bpm in first week.
   b. Normal sinus rhythm: P wave precedes QRS complex.
   c. P wave: duration 0.04 to 0.08 second.
   d. PR interval: 0.09 to 0.12 second. Prolonged interval is seen in first-degree heart block and is usually benign (Park, 2002).
   e. Rightward deviation of the QRS complex with a maximum of minus 180 degrees and duration of 0.03 to 0.07 second. Prolonged complex indicates interventricular conduction delay (Park, 2002).
   f. Occasional Q waves in V1 (~10% of newborns).

g. Premature infants have higher resting heart rates with greater variation. Duration of P wave is shorter. PR and QRS intervals are decreased (0.10 and 0.04 second, respectively).

D. Echocardiography.

1. Provides rapid, noninvasive, and painless evaluation of heart anatomy and flow by use of ultrasonic sound waves. Used to estimate pressures, measure gradients, and evaluate cardiac function (Montoya and Washington, 2002).
   - **a.** M-mode (single-dimension) echocardiography permits evaluation of anatomic relationships of heart and vessels, including relative sizes of each. It is also used to evaluate the motion of the cardiac valves and detect pericardial fluid.
   - **b.** Two-dimensional (real-time) echocardiography has greater versatility, providing more specific information regarding anatomic relationships. This mode is used to diagnose PDA, or ventricular dysfunction in premature infants (Park, 2002).
   - **c.** Color-flow Doppler echocardiography shows:
     - (1) Patterns of blood flow (i.e., right-to-left versus left-to-right shunting).
     - (2) Location of restrictions and/or regurgitation.
   - **d.** Continuous-wave Doppler echocardiography shows the quantity of flow across an obstruction, giving an estimate of pressure gradients. It is used to detect the direction of shunting, to estimate cardiac output, and to assess ventricular diastolic function.
   - **e.** Contrast echocardiography is accomplished by rapid injection of saline or dextrose in water solution in a vein while conducting an ultrasonographic examination. It allows for greater evaluation of flow patterns throughout the heart and identifies the presence of shunts.
2. Although echocardiography allows for rapid bedside diagnosis of cardiac lesions and differentiation from other abnormalities (e.g., sepsis, persistent fetal circulation), it does not replace cardiac catheterization as a diagnostic tool.

E. Magnetic resonance imaging.

1. Three-dimensional, providing high-resolution images of the heart and great vessels. Used to evaluate arch anomalies, vascular rings and pulmonary arteriovenous malformations (Montoya and Washington, 2002).

F. Cardiac catheterization.

1. An invasive procedure to obtain data (e.g., oxygen saturation and pressure measurements) for definitive diagnosis or in preparation for cardiac surgery. Over the last decade, the focus has changed from diagnostic to therapeutic (Pihkala et al., 1999).
   - **a.** May be used in palliative treatment (e.g., in the use of balloon atrial septostomy to treat TGV).
   - **b.** Usually reserved for cyanotic heart lesions.
   - **c.** For acyanotic heart lesions, can be delayed until full effect of medical management of CHF is seen.
   - **d.** Treatment modalities during catheterization have included placement of stents, angioplasty, and implanting of devices for closure of an ASD.
2. Procedure: advancement of a catheter through the umbilical, subclavian, femoral, or right internal jugular vessels and into the heart.
   - **a.** If balloon septostomy is anticipated, a large vessel will be needed.
   - **b.** Pressure measurements are made of all chambers and outlet tracts.
3. Concomitant angiography (injection of contrast medium): often performed to achieve maximal cardiac information.

4. Interventional techniques have replaced conventional surgery for many lesions.
   a. Objective is improvement or preservation of cardiac function, improvement in quality and quantity of life.
   b. Common procedures.
      (1) Dilation of valvular lesions (mitral stenosis).
      (2) Balloon valvuloplasty for critical aortic or pulmonary valve stenosis.
      (3) Dilation of coarctation of the aorta.
      (4) Dilation of pulmonary artery stenosis.
      (5) Balloon atrial septostomy.
      (6) Transcatheter defect occlusion for PDA.
      (7) Catheter delivered devices for ASD closure and certain muscular VSD closures.
5. Complications.
   a. Mortality risk is approximately 1% to 5% in the newborn period and is related to the defect, severity of symptoms, and the patient's condition (Park, 2002).
   b. High sodium content of contrast medium contributes to myocardial depression and exerts an osmotic effect, temporarily increasing intravascular volume.
   c. Hemorrhage with catheter insertion or removal may lead to:
      (1) Hypotension.
      (2) Shock.
      (3) Cardiac tamponade if bleeding is in the pericardial sac.
   d. Dysrhythmias are not uncommon (e.g., premature atrial and ventricular beats, heart block, and tachycardia), because of catheter manipulation.
   e. In infants younger than 4 months of age, the rate of nonfatal serious complications is 12%.

G. Laboratory data.
1. Complete blood cell count with differential cell count.
   a. Rules out anemia or polycythemia as cause of CHF.
   b. Decreased number of neutrophils and presence of left shift: possible indication of sepsis. Group B β-hemolytic streptococci can mimic hypoplastic left heart syndrome.
2. Blood glucose concentration. Used to evaluate hypoglycemia as potential cause of cardiomyopathy.
3. Electrolytes (especially potassium and calcium). Both potassium and calcium are major cations in electrical conductivity. Alterations can adversely affect cardiac contractility.

DEFECTS WITH INCREASED PULMONARY BLOOD FLOW

Patent Ductus Arteriosus (PDA)

A. Incidence (fourth most common lesion).
1. Isolated PDA in term gestations: 1:2000 live births.
2. In preterm gestations:
   a. Incidence is inversely related to gestational age.
   b. Appears in 45% of infants weighing less than 1750 g at birth.
   c. Is apparent in 80% of infants weighing less than 1200 g at birth.

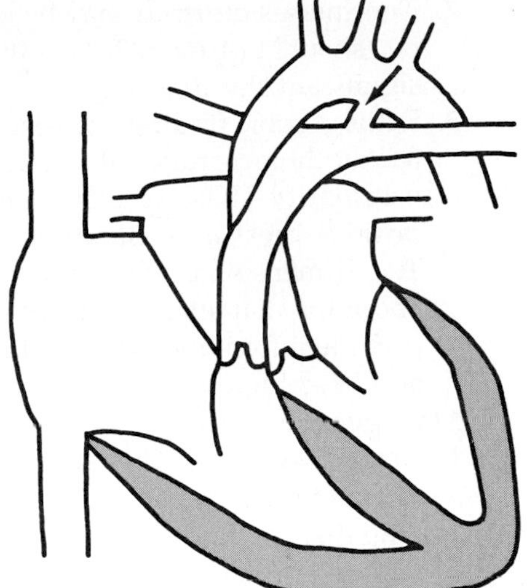

FIGURE 27-9 ■ Patent ductus arteriosus (PDA). (Redrawn courtesy G.G. Janos, M.D., 1989.)

   d. Significant PDA with CHF in 15% of premature infants with a birthweight (BW) less than 1750 g and 40% to 50% of those less than 1500 g BW (Park, 2002).
  3. Occurs three times more commonly in females than in males.

B. **Anatomy:** persistent patency of the ductus arteriosus after birth (Fig. 27-9).
  1. In utero patency of this structure is functional, diverting blood to the placenta for oxygen gas exchange.
  2. Persistent patency is influenced by several factors.
     a. Improvement in oxygenation causes the pulmonary vascular resistance to drop rapidly. Although increased oxygen tension is a potent stimulant of smooth muscle contraction, which should decrease patency, premature infants have an immature response to oxygen, thus the PDA remains open.
     b. Lack of ductal smooth muscle (e.g., in premature infants) prolongs patency.
     c. Prostaglandins inhibit closure of ductus.

C. **Hemodynamics.**
  1. As PVR falls and SVR rises, a left-to-right shunt via the PDA results in blood flow from the aorta into the pulmonary artery, increasing pulmonary blood flow. The increased pulmonary artery pressure and increased left ventricular pressure and volume lead to bilateral CHF.
  2. Because left-to-right flow is dependent on a drop in PVR, infants with pulmonary disease (e.g., hyaline membrane disease) will show symptoms when lung disease improves. Before this time, PVR greater than SVR leads to a right-to-left shunt via the patent ductus (commonly referred to as persistent pulmonary hypertension of the neonate).

D. **Clinical manifestations.**
  1. Presents at 4 to 7 days of life with inability to wean from the ventilator or has a need for increased ventilatory and oxygen support. May present with apneic and/or bradycardic spells if not on a ventilator.
     a. Increased pulmonary vasculature and cardiomegaly.
     b. Bounding peripheral pulses and hyperactive precordium.
     c. Widening pulse pressure (>20 mm Hg).

2. Continuous murmur may be present at the upper left sternal border but may be "silent" in 10% to 20% of the preterm infants despite hemodynamically significant shunt.
3. Radiographic findings consist of normal size or mild cardiomegaly (cardiothoracic ratio >0.60), pulmonary edema, and increased pulmonary vascularity. These "typical" signs may be absent if the infant is receiving positive-pressure ventilation.
4. Two-dimensional echocardiography will provide anatomic information about the diameter, length and shape of the ductus. Doppler flow will provide information on the ductal shunt magnitude and patterns (Montoya and Washington, 2002).

E. **Management.**
1. Dependent on whether shunt is hemodynamically significant. In premature infants the PDA may prolong ventilator use beyond the dictates of the initial lung disease. Early intervention may prevent lung complications of ventilator use (Corbet, 1998).
2. Hemodynamically significant ductus arteriosus includes the following:
   a. Heart rate greater than 170 bpm.
   b. Respiratory rate greater than 70 per minute.
   c. Hepatomegaly greater than 3 cm below costal margin.
   d. Bounding pulses.
3. Conservative measures are generally employed initially.
   a. Fluid restriction.
   b. Diuretics: if employed with fluid restriction, may lead to electrolyte imbalance, dehydration, and caloric deprivation.
   c. Positive end-expiratory pressure: useful in reducing left-to-right shunt via PDA.
4. Indomethacin management includes the following:
   a. As a prostaglandin inhibitor, indomethacin can constrict and close the PDA in some premature infants.
   b. Dosage is 0.1 to 0.2 mg/kg/dose, given every 8 hours for a total of three doses (Montoya and Washington, 2002).
   c. Less effective if given after 7 days.
   d. Prophylactic indomethacin, given within 15 hours of birth, provides an increase in permanent closure of the ductus (Narayanan-Sankar and Clyman, 2003).
   e. Complications are as follows:
      (1) Transient decreased renal function.
      (2) Increased incidence of gastrointestinal bleeding.
      (3) Inhibition of platelet aggregation for 7 to 9 days, with potential for intracerebral hemorrhage.
   f. Ductus recurrence rate was high in infants weighing less than 1000 g who were treated with indomethacin (Corbet, 1998).
   g. Contraindications are as follows (Takemoto et al., 1999):
      (1) Renal failure (blood urea nitrogen [BUN] concentration >30 mg/dl, serum creatinine concentration >1.8 mg/dl, urine output <0.6 ml/kg/hour).
      (2) Active gastrointestinal bleeding.
      (3) Necrotizing enterocolitis: not a contraindication. However, surgical ligation is more rapid, and certain resolution of PDA results in prompt decrease in bowel ischemia from the PDA.
      (4) Platelet count less than 60,000/mm^3.

(5) Sepsis: proved or strongly suspected.
(6) Severe pulmonary hypertension with irreversible pulmonary vascular disease.

5. Ibuprofen administration (currently undergoing investigation).
   a. Initial dose 10 mg/kg IV followed by two doses of 5 mg/kg every 24 hours.
   b. Significantly lower incidence of oliguria.
   c. Does not appear to affect cerebral blood flow.
   d. Does not appear to affect mesenteric blood flow (Narayanan-Sankar and Clyman, 2003).
   e. May prove to be a better choice than indomethacin (Park, 2002).
6. Surgical management involves ligation of the PDA.
   a. Standard approach is surgical ligation via posterolateral thoracotomy incision risk.
   b. New techniques include minimally invasive video-assisted thoracoscopic surgery, allowing for PDA interruption without cutting muscles or spreading ribs (Montoya and Washington, 2002). Surgery carries potential for complications of bleeding with prior indomethacin therapy (risk dependent on time from dose to surgical intervention).
7. Cardiac catheterization and insertion of a vascular occlusion device, consisting of a coil-filled sac that releases from the catheter (Montoya and Washington, 2002).

F. **Prognosis.** Surgical mortality is less than 1%. If the defect is asymptomatic or medically or surgically ligated, prognosis is excellent.

Ventricular Septal Defect (VSD)

A. **Incidence.** At 1:3000 live births, VSDs are the most common of all CHDs.

B. **Anatomy:** abnormal opening in the septum between the right and left ventricle. Sizes range from pinhole to almost complete absence of the ventricular septum (Fig. 27-10).

C. **Hemodynamics.**
   1. The degree of hypertrophy of ventricles and the pressure relationships are dependent on the size of the defect. A small defect allows pressure differences between ventricles.

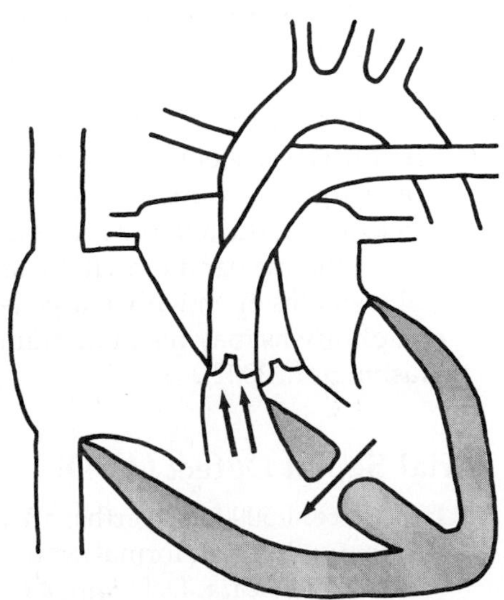

FIGURE 27-10 ■ Ventricular septal defect (VSD). (Redrawn courtesy G.G. Janos, M.D., 1989.)

2. PVR less than SVR results in a left-to-right shunt, producing increased pulmonary blood flow and leading to decreased pulmonary compliance and pulmonary edema.
3. Excessive pulmonary artery blood flow eventually results in pulmonary artery hypertrophy and stenosis.
4. High pulmonary artery pressure can delay maturation of pulmonary arterioles.

D. **Clinical manifestations.**
1. Size dependent.
2. Small VSD.
   a. Asymptomatic.
   b. High-pitched pansystolic murmur along left sternal border.
3. Moderate VSD: asymptomatic except for murmur and recurrent respiratory infection.
4. Large VSD.
   a. Present at 1 to 2 months of age with CHF, pulmonary infection, and increased precordial activity.
   b. Loud, blowing pansystolic murmur at left lower sternal border.
   c. Chest x-ray examination: cardiomegaly and increased pulmonary vascular markings.
   d. Two-dimensional echocardiography is capable of identifying 90% of VSDs. Doppler and/or color flow mapping increases the accuracy of diagnosis of VSD and color flow is extremely useful in identifying multiple VSDs and the direction of blood flow across the VSD.

E. **Management.**
1. 50% to 75% of small defects will close spontaneously; 20% of large defects become smaller or close.
2. With mild CHF, treatment consists of digoxin and diuretics.
3. Surgery is indicated if patient has failure to thrive or intractable CHF.
   a. Palliative: surgical banding of pulmonary artery to reduce pulmonary blood flow, decrease CHF, and prevent pulmonary vascular resistance.
   b. Surgical: repair by suturing defect or patching defect through a median sternotomy. The defect is approached via the right atrium and tricuspid valve. If the infant is less than 2000 g, it may be necessary to perform pulmonary artery banding to decrease blood flow to the lungs. Surgical closure is then done when the infant is greater than 2000 g.
   c. Transcatheter devices such as the clamshell, double-umbrella, and buttoned devices are used but further experience is needed (Pihkala et al., 1999).

F. **Prognosis:** excellent. Mortality rate is less than 5% in infants. Complications from surgical closure may include right bundle-branch block, third-degree heart block, and aortic and/or tricuspid insufficiency. Earlier surgical repair, rather than palliative banding with delayed repair is associated with better results. If VSD remains open with a large left-to-right shunt after 9 months of age, complications may result in pulmonary vascular disease (Montoya and Washington, 2002).

Atrial Septal Defect (ASD)

A. **Incidence:** 1:5000 live births, 5% to 10% of all cardiac defects.

B. **Anatomy:** defect in formation of septum, resulting in a communication between right and left atria. Defect may be an ostium primum defect, an ostium secundum defect (most common), or a partial endocardial cushion defect (Fig. 27-11). By definition, a patent foramen ovale is generally excluded, although symptoms can be the same.

C. **Hemodynamics.**
   1. Immediately after birth, right ventricular pressure is greater than left ventricle pressure, so there is no shunt or only a small right-to-left shunt.
   2. As PVR decreases, left-to-right shunt develops with concomitant right ventricular volume overload and hypertrophy.

D. **Clinical manifestations.**
   1. In isolated defect, generally asymptomatic and unrecognized. If ASD is diagnosed in infancy, greater than 50% of the patients will be symptomatic.
   2. CHF from left-to-right shunt with mitral valve insufficiency.
   3. Failure to thrive.
   4. Recurrent respiratory infections.
   5. Systolic murmur at second intercostal space at left sternal border, persistent split S_2 if shunt is large, diastolic murmur heard at left lower sternal border.
   6. Chest x-ray examination: increased pulmonary vascular markings with enlarged right atrium and ventricle (Park, 2002).

E. **Management.**
   1. If defect is small, clinical follow-up is indicated; the defect may close spontaneously.
   2. ASD with CHF: medical treatment of CHF and delay surgical repair.
   3. ASD with intractable CHF: early surgical repair (i.e., suturing or patching of defect).
   4. Surgical repair may be done by placement of a variety of catheter-introduced occlusion devices (button, disk, double umbrella) or by traditional patching or suturing the defect. Complications include residual shunting and embolization of the device (Pihkala et al., 1999).

F. **Prognosis.**
   1. Spontaneous closure occurs in up to 40% of ASDs during the first 5 years of life (Kenner et al., 1998).
   2. Perioperative mortality rate is less than 1%, with good long-term results in survivors. Survival at 5 years of age is 97% and at 10 years, 90%.

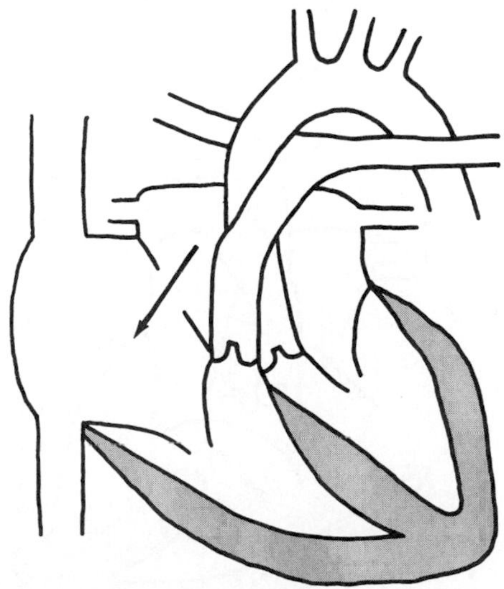

FIGURE 27-11 ■ Atrial septal defect (ASD). (Redrawn courtesy G.G. Janos, M.D., 1989.)

Endocardial Cushion Defect (Atrioventricular Canal)

A. **Incidence:** 1:9000 live births. Most common heart defect found in Down syndrome.

B. **Anatomy.**
   1. Endocardial cushions form the lower portion of the atrial septum, the upper portion of the ventricular septum, and septal portions of the mitral and tricuspid valves.
   2. A wide range of defects is possible, from simple cleft of the mitral and/or tricuspid valves to complete absence of the lower atrial and upper ventricular septa with common atrioventricular valve (i.e., atrioventricular canal) (Fig. 27-12).

C. **Hemodynamics.**
   1. With PVR less than SVR, blood dependently shunts left to right via the ASD and the VSD.
   2. Higher pressure of the left ventricle creates obligatory left-to-right shunting via the atrioventricular valve (atrioventricular valve regurgitation). Blood flows from the left ventricle to the mitral portion of the atrioventricular valve to the left atrium to the ASD, and to the right atrium.

D. **Clinical manifestations.**
   1. Isolated ostium primum atrial defect: rarely identified in the neonatal period.
   2. Isolated ventricular defect: see clinical features of VSD, p. 610.
   3. Complete atrioventricular canal.
      a. Atrioventricular valve regurgitation controls age at presentation.
         (1) Severe: seen at 1 to 2 weeks of age with CHF.
         (2) Valves competent: seen in first or second month of life.
      b. Respiratory distress.
      c. Active precordium, with a thrill at the left lower sternal border.
      d. Variable murmurs; usually loud pansystolic murmur at the lower left sternal border, radiating to left back.
      e. Recurrent respiratory infections.
      f. Chest x-ray examination: cardiomegaly, bilateral atrial and ventricular hypertrophy, increased pulmonary markings.

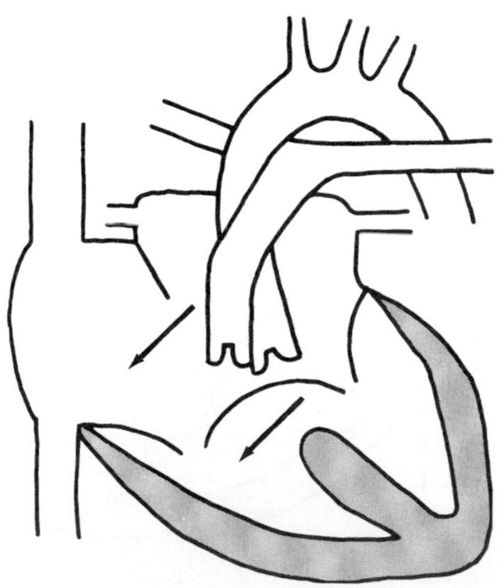

FIGURE 27-12 ■ Atrioventricular canal (AVC). (Redrawn courtesy G.G. Janos, M.D., 1989.)

E. **Management.**
   1. Objective: to avoid development of pulmonary vascular obstructive disease.
   2. Medical management: to prevent or control CHF with digoxin and diuretics.
   3. Palliative pulmonary artery banding to decrease pulmonary overload. Does not influence obligatory shunting of the atrioventricular valve.
   4. Primary repair with closure of atrial and ventricular septal defects and mitral and tricuspid valve reconstruction (Vick, 1998). Usually done between 6 months and 2 years of age.

F. **Prognosis.**
   1. Prognosis is dependent on details of anatomic form and on the presence of significant associated noncardiac anomalies and significant pulmonary obstructive vascular disease.
   2. Best results are seen with ostium primum defect or common atrium; long-term prognosis is good.
   3. Outlook for complete atrioventricular canal without operation is poor.
   4. Mortality rate for surgical repair is 5% to 10%. However, this increases to 15% for those infants who undergo pulmonary artery banding (Kenner et al., 1998).

OBSTRUCTIVE DEFECTS WITH PULMONARY VENOUS CONGESTION

Coarctation of the Aorta

A. **Incidence:** 8% of congenital heart lesions.
   1. Most common congenital heart defect presenting in week 2 of life.
   2. Male dominance: 2:1.
   3. 30% of those with Turner syndrome will have this defect.

B. **Anatomy:** constriction of aorta at the junction or the transverse aortic arch or the vicinity of the ductus arteriosus (Fig. 27-13).
   1. Most common site is below the origin of the left subclavian artery.
   2. Preductal coarctation is associated with hypoplasia of the aortic arch and defects such as VSD, PDA, and transposition of the great arteries (TGA) will be found in 40%.
   3. More than 50% of infants with coarctation will have a bicuspid aortic valve.

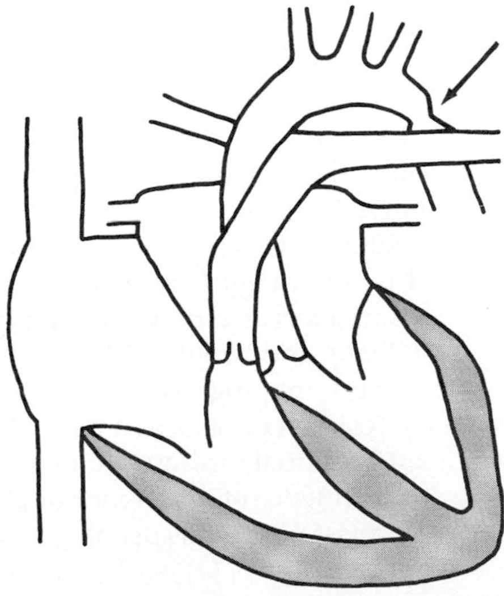

FIGURE 27-13 ■ Coarctation of aorta. (Redrawn courtesy G.G. Janos, M.D., 1989.)

C. **Hemodynamics.**
   1. Isolated coarctation: obstruction to left ventricular outflow, leading to increased left ventricular, left atrial, and pulmonary venous pressures. Pulmonary venous congestion develops.
   2. Coarctation with VSD: elevated left ventricular pressure, shunting blood left to right via VSD and causing pulmonary overload.
   3. Preductal coarctation: dependent on PDA for distal aorta and lower body blood flow.

D. **Clinical manifestations.**
   1. CHF as a result of pressure overload on the left ventricle.
   2. Decreased or absent pulses in the lower extremities.
   3. Higher blood pressure (>15 mm Hg) in upper extremities is the most consistent factor in critical coarctation. If blood pressures are lower in the upper extremities, the following applies:
      a. Decreased blood pressure in left arm, indicative of left subclavian artery as site of coarctation.
      b. Decreased blood pressure in right arm: right subclavian artery arises below coarctation (rare).
      c. Pulses that "wax and wane": related to increase or decrease in PDA blood flow.
   4. Heart sounds.
      a. Postductal: no murmur or short systolic ejection click in axilla or back.
      b. Preductal with VSD: harsh pansystolic murmur at left lower sternal border.
      c. Gallop rhythm possible.
   5. Systolic thrill **heard** at the suprasternal notch.
   6. Chest x-ray examination: enlarged heart with left ventricular hypertrophy and increased pulmonary vascular markings.
   7. Cardiac catheterization is diagnostic and usually performed prior to surgical management to evaluate for other anomalies (Kenner et al., 1998).

E. **Management.**
   1. Aggressive medical management of CHF.
   2. Prostaglandin E_1 (PGE_1) to dilate ductus arteriosus (preductal lesion).
   3. Isolated postductal coarctation: control of CHF first, then delayed surgical correction.
   4. Surgical correction: two common repairs.
      a. Either resection of abnormal segment and reanastomosis.
      b. *Or* subclavian patch across area of obstruction.
      c. With associated anomalies, variable approaches according to type of defect.
   5. Balloon angioplasty is the treatment of choice for recoarctation with success rate 65% to 100% (Pihkala et al., 1999).

F. **Prognosis.**
   1. Outcome is dependent on complexity of coarctation, with mortality rates at 1 month ranging from zero for simple coarctation to 13%; can be higher for complex coarctation associated with VSD or other left-sided obstruction (Chang and Vaughn, 1998).
   2. Long-term prognosis after coarctation repair is determined by the presence of residual or recurrent coarctation, persistence of pulmonary hypertension, and residual cardiovascular lesions (Montoya and Washington, 2002).
      a. Incidence of recurrence of 25% to 60% after resection and end-to-end anastomosis has been reported after repair in infancy.

b. Overall surgical mortality is less than 20% in infancy; however, earlier detection and use of PGE_1 may reduce mortality.
c. Potential residual complications include persistent hypertension, Horner syndrome, and mesenteric vasculitis.

Aortic Stenosis

A. **Incidence:** 1:24,000 live births, accounts for 3% to 5% of all cardiac anomalies.
 1. Four times more likely in males.
B. **Anatomy:** may be subvalvular, valvular, or supravalvular, with valvular stenosis being the most common form. The myocardium of the left ventricle is hypertrophied (Fig. 27-14).
 1. Valvular stenosis usually has a bicuspid aortic valve.
 2. Supravalvular stenosis is the least common and is seen with Williams syndrome.
C. **Hemodynamics.** Obstruction to left ventricular outflow leads to increased left ventricular pressures and hypertrophy. If aortic stenosis is severe in utero, blood flow through the ventricle is decreased, resulting in left ventricular hypoplasia and left-sided heart syndrome.
D. **Clinical manifestations.**
 1. Usually asymptomatic at birth (Montoya and Washington, 2002).
 2. Acrocyanosis.
 3. Heart sounds include a grade II to IV/VI harsh systolic murmur in upper right sternal border, radiating to the neck and lower left sternal border.
 4. Suprasternal notch thrill may be present.
 5. CHF symptoms may be delayed by weeks but progress rapidly after onset.
 6. Chest x-ray examination shows cardiomegaly with normal pulmonary vascular markings.
 7. If critical aortic stenosis is present, the infant will suddenly deteriorate when the ductus arteriosus closes (Westmoreland, 1999).
E. **Management.**
 1. Medical management is usually not successful.
 2. Initially, CHF is treated with fluid restriction, diuretics, digoxin, acidosis management, and antibiotic prophylaxis.

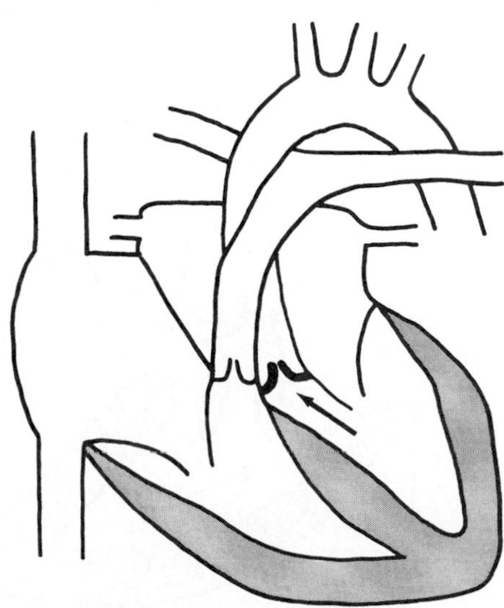

FIGURE 27-14 ■ Aortic stenosis. (Redrawn courtesy G.G. Janos, M.D., 1989.)

3. If stenosis is critical, use PGE_1 to prevent hypoxia.
4. In recent studies, percutaneous balloon dilation has been shown to be as effective and safe as surgical dilation in the treatment of the newborn according to Pihkala and coworkers (1999). Early mortality rate is 11%. Most newborns will require further intervention within 10 years.
5. Surgery involves aortic valvotomy or valve replacement.

F. **Prognosis.**
1. Success rate of balloon valvuloplasty is 87% to 97% (Pihkala et al., 1999).
2. Mortality rate is 19% with death resulting from sudden death. Operative risk is high as a result of ventricular hypoplasia and myocardial hypertrophy. Late potential complications include calcification and endocarditis.
3. Aortic stenosis is the most common cause of sudden death in children with heart disease.

OBSTRUCTIVE DEFECTS WITH DECREASED PULMONARY BLOOD FLOW

Tetralogy of Fallot (TOF)

A. **Incidence:** 1:5000 live births. Most common cyanotic heart lesion, accounting for 10% of all defects.

B. **Anatomy:** classified as a combination of four defects, although numbers 3 and 4, below, are consequences of numbers 1 and 2 below (Fig. 27-15).
1. Pulmonary stenosis: obstruction of outflow tract.
2. VSD.
3. Aorta overriding VSD.
4. Right ventricular hypertrophy.

C. **Hemodynamics.**
1. Dependent primarily on degree of pulmonary stenosis and to a lesser extent on VSD size.
2. In severe pulmonary stenosis, blood flow passes from right to left via the VSD, with resulting hypoxia and cyanosis.

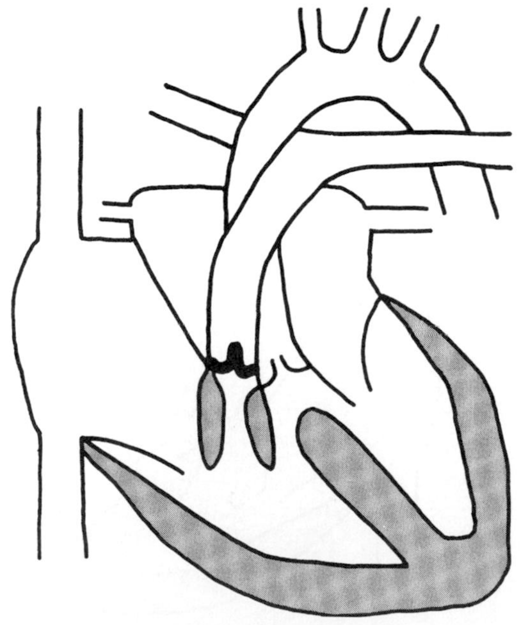

FIGURE 27-15 ■ Tetralogy of Fallot (TOF). (Redrawn courtesy G.G. Janos, M.D., 1989.)

3. In mild pulmonary stenosis, blood flows from left to right via the VSD, with CHF resulting.
4. In mild to moderate pulmonary stenosis, blood flow via VSD may be minimal as long as PVR and SVR are balanced. With crying, right-to-left shunting occurs.

D. Clinical manifestations.

1. Presentation is a function of the degree of pulmonary stenosis.
2. Severe obstruction presents in the first days of life with severe cyanosis, hypoxia, and dyspnea.
3. Milder pulmonary obstruction presents in the first days of life with mild cyanosis.
4. Harsh grades II to IV/VI systolic murmur with thrill present at mid- to upper left sternal border.
5. Chest x-ray examination shows normal-sized boot-shaped heart with normal or decreased pulmonary vascular markings.
6. Traditional "TET spells" (paroxysmal dyspnea and severe cyanosis) are common in infants and can occur in neonates (Kenner et al., 1998).

E. Management.

1. Medical (Montoya and Washington, 2002).
   a. Propranolol is the drug of choice for treating hypercyanotic infants.
   b. PGE_1 is used to maintain patency of the ductus arteriosus until the infant can be taken to surgery in severe TOF.
2. Corrective surgery involves closure of the VSD with a patch and eliminating the pulmonary stenosis by resection. The pulmonary outflow tract may be enlarged by a patch. This procedure is done while the infant is on cardiopulmonary bypass.
   a. Surgical correction is performed after 6 months of age and may be delayed to 2 to 4 years of age in symptom-free children.
   b. If child has symptoms before 6 months of age, a Blalock-Taussig procedure is generally performed, with full correction at a later time.
3. Prognosis.
   a. Prognosis without surgery is very poor. Mortality rate in infancy is less than 10% (Montoya and Washington, 2002).
   b. Complications/residual effects include decreased or absent pulses in affected arm, inadequate shunt, and CHF resulting from large shunt.
   c. Postoperative mortality is less than 10% for uncomplicated TOF. This rate increases with the more severe forms of TOF.

Pulmonary Stenosis

A. Incidence: 1:14,000 live births, 5% to 8% of all congenital heart defects.

B. Anatomy: narrowed opening either in pulmonary valve as a consequence of pulmonary valve cusp fusions (Fig. 27-16) or above or below the valve because of tissue hypertrophy.

C. Hemodynamics.

1. In utero, right ventricular hypoplasia can develop, depending on the degree of pulmonary valve stenosis and subsequent decrease in right ventricular blood flow.
2. After birth, the combination of right ventricular hypoplasia and severe pulmonary valve stenosis redirects blood flow from right to left at the atrial level via the foramen ovale. Pulmonary blood becomes dependent on a left-to-right flow via the PDA.

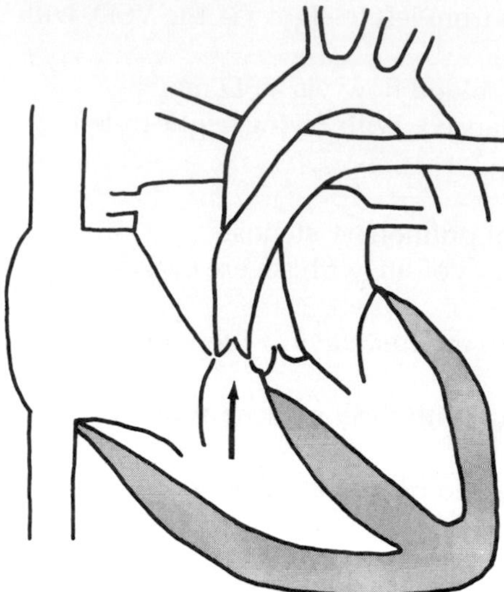

FIGURE 27-16 ■ Pulmonary stenosis (PS). (Redrawn courtesy G.G. Janos, M.D., 1989.)

3. In mild stenosis, the pulmonary blood flow is not excessively restricted and is PDA independent. As PVR decreases, atrial right-to-left shunt will decrease, improving systemic hypoxia.

D. **Clinical manifestations.**
   1. Mild pulmonary stenosis: loud systolic murmur at left upper sternal border is the only finding.
   2. Moderately severe stenosis.
      a. Murmur is less prominent. Murmur of tricuspid insufficiency may be noted.
      b. Cyanosis is present and increases with PDA closure.
      c. Generally, hepatomegaly is present.
   3. Chest x-ray examination: mild cardiomegaly with bulging right heart border and decreased pulmonary vascular markings.
   4. Two-dimensional echocardiography used to make anatomic and physiologic diagnosis (Waldman and Wernly, 1999).

E. **Management.**
   1. Cyanotic neonate.
      a. Initial management: oxygen, bicarbonate, and PGE_1.
      b. Nonsurgical treatment with catheter-introduced balloon valvuloplasty or angioplasty.
         (1) Few complications; effective.
         (2) Treatment of choice for discrete valvular lesion.
      c. Surgical valvotomy or tissue excision if valvuloplasty fails and patient is symptomatic.
   2. Noncyanotic neonate: conservative management includes catheterization at 6 to 12 months if stenosis is severe, with subsequent surgery if right ventricular pressure exceeds systemic.

F. **Prognosis.** Excellent. Operative mortality rate for valvuloplasty is less than 5%; however, acute complications in the neonate are 10% to 30% (Pihkala et al., 1999).

Pulmonary Atresia

A. **Incidence:** 1:14,000 live births, accounting for less than 1% of cardiac defects.

B. Anatomy: complete obstruction of the pulmonic valve, resulting in a hypoplastic right ventricle and tricuspid valve (Fig. 27-17). In the presence of a VSD the right ventricle may be of adequate size.

C. Hemodynamics.

1. Venous blood returning to the right atrium goes across the foramen ovale into the left atrium, into the left ventricle, and out the aorta.
2. Blood flow to the lungs is derived entirely from a left-to-right shunt at the ductus arteriosus, which is generally small and tortuous. As the PDA closes, severe hypoxemia ensues.
3. Regurgitant blood flow occurs at the tricuspid valve.

D. Clinical manifestations.

1. Mild cyanosis at birth, progressing to intense cyanosis by 24 hours.
2. Tachypnea.
3. Heart sounds.
   a. PDA murmur is present.
   b. Soft systolic murmur is heard at the upper left sternal border, harsh systolic murmur at lower right and upper left sternal border if tricuspid insufficiency present.
4. Chest x-ray examination shows increased heart size with decreased pulmonary markings; right atrial hypertrophy is seen in 70%.
5. Two-dimensional echocardiography with Doppler and color flow mapping is used to determine absence of blood flow across the pulmonary valve and is diagnostic (Kenner et al., 1998).

E. Management.

1. Initial treatment is use of oxygen and bicarbonate for metabolic acidosis and PGE_1 to maintain patency of the ductus arteriosus.
2. Cardiac catheterization is done with balloon atrial septostomy in infants with pulmonary atresia.
3. Mild right ventricle hypertrophy: surgical valvotomy may be effective.
4. With severe hyperplasia of right ventricle and tricuspid valve, is usually a Blalock-Taussig shunt to provide systemic-to-pulmonary shunting in the neonatal period. These infants will later require definitive repair via single or staged Fontan resulting in communication between the right atrium and pulmonary artery. Closure of ASD or VSD is done at this time (Montoya and Washington, 2002).

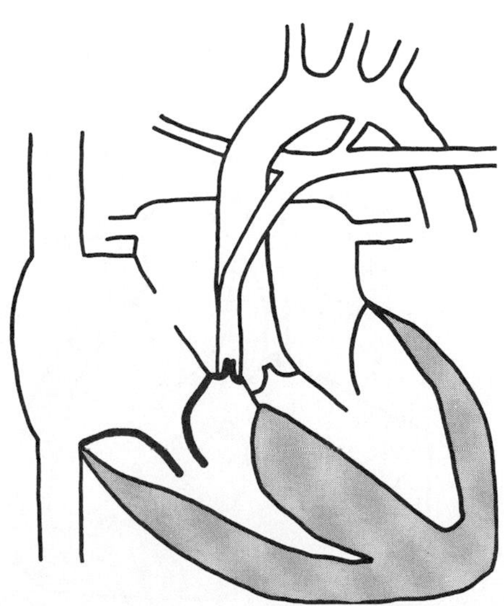

FIGURE 27-17 ■ Pulmonary atresia. (Redrawn courtesy G.G. Janos, M.D., 1989.)

F. **Prognosis.**
   1. Without surgery, mortality rate is 100%. If reconstruction of the right ventricular outflow tract is needed, the mortality rate is 25%. If Fontan procedure is done, the mortality rate jumps to 40%. Operative outlook for pulmonary atresia with intact ventricular septum is poor (Kenner et al., 1998).
   2. Reported survival rates range from 20% to 36%, depending on extent of defect, size of right ventricle, and operative procedure (Reddy et al., 1998).

Tricuspid Atresia

A. **Incidence:** 1:18,000 live births.
B. **Anatomy:** agenesis of the tricuspid valve development with associated patent foramen ovale or ASD (Fig. 27-18).
   1. VSD is often associated with the hypoplastic right ventricle.
   2. Pulmonary atresia or stenosis is possible.
   3. Transposition of the great vessels occurs in 30% of the cases.
C. **Hemodynamics.**
   1. Systemic venous blood is shunted from the right atrium across the foramen ovale or ASD into the left atrium. With an isolated defect the pulmonary blood flow is supplied by the left ventricular outflow via the PDA.
   2. In the presence of a VSD, some of the blood entering the left ventricle shunts across into the hypoplastic right ventricle and out the pulmonary artery—or out the aorta in the case of coexisting transposition. If severe pulmonary stenosis or atresia is present, blood does not flow through the VSD. (See also item C.1, above.)
D. **Clinical manifestations.**
   1. Cyanosis usually presents soon after birth with an isolated defect or coexisting VSD and pulmonary outflow tract obstruction. Increasing cyanosis occurs with closure of the ductus.
   2. Dyspnea, tachypnea may be present.
   3. CHF ensues with large VSD and absent pulmonary stenosis (usually in the first month of life).

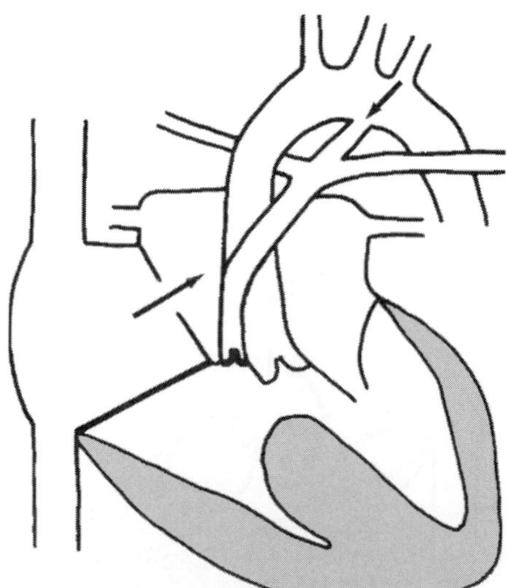

FIGURE 27-18 ■ Tricuspid atresia. *Arrows* identify shunting through patent foramen ovale and patent ductus arteriosus. (Redrawn courtesy G.G. Janos, M.D., 1989.)

4. Murmur is absent unless associated with pulmonary stenosis, VSD, or PDA.
5. Chest x-ray examination shows variable heart size, depending on the degree of pulmonary stenosis; size is generally nondiagnostic.
6. Cardiac catheterization to perform a balloon septostomy to improve intraatrial mixing of blood.

E. **Management.**
1. Primary treatment: oxygen, bicarbonate, and PGE_1 for severe hypoxia.
2. Palliative treatment.
   a. Systemic–pulmonary artery shunt including Blalock-Taussig procedure.
   b. Large VSD with no pulmonary stenosis. Pulmonary artery banding is performed to control CHF.
3. Reparative surgery.
   a. Right atrium is connected to either the right ventricular outflow track or the pulmonary artery (Fontan or modified Fontan), so that the right atrium forces blood into the lungs. Closure of the ASD and VSD is done at this time if they are present.
   b. Modified Fontan procedure separates oxygenated and unoxygenated blood inside the heart but does not restore normal hemodynamics or anatomy.

F. **Prognosis.** Mortality rates in older children are 10% to 25%. Complications include heart failure, persistent shunts, and dysrhythmias (Montoya and Washington, 2002).

MIXED DEFECTS

Transposition of the Great Vessels (TGV)

A. **Incidence:** 1:5000 live births; male predominance: 2:1. Most common cardiac cause of cyanosis in neonates (Grifka, 1999).

B. **Anatomy:** positions of the great arteries are reversed (i.e., the pulmonary artery arises from the left ventricle and the aorta from the right ventricle). Without other intracardiac defects (e.g., VSD, ASD), an independent, parallel circuit exists (Fig. 27-19). In dextroposition ("D" presentation), aorta is situated to the left of the pulmonary artery.

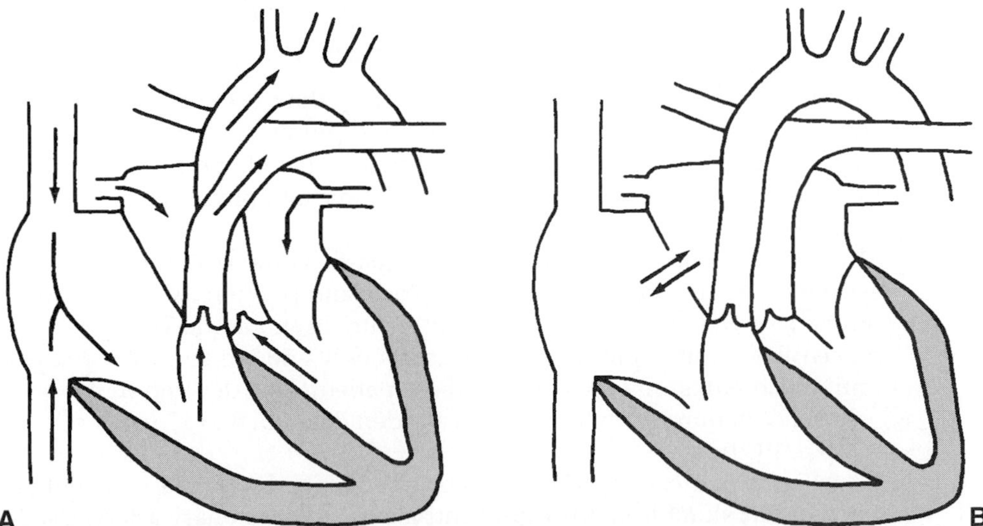

FIGURE 27-19 ■ Transposition of great vessels (TGV). **A,** Normal anatomy. **B,** Appearance of heart with TGV. (Redrawn courtesy G.G. Janos, M.D., 1989.)

C. Hemodynamics.

1. Oxygenated blood returns from the lungs to enter the left atrium and ventricle, then recirculates to the lungs by way of the pulmonary artery.
2. Unoxygenated blood returns to the right atrium and ventricle and is returned through the aorta to the body.
3. Mixing of oxygenated and unoxygenated blood occurs at the ductus arteriosus (as long as patency exists) or through any existing septal defects (ASD, VSD).
   a. Mixing is required for survival.
   b. Shunting occurs from left to right through septal defects or the PDA, ameliorating degree of cyanosis and hypoxia.

D. Clinical manifestations.

1. Cyanosis is present within the first 24 hours of life and becomes progressively more intense.
2. Prominent murmurs are uncommon; VSD (if present) will have a loud murmur.
3. Chest x-ray findings are usually normal; the heart may have an "egg on a string" appearance. Pulmonary vasculature may be increased or decreased.
4. Echocardiography is the standard diagnostic test (Westmoreland, 1999).

E. Management. TGA is a cardiac emergency.

1. Correction of metabolic acidosis.
2. PGE_1 to maintain patency of the PDA until palliative surgery can be performed.
3. Palliation of choice: catheter-introduced balloon septostomy.
   a. Balloon catheter is inserted into the femoral or umbilical vein; it is advanced across the foramen ovale into the left atrium, and the balloon is inflated and pulled across the atrium, creating an ASD.
   b. Procedure rapidly improves systemic and pulmonary circulation admixing, thus increasing PaO_2 (30s) and saturation (70s).
4. Blade septostomy: if atrial septum is too thick to be torn by balloon septostomy or balloon septostomy is unsuccessful. A catheter with a blade is introduced into the left atrium with standard catheterization technique, and a hole is excised in the atrial septum (Neches et al., 1998).
5. Pulmonary artery banding: to prevent pulmonary vascular disease, to decrease CHF, or to exercise the left ventricle before surgery by increasing the ventricular workload.
6. Corrective surgery.
   a. Arterial switch operation (Jatene procedure) is the treatment of choice: detaches aorta, coronary arteries, and pulmonary artery, reattaching to correct ventricles. Procedure is generally performed within first 2 weeks of life and provides both anatomic and physiologic correction.
   b. Mustard or Senning Procedures: creates a baffle at the atrium to divert systemic venous blood into the left ventricle and pulmonary artery and pulmonary venous blood into the right ventricle and aorta. These procedures result in physiologic correction only and are generally delayed until the infant is 6 months of age. These patients will develop right ventricular failure, arrhythmias, and sudden death in 8 to 15 years (Grifka, 1999).
   c. Rastelli procedure: intraventricular repair combined with placement of an extracardiac shunt from the right ventricle to the pulmonary artery. Used for TGV with large VSD and extensive left ventricular outflow tract obstruction.

F. Prognosis.
1. Changes in medical operative management make short-term data potentially misleading and long-term data out of date.
2. Without surgery, 90% will die within the first year.
3. Survival outcomes are 95%, if arterial switch is performed (Grifka, 1999).
4. Complications and other residual effects of the Mustard and Senning procedures are dysrhythmias, myocardial ischemia, and aortic and/or pulmonic supravalvular stenosis.
5. The incidence of neurologic and developmental complications is relatively high after neonatal arterial switch. These complications include gross motor deficits, fine motor deficits, sensory dysfunction, and speech and language difficulties (Hövels-Gürich et al., 2002).

Truncus Arteriosus

A. Incidence: 1:33,000 live births, less than 1% of cardiac defects.

B. Anatomy: a single great artery arises from both ventricles, overriding a VSD (Fig. 27-20).
1. Type I: short pulmonary artery arising from the base of the common trunk, then divides into the right and left arteries.
2. Type II: right and left pulmonary arteries arise from the posterior surface of the common trunk.
3. Type III: right and left pulmonary arteries have separate origins in the lateral walls of the common trunk (Montoya and Washington, 2002).

C. Hemodynamics.
1. Both ventricles pump blood into the common trunk supplying the systemic and pulmonary circulation. As PVR drops, preferential shunting to the pulmonary circulation occurs, increasing blood flow to the lungs and workload of the left ventricle.
2. If pulmonary arteries are stenotic or hypoplastic, blood flow to the lungs is restricted.

D. Clinical manifestations.
1. CHF with bounding pulses and widened pulse pressure.
2. Intermittent cyanosis: severe cyanosis with pulmonary artery stenosis.

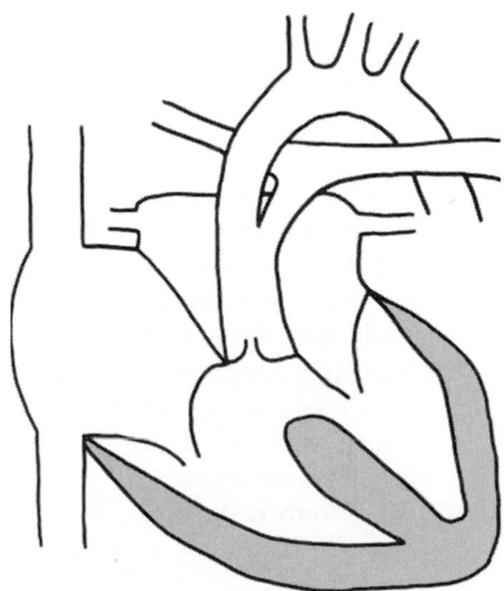

FIGURE 27-20 ■ Truncus arteriosus. (Redrawn courtesy G.G. Janos, M.D., 1989.)

3. Heart sounds: harsh systolic murmur at mid- to lower left sternal border and systolic ejection click with single S_2.
4. Chest x-ray examination: cardiomegaly with increased pulmonary vascular markings. (Exception: if pulmonary artery stenosis exists, decreased pulmonary markings are seen.)
5. Echocardiography is the standard diagnostic test and is used to identify the number of truncal valve leaflets, presence of pulmonary stenosis, and to assess the aortic arch (Westmoreland, 1999).

E. **Management.**
1. Medical management is temporary and is directed toward treating CHF.
   a. Diuretics, digoxin, and angiotensin-converting enzyme (ACE) inhibitors are used to control pulmonary overload and decrease systemic resistance, which leads to decrease in pulmonary vascular resistance.
2. Surgical repair at 6 to 8 weeks is the treatment of choice (Rastelli procedure).
   a. Homograft between the right ventricle and the pulmonary artery.
   b. VSD closure using a patch.
   c. Separation of the pulmonary arteries from the truncus (Westmoreland, 1999).
3. Homografts are preferred to synthetic because they are more flexible, easier to use during surgery, and less prone to obstruction.

F. **Prognosis.**
1. Mortality rate ranges from 10% to 50% in infancy (Montoya and Washington, 2002).
2. Multiple reoperations for conduit or homograft, truncal valve replacement due to lack of homograft growth. These reoperations are usually performed at 3 to 6 years of age and again in adolescence (Grifka, 1999).

Total Anomalous Pulmonary Venous Return (TAPVR)

A. **Incidence:** 1:17,000 live births, 1% of all cardiac defects.

B. **Anatomy.** In TAPVR, pulmonary veins drain into the right atrium either directly or indirectly via a systemic venous channel (Fig. 27-21).
1. Presence of a patent foramen ovale or true ASD is required for survival.
2. Varying degrees of pulmonary venous obstruction occur.
3. Three types of TAPVR occur.
   a. Supracardiac. Pulmonary veins attach above the diaphragm, often to the superior vena cava (common form).
   b. Cardiac. Pulmonary veins attach directly to the coronary sinus and drain into the right atrium.
   c. Infracardiac. Pulmonary veins attach below the diaphragm into the portal venous system, draining into the inferior vena cava (most severe form).

C. **Hemodynamics.**
1. Oxygenated blood from the lungs drains into the right atrium, mixing with the systemic venous return. Part of this flow passes into the left atrium via the patent foramen ovale or ASD, into the left ventricle, and out the aorta. With the normal decrease in PVR, pulmonary blood flow will increase.
2. If obstruction to pulmonary venous return exists, the resulting increase in PVR leads to pulmonary edema and diversion of blood from the pulmonary artery to the aorta via the PDA. Closure of the PDA then increases right-to-left atrial shunting.

D. **Clinical manifestations.**
1. Nonobstructed.
   a. CHF.
   b. Mild cyanosis.

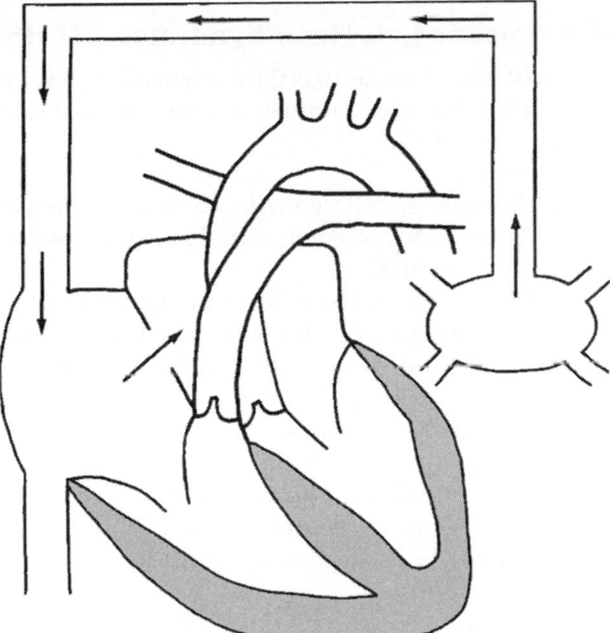

FIGURE 27-21 ■ Total anomalous pulmonary venous connection (TAPVR). (Redrawn courtesy G.G. Janos, M.D., 1989.)

c. Heart sounds: systolic murmur at upper left sternal border, diastolic rumble at the lower left sternal border. Wide split S_2 may be present but is generally nonspecific.
d. Chest x-ray examination: right ventricle dilation, increased pulmonary vascular markings, "snowman" appearance after 4 months of age.

2. Obstructed.
   a. Profound cyanosis present.
   b. Respiratory distress, may not respond to mechanical ventilation.
   c. Chest x-ray examination: normal size with pulmonary edema.
3. Echocardiography with color flow mapping reveals an extra cavity behind the left atrium, a right-to-left shunt across the atrial septum and the anomalous return as the blood enters the atrium, superior vena cava, or coronary sinus. It may be difficult to visualize the pulmonary veins (Montoya and Washington, 2002).

E. **Management:** Surgical treatment of obstructed TAPVR is an emergency.
   1. Medical management of nonobstructed TAPVR is only a temporary measure and is aimed at preventing or treating CHF.
   2. Cardiac catheterization may be omitted to speed time to operation, with surgery based on echocardiography.
   3. Anomalous veins are detached and transplanted to the left atrium; the ASD is repaired.

F. **Prognosis.**
   1. Mortality rate for infants with TAPVR who undergo surgery is 10% to 25% in infancy (Montoya and Washington, 2002); the highest mortality is in the infracardiac type.
   2. Long-term prognosis is excellent because TAPVR is closer to a surgically "curable" condition than are most congenital cardiac lesions.

Hypoplastic Left Heart Syndrome (HLHS)

A. **Incidence:** 2 to 2.6:10,000 live births. 28% have chromosomal abnormalities. HLHS is the most common cardiac cause of death in the first week of life (Strife and Sze, 1999).
B. **Anatomy.**
   1. Hypoplastic left ventricle, aortic arch and ascending aorta.
   2. Atretic or hypoplastic mitral and aortic valves (Fig. 27-22).
C. **Hemodynamics.**
   1. Obstruction of blood flow through the left side of the heart due to hypoplastic aorta and ventricle leads to pulmonary venous congestion and edema.
   2. Blood supply to the descending aorta and to the aortic arch and coronary arteries (retrograde flow) is dependent on the PDA.
D. **Clinical manifestations.**
   1. Asymptomatic at birth.
   2. Tachypnea and dyspnea with increasing pulmonary blood flow.
   3. CHF: usually presents at 24 to 48 hours of life.
   4. Cyanosis: rarely permanent despite mixing of systemic and pulmonary circulations.
   5. Rapid deterioration as PDA closes (Westmoreland, 1999).
      a. Severe mottling.
      b. Gray pallor of skin.
      c. Markedly diminished pulses.
      d. Cardiovascular collapse and shock.
      e. Systolic murmur present in two thirds.
   6. Chest x-ray examination: cardiomegaly with increased pulmonary blood flow and pulmonary edema.
   7. Diagnosis can be made by echocardiography.
E. **Management.**
   1. Treatment options include comfort care, a multistaged surgical approach, or cardiac transplantation.
   2. Initial management.
      a. PGE_1 to maintain ductus arteriosus patency and systemic circulation.
      b. Use of inhaled O_2 and nitrogen combination for an inspired O_2 of less than 21%. Nitrogen therapy creates pulmonary hypoxia and vasoconstriction, which may maximize right-to-left shunting and systemic

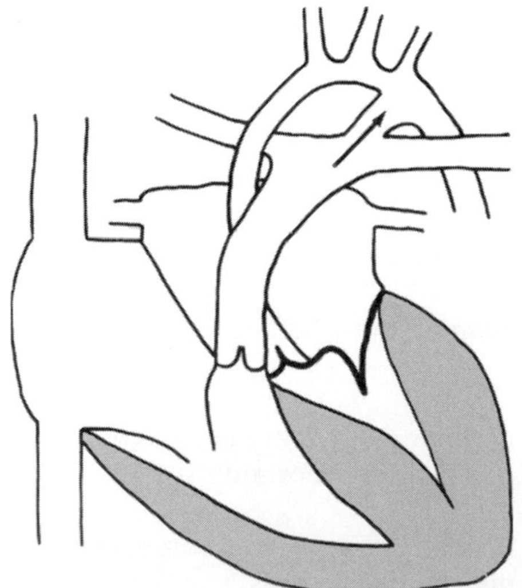

FIGURE 27-22 ■ Hypoplastic left heart syndrome. (Redrawn courtesy G.G. Janos, M.D., 1989.)

blood flow, with a resulting increase in systemic oxygen saturation (Green et al., 2002).

c. Transcatheter balloon atrial septostomy to decompress the left atrium.

3. Staged surgical repair "Norwood" procedure has an overall mortality rate of 23% to 46% (Gutgesell and Gibson, 2002).
   a. First (Norwood) stage has a greater than or equal to 35% mortality, with 12-month survival around 45%.
      (1) Division of the main pulmonary artery and ligation of the ductus arteriosus.
      (2) Gore-Tex shunt is placed to maintain pulmonary blood flow and prevent CHF.
      (3) Atrial septectomy to ensure pulmonary venous return to the right atrium.
      (4) Connection of the right pulmonary artery and the aorta using an aortic allograft.
   b. Second stage: bidirectional Glenn procedure (anastomosis of the superior vena cava to the right pulmonary artery) done at 6 to 12 months of age to reduce volume overload to the right ventricle. Mortality rate for this stage is less than 5% (Park, 2002).
   c. Third stage, or modified Fontan procedure with a mortality rate of 15% to 20% (Park, 2002).
      (1) Involves completion of Fontan procedure between 12 and 24 months of age to connect the inferior vena cava to the pulmonary artery and close the atrial communication.
      (2) Completion of stages 2 and 3 separates the pulmonary from the systemic circulation.
   d. Disadvantages.
      (1) Two or three open surgeries in first 2 years of life.
      (2) Single right ventricle supplies the systemic circulation.
   e. Contraindication: significant tricuspid valve or pulmonic valve dysplasia associated with functional disturbances.
4. Cardiac transplantation.
   a. Provides a structurally and physiologically normal heart in one operation.
   b. 30% of infants die while waiting for a donor heart (Boucek and Shady, 2001).
   c. Complications include (Suddaby, 1999):
      (1) Increased susceptibility to infections as result of immunosuppression.
      (2) Allograft rejection with acute rejection as the leading cause of death in the first year after transplant.
      (3) Systemic hypertension: usually seen only in first year after transplantation.
      (4) Recurrent or residual coarctation: managed with angioplasty or surgical repair.
      (5) Abnormal neurologic findings in as many as 19%, including seizures.
5. Prognosis.
   a. Comparison of staged repair versus heart transplantation outcomes requires evaluation of numbers of surviving children who completed procedures and numbers of those "lost" through death awaiting procedure or death between stages of the procedure.
   b. According to a compilation of data by Gutgesell and Gibson (2002), neonatal cardiac transplant mortality in the 1990s was around 38%.
   c. Staged repair survival after completion of the Norwood procedure is reported at 42% (Green et al., 2002). Overall survival after completion of the staged procedure is 42% to 71% (Strife and Sze, 1999).

CONGESTIVE HEART FAILURE (CHF)

Etiology

A. **CHF is a set of clinical signs and symptoms that reflect the heart's inability to deliver adequate oxygen to meet the metabolic requirements of the body.**
   1. Cardiac output is unable to meet the body's metabolic requirements.
   2. Right and/or left ventricular end-diastolic pressures are elevated, impeding systemic and/or pulmonary venous returns.

B. **Although structural heart defects are the most common cause of CHF in neonates, other causes such as birth asphyxia, severe anemia, dysrhythmias, and sepsis should be considered.**
   1. Timing of detection is often helpful in predicting causes because the diseases causing CHF characteristically show up at certain ages. Table 27-4 indicates conditions associated with CHF and their time of onset.
   2. CHF in utero that is detected at birth may be due to the following:
      a. Profound anemia: erythroblastosis fetalis or twin-to-twin transfusion.
      b. Arrhythmia: supraventricular tachycardia or congenital heart block.
      c. Intrauterine infection with myocarditis.
      d. Arteriovenous malformations.
      e. Absent pulmonary valve.
      f. Premature ductus arteriosus closure: maternal use of prostaglandin inhibitor (e.g., aspirin, ibuprofen).
      g. Volume overload: twin-to-twin or mother-to-infant transfusion.

Clinical Manifestations

A. **Common signs.**
   1. Tachypnea (60-100 respirations per minute at rest) is the first clinical sign of pulmonary edema.
   2. Tachycardia (160-180 bpm at rest) from compensation for decreased cardiac output.
   3. Arrhythmias.
   4. Cardiomegaly on x-ray.
      a. Dilational or hypertrophic cardiomyopathy.
      b. Diminished or engorged pulmonary vasculature.

TABLE 27-4
Causes of Congestive Heart Failure and Time of Onset

Age at Onset of Symptoms	Underlying Cause
At birth	Hypoplastic left heart syndrome (HLHS) Severe tricuspid or pulmonary regurgitation Systemic arteriovenous fistula
In first week of life	Patent ductus arteriosus (PDA) in premature infants Transposition of the great vessels (TGV) Total anomalous pulmonary venous return (TAPVR) with pulmonary venous obstruction
1 to 4 weeks after birth	Coarctation of the aorta Critical aortic or pulmonary stenosis All other lesions listed above

Data from Park, M.K.: *Pediatric cardiology for practitioners* (4th ed.). St Louis, 2002, Mosby.

5. Hepatomegaly (3-5 cm below coastal margin): one of the most useful signs.
6. Pulmonary fine rales and coarse rales (rhonchi).
7. Fatigue or difficulty with feeding.

B. Less common signs.

1. Peripheral edema: usually not obvious unless CHF is present for some time.
2. Diaphoresis.
3. Gallop rhythm.
4. Altered pulses (variable, depending on underlying cause).
5. May have mottling of the extremities from redistribution of blood flow to vital tissues.
6. ECG indicating the following:
   a. Hypertrophy of one or more chambers.
   b. Abnormal mean QRS axis.
   c. Rhythm disturbances.
7. New York University Pediatric Heart Failure Index (NYUPHFI).
   a. New tool to assess degree of heart failure developed by the New York University School of Medicine.
   b. Reliability of tool documented by Connolly and colleagues (2001).
   c. Further testing is recommended.

Management of Congestive Heart Failure

A. General measures (appropriate for any heart disease).

1. Use semi-Fowler or prone position to achieve maximal diaphragmatic excursion and lung expansion.
2. Decrease oxygen consumption.
   a. Maintain neutral thermal environment.
   b. Minimize stimulation (e.g., heel sticks, radial sticks).
   c. Provide sedation with morphine or fentanyl for agitated infant.
   d. Consider assisted ventilation to reduce work of breathing and decrease pulmonary edema if present.
3. Provide supplemental oxygen. The amount is dictated by the PaO_2 and the presence of CHD with admixing of arterial and venous blood.
4. Correct acidosis and any metabolic derangements (e.g., hypoglycemia or hypocalcemia).

B. Specific measures.

1. Fluid and nutritional support.
   a. During acute phase, volume intake is reduced, generally to two thirds of maintenance levels.
   b. Use of glucose polymers (Polycose) or medium-chain triglycerides (MCT oil) enhances caloric content without significant volume increase.
   c. IV infusions of up to 50% fat emulsions can also be used to increase caloric intake with minimal intake volume.
2. Pharmacologic therapy.
   a. Digoxin therapy (Table 27-5).
      (1) Achieve maximal cardiac output; use is controversial in preterm and term newborns (Kenner et al., 1998).
      (2) Digitalize patient (Table 27-5) and observe for bradycardia (discontinue if heart rate <100 bpm).
         (a) Arrhythmias or heart block.
         (b) Hypokalemia.

■ TABLE 27-5
■ ■ **Use of Digoxin for Congestive Heart Failure**

	Total Dose (μg/kg)		Maintenance Dose (μg/kg)	
Age	**Oral**	**IV**	**Oral**	**IV**
Newborn				
Preterm	20-30	15-25	5-7.5	4-6
Term	25-35	20-30	6-10	5-8
1 month to 2 years	35-60	30-50	10-15	7.5-12

Data from Takemoto, C.K., Hodding, J.H., and Kraus, D.M.: *Pediatric dosage handbook: Including neonatal dosing drug administration and extemporaneous preparations* (6th ed.). Cleveland, 1999, Lexi-Comp.

(c) Toxic effects: increased in premature infants because of a longer serum half-life (61-170 hours) for digoxin than in term or older infants (18-45 hours) (Takemoto et al., 1999).

b. Diuretic therapy.
(1) Used to eliminate excess intravascular fluid.
(2) Furosemide (Lasix), 1 to 2 mg/kg every 12 hours IV, or 1 to 3 mg/kg every 12 hours by mouth.
(a) In severe CHF the IV route is preferable for its rapid onset of action.
(b) Hypokalemia and hypochloremia are side effects that can result in metabolic alkalosis.
(c) May cause hypocalcemia with urinary loss of calcium leading to nephrocalcinosis.
(d) Use is contraindicated in renal failure.
(3) Ethacrynic acid (Edecrin), 1 mg/kg/dose IV or 2 to 3 mg/kg/day by mouth (Park, 2002).
(a) Has renal action similar to that of furosemide.
(b) Complications include gastrointestinal side effects and ototoxic effects.
(4) Chlorothiazide (Diuril), 20 to 40 mg/kg/day in two oral doses (Hay et al., 2003).
(a) Administered when less acute oral diuresis is required.
(b) Does not produce the profound potassium losses seen with furosemide; may reduce urinary calcium losses seen with furosemide.
(5) Spironolactone (Aldactone), 1 to 3 mg/kg/day by mouth.
(a) Potassium sparing; must monitor for hyperkalemia.

c. Inotropic agents.
(1) May be necessary in severe CHF or cardiogenic shock.
(2) Most commonly used are dopamine, dobutamine, and isoproterenol.

C. Cardiology consultation to rule out or establish presence of congenital heart lesion. Cardiac catheterization, angiocardiography, and surgery may be indicated.

POSTOPERATIVE CARDIAC MANAGEMENT

Noninvasive Monitoring

A. Electrocardiography.

1. Continuous display of a limb lead, which shows P wave and QRS complex should be monitored (Feltes, 1998).
a. Tachycardia.
b. Bradycardia.

   c. Fibrillation.
   d. Asystole.
2. Lead II: assessment of amplitude, axis, and presence and absence of P waves.
3. Lead V_5 changes: septal or lateral wall ischemia.

B. **Blood pressure: manual.**
1. Cuff can be used to occlude an arterial catheter leak.
2. Measurement of upper and lower extremities after repair of coarctation of the aorta gives pressure gradient across repair site.
3. Avoid extremity for blood pressure measurement when an artery has been used for surgical repair (e.g., subclavian patch for coarctation of the aorta, Blalock-Taussig shunt).

C. **Pulse oximetry.**
1. Decreasing oxygen saturations may indicate:
   a. Decreased cardiac output.
   b. Increasing intracardiac shunting.
   c. Increased intrapulmonary shunting.
2. Continuous monitoring is useful in pulmonary hypertension. Small decrease in saturation may be the first sign of increased pulmonary artery pressure with onset of right-to-left shunting.

D. **Urinary output.**
1. Hourly output rate of 1 to 2 ml/kg/hour is a good clinical indicator of renal perfusion (Polak, 2003).
   a. Invalid in first 2 hours postoperatively after diuretic administration.
   b. Urinary retention can be induced by analgesics.
   c. A sudden decrease in urine output may indicate renal failure.
2. Oliguria may persist for up to 48 hours following cardiopulmonary bypass.
3. It is common to see increased urine output secondary to osmotic diuresis in the initial postoperative period, followed by decreased urine output after 6 to 8 hours (Pike and Falco, 2002).
4. Indwelling catheter is generally not required in those with uncomplicated procedures, stable vital signs, and good peripheral perfusion.

Invasive Monitoring

For pressure values from cardiac catheterization, see Table 27-6.

A. **Arterial pressure.**
1. Mandatory for timely vasoactive medication adjustments.
2. Arterial tracing provides information for analysis of waveform and calculation of pulse pressure.

TABLE 27-6
Pressure Values from Cardiac Catheterization

Pressure	Normal Neonatal Values
Systemic arterial pressure	60-90/20-60 mm Hg (birth to 5 days of age)
Right atrial pressure	3 mm Hg
Right ventricular pressure	30/3 mm Hg
Pulmonary artery occlusion pressure/pulmonary wedge pressure	6-10 mm Hg
Left atrial pressure	8 mm Hg
Left ventricular pressure	100/6 mm Hg

3. Dampened waveforms during mechanical ventilation may indicate hypovolemia or heart failure (Feltes, 1998).

B. Right-sided cardiac pressures.

1. In patients with normal cardiac anatomy: right atrial pressure = right ventricular end-diastolic pressure = central venous pressure.
2. Increasing values seen with (Artman et al., 2002):
   a. Right ventricular overload.
   b. Poor ventricular function.
   c. Elevated pulmonary artery pressure, resulting from reactive pulmonary hypertension.
   d. Tricuspid regurgitation.
   e. Cardiac tamponade.
   f. Residual shunting.
3. Particularly useful for evaluating:
   a. Right-sided cardiac lesions.
      (1) Pulmonic stenosis.
      (2) Tetralogy of Fallot.
   b. Those lesions requiring high right atrial pressures, such as in the Fontan procedure.

C. Pulmonary artery pressure.

1. Surgical placement using a pursestring structure or transthoracic placement of a pulmonary artery catheter into the right ventricular outflow tract is indicated for those neonates at risk for pulmonary hypertension (Artman et al., 2002; Hill et al., 2002).
2. Measurements guide the medical management of pulmonary hypertension and are most frequently used in conditions in which postoperative pulmonary hypertension is anticipated, as in endocardial cushion repair. Lindberg and coworkers (2002) found the incidence of severe pulmonary hypertension following pediatric cardiac surgery to be 2%.
3. Mixed venous oxygen saturation ($S\bar{v}O_2$) monitoring can be obtained from newer pulmonary artery catheters with continuous oximetry capabilities.
   a. $S\bar{v}O_2$ reflects a balance between oxygen delivery and consumption.
   b. Alterations are seen in:
      (1) Anemia.
      (2) Shock.
      (3) Left-to-right or right-to-left shunts.
   c. Change in $S\bar{v}O_2$ generally precedes detectable hemodynamic changes by several minutes.

D. Left-sided cardiac pressures are monitored using a left atrial line.

1. In patients with normal cardiac anatomy: left ventricular end-diastolic pressure = left atrial pressure = pulmonary artery occlusion pressure = pulmonary artery wedge pressure.
2. Used to monitor systemic ventricular function and pulmonary shunting (Pike and Falco, 2002).
3. Useful in patients with mitral valve dysfunction, as seen in postendocardial cushion repair.
4. Requires meticulous line care because the risk of air or particulate embolization is high.

E. Epicardial pacing wires.

1. Usually attached to right atrium and/or right ventricle.
2. Provides temporary back-up pacing for up to 10 days (Dubin and Van Hare, 2002).

3. Access to pacing is most important after surgical repairs near the cardiac conduction system. For example:
   a. VSD.
   b. Transposition of the great arteries.
   c. Truncus arteriosus.
   d. Endocardial cushion defects.

Hemodynamic Management

A. **Bradycardia.**
   1. Common result of intraoperative cooling; proportional to degree of hypothermia.
   2. After extensive atrial surgery, such as arterial switch procedure, TAPVR repair.
   3. After injury to sinoatrial node.
   4. With conducting problems:
      a. Sinoatrial block.
      b. Sinus asystole.
      c. Atrioventricular block is of most concern in the postoperative period (Dubin and Van Hare, 2002).
   5. As a consequence of edema around conduction system (generally resolves in 3-4 days).

B. **Tachycardia.** Observed as a consequence of or in response to (Dubin and Van Hare, 2002):
   1. Pain.
   2. Anxiety/agitation.
   3. Fever.
   4. Hypovolemia.
   5. Junctional conduction disturbance.

Postoperative Disturbances

Heart Failure

ETIOLOGY

A. **Most common postoperative event resulting from decreased neonatal cardiac reserve, limited by:**
   1. Decreased myofilament numbers.
   2. Decreased ventricular compliance.
   3. Greater oxygen consumption, cardiac output, and resting heart rate in the neonate.
   4. Nearly maximal neonatal cardiac performance in the absence of stress.

B. **Causes (Artman et al., 2002).**
   1. Cardiopulmonary bypass adversely affects myocardial performance.
      a. Peak effect is 6 to 12 hours postoperatively.
   2. Residual anatomic lesions.
      a. Transesophageal echocardiography in the operating room has minimized the incidence.
   3. Pulmonary artery hypertensive crisis.
      a. Life-threatening right heart failure may be caused by an acute increase in pulmonary artery pressure.
   4. Arrhythmias.

C. Preload or diastolic filling.
   1. Hypovolemia.
      a. Inadequate volume replacement.
      b. Inadequate mechanical hemostasis.
      c. Impaired clotting.
   2. Iatrogenic volume overload.
   3. Left ventricular dysfunction.
   4. Cardiac compression.

D. Afterload (Feltes, 1998).
   1. In the postoperative period, the neonatal heart is extremely sensitive to increased afterload.
   2. Evidenced by peripheral vasoconstriction.
      a. Vasodilators are used to enhance the reduction of ventricular afterload.

E. Contractility (Feltes, 1998).
   1. Decreased peripheral perfusion.
   2. Decreased urine output.
   3. Treat with inotropic medications.

F. Inadequate systemic venous return.
   1. Excessive positive end-expiratory pressure.
   2. Tension pneumothorax.
   3. Atrial baffle obstruction.
   4. Postpericardial effusions.

G. Increased pulmonary vascular resistance.

H. Decreased cardiac contractility, resulting from:
   1. Accidental discontinuation of vasoactive drugs.
   2. Electrolyte disturbances.
   3. Hypoglycemia.
   4. Surgical manipulation or damage.

RECOGNITION OF LOW CARDIAC OUTPUT

A. Frequently seen with changes in preload, afterload, and contractility in the postoperative period (Cuadrado, 2002).

B. Factors that influence the severity of low cardiac output:
   1. Age less than 1 month.
   2. Weight less than 2.5 kg.
   3. Preoperative condition.
   4. Type of defect (Cuadrado, 2002).

C. Observation: "just not doing well."
   1. Noninteractive or becoming less interactive with environment.
   2. Lack of/or decreasing vigor of cry.
   3. Awake but "floppy."

D. Color.
   1. Violet color of mucosa.
   2. Gray skin or mottling of skin.

E. Extremities.
   1. Cool to touch (Rodgers, 2001).
   2. Lack of or decrease in pedal pulses.
   3. Capillary refill time longer than 3 seconds.
   4. Edema: often seen postoperatively as third spacing, but also indicative of fluid overload (Polak, 2003).

F. Oliguria (urine output <0.5-1 ml/kg/hour).
   1. Transient acute renal failure may occur in 5% of neonates who require cardiopulmonary bypass during cardiac surgery (McElhinney and Wernovsky, 2001).

G. **Tachycardia.**
   1. Gallop rhythm.
   2. Distant heart sounds: possible indication of pericardial effusions.

H. **Low arterial blood pressure.**

I. **Respiratory distress.**
   1. Retractions, tachypnea, grunting, and/or stridor in infant after extubation.
   2. Rales: often heard after bypass procedure.

J. **Weight gain disproportionate to caloric intake.**
   1. May be early indicator of fluid retention.

K. **X-ray findings.**
   1. Excessive cardiac size or enlargement of specific chamber.
   2. Large cardiac silhouette or "bag of waters" appearance may indicate pericardial effusions.
   3. Increased fluffy densities; these are not seen if elevated positive end-expiratory pressure is used in ventilation.

L. **Metabolic derangement.**
   1. Metabolic acidosis, generally resulting from low bicarbonate levels and lactic acid buildup that results from diminished tissue perfusion.
   2. Low sodium value, in part due to excessive free water.

MANAGEMENT OF LOW CARDIAC OUTPUT

A. **Use blood for volume replacement.**
   1. Maintain hemoglobin greater than 12 g/dl for noncyanotic lesions and greater than 15 g/dl for cyanotic lesions (Cuadrado, 2002).

B. **Volume challenge is appropriate in light of cardiopulmonary bypass third spacing.**
   1. Close monitoring required.
   2. Strict intake and output.
   3. Neonates are easily fluid overloaded when given excessive fluids (Polak, 2003).

C. **Provide correction of metabolic disorders.**
   1. Hypocalcemia, hyponatremia, and hypoglycemia.
   2. Acid-base balances.
      a. Acidosis may result from poor tissue perfusion, prolonged hypovolemia, or impaired renal function (Polak, 2003). Correction depends on the underlying cause.
      b. Serial serum lactate levels may prove useful in predicting poor outcomes following neonatal cardiac surgery (Charpie et al., 2000), with only minimal correlation between bicarbonate levels and the lactate levels.

D. **Reduce right ventricular afterload.**
   1. Hyperventilation.
   2. Pulmonary vasodilating agents.
      a. PGE_1.
      b. Nitroglycerin.
      c. Nitroprusside is a mixed vasodilator frequently used with dopamine or dobutamine (Park, 2002).
      d. Inhaled nitric oxide.
   3. Provide sedation and analgesia (Cuadrado, 2002).

E. **Treat rate or rhythm disturbance.**
   1. Increased heart rate.
      a. Rate of 200 to 210 bpm is tolerated well, with acceptable myocardial work and oxygen consumption.
      b. Cardioversion can be used for supraventricular tachycardia, atrial flutter/fibrillation, and ventricular tachycardia (Hay et al., 2003).
   2. Atrial or atrioventricular pacing is often necessary.

F. **Consider pharmaceutical agents.**
   1. Isoproterenol (Isuprel): acts to decrease pulmonary and systemic vascular resistance (decreases afterload).
   2. Nitroprusside or nitroglycerin: a venodilator that reduces afterload.
   3. Milrinone: increases heart rate and contractility with some vasodilatory properties. Does not affect platelet function (Cuadrado, 2002).
   4. Volume replacement: possibly necessary because of vasodilation (maintain preload). Central venous pressure is useful in determining volume needs.
   5. Vasopressors (i.e., dopamine >10 μg/kg/min, or dobutamine). Potential for increasing PVR. Careful monitoring of effects is necessary.

G. **Monitor blood pressure.**

BLEEDING

A. **Provide sedation.** Keep infant sedated, avoiding agitation, to prevent hypertension and pressure at active and potential bleeding sites, which may aggravate or disrupt clot formation.

B. **Assess and treat coagulopathy (Miller and Spitzer, 2002).**
   1. Coagulation factors are 30% to 40% lower in neonates with congenital heart defects than in neonates without defects (Pike and Falco, 2002).
   2. Use fresh whole blood less than 48 hours old for volume and clotting.
      a. Maintain hematocrit greater than 40% to 45% (Artman et al., 2002).
   3. Use cryoprecipitate for fibrinogen (aids clotting).
   4. Evaluate platelets: count is low and function is inadequate because of "bypass" and deep hypothermia.
      a. Give platelet infusion.
      b. Give desmopressin (DDAVP), 0.3 μg/kg, to increase levels of von Willebrand factor (vWF) which stimulates platelets to aggregate.

Pulmonary Hypertension/Pulmonary Vasospasm

A. **Avoid hypoxemia and acidosis.**
   1. Hypoxia increases PVR and acidosis.
   2. Neonates at risk for postoperative pulmonary hypertension need to be identified upon return from the recovery room (Pike and Falco, 2002).
      a. Large VSD.
      b. Complete AV canal.
      c. Truncus arteriosus.
      d. Total anomalous venous return.
      e. *D*-transposition of the great arteries.
   3. Hyperoxygenate before suctioning; increase fractional inspired oxygen (FiO_2) and hyperventilate; keep suctioning time to minimum.
      a. Pain management, sedation, and/or paralysis.
      b. Do not disconnect ventilator when suctioning; inline suctioning system is recommended.

B. **Minimize handling.**
   1. Group noxious stimuli when possible; cluster care activities.
   2. Provide adequate pain relief (Anand and the International Evidence-Based Group for Neonatal Pain, 2001).
      a. Neonates have an increased sensitivity to pain.
      b. Give fentanyl or morphine for pain relief.
      c. Midazolam (Versed) is not recommended.
   3. In addition to analgesia, infant may require sedation for agitation, or paralytic agent to assist in adequate oxygenation and ventilation (Polak, 2003).

Maintenance of Fluid and Electrolyte Balance

A. **Hypoglycemia, hypokalemia, and hypocalcemia are potential problems.**
   1. All result in decreased myocardial function.
   2. Potential for seizures is present.
      a. Poor cardiac output to the brain may cause seizures.
      b. Cardiopulmonary bypass and circulatory arrest also predispose an infant to seizures.
   3. Monitor laboratory values and replace electrolytes as needed.

B. **Avoid acidosis.**
   1. Metabolic acidosis is common in tissue hypoxia and suboptimal perfusion from lowered cardiac output.
   2. Management includes:
      a. Maintenance of slight alkalosis by means of hyperventilation and sodium bicarbonate.
      b. Hyperoxygenation.
   3. Respiratory acidosis may be caused by poor pulmonary compliance, decreased respiratory drive, pulmonary disease, or inadequate mechanical ventilation (Feltes, 1998).

C. **Avoid fluid overload.**
   1. Meticulous monitoring of infusion rates.
   2. Monitor urine output; may require catheter for accuracy, especially if output is minimal.

Shock

ETIOLOGY

A. **Shock is a state of inadequate circulating blood volume, resulting in reduced perfusion and oxygenation to the tissues.** Several varieties of shock are recognized.

B. **Hypovolemic shock may be caused by the following (Karlsen, 2001):**
   1. Blood loss from placental abnormalities (e.g., umbilical cord rupture, abruptio placentae, placenta previa, and twin-to-twin transfusion syndrome).
   2. Acute blood loss postnatally (such as intracranial or pulmonary hemorrhage).
   3. Plasma and fluid losses.
      a. Skin integrity losses (e.g., myelomeningocele, gastroschisis).
      b. Pleural effusions (e.g., erythroblastosis fetalis or nonimmune hydrops).
      c. Body water loss from persistent vomiting, diarrhea, or evaporative skin losses.
      d. Capillary leak syndrome resulting in third spacing.

C. **Cardiogenic shock may be caused by the following (Artman et al., 2002):**
   1. Myocardial failure may be from severe hypoxemia, hypoglycemia, hypocalcemia, or acidosis.
   2. Congenital heart lesions.
   3. Cardiac arrhythmias.
      a. Sustained supraventricular tachycardia (SVT).
      b. Complete atrioventricular block (third degree).
   4. Restriction of cardiac function by:
      a. Tamponade.
      b. Tension pneumothorax.
      c. Excessive levels of ventilatory distending pressures.
   5. Myocarditis: often associated with sepsis.

D. **Distributive shock:** also known as septic shock.
   1. Results from impaired peripheral arterial resistance usually caused by sepsis (i.e., release of bacterial toxins).
   2. Typically is associated with gram-negative organisms; however, gram-positive organisms may be the causative agent.

CLINICAL INDICATORS

A. **Signs of shock are frequently nonspecific.** (Cardiogenic shock may be indistinguishable from CHF.)
B. **Cardiopulmonary status changes.**
   1. Tachycardia at rest.
   2. Bradycardia.
   3. Increased work of breathing, may have tachypnea.
   4. Poor peripheral perfusion.
      a. Pallor (especially with blood loss).
      b. Capillary refill time longer than 3 seconds.
      c. Mottling.
   5. Hypotension.
C. **Decreased urinary output.**
D. **Metabolic disturbances.**
   1. Metabolic acidosis.
   2. Hypoglycemia.
   3. Hypothermia.
E. **Evidence of coagulation defects.**
F. **Indicators of blood volume** (or effective blood volume) are as follows:
   1. Change in hemoglobin and hematocrit values.
   2. Response to fluid challenge of 10 ml of saline solution per kilogram of body weight, while blood pressure and urine output are monitored.
   3. Positive Betke-Kleihauer test result indicates fetal-to-maternal transfusion in utero. This test examines the maternal blood for the presence of fetal erythrocytes.
G. **Indicators of cardiac function.**
   1. See Cardiopulmonary Status Changes, point B, above.
   2. Echocardiogram establishes anatomic defects and/or specific myocardial function abnormalities.
   3. Central venous pressure is generally elevated, except during hypovolemic shock.
H. **Indicators of septic shock.**
   1. Clinical signs of sepsis or positive culture results.
   2. Normal blood pressure in the face of prominent hypoperfusion.
   3. Edema or sclerema from capillary protein and fluid leakage.
   4. Oliguria, proteinuria.
   5. Persistent pulmonary hypertension of the neonate (common).

MANAGEMENT

A. **Shock management: depends largely on prevailing pathogenesis.** A large proportion of the care is supportive.
B. **Supportive care.**
   1. Maintain oxygenation and ventilation as dictated by arterial blood gas values.
      a. Give ventilatory support if concurrent pulmonary disease exists.
      b. Provide neutral thermal environment to decrease oxygen consumption.
      c. Decrease external stress (i.e., handling, peripheral blood sampling).
      d. Consider sedatives, analgesics, and paralytics to decrease stress.

2. Promptly treat acidosis to avoid adverse effects on myocardial contractility. Sodium bicarbonate is often necessary.
3. Maintain fluid and electrolyte balance.

C. **Specific therapies.**
1. Increase blood volume and erythrocyte mass.
   a. Maintain blood pressure and maximize oxygen content.
   b. Treatment of acute blood loss may require large volume transfusion.
   c. Monitoring arterial blood pressure is essential; monitoring of central venous pressure ideally should be included.
   d. *Caution:* In cardiogenic shock, added volume may increase the myocardial workload.
2. Treat the infectious process in septic shock.
   a. Antibiotic therapy should be initiated.
   b. Consider use of granulocyte colony-stimulating factor (G-CSF), giving 5 to 10 µg/kg/day for 3 to 5 days for infants who are in septic shock and have an absolute neutrophil count less than 1000/mm^3 (Takemoto et al., 1999).
3. Maximize cardiac output.
   a. Inotropic agents such as epinephrine are useful in cardiogenic shock to increase cardiac output and support circulation. Start early in septic shock if evidence of oliguria, hypotension, or acidosis exists. Monitor for hypertension and edema (Takemoto et al., 1999). Norepinephrine may prove useful in dopamine-resistant shock (Carcillo and Fields, 2002). According to Takemoto and colleagues (1999), the usual dose is 0.5 µg/kg/minute.
   b. Isoproterenol (Isuprel): increases heart rate and contractility (β_1-adrenergic effects). Simultaneous effects produce bronchodilation and smooth muscle relaxation (β_2-effects). Usual dose is 0.05 to 2 µg/kg/minute. Observe for ventricular arrhythmias and tachycardia.
   c. Dopamine (Intropin): increases cardiac contractility and cardiac output. Effects are dose dependent. At low doses (1-3 µg/kg/min, IV), selective vasodilation of the renal, mesenteric, cerebral, and coronary vascular beds occurs with little effect on heart rate or blood pressure. With moderate doses (5-10 µg/kg/min), increased blood pressure and improved tissue perfusion can be observed. Beneficial effects are dependent largely on adequate blood volume. Correct hypovolemia before the dopamine infusion. At higher doses (>10 µg/kg/min, IV), vasoconstriction occurs and consists of vasoconstriction of the pulmonary vasculature, increased right ventricular afterload, reduction in pulmonary blood flow, right-to-left shunting through fetal structures, increased blood pressure, and increased hypoxemia. Tachycardia, dysrhythmias, and ectopic beats can occur as a consequence of dopamine infusion.
   d. Dobutamine (Dobutrex): increases cardiac contractility and heart rate while exerting limited effects on vasculature. Cardiac output increases, depending on myocardial catecholamine stores. A dose of 2 to 15 µg/kg/minute, continuous IV infusion (Takemoto et al., 1999).
   e. Amrinone and/or milrinone can prove beneficial in pediatric patients who continue to have increased vascular resistance after cardiac output is corrected to a low normal state (Carcillo and Fields, 2002).
   f. Digitalis should be considered and used selectively, especially in the face of hypoxia or toxic myocardiopathy (see Table 27-5).
4. Correct any tension pneumothorax or cardiac tamponade.

D. Treatment goals.
1. Reduce morbidity (Artman et al., 2002).
2. Normalization of hemodynamic status.
3. Halt progression of the shock state.

REFERENCES

Anand, K.J.S. and the International Evidence-Based Group for Neonatal Pain: Consensus statement for the prevention and management of pain in the newborn. *Archives of Pediatrics and Adolescent Medicine, 155*(2):173-180, 2001.

Artman, M., Mahony, L., and Teitel, D.F.: *Neonatal cardiology*. New York, 2002, McGraw-Hill, pp. 196-199, 231-243.

Ayres, N.: Fetal cardiology. In A. Garson, J. Bricker, D. Fisher, and S. Neish (Eds.): *The science and practice of pediatric cardiology* (2nd ed., vol. 2.). Baltimore, 1998, Williams & Wilkins, pp. 2281-2300.

Baraitser, M. and Winter, R.M.: *Color atlas of congenital malformation syndromes*. London, 1996, Mosby-Wolfe, pp. 212-214.

Bell, S.: Neonatal cardiovascular pharmacology. *Neonatal Network, 17*(2):7-15, 1998.

Boucek, M.M. and Shady, R.E.: Pediatric heart transplantation. In H.D. Allen, G. Emmanouilides, T. Riemenschneider, et al. (Eds.): *Moss and Adams heart disease in infants, children, and adolescents* (6th ed.). Philadelphia, 2001, Williams & Wilkins.

Brent, R.L.: Addressing environmentally caused birth defects. *Pediatrics in Review, 22*(5):153-165, 2001.

Carcillo, J.A. and Fields, A.I.: Clinical practice parameters for hemodynamic support of pediatric and neonatal patients in septic shock. *Critical Care Medicine, 30*(6):1365-1378, 2002.

Carey, B.: Incidence and epidemiology of congenital cardiovascular malformations in the newborn and infant. *Newborn and Infant Nursing Reviews*, 2(2):54-59, 2002.

Chang, A. and Vaughn, A.: Coarctation of the aorta. In A. Chang, F. Hanley, G. Wernovsky, and D. Wessel (Eds.): *Pediatric cardiac intensive care*. Baltimore, 1998, Williams & Wilkins, pp. 247-256.

Charpie, J.R., Dekeon, M.K., Goldberg, C.A., et al.: Serial blood lactate measurements predict early outcome after neonatal repair or palliation for complex congenital heart disease. *Journal of Thoracic and Cardiovascular Surgery, 120*(1):73-80, 2000.

Collins-Nakai, R. and McLaughlin, P.: How congenital heart disease originates in life. *Cardiology Clinics, 20*(3):367-383, 2002.

Connolly, D., Rutkowski, M., Auslender, M., and Artman, M.: The New York University Pediatric Heart Failure Index: A new method of quantifying chronic heart failure in children. *Journal of Pediatrics, 138*(5):644-648, 2001.

Corbet, A.: Medical manipulation of the ductus arteriosus. In A. Garson, J. Bricker, D. Fisher, and S. Neish (Eds.): *The science and practice of pediatric cardiology* (2nd ed., vol. 2.). Baltimore, 1998, Williams & Wilkins, pp. 2489-2513.

Cuadrado, A.R.: Management of postoperative low cardiac output syndrome. *Critical Care Nursing Quarterly, 25*(3):63-71, 2002.

Cuneo, B.F.: Perinatal cardiology. *Newborn and Infant Nursing Reviews*, 2(2):90-104, 2002.

del Nido, P.J.: Developmental and neurologic outcomes late after neonatal corrective surgery. *Journal of Thoracic and Cardiovascular Surgery, 124*(3):425-427, 2002.

Dubin, A.M. and Van Hare, G.: Postoperative arrhythmias. In B.A. Reitz, and D.D Yuh (Eds.): *Congenital cardiac surgery*. New York, 2002, McGraw-Hill, pp. 203-215.

Duff, D. and McNamara, D.: *History and physical examination of the cardiovascular system*. In A. Garson, J. Bricker, D. Fisher, and S. Neish (Eds). *The science and practice of pediatric cardiology* (2nd ed., vol.1). J. Baltimore, 1998, Williams & Wilkins, pp. 693-713.

Feltes, T F.: Post-operative recovery from congenital heart disease. In A. Garson,

J. Bricker, D. Fisher, and S. Neish (Eds.): *The science and practice of pediatric cardiology* (2nd ed., vol. 2.). Baltimore, 1998, Williams & Wilkins, pp. 2390-2403.

Green, A., Pye, S., and Yetman, A.: The physiologic basis for and nursing considerations in the use of subatmospheric concentrations of oxygen in HLHS. *Advances in Neonatal Care, 2*(4):177-186, 2002.

Grifka, R.: Cyanotic congenital heart disease with increased pulmonary blood flow. *Pediatric Clinics of North America, 46*(2):405-425, 1999.

Gutgesell, H.P. and Gibson, J.: Management of hypoplastic left heart syndrome in the 1990s. *American Journal of Cardiology, 89*(7):842-846, 2002.

Guyton, A. and Hall, J.: *Textbook of medical physiology* (9th ed.). Philadelphia, 1996, Saunders, pp. 107-127.

Hay, W.W., Hayward, A.R., Levin, M.J., and Sondheimer, J.M.: Cardiovascular diseases. In S. Reinhardt, H. Lebowitz, and L.A. Sheinis (Eds.): *Current pediatric diagnosis and treatment* (16th ed.). New York, 2003, McGraw-Hill.

Hegyi, T., Anwar, M., Carbone, M.T., et al.: Blood pressure ranges in premature infants: II. The first week of life. *Pediatrics, 97*(3):336-342, 1996.

Hill, L.L., Lammers, C.R., and Boltz, M.G.: Pediatric cardiac anesthesia. In B.A. Reitz and D.D. Yuh (Eds.): *Congenital cardiac surgery*. New York, 2002, McGraw-Hill, pp. 81-85.

Hövels-Gürich, H.H., Seghaye, M.C., Schnitker, R., et al.: Long-term neurodevelopmental outcomes in school-aged children after neonatal arterial switch operation. *Journal of Thoracic and Cardiovascular Surgery, 124*(3):448-458, 2002.

Ivy, D., Neish, S., and Abman, S.: Regulation of pulmonary circulation. In A. Garson, J. Bricker, D. Fisher, and S. Neish (Eds.): *The science and practice of pediatric cardiology* (2nd ed., vol. 1). Baltimore, 1998, Williams & Wilkins, pp. 328-347.

Karlsen, K.A.: Transporting newborns the S.T.A.B.L.E. way. A manual for community hospital caregivers: Pre-transport stabilization of sick newborns. In *The S.T.A.B.L.E. program instructor manual*. Park City, UT, 2001, S.T.A.B.L.E. Program, pp. 51-57.

Kenner, C., Amlung, S.R., and Flandermeyer, A.A.: Assessment and management of cardiovascular dysfunction. In Kenner, Amlung, and Flandermeyer. *Protocols in neonatal nursing*. Philadephia, 1998, Saunders, pp. 145-175.

Lee, J., Rajadurai, V.S., and Tan, K.W.: Blood pressure standards for very low birthweight infants during the first day of life. *Archives of Disease in Childhood, 81*(3):F168-F170, 1999.

Limperopoulos, C., Majnemer, A., Shevell, M., et al.: Functional limitations in young children with congenital heart defects after cardiac surgery. *Pediatrics, 108*(6):1325-1331, 2001.

Lindberg, L., Olsson, A.K., Jögi, P., and Jonmarker, C.: How common is severe pulmonary hypertension after pediatric cardiac surgery? *Journal of Thoracic and Cardiovascular Surgery, 123*(6):1155-1163, 2002.

McElhinney, D.B. and Wernovsky, G.: Outcomes of neonates with congenital heart disease. *Current Opinion in Pediatrics, 13*(2):104-110, 2001.

Miller, B.E., and Spitzer, K.K.: Anesthetic and perfusion issues in contemporary pediatric cardiac surgery. *Critical Care Nursing Quarterly, 25*(3):48-62, 2002.

Montoya, K.D., and Washington, R.L.: Cardiovascular diseases and surgical interventions. In G.B. Merenstein and S.L. Gardner (Eds.): *Handbook of neonatal intensive care* (5th ed.). St Louis, 2002, Mosby, pp. 576-608.

Narayanan-Sankar, M. and Clyman, R.I.: Pharmacology review: Pharmacologic closure of patent ductus arteriosus in the neonate. *NeoReviews, 4*(8):e215, 2003.

Neches, W., Park, S., and Eltedgin, J.: Transposition of the great arteries. In A. Garson, J. Bricker, D. Fisher, and S. Neish (Eds.): *The science and practice of pediatric cardiology* (2nd ed., vol. 1). Baltimore, 1998, Williams & Wilkins, pp. 1463-1503.

O'Laughlin, M.P.: Congestive heart failure in children. *Pediatric Clinics of North America, 46*(2):263-273, 1999.

Park, M.K.: *Pediatric cardiology for practitioners* (4th ed.). St Louis, 2002, Mosby.

Patterson, S.W. and Starling, J.: On the mechanical factors which determine the output of the ventricles. *Journal of Physiology*, 48:357, 1914.

Pelech, A.N.: Evaluation of the pediatric patient with a cardiac murmur. *Pediatric Clinics of North America, 46*(2):167-188, 1999.

Penny, D.J. and Shekerdemian, L.S.: Management of the neonate with symptomatic congenital heart disease. *Archives of Disease in Childhood, 84*(3), F141-F145, 2001.

Pihkala, J., Nykanen, D., Freedon, R.M., and Benson, L.N.: Interventional cardiac catheterization. *Pediatric Clinics of North America, 46*(2):441-464, 1999.

Pike, N.A. and Falco, D.A.: Postoperative care of the neonate/infant after cardiac surgery. In B.A. Reitz and D.D. Yuh (Eds.): *Congenital cardiac surgery*. New York, 2002, McGraw-Hill, pp. 193-202.

Polak, J.: Assessment and management of the surgical newborn and infant. In C. Kenner and J.W. Lott (Eds.). *Comprehensive neonatal nursing: A physiologic perspective* (3rd ed.). St Louis, 2003, Saunders, pp. 758-761.

Reddy, V., Ungerleider, R., and Hanley, F.: Pulmonary valve atresia with intact ventricular septum. In A. Garson, J. Bricker, D. Fisher, and S. Neish (Eds.): *The science and practice of pediatric cardiology* (2nd ed., vol. 1). Baltimore, 1998, Williams & Wilkins, pp. 1563-1577.

Rodgers, B.: Perioperative nursing. In S.M. Nettina (Ed.): *The Lippincott manual of nursing practice*. Baltimore, 2001, Lippincott Williams & Wilkins.

Sansoucie, D.A. and Cavaliere, T.A.: Newborn and infant assessment. In C. Kenner and J.W. Lott (Eds.): *Comprehensive neonatal nursing: A physiologic perspective* (3rd ed.). St Louis, 2003, Saunders, pp. 316-322.

Seri, I. and Evans, J.: Controversies in the diagnosis and management of hypotension in the newborn infant. *Current Opinion in Pediatrics, 13*(2):116-123, 2001.

Strife, J.L. and Sze, R.W.: Neonatal imaging: Radiographic evaluation of the neonate with congenital heart disease. *Radiology Clinics of North America, 37*(6):1093-1107, 1999.

Suddaby, E.C.: The state of pediatric heart transplantation. *Advanced Practice in Acute Critical Care, 10*(2):202-216, 1999.

Takemoto, C.K., Hodding, J.H., and Kraus, D.M.: *Pediatric dosage handbook: Including neonatal dosing drug administration and extemporaneous preparations* (6th ed.). Cleveland, 1999, Lexi-Comp.

Theorell, C.: Cardiovascular assessment of the newborn. *Newborn and Infant Nursing Reviews, 2*(2):111-127, 2002.

Vick, G.: Defects of the atrial septum including atrioventricular septal defects. In A. Garson, J. Bricker, D. Fisher, and S. Neish (Eds.): *The science and practice of pediatric cardiology* (2nd ed., vol. 1). Baltimore, 1998, Williams & Wilkins, pp. 1141-1179.

Waldman, J.D. and Wernly, J.A.: Pediatric cardiology: Cyanotic congenital heart disease with decreased pulmonary blood flow in children. *Pediatric Clinics of North America, 46*(2):385-404, 1999.

Westmoreland, D.: Critical congenital cardiac defects in the newborn. *Journal of Perinatal and Neonatal Nursing, 12*(4):67-87, 1999.

Witt, C.: Cardiac embryology. *Neonatal Network, 16*(1):43-49, 1997.

CHAPTER

28 Gastrointestinal Disorders

ROBIN L. WATSON

OBJECTIVES

1. Discuss normal and abnormal abdominal assessment findings.
2. Discuss common laboratory and diagnostic tests used to evaluate the gastrointestinal system.
3. Differentiate between omphalocele and gastroschisis.
4. Describe immediate management for a newborn infant with an abdominal wall defect.
5. Identify four common associations in infants with intestinal obstruction.
6. Identify the clinical presentation of a neonate with tracheoesophageal fistula.
7. Describe x-ray findings in an infant with duodenal atresia.
8. Identify one gastrointestinal disorder that is considered a surgical emergency.
9. Identify the gastrointestinal presentation of infants with cystic fibrosis.
10. Describe the defect in Hirschsprung disease.
11. Identify the three mechanisms involved in the pathogenesis of necrotizing enterocolitis.
12. Identify the single most important risk factor for the development of necrotizing enterocolitis.
13. Identify the two most important factors in determining prognosis in infants with short bowel syndrome.
14. Describe the clinical presentation of an infant with biliary atresia.
15. Identify at least three management strategies for the infant with cholestasis.
16. Identify at least three management strategies for the infant with gastroesophageal reflux.
17. Identify the triad of anomalies occurring in prune-belly syndrome.
18. Describe the symptoms of diaphragmatic hernia.
19. Differentiate between unconjugated and conjugated bilirubin.
20. Identify limitations in the normal newborn infant that lead to physiologic jaundice.
21. Compare and contrast physiologic and nonphysiologic jaundice.
22. Describe management of an infant receiving phototherapy.
23. Define "hydrops."
24. Identify four causes of nonimmune hydrops.

Unique embryologic features of the gastrointestinal (GI) tract, such as the obliteration and recanalization of the GI tract, midgut herniation into the umbilical cord, and rotation of the intestines, make the GI tract prone to a variety of congenital anomalies. The majority of neonatal GI disorders involve anomalies that may affect any part of the GI tract, from the mouth to the anus. Atresias, stenoses, and functional obstructions account for the vast majority of defects. As for acquired defects, necrotizing enterocolitis is the most common serious GI illness in neonates. This chapter will review the more common GI obstructions, in addition to a variety of multisystem disorders that have significant GI involvement, such as prune-belly syndrome, congenital diaphragmatic hernia, hyperbilirubinemia, and hydrops.

GASTROINTESTINAL EMBRYONIC DEVELOPMENT

A. **Week 3.** Liver bud is present; mesentery is forming.
B. **Week 4.** Intestine is present; esophagus and stomach become distinct.
C. **Weeks 5 and 6.** Intestine elongates into a loop and begins to rotate.
D. **Week 7.** Duodenum is temporarily occluded; intestinal loops herniate into umbilical cord, lengthen, and rotate; and urorectal septum fuses with cloacal membrane, separating rectum from developing urinary bladder.
E. **Week 8.** Small intestine recanalizes; villi are present.
F. **Weeks 9 and 10.** Intestines begin to reenter abdominal cavity and continue counterclockwise rotation around the axis of the superior mesenteric artery.
G. **Week 12.** Muscular layers of intestine are present; active transport of amino acids begins; pancreatic islet cells appear; bile appears.
H. **Week 16.** Meconium is present; swallowing is observed.
I. **Week 24.** Ganglion cells are detected in the rectum.
J. **Week 26.** Random peristalsis begins.
K. **Weeks 34 to 36.** Sucking and swallowing become coordinated.
L. **Weeks 36 to 38.** Maturity of GI system completed.
M. **Weeks 5 to 40.** Intestine elongates approximately 100-fold (small intestine is six times the length of the colon).

FUNCTIONS OF THE GASTROINTESTINAL TRACT

A. **Absorption and digestion of nutrients.**
B. **Maintenance of fluid and electrolyte balance.**
C. **Protection of host from toxins and pathogens.**

ASSESSMENT OF THE GASTROINTESTINAL SYSTEM

A. **History.**
   1. Presence of GI disease in family.
   2. Presence of genetic syndrome. Major syndromes associated with GI defects include (Thigpen and Kenner, 2003):
      a. Apert syndrome.
      b. Beckwith-Wiedemann syndrome.
      c. Fetal hydantoin syndrome
      d. Meckel-Gruber syndrome.
      e. Sirenomelia.
      f. Trisomy 13.
      g. Trisomy 18.

h. Trisomy 21.
i. VATER association (*v*ertebral defects, imperforate *a*nus, *t*racheo*e*sophageal fistula, and *r*adial and *r*enal dysplasia); VACTERL association (*v*ertebral abnormalities, *a*nal atresia, *c*ardiac abnormalities, *t*racheo*e*sophageal fistula and/or esophageal atresia, *r*enal agenesis and dysplasia, and *l*imb defects).

3. Fetal ultrasonography.
   a. Abdomen can be seen by 10 weeks' gestation, stomach by 13 weeks.
   b. Abdomen can be assessed for intactness of abdominal wall, umbilical cord insertion, stomach as fluid-filled chamber, bowel dilation, or indication of obstruction.
   c. Maternal polyhydramnios (>2000 ml) may indicate interference with fetal swallowing or intestinal obstruction.

B. Abdominal assessment.

1. Inspection.
   a. Size and shape.
      (1) Should be slightly round, soft, symmetric.
      (2) Distended: intestinal obstruction, infection, enlarged abdominal organ.
      (3) Scaphoid: associated with congenital diaphragmatic hernia.
      (4) Asymmetric: mass, organomegaly, intestinal obstruction.
   b. Muscular development.
      (1) Flat, flabby: prune-belly syndrome.
      (2) Gap between rectus muscles: diastasis recti.
      (3) Externalization of abdominal contents: omphalocele, gastroschisis, bladder exstrophy.
      (4) Hernias: protrusions of peritoneum and intestine through a weakened spot in abdominal wall. Common in three areas:
         (a) Umbilical: common in black males, Down syndrome, hypothyroidism, Hurler syndrome, or other mucopolysaccharidosis.
         (b) Inguinal.
            (i) More common in males.
            (ii) Frequently bilateral.
            (iii) May not be evident until second or third month of life.
            (iv) Usually readily reducible.
         (c) Femoral.
            (i) More common in females.
            (ii) Located just below inguinal ligament on anterior aspect of thigh.
   c. Umbilicus/umbilical cord.
      (1) Normally is pearly white.
      (2) Green or yellow staining suggests in utero meconium passage.
      (3) Wet, foul smelling, or red: infection.
      (4) Persistent clear drainage: patent urachus.
      (5) Ileal fluid drainage: omphalomesenteric duct.
      (6) Serous or serosanguineous drainage: granuloma.
      (7) Abnormally thick: single herniated loop of intestine.
      (8) Thick, gelatinous: large for gestational age.
      (9) Thin, small: intrauterine growth restriction.
      (10) Normally three vessels: two ventrally situated arteries, one dorsally situated vein.
      (11) Usually falls off after 10 to 14 days.

d. Bowel loops.
   (1) Normally not visible.
   (2) Presence: obstruction.
e. Movements.
   (1) Should move in synchrony with respirations.
   (2) Movements not in synchrony may represent respiratory distress, peritoneal irritation, central nervous system (CNS) disease.
   (3) Peristalsis: not normally seen.
      (a) May be seen in premature infants with thin abdominal walls.
      (b) Presence: associated with hypertrophic pyloric stenosis.
f. Veins.
   (1) Superficial veins become more prominent with abdominal distention.
   (2) Dilated veins: venous obstruction.
g. Perineum: inspected for patency of anus and presence of fistulas.

2. Auscultation.
   a. Done before palpation (to avoid altering sounds).
   b. Bowel sounds.
      (1) Become audible within 15 to 30 minutes after birth (Thigpen and Kenner, 2003).
      (2) Should have a metallic clicking quality.
      (3) Hyperactive or hypoactive does not necessarily represent pathologic change. Other historical or clinical finding should be taken into consideration when interpreting bowel sounds.
      (4) Increased sounds.
         (a) Malrotation.
         (b) Hirschsprung disease.
         (c) Diarrhea.
      (5) Decreased or absent sounds.
         (a) Ileus.
         (b) Starvation.
   c. Vascular sounds: bruit, similar to murmur. Caused by turbulent blood flow through the abdominal circulatory system, especially if heard despite position change of infant.
   d. Friction rub: peritoneal inflammation, splenic involvement, hepatic tumor, abscess.
3. Percussion.
   a. Provides information regarding size of organs, presence of masses, fluids, gases. Not significantly useful tool in newborn infant.
   b. Two main sounds to listen for:
      (1) Tympanic: low pitched, heard over gas-filled structures (stomach).
      (2) Dullness: high pitched, short, heard over dense or solid organs (liver, spleen).
4. Palpation.
   a. Performed to assess:
      (1) Abdominal tone.
      (2) Masses.
      (3) Pulsations.
      (4) Fluid.
      (5) Organ enlargement.
      (6) Organ position.
         (a) Liver should be 1 to 2 cm below right costal margin, midclavicular line.

(b) Spleen rarely palpable. Tip should not be more than 1 cm below left costal margin.
(c) Kidneys are about 4 to 5 cm in length. Left kidney is easier to palpate.

b. Technique: start in lower quadrants and progress to upper quadrants, using slow, gentle pressure. Place one hand directly behind palpating hand on infant's back. Start with light palpation, then progress to deep palpation.

c. Hints to relax infant.
(1) Flex legs.
(2) Use warm hands.
(3) Palpate any known areas of tenderness last.
(4) Use gentle circular motion.
(5) Slowly increase depth of palpation.

C. Diagnostic tests.

1. Gastric aspirate. Measure pH of gastric contents.

2. Apt test.
a. Differentiates maternal from fetal blood.
b. Can be done on gastric fluid or stool.
c. Fluid is centrifuged in 5 ml water; 1 part 0.25 NaOH is added to supernatant. Fluid that remains pink indicates blood is from infant; fluid that turns brown indicates blood is maternal.

3. Stool examination.
a. Usually examined for color, consistency, odor, blood, mucus, pus, tissue fragments, bacteria, parasites.
b. Color may be influenced by diet, dyes, drugs, pathologic change.
(1) Green: indomethacin, meconium.
(2) Greenish black: iron, meconium.
(3) Black: iron.
(4) Pale: biliary atresia.
(5) White: antacids, barium.
c. Odor.
(1) Sweet, yeasty, or acidic in odor suggests carbohydrate malabsorption typical of osmotic diarrhea of viral enteritis.
(2) Stool with purulent odor suggests colitis.
d. pH less than 5 in infants suggests carbohydrate malabsorption.
e. Guaiac.
(1) Detects occult blood.
(2) Based on the oxidation of guaiac by hydrogen peroxide in the Hemoccult solution, resulting in an alkaline compound, which turns the test paper blue.
(3) False-positive results: indomethacin, salicylates, steroids.
(4) False-negative results: high doses of vitamin C.
f. Reducing substances. Use of reagent tablets (Clinitest) for evaluation of reducing substances in any fluid other than urine is not supported or approved by the manufacturer.

4. pH probe test: 24-hour pH probe study to diagnose GI reflux. Detects acid reflux only; does not detect nonacid or gas reflux.

5. Radiologic studies.
a. X-ray examination (see Chapter 14 for further information).
(1) Bowel gas pattern (Thigpen and Kenner, 2003).
(a) At birth, gut is fluid filled.
(b) Within 30 minutes, gas should be in stomach.

(c) By 3 to 4 hours, gas should be in small intestine.
(d) After 6 to 8 hours, gas should be in entire intestine.
(2) Absence of gas below pylorus: possible indication of obstruction.

b. Upper GI series: done to assess structure and function of esophagus, hypertrophic pyloric stenosis, malrotation.
(1) Contrast material such as barium or Gastrografin is administered via nasogastric tube and observed by fluoroscopy.
(2) Water-soluble Gastrografin is preferred in cases of suspected perforation.

c. Lower GI series: may be used to detect presence of malrotation, Hirschsprung disease, meconium ileus, and meconium plug syndrome. May be therapeutic in meconium ileus and meconium plug syndrome.

6. Ultrasonography: may be used to diagnose suspected cases of pyloric stenosis, duplications, gastroesophageal reflux, or biliary atresia.

7. Scintigraphy (nuclear scan): used to evaluate gastric emptying, aspiration with swallowing, reflux with aspiration, and liver excretory function. Radionuclide tagged formula is fed to the infant and recorded by a gamma camera.

8. Endoscopy: used to directly visualize the upper or lower GI mucosa. Endoscopic retrograde cholangiopancreatography (ERCP) visualizes the biliary pancreatic ducts.

9. Fecal fat: used to diagnosis malabsorption syndromes. Fecal fat content greater than 6 g/24 hours is associated with malabsorption syndrome.

10. Culture: helpful in differentiating bloody diarrhea caused by infection vs. insult to intestine.

D. Laboratory tests (Table 28-1).

1. Aminotransferase activity.

a. Alanine aminotransferase (ALT) catabolizes the reversible transfer of the α-amino group of aspartic acid to the α-keto group of α-ketoglutaric acid, leading to the formation of pyruvic acid (D'Agata and Balistreri, 1999).

b. Aspartate aminotransferase (AST) catabolizes the reversible transfer of the α-amino group of aspartic acid to the α-keto group of α-ketoglutaric acid, leading to the formation of oxaloacetic acid (D'Agata and Balistreri, 1999).

c. ALT and AST are the most sensitive tests of hepatocyte necrosis. ALT is more specific than AST because it is not found in high concentrations in other tissues.

d. High elevations occur in hepatocellular injury. Slight elevations occur in cholestasis.

e. ALT-to-AST ratio is often performed to help differentiate among different forms of liver disease.

2. Alkaline phosphatase (ALP).

a. ALP is derived from the epithelium of the intrahepatic bile ducts and excreted into the bile. It is also found in the bone, kidney, and small intestine.

b. Elevated levels occur in obstructive liver disease (e.g., biliary atresia) as well as in bone disease

3. Serum bile acids.

a. In the absence of abnormalities of the ileum, normal serum values reflect functioning of the enterohepatic circulation.

b. Elevations occur in acute or chronic liver disease.

4. Gamma-glutamyl-transferase (GGT).

a. GGT assists in the transfer of amino acids across cell membranes.

■ TABLE 28-1
■ ■ **Laboratory Tests Used to Evaluate the Gastrointestinal System**

Test	Preterm	Term	Reference
Alanine aminotransferase (ALT) (units/L)	——	10-33	1
Aspartate aminotransferase (AST) (units/L)		24-81	1
Alkaline phosphatase (ALP) (units/L)	207 ± 60 to 320 ± 142	164 ± 68	1
Albumin	——	2.8-4.4 g/dl	2
Bile acids	⅙ adult value	½ adult value	3
Bilirubin, total (mg/dl)			1
Cord	<2.8	<2.8	
24 hours	1-6	2-6	
48 hours	6-8	6-7	
3-5 days	10-12	4-6	
≥1 month	<1.5	<1.5	
Bilirubin, direct (mg/dl)	<0.5	<0.5	
Ammonia (μg/dl)	——	90-150	1
Gamma-glutamyl-transferase (GGT) (units/L)	——	14-131	1
5′nucleotidase (5′N, 5′NT) (units/L)	——	5-10	4
Prothrombin (PT) (sec)	——	13-18	2

Adapted from Blackburn, S.T.: *Maternal, fetal, and neonatal physiology: A clinical perspective* (2nd ed.). St. Louis, Saunders, 2003, p. 447; Fanaroff, A.A. and Martin, R.J. (Eds.): *Neonatal-perinatal medicine: Diseases of the fetus and infant* (7th ed.). St Louis, 2002, Mosby; Malarkey, L.M. and McMorrow, M.E.: *Nurse's manual of laboratory tests and diagnostic procedures* (2nd ed.). Philadelphia, 2000, Saunders; Simone, S.: Gastrointestinal critical care problems. In M.C. Curley and P.A. Moloney-Harmon (Eds.): *Critical care nursing of infants and children* (2nd ed.). Philadelphia, 2001, Saunders, pp. 765-804.

   b. GGT is present in the small bile ductule epithelium of the liver and in hepatocytes.
   c. Because GGT is also found in the pancreas, spleen, brain, breast, small intestine and kidney, it is not specific for hepatocellular injury.
   d. Often used along with ALP to evaluate for biliary tract disease.
5. 5′nucleotidase (5′N, 5′NT).
   a. 5′N is an enzyme found in the plasma membrane of all cells.
   b. It assists in the catabolism of nucleic acids.
   c. Often used with ALP to evaluate for biliary tract disease. Unlike ALP, 5′N does not increase in bone disease.
6. Albumin.
   a. Synthesized in the liver and is the most abundant plasma protein.
   b. Decreased levels occur in hepatocellular injury; usually a late finding.
7. Bilirubin.
   a. By-product of heme breakdown.
   b. Increased indirect bilirubin occurs when liver is unable to conjugate bilirubin or when there is an excessive load of unconjugated bilirubin.
   c. Increased direct bilirubin occurs when the liver cannot excrete conjugated bilirubin into the bile ducts or biliary tract.
8. Ammonia.
   a. Produced from the deamination of amino acids during protein metabolism and is a by-product of colonic bacteria protein breakdown. Liver is responsible for metabolizing ammonia.
   b. Elevated in liver failure.

9. Prothrombin time (PT).
   a. Measures the time required for prothrombin (factor II) to be converted to thrombin.
   b. Coagulation factors II, VII, IX, and X require fat-soluble vitamin K.
   c. In cases of obstructive liver disease in which bile acids do not reach the intestine, fat-soluble vitamins are not absorbed.
   d. Prolonged PT occurs in patients with hepatocellular injury and biliary obstruction.

ABDOMINAL WALL DEFECTS

A. Omphalocele.

1. Definition: herniation of abdominal viscera into umbilical cord, usually covered by a peritoneal sac and with umbilical arteries and veins inserting into apex of defect (Fig. 28-1).
2. Etiology: uncertain, but condition may be caused by incomplete closure of anterior abdominal wall or incomplete return of bowel into abdomen.
3. Incidence: 1:5000 to 1:6000 live births (Thigpen and Kenner, 2003).
4. Associated conditions: 50% to 70% will have associated anomalies (Thigpen and Kenner, 2003).
   a. Prematurity (33%); small for gestational age (19%) (Thigpen and Kenner, 2003).
   b. Cardiac defects (15%-25%) (Ryckman, 2002).
   c. Intestinal malrotation and/or atresia.
   d. Pentalogy of Cantrell (omphalocele, diaphragmatic hernia, sternal cleft, pericardial defect, intracardiac defect).
   e. Neurologic anomalies.
   f. Genitourinary anomalies.
   g. Skeletal anomalies.

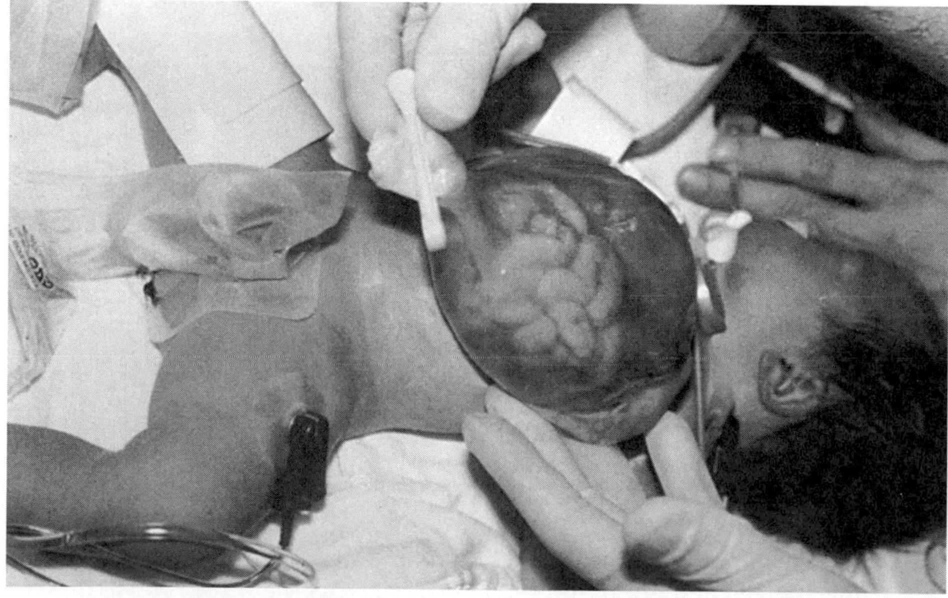

FIGURE 28-1 ■ Omphalocele.

h. Chromosomal anomalies (45%-55%) (Berseth, 1998b). Common anomalies include trisomy 13, 18, and 21.
i. Beckwith-Wiedemann syndrome.

5. Diagnosis.
a. Prenatal ultrasonography.
b. Elevated levels of maternal serum α-fetoprotein.
c. Inspection at birth.
(1) Omphaloceles differ in size; large defects may include stomach, liver, spleen, bladder, ovaries and fallopian tubes or testicles, as well as intestines.
(2) Defect can be small; therefore, any umbilical cord that is unusually fat should be inspected carefully before clamping to be certain it is not a very small omphalocele.
(3) Sac may rupture before or at time of delivery, exposing the viscera to amniotic fluid.

6. Prognosis.
a. Mortality rate is related to size of defect and severity of other defects.
b. Mortality rate with associated heart disease is 80% but only 30% in absence of heart disease (Berseth, 1998b).

B. Gastroschisis.

1. Definition: herniation of abdominal contents through an abdominal wall defect, usually to right of umbilicus. See Table 28-2 for a comparison of omphalocele and gastroschisis.
2. Etiology: unclear; theories include right periumbilical ischemia due to atropy or persistence of the right umbilical vein, or a vascular accident of the right omphalomesenteric artery (Robinson and Abuhamad, 2000).
3. Incidence: 1:4000 to 1:10,000 live births (Howell, 1998). There is an association between gastroschisis and young maternal age and low socioeconomic status (Gaines et al., 2000).
4. Diagnosis.
a. Prenatal ultrasonography.
b. Elevated levels of maternal serum α-fetoprotein.
c. Inspection at birth.
(1) No sac covers the gastroschisis.
(2) Usually placed to right of umbilicus (Fig. 28-2).

TABLE 28-2
Comparison of Omphalocele and Gastroschisis

	Omphalocele	Gastroschisis
Incidence	1:5000 to 1:6000	1:30,000 to 1:50,000
Covering	Present, may be ruptured	None
Site	Umbilical	Paraumbilical, usually to the right
Fascial defect	Small or large	Small
Herniated organs	Intestines; stomach, liver, spleen sometimes	Intestines; rarely liver
Appearance of herniated bowel	Normal, unless sac is ruptured	Often edematous, matted
Associated anomalies	45% to 55%	10% to 15%
IUGR	Less common	Common

IUGR, Intrauterine growth restriction.

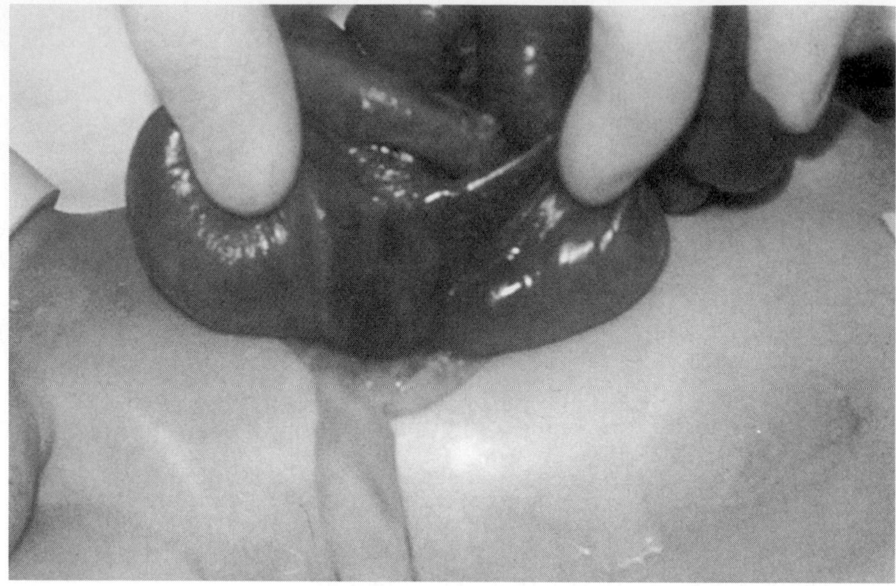

FIGURE 28-2 ■ Gastroschisis.

(3) Gastroschisis usually includes small and large intestines and rarely the liver.
(4) Intestine may be thickened, edematous, and inflamed because it has been exposed to amniotic fluid.
(5) Fascial defect is smaller than the omphalocele.
(6) Umbilical cord is intact.

5. Associated conditions.
  a. 58% of infants are premature; 92% are low birth weight (Thigpen and Kenner, 2003).
  b. Intestinal malrotation and atresia.
  c. Other anomalies are uncommon.

6. Prognosis. Mortality rate ranges from 10% to 30% (Berseth, 1998b). Malabsorption is a common prolonged problem postoperatively. Preterm delivery to improve neonatal outcome has not shown beneficial (Dunn et al., 1999). Recommended mode of delivery remains controversial.

C. Care of the neonate with an abdominal wall defect (omphalocele and gastroschisis).

1. Goal of initial management is to prevent hypothermia, maintain sterile environment, and maintain perfusion to the eviscerated contents.

2. At the time of delivery, place infant in a sterile bowel bag from the feet to the axilla. The bag has a drawstring at the open end that can be secured around the infant's torso. Infants with a ruptured omphalocele or gastroschisis are at higher risk of having fluid, electrolyte, and temperature loss because of exposed bowel. If bowel bag is not available, cover the exposed bowel with warm, moist dressings. (Sterile normal saline solution is recommended. In addition, cover the dressing in plastic to prevent evaporated heat loss.) The bowel bag has the advantage of maintaining a sterile environment for the exposed contents and allowing visualization of contents. Gauze dressings require rehydration to prevent adherence to the bowel and tissue trauma and may contribute to hypothermia as the gauze cools over time.

3. To prevent intestinal vascular compromise from torqued abdominal contents, either position the infant on his or her side or support the defect with a small roll. Handling should be kept to a minimum and done only with sterile gloves.
4. Place infant on a regimen of nothing by mouth (NPO) and insert a sump tube. Place sump tube on intermittent low suction for gastric decompression. Bowel distended with air can restrict normal blood flow and further compromise the bowel.
5. Begin IV fluid-and-electrolyte therapy and antibiotic therapy as soon as possible. IV fluids are usually increased to approximately 150 ml/kg/day because of increased fluid loss through exposed bowel.
   - a. When a sac covers the defect, fluid losses are not as great.
   - b. Ideally, IV infusions should not be started in the lower extremities because postoperative venous stasis results from increased abdominal pressure (Brandt, 1998).
6. Blood studies should be performed: hematocrit, electrolyte values, blood type and cross-match, pH and blood gas values, and clotting times.
7. Assess the infant carefully for associated anomalies, syndromes, or deformations.
8. Most newborn infants with abdominal wall defects require surgical repair. The types of repair include the following:
   - a. Primary repair. All contents are returned to the abdominal cavity, and the fascia and skin are closed. The infant may require prolonged respiratory support because of increased intraabdominal pressure. Preferred repair, but not possible in all cases.
   - b. Staged reduction. Not all the organs are returned to the abdominal cavity during the first surgery; the organs remaining outside the cavity are covered by a mesh-reinforced Silastic sac (silo). The sac is either sutured to the edge of the defect or secured underneath the fascia, allowing gradual reduction of the intestines on a daily basis in the neonatal intensive care unit (NICU). This technique is employed with infants with large defects and for those who cannot tolerate primary repair. A variation of this technique is the insertion of a spring-loaded silo over the exposed viscera under the fascia performed in the delivery room or NICU and subsequent closure on an elective basis. This latter technique is gaining in popularity and has been associated with fewer complications, fewer ventilator days, and shorter hospital stays (Minkes et al., 2000).
     - (1) Reduction minimizes the stress on the respiratory and vascular systems by allowing these systems to adjust slowly to the increased pressure of the organs as they are slowly returned to the abdominal cavity.
     - (2) Reduction can usually be accomplished during a period of 10 days, after which infection becomes a major consideration.
     - (3) Assess perfusion of herniated contents frequently through the opaque silo. Compromise of mesenteric vasculature can occur within the silo.
     - (4) Topical antibacterial agent may be applied to silo and the suture lines to prevent infection.
     - (5) The abdominal wall is closed after the reduction is completed.
   - c. Skin flap closure. Only the skin is pulled over the exposed organs. This method is not a long-term solution and is used when the fascia cannot be initially repaired.

(1) Definitive repair done at 6 to 12 months of age.
(2) Positioning infant prone while awaiting definitive repair may facilitate growth of peritoneal cavity (Ryckman, 2002).

d. Nonsurgical repair. The defect is painted with an escharotic agent such as merbromin solution (Mercurochrome), silver nitrate, or silver sulfadiazine and allowed to air dry and epithelialize.
(1) This uncommon procedure is used only if the defect is large, if the infant cannot tolerate surgery or has uncorrectable congenital anomalies, or if the reduction fails.
(2) Systemic side effects are associated with most of the escharotic agents. The health care team should be aware of such effects and assess the infant for them.

9. Postoperative care.

a. Pain management (see Chapter 16).

b. Dressing changes are performed with aseptic technique; IV antibiotic therapy is continued postoperatively.

c. Oxygen saturation, urine output, and blood pressure are monitored continuously. Other parameters to watch closely include fluid-and-electrolyte balance, pH, and clotting times.

d. Observe the following for complications: sepsis, intestinal obstruction, respiratory distress, skin necrosis over repaired defect, and venous stasis.

e. When staged reduction is employed, the silo must be supported to prevent tilting or torsion of the enclosed viscera. Sterile gauze may be wrapped around the base of the silo for this purpose.

f. Infant will require gastric suction after surgery until gastric output is minimal. Gastric losses should be replaced with physiologic IV solutions (i.e., suctioned gastric contents should be measured every 4 hours and parenteral fluids increased an equal amount).

g. Total parenteral nutrition is provided until infant can tolerate feedings.

h. Bowel sounds are assessed to determine readiness to feed. A prolonged ileus is a common complication in gastroschisis, but relatively uncommon in omphalocele (Gaines et al., 2000).

i. Feeding is begun very slowly when gastric output is minimal and bowel sounds are active.
(1) Low osmolality feeding, such as half-strength formula, breast milk, or mineral-electrolyte solution (Pedialyte) is usually preferred. Feedings are frequently stopped and started for a time.
(2) Soy-based and elemental formulas are used for infants who exhibit signs of feeding intolerance or malabsorption.

j. Parents should be supported through the often long recovery process.

OBSTRUCTIONS OF THE GASTROINTESTINAL TRACT

A. General considerations.

1. Obstructions may be either mechanical (in which there is a specific point of obstruction) or functional (usually related to motility) in nature and can be found anywhere from the esophagus to the anus.

2. Obstruction occurs because of an intrinsic or extrinsic blockage (Table 28-3).

3. Common associations in infants with intestinal obstruction.

a. History of polyhydramnios.
(1) Occurs more often in proximal obstructions.
(2) 15% to 20% of polyhydramnios is associated with fetal GI obstructions.

■ TABLE 28-3
■ ■ **Causes of Intestinal Obstruction in the Newborn Infant**

Mechanical		
Congenital	**Acquired**	**Functional**
Intrinsic Atresias Stenoses Meconium ileus Anorectal malformations Enteric duplications	Necrotizing enterocolitis Intussusception Peritoneal adhesions	Hirschsprung disease Meconium plug syndrome Ileus Peritonitis
Extrinsic Volvulus Peritoneal bands Annular pancreas Cysts and tumors Incarcerated hernias		Intestinal pseudo-obstruction syndrome

From Berseth, C.L.: Disorders of the intestines and pancreas. In W.H. Taeusch, and R.A. Ballard (Eds.): *Avery's diseases of the newborn* (7th ed.). Philadelphia, 1998c, W.B. Saunders, p. 919.

b. Failure to pass meconium within 24 to 48 hours: 94% of term infants pass meconium by 24 hours, and 99.8% pass meconium by 48 hours (Berseth, 1998a).
c. Abdominal distention: occurs more often in distal obstructions and tracheoesophageal fistula.
d. Bilious vomiting: occurs when obstruction is distal to the ampulla of Vater, located in the duodenum.

4. General preoperative management.
   a. NPO.
   b. Gastric decompression.
   c. IV therapy and replacement of fluid losses.
   d. Antibiotics.

B. Esophageal atresia (EA) and tracheoesophageal fistula (TEF).

1. Definitions: EA, an interruption in the esophagus; TEF, an abnormal communication between the esophagus and trachea. EA and TEF may occur as separate defects or, more commonly, in association with each other.
2. Incidence: approximately 1:4500 live births (Ryckman and Balistreri, 2002).
3. Associated anomalies: 30% to 40% of affected infants. The most common associated anomalies include the following (Ryckman and Balistreri, 2002):
   a. Low birth weight (30%-40%) (Filston and Shorter, 2000).
   b. Cardiac defects: primarily atrial septal defects and ventricular septal defects.
   c. GI anomalies: pyloric stenosis, duodenal obstruction, and imperforate anus.
   d. Esophageal atresia is a frequent component of the VATER or VACTERL association. Infants with TEF should have a cardiac evaluation, renal ultrasound, and skeletal x-rays.
   e. Esophageal abnormalities are also seen in the CHARGE (*c*olobomata, *h*eart disease, choanal *a*tresia, mental *r*etardation, *g*enital hypoplasia, and *e*ar anomalies with deafness) association.

4. Etiology: incomplete elongation and separation of esophagus and trachea during fourth week of gestation.
5. Types of TEFs include the following (Fig. 28-3):
   a. Blind proximal pouch (esophageal atresia) with distal tracheoesophageal fistula (most common; 85% of cases) (Ryckman and Balistreri, 2002).
   b. Isolated esophageal atresia without tracheoesophageal fistula (3%-5% of cases) (Filston and Shorter, 2000).
   c. Isolated tracheoesophageal fistula without esophageal atresia (H type of TEF) (3%-6% of cases) (Filston and Shorter, 2000).
   d. Esophageal atresia with fistula between upper pouch and trachea (rare).
   e. Esophageal atresia with fistulas between upper pouch and lower pouches and trachea (rare).
6. Clinical presentation.
   a. Clinical presentation is dependent on the type of tracheoesophageal anomaly.
   b. Accumulation of oral secretions in mouth, drooling.
   c. Inability to pass gastric tube.
   d. Coughing, choking, or cyanosis with feedings.
   e. Abdominal distention if fistula between distal esophagus and trachea.
   f. Recurrent pneumonia (more common in infants with isolated TEF without EA).
7. Diagnosis.
   a. History of polyhydramnios is present.
   b. Fetal ultrasound.
   c. Gastric tube will stop in the esophageal pouch (will most likely not pass beyond 10 cm).
   d. On x-ray film the gastric tube appears coiled in the upper esophageal pouch. In addition, air in the GI tract indicates the presence of a TEF. A gasless abdomen indicates an isolated EA (refer to Chapter 14).
   e. Use of contrast studies is not recommended because of the risk of aspiration and subsequent chemical pneumonitis.
8. Preoperative care.
   a. See section A, "General Considerations," p. 654-655.
   b. The head of the bed should be in a 30- to 45-degree upright position to avoid reflux and aspiration of gastric secretions. If EA is present without a fistula, preferred position may be flat or head down to facilitate drainage of saliva out of esophageal pouch.

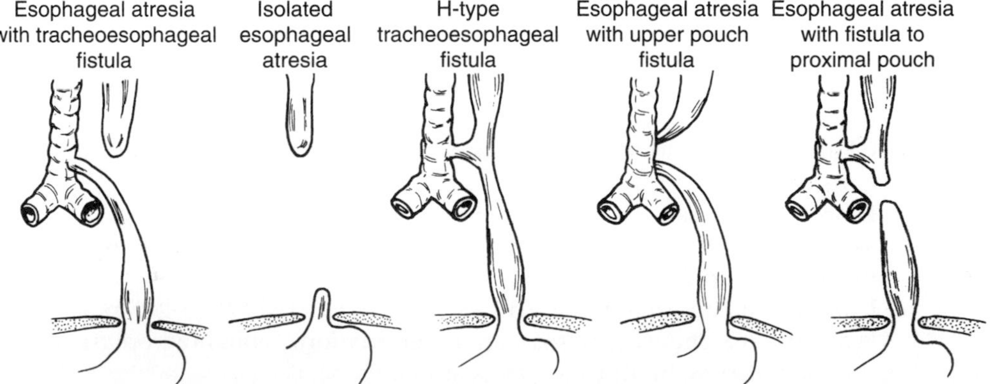

FIGURE 28-3 ■ Esophageal malformations.

c. A sump catheter on low constant suction should be left in the upper pouch to suction oral secretions.
   (1) The holes in the Replogle tube (Sherwood Medical, Norfolk, Nebraska) are down close to the end of the tube, making this the desired sump tube for use in TEF.
   (2) Assess and maintain patency of the sump tube.
   (3) Do not irrigate sump tube because this may lead to aspiration.
d. Use comfort measures to prevent crying, which leads to increased swallowed air, abdominal distention, and increased risk of reflux.

9. Surgical repair.
   a. Primary repair is ligation of the TEF and anastomosis of the proximal and distal portions of the esophagus.
   b. Staged repair is used with infants who are very premature, who have pneumonia or other coexisting life-threatening problems, or in whom the gap between the two esophageal pouches is great.
      (1) Ligation of TEF is performed at initial surgery.
      (2) Gastrostomy tube is placed at the first surgery to allow gastric decompression, minimize pulmonary aspiration, and provide route for enteral feedings.
      (3) Suction to proximal pouch is continued until second surgery.
      (4) Final surgery is usually delayed for 6 to 12 months in infants with a long gap between pouches. To allow a portal of exit for swallowed saliva, the surgeon creates a spit fistula at the initial procedure, exteriorizing the proximal esophageal pouch to the neck.
   c. When end-to-end anastomosis is impossible because the gap between the esophageal pouches is too great, either some other structure must be used to connect the pouches or the upper pouch must undergo an elongation procedure (rarely successful).

10. Postoperative care.
   a. Provide pain management (see Chapter 16).
   b. Maintain elevation of head of bed.
   c. Intubation with low-pressure ventilation protects the tracheal suture line.
   d. Suction endotracheal tube only the length of the endotracheal tube to avoid damage to the tracheal suture line.
   e. Suction posterior pharynx carefully and gently with a measured catheter.
   f. There is usually a thoracic drain in place postoperatively; note the color, consistency, and amounts of fluid drainage. Saliva indicates an esophageal leak.
   g. Gastrostomy tube care.
   h. Because of the potential for perforating or damaging the repair, a gastric tube should not be passed.
   i. Hyperalimentation and antibiotics are commonly used postoperatively until the anastomosis is proven intact and patent.
   j. Gastrostomy feedings may be started 2 days postoperatively. Oral feedings are usually started 7 to 10 days postoperatively. Contrast esophagram is frequently obtained before oral feedings to confirm that there are no leaks at the esophageal anastomosis.

11. Postoperative complications.
   a. Leaking at site of anastomosis, which may lead to sepsis and thoracic empyema. Commonly occurs at days 2 through 6 postoperatively.
   b. Stricture at site of anastomosis. Stricture should be suspected if feeding difficulties exist after the third postoperative week (Ryckman and Balistreri, 2002).

c. Dysmotility of lower esophageal segment. Most often a problem with long gap atresia and when oral intake is delayed for a prolonged period of time (Filston and Shorter, 2000).
d. Recurrent fistula, usually resulting from a leak.
e. Pneumonia.
f. Sepsis.
g. Unilateral diaphragmatic paralysis.
h. Tracheomalacia. This complication is occasionally severe enough to require a tracheostomy.
i. "TEF cough." Characterized by stridor, brassy cough, and bronchospastic airway symptoms. Caused by deformation and softening of tracheal cartilages from compression of posterior trachea by enlarged proximal esophageal pouch.
j. Gastroesophageal reflux is common.

12. Prognosis: survival rate excellent for healthy term infants. Prognosis is dependent on birth weight, presence of other congenital anomalies, especially cardiac, and preoperative condition. Highest mortality occurs in infants less than 1500 g and those associated with cardiac or chromosomal abnormalities (Cass and Wesson, 2002)

C. **Hypertrophic pyloric stenosis.**

1. Definition: hypertrophy of the pyloric musculature.
2. Incidence: 1:1000 to 3:1000 births (Dillon and Cilley, 2000).
   a. Males more likely to be affected than females (4:1 ratio).
   b. More common in white infants.
   c. First born more often affected; at highest risk is the first-born male of an affected mother.
3. Etiology: exact cause unknown. Hereditary component exists because incidence is increased if parent has history of pyloric stenosis.
4. Associated conditions: uncommon. Three major malformations associated with pyloric stenosis are intestinal malrotation, obstructive uropathy, and esophageal atresia.
5. Symptoms usually occur at 3 to 4 weeks of age but may present up to 5 months after birth. Pyloric stenosis may be congenital or acquired.
6. Clinical presentation.
   a. Nonbilious vomiting that becomes projectile with time.
   b. Hypochloremia.
   c. Hypokalemia.
   d. Metabolic alkalosis.
   e. Dehydration.
   f. Visible peristaltic waves in epigastrium.
   g. Palpable pyloric "olive."
   h. Failure to thrive.
7. Diagnosis.
   a. Presence of signs and symptoms.
   b. Confirmation by ultrasonography.
   c. Upper GI tract contrast study.
8. Preoperative care.
   a. Primary concern is correcting the hypokalemia, hypochloremia, and dehydration.
   b. Gastric decompression to prevent vomiting and risk of aspiration.
9. Surgical repair is a pyloromyotomy via laparascopy or laparotomy.

10. Postoperative care.
    a. Pain management (see Chapter 16).
    b. Routine wound care.
    c. NPO regimen for 6 to 8 hours after surgery.
    d. Prevention of perforation of the mucosa at the pyloromyotomy site by avoiding placement of a gastric tube postoperatively.
11. Prognosis: excellent. Generally, complete recovery with no residual effects; some continued vomiting possible in first few days after surgery, followed by quick resolution.

D. Duodenal atresia.

1. Definition: congenital obstruction of the duodenum. The atresia usually occurs distal to the ampulla of Vater.
2. Other types of duodenal obstruction.
    a. Annular pancreas.
    b. Preduodenal portal vein.
    c. Peritoneal (Ladd) band due to intestinal malrotation.
3. Incidence: approximately 1:2500 live births (Millar et al., 2000). Females are more commonly affected than males.
4. Etiology: unknown, but cause may be from a failure of recanalization of the duodenum during weeks 8 to 10 of fetal life.
5. Associated conditions (other anomalies found in 60%-70% of all cases) (Thigpen and Kenner, 2003).
    a. Intestinal malrotation. Up to 50% of infants with duodenal atresia have malrotation (Clark and Oldham, 2000).
    b. Down syndrome. More than 25% of infants with duodenal atresia have Down syndrome (Thigpen and Kenner, 2003).
    c. Prematurity.
    d. Congenital heart disease.
    e. Tracheoesophageal abnormalities.
    f. Anorectal lesions.
6. Clinical presentation.
    a. Bilious vomiting. Nonbilious vomiting does not rule out duodenal atresia or obstruction.
    b. Abdominal distention, generally confined to upper abdomen.
    c. Possible passage of meconium in first 24 hours of life. Bowel movements then cease.
    d. Jaundice.
7. Diagnosis.
    a. History of polyhydramnios.
    b. Prenatal diagnosis by ultrasonography.
    c. X-ray film showing "double bubble" pattern (see Chapter 14).
8. Preoperative care. See section A, "General Considerations," on p.654-655.
9. Surgery is performed to remove the atretic portions and reanastomose the remaining ends.
10. Postoperative care.
    a. Pain management (see Chapter 16).
    b. NPO regimen for 3 to 10 days; delayed gastric emptying is common.
    c. Gastric decompression.
    d. Most infants will have a gastrostomy tube in place postoperatively.
    e. Continue total parenteral nutrition (TPN) and antibiotics.
11. Prognosis: excellent. Long-term outcome is primarily dependent on associated anomalies and malformations.

E. Jejunal or ileal atresia.

1. Incidence: 1:1000 live births (Millar et al., 2000). Males and females are equally affected; of all jejunoileal atresias, approximately 31% are in the proximal jejunum, 20% in the distal jejunum, 13% in the proximal ileum, and 36% in the distal ileum (Ryckman, 2002).
2. Etiology: unknown, believed to result from a mesenteric vascular insult to the small bowel during fetal life with subsequent necrosis and resorption of the affected segment or segments (Millar et al., 2000).
3. Associated conditions.
   a. Intestinal malrotation. Up to one third of infants with jejunal atresia have malrotation (Clark and Oldham, 2000).
   b. Small for gestational age.
   c. Low birth weight.
4. Five types of jejunal or ileal atresia (Fig. 28-4) (Ryckman, 2002).
   a. Type I: bowel intact, but lumen is obstructed by a septum of tissue (20%).
   b. Type II: blind ends of bowel joined by a fibrous cord; mesentery is intact (35%).
   c. Type IIIa: blind ends separated by V-shaped mesenteric defect; most common type (35%).
   d. Type IIIb ("apple peel" or "Christmas tree"): blind ends separated by V-shaped mesenteric defect; the proximal intestine coils around a single distal ileal vessel (11%). This form is usually familial and carries the highest mortality rate.
   e. Type IV: Bowel has multiple atresias separated by V-shaped mesenteric defects (6%).
5. Clinical presentation.
   a. Bilious vomiting.

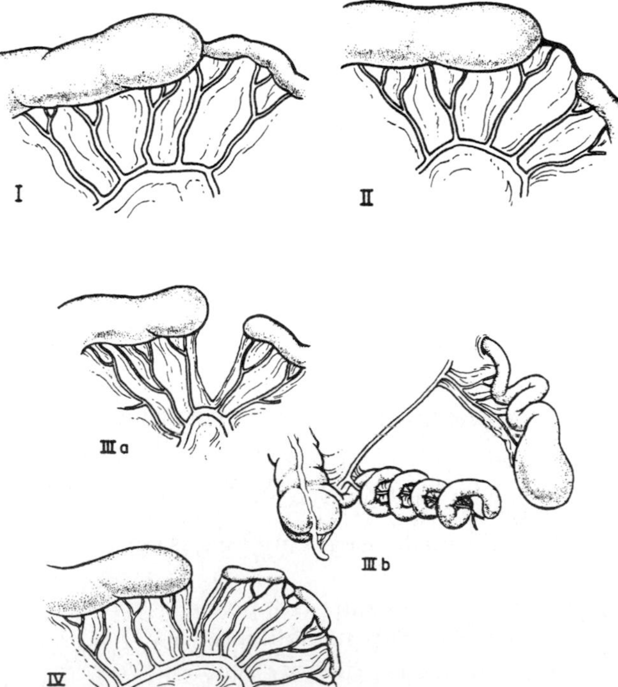

FIGURE 28-4 ■ Types of jejunal atresia. Type I—mucosal atresia with intact muscularis. Type II—atretic ends are separated by a fibrous band. Type IIIa—atretic ends are separated by a V-shaped gap defect. Type IIIb—apple-peel deformity of the distal atretic segment with retrograde blood supply from the ileocolic or right colic artery. Type IV—multiple astresias (string-of-sausage effect). (From Rowe, M.I., O'Neill, J.A., Grosfeld, J.L., et al.: *Essentials of pediatric surgery*. St Louis, 1995, Mosby, p. 511.)

b. Abdominal distention that usually progresses over the first 12 to 24 hours after birth. The lower the obstruction, the greater the abdominal distention.
c. Failure to pass meconium.
d. Prematurity (25%-38%) (Thigpen and Kenner, 2003).
e. Jaundice; more common in proximal atresias.

6. Diagnosis.
   a. Presence of symptoms.
   b. History of polyhydramnios.
      (1) Present in about one third of cases with jejunal atresia (Thigpen and Kenner, 2003).
      (2) Rare in ileal atresia (Thigpen and Kenner, 2003).
   c. X-ray films showing dilated loops of bowel and multiple air-fluid levels (refer to Chapter 14). Infants with proximal jejunal atresia have characteristic "triple bubble" on x-ray. If in utero perforation occurred, peritoneal calcifications may be visible.
   d. Barium-enema x-ray film shows a microcolon.
7. Preoperative care: see section A, "General Considerations," on p. 654-655.
8. Surgery.
   a. Surgical procedure depends on location of atresia and amount of intestine involved.
   b. Atretic intestinal portion is often resected proximally to the point of normal bowel dimensions and then connected to distal segment using an end-to-oblique-side anastomosis.
   c. Occasionally, exteriorization of the proximal and even distal ends may be necessary with reanastomosis later.
9. Postoperative care.
   a. Pain management (see Chapter 16).
   b. Continue NPO regimen until normal bowel function is restored (usually 3-7 days).
   c. Continue TPN and antibiotic therapy.
   d. Feedings are often initiated with elemental formulas until standard formulas can be tolerated. Feedings can be started 24 hours postoperatively via a Silastic transanastomotic tube (TAT) inserted through the lumen of a gastrostomy tube or transnasally (Millar et al., 2000).
   e. Assess feeding tolerance once feedings are begun.
10. Complications.
   a. Ileus.
   b. Peritonitis.
   c. Prolonged intestinal dysfunction, especially with type IIIb ("apple peel") and IV varieties.
11. Prognosis: very good, with return to normal bowel function usually within 10 days. Deaths, when they do occur, are usually related to prematurity, postoperative short bowel syndrome, or infarction (Thigpen and Kenner, 2003). Survival decreased in infants with proximal atresias, complex type IIIb and type IV atresias, short bowel syndrome and cystic fibrosis.

F. Malrotation.

1. Definition: an assortment of intestinal anomalies of rotation and fixation.
2. Etiology: exact cause unknown. Occurs when the intestines do not rotate and/or the mesentery does not fixate appropriately during weeks 6 to 10 of gestation. Intestines may twist on themselves (midgut volvulus), occluding

the intestinal lumen, or around the superior mesenteric artery, occluding intestinal blood supply. Ischemia and bowel necrosis then results.

3. Incidence: unknown; true incidence of malrotation is much higher than cases with clinically significant symptoms. More males affected than females.
4. Associated anomalies.
   a. Intestinal atresia.
   b. Diaphragmatic hernia.
   c. Duodenal obstruction due to peritoneal (Ladd) bands encircling the duodenum.
   d. Omphalocele.
   e. Gastroschisis.
5. Clinical presentation of acute cases.
   a. 75% of patients who become symptomatic do so within the first month of life. Approximately 90% of clinical symptoms appear in children in the first year of life (Clark and Oldham, 2000).
   b. Bilious vomiting, suggestive of malrotation with volvulus formation; needs immediate confirmation.
   c. Abdominal distention.
   d. Diarrhea.
   e. Rectal bleeding.
   f. Abdominal pain.
   g. Signs of shock and sepsis.
6. Clinical presentation of "less acute cases."
   a. Failure to thrive.
   b. Intermittent bilious vomiting.
   c. Abdominal tenderness.
7. Diagnosis.
   a. Presence of symptoms.
   b. Classic early x-ray of malrotation with volvulus showing distended stomach and proximal duodenum and scanty gas distributed throughout remainder of bowel. An airless abdomen is an ominous sign. X-ray may be normal.
   c. Contrast upper GI tract x-ray film showing distended stomach and a beaklike narrowing at the pylorus; gastric mucosa folds are also seen on the x-ray film.
8. Preoperative care.
   a. See section A, "General Considerations," on p. 654-655.
   b. In addition, the infant with malrotation with volvulus will likely need fluid resuscitation, ventilatory support, electrolyte maintenance, and broad-spectrum antibiotics.
   c. Malrotation with volvulus is considered a surgical emergency; the primary goal of preoperative care is to get the infant to the operating room as fast as possible to prevent intestinal infarction. Infant is particularly at risk for hypovolemia and metabolic acidosis.
9. Surgical repair. Surgery is aimed at release of strangulation of the bowel.
   a. Operative repair is the Ladd procedure:
      (1) Intestines are untwisted in a counterclockwise fashion.
      (2) If present, peritoneal (Ladd) bands are divided, relieving duodenal obstruction; the small bowel is placed on right side of abdomen, and colon is placed on left side.
      (3) Base of the mesentery is widened.

(4) Appendectomy is performed to eliminate appendicitis as a differential diagnosis in the future when the child has abdominal pain.

10. Postoperative care.
    a. Pain management (see Chapter 16).
    b. The infant should remain on NPO regimen until the return of bowel function (usually in 3-7 days).
    c. IV therapy and antibiotics, parenteral nutrition.
    d. Feedings are often initiated with elemental formulas until standard formulas can be tolerated.
    e. Routine wound and stoma care.
11. Prognosis: excellent if uncomplicated by infarction or associated anomalies. Operative mortality rate is less than 9% (Clark and Oldham, 2000). Mortality increases with intestinal necrosis, prematurity, or other abnormalities. Amount of intestinal resection is an important predicting factor in outcome. Major postoperative complication is short bowel syndrome.

G. Meconium ileus.

1. Definition: mechanical obstruction of the distal ileum due to intraluminal accumulation of thick, inspissated meconium. Although meconium ileus has been reported in a few patients without cystic fibrosis, it is the predominant cause of meconium ileus in infants.
2. Incidence. Cystic fibrosis occurs in 1:2000 live births of white infants; 10% to 15% of children with cystic fibrosis have meconium ileus (Ryckman, 2002).
3. Etiology: exact cause unknown. Two implicating factors are:
    a. Hyposecretion of pancreatic enzymes, which may play a part in some but not all meconium ileus. As a result, meconium contains an abnormal amount of proteins and glycoproteins, making the meconium thick and viscid.
    b. Abnormal viscid secretions from the mucous glands of the small intestine.
4. Two types of meconium ileus.
    a. Simple meconium ileus.
        (1) More common.
        (2) Distal segment of small bowel is obstructed with thick, tarlike tenacious meconium, and proximal segment of small bowel is dilated.
        (3) Clinical presentation is usually within 48 hours.
    b. Complicated meconium ileus.
        (1) This type of meconium ileus is complicated because of its association with the following:
            (a) Volvulus.
            (b) Intestinal necrosis and perforation.
            (c) Meconium peritonitis or pseudocyst formation.
        (2) Clinical presentation is usually within 24 hours.
5. Clinical presentation.
    a. Abdominal distention at birth.
    b. Bilious vomiting.
    c. Failure to pass meconium within 12 to 24 hours.
    d. Palpable, rubbery loops of bowel. Small grapelike pellets of meconium may be palpated distally.
    e. Complicated form has earlier presentation, and these infants appear sicker, with signs of sepsis and respiratory distress.
6. Diagnosis.
    a. Distended bowel loops without air-fluid levels.
    b. X-ray film showing "soap bubble" appearance of distal intestine created by the mixture of air and meconium.

c. Scattered calcifications on x-ray due to intrauterine intestinal perforations may be seen in complicated form.
d. Possible microcolon on contrast radiograph.
e. Family history of cystic fibrosis: highly suggestive of meconium ileus.
f. Definitive diagnosis based on diagnosis of cystic fibrosis by a sweat chloride test (sodium and chloride concentrations >60 mEq/L).

7. Management.
a. Simple meconium ileus.
(1) Nonsurgical management.
(a) A hypertonic contrast enema (Gastrografin or Hypaque) may be successful in dislodging the meconium by drawing fluid into the intesting and allowing for normal intestinal activity. Successful in up to 60% of patients (Ryckman, 2002). Usually meconium pellets are passed quickly, followed by liquid meconium for 24 hours after the procedure. A second enema may be required.
(b) Pre-enema management.
(i) Volvulus, atresia, perforation, and peritonitis must be ruled out.
(ii) Broad-spectrum antibiotics.
(iii) Evaluation by pediatric surgeon who remains in attendance during the procedure.
(iv) Fluid resuscitation as necessary.
(v) Patient should be prepared for surgery should complications occur during nonoperative therapy.
(c) Management after enema includes:
(i) Fluids at one-and-one-half times maintenance.
(ii) Careful monitoring of urine output, urine specific gravity or osmolality, blood urea nitrogen, creatinine, and serum osmolality.
(iii) Broad-spectrum antibiotics.
(iv) Continued gastric decompression.
(d) Complications of nonsurgical management include the following:
(i) Hypovolemic shock secondary to rapid fluid shift resulting from hypertonic solution used for enema.
(ii) Intestinal perforation which may occur up to 48 hours after administration of enema.
(iii) Risk of intestinal perforation increases with successive attempts at nonoperative techniques.
(2) Surgical management.
(a) Used when nonsurgical intervention has failed.
(b) A T-tube (Fig. 28-5) is inserted into the ileum which is irrigated postoperatively with *N*-acetylcysteine or pancreatic enzymes.

b. Complicated meconium ileus.
(1) Always requires surgical intervention.
(2) Compromised intestine is resected.
(3) If bowel is viable, end-to-end anastomosis performed.
(4) In extreme cases in which bowel necrosis has occurred, all compromised intestine is resected and the proximal and/or distal segment is exteriorized.
(5) Preoperative care. See section A, "General Considerations," above.
(6) Postoperative care.
(a) Pain management (see Chapter 16).

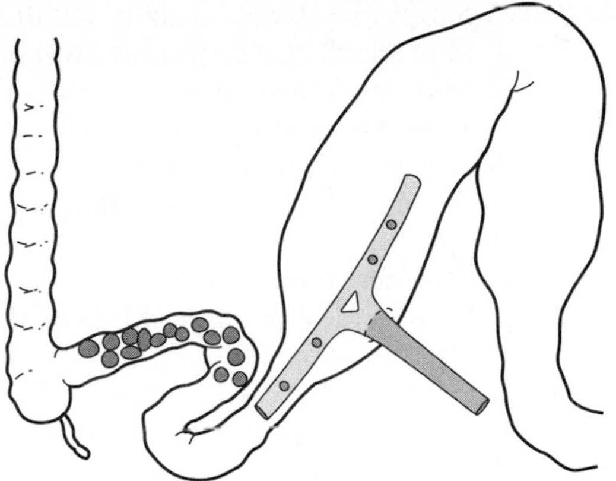

FIGURE 28-5 ■ T-tube. (From Mak G.Z., Harberg F.J., Hiatt P, Deaton A., Calhoon R., Brandt M.: (2000). T-tube ileostomy for meconium ileus: Four decades of experience. *Journal of Pediatric Surgery, 35*(2): 349-352).

(b) Continuation of NPO regimen and gastric decompression until normal bowel function is restored (approximately 3-7 days).
(c) Begin feedings with elemental formula, supplemented with pancreatic enzymes.
(d) Antibiotics.
(e) Irrigation of distal stoma or T-tube with *N*-acetylcysteine or pancreatic enzymes around postoperative day 3.
(f) Chest physiotherapy, aerosolized acetylcysteine sodium (Mucomyst), and supplemental humidity to prevent atelectasis and pneumonia, which infants with cystic fibrosis are prone to develop.
(g) Genetic counseling for the parents.
(h) Parental education on pulmonary hygiene.

8. Postoperative complications.
   a. Volvulus.
   b. Gangrene.
   c. Perforation.

9. Prognosis: operative mortality rate 10% (Ryckman, 2002). Morbidity is primarily related to pulmonary disease associated with cystic fibrosis.

H. Meconium plug syndrome.

1. Definition: a mechanical obstruction, usually of the distal segment of the colon and the rectum, that occurs from thick, inspissated meconium in the absence of an abnormality of ganglion cells or enzymatic deficiency.

2. Etiology: unclear; results from diminished colonic motility and meconium clearance.

3. Incidence: 1:100 newborns; 75% of newborns are able to expel the plug spontaneously, avoiding the complication of intestinal obstruction (Thigpen and Kenner, 2003).

4. Risk factors.
   a. Maternal diabetes, probably due to the increased fetal glycogen production leading to decreased bowel motility.
   b. Neonatal hypermagnesemia: usually occurs after mother has been treated with magnesium sulfate for pregnancy-induced hypertension; the decreased bowel motility is secondary to myoneural depression.
   c. Prematurity.
   d. Hypotonia in infant with CNS disease.
   e. Sepsis.

5. Clinical presentation: usually within first 3 days of life.
   a. Multiple dilated loops of bowel on physical examination.
   b. Abdominal distention.
   c. Failure to pass meconium.
   d. Hyperactive bowel sounds.
   e. Bilious vomiting (late finding).
6. Diagnosis.
   a. Presence of symptoms.
   b. X-ray film showing multiple distended loops of bowel (refer to Chapter 14).
   c. Water-soluble contrast enema often outlines an intraluminal plug. Such an enema will commonly dislodge the plug, and no further interventions will be required.
7. Differential diagnosis. A biopsy for Hirschsprung disease and a sweat test for cystic fibrosis will rule out these disorders and are commonly recommended for infants with meconium plug.
8. Management.
   a. Gastric decompression.
   b. Hydration.
   c. Electrolyte balance.
   d. Rectal examination may expel plug in some circumstances.
   e. Enemas of warm saline, meglumine diatrizoate, or actylcysteine (Thigpen and Kenner, 2003).
      (1) Meglumine diatrizoate is hyperosmolar, drawing fluid into the bowel from interstitial space. Careful assessment and management of fluid status are important.
      (2) Because the meconium plug is formed primarily by mucous and intestinal secretions, the plug appears as yellowish white and is gelatinous.
   f. Surgery rarely necessary.

I. Hirschsprung disease (congenital megacolon, aganglionic megacolon).

1. Definition: congenital absence of parasympathetic innervation to the distal intestine in association with absence of ganglionic cells in the submucosal and myenteric plexuses of the colon.
   a. Length of bowel involvement is dependent on the time during which migration of neuroblasts ceased.
   b. Agangliosis commonly involves rectum or rectosigmoid portion of colon only.
   c. Agangliosis may extend to proximal colon. Total colon agangliosis is rare (Quinn and Shannon, 2000).
2. Incidence: 1:5000 live births. Males are affected four times more often than females (Ryckman, 2002). More than one third of affected patients have a relative with Hirschsprung.
3. Etiology: thought to be related to interrupted migration of ganglionic cell precursors before week 12 of gestation. Three genes on three separate chromosomes have been identified and implicated in the development of Hirschsprung.
4. Pathophysiology: The lack of intestinal ganglion cells prevents the inhibitory relaxation normally regulated by parasympathetic nerves. The affected segment is unable to relax, and functional obstruction ensues. The normally innervated proximal colon becomes hypertrophied from its attempts to overcome the functional obstruction.

5. Associated anomalies: not common but may include colonic atresia or imperforate anus; 3% to 10% of children with Down syndrome have Hirschsprung disease. Congenital deafness and ocular neuropathies found in small number of affected infants. The oral, facial, and cranial ganglia arise from the same craniocervical neural crest as the ganglionic plexus of the bowel.
6. Clinical presentation.
   a. Early symptom is failure to pass meconium within 24 to 48 hours after birth.
   b. Bilious vomiting.
   c. Late symptom is the inability to stool normally. Abnormal stooling since birth is a common symptom of Hirschsprung disease. As the obstruction continues, enterocolitis may develop, with fever, abdominal distention, and diarrhea. The infant usually has symptoms in the first several weeks and then has diarrhea, abdominal distention, and/or vomiting. In advanced cases, urinary obstruction may occur secondary to mechanical compression of the ureters and bladder.
   d. Failure to thrive.
7. The most common complication is acute enterocolitis caused by:
   a. Bowel wall distention and ischemia.
   b. Bacterial invasion leading to sepsis.
8. Diagnosis.
   a. X-ray showing diffuse intestinal and bowel dilation along with an absence of air in the rectum is suggestive.
   b. Contrast studies showing a nondistensible rectal ampulla, with a dilated bowel above and a transition zone (an area between the normal and abnormal aganglionic intestine having a conical tapering appearance) is suggestive.
   c. Retained barium in the rectum for more than 24 hours after the procedure is suggestive of Hirschsprung disease.
   d. Anal manometry is useful in very-short-segment agangliosis or in patients who have normal findings on contrast studies.
   e. Confirmed by rectal biopsy showing the absence of ganglion cells. Punch or suction biopsy may be done in the nursery in which case the nurse should ensure appropriate analgesia and sedation. Full-thickness biopsy under general anesthesia is rarely needed. Increased acetylcholinesterase content in rectal tissue is identified by histochemical staining.
   f. Age at diagnosis has decreased significantly with some reports indicating 90% of cases identified in the neonatal period (Teitelbaum et al., 1998).
9. Preoperative care: see section A, "General Considerations," p. 654-655.
   a. In addition to routine preoperative management, rectal irrigation is routinely performed to allow repeated emptying of colon.
10. Treatment is surgery. Goal of surgery is to bring the normal ganglionated bowel down to the anus. Traditional repair involves creation of a colostomy just above the transition zone followed by a definitive pull through procedure performed at 6 months to 1 year of age. Although there is growing experience with a complete pull through repair done laparoscopically or via a perineal approach in the neonatal period, a staged repair is most common.
11. Postoperative care.
    a. Pain management (see Chapter 16).
    b. Gastric decompression.

c. Careful monitoring of fluid and electrolyte balance.
d. Administration of maintenance fluid and electrolytes; replacement of gastric losses.
e. NPO regimen and parenteral nutrition until oral feedings can be begun.
f. Close observation for shock and recurrent enterocolitis.
g. Routine ostomy care.
h. Routine rectal irrigations with normal saline to decrease risk of postoperative enterocolitis.
i. If frequent and liquid stools cause perineal irritation, loperamide may be administered to reduce stool frequency and kaolin-pectin suspension can solidify stools.
j. Special diets may be necessary to improve stool consistency.
k. Genetic counseling should be offered to infant's family.

12. Complications.
    a. Fecal incontinence
    b. Persistent constipation.
    c. Anastomotic leakage with subsequent stricture formation.
    d. Rectal stenosis.
13. Prognosis: excellent. Mortality rate increases when diagnosis is delayed and enterocolitis occurs. Enterocolitis is the leading cause of death. Approximately 10% of patients will have subsequent elimination problems such as constipation and delayed toilet training (Holschneider and Ure, 2000).

J. Imperforate anus (anorectal agenesis).

1. Definition: a broad spectrum of anorectal malformations characterized by a stenotic or atretic anal canal. A fistula between the rectum and the perineum, vagina in females or urethra in males, may also occur.
2. Incidence: 1:5000 live births (Ryckman, 2002).
3. Etiology: failure of differentiation of the urogenital sinus and cloaca during embryologic development.
4. Common associations: anomalies, including vertebral, genitourinary, cardiovascular, and GI malformations, in 20% to 75% of infants (Thigpen and Kenner, 2003). Specific anomalies include cryptorchidism, congenital heart defects, esophageal atresia, spinal dysraphrism.
5. Classification: high or low, depending on level of defect (i.e., above or below a line drawn from the symphysis pubis to the coccyx [pubococcygeal line]). Level of defect significantly influences outcome regarding fecal continence (Fig. 28-6).

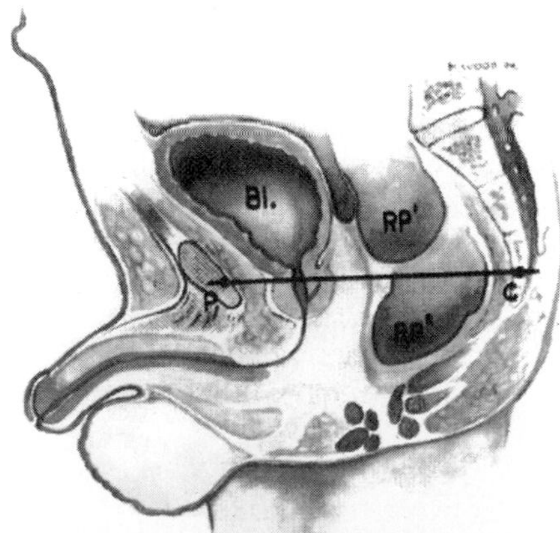

FIGURE 28-6 ■ Imperforate anus. Rectal pouch 1 (*RP*[1]) sits above the pubococcygeal line (*PC*) and would be classified as a "high type" anomaly. Rectal pouch 2 (*RP*[2]) sits below the PC line and represents a "low type" anomaly. The level of the rectal pouch is crucial in decisions of management. *Bl,* Bladder. (From Ross, A.J.: Intestinal obstruction in the newborn. *Pediatrics in Review,* 15[9]:338-347, 1994.)

a. High imperforate anus.
   (1) More common and generally more complex.
   (2) Occurs more frequently in males.
   (3) Rectourinary and rectovaginal fistulas are common associations.
   (4) High imperforate anus with sacral anomaly can be associated with lack of innervation of the bowel and/or bladder, causing incontinence.
   (5) Diagnosis is made by physical inspection, x-ray, contrast x-ray, and ultrasonography. An inverted lateral radiograph may be obtained to determine the level of the air-filled rectal pouch in relation to the pubococcygeal line.
   (6) Infants with a fistula are at risk for hyperchloremic acidosis as a result of colonic absorption of urine.
   (7) Surgical intervention is always necessary, with the procedure dependent on the level of the anorectal pouch. High and intermediate pouches are treated with a colostomy and a definitive pull-through procedure performed after the infant is approximately 8 months of age and weighs 18 pounds.

b. Low imperforate anus.
   (1) Male/female ratio closer to 1:1.
   (2) Perineal fistula is a common association.
   (3) Diagnosis is made by physical inspection, x-ray and contrast x-ray examination, and ultrasonography. An infant with anal stenosis or imperforate anal membrane may have a normal-appearing rectum, with the condition detected only after the absence of stooling is noted.
   (4) Surgical intervention is always necessary, with the procedure dependent on the level of the anorectal pouch. A low pouch can usually be repaired by anoplasty with good results.

6. Preoperative care: see section A, "General Considerations," p. 654-655.
7. Postoperative care.
   a. Pain management (see Chapter 16).
   b. NPO regimen and gastric decompression continued until normal bowel function is restored.
   c. Routine ostomy care if applicable.
8. Postoperative complications: dependent on the level of the defect, whether there is innervation of the bowel, and what type of repair is performed.
   a. Postoperative colostomy complications include ostomy prolapse, intestinal obstruction, skin dehiscence and excoriation, and stomal ulceration and bleeding.
9. Prognosis: generally excellent with low imperforate anus although there is an association with constipation. High imperforate anus is associated with bowel incontinence.

K. Necrotizing enterocolitis (NEC).

1. Definition: an acquired disease that affects the GI system, particularly that of premature infants. It is characterized by areas of necrotic bowel, most commonly in the terminal ileum but may affect both small and large intestine.
2. Incidence: up to 10% of all admissions to the NICU; approximately 90% of cases occur in preterm infants (Kaul and Balistreri, 2002). Occurs sporadically and in clusters.
3. Single most important risk factor: prematurity. The following factors may contribute to the preterm infant's susceptibility to NEC:
   a. Decreased immunologic factors in the intestinal tract.
   b. Increased gastric pH.

c. Immature intestinal barrier.
d. Decreased intestinal motility.

4. Etiology: unclear and multifactorial. A combination of three mechanisms has been suggested as the pathogenesis of NEC:
   a. Intestinal ischemia. Generally occurs in response to asphyxia or hypoxia. A redistribution of blood flow occurs, shunting of blood away from the mesenteric, renal and peripheral vasculature beds to the cerebral and myocardial circulation. Conditions that may cause mucosal ischemia include the following:
      (1) Asphyxia or hypoxia.
      (2) Hypotension.
      (3) Hypovolemia.
      (4) Hypothermia.
      (5) Umbilical line.
      (6) Polycythemia.
      (7) Exchange transfusion.
      (8) Patent ductus arteriosus.
      (9) Severe stress.
   b. Bacterial colonization of the intestinal tract. The occurrence of NEC in clusters suggests a role for microorganism involvement. Fetal GI tract is sterile. Intestinal flora established by about 10 days in full-term newborn infants. May be delayed in preterm infants and high-risk infants who have been NPO. Organisms commonly associated with NEC include *Klebsiella, Escherichia coli, Clostridia* species.
   c. Enteral feedings.
      (1) Of all infants who have NEC, 90% to 95% have had enteral feedings.
      (2) Mechanism is unclear; formula may provide a substrate for bacterial proliferation; feeding may increase intestinal oxygen demand during nutrient absorption, resulting in tissue hypoxia.
      (3) Breast milk may have protective effect against development of NEC. Protective ingredients include secretory immunoglobulin (IgA), lactobacilli, which is an antistaphylococcal agent, complement components, lysozymes, lactoferrins, macrophages, and lymphocytes. However, NEC can occur in infants who have received breast milk (Kaul and Balistreri, 2002).
      (4) An increase in enteral feedings of greater than 20 ml/kg/day has been associated with an increased incidence of NEC (Berseth et al., 2003).
      (5) Hyperosmolar formula and medications cause fluid shifts into the intestine, leading to decreased gastrointestinal blood flow and intestinal ischemia (Thigpen and Kenner, 2003). Medications implicated in the development of NEC include aminophylline and vitamin E.
5. Onset is usually between days 3 and 10 of life. Preterm infants are more likely than term infants to develop NEC at an older age (Caty and Azizkhan, 2000).
6. The distal ileum and proximal colon are most commonly affected, although NEC can affect any or all of the small and large bowel.
7. Clinical presentation varies and includes any or all of the following findings:
   a. Abdominal distention.

b. Gastric residuals.
c. Bilious vomiting.
d. Bloody stools.
e. Lethargy.
f. Abdominal tenderness.
g. Apnea and bradycardia.
h. Hypoperfusion.
i. Hypotension due to third-space fluid loss from the intravascular space into the extracellular (third-space) compartment.
j. Temperature instability.
k. Visible loops of bowel.
l. Abdominal erythema (usually indicates peritonitis).

8. Laboratory findings include the following:
   a. Leukocytosis or leukopenia.
   b. Thrombocytopenia.
   c. Electrolyte imbalances.
   d. Metabolic acidosis.
   e. Hypoxemia.
   f. Hypercapnia.
   g. Presence of blood in stools.
   h. Carbohydrate malabsorption; may be an early sign of NEC.
   i. Disseminated intravascular coagulation (DIC).
9. X-ray findings.
   a. Diffuse gaseous distention of intestines is an early but nonspecific sign.
   b. Asymmetric bowel gas pattern and a relative lack of gas in a certain area with dilation in another area.
   c. Persistently dilated loop of bowel (usually represents advanced disease).
   d. Pneumatosis intestinalis (air within the wall of the intestine) is pathognomonic of NEC (see Chapter 14).
   e. Air in the portal venous system (see Chapter 14).
   f. Pneumoperitoneum (free air in the abdomen; represents intestinal perforation) (see Chapter 14). Absence of free air does not rule out intestinal perforation. Only about 63% of cases with perforation have radiographic evidence (Kaul and Balistreri, 2002).
10. Nonsurgical medical treatment for necrotizing enterocolitis includes the following:
   a. Pain management.
   b. NPO regimen; duration depends on clinical status.
   c. Gastric decompression.
   d. Antibiotics, 3 to 14 days, depending on clinical status.
   e. Frequent complete blood cell counts (CBC) and electrolytes to evaluate infant for thrombocytopenia and electrolyte imbalances.
   f. Serial x-ray films (usually every 6-8 hours).
   g. Respiratory and ventilatory support as needed.
   h. Circulatory support as needed to prevent hypotension. Fresh-frozen plasma, dopamine, and/or dobutamine should be considered.
   i. Platelet transfusions for thrombocytopenia.
   j. Fresh-frozen plasma for DIC; consider use of vitamin K.
   k. Careful monitoring of intake and output. "Third-spacing" of fluids is common.
   l. Frequent abdominal girth measuring.
   m. Close watch of blood glucose.

11. Surgical management.
    a. Used if medical management is not possible or fails. Indications for surgery include the following:
        (1) Absolute indication.
            (a) Pneumoperitoneum
        (2) Relative indications.
            (a) Intestinal gangrene.
            (b) Progressive clinical deterioration.
            (c) Portal vein gas.
            (d) Persistent fixed dilated loop of bowel.
            (e) Abdominal wall edema or erythema.
            (f) Progressive pneumatosis.
            (g) Progressive acidosis.
            (h) Progressive thrombocytopenia.
            (i) Leukopenia or leukocytosis.
    b. Principles of surgery for NEC are to decompress the bowel, resect necrotic bowel, and divert the proximal fecal stream.
    c. Actual procedures performed are dependent on condition and age of infant and amount of bowel necrosis.
    d. In a stable infant who has isolated necrosis with remaining bowel looking good, resection of necrotic bowel and primary anastomosis is appropriate.
    e. Placement of peritoneal drains without surgery has been very successful for the initial management of extremely low birth weight infants with perforated NEC (Lessin et al., 1998). Up to one third of these patients will not require any further surgery (Bensard et al., 2002).
    f. When there is less than 25% viable bowel, options include simple closure of abdomen (always fatal), resection of all necrotic bowel and creation of stomas (frequently results in short bowel syndrome), and proximal diversion without bowel resection (may allow healing of part of bowel). Subsequent operations are usually required to resect gangrenous bowel, but there may be enough remaining bowel for survival (Caty and Azizkhan, 2000).
12. Postoperative care includes the following:
    a. Pain management (see Chapter 16).
    b. Placement of a central venous line for TPN.
    c. Maintenance of fluid and electrolyte balance.
    d. Antibiotic therapy (both a penicillin derivative and an aminoglycoside).
    e. Gastric decompression.
    f. NPO and TPN regimens until the bowel is functioning, followed by the slow resumption of feedings with a diluted formula.
    g. Observation of stomas for color and drainage.
13. Prevention.
    a. Emphasis is on minimizing the factors contributing to NEC.
    b. Prevent/correct asphyxia, hypoxia, hypovolemia, hypotension.
    c. Correct hyperviscosity.
    d. Cautious initiation of enteral feedings in small premature infants and in infants who have had perinatal asphyxia.
    e. Careful monitoring of feeding tolerance.
    f. Oral administration of immunoglobulins and bifidobacterium may be beneficial (Kaul and Balistreri, 2002).

14. Complications.
    a. Strictures occur in approximately a third of infants with resection and creation of stomas (Thigpen and Kenner, 2003). Signs of strictures include bloody stools, failure to thrive, feeding abnormalities, and diarrhea.
    b. Other GI sequelae include enteric fistulas and short bowel syndrome (malabsorption and diarrhea).
    c. Recurrent NEC is not common but can occur.
15. Prognosis: overall survival rate for all cases is 78% to 92% (Thigpen and Kenner, 2003).
16. Focal intestinal perforation vs. NEC (Caty and Azizkhan, 2000).
    a. Focal bowel perforation can occur in the absence of NEC.
    b. Factors distinguishing focal perforation from NEC:
        (1) Less hemodynamic instability.
        (2) Less metabolic acidosis.
        (3) Improved survival rate.
        (4) Use of umbilical artery catheters and indomethacin more common.
        (5) Pathologic finding of coagulation necrosis found in NEC is absent in focal intestinal perforations.

SHORT BOWEL SYNDROME

A. **Definition:** syndrome of malabsorption and malnutrition as a result of bowel shortening.
B. **Etiology.**
    1. Surgery requiring extensive resection of bowel
        a. NEC (most common, as high as 50%) (Georgeson, 1998).
        b. Jejunal or ileal atresia.
        c. Midgut volvulus.
        d. Extensive Hirschsprung disease.
        e. Omphalocele or gastroschisis.
C. **Pathophysiology.**
    1. Depends on length of intestine, segment of remaining intestine, and whether or not the ileocecal valve is intact.
    2. Consequences are related to malabsorption due to decreased surface area and loss of specific functions of resected segments (Hwang and Shulman, 2002).
    3. Following bowel resection, the remaining bowel has the ability to adapt to increase its digestive and absorptive capabilities. Villi and crypts elongate and muscle hypertrophy occurs. Adaptive process is greater in the ileum than in the jejunum.
D. **Clinical presentation:** in general, infants experience diarrhea and malabsorption; specific problems are dependent on length of small bowel and site of intestinal loss.
    1. Loss of stomach is well tolerated if vitamin B_{12} is periodically given parenterally to prevent anemia.
    2. Jejunum is the primary site of digestion and absorption; however, these functions can be performed in other areas of the intestine after adaptation occurs. Infants with loss of jejunum tend to do much better than those whose ileum is removed. Loss of jejunum can result in nutritional deficiencies, steatorrhea, and cholestasis.

3. Ileum is responsible for absorption of fat-soluble vitamins, vitamin B_{12}, and bile salts. Loss of ileum has significant metabolic and nutritional consequences.
   a. Vitamin deficiencies (especially fat-soluble vitamins A, B_{12}, D, E, and K).
   b. Watery or fatty diarrhea.
   c. Cholelithiasis, due to depletion of bile acids.
4. Ileocecal valve delays intestinal transit time and prevents overgrowth of colonic bacteria in the small intestine. Loss of ileocecal valve results in small bowel colonization with colonic bacteria and less time for digestion and absorption of nutrients in the small intestine.
5. Loss of the colon may result in hypovolemia, dehydration, and electrolyte disturbances.

E. **Treatment.**
1. TPN regimen; cyclic administration often used.
2. Careful monitoring of complications of TPN.
3. Slow introduction of feedings, beginning with elemental formulas.
4. Provision of nonnutritive sucking.
5. Prevention of skin breakdown due to diarrhea and infection.
6. H_2 antagonists for gastric hypersecretion.
7. Cholestyramine for steatorrhea.
8. Antiperistaltic agents for persistent diarrhea.
9. Trimethoprim-sulfamethoxazole, metronidazole, or other nonabsorbable antibiotics for bacterial overgrowth.
10. Somatostatin is used to suppress intestinal hormones, decrease gastric and pancreatic secretions, and decrease splanchnic blood flow.
11. Octreotide to decrease stool output.
12. Vitamin B_{12} may be given every 6 months if ileum is lost.
13. Any of a variety of surgical procedures to increase intestinal surface area or decrease intestinal motility.
14. Intestinal transplantation: successful for only a small number of infants; reserved for infants in whom medical and other surgical management has been unsuccessful or who have life-threatening complications of TPN.
    a. Indications (Kaufman et al., 2001).
       (1) Parenteral nutrition associated liver disease.
       (2) Recurrent sepsis.
       (3) Threatened loss of central venous access.
    b. Contraindication to small bowel transplant.
       (1) Profound neurologic disabilities.
       (2) Life-threatening and other noncorrectable illnesses not directly related to the digestive system.
       (3) Severe congenital or acquired immunologic deficiencies.
       (4) Nonresectable malignancies.
       (5) Insufficient vascular patency to guarantee easy central venous access for up to 6 months following transplant.
    c. Survival.
       (1) Center specific.
       (2) 1-year survival of 70%, declining to 55% at 3 years has been reported (Reyes, 2001).

F. **Prognosis.** Both the length of small bowel and site of intestinal loss influence survival of infants receiving enteral nutrition.
1. Overall survival rate 80% to 94% (Hwang and Shulman, 2002). Long-term survival of patients treated with long-term parenteral nutrition is

significantly longer than for patients with small bowel transplant (Hwang and Shulman, 2002).

2. With an intact ileocecal valve, infants with as little as 15 cm of small bowel can survive (Cohen and Balistreri, 2002).
3. Without an intact ileocecal valve, infants require about 30 to 45 cm of small bowel for survival (Cohen and Balistreri, 2002).

BILIARY ATRESIA

A. **Definition:** obstruction of bile flow in the extrahepatic bile duct system.

B. **Incidence:** 1:10,000 live births, with a slight preponderance in females (Thigpen and Kenner, 2003).

C. **Etiology:** exact mechanism unknown. Suggested theories: alteration in embryologic development, association to viral infections, and immunologic mechanisms (Fischler et al., 2002).

D. **Associated anomalies:** occurrence in 10% to 15% of infants; include cardiovascular disorders, polysplenia, preduodenal or absent portal vein, malrotation, situs inversus, and intestinal atresias (Halamek and Stevenson, 2002).

E. **Pathophysiology.**
1. Obstruction to bile flow prevents bile from entering duodenum.
2. Deficiencies of fat-soluble vitamins and vitamin K ensue to alterations in fat digestion and absorption.
3. Bleeding tendencies can occur due to vitamin K deficiency.
4. Bile accumulates in bile ducts and gallbladder causing distention of these structures.
5. Progressive disease leads to cirrhosis of the liver and subsequent portal hypertension.

F. **Clinical presentation.**
1. Normal appearance at birth, with gradual manifestation during first month of life.
2. Jaundice; usually becomes apparent between second and sixth week of life.
3. Skin green-bronze color (because of increased direct bilirubin concentration).
4. Acholic stools (meconium is normal in color).
5. Enlarged and hard liver.
6. Portal hypertension.
   a. Hemorrhoids.
   b. Engorged abdominal and rectal veins.
   c. Splenomegaly.
   d. Ascites.
   e. Bloody stools.
7. Conjugated hyperbilirubinemia.
8. Elevated serum levels of aminotransferase, alkaline phosphatase, gamma-glutamyltranspeptidase, and 5′-nucleotidase.

G. **Diagnosis.**
1. Liver ultrasonography.
2. Liver biopsy.
3. Operative cholangiography.

H. **Surgical management.**
1. Resection of atretic segments and end-to-end anastomosis: possible in only a few cases.

2. Hepatic portoenterostomy (Kasai procedure). Intestinal conduit is created between the liver surface and small intestine. This is most successful when performed by 2 months of age (Sigalet, 2000). The conduit is sometimes exteriorized temporarily to allow assessment of bile flow.
3. Liver transplant.

I. Postoperative management.

1. Pain management (see Chapter 16).
2. NPO and parenteral nutrition regimens.
3. Gastric decompression.
4. Assessment of bile flow and replacement as appropriate (if exteriorized).
5. Careful monitoring of fluids and electrolytes.

J. Long-term management.

1. Administration of fat-soluble vitamins.
2. Administration of prophylactic antibiotics to decrease risk of cholangitis.
3. Use of formulas with medium-chain triglycerides.
4. Choleretic agents such as ursodiol (Actigall) may be given to increase bile flow.
5. Steroids are commonly given for a month, then tapered. Used for their choleretic effect and to decrease scarring at the site of anastomosis.
6. Careful monitoring for hemorrhage secondary to portal hypertension and bleeding tendencies.

K. Complications of Kasai procedure.

1. Cholangitis is the most common complication of infants undergoing the Kasai procedure. It results from bile stasis and bacterial contamination of the intestinal conduit. Cholangitis presents with fever, leukocytosis, increased serum bilirubin, and nonspecific signs of infection.
2. Cessation of bile flow.
3. Portal hypertension.

L. Prognosis.

1. Without treatment, most infants will die by 2 years of age (Thigpen and Kenner, 2003).
2. Less than 20% of patients who had a portoenterostomy survive to adulthood without a liver transplant (Sigalet, 2000).
3. Survival is improved for patients who initially undergo the Kasai procedure, later to be followed by a liver transplant.

CHOLESTASIS

A. Definition: marked impairment in bile flow.

B. Incidence: overall incidence is not reported. Incidence of cholestasis associated with TPN varies; 7% to 50%. Frequency increases with younger gestational age and longer duration of TPN. Most cases occur within 2 to 10 weeks after starting TPN; 90% of infants develop cholestasis within 13 weeks (Siafakas and Jonas, 1999).

C. Etiology: the main determinant of bile flow is the enterohepatic circulation, with the rate-limiting step being secretion of bile by the hepatocyte. The neonatal liver is prone to cholestasis because its bile acid pool size is diminished and hepatic uptake and excretion mechanisms are immature. Causes of cholestasis by anatomic location (Karpen, 2002):

1. Extrahepatic bile duct.
   a. Biliary atresia.
   b. Choledochal cyst.

   c. Choledocholithiasis.
   d. Bile duct perforation.
2. Intrahepatic bile duct.
   a. Syndrome paucity (Alagille syndrome).
   b. Nonsyndromic paucity of intrahepatic ducts.
   c. Bile duct dysgensis.
   d. Cystic fibrosis.
   e. Langerhans' cell histiocytosis.
   f. Hyper-IgM syndrome.
3. Hepatocyte.
   a. Sepsis associated.
   b. Neonatal hepatitis.
   c. Viral infections.
   d. Toxoplasmosis.
   e. Syphillis.
   f. Progressive familial intrahepatic cholestasis syndromes.
   g. Inborn errors of metabolism.
   h. Neonatal hemachromatosis.
   i. Total parenteral nutrition-associated cholestasis (TPNAC).

D. **Clinical presentation.**
1. Hepatomegaly.
2. Pruritus.
3. Clay-colored stools.
4. Laboratory findings.
   a. Direct bilirubin greater than 2 mg/dl.
   b. Direct to total bilirubin ratio greater than 15%.
   c. Elevated aminotransferase concentrations (in cases involving hepatocellular damage).
   d. Elevated alkaline phosphatase, 5′-nucleotidase or γ-glutamyl transpeptidase (GGTP) (in cases involving biliary injury or obstruction).

E. **Diagnostic evaluation:** there is no one test for cholestasis. Once it is established that the infant has conjugated hyperbilirubinemia, the diagnostic evaluation should be individualized. Work-up may include the following (Siafakas and Jonas, 1999):
1. History.
2. Stool examination.
3. Bilirubin fractionation.
4. Bacterial cultures of blood and urine.
5. Liver enzymes.
6. Assessment of synthetic liver function: serum albumin, glucose, ammonia, cholesterol, prothrombin time.
7. Urinalysis.
8. Ultrasound.
9. Serology for vital hepatitides, human immunodeficiency virus (HIV), *t*oxoplasmosis, *o*ther (congenital syphilis and viruses), *r*ubella, *c*ytomegalovirus, *h*erpes simplex virus (TORCH) infections, Venereal Disease Research Laboratory (VDRL) test.
10. Viral cultures.
11. Ophthalmologic examination.
12. Test for inborn errors of metabolism.
13. Sweat chloride test.
14. Radiographs of long bones and skull for congenital infections.

15. Hepatobiliary scintigraphy (HIDA scan).
16. Percutaneous or endoscopic cholangiography.
17. Liver biopsy.

F. **Management:** no specific therapy reverses cholestasis or prevents its progression. Goals of therapy are to improve nutritional status, maximize growth, and minimize discomfort (Dellert and Balistreri, 2000).
1. TPN management.
   a. Decrease parenteral protein to 1 to 2 g/kg/day.
   b. Decrease parenteral dextrose concentration to 10%.
   c. Eliminate copper and manganese from trace minerals in TPN.
2. Enteral feeding management.
   a. Increase enteral feedings as tolerated. Caloric intake should be 125% to 150% of recommended dietary additives (RDA).
   b. Administer formulas with medium chain triglycerides (e.g., Pregestimil, Alimentum).
   c. Encourage breast-feeding as long as infant grows appropriately.
3. Pharmacologic management.
   a. Supplemental fat-soluble vitamins. TPGS-tocopherol (Liqui-E or Nutr-E-Sol) is the preferred vitamin E preparation, to be given with a multivitamin supplement (e.g., Poly-Vi-Sol) and vitamin K. These preparations should all be mixed together for administration (Karpen, 2002).
   b. Cholestyramine to increase fecal excretion of bile acids. The decrease in bile acids returning to the liver stimulates the production of new bile acids from cholesterol, resulting in the reduction of toxic bile acids in the liver and a decrease in cholesterol. May help decrease pruritus.
   c. Rifampin for pruritus.
   d. Ursodeoxycholic acid for pruritus and to increase intestinal excretion of bile acids.
   e. Phenobarbital to decrease bile acid pool size.

G. **Complications:** related to reduction of intestinal bile acids.
1. Malabsorption of fat- and lipid-soluble vitamins: steatorrhea, growth failure, fat-soluble vitamin deficiency, mineral and trace mineral deficiency.
2. Retention of bile acids and cholesterol: pruritus, xanthomas, jaundice.
3. Hepatocellular damage: portal hypertension, variceal bleeding.
4. Liver failure.

H. **Prognosis:** related to underlying cause of cholestasis.

GASTROESOPHAGEAL REFLUX (GER)

A. **Definitions.**
1. GER: retrograde movement of gastric contents into the esophagus and above.
2. Gastroesophageal reflux disease (GERD): the symptoms of disease resulting from GER events. GERD has not been well defined in neonates.
3. Regurgitation: movement of gastric contents into the mouth. Regurgitation may be a sign of GER, but GER can occur without regurgitation (Blackburn, 1999).

B. **Incidence:** varied; 40% to 50% of infants regurgitate more than once a day (Blackburn, 1999). GER with symptoms has been noted in 3% to 10% of premature infants less than 1500 g (Orenstein, 1997).

C. **Spectrum of GER.**
1. Reflux episodes occur to some extent in all individuals, especially after meals.

2. Reflux is considered physiologic as long as the individual continues to thrive and has no complications.
3. Complications generally do not occur as long as the frequency and duration of reflux are in the normal range.
4. Infants who have regurgitation as their only sign of reflux are considered to have physiologic gastroesophageal reflux and are referred to as "happy spitters" (Orenstein et al., 1999).
5. Pathologic GER usually manifests as malnutrition, respiratory disorders, or esophagitis.

D. **Risk factors.**
1. Prematurity.
2. Birth asphyxia.
3. Neurodevelopmental delay.
4. Esophageal atresia/tracheoesophageal fistula.
5. Gastroschisis/omphalocele.
6. Duodenal atresia
7. Hiatus hernia.
8. Malrotation.
9. Esophagitis.
10. Pyloric stenosis.
11. Diaphragmatic hernia/paralysis.
12. Chronic lung disease.
13. Medications: xanthines, betamimetics, prostaglandin E_1, dopamine.
14. Extracorporeal membrane oxygenation (ECMO).

E. **Pathophysiology.** Mechanisms for reflux in infants include a transient relaxation of the lower esophageal segment (LES), delay in esophageal clearance of contents, air entry into stomach during swallowing, excessive swallowing, delayed gastric emptying, and decreased esophageal motility (Blackburn, 1999; Jadcherla, 2002). A complete understanding of the pathophysiology of GER remains unclear.

F. **Clinical presentation.**
1. Regurgitation; most common presentation in infants.
2. Fussiness.
3. Irritability.
4. "Colic."
5. Apnea.
   a. Protective airway reflexes may respond to refluxed pharyngeal material, causing laryngospasm and obstructive apnea.
   b. Reflux related apnea most commonly occurs after a meal, with the infant supine or seated. The infant may not cough, choke, or gag prior to the apneic episode.
6. Aspiration.
7. Stridor.
8. Failure to gain weight.
9. Feeding refusal.
10. Back arching with feeding.
11. Gagging.

G. **Diagnosis.**
1. Esophageal pH probe study. Detects acid reflux only; does not detect nonacid or gas reflux.
2. Intraesophageal electrical impedance study (pH independent).
3. Fluoroscopy or upper GI series.

4. Esophageal manometry study.
5. Scintigraphy.
6. Endoscopy.

H. Management.

1. Conservative measures.
   a. Interventions to minimize simple regurgitation (Blackburn, 1999).
      (1) Frequent burping.
      (2) Feeding slowly.
      (3) Small frequent feedings.
   b. Minimize/eliminate provoking and aggravating factors (Jadcherla, 2002).
      (1) Provoking factors: frequent suctioning, chest physical therapy, supine position.
      (2) Aggravating factors: xanthine and betamimetic agents (increase LES relaxation).
   c. Position infant prone or in left lateral position with 30-degree elevation.
      (1) May reduce reflux, improve gastric emptying, and decrease the risk of aspiration.
      (2) Supine, right lateral position, and upright position in a car seat can make reflux worse.
      (3) Infants with GER are exempt from the American Academy of Pediatrics (AAP) recommendations for supine positioning (AAP, 1996).
      (4) The surface on which the infant is placed prone should be firm and without soft bedding or gas-trapping objects.
   d. Thickening feedings with rice cereal, carob bean gum, or sodium alginate may be helpful.
      (1) Standard thickening instructions are to mix 1 tablespoon of dry rice cereal per ounce of formula (Orenstein, 2001).
      (2) Standard thickening mixture increases viscosity 100-fold.
      (3) Thickened formula has 150% of the caloric density of unthickened formula, thus only 65% of the volume needs to be fed.
   e. Position infant at a 45- to 60-degree angle during feeding.
   f. Avoid pressure on abdomen during feeding.
   g. Avoid jiggling or bouncing the infant during feeding.
2. Pharmacologic measures.
   a. Prokinetics. These are used to increase gastric motility. Commonly used agents include bethanechol, metoclopramide, and erythromycin.
   b. H_2 antagonists or proton pump inhibitors. These are used to reduce gastric acid when complications such as esophagitis occur. Commonly used agents include ranitidine, famotidine, and omeprazole.
   c. Acid-neutralizing agents (e.g., calcium- and aluminum-containing antacids). These are used to facilitate healing of esophagitis but are infrequently given to neonates because of the side effect of constipation.
3. Surgical measures: initiated when conservative and medical management has failed and the infant has developed or is anticipated to develop sequelae and complications (Jadcherla, 2002).
   a. Nissen fundoplication (Fig. 28-7). Stomach fundus is wrapped 360 degrees around the LES.
   b. Thal procedure. Stomach fundus is wrapped 270 degrees around the LES.

I. Complications.

1. Worsening of chronic lung disease.
2. Esophagitis; occurs in 61% to 83% of infants with clinically significant reflux (Orenstein, 1999).

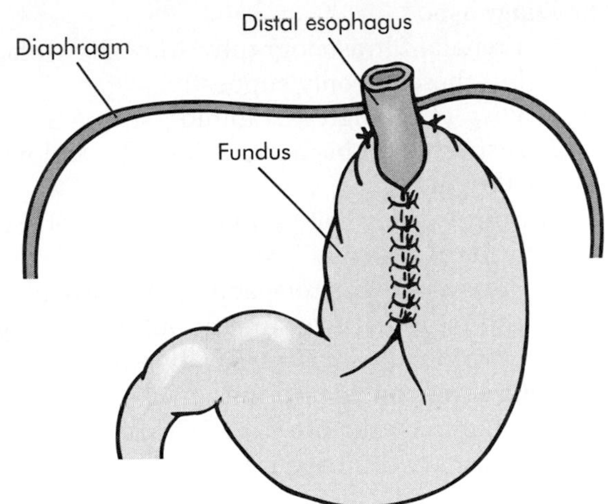

FIGURE 28-7 ■ Nissen fundoplication for repair of hiatal hernia. Fundus of stomach is wrapped around distal esophagus and sutured to itself. (From Lewis, S.M., Heitkemper, M.M., and Dirksen, S.R.: *Medical-surgical nursing: Assessment and management of clinical problems* [6th ed.]. St Louis, 2004, Mosby.)

3. Esophageal bleeding.
4. Esophageal strictures.
5. Anemia from chronic bleeding.
6. Bronchospasm and pneumonia more commonly occur in older children.

J. **Prognosis.** Resolves in almost all infants by 12 to 18 months of age (Orenstein et al., 1999); 10% to 15% require prolonged medical management; 10% to 15% also require surgery (Thigpen and Kenner, 2003). Success after fundoplication varies.

MULTISYSTEM DISORDERS WITH GASTROINTESTINAL INVOLVEMENT

Prune-Belly Syndrome

A. **Definition:** triad of congenital anomalies consisting of absence of abdominal musculature, genitourinary tract abnormalities, and cryptorchidism (undescended testes). Most common genitourinary defects are:
   1. Megaloureter.
   2. Cystic renal dysplasia.
   3. Urethral obstruction.
   4. Megacystitis.

B. **Incidence:** 1:35,000 to 1:50,000 live births (Keating and Rich, 2000). Approximately 95% of affected infants are male.

C. **Etiology:** unclear, but may be the result of a generalized developmental defect of abdominal parietes and mesenchyma. The condition is rarely familial, and no cytogenic abnormality has been discovered.

D. **Associated anomalies.**
   1. Pseudohermaphroditism in females.
   2. GI tract anomalies (30%) (Berseth, 1998b): malrotation, atresias, gastroschisis, imperforate anus, splenic torsion, persistent cloaca, Hirschsprung disease.
   3. Cardiac anomalies (10%) (Keating and Rich, 2000): patent ductus arteriosus (PDA), atrial and ventricular septal defects, tetralogy of Fallot.
   4. Pulmonary hypoplasia.
   5. Patent urachus.
   6. Musculoskeletal anomalies: clubfoot, scoliosis, congenital dislocated hips.

E. **Diagnosis.**
   1. Prenatal ultrasonography. May show bladder distention and dilated ureters, but these are only suggestive.
   2. History of oligohydramnios: suggestive of renal pathologic changes.
   3. Inspection at birth: shapeless, flat abdomen with wrinkled skin.

F. **Treatment.**
   1. Surgery may be required for repair of associated defects in the renal and urinary systems.
   2. Measures to improve abdominal musculature include use of abdominal binders and reconstructive surgery, but these are only palliative and cosmetic.
   3. Cryptorchidism is surgically repaired by orchiopexy.

G. **Long-term considerations.**
   1. Infant may require use of Credé method to empty bladder.
   2. If urinary drainage is compromised, nephrostomy or uretostomy may be performed.
   3. Constipation is a common problem.
   4. Long-term antibiotic therapy may be necessary to prevent infection.
   5. Respiratory secretions are difficult to expectorate due to the weak abdominal muscles. Respiratory infections are common. This risk is increased after general anesthesia.

H. **Prognosis:** directly related to degree of renal dysfunction. Approximately 20% of infants die during the first month of life from renal dysplasia or hypoplasia. Renal failure develops in childhood in approximately 30% of the infants who survive (Berseth, 1998b).

Congenital Diaphragmatic Hernia

A. **Definition:** herniation of abdominal organs into the thoracic cavity through a defect in the diaphragm. Severity is related to timing and degree of prenatal herniation. Early herniation through a large defect can produce bilateral pulmonary hypoplasia, resulting in death.

B. **Etiology:** failure of the pleuroperitoneal membranes to fuse. Congenital diaphragmatic hernia (CDH) may occur sporadically or be a familial disorder (Arensman and Bambini, 2000).

C. **Incidence:** 1:1000 to 1:6000 live births (Berseth, 1998b).

D. **Associated findings and anomalies.**
   1. Herniation of the intestine into the chest results in hypoplasia of the ipsilateral lung. Displacement of the mediastinum into the chest may also cause hypoplasia of the contralateral lung.
   2. Pulmonary vascular bed may be hypoplastic due to lung hypoplasia, resulting in pulmonary hypertension.
   3. Ductus arteriosus or foramen ovale usually remains patent because of pulmonary hypertension and right-to-left shunting.
   4. Associated anomalies are reported to be greater than 40% (Braby, 2001) and include CNS, cardiovascular, skeletal, GI, and genitourinary defects. Intestinal malrotation is present in all cases.
   5. Of diaphragmatic hernias, 85% to 90% occur on the left (Holland et al., 2002).
   6. The defect can vary from a small slit to the complete absence of the diaphragm on the affected side.

E. **Clinical presentation.**
   1. Respiratory distress and cyanosis at birth or shortly after birth.
   2. Decreased breath sounds on ipsilateral side of the chest.

3. Hypoxemia, hypercapnia, and respiratory acidosis.
4. Hypoperfusion and hypoxia due to right-to-left shunting through the ductus arteriosus, foramen ovale, and intrapulmonary shunts.
5. Heart tones may be shifted from their normal point of maximal intensity.
6. Barrel chest.
7. Scaphoid abdomen.

F. **Diagnosis.**
1. Prenatal ultrasonography.
2. History of polyhydramnios.
3. X-ray films showing air-filled loops of intestine within the chest and a mediastinal shift (see Chapter 14).

G. **Prenatal treatment.**
1. Prenatal surgery: Procedures to ligate the trachea have been used successfully in fetuses via both hysterotomy and endoscopic techniques. These procedures were developed based on observations that upper airway obstructions spontaneously occurring in fetal life are associated with increased lung mass. Such techniques remain highly experimental.
2. In utero repair of CDH has been performed successfully for fetuses without hepatic herniation. But infants without hepatic herniation also have good prognosis for survival with conventional treatment. In utero repair has not been shown to improve survival (Arensman and Bambini, 2000).

H. **Postnatal treatment and preoperative care.**
1. Gastric decompression should be performed as soon as possible to prevent entrance of air into the herniated intestine.
2. Intubation and positive-pressure ventilation. Bag-mask ventilation should be avoided to prevent gastric distention.
3. Prophylactic surfactant treatment at birth has had some success in improving oxygenation in infants with CDH but its effectiveness is still investigational (Arensman and Bambini, 2000).
4. CDH is no longer considered a surgical emergency (Adzick and Nance, 2000). Optimal timing of repair remains controversial. Primary concerns immediately after birth are pulmonary hypoplasia and pulmonary hypertension. Immediate treatment must be prompt and aggressive. Two primary considerations are:
   a. Establishment of adequate perfusion and oxygen status.
   b. Correction of acid-base imbalances.
5. Carefully monitor infant for pneumothorax, which is more common in the contralateral side of the chest.
6. Inotropes are used to increase systemic blood pressure and decrease right-to-left shunting.
7. Mechanical ventilation.
   a. Hyperventilation is controversial. Although hyperventilation induces respiratory alkalosis and pulmonary artery vasodilation, it may result in ventilation-induced lung injury. Sensorineural hearing loss has also been associated with hyperventilation.
   b. In a multicenter observational study on infants with persistent pulmonary hypertension of the newborn, treatment with hyperventilation was clearly shown to not be equivalent to treatment with alkali infusion. Infants treated with alkali infusion had a much greater chance of treatment with ECMO compared with those treated with hyperventilation, and an increased rate of supplemental oxygen administration at 28 days (Walsh-Sukys et al., 2000).

c. Permissive hypercapnia may minimize ventilator-induced lung injury and result in improved survival (Braby, 2001).
d. High-frequency oscillatory ventilation (HFOV) is often used. There are reports of improved survival of infants with CDH treated with HFOV; however, its benefits over conventional ventilation still need to be investigated (Cacciari et al., 2001; Reyes et al., 1998).

8. Inhaled nitric oxide (iNO) may be considered.
   a. iNO has been used in neonates with severe hypoxemia to improve oxygenation. iNO dilates the pulmonary arteries, decreases pulmonary vascular resistance, and decreases a right-to-left shunt across the ductus arteriosus.
   b. iNO has not been shown to reduce the need for ECMO or improve survival in infants with CDH (Clark et al., 2000)
   c. May be helpful in stabilizing infants for transport and initiation of ECMO.
9. ECMO is instituted if ventilation does not effectively stabilize infant's pulmonary status. ECMO may be used preoperatively to stabilize the patient for surgery, intraoperatively if the infant cannot be weaned from ECMO, and/or postoperatively to rest the lungs.
   a. Approximately 50% of infants with CDH are treated with ECMO (Stevens et al., 2002).
   b. 58% of infants placed on ECMO for CDH survive to discharge or transfer (Extracorporeal Life Support Organization, 2000).
   c. A recent retrospective analysis of full-term infants treated with ECMO showed that late-term delivery ($40\frac{0}{7}$-$41\frac{6}{7}$) had improved survival, shorter ECMO duration, shorter hospital length of stay, and fewer complications on ECMO compared with infants delivered at $38\frac{0}{7}$ to $39\frac{6}{7}$ weeks (Stevens et al., 2002).

I. Surgical repair.

1. Primary closure of the diaphragmatic defect is usually possible.
2. When primary closure is not possible, a synthetic patch or muscle flap can be used to close the diaphragmatic defect.

J. Postoperative special considerations.

1. Appropriate pain management should be initiated (see Chapter 16).
2. Gastric decompression should continue until the bowel is functioning (approximately 7-10 days).
3. A chest tube for drainage should be placed on water seal (without suction) to prevent acute mediastinal shift.
4. Pulmonary management should be carried out very carefully because of hypoplastic lungs and potential for pulmonary hypertension and pneumothorax. If pulmonary management fails, ECMO or iNO may be considered.
5. Blood pressure and perfusion may be especially problematic, and vasopressors such as dopamine and/or dobutamine may be required.

K. Prognosis: survival has recently been reported to be 63% in a multicenter series. However, this information does not reflect infants who did not reach a tertiary care center for management (Clark et al., 1998).

1. Onset of symptoms after 1 day of age increases the survival rate (Holland et al., 2002).
2. Increased mortality rates have been associated with prenatal diagnosis, right-sided diaphragmatic hernia, and the 1-minute Apgar score (Skari et al., 2002). However, there is no absolutely reliable predictor of mortality.
3. Prognosis most often related to degree of pulmonary hypoplasia.

HYPERBILIRUBINEMIA

A. Natural history.

1. Visible jaundice develops in more than 60% of all term newborn infants (AAP, 1994).
2. Most newborn infants will appear jaundiced when their serum bilirubin concentration is greater than 6 to 7 mg/dl. Jaundice first appears on the face and progresses caudally as serum bilirubin levels increase.

B. Bilirubin metabolism (Fig. 28-8).

1. Synthesis.
   a. Bilirubin is produced from the breakdown of heme-containing proteins.
      (1) Major heme-containing protein is erythrocyte hemoglobin (produces 75% of all bilirubin). Catabolism of 1 g of hemoglobin produces 34 mg of bilirubin.
      (2) A small percentage (approximately 25%) of bilirubin comes from the breakdown of other proteins, such as myoglobin, cytochromes, catalase, and peroxidases.
   b. Normal neonates will produce 6 to 10 mg of bilirubin per kilogram per day.
   c. Newborn infants produce twice as much bilirubin per day as adults do.

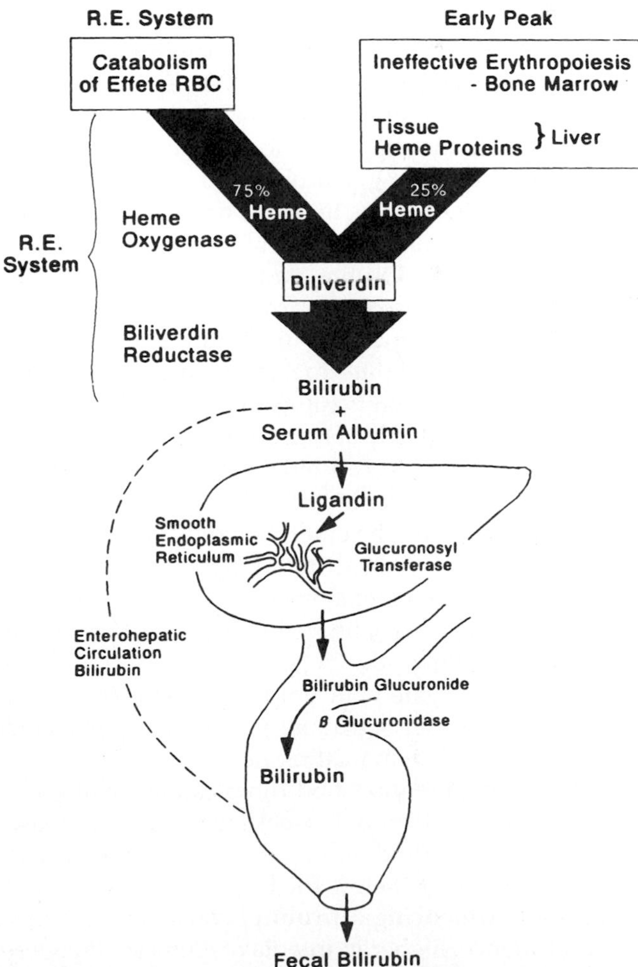

FIGURE 28-8 ■ Neonatal bile pigment metabolism. *RE,* Reticuloendothelial; *RBC,* red blood cells. (From Maisels, M.J.: Jaundice. In G.B. Avery, M.A. Fletcher, and M.G. MacDonald (Eds.): *Neonatology: Pathophysiology and management of the newborn* [5th ed.]. Philadelphia, 1999, Lippincott Williams & Wilkins, p. 767.)

2. Transport.
   a. Newly synthesized bilirubin is referred to as unconjugated, is measured as indirect bilirubin, and is fat soluble. The last reason explains its propensity for fatty tissues such as subcutaneous and brain tissue.
   b. Bilirubin binds to albumin for transport in the blood to the liver.
   c. Each gram of albumin can bind with approximately 8.5 to 10 mg of bilirubin.
   d. The binding of bilirubin to albumin is reversible; factors that can decrease albumin-bilirubin binding include:
      (1) Metabolic derangements: acidosis, hypoxia.
      (2) Hypothermia.
      (3) Infection.
      (4) Drugs: salicylates, sulfonamides, sodium benzoate, indomethacin, ampicillin (when rapidly injected).
      (5) Free fatty acids: from emulsified fats (Intralipid), starvation, hypothermia, hypoglycemia, and anoxia.
   e. Bound bilirubin does not usually enter the CNS and is nontoxic.
   f. When available albumin binding sites are saturated, unconjugated bilirubin circulates as free bilirubin and can cross the blood-brain barrier, causing kernicterus.
3. Liver uptake, conjugation, and excretion.
   a. Once in the liver, bilirubin detaches from albumin and enters the hepatocyte.
   b. Within the hepatocytes, bilirubin binds to protein Y (ligandin), protein Z, and glutathione S-transferase for transport to the smooth endoplasmic reticulum for conjugation.
   c. Inside the smooth endoplasmic reticulum of the hepatocyte, bilirubin is converted to glucuronic acid with the aid of glucuronyl transferase.
      (1) This process depends on adequate amounts of glucose and oxygen.
      (2) The converted bilirubin is referred to as conjugated, is measured as direct bilirubin, and is water soluble.
   d. This water-soluble form of bilirubin is then excreted into the bile and eventually into the duodenum to be excreted later in the stool.
   e. In the small intestine, the high concentration of beta-glucuronidase in newborn infants can convert this bilirubin back into the fat-soluble form, which is easily absorbed from the small intestine into the portal circulation. Because the venous blood supply leaving the intestines goes directly to the liver, this process is referred to as the enterohepatic circulation. The enterohepatic circulation may explain why infants with GI obstructions distal to the ampulla of Vater have hyperbilirubinemia.
4. Fetal bilirubin metabolism.
   a. Conjugation is limited in the fetus because there is limited fetal hepatic blood flow.
   b. Unconjugated bilirubin in the fetus is cleared by the placenta.
   c. Conjugated bilirubin in the fetus is not cleared by the placenta and may accumulate in fetal tissue.
   d. Small amounts of bilirubin can normally be found in amniotic fluid between 12 and 37 weeks' gestation. Increased amounts of bilirubin in the amniotic fluid may indicate hemolytic disease or fetal intestinal obstruction below the bile ducts.

C. Factors influencing bilirubin levels.

1. Incidence: higher in infants of Chinese, Japanese, Korean, Native American, and Greek descent.

2. Perinatal events.
   a. Delayed cord clamping, which increases erythrocyte volume.
   b. Breech presentation and delivery with the use of vacuum extraction or forceps, which produce bruising and subsequent erythrocyte destruction.
   c. Use of oxytocin. The mechanism is unclear but may involve hemolysis.
   d. Use of epidural bupivacaine. The mechanism is unclear but may involve hemolysis due to changes in erythrocyte deformability.
   e. Asphyxia.
      (1) Inability of liver to process bilirubin.
      (2) Intracranial hemorrhage.
3. Maternal diabetes. Possibly related to hypoxia, polycythemia, or delayed hepatic uptake of bilirubin.
4. Early feeding, which decreases serum bilirubin by decreasing the reabsorption of bile caused by increased gut motility. Feeding introduces bacteria into the gut, which contributes to the conversion of bilirubin to urobilin, a substance that cannot be reabsorbed.

D. Physiologic jaundice.

1. Jaundice is the clinical manifestation of hyperbilirubinemia. Jaundice is usually visible when the bilirubin level reaches 5 to 7 mg/dl (Blackburn, 2003).
2. Physiologic jaundice is the manifestation of the normal hyperbilirubinemia seen in newborn infants and is a diagnosis of exclusion.
3. Chemical hyperbilirubinemia (bilirubin ≥2 mg/dl) is present in essentially all newborn infants during the first week of life because of the limitations and abnormalities of bilirubin metabolism (MacMahon et al., 1998).
4. Physiologic jaundice occurs in 50% to 60% of term infants and up to 80% of preterm infants (Blackburn, 2003).
5. Physiologic jaundice is due to a combination of the following:
   a. Increased bilirubin load to liver.
      (1) Newborn infants have a larger red blood cell mass.
      (2) The life span of red blood cells is shorter in neonates (70-90 days vs. 120 days in adults).
      (3) Newborn infants produce a greater amount of bilirubin from sources other than red blood cells.
      (4) Neonates have an increased reabsorption of bilirubin from the intestine (enterohepatic circulation) secondary to decreased GI motility, increased β-glucuronidase activity, and decreased intestinal flora.
   b. Decreased hepatic uptake secondary to decreased ligandin and binding of Y- and Z-proteins by other anions.
   c. Defective conjugation secondary to decreased glucuronyl transferase activity.
   d. Decreased excretion of bilirubin.
6. Bilirubin levels generally peak on day 3 of life in full-term infants and days 5 to 6 in preterm infants.
7. Hyperbilirubinemia in preterm infants is an exaggerated form of physiologic jaundice, mainly because of increased red blood cell breakdown from a short red blood cell life span and decreased glucuronyl transferase activity in the liver cell (Shaw, 2003).
8. Bilirubin is a potent antioxidant and may have protective properties against oxygen-free radicals during the newborn period (Halamek and Stevenson, 2002).

E. Breast-feeding and jaundice.
1. Breast-fed infants have higher bilirubin levels than bottle-fed infants.
2. Breast-feeding vs. breast milk jaundice.
   a. Breast-feeding jaundice.
      (1) Early onset, starting at 2 to 4 days of life.
      (2) Related to inadequate frequency of breast-feeding during early days of lactation and subsequent decreased fluid and caloric intake.
      (3) Can be avoided by frequent breast-feeding and avoiding glucose water supplementation.
   b. Breast milk jaundice.
      (1) Late onset, usually starting at 4 to 7 days of life.
      (2) Occurs in 10% to 30% of breast-fed newborn infants in weeks 2 to 6 of life.
      (3) Bilirubin levels can reach 12 to 20 mg/dl and remain elevated for up to 2 months.
      (4) Recognized as prolonged physiologic jaundice.
      (5) Related to the ingredients in breast milk. Mechanisms may include the following:
         (a) Decreased conjugation secondary to inhibition of glucuronyl transferase by pregnanediol and nonesterified fatty acids (Shaw, 2003).
         (b) Increased enterohepatic circulation due to increased β-glucuronidase activity in breast milk (Frank et al., 2002).
         (c) Increased fat absorption from breast milk, which results in decreased unabsorbed fat in intestinal lumen and subsequent decreased capacity to excrete unconjugated bilirubin in fecal fat (Verkade, 2002).
3. Treatment.
   a. The AAP does not encourage the interruption of breast-feeding in healthy term infants (AAP, 1994).
   b. Mother's preference and physician's judgment are important considerations.
   c. The following options are acceptable (AAP, 1994):
      (1) Observe.
      (2) Continue breast-feeding; start phototherapy.
      (3) Supplement breast-feeding with bottle feeding, with or without phototherapy.
      (4) Temporarily discontinue breast-feeding; substitute bottle feeding.
      (5) Temporarily discontinue breast-feeding; substitute bottle feeding and start phototherapy.
   d. Bilirubin levels should decrease rapidly after discontinuance of breast-feeding. If levels do not decrease by 72 hours, breast milk jaundice is not the diagnosis.
   e. When breast-feeding is begun again, bilirubin levels may increase slightly but not to previous high levels.
   f. Provision of water or dextrose supplements to healthy breast-fed infants does not seem to be beneficial and is not recommended (Shaw, 2003).

F. Transcutaneous bilirubinometry.
1. Use of devices to measure transcutaneous bilirubin (TcB) remain controversial.
   a. Minolta Jaundice Meter (Hill-Rom/Airshield, Hatboro, PA) provides a numerical index based on spectral reflectance. Measurements have been shown to be affected by skin pigmentation (Bhutani et al., 2000).

b. BiliCheck (SpectRx Inc., Norcross, GA) provides a numerical index based on multiwavelength spectral analysis. This device does not appear to be affected by skin pigmentation. There are conflicting reports on its ability to accurately reflect total serum bilirubin in term and near-term infants (Bhutani et al., 2000; Engle et al., 2002).
2. These devices help establish a risk assessment about an infant, but not necessarily determine the exact serum bilirubin concentration (Schumacher, 2002).
3. Usefulness of these devices in preterm infants, infants receiving phototherapy, and those with total serum bilirubin values greater than or equal to 15 mg/dl needs further study.

G. **Pathologic unconjugated hyperbilirubinemia.** (For blood incompatibilities, see Chapter 30.)
1. A pathologic reason for unconjugated hyperbilirubinemia is suggested by any of the following criteria (Frank et al., 2002):
   a. Jaundice that appears in the first 24 hours of life.
   b. Total serum bilirubin level that increases by more than 5 mg/dl per day.
   c. Total serum bilirubin level that exceeds 12.9 mg/dl in a term infant or 15 mg/dl in a preterm infant.
   d. Direct serum bilirubin level that exceeds 1 to 2 mg/dl.
   e. Jaundice lasting for more than 1 week in a term infant or 2 weeks in a preterm infant.
2. Etiology.
   a. Hemolysis.
      (1) ABO/Rh incompatibilities.
      (2) Bacterial and viral sepsis (especially TORCH infections).
      (3) Inherited disorders of red blood cell (RBC) metabolism.
         (a) RBC membrane defects (e.g., spherocytosis, elliptocytosis).
         (b) RBC enzyme defects (e.g., glucose-6-phosphate dehydrogenase deficiency).
      (4) Inherited disorders of bilirubin metabolism (e.g., Crigler-Najjar syndrome types I and II, Gilbert disease).
      (5) Conditions acquired secondary to maternal drug use and microangiopathies.
   b. Extravasation of blood.
      (1) Cephalohematoma.
      (2) Pulmonary, cerebral, or retroperitoneal hemorrhage.
   c. Swallowed blood.
   d. Increased enterohepatic circulation.
      (1) Delayed feeding.
      (2) Intestinal obstructions.
   e. Decreased hepatic function and perfusion.
      (1) Hypoxia.
      (2) Asphyxia.
      (3) Sepsis.
   f. Hypothyroidism.
   g. Hypopituitarism.
   h. Inborn errors of metabolism (with both unconjugated and conjugated hyperbilirubinemia).
      (1) Galactosemia.
      (2) α_1-antitrypsin deficiency.
      (3) Tyrosinosis.

(4) Hypermethioninemia.
(5) Cystic fibrosis.

H. Bilirubin toxic effects.

1. Definition.

a. Acute bilirubin encephalopathy (kernicterus): bilirubin staining of neurons and neuronal injury, particularly in the basal ganglia (Volpe, 2001).

2. Incidence: rare. There are no data on the incidence of kernicterus in the U.S. population; however, recent reports indicate that it is still occurring (AAP, 2001).

3. Etiology.

a. Unbound (free) bilirubin can cross the blood-brain barrier, where it stains and injures brain cells.

b. Mechanism by which neuronal injury occurs is unclear.

c. Factors that decrease albumin-bilirubin binding or alter the integrity of the blood-brain barrier put the infant at risk of having bilirubin toxic effects.

(1) Hypoproteinemia.
(2) Drugs that compete with bilirubin for binding sites on albumin: sulfisoxazole, salicylates, sodium benzoate, indomethacin).
(3) Sepsis.
(4) Acidosis.
(5) Hypoxia.

4. Risk assessment.

a. When early follow-up as recommended by the AAP cannot be ensured, timing of discharge or other follow-up should be based upon risk assessment (AAP, 2001).

b. Strategies for identifying infants at risk for developing severe hyperbilirubinemia (AAP, 2001):

(1) Use of common clinical risk factors.
  (a) Jaundice in the first 24 hours.
  (b) Visible jaundice before discharge.
  (c) Previous jaundiced sibling.
  (d) Gestation 35 to 38 weeks.
  (e) Exclusive breast-feeding.
  (f) East Asian race.
  (g) Bruising, cephalohematoma.
  (h) Maternal age greater than or equal to 25 years.
  (i) Male sex.
(2) Calculation of a risk index score (Fig. 28-9).
(3) Measuring serum or transcutaneous bilirubin level before discharge. Bhutani and colleagues (1999) have developed an hour-specific nomogram in which a predischarge total serum bilirubin is plotted (Fig. 28-10). From this, the infant is assigned a low, intermediate, or high risk for developing clinically significant hyperbilirubinemia.

5. Clinical presentation. Major neurologic features involve abnormalities of level of consciousness, tone and movement, and brainstem function, especially related to feeding and cry (Volpe, 2001).

a. Initial phase: slight stupor (lethargy), hypotonia, paucity of movement, poor suck, high-pitched cry.

b. Intermediate phase: moderate stupor often with irritability, increased tone, especially with stimulation, backward arching of neck (retrocollis), or back (opisthotonos), fever.

VARIABLE	SCORE
Exclusive breast-feeding	6
Family history of jaundice in a newborn	6
Bruising noted	4
Asian race	4
Cephalohematoma noted	3
Maternal age ≥25 years	3
Male sex	1
Black race	−2
Gestational age, weeks	2 (40-GA)

*Risk index score is calculated as the sum of all characteristics that apply to the patient, except that points for gestational age (GA) are assigned based on twice the difference of GA from 40 weeks. For example, a 37-week bottle-fed Asian male newborn whose mother was 30 years old would receive a score of 14: 6 (2 × [40-37]) + 4 (Asian) + 1 (male) + 3 (mother >25 y).

FIGURE 28-9 ■ Risk index for predicting total serum bilirubin (TSB) greater than or equal to 428 μmol/L (25 mg/dl) in newborns who do not have early jaundice.* (From Newman, T.B., Xiong, B., Gonzales, V.M., and Escobar, G.J.: Prediction and prevention of extreme neonatal hyperbilirubinemia in a mature health maintenance organization. *Archives of Pediatric and Adolescent Medicine, 154*[11]:1144-1147, 2000.)

c. Advanced phase: deep stupor to coma, pronounced retrocollis/opisthotonos, no feeding.

d. Chronic bilirubin encephalopathy.

(1) During the first year of life, characteristic findings are hypotonia, active deep tendon reflexes, persistent tonic neck reflex, and delayed acquisition of motor skills. These findings are usually not apparent until after 6 months to 1 year of age.

(2) Characteristics of fully developed encephalopathy may not be clearly evident for several years. These include hearing loss, choreoathetoid cerebral palsy, and gaze abnormalities, especially upward gaze. Intellectual deficits are common but usually not severe.

6. Treatment. There is no treatment for kernicterus. Prevention of hyperbilirubinemia, early detection, and management are the most effective strategies.

I. Management of unconjugated hyperbilirubinemia.

1. The goal of treating hyperbilirubinemia is to prevent bilirubin toxic effects.

2. Although kernicterus is rare, there is evidence that healthy term infants are at risk (Johnson et al., 2002).

3. Guidelines for treating hyperbilirubinemia in healthy term infants are listed in Table 28-4. The AAP (2001) has recently given emphasis to the following:

a. Any infant who is jaundiced before 24 hours requires a measurement of serum bilirubin, and if it is elevated the infant should be evaluated for possible hemolytic disease.

b. Follow-up should be provided within 2 to 3 days of discharge to all neonates discharged at less than 48 hours after birth. Early follow-up is particularly important for infants greater than 38 weeks' gestation. Timing of follow-up depends on the age at discharge and the presence of risk factors.

4. Management of hyperbilirubinemia in low birth weight infants is determined by clinical status, age, weight, and history (Table 28-5).

5. In hemolytic disease, phototherapy is begun immediately.

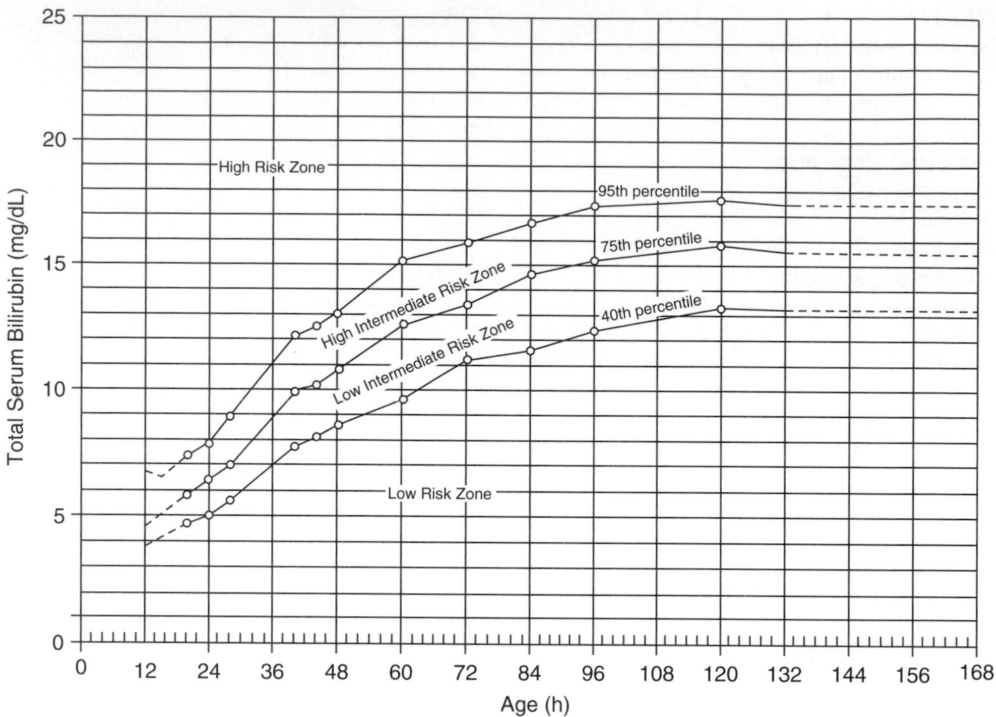

FIGURE 28-10 ■ Risk designation of term and near-term well newborns based on their hour-specific serum bilirubin values. The high-risk zone is designated by the 95th percentile track. The intermediate-risk zone is subdivided to upper- and lower-risk zones by the 75th percentile track. The low-risk zone has been electively and statistically defined by the 40th percentile track. (Dotted extensions are based on <300 total serum bilirubin (TSB) values/epoch.) (From Bhutani, V.K., Johnson, L., and Sivieri, E.M.: Predictive ability of a predischarge hour-specific serum bilirubin for subsequent significant hyperbilirubinemia in healthy term and near-term newborns, *Pediatrics, 103*[1]:6-14, 1999.)

J. Phototherapy.

1. Most effective in decreasing nonhemolytic hyperbilirubinemia.
   a. Decreases serum bilirubin 20% to 30% by day 2 of life and 41% to 55% by day 4 of life (Shaw, 2003).
2. Mechanism for phototherapy action.
   a. Photo-oxidation.
      (1) Accounts for only 15% of photodecomposition of bilirubin (Shaw, 2003).
      (2) Involves oxidation of bilirubin to water-soluble products excreted in urine.
   b. Photoisomerization.
      (1) Major mechanism of phototherapy action.
      (2) Involves the conversion of bilirubin to water-soluble structural and configurational isomers that can be excreted by the liver without conjugation.
   c. Increased hepatic excretion of unconjugated bilirubin and increased bowel transit time are also believed to result from phototherapy (Shaw, 2003).
3. Effectiveness: influenced by energy output of phototherapy unit, spectrum of light, and amount of infant's body surface area exposed to light.

■ TABLE 28-4
■ ■ **Management of Hyperbilirubinemia in Healthy Term Neonate***

	TSB Level, mg/dl (Φmol/l)			
Age (hr)	**Consider Phototherapy***	**Phototherapy**	**Exchange Transfusion If Intensive Phototherapy Fails†**	**Exchange Transfusion and Intensive Phototherapy**
≤24‡	C	C	C	C
25-48	∃12 (170)	∃15 (260)	∃20 (340)	∃25 (430)
49-72	∃15 (260)	∃18 (310)	∃25 (430)	∃30 (510)
>72	∃17 (290)	∃20 (340)	∃25 (430)	∃30 (510)

TSB, Total serum bilirubin.
*Phototherapy at these TSB levels is a clinical option, meaning that the intervention is available and may be used *on the basis of individual clinical judgment.*
†Intensive phototherapy should produce a decline of TSB of 1 to 2 mg/dl within 4 to 6 hours and the TSB level should continue to fall and remain below the threshold level for exchange transfusion. If this does not occur, it is considered a failure of phototherapy.
‡Term infants who are clinically jaundiced at ≤24 hours old are not considered healthy and require further evaluation.
From American Academy of Pediatrics Provisional Committee for Quality Improvement and Subcommittee on Hyperbilirubinemia: Practice parameter: Management of hyperbilirubinemia in the healthy term newborn. *Pediatrics, 94* (4 pt1):558-565, 1994. Used with permission.

4. Delivery methods.
   a. Bilirubin can absorb light of only certain wavelengths (blue, violet, green). Photodecomposition of bilirubin occurs most effectively with lights having an output close to the maximum absorption peak of bilirubin (450-460 nm). Lights that emit blue wavelengths of approximately 425 to 475 nm achieve this most effectively.
   b. Not all blue lights are equally effective. Only "special blue" lights (labeled F20 T12/BB) are more effective than white lamps. Disadvantages of these lights are that they create a difficult environment in which to work, and they distort an infant's color.
   c. White lamps, tungsten-halogen lamps, and fiberoptic "blankets" are effective alternatives and do not make the infant look cyanotic. Halogen lamps cannot be placed as close to the infant due to the risk of burning the infant.

■ TABLE 28-5
■ ■ **Management of Hyperbilirubinemia in the Low Birth Weight Infant**

	Total Serum Bilirubin Level, mg/dl			
	Healthy		Sick	
Gestational Age	**Phototherapy**	**Exchange Transfusion**	**Phototherapy**	**Exchange Transfusion**
Premature				
<1000 g	5-7	Variable	4-6	Variable
1001-1500 g	7-10	Variable	6-8	Variable
1501-2000 g	10-12	Variable	8-10	Variable
2001-2500 g	12-15	Variable	10-12	Variable

From Halamek, L.P. and Stevenson, D.K: Neonatal Jaundice and liver disease. In A.A. Fararoff and R.J. Martin, (Eds.): *Neonatal-perinatal medicine: Diseases of the fetus and infant (7th ed.).* St Louis, 2002, Mosby, p. 1335.

d. Advantages of the fiberoptic "blankets" are that eyepatches are not needed, the infant can be held while phototherapy is maintained, and phototherapy can be administered outside of the nursery with less interference on maternal-infant bonding.

5. Management of phototherapy and of the infant receiving phototherapy.
   a. Fluorescent lights should be at a distance of 45 to 50 cm from the infant to provide optimal irradiance.
   b. Manufacturer's instructions should be followed for appropriate distance of spotlights.
   c. When bank lights are used, lamps should be covered with Plexiglas to protect the infant from ultraviolet light.
   d. Fluorescent lights should be placed at least 2 inches from the top of an incubator.
   e. Recommendations for changing lamp bulbs range from 200 to 2000 hours of use because of decreased energy output. Use of a spectroradiometer is probably a more useful strategy to ensure optimal irradiance. Light irradiance of 4 to 6 $\mu W/cm^2/nm$, as measured by spectroradiometer is required for optimal phototherapy efficacy (Shaw, 2003).
   f. Infants receiving phototherapy need to have as much skin exposed as possible.
   g. Infants receiving phototherapy via bank lights or halogen lights need to have their eyes covered with eyepatches to protect them from the strong light. Phototherapy should be temporarily discontinued to remove eyepatches, provide visual stimulation, and allow the parents to hold and feed the infant.
   h. Turn the infant frequently to allow all areas of the skin to be exposed.
   i. Temperature control is important to monitor whether the infant is in an open crib, an incubator, or an overhead warmer.
   j. Monitor fluids carefully.
      (1) Phototherapy increases insensible water loss. Fluid intake should be increased appropriately.
      (2) Phototherapy may cause diarrhea with further fluid loss.
   k. Monitor bilirubin levels after phototherapy is discontinued. A rebound of 1 to 2 mg/dl can be expected.
6. Side effects.
   a. Loose stools.
   b. Hyperthermia.
   c. Bronze baby syndrome: thought to be caused by skin deposition of copper porphyrins, a photoproduct of bilirubin degradation, leading to bronze colored skin and urine (Shaw, 2003).
   d. Dehydration.
   e. Skin rashes.
   f. Lethargy.
   g. Abdominal distention.
   h. Hypocalcemia.
   i. Lactose intolerance.
   j. Eye damage.
   k. Thrombocytopenia.
7. Home phototherapy: an option that decreases hospitalization time for an otherwise healthy newborn infant. Temperature control and fluid intake need to be monitored carefully.

K. Exchange transfusion.

1. The decision to perform an exchange transfusion should be made while taking into consideration the bilirubin level, how quickly the level is rising, the gestational age of the infant, and the age (in hours and days) of the infant.
2. Early exchange transfusion is indicated in infants with significant hemolytic disease such as hydrops fetalis, particularly with cord bilirubin levels greater than 4.5 mg/dl and cord hemoglobin less than 11 g/dl.
3. A double-volume exchange transfusion removes 85% to 90% of the infant's RBC volume and 25% of the infant's total bilirubin.
4. Administration of 25% albumin, 1 g/kg 1 to 2 hours to infants with low serum albumin before the transfusion, may increase albumin-bilirubin binding and facilitate movement of bilirubin from the tissues into the intravascular space, thereby increasing the amount of bilirubin exchanged. This therapy remains controversial, because the albumin equilibrates with extravascular albumin quickly and may facilitate movement of bilirubin from the intravascular space into the extravascular space (Shaw, 2003). Albumin administration is contraindicated in neonates with severe anemia, hydrops, or congestive heart failure.
5. Infant should be NPO prior to procedure; if NPO status has not been maintained, remove gastric contents with orogastric tube.
6. Selection of blood.
   a. If performing exchange transfusion for Rh incompatibility, use type-specific and Rh-negative blood. O-negative blood cross-matched with mother's blood may also be used.
   b. If performing exchange transfusion for ABO incompatibility, use O-type Rh-specific or low-titer (low anti-A and anti-B) O-type cells suspended in AB plasma.
   c. If infant is immunocompromised or has received an intrauterine transfusion, use irradiated blood to minimize the risk of graft-versus-host disease.
   d. Blood less than 48 hours old should be used to minimize problems with elevated potassium that occurs in older blood.
   e. Cytomegalovirus (CMV)-negative blood is always used for neonatal transfusions.
7. Procedure for exchange transfusion.
   a. Treat hypoglycemia, acidosis, hypotension, and temperature control before the start of an exchange transfusion.
   b. The infant is secured on a radiant warmer and placed on a cardiorespiratory monitor. Oxygen and suction should be available at the bedside. Vital signs should be assessed frequently during transfusion.
   c. Ideally, an umbilical artery catheter and umbilical venous catheter are placed (see Chapter 15 for procedure).
   d. The initial blood removed should be sent to the laboratory for CBC, bilirubin and calcium, and blood cultures.
   e. The exchange should be done slowly. Procedure usually lasts 1 to 2 hours. Small aliquots, e.g., 3 to 5 ml/kg, should be used in preterm or critically ill patients; larger aliquots, e.g., 10 ml/kg, can be used in full-term infants.
   f. Accurate recording of blood volumes exchanged is essential during the procedure.

g. Watch carefully for hypocalcemia. The citrates found in the anticoagulants (acid-citrate-dextrose and citrate-phosphate-dextrose negative [CPD-] adenosine) bind to calcium. Symptoms of hypocalcemia include the following:
(1) Irritability.
(2) Tachycardia.
(3) Prolonged QT interval.
h. Calcium gluconate should be administered if the infant has hypocalcemia. Normal dose is 1 ml of 10% solution.
i. Always have a resuscitation cart nearby during an exchange transfusion.
j. Evaluate medications. Medications known to decrease significantly during exchange transfusions should be administered after the transfusion (e.g., ampicillin, gentamicin, digoxin, phenobarbital, vancomycin).
8. Complications of exchange transfusions.
a. Embolization.
b. Thrombosis.
c. Hyperglycemia or hypoglycemia.
d. Hyperkalemia.
e. Hypocalcemia.
f. Hypomagnesemia.
g. Acidosis.
h. NEC.
i. Overheparinization.
j. Thrombocytopenia.
k. Infection.
l. Cardiac arrhythmias and arrest.
m. Heart failure.
9. Postexchange care. Phototherapy should be continued after exchange transfusion.
a. Recheck bilirubin levels every 4 hours. Rebound usually occurs within 1 hour after the exchange.
b. Check blood glucose levels frequently. Rebound hypoglycemia can occur because the dextrose concentration in the blood preservatives is equivalent to 300 mg of glucose per liter of blood (Shaw, 2003). In response to the high dextrose concentration, the infant secretes insulin, which will require supplemental glucose if hypoglycemia is to be avoided.
c. Observe closely for signs of complications, such as infection, electrolyte imbalance, NEC, and thrombosis.

L. Alternative therapies.
1. Early feeding: decreases the enterohepatic circulation.
2. Binding agents: agar and activated charcoal bind bilirubin in the gut and decrease the enterohepatic circulation.
3. Phenobarbital: increases hepatic ligandin concentration.
4. Metalloporphyrins: inhibit heme oxygenase, the enzyme that catalyzes the conversion of heme to biliverdin, thereby decreasing bilirubin production. Tin mesoporphyrin and tin protoporphyrin are the two metalloporphyrins most commonly used; however, their use is still investigational.

M. Conjugated hyperbilirubinemia (direct).
1. Causes of elevated conjugated bilirubin.
a. Liver cell injury.

(1) Cholestatic jaundice related to use of parenteral nutrition.
(2) Infection.
(a) Viral.
(b) Bacterial.
(c) Parasitic.
(3) Hepatitis.
(4) Drugs.
b. Bile flow obstruction.
(1) Biliary atresia.
(2) Extrahepatic obstruction (choledochal cyst, trisomy 13 or 18, or polysplenia).
(3) Intrahepatic obstruction (choledochal cyst, bile duct stenosis, bile duct rupture, tumors, cystic fibrosis).
c. Excessive bilirubin load.
d. Maternal-fetal blood group incompatibility (i.e., ABO, Rh; see Chapter 30).
2. Management of conjugated hyperbilirubinemia.
a. A thorough examination to evaluate for hepatomegaly, splenomegaly, petechiae, chorioretinitis, and microcephaly should be performed.
b. Assess liver function (aspartate aminotransferase, activated clotting time), prothrombin time, partial thromboplastin time, and serum albumin levels.
c. Test for ABO and Rh incompatibility (see Chapter 30).
d. Management is related to the causative factor(s).

HYDROPS

A. Definition: generalized subcutaneous edema in fetus and neonate. Usually accompanied by ascites and pleural and/or pericardial effusions.
B. Incidence: 1:2500 to 3700 pregnancies (Bukowski and Saade, 2000).
C. Classification.
1. Alloimmune hydrops occurs when maternal antibodies cross the placenta and destroy fetal erythrocytes. Alloimmune hydrops is also referred to as hydrops fetalis. ABO and Rh incompatibilities are the most common causes of alloimmune hydrops.
2. Nonimmune hydrops occurs for reasons other than those cited above (see section D, Etiology of Nonimmune Hydrops, below).
D. Etiology of nonimmune hydrops (NIH). Most conditions associated with hydrops cause edema through either anemia with hypoxia and subsequent capillary leak or through cardiovascular anomalies with heart failure and subsequent tissue hypoxia, vascular permeability, and decreased lymphatic flow.
1. Cardiovascular (most frequent cause).
a. Supraventricular tachycardia.
b. Complete heart block.
c. Atrial flutter.
d. Cardiac malformation: hypoplastic left heart syndrome and endocardial cushion defects are the most common heart defects associated with NIH.
e. Myocarditis.
2. Chromosomal.
a. Achondroplasia.
b. Turner syndrome.
c. Trisomy 13, 18, and 21.
d. Triploidy.
e. Aneuploidy.

3. Infection.
    a. CMV.
    b. Parvovirus.
    c. Syphilis.
    d. Rubella.
    e. Congenital hepatitis.
    f. Toxoplasmosis.
4. Hematologic.
    a. α-thalassemia.
    b. Glucose-6-phosphate dehydrogenase deficiency.
    c. Chronic fetal-maternal or twin-to-twin transfusion.
    d. Hemorrhage.
    e. Bone marrow failure.
5. Renal.
    a. Nephrosis.
    b. Renal vein thrombosis.
    c. Renal hypoplasia.
    d. Urinary obstruction.
6. Pulmonary.
    a. Pulmonary hypoplasia.
    b. Cystic adenomatoid malformations.
    c. Pulmonary lymphangiectasis.
    d. Congenital diaphragmatic hernia (Bukowski and Saade, 2000).
7. Placenta and cord (uncommon).
    a. Chorioangioma.
    b. Umbilical vein thrombosis.
    c. Arteriovenous malformation.
8. Maternal.
    a. Toxemia.
    b. Diabetes.
    c. Systemic lupus erythematosus
9. Gastrointestinal.
    a. In utero volvulus.
    b. Meconium peritonitis.
    c. Prune-belly syndrome.
10. Idiopathic. Approximately 22% to 35% of cases have no identifiable cause. Incidence of idiopathic NIH is dependent on the thoroughness of the diagnostic work-up of the populations studied (Bukowski and Saade, 2000).

E. Clinical presentation.

1. Prenatal findings in NIH include uterine size greater than normal for gestational age, sudden increase in abdominal girth or weight gain, and abdominal pain.
2. Massive edema, often restricting joint movement.
3. Ascites.
4. Hepatosplenomegaly.
5. Cardiomegaly.

F. Associated laboratory findings.

1. Anemia.
2. Hypoalbuminemia.
3. Reticulocytosis.
4. Thrombocytopenia.

G. Diagnosis.
1. Vigorous prenatal diagnosis with ultrasonography is essential.
2. Echocardiography.
3. Serologic testing for isoimmunization and infection.
4. Chromosomal testing.

H. Management.
1. Antenatal: treatment depends on underlying cause and includes:
   a. Intrauterine transfusion (for isoimmune hemolytic anemia).
   b. Maternal medication administration (e.g., flecainide or digoxin for tachyarrhythmias).
   c. Fetal medication administration.
   d. Thoracoamniotic shunt placement.
   e. Thoracentesis.
   f. Delivery.
2. Neonatal.
   a. Resuscitation is frequently required.
   b. Paracentesis may be required for difficulties with ventilation.
   c. Thoracentesis or chest tubes may be required for pleural effusions.
   d. Frequent monitoring of breath sounds and chest movement, and x-rays are essential.
   e. Partial exchange transfusion may be necessary if the hematocrit is less than 30%.
   f. Fresh frozen plasma may be given for hypoalbuminemia.
   g. Inotropes may be given to improve cardiac output.
   h. A complete head-to-toe neonatal assessment should be performed to determine the etiology of the hydrops if it is unknown (including echocardiogram, ultrasound of GI and renal systems).
   i. Provide phototherapy when indicated.

I. Prognosis. Immune hydrops is associated with a survival rate of 74% (Bukowski and Saade, 2000). Prognosis in NIH is very poor and is related to the underlying cause. NIH due to a cardiac cause carries the best survival rate.

REFERENCES

Adzick, N.S. and Nance, M.L: Pediatric surgery: First of two parts. *New England Journal of Medicine, 342*(22):1651-1657, 2000.

American Academy of Pediatrics Provisional Committee for Quality Improvement and Subcommittee on Hyperbilirubinemia: Practice parameter: Management of hyperbilirubinemia in the healthy term newborn. *Pediatrics, 94*(4 Pt 1):558-565, 1994.

American Academy of Pediatrics Subcommittee on Neonatal Hyperbilirubinemia: Neonatal jaundice and kernicterus. *Pediatrics, 108*(3):763-765, 2001.

American Academy of Pediatrics Task Force on Infant Positioning and SIDS. Positioning and sudden infant death syndrome (SIDS): Update. *Pediatrics, 98*(6 Pt 1):1216-1218, 1996.

Arensman, R.M. and Bambini, D.A.: Congenital diaphragmatic hernia and eventration. In K.W. Ashcraft (Ed.): *Pediatric surgery* (3rd ed.). Philadelphia, 2000, Saunders, pp. 300-317.

Bensard, D.D., Calkins, C.M., Partrick, D., and Price, F.N.: Neonatal surgery. In G.B. Merenstein and S.L. Gardner (Eds.): *Handbook of neonatal intensive care* (5th ed.). St Louis, 2002, Mosby, pp. 702-724.

Berseth, C.L.: Developmental anatomy and physiology of the gastrointestinal tract. In W.H. Taeusch and R.A. Ballard (Eds.):

Avery's diseases of the newborn (7th ed.). Philadelphia, 1998a, Saunders, pp. 893-904.

Berseth, C.L.: Disorders of the umbilical cord, abdominal wall, urachus, and omphalomesenteric duct. In W.H. Taeusch and R.A. Ballard (Eds.): *Avery's diseases of the newborn* (7th ed.). Philadelphia, 1998b, Saunders, pp. 933-940.

Berseth, C.L., Bisquera, J.A., and Paje, V.U.: Prolonging small feeding volumes early in life decreases the incidence of necrotizing enterocolitis in very low birth weight infants. *Pediatrics, 111*(3):529-534, 2003.

Bhutani, V.K., Gourley, G.R., Adler, S., et al.: Noninvasive measurement of total serum bilirubin in a multiracial predischarge newborn population to assess the risk of severe hyperbilirubinemia. *Pediatrics, 106*(2):E17, 2000.

Bhutani V.K., Johnson, L., and Sivieri, E.M.: Predictive ability of a predischarge hour-specific serum bilirubin for subsequent significant hyperbilirubinemia in healthy term and near-term newborns. *Pediatrics, 103*(1):6-14, 1999.

Blackburn, S.: Understanding gastroesophageal reflux in infants. *Central Lines, 15*(1):1,16-22, 1999.

Blackburn, S.T.: *Maternal, fetal, and neonatal physiology: A clinical perspective* (2nd ed.). St Louis, 2003, Saunders.

Braby, J.: Current and emerging treatment for congenital diaphragmatic hernia. *Neonatal Network, 20*(2):5-15, 2001.

Brandt, M.L.: Gastrointestinal surgical emergencies of the newborn. In W.H. Taeusch and R.A. Ballard (Eds.): *Avery's diseases of the newborn* (7th ed.). Philadelphia, 1998, Saunders, pp. 979-994.

Bukowski, R., Saade, G.R.: Hydrops fetalis. *Clinics in Perinatology, 27*(4):1007-1031, 2000.

Cacciari, A., Ruggeri, G., Mordenti, M., et al.: High-frequency oscillatory ventilation versus conventional mechanical ventilation in congenital diaphragmatic hernia. *European Journal of Pediatric Surgery, 11*(1):3-7, 2001.

Cass, D.L. and Wesson, D.E.: Advances in fetal and neonatal surgery for gastrointestinal anomalies and disease. *Clinics in Perinatology, 29*(1):1-21, 2002.

Caty, M.G. and Azizkhan, R.G.: Necrotizing enterocolitis. In K.W. Ashcraft (Ed.): *Pediatric surgery* (3rd ed.). Philadelphia, 2000, Saunders, pp. 443-452.

Clark, L.A. and Oldham, K.T.: Malrotation. In K.W. Ashcraft (Ed.): *Pediatric surgery* (3rd ed.). Philadelphia, 2000, Saunders, pp. 425-434.

Clark, R.H., Hardin, W.D. Jr., Hirschl, R.B., et al.: Current surgical management of CDH: A report from the CDH study group. *Journal of Pediatric Surgery, 33*(7):1004-1009, 1998.

Clark, R.H., Kueser, T.J., Walker, M.W., et al.: Low dose nitric oxide therapy for persistent pulmonary hypertension of the newborn. *New England Journal of Medicine, 342*(7): 469-474, 2000.

Cohen, M.B. and Balistreri, W.F.: Part three: Disorders of digestion. In A.A. Fanaroff and R.J. Martin (Eds.): *Neonatal-perinatal medicine: Diseases of the fetus and infant* (7th ed.). St Louis, 2002, Mosby, pp. 1268-1276.

D'Agata, I.D. and Balistreri, W.F.: Evaluation of liver disease in the pediatric patient. *Pediatrics in Review, 20*(11):376-390, 1999.

Dellert, S.F. and Balistreri, W.F.: Neonatal cholestasis. In W.A. Walker, P.R. Durie, J.R. Hamilton, et al. (Eds.): *Pediatric gastrointestinal disease: Pathophysiology, diagnosis, management* (3rd ed.). Hamilton, Ontario, B.C., 2000, Decker, pp. 880-894.

Dillon, P.W. and Cilley, R.E.: Lesions of the stomach. In K.W. Ashcraft (Ed.): *Pediatric surgery* (3rd ed.). Philadelphia, 2000, Saunders, pp. 391-405.

Dunn J.C.Y., Fonkalsrud, E.W., and Atkinson, J.B.: The influence of gestational age and mode of delivery on infants with gastroschisis. *Journal of Pediatric Surgery, 34*(9):1393-1395, 1999.

Engle, W.D., Jackson, G.L., Sendelbach, D., et al.: Assessment of a transcutaneous device in the evaluation of neonatal hyperbilirubinemia in a primarily Hispanic population. *Pediatrics, 110*(1 Pt 1):61-67, 2002.

Extracorporeal Life Support Organization: ECLS Registry Report. Ann Arbor, Michigan, 2000, ELSO. Retrieved April 12, 2003, from www.med.umich.edu/ecmo/registry.htm.

Filston, H.C. and Shorter, N.A.: Esophageal atresia and tracheoesophageal malformations. In K.W. Ashcraft (Ed.): *Pediatric surgery* (3rd ed.). Philadelphia, 2000, Saunders, pp. 348-369.

Fischler, B., Hadlund, B., and Hjern, A.: A population-based study on the incidence and possible pre- and perinatal etiologic risk factors of biliary atresia. *Journal of Pediatrics, 141*(2):217-222, 2002.

Frank, C.G., Cooper, S.C., and Merenstein, G.B.: Jaundice. In G.B. Merenstein, G.B and S.L. Gardner (Eds.): *Handbook of neonatal intensive care* (5th ed.). St Louis, 2002, Mosby, pp. 443-461.

Gaines, B.A., Holcomb, G.W., and Neblett, W.W.: Gastroschisis and omphalocele. In K.W. Ashcraft (Ed.): *Pediatric surgery* (3rd ed.). Philadelphia, 2000, Saunders, pp. 639-649.

Georgeson, K.E.: Short-bowel syndrome. In J.A. O'Neill, M.I. Rowe, J.L. Grosfeld, et al. (Eds.): *Pediatric surgery* (5th ed.). St Louis, 1998, Mosby, pp. 1223-1232.

Halamek, L.P. and Stevenson, D.K.: Neonatal jaundice and liver disease. In A.A. Fanaroff and R.J. Martin (Eds.): *Neonatal-perinatal medicine: Diseases of the fetus and infant* (7th ed.). St Louis, 2002, Mosby, pp. 1309-1350.

Holland, R.M., Price, F.N., and Bensard, D.D.: Neonatal surgery. In G.B. Merenstein, and S.L. Gardner (Eds.): *Handbook of neonatal intensive care* (5th ed.). St Louis, 2002, Mosby, pp. 625-646.

Holschneider, A. and Ure, B.M.: Hirschprung's disease. In K.W. Ashcraft (Ed.): *Pediatric surgery* (3rd ed.). Philadelphia, 2000, Saunders, pp. 453-472.

Howell, K.K.: Understanding gastroschisis: An abdominal wall defect. *Neonatal Network, 17*(8):17-25, 1998.

Hwang, S.T. and Shulman, R.: Update on management and treatment of short gut. *Clinics in Perinatology, 29*(1):181-194, 2002.

Jadcherla, S.R.: Gastroesophageal reflux in the neonate. *Recent Advances in Neonatal Gastroenterology, 29*:135-157, 2002.

Johnson, L.H., Bhutani, V.K., and Brown, A.K.: System-based approach to management of neonatal jaundice. *Journal of Pediatrics, 140*(4):396-403, 2002.

Karpen, S.J.: Update on the etiologies and management of neonatal cholestasis. *Clinics in Perinatology, 29*(1):159-180, 2002.

Kaufman, S.S., Atkinson, J.B., Bianchi, A., et al.: Indications for pediatric intestinal transplantation: A position paper of the American Society of Transplantation. *Pediatric Transplantation, 5*(2):80-87, 2001.

Kaul, A.J. and Balistreri, W.F.: Part five: Necrotizing enterocolitis. In A.A. Fanaroff and R.J. Martin (Eds.): *Neonatal-perinatal medicine: Diseases of the fetus and infant* (7th ed.). St Louis, 2002, Mosby, pp. 1299-1303.

Keating, M.A. and Rich, M.A.: Prune-belly syndrome. In K.W. Ashcraft (Ed.): *Pediatric surgery* (3rd ed.). Philadelphia, 2000, Saunders, pp. 787-805.

Lessin, M.S., Luks, F.I., Wesselhoeft, C.W., et al.: Peritoneal drainage as definitive treatment for intestinal perforation in infants with extremely low birth weight (<750 g). *Journal of Pediatric Surgery, 33*(2):370-372, 1998.

MacMahon, J.R., Stevenson, D.K., and Oski, F.A.: Physiologic jaundice. In W.H. Taeusch and R.A. Ballard (Eds.): *Avery's diseases of the newborn* (7th ed.). Philadelphia, 1998, Saunders, pp. 1003-1007.

Millar, A.J.W., Rode, H., and Cywes, S.: Intestinal atresia and stenosis. In K.W. Ashcraft (Ed.): *Pediatric surgery* (3rd ed.). Philadelphia, 2000, Saunders, pp. 406-424.

Minkes, R.K., Langer, J.C., Mazziotti, M.V., et al.: Routine insertion of a Silastic spring-loaded silo for infants with gastroschisis. *Journal of Pediatric Surgery, 35*(6):843-846, 2000.

Orenstein, S.R.: Infantile reflux: Different from adult reflux. *American Journal of Medicine, 103*(3A):114S-119S, 1997.

Orenstein, S.R.: Gastroesophageal reflux. In R. Wyllie and J.S. Hyams (Eds.): *Pediatric gastrointestinal disease: Pathophysiology, diagnosis, and management*. Philadelphia, 1999, Saunders, pp. 164-187.

Orenstein, S.R.: An overview of reflux-associated disorders in infants: Apnea, laryngospasm, and aspiration. *American Journal of Medicine, 111*(8A):60S-63S, 2001.

Orenstein, S.R., Izadnia, F., and Khan, S.: Gastroesophageal reflux disease in children. *Gastroenterology Clinics of North America, 28*(4):947-969, 1999.

Quinn, D. and Shannon, L.: Radiology basics: The colon and rectum. *Neonatal Network, 19*(6):48-52, 2000.

Reyes, C., Chang, L.K., Waffarn, F., et al.: Delayed repair of congenital diaphragmatic hernia with early high-frequency oscillating ventilation during preoperative stabilization. *Journal of Pediatric Surgery, 33*(3):1010-1016, 1998.

Reyes, J: Intestinal transplantation for children with short-bowel syndrome. *Seminars in Pediatric Surgery, 10*(2): 99-104, 2001.

Robinson, J.N. and Abuhamad, A.Z.: Abdominal wall and umbilical cord anomalies. *Clinics in Perinatology, 27*(4):947-978, 2000.

Ryckman, R.C.: Part four: Selected anomalies and intestinal obstruction. In A.A. Fanaroff and R.J. Martin (Eds.): *Neonatal-perinatal medicine: Diseases of the fetus and infant* (7th ed.). St Louis, 2002, Mosby, pp. 1276-1298.

Ryckman, R.C. and Balistreri, W.F.: Part two: Upper gastrointestinal disorders. In A.A. Fanaroff and R.J. Martin (Eds.): *Neonatal-perinatal medicine: Diseases of the fetus and infant* (7th ed.). St Louis, 2002, Mosby, pp. 1263-1268.

Schumacher, R.E.: Transcutaneous bilirubinometery and diagnostic tests: The right job for the tool. *Pediatrics, 110*(2 Pt 1): 407-498, 2002.

Shaw, N.M.: Assessment and management of the hematologic system. In C. Kenner and J.W. Lott (Eds.): *Comprehensive neonatal nursing: A physiologic perspective* (3rd ed.). Philadelphia, 2003, Saunders, pp. 580-623.

Siafakas, C.G. and Jonas, M.M.: Neonatal hepatitis. In R. Wyllie and J.S. Hyams (Eds.): *Pediatric gastrointestinal disease: Pathophysiology, diagnosis, and management*. Philadelphia, 1999, Saunders, pp. 553-567.

Sigalet, D.L.: Biliary tract disorders and portal hypertension. In K.W. Ashcraft (Ed.): *Pediatric surgery* (3rd ed.). Philadelphia, 2000, Saunders, pp. 580-596.

Skari, H., Bjornland, K., Frenckner, B., et al.: Congenital diaphragmatic hernia in Scandinavia from 1995 to 1998: Predictors of mortality. *Journal of Pediatric Surgery, 37*(9):1269-1275, 2002.

Stevens, T.P., Chess, P.R., McConnochie, K.M., et al.: Survival in early- and late-term infants with congenital diaphragmatic hernia treated with extracorporeal membrane oxygenation. *Pediatrics, 110*(3):590-596, 2002.

Teitelbaum, D.H., Coran, A.G., Weitzman, J.J., et al.: Hirschprung's disease and related neuromuscular disorders of the intestine. In J.A. O'Neill, M.I. Rowe, J.L. Grosfeld, et al. (Eds.): *Pediatric surgery* (5th ed.). St Louis, 1998, Mosby, pp. 1381-1424.

Thigpen, J.L. and Kenner, C.: Assessment and management of the gastrointestinal system. In C. Kenner and J.W. Lott (Eds.): *Comprehensive neonatal nursing: A physiologic perspective* (3rd ed.). Philadelphia, 2003, Saunders, pp. 448-485.

Verkade, H.J.: A novel hypothesis on the pathophysiology of neonatal jaundice. *Journal of Pediatrics, 141*(4):594-595, 2002.

Volpe, J.J.: *Neurology of the newborn* (4th ed.). Philadelphia, 2001, Saunders.

Walsh-Sukys, M.C., Tyson, J.E., Wright, L.L., et al.: Persistent pulmonary hypertension of the newborn in the era before nitric oxide: Practice variation and outcomes. *Pediatrics, 105*(1 Pt 1):14-20, 2000.

CHAPTER

29 Endocrine Disorders

LAURA STOKOWSKI

OBJECTIVES

1. Define the endocrine system.
2. Describe endocrine system regulation.
3. Identify and discuss endocrine disorders that manifest in the neonatal period, including disorders of thyroid function, adrenal gland, and genital development.
4. List effective ways to help parents cope with the birth of an infant with ambiguous genitalia.

THE ENDOCRINE SYSTEM

The classic endocrine system is a group of nine ductless glands (Table 29-1) but in reality includes every organ and cell in the body that produces and responds to hormones (Chrousos, 2002). Regulation of growth and development, metabolic homeostasis, reproduction, and response to environmental changes are only a few of the tasks of this complex system.

A. **Hormones.**

1. Hormones are the molecular messengers of the endocrine system, allowing communication between organs, tissues, and cells throughout the body. In composition, hormones are steroids, proteins, glycoproteins, peptides, or amines.
2. To act physiologically, a hormone must bind to a specific receptor on a target cell. Sensitivity of a target cell to its hormones is critical to normal function.
3. Many hormones are secreted directly into the circulation and thus transported to various target tissues. Hormones can also act on cells in the immediate vicinity of their release *(paracrine action)* or on the cell that produced the hormone (*autocrine* or *intracrine action*).
4. Some hormones circulate partly in free form and partly bound to transport proteins. It is the free form that is available for receptor binding and that dictates the regulatory influences on hormone release. Clinical states of hormone excess and deficiency correlate best with free hormone levels.
5. Most hormones are secreted in their biologically active form, but some must be converted to the final active form in peripheral tissues.

B. **Endocrine system regulation (Fig. 29-1).**

1. Many hormones are regulated by a negative-feedback loop involving the hypothalamic-pituitary axis and the target endocrine gland. This type of control begins with hormonal or neural input to the hypothalamus, which produces two substances: *releasing hormones* and *inhibiting hormones*. These are transported via the pituitary portal system to the anterior pituitary. Tropic hormones secreted by the anterior pituitary then regulate the secretions of target organs. As blood concentrations of target hormones reach required levels, a negative message sent to the anterior pituitary inhibits further release of tropic hormones. Examples of hormones regulated by negative feedback are thyroid hormone and cortisol.

TABLE 29-1
Major Glands and Hormones of the Endocrine System

Endocrine Gland	Hormones Produced
Hypothalamus	Corticotropin-releasing hormone (CRH)
	Thyrotropin-releasing hormone (TRH)
	Gonadotropin-releasing hormone (GnRH)
	Somatostatin
	Growth hormone-releasing hormone (GHRH)
	Prolactin-releasing factor (PRF)
	Prolactin release–inhibiting hormone (PIH; dopamine)
Anterior pituitary	Adrenocorticotropic hormone (ACTH)
	Thyroid-stimulating hormone (TSH; thyrotropin)
	Follicle-stimulating hormone (FSH)
	Growth hormone (GH)
	Luteinizing hormone (LH)
	Prolactin (PRL)
Posterior pituitary	Antidiuretic hormone (ADH; arginine vasopressin)
	Oxytocin (OCT)
Thyroid gland	Thyroxine (T_4)
	Triiodothyronine (T_3)
	Calcitonin
Parathyroid gland	Parathyroid hormone (PTH)
Adrenal medulla	Epinephrine (adrenaline)
	Norepinephrine (noradrenaline)
Adrenal cortex	Cortisol (hydrocortisone)
	Aldosterone
Pancreas	Insulin
	Glucagon
	Somatostatin
Pineal gland	Melatonin

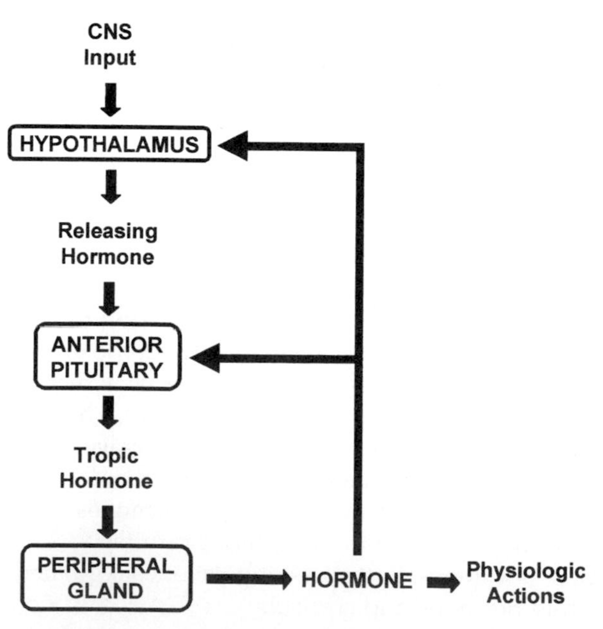

FIGURE 29-1 ■ Negative feedback-loop control of endocrine gland function. Hypothalamic-releasing hormones stimulate pituitary tropic hormones, which in turn act on peripheral glands to release hormones. Levels of circulating hormones then exert feedback control on the pituitary and hypothalamus, modulating further output by these glands.

2. Other endocrine glands, such as the parathyroids and the pancreatic islets, are not part of the hypothalamic-pituitary axis, but have a "freestanding" control mechanism. These glands release hormones that stimulate a target tissue to produce an effect, which in turn directly modifies the output of the gland.
3. In the neuroendocrine relationship, the endocrine and autonomic nervous systems are closely linked in the control of body homeostasis. Hormones act as neurotransmitters, and neurotransmitters are involved in regulating endocrine function. Endocrine glands such as the hypothalamus, the pituitary, and the adrenal cortex respond to neural stimulation. The neuroendocrine system is important in the smooth adaptation of the neonate to the stresses of extrauterine life.

C. **Endocrine disorders in the neonate.** In addition to well-described neonatal endocrine disorders (hypothyroidism, congenital adrenal hyperplasia), endocrine dysfunction can affect the preterm infant in a variety of ways as a function of maturation. Some of the more common endocrine alterations seen in term and preterm infants will be addressed here.

THYROID GLAND DISORDERS

The Thyroid Gland

A. **Normal physiology.**
1. Functions of the thyroid gland.
   a. Concentrates and stores iodide, a trace element required for thyroid hormone synthesis.
   b. Synthesizes *thyroglobulin* (Tg), a thyroid hormone precursor.
   c. Synthesizes and releases the thyroid hormones *thyroxine* (T_4) and *triiodothyronine* (T_3).
2. Thyroid hormone metabolism.
   a. The thyroid gland produces T_4 and a small amount of T_3. Most of plasma T_3 (the more potent hormone) is derived from peripheral metabolism *(deiodination)* of T_4.
   b. T_4 enters the cell and is converted to T_3 by enzymes (deiodinases).
   c. Deiodination of the outer ring of T_4 produces T_3. Deiodination of the inner ring of T_4 produces *reverse* T_3 (rT_3), a biologically inactive product.
3. Thyroid hormone transport.
   a. Thyroid hormones circulate in the blood bound to *thyroid-binding globulin* (TBG) and other albumins. Only a tiny fraction is in equilibrium as free hormone, but it is this free fraction that is responsible for hormonal activity.
   b. TBG, which is synthesized in the liver, has a high affinity for T_3 and T_4, carrying 70% of circulating hormone. When TBG is deficient, total thyroid hormone concentrations may be lower but free hormone levels are normal.
4. Mechanisms of thyroid gland regulation.
   a. Hypothalamic-pituitary-thyroid (HPT) axis.
      (1) Hypothalamic thyrotropin-releasing hormone (TRH) is secreted in response to neural input, such as cooling of the skin. TRH stimulates synthesis and release of thyroid-stimulating hormone (TSH; thyrotropin) by the anterior pituitary.
      (2) TSH binds to receptors on thyroid cell membranes and stimulates production of thyroid hormones.

(3) As thyroid hormone levels rise, further secretion of TSH and TRH is inhibited.

b. Deiodinase enzymes in the anterior pituitary, brain, heart, liver, and other tissues regulate intracellular T_3 availability.

c. Autoregulation of hormone synthesis by the thyroid gland itself in relationship to its iodine supply.

d. Stimulation or inhibition of thyroid function by TSH receptor antibodies.

5. Physiologic effects of thyroid hormones.

a. Metabolic processes such as those involved in oxygen consumption, thermogenesis, cardiac output, erythropoiesis, respiratory drive, gut motility, and carbohydrate, protein, and lipid metabolism.

b. Growth and differentiation of organs and tissues, including the bones, lungs, and central nervous system (CNS). Sufficient thyroid hormones are mandatory for normal brain development.

B. Fetal thyroid development.

1. Fetal thyroid activity begins with synthesis of Tg (week 8), followed by trapping of iodide and limited synthesis of T_4 and T_3 (weeks 10-12).
2. The HPT axis begins to function at midgestation (weeks 18-20), when iodide uptake increases and the fetal thyroid gland begins to release T_4. Total and free T_4, TSH, and TBG increase steadily until term. The T_3 level remains low until 30 weeks' gestation, rising only in the last 10 weeks as mechanisms for deiodination of T_4 in fetal tissues mature.
3. The placenta is permeable to TRH, iodide, thyroid autoantibodies, and antithyroid drugs but impermeable to TSH. Maternal T_4 crosses the placenta in limited but significant quantities essential for normal CNS maturation in the fetus.
4. The fetus is also dependent on the maternal-placental system for adequate supply of iodide, a critical substrate for fetal thyroid hormone synthesis. Autoregulation of iodide uptake is not yet mature, so the fetal thyroid is susceptible to inhibitory effects of both iodide deficiency and iodide excess.

C. Neonatal thyroid physiology.

1. At birth in term and near-term neonates, the cooling of the skin and a surge of circulating catecholamines stimulate a sharp rise in the serum TSH level. TSH peaks in the 70 to 100 mU/L range at 30 minutes of age and then falls to a normal (<20 mU/L) level during the first 3 days of life.
2. The TSH surge stimulates an abrupt rise in thyroid hormone levels. T_4 and T_3 both increase in response to TSH, peaking at 24 to 36 hours after birth. It is speculated that this physiologic hyperthyroid state is important in stimulating thermogenesis of brown adipose tissue and in the cardiovascular and pulmonary adaptation to extrauterine life
3. Postnatal changes in TSH, T_4 and T_3 occur in some less mature infants as well, but are quantitatively lower. In infants less than 30 weeks' gestation, the postnatal surge of thyroid hormones does not occur (Biswas et al., 2002).

Hypothyroidism

Hypothyroidism in the neonate is classified in several ways. It can be considered either permanent (lifelong therapy required) or transient (spontaneously resolving in weeks or months; treatment is temporary or not required at all). Hypothyroidism can also be termed *congenital* (existing at birth) or *acquired*. Other labels indicate the origin of the hypothyroidism:

1. *Primary*. A disorder involving the thyroid gland or some aspect of thyroid hormone synthesis, metabolism, or transport.
2. *Central* (also called secondary/tertiary). Deficient thyroid hormone secretion due to a disorder affecting pituitary control (TSH production) or hypothalamic control (TRH production).

A. Etiology of permanent congenital hypothyroidism (CH).

1. Thyroid abnormalities.
   a. *Thyroid dysgenesis:* absent *(thyroid agenesis)*, hypoplastic, or ectopic gland.
   b. *Familial dyshormonogenesis:* inborn errors of thyroid hormone biosynthesis or metabolism, of which the most common is an organification defect.
2. Extrathyroid abnormalities.
   a. Defects of the pituitary gland (e.g., hypopituitarism) or the hypothalamus.
   b. *TBG deficiency:* X-linked disorder; more common than CH in males.

B. Etiology of transient hypothyroid states.

1. Prenatally acquired:
   a. Maternal autoimmune thyroid disorders characterized by transplacental passage of TSH-receptor blocking antibodies, which inhibit the binding of TSH to the thyroid cell.
   b. Drugs given to the mother that cross the placenta and affect fetal thyroid production. These include propylthiouracil, methimazole, lithium, phenytoin, amiodarone, and radioiodine.
   c. Ingestion of excess iodide or severe deficiency of dietary iodide.
2. Postnatally acquired: transiently impaired thyroid hormone production from exposure to iodine-containing topical disinfectants, ointments, or intravenously administered contrast media. Preterm infants can absorb and excrete large amounts of iodine during exposure to these products. Until it is clear that this exposure does not affect thyroid function, minimal use of iodinated substances in the preterm population is usually recommended.

C. The preterm infant. Preterm infants have the same incidence of permanent congenital hypothyroidism as full-term infants. In addition, several transient hypothyroid states have been described in this population. Because these transient conditions can coexist, it is not always possible to determine the precise cause of low thyroid hormone levels in preterm infants.

1. *Hypothyroxinemia of prematurity*. Serum levels of thyroid hormones in preterm neonates are significantly lower than those of term neonates. T_4 levels of most preterms decline to a nadir at 7 to 14 days of age and then climb to normal within 4 to 8 weeks (Oden and Freemark, 2002). The severity of hypothyroxinemia is inversely related to gestational age. TSH is not elevated, suggesting relative lack of hypothalamic response to the declining T_4 level. It is generally believed that this condition is a developmental phenomenon caused by one or more of the following:
   a. Immaturity of thyroid hormone metabolism and the HPT axis.
   b. Loss of maternal contributions to the thyroid hormone pool at birth.
   c. Low TBG levels.
   d. Increased use of T_4 to meet the demands of extrauterine life.
   e. Insufficient enteral or parenteral iodine intake.
2. *Atypical primary hypothyroidism*. Infants weighing less than 1500 g at birth have 20 times the incidence of a low T_4/high TSH profile (consistent with primary hypothyroidism) compared with those weighing more than 2500 g

(Mandel et al., 2000). The majority of these very low birth weight (VLBW) infants will have a normal TSH on initial screening, followed by an elevated TSH on repeat screening (delayed TSH rise). In addition to immaturity of the HPT axis, possible etiologies include:

a. Exposure to iodine.
b. Exposure to dopamine (which suppresses TSH and the thyroid axis).
c. Exposure to glucocorticoids.
d. Effects of concurrent illness on thyroid function (see below).

3. *Nonthyroidal illness (NTI) syndrome*. Nonthyroidal illnesses (e.g., respiratory distress syndrome or sepsis) can affect thyroid function in the neonate. NTI can lower serum TBG and total T_4 and T_3, and inhibit extrathyroidal conversion of T_4 to T_3 (Rapaport et al., 2001). Thus the small, sick infant who already has a low T_4 related to prematurity may suffer a further fall in T_4 levels as a result of concurrent illness. It is hypothesized that cytokines produced in response to illness and inflammation inhibit thyroid function, metabolism, and thyroid hormone action (Kok et al., 2000).

D. **Clinical presentation and assessment.**

1. Few neonates are diagnosed with CH on clinical grounds, but 15% to 20% will have suggestive signs when carefully examined (Fisher, 2000). Early signs and symptoms reflect the wide-ranging actions of thyroid hormones on metabolism, intestinal motility, cardiac function, temperature regulation, neurologic function, and bone maturation:
   a. Large, open posterior fontanelle (>1 cm).
   b. Birth weight greater than 4 kg; gestation longer than 42 weeks.
   c. Hypothermia.
   d. Abdominal distention.
   e. Poor feeding.
   f. Prolonged hyperbilirubinemia.
   g. Hoarse cry.
   h. Umbilical hernia.
   i. Goiter.
2. Other features typical of hypothyroidism (e.g., macroglossia, dry skin, coarse hair, constipation) are not usually seen for several weeks after birth.
3. Most preterm/VLBW infants will not have clinical signs and symptoms readily associated with hypothyroidism.
4. Infants with hypopituitary hypothyroidism may present with midline facial defects (cleft lip and palate), microphallus, and hypoglycemia.
5. Palpation of the neck will identify thyroid enlargement *(goiter)*. A goiter indicates functional thyroid tissue with regard to iodine uptake and is associated with thyroid dyshormonogenesis. Small goiters can be difficult to detect in the short neck of the neonate; extending the neck is helpful.

E. **Diagnostic studies in hypothyroidism (Table 29-2).** Unless the infant is born to a mother with a history of thyroid dysfunction or has obvious clinical signs of hypothyroidism at birth, the diagnosis is usually made after the infant is identified by neonatal screening.

1. Newborn screening for hypothyroidism.
   a. Screening for congenital hypothyroidism utilizes either a two-tiered T_4-TSH testing approach, or primary TSH testing. In the two-tiered system, TSH is measured only if the T_4 is low. Many screening programs are transitioning to primary TSH testing for CH.
   b. An elevated TSH level is presumed to be CH until further testing proves otherwise. Rapid confirmation is essential.

TABLE 29-2
Summary of Low Thyroid States in the Newborn Infant

Screening Results	Possible Conditions	Further Diagnostic Tests	Treatment
T_4 low[*] TSH elevated[†]	Congenital hypothyroidism (thyroid agenesis, ectopia dyshormonogenesis)	Serum TFTs[‡], Tg[§] level; thyroid scan; ultrasonography; bone age radiography	Thyroid replacement
	Transient hypothyroidism Maternal (autoimmune, drugs)	TSI, TBA	Monitoring
	iodine exposure	Urinary iodine level	
T_4 low, TSH normal or low-normal, TSH slightly elevated (borderline)	Congenital hypothyroidism	Repeat screen, other tests as for congenital hypothyroidism (above)	Thyroid replacement
	Early specimen collection (<24 hours) or false-positive	Repeat screen	
T_4 low, TSH normal	Hypothyroxinemia of prematurity	Serum TFTs or repeat screen to detect delayed TSH rise	Monitoring
	TBG deficiency	Serum TFTs; TBG level; T_3, resin uptake level[‖]	None
	Early specimen collection (<24 hours) or false-positive	Repeat screen	
T_4 low, delayed TSH rise	Atypical hypothyroidism Some VLBW infants (nonthyroidal Illness?)	Serum TFTs	Close monitoring; possible treatment
	Congenital hypothyroidism (some functional thyroid; ectopic or hypoplastic)	Serum TFTs and other tests as for congenital hypothyroidism (above)	Thyroid replacement
T_4 low, TSH low	Central hypothyroidism (hypothalamic-pituitary)	Serum TFTs; TRH stimulation test[¶]; other tests of pituitary function (cortisol, growth hormone)	Thyroid replacement; other hormonal therapy

TFTs, Thyroid function tests; *TSH,* thyroid-stimulating hormone; *TBG,* thyroid-binding globulin; *TSI,* thyroid-stimulating immunoglobulins; *TBA,* thyroid-blocking antibodies; *VLBW,* very low birth weight.

*T_4 low: <6 mcg/dl

†TSH elevated: >40 mU/L; TSH normal: <10 mU/L; TSH borderline: 20-40 mU/L. Note that a slightly elevated TSH level may be normal in the first 2 days of life.

‡TFTs: May include assays of total and free T_4 and T_3 along with TSH.

§Tg: Thyroglobulin, a thyroid hormone precursor produced by the thyroid gland. A low level suggests thyroid agenesis.

‖T_3, resin uptake level: An Indirect measure of protein binding. A high level suggests low binding capacity as in TBG deficiency.

¶TRH stimulation is a test of hypothalamic or pituitary control of thyroid function. A dose of TRH is administered and TSH is measured serially. A subnormal TSH response suggests a deficient pituitary gland, and a delayed response suggests hypothalamic congenital hypothyroidism.

c. Incidence of CH by screening: 1:4000, with a 2:1 female/male ratio.
d. False-positive results can occur when samples are drawn during the first 24 hours, when TSH levels are still physiologically elevated.
e. Approximately 10% of infants with CH are missed on initial screening; they are detected only through routine second screening in states where this is required or on clinical grounds. Some of these infants have compensated hypothyroidism or delayed rise in the TSH level; most seem to have milder forms of hypothyroidism but still require treatment.
f. Infants at risk of a missed or delayed diagnosis are those born at home, those who are extremely ill in the neonatal period, and those who are transferred to another hospital at an early age.

2. Thyroid function tests.
   a. When CH is suspected clinically or suggested by initial screening results, confirmatory serum T_4 and TSH measurements are obtained. Free T_4 and T_3 may also be measured, along with other tests, as needed, to determine the cause of abnormal screening results (see Table 29-2).
   b. Maternal serum may be analyzed for the presence of TSH receptor–blocking antibodies to rule out transient hypothyroidism in the neonate.
3. Further evaluation for the cause of a CH blood profile includes ultrasonography of the neck, thyroid radionuclide imaging (to identify normal or ectopic thyroid tissue), and bone age radiography of the knee or foot (delayed bone ossification suggests long-standing thyroid deprivation).

F. Patient care management.

1. CH.
   a. Thyroid replacement with synthetic T_4 (L-thyroxine), initially 12 to 17 μg/kg/day (Selva et al., 2002). The early goals of treatment are to raise the serum T_4 concentration into the upper half of the normal range as quickly as possible, and then normalize the TSH.
   b. Close monitoring of serum T_4 levels and clinical response is needed to prevent overtreatment or undertreatment.
      (1) Overtreatment can lead to advanced bone age, craniosynostosis, and thyrotoxicosis (tachycardia, irritability, hyperactivity, poor weight gain, and loose stools).
      (2) Undertreatment leads to clinical hypothyroidism, delayed bone maturation, and neurologic damage.
2. Transient hypothyroidism.
   a. Hypothyroxinemia of prematurity is not routinely treated with T_4 supplementation. Despite evidence of associations between low thyroxine levels and higher mortality and severity of lung disease (Biswas et al., 2002), intraventricular hemorrhage (Paul et al., 2001), cerebral white matter damage (Leviton et al., 1999), and worse cognitive and neuromotor outcome (van Wassenaer et al., 2002), causal relationships have not been established (Oden and Freemark, 2002). Furthermore, research to date has not demonstrated clear clinical or developmental benefits of T_4 supplementation in all infants. Some neurodevelopmental benefits of thyroid supplementation have been demonstrated in the most immature (25-26 weeks) neonates (van Wassenaer et al., 1999), but more research is needed to confirm these findings (Ogilvy-Stuart, 2002).
   b. Because transient hypothyroidism is not always recognized as such in the neonate, replacement therapy for a low T_4–high TSH profile is begun just as it is for established permanent hypothyroidism. Evaluation of the

permanence of the disease is conducted after the child is 2 to 3 years of age.

c. Infants who are not treated are reevaluated by repeated filter-paper specimen or thyroid function tests, to ensure that thyroid function becomes normal. The late-onset TSH rise of atypical hypothyroidism that can occur in extremely preterm infants will only be detected if thyroid function is closely monitored (Rapaport, 2002).

G. Outcome.

1. Congenital hypothyroidism (CH).
   a. CH is one of the most preventable causes of mental retardation. The majority of infants with early diagnosis and early and adequate treatment will have normal IQs. A delay in treatment after birth can lower IQ by several points per week (Fisher, 2000).
   b. Lifelong thyroid replacement therapy is necessary for normal growth and development.
2. Transient hypothyroidism.
   a. Hypothyroxinemia of prematurity is transient, correcting spontaneously over 6 to 10 weeks as the infant matures.
   b. More research is needed to determine whether hypothyroxinemia of prematurity is a benign physiologic phenomenon or a cause of psychomotor and neurodevelopmental sequelae in the preterm population.

Hyperthyroidism

A. Etiologies.

1. Maternal *Graves disease* (either active or inactive) causes *neonatal Graves disease* in 1 of 70 affected pregnancies.
2. Rare causes of neonatal hyperthyroidism include McCune-Albright syndrome and activating mutations in the TSH receptor.

B. Pathophysiology of Graves disease.

1. Graves disease is an autoimmune disorder that results in the production of TSH receptor antibodies. The mother produces *thyroid-stimulating immunoglobulins* (TSI) that mimic the action of TSH in stimulating fetal and neonatal thyroid growth and function. Some mothers also produce *thyroid-blocking antibodies* (TBA), which inhibit the binding of TSH to the thyroid receptor. The effects on the fetus and neonate can therefore be highly variable, depending on the concentration and potency of the two opposing types of antibodies. The clinical picture also differs between untreated (active) and treated (inactive) maternal Graves disease.
2. Effects of active maternal Graves disease. Maternal TSI cause fetal hyperthyroidism with tachycardia and, in some cases, development of a fetal goiter detectable by ultrasound. The neonate can exhibit early or delayed signs of hyperthyroidism, but these effects are usually self-limiting and disappear as the TSI are degraded in the first 3 to 12 weeks of life.
3. Effects of treated maternal Graves disease. Treatment of the mother is aimed at correcting her elevated thyroid hormone levels with antithyroid drugs, but this does not necessarily halt the production of thyroid antibodies. Antithyroid drugs cross to the fetus and block fetal thyroid production. Thus the neonate may actually be hypothyroid at birth, with a delayed onset (up to 10 days) of hyperthyroidism. As maternal antithyroid drugs leave the neonate's circulation, residual TSI stimulate the neonate's thyroid, and

thyrotoxicosis can ensue. If there are coexisting TBA, even longer delays (up to 4-6 weeks) are possible before the onset of hyperthyroidism in the infant.

C. Clinical presentation and assessment.

1. Many affected infants are born prematurely and/or exhibit intrauterine growth restriction.
2. Signs and symptoms include irritability, tremor, hyperactivity, flushing of the skin, hyperthermia, sweating, gastrointestinal dysfunction (vomiting, diarrhea), and signs of cardiac stimulation (tachycardia, arrhythmias, congestive heart failure). Eye signs include exophthalmos, eye stare, and lid retraction.
3. Thyromegaly, if present, can worsen during the neonatal period.
4. In severely affected infants, evidence of advanced skeletal maturation (craniosynostosis, frontal bossing) is seen.

D. Diagnostic studies.

1. Total and free T_4 and T_3 are elevated (may initially be normal or low in neonates born to mothers with treated Graves disease).
2. The TSH is low because of feedback-loop suppression.
3. Levels of TSI, TBII (thyroid binding inhibitory immunoglobulins) and TBA in the mother and infant are measured as indicated by clinical circumstances.

E. Patient care management. Clinical and biochemical hyperthyroidism is a medical emergency; the use of some or all of the following can be anticipated:

1. β-adrenergic blockers, such as propranolol, to treat cardiovascular overstimulation. Digitalization may also be necessary.
2. Agents to suppress hypersecretion of thyroid hormone:
   - **a.** Propylthiouracil may be administered but will not be effective for 24 to 36 hours.
   - **b.** Lugol iodine solution has been used for acute inhibition of thyroid hormone release.
   - **c.** Radiographic contrast agents (ipodate sodium and iopanoic acid) block peripheral conversion of T_4 to T_3 and inhibit thyroidal secretion of T_4 and T_3.
   - **d.** Glucocorticoids are used to inhibit thyroid hormone secretion.
3. A hypothyroid state could be induced by use of the agents mentioned above, making replacement with T_4 necessary.
4. Sedatives are given for neurologic symptoms.
5. If an enlarged thyroid gland is compressing the trachea, as evidenced by respiratory distress, elevation and extension of the infant's head will help maintain a patent airway. In very rare cases, surgery is necessary to relieve the obstruction.
6. Infants with nonimmune hyperthyroidism related to an activating TSH receptor mutation are treated with thyroid ablation.

F. Complications: more severe manifestations of thyrotoxicosis, such as congestive heart failure, hepatosplenomegaly, thromobocytopenia, and hyperviscosity syndrome.

G. Outcome.

1. The mortality rate is 12% to 16%.
2. Survivors of severe, prolonged thyrotoxicosis often have permanent neurologic impairment from premature craniosynostosis and the direct effects of excess thyroid hormones on the brain (Buckingham, 2000).

ADRENAL GLAND DISORDERS

The Adrenal Gland

A. Anatomy and physiology.

1. The adrenal glands are located at the superior poles of the kidneys. Each highly vascular gland is composed of two endocrine organs: the inner *adrenal medulla* and the outer *adrenal cortex.*
2. The adrenal medulla produces and stores catecholamines (epinephrine, norepinephrine, dopamine) and is linked to the sympathetic nervous system.
3. The adrenal cortex produces steroid hormones derived from cholesterol (*glucocorticoids, mineralocorticoids,* and *androgens*), known as *adrenocortical hormones.*

B. Adrenocortical hormones.

1. *Cortisol,* the primary glucocorticoid, has a major role in glucose homeostasis and key regulatory roles in development, growth, inflammatory responses, cardiovascular function, and response to stress.
2. Cortisol is closely regulated by adrenocorticotropic hormone (ACTH) and the hypothalamic-pituitary-adrenal (HPA) axis via a negative-feedback loop. Increased plasma cortisol inhibits secretion of corticotropin-releasing hormone and ACTH, whereas decreased plasma cortisol permits their release. Cortisol is also released in response to stress, hypoglycemia, surgery, extreme heat or cold, decreased oxygen concentration, infection, or injury.
3. *Aldosterone,* the most important mineralocorticoid, regulates renal sodium and water retention and potassium excretion, thus affecting not only electrolyte balance but blood pressure and intravascular volume as well. Aldosterone is regulated by the plasma renin-angiotensin system and by plasma potassium concentrations. A drop in intravascular volume or the sodium concentration or a rise in the potassium level stimulates the renin-angiotensin system, which in turn stimulates production of aldosterone.
4. Adrenal androgens include dehydroepiandrosterone (DHEA), DHEA sulfate, and androstenedione and are regulated by ACTH. These steroids have minimal androgenic activity but are converted in the peripheral tissues to two more potent androgens: testosterone and dihydrotestosterone.

C. Fetal adrenocortical development.

1. Early in gestation, the fetal adrenal cortex begins to differentiate into distinct zones: a large, unique *fetal zone* and a smaller *definitive zone.* The fetal zone is responsible for most of the steroids produced during fetal life. Fetal adrenal growth is rapid; at term the gland is twice the size of the adult's but begins to shrink after birth as the fetal zone involutes.
2. The fetal adrenal gland and the placenta are an integrated endocrine organ known as the fetoplacental unit. The fetal zone, deficient in a critical enzyme for cortisol synthesis, produces mostly DHEA and DHEA sulfate. These are the precursors for placental estrogen, which is vital to maintenance of the pregnancy and fetal well-being. In turn, the placenta provides substrates for fetal cortisol production.
3. Until about 30 weeks' gestation fetal cortisol comes from both the fetal gland and transplacental transfer. Its rapid metabolism to inactive cortisone protects the fetus from very high cortisol levels. Near term, maturation of enzyme systems allows greater conversion of cortisone back to cortisol and synthesis of cortisol from cholesterol. Increases in circulating cortisol during the last 10 weeks of gestation (the prenatal cortisol surge) induce critical

physiologic changes that prepare the fetus for extrauterine life, including maturation of pulmonary surfactant.
4. Aldosterone production increases throughout pregnancy, preparing the fetus to assume control of salt and water balance after birth.

D. **Neonatal adrenocortical function.**
1. Plasma cortisol levels are high at the time of birth but begin to fall in the first few days of life. In term infants a nadir is seen on day 4. Likewise, levels of a cortisol precursor, *17-hydroxyprogesterone* (17-OHP), are high at birth but decrease to normal neonatal levels by 12 to 24 hours of age.
2. In the neonate, aldosterone concentration and plasma renin activity are elevated compared with values for older infants, allowing for positive sodium balance until the kidneys fully mature. The hyponatremia and urinary sodium loss often seen in preterm infants during the early postnatal weeks are due to a relative mineralocorticoid deficiency as a consequence of immaturity of both the kidneys and the adrenal glands.

E. **Adrenal disorders in the neonate.**
1. *Congenital adrenal hyperplasia* (see following section).
2. Adrenal hemorrhage (from hemorrhagic diathesis, shock, anoxia, birth trauma).
3. *Hypopituitarism.* The pituitary fails to produce ACTH, and the consequent lack of cortical stimulation results in hypoplasia of the adrenal cortex and adrenal insufficiency.
4. Adrenocortical insufficiency in ill extremely low birth weight (ELBW) infants.
   a. Low cortisol levels, seen in preterm infants, are most likely related to hypothalamic-pituitary-adrenal immaturity. Some ELBW (<1000g) infants show symptoms that suggest adrenocortical insufficiency, including hypotension unresponsive to inotropes, oliguria with edema, hyponatremia, and hyperkalemia (Jett et al., 1997).
   b. An inappropriately low cortisol level in the presence of significant stress (respiratory illness, mechanical ventilation, invasive procedures, etc.) indicates an inability to recognize stress owing to immaturity of brain regions involved in the stress response (Bolt et al., 2002).

Congenital Adrenal Hyperplasia (CAH)

A. **Definition:** a group of autosomal recessive genetic disorders resulting from deficient activity of one of the enzymes needed for cortisol biosynthesis. A deficiency of the enzyme P-450_{c21} is the most common type of CAH and is known as *21-hydroxylase deficiency* (21-OHD). Deficiencies of 11-β-hydroxylase and 3-β-hydroxysteroid dehydrogenase are less common; the remainder are very rare. CAH refers to the end result of these disorders, hypertrophy of the adrenal gland, which is the most prominent finding at autopsy (Miller, 2002). CAH has a worldwide incidence of 1:15,000 to 1:16,000 (Therrell, 2001).

B. **Pathophysiology (Fig. 29-2).** Because 21-OHD represents 95% of cases, the remainder of the discussion will pertain to this form of CAH.
1. Lack of fetal P-450_{c21} (21-hydroxylase) prevents conversion of progesterone to its two end products: cortisol and aldosterone.
2. By reduced negative-feedback regulation, the absence of cortisol causes oversecretion of ACTH, which chronically stimulates the adrenal cortex, resulting in hyperplasia.

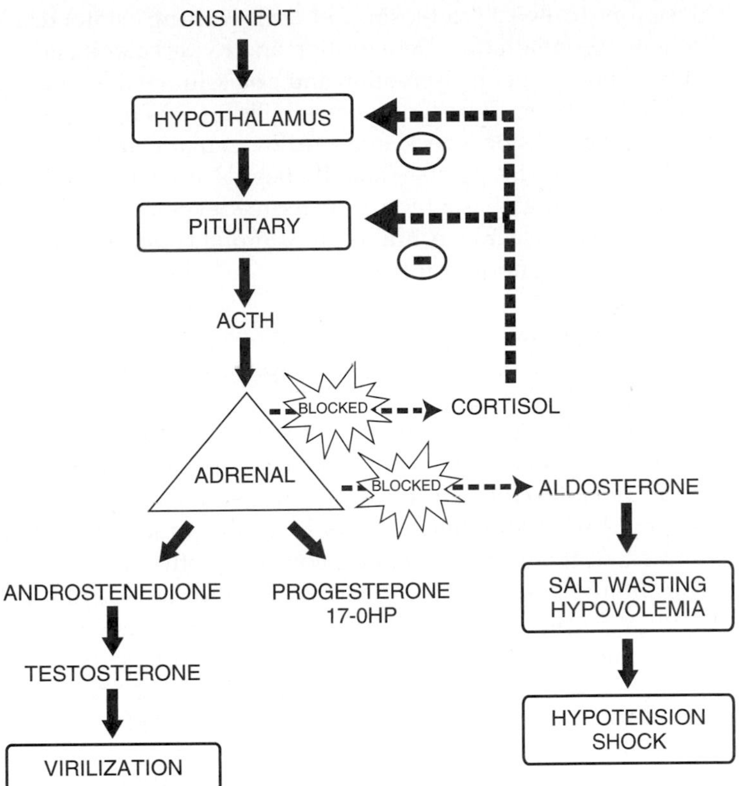

FIGURE 29-2 ■ Pathophysiology of congenital adrenal hyperplasia (CAH) caused by 21-hydroxylase deficiency. In the absence of cortisol, adrenocorticotropic hormone (ACTH) stimulates the adrenal cortex to produce virilizing androgens. Diminished production of aldosterone leads to salt wasting and hypovolemia. (Adapted from Fanaroff, A.A. and Martin, R.J.: *Neonatal-perinatal medicine: Diseases of the fetus and infant* [7th ed.]. St Louis, 2002, Mosby, p. 1448.)

3. The cortisol precursor 17-OHP accumulates in the blood because its conversion to cortisol is blocked.
4. The excess 17-OHP enters the unblocked androgen metabolic pathway, which results in an overproduction of androgens. At a critical stage in fetal development, these androgens cause virilization of the external genitalia in female fetuses. Equally important may be the effects of this androgen exposure on the developing CNS.

C. **Clinical presentation.** Three subtypes of CAH related to 21-OHD are traditionally recognized, each of which can give rise to a different clinical picture. Two are known as "classic" CAH: a simple virilizing form and a salt-wasting form. A third, "nonclassic" CAH, a milder subtype, presents later in life. It has been proposed that rather than dividing CAH into types, this complex disorder is best viewed as a disease continuum that reflects the severity of enzyme deficiency (Therrell et al., 1998).
   1. *Simple virilizing* (25% of patients). An incomplete enzymatic block allows enough aldosterone production to maintain fluid and electrolyte homeostasis. In these infants, clinical signs are few or absent, depending on the degree of enzyme deficiency.
   2. *Salt-wasting disease* (75% of patients).
      a. A complete deficiency of P-450_{c21} activity eliminates both cortisol and aldosterone synthesis. High sodium excretion occurring in the absence of

aldosterone (called a "salt-losing" or "salt-wasting" state) results in profound hyponatremia. Dehydration and hyperkalemia are related to failure of both water conservation and potassium excretion. Glucocorticoid deficiency impairs carbohydrate metabolism (causing hypoglycemia) and leads to hypotension, shock, and cardiovascular collapse.

b. Onset of the salt-losing state usually begins after day 7 of life. The newborn normally has a high aldosterone level in the first week because of slow hepatic clearance, but as aldosterone is depleted, the deficient adrenal cortex cannot restore it.

D. **Assessment.**

1. The earliest signs and symptoms are lethargy, poor feeding, vomiting, diarrhea, dehydration, failure to thrive, apnea, and seizures.
2. Appearance of the genitalia.
   a. In girls with 21-OHD (female karyotype, 46,XX) the external genitalia are virilized. The phenotype is mild to moderate clitoral hypertrophy, varying degrees of labioscrotal fusion, and a urogenital sinus. In the most severe cases, marked clitoral hypertrophy gives the appearance of a penile urethra, and labioscrotal folds are completely fused (Prader stage V virilization). These infants can be mistaken for boys with bilateral cryptorchidism (undescended testes). There can also be hyperpigmentation of the genital skin resulting from excessive pituitary ACTH secretion.
   b. In boys with 21-OHD (male karyotype, 46,XY), external genitalia are male.

E. **Diagnosis of CAH related to 21-OHD.** In the past, CAH was not always diagnosed in the neonatal period unless atypical genitalia were noted at birth or the infant had an early salt-wasting adrenal crisis. With neonatal screening, however, CAH is increasingly diagnosed before clinical recognition of the disorder (Therrell et al., 1998).

1. Common diagnostic tests and findings in 21-OHD CAH are:
   a. 17-OHP level is markedly elevated and is hyperresponsive to ACTH stimulation; levels of testosterone and its precursors are increased.
   b. Serum aldosterone and plasma renin activity are measured to detect salt-losing states. The aldosterone level is low and plasma renin activity is high.
   c. Serum and urine electrolytes reveal hyponatremia, hyperkalemia, and high urine sodium excretion. Other metabolic disturbances include hypoglycemia and metabolic acidosis.
   d. Fluorescence in situ hybridization (FISH) studies or karyotyping to establish genetic sex.
   e. Ultrasonography and/or magnetic resonance imaging is done to visualize the uterus and adrenal glands.
2. Neonatal screening for CAH is currently performed in 32 states (for current list refer to www.genes-r-us.uthscsa.edu/resources/newborn/screenstatus.htm).

The basis of screening is measurement of 17-OHP, which is elevated in CAH. Some preterm infants and other sick infants have false-positive results because their 17-OHP levels are typically higher. Blood samples drawn early in life (before 24 hours of age) can also give a false-positive screening result because 17-OHP is still physiologically elevated.

F. **Management of CAH.**

1. Restore physiologic levels of cortisol, suppress ACTH and androgen overproduction, and maintain fluid and electrolyte homeostasis.

2. Administer *hydrocortisone* (glucocorticoid) and *9-α-fludrocortisone* (mineralocorticoid). New drugs such as androgen-blockers and aromatase inhibitors are currently under study.
3. Dietary sodium supplementation to prevent hyponatremia, if needed.
4. Additional measures. In a salt-losing state/adrenal crisis, these may include intravenous (IV) administration of fluids (glucose and sodium to correct dehydration and metabolic imbalances), treatment of shock, and correction of acidosis.
5. Genetic counseling.
   a. Prenatal diagnosis for subsequent pregnancies using direct analysis of the CYP_{21} gene using DNA samples extracted from chorionic villus sampling or amniocentesis (Hughes, 2002)
   b. Intrauterine treatment can prevent some or all of the virilization of female fetuses. Dexamethasone given to the mother crosses the placenta and suppresses fetal ACTH. Treatment must begin before 8 weeks' gestation and continue to term in affected female fetuses.
6. Parent education. Discuss immediate and long-term management of the disorder, the importance of compliance with therapy, and the need for follow-up of growth and development.

G. **Management of virilized genitalia in female neonates with CAH.** There are two issues regarding the management of the neonate with virilizing CAH. One is gender of rearing, the other is the type of surgery that will be needed, if any, and the timing of that surgery.

1. Gender of rearing.
   a. The genetic female (46,XX) with 21-OHD, regardless of the degree of virilization of the external genitalia, has normal female reproductive structures: ovaries, uterus, fallopian tubes, and upper vagina, and is potentially fertile. The lower vagina is foreshortened, conjoining with the urethra to form a high urogenital sinus defect where the vagina enters the urethra (Schnitzer and Donahoe, 2001). Most 46,XX neonates with CAH are assigned to the female gender to preserve endogenous sex hormone production and fertility (Meyer-Bahlburg, 2001).
   b. Occasionally as a result of missed or delayed diagnosis, 46,XX neonates with severe virilization (complete fusion of the labia and a penile urethra) are raised as males, despite potential fertility as females. Choosing male sex of rearing at birth for similarly affected neonates has been suggested, based on the theory that significant prenatal brain virilization might have occurred, leading to the later adoption of a male gender identity. No studies have been done yet to evaluate this approach (Blizzard, 2002).
2. Surgical considerations.
   a. Typically, feminizing genitoplasty (clitoral recession and labioscrotal reduction) is performed early in life, often combined with vaginal exteriorization in a one-stage procedure to "normalize" the genitalia and spare the child the trauma of later genital surgeries. Some data suggest, however, that this has not always had the desired outcome. Some girls and women who have undergone surgical correction of their virilized genitalia in infancy have had poor results, including clitoral atrophy, vaginal stenosis, scarring, and persistent urogenital sinus. Virtually all required additional procedures after puberty (Alizai et al., 1999). Newer surgical techniques now in use might avoid these problems, but objective long-term outcome studies for these patients are not yet available (Schnitzer and Donahoe, 2001).

b. Lee and Witchel (2002) documented a shift away from early surgery, by parental choice, for female infants with CAH. They speculate that this might be the result of increased parental awareness of the variation of clitoral size and a desire to avoid unnecessary surgery.

c. Many surgeons now agree that infants with mild clitoromegaly should not undergo early surgery in anticipation that as the hormonal milieu normalizes with therapy, clitoral size will decrease and labial appearance will improve (Aaronson, 2001).

H. **Complications of CAH.**

1. Adrenal crisis can occur with sudden signs of cortisol insufficiency (shock, hypotension, acidosis, hypoglycemia, seizures) plus sodium depletion. This can be triggered by episodes of illness or stress (such as systemic infection or surgery) in the neonatal period. Stress therapy to prevent this complication requires two or three times the usual dosage of hydrocortisone.

2. Consequences of poorly controlled CAH:

a. Failure to suppress ACTH and androgen production can result in signs of virilization and accelerated growth or bone maturation.

b. Overtreatment, resulting in hypertension, pulmonary edema, congestive heart failure, growth failure, adrenal atrophy, and lowered resistance to infection.

I. **Outcome.**

1. Lifelong hormonal replacement is usually necessary to improve chances for normal growth, pubertal development, and fertility.

2. Missed or delayed diagnosis can result in sudden deterioration or death in infants with undiagnosed CAH.

3. Hyperandrogenemia in the fetus with CAH has a masculinizing effect on the fetal brain during a critical period of development (Hrabovzky and Hutson, 2002). It is believed that this accounts for later differences in gender role behavior seen in females with CAH, compared with those without CAH, including toy preferences, rough-and-tumble play, aggressiveness, interest in sports, maternal behavior, and vocational preferences (Meyer-Bahlburg, 2001). In spite of this, females with CAH generally grow up with a female gender identity, provided that steroid treatment is started early and suppression of adrenal androgens is maintained (Warne and Kanumakala, 2002).

DISORDERS OF SEXUAL DEVELOPMENT

Sexual Differentiation

At every stage of fetal sexual differentiation there is a tendency for the internal and external sexual structures to develop along female lines. Development along male lines requires the expression of specific genes and the secretion of hormones at precise times. Appreciation of the bipotentiality of embryologic tissues is fundamental to understanding disorders of sexual development.

A. **Fertilization:** determination of genetic sex based on X or Y chromosome, contained in the spermatozoon.

B. **Primitive gonad development** beginning at about 6 weeks of gestation.

1. Embryonic gonads form on the genital ridge near the kidneys and are seeded by germ cells that migrate from the yolk sac.

2. At this stage gonads of male and female embryos are indistinguishable.

C. **Gonadal differentiation:** beginning about week 6 or 7 of gestation.

1. Tendency of the primitive gonad is to become an ovary. Two intact X chromosomes are required for differentiation to a normal ovary.

2. Differentiation to a testis is thought to be activated principally by the testis-determining gene SRY (sex-determining region Y) on the Y chromosome. SRY initiates the testicular developmental cascade along with other early development genes including SF-1, WT-1, SOX-9, and DAX-1 (Dewing et al., 2002)
3. Primitive Sertoli cells of the testes begin to develop first, followed by the Leydig cells. The testes begin secreting hormones necessary for further male differentiation. Ovaries differentiate more slowly and do not play an active role in controlling subsequent sexual development.

D. **Genital duct differentiation:** begins at about week 7 of gestation.
1. Before differentiation, two pairs of primordial ducts form in all embryos: the müllerian ducts and the wolffian ducts.
2. In the absence of further hormonal influence, the müllerian ducts become the female urogenital structures (fallopian tubes, uterus, cervix, and upper portion of the vagina) and the wolffian ducts regress.
3. Differentiation of the wolffian ducts into male urogenital structures requires secretion of müllerian inhibiting substance (MIS) by the Sertoli cells and of testosterone, produced by the Leydig cells. These hormones act in a paracrine fashion, causing the adjacent müllerian ducts to regress and the wolffian ducts to persist, forming the excretory ducts to the testes, seminal vesicles, and prostatic glands.
4. The fetal testes begin to descend in the first trimester but do not appear in the scrotum until the last 12 weeks of gestation.

E. **External genital differentiation (Fig. 29-3):** begins about week 8.
1. Early undifferentiated structures are identical in both sexes: a small genital tubercle, central urogenital slit surrounded by genital folds, and lateral genital swellings.
2. Tendency is for external genitalia to feminize: the genital tubercle forms the clitoris, genital folds become the labia minora, genital swellings form the labia majora, and the genital slit remains open to the vagina.
3. In the presence of testosterone and its metabolite, dihydrotestosterone (DHT), genital structures are masculinized: the genital tubercle becomes the glans penis, genital folds form the ventral surface of the urethra and penile shaft, genital swellings become the scrotum, and the genital slit fuses. The enzyme 5-α-reductase is required for conversion of testosterone to DHT. The presence of testosterone at this time will also induce virilization in a female fetus, because the genital tubercle and genital folds are rich in androgen receptors and 5-α-reductase, and are highly sensitive to DHT (Warne and Kanumakala, 2002).
4. Penile growth continues to term under the influence of the pituitary gland. Pituitary luteinizing hormone stimulates the Leydig cells to produce testosterone, which promotes growth of the differentiated penis.

Sexual Differentiation (Intersex) Disorders

Intersex conditions arise when there is either a failure in one of the steps along the male developmental pathway, or when a genetically female fetus is exposed to an excess of androgens early in development (Aaronson, 2001). Most intersex conditions are very rare. The more common disorders will be presented here; for a more comprehensive review the reader is referred to a textbook of pediatric endocrinology.

A. **Disorders of gonadal differentiation.**
1. *Pure gonadal dysgenesis* (46,XY). Complete or partial failure of testicular differentiation; affected neonates often have female internal genitalia.

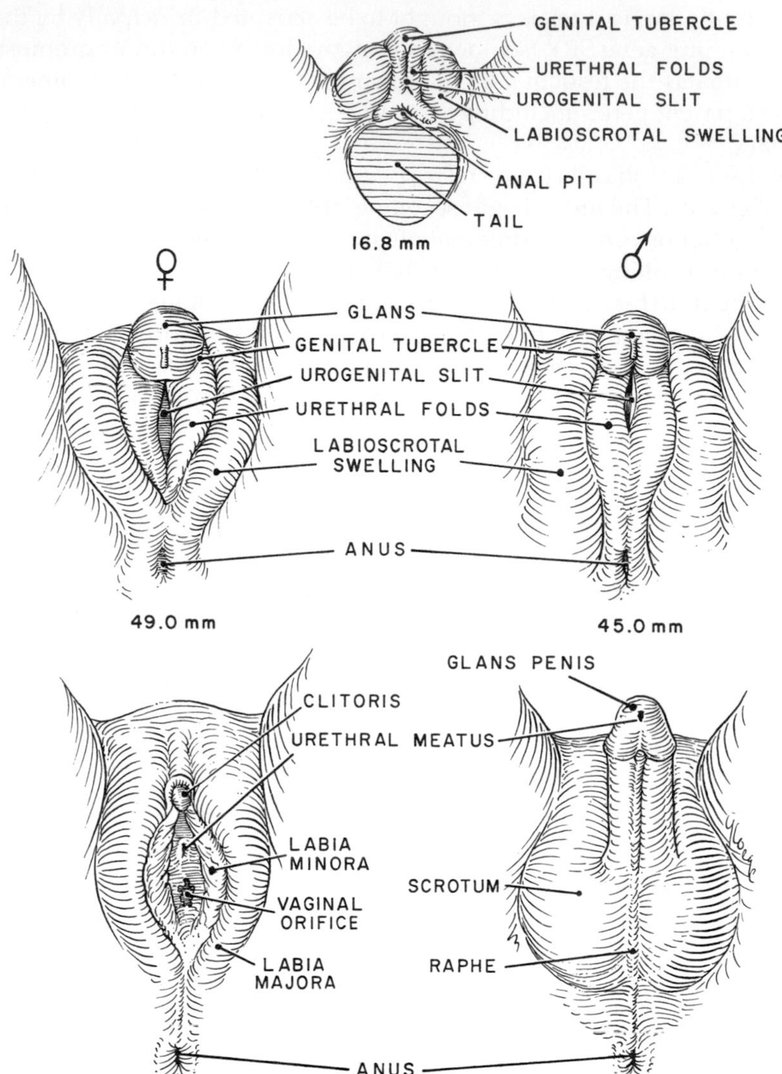

FIGURE 29-3 ■ Development and differentiation of male and female external genitalia. (Adapted from Spaulding, M.H.: The development of the external genitalia in the human embryo. *Contrib Embryol Carnegie Inst*, *13*:69-88, 1921; In P.R. Larsen, H.M. Kronenberg, S. Melmed, and K.S. Polonsky: *Williams textbook of endocrinology* [10th ed.]. Philadelphia, 2003, Saunders, p. 873.)

2. *Mixed gonadal dysgenesis* (45,XO/46,XY). These infants have ambiguous genitalia that are asymmetric, such as a scrotum on one side only.
3. *Klinefelter syndrome* (usually 47,XXY), involving dysgenesis of the seminiferous tubules. This common disorder affects 1 in 1000 newborn male infants but is not generally diagnosed in the neonatal period.
4. *Turner syndrome* (45,X or variation), a type of gonadal dysgenesis. Affected infants have the female phenotype, with classic somatic features and bilateral streak gonads. Affects 1 in 2500 live female births.

B. True hermaphroditism.

1. Karyotype varies (46,XX, 46,XY mosaicism, or 46,XX/46,XY chimerism). Both ovarian and testicular tissues are present, either separately or combined in an ovotestis.

2. The internal ducts parallel the ipsilateral gonadal histology. The appearance of the external genitalia reflects the amount of testicular tissue in the gonads (Aaronson, 2001).

C. **Disorders of differentiation of the genital ducts/external genitalia.**
   1. Genetic female (46,XX) with virilized external genitalia (also known as *female pseudohermaphroditism*). Internal organs (gonads, genital ducts) are normal female structures. The degree of masculinization depends on the point during gestation when development was influenced by androgens. Etiologies include:
      a. *CAH*, caused by 21-hydroxylase deficiency, 11-β-hydroxylase deficiency, or 3-β-hydroxysteroid dehydrogenase deficiency. 21-OHD is the most common cause of genital ambiguity in the 46,XX neonate.
      b. *Placental aromatase deficiency*. The enzyme aromatase normally catalyzes the conversion of androgens to estrogens. In its absence, excess androgens can virilize both mother and fetus.
      c. Excessive androgen production by the mother (maternal CAH, androgen-producing tumors), ingestion of certain drugs, such as danazol.
   2. Genetic male (46,XY), with incomplete masculinization of external genitalia (also known as *male pseudohermaphroditism*), as a result of defects in the synthesis, metabolism, or receptor sensitivity of androgens. Gonads are normal, but genital ducts may fail to fully develop and external genitalia are ambiguous. Etiologies include:
      a. *Androgen insensitivity syndrome* (AIS). This X-linked recessive disorder is characterized by defects in androgen receptors, preventing binding of testosterone and DHT to genital tissues. DHT is present but is unable to effect its masculinizing action. There are complete and partial forms.
         (1) Partial AIS is the most common intersex disorder in the 46,XY neonate. PAIS is extremely heterogeneous. Depending on the degree of androgen receptor function, a wide range of genital phenotypes, from a small phallus or hypospadias to extreme hypovirilization, can be seen.
         (2) Complete AIS may not be recognized at birth because the infant's genitalia are female. Many infants will present with an inguinal or labial hernia.
      b. *Deficiency of 5-α-reductase*. This enzyme is required for conversion of testosterone to DHT. Internal structures are normal male, but because of variable degrees of enzyme activity, the external phenotype ranges from ambiguous to female.
      c. *Defect of testosterone biosynthesis*. The most common disorder of testosterone biosynthesis causing ambiguous genitalia in the 46,XY neonate is 17-β-hydroxysteroid dehydrogenase deficiency (also termed 17-ketosteroid reductase deficiency).
      d. *Persistent müllerian duct*. The uterus and fallopian tubes fail to regress in an otherwise normal male fetus because of a defect in synthesis, secretion, or response to müllerian inhibiting substance.
   3. Other conditions associated with disorders of sexual development:
      a. *Cryptorchidism:* unilateral or bilateral absence of testes in the scrotum, caused by failure of testicular descent. Occurring in 5% of term infants, it is one of the most common urogenital abnormalities of childhood.
      b. *Hypospadias:* incomplete fusion of the penile urethra. The urethral meatus is found proximal to the glans penis, somewhere along the ventral surface of the penis or, in severe cases, on the perineum. Hypospadias occurs in

approximately 1 of 125 newborn male infants. Perineoscrotal hypospadias is frequently a feature of abnormal sexual differentiation.

   c. *Micropenis:* an otherwise normally formed penis that measures less than 2.5 cm in stretched length from the pubic bone to the tip of the glans. Micropenis results from reduced androgen and/or growth hormone effects during the second or third trimester. Major causes of isolated micropenis include *primary hypogonadism* and *hypopituitarism*. With congenital hypopituitarism, neonates may have persistent hypoglycemia, hypothyroidism, hyperbilirubinemia, and midline craniofacial defects (cleft lip and palate) or septo-optic dysplasia.

D. Clinical presentation.

1. Often, but not always, neonates with disorders of sexual development present with ambiguous genitalia, a term that refers to genitals that are anatomically in between what is typically considered male and typically considered female. In some intersex disorders, there may be only a single atypical genital feature; in still others, genitalia appear "normal" at birth.
2. Other presenting signs and symptoms may relate to a primary endocrine disorder (adrenal insufficiency, hypopituitarism, growth hormone deficiency).
3. Dysmorphic features, such as those of Turner syndrome, can be associated with cases of gonadal dysgenesis. Many malformation syndromes and other nonendocrine conditions can be associated with genital ambiguity; among these are trisomy 13, cloacal exstrophy, Smith-Lemli-Opitz syndrome and camptomelic dysplasia.

E. Assessment and physical examination.

1. Examination of the genitalia: close scrutiny not only of infants with clearly atypical genitalia but also of apparent "girls" with inguinal masses, hernias, or clitoromegaly and of apparent "boys" with nonpalpable testes, hypospadias, or unusually small genitalia.
   a. Phallus: size (length and width), presence of *chordee* (downward curvature of the penis, found in some forms of hypospadias), and location of the urethral meatus relative to normal position (may require observation of voiding).
   b. Perineal openings (separate vaginal and urethral openings or a single urogenital sinus): presence of a vagina or a blind vaginal pouch.
   c. Gonads: presence, location (scrotal sac, inguinal canal, groin), size, and symmetry.
   d. Labioscrotal folds: location (posterior or anterior) and degree of fusion (partial or complete), rugosity.
   e. Pigmentation of the genitalia.
2. Assessment findings. Possibilities include:
   a. Virilization of a female neonate (Fig. 29-4) can be expressed by degrees of clitoral hypertrophy, partial or complete fusion of the posterior labia, a single urogenital orifice, and hyperpigmentation of the labia, which may also be rugose. Because complete virilization can be mistaken for a male with bilateral cryptorchidism, any term infant with bilateral undescended testes should receive further evaluation.
   b. Hypovirilization of a male neonate (Fig. 29-5) may be expressed by a micropenis (with or without chordee), absence of testes in the scrotum, or incomplete fusion of the genital folds (bifid scrotum, resembling labia majora). A urogenital orifice on the perineum may have a small vaginal

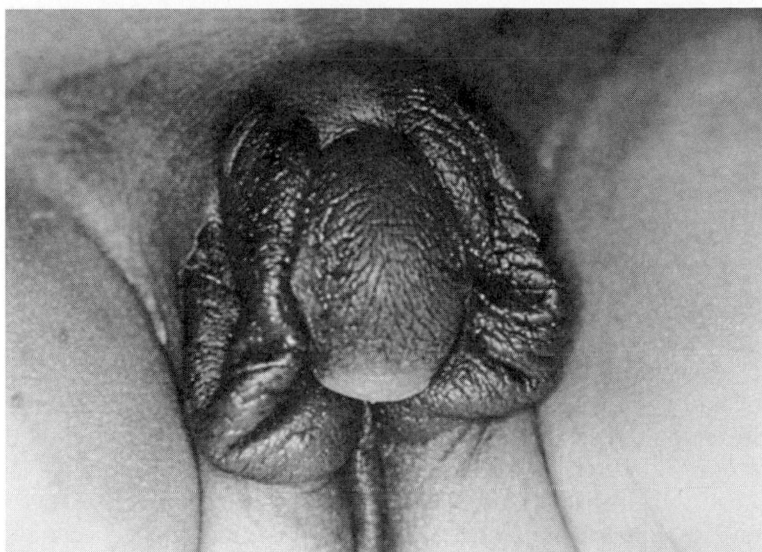

FIGURE 29-4 ■ Virilization in a 46,XX infant with 21-hydroxylase deficiency. Note clitoral hypertrophy and hyperpigmented and rugated labiosacral folds, resembling an empty scrotum. (Courtesy Michael S. Kappy, M.D., PhD.)

pouch. A presumed female infant with unilateral or bilateral inguinal hernia(s) should be tested for complete AIS.

c. True hermaphrodites and infants with mixed gonadal dysgenesis may present with marked ambiguity that is asymmetric.

F. **Diagnosis:** a combination of genetic evaluation, clinical and biochemical findings, and examination of internal structures.

1. Family history: a similarly affected infant or family member, ingestion of androgens during pregnancy, maternal virilization, or uncontrolled CAH.

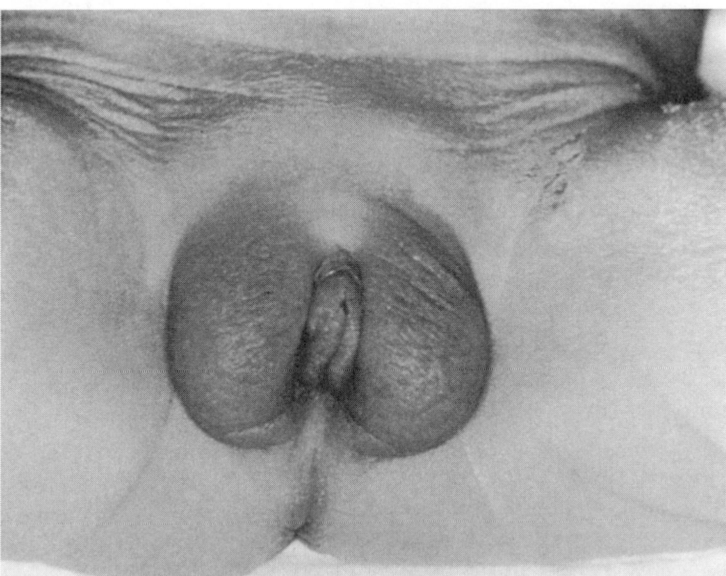

FIGURE 29-5 ■ Infant with karyotype 46,XY and ambiguous genitalia caused by 5-α-reductase deficiency. Note absence of a penis and lack of fusion of labiosacral folds, indicating incomplete virilization. (Courtesy Michael S. Kappy, M.D., PhD.)

2. Karyotype, fluorescence in situ hybridization (FISH) testing.
3. Hormonal studies for a possible underlying endocrine disorder and/or to evaluate response to exogenously administered human chorionic gonadotropin (hCG) or testosterone.
4. Evaluation of internal structures with ultrasonography, magnetic resonance imaging, radiographic studies (genitography).
5. Laparoscopy/surgical exploration and gonadal biopsy.
6. More extensive tests (molecular genetic studies, enzyme assays of genital skin) for a definitive diagnosis.

G. **Care of the parents.** With advances in prenatal sonography and testing, some infants with genital anomalies are now being identified prior to birth and parents have already been counseled about their infant's condition (Pinhas-Hamiel et al., 2002). In another scenario, determination of fetal gender by routine prenatal ultrasound leads to delivery room confusion when the actual gender of the newborn is uncertain. And finally, parents who wish to be surprised by their infant's gender at birth might find it incomprehensible that doctors and nurses cannot immediately tell them the sex of their newborn infant. With very little time to consider their reply, caregivers must respond to the "simple" question, "Is it a boy or a girl?"

1. Communication and education.
   a. When faced with an infant of uncertain sex, staff in the delivery room should not announce a gender, no matter how much pressure they feel to do so, because reversing this gender assignment at a later time will be even more difficult for the parents. An alternative is to tell the parents that a difference in their infant's development prevents determination of the sex in the usual way (i.e., by examining the external genitalia).
   b. Parents should be shown the infant while the differences from more typical features are explained. Open communication regarding planned tests to determine the infant's sex, and when they may expect to hear results, is advocated.
   c. Later, explanations of fetal sexual development, the bipotential nature of developing sexual organs, and critical influences during development are used to help parents understand what caused their infant's development to follow a different path.
2. Emotional support.
   a. Anticipate parents' reactions, which may include shock, grief, anger, confusion, and disbelief. Frustration with long waits for test results may be expressed.
   b. Provide guidance in dealing with friends and relatives, a significant source of distress for most parents.
   c. It is suggested that parents delay naming the infant and registering the birth.
   d. Every effort must be made to encourage parent-infant bonding from the moment of birth.
   e. Counseling for the parents should begin immediately.
3. Decision making.
   a. In the past, decisions regarding gender assignment and surgery for neonates with intersex disorders were often made primarily by teams of physicians. With parents excluded from full participation, such decisions could have reflected physicians' preferences, customs or even biases, and perpetuated a morally and legally unacceptable paternalism (Daaboul and Frader, 2001).

b. Increasingly, experts are advocating complete disclosure of information to parents to allow them to make fully informed decisions regarding gender assignment and surgery that are in the best interests of their child and family (Blizzard, 2002; Lee and Witchel, 2002).

H. Care of the infant.

1. Information gathering.
   a. The birth of an infant with ambiguous genitalia is treated with urgency; diagnostic testing begins immediately. A multidisciplinary team (pediatric endocrinologist, geneticist, pediatric urologic surgeon, radiologist, psychiatrist) may be called on to evaluate the infant or consult on the case.
   b. It can take several days to get the information needed for some sex-of-rearing decisions. In the interim, sex assignment should not be made or guessed at on the basis of external features alone.
   c. Sex assignment is not determined by any one factor in isolation, such as the chromosomes, gonads, or external anatomy. These and many other factors (e.g., underlying pathophysiology, prognosis for pubertal development, future sexual function and sensation, fertility, chances for a satisfactory surgical repair and need for additional procedures, cultural beliefs and values of the family) are considered when sex-of-rearing decisions are made.
2. Gender assignment.
   a. The majority of 46,XX neonates with CAH are raised as girls, regardless of the degree of virilization, because internal structures are female, fertility is possible, and most develop a female gender identity. (See Congenital Adrenal Hyperplasia on p. 714-718.)
   b. 46,XY neonates with defects of testosterone synthesis or gonadotropin deficiencies are usually raised as boys because they may respond to hormonal treatment with phallic growth and testicular descent. A stimulation test (hCG) may be given to evaluate this response. Neonates with 5-α-reductase deficiency are also assigned the male gender because they will virilize at puberty.
   c. Gender assignment of 46,XY neonates with partial androgen insensitivity depends on the individual phenotype and in some cases, the results of additional testing conducted in the newborn period.
   d. Occasionally, a severely undervirilized 46,XY neonate is assigned to the female sex of rearing after considerable testing, consultation with experts, and discussion with the parents. At the present time, data are insufficient to predict a child's eventual gender identity based on underlying condition or appearance of the genitalia, rendering these decisions difficult for parents and professionals alike.
3. Surgical considerations.
   a. Decisions regarding surgery might not be finalized in the neonatal period, but the same issues faced during gender assignment decisions will have to be addressed when discussing surgical management. While it is hoped that the child will adapt to the chosen sex of rearing, if surgery is carried out too early and a different gender identity becomes apparent, the outcome can be disastrous (Warne and Kanumakala, 2002).
   b. Controversy exists regarding the performance of genital surgery on neonates with intersex conditions unless it is medically necessary. Former patients who believe they were irreversibly harmed by gender

reconstruction in infancy point out that such procedures are often done for cosmetic purposes only, and should be deferred until the child is old enough to give consent (ISNA, 1994). This remains a matter of debate (Daaboul and Frader, 2001); however, it has been recommended that in discussing all options with parents they be informed that delaying surgery is an alternative available to them (Warne and Kanumakala, 2002).

c. Early surgery may be medically necessary for some infants to reduce the risk of gonadal cancer or to prevent recurrent urinary tract infections (Warne and Kanumakala, 2002).

I. **Complications.**

1. Inappropriate sex assignment when the ambiguity was not detected in the neonatal period.
2. Gonadal or genital duct malignancy.

J. **Outcome.**

1. Some children undergoing genital surgery will require staged reconstructive procedures and, at puberty, hormonal therapy to induce development of gender-appropriate secondary sexual characteristics.
2. Reproductive capacity varies according to the condition. Fertility is possible in some circumstances (e.g., in a woman with CAH) but is rare or impossible in others (complete AIS, some forms of gonadal dysgenesis).
3. Outcome studies of intersex disorders are limited. Available data reveal that the affected child and the family face difficulties that extend well beyond the initial crisis in the neonatal period (Slijper et al., 1998). With patients sometimes "lost to follow-up," professionals may not always be fully aware of the lifelong implications of decisions that were made in the first days of life.

REFERENCES

Aaronson, I.A: The investigation and management of the infant with ambiguous genitalia: A surgeon's perspective. *Current Problems in Pediatrics, 31*(6): 168-194, 2001.

Alizai, N.K., Thomas, D.F.M., Lilford, R.J., et al.: Feminizing genitoplasty for congenital adrenal hyperplasia: What happens at puberty? *Journal of Urology, 161*(5): 1588-1591, 1999.

Biswas, S., Buffery, J., Enoch, H., et al.: Longitudinal assessment of thyroid hormone concentrations in preterm infants younger than 30 weeks gestation during the first 2 weeks of life and their relationship to outcome. *Pediatrics, 109*(2): 222-227, 2002.

Blizzard, R.M.: Intersex issues: A series of continuing conundrums. *Pediatrics, 110*(3):616-621, 2002.

Bolt, R.J., van Weissenbruch, M.M., Lafeber, H.N., and Delemarre-van de Waal, H.A.: Development of the hypothalamic-pituitary-adrenal axis in the fetus and preterm infant. *Journal of Pediatric Endocrinology and Metabolism, 15*(6): 759-769, 2002.

Buckingham, B.: The hyperthyroid fetus and infant. *NeoReviews, 1*(6):e103-e109, 2000. Retrieved February 28, 2003 from http://neoreviews.aapjournals.org.content/vol1/issue6/index.shtml.

Chrousos, G.P.: Organization and integration of the endocrine system. In M.A. Sperling (Ed.): *Pediatric endocrinology* (2nd ed.). Philadelphia, 2002, Saunders.

Daaboul J. and Frader, J.: Ethics and management of the patient with intersex: A middle way. *Journal of Pediatric Endocrinology and Metabolism, 14*(9):1575-1583, 2001.

Dewing, P., Bernard, P., and Vilain, E.: Disorders of gonadal development. *Seminars in Reproductive Medicine, 20*(3):189-197, 2002.

Fisher, D.A.: The importance of early management in optimizing IQ in infants with congenital hypothyroidism. *Journal of Pediatrics, 136*(3):273-274, 2000.

Hrabovszky, Z. and Hutson, J.M.: Androgen imprinting of the brain in animal models and humans with intersex disorders: Review and recommendations. *Journal of Urology, 168*(5):2142-2148, 2002.

Hughes, I.: Congenital adrenal hyperplasia: Phenotype and genotype. *Journal of Pediatric Endocrinology and Metabolism, 15*(Suppl 5):1329-1340, 2002.

Intersex Society of North America: Recommendations for Treatment. San Francisco, 1994. Retrieved February 28, 2003 from www.isna.org.

Jett, P.L., Samuels, M.H., McDaniel, P.A., et al.: Variability of plasma cortisol levels in extremely low birth weight infants. *Journal of Clinical Endocrinology and Metabolism, 82*(9):2921-2925, 1997.

Kok, J.H., Briet, J.M., and van Wassenaer, A.G.: Postnatal thyroid hormone replacement in very low birth weight infants. *Seminars in Perinatology, 25*(6):417-425, 2001.

Lee, P.A. and Witchel, S.F.: Genital surgery among females with congenital adrenal hyperplasia: changes over the past five decades. *Journal of Pediatric Endocrinology and Metabolism, 15*(9): 1473-1477, 2002.

Leviton, A., Paneth, N., Reuss, M.L., et al. Hypothyroxinemia of prematurity and the risk of cerebral white matter damage. *Journal of Pediatrics, 134*(6):706-711, 1999.

Mandel, S.J., Hermos, R.J., Larson, C.A., et al.: Atypical hypothyroidism and the very low birth weight infant. *Thyroid, 10*(8):693-695, 2000.

Meyer-Bahlburg, H.F.L.: Gender and sexuality in classic congenital adrenal hyperplasia. *Endocrinology and Metabolism Clinics of North America, 30*(1):155-171, 2001.

Miller, W.: The adrenal cortex. In M.A. Sperling (Ed.): *Pediatric endocrinology* (2nd ed.). Philadelphia, 2002, Saunders.

Oden, J. and Freemark, M.: Thyroxine supplementation in preterm infants. *Current Opinion in Pediatrics, 14*(4):447-452, 2002.

Ogilvy-Stuart, A.L.: Neonatal thyroid disorders. *Archives of Disease in Childhood Fetal Neonatal Edition, 87*(3):F165-F171, 2002.

Paul, D.A., Leef, K.H., Voss B., et al.: Thyroxine and illness severity in very low-birth-weight infants. *Thyroid, 11*(9):871-875, 2001.

Pinhas-Hamiel, O., Zalel, Y., Smith, E., et al.: Prenatal diagnosis of sex differentiation disorders: The role of fetal ultrasound. *Journal of Clinical Endocrinology and Metabolism, 87*(10):4547-4553, 2002.

Rapaport, R.: Thyroid function in the very low birth weight newborn. Rescreen or reevaluate? *Journal of Pediatrics, 140*(3):287-289, 2002.

Rapaport, R., Rose, S., and Freemark, M.: Hypothyroxinemia in the preterm infant: The benefits and risks of thyroxine treatment. *Journal of Pediatrics, 139*(2):182-188, 2001.

Schnitzer J.J. and Donahoe, P.K.: Surgical treatment of congenital adrenal hyperplasia. *Endocrinology and Metabolism Clinics of North America, 30*(1):137-154, 2001.

Selva, K.A., Mandel, S.H., Rien, L.R., et al.: Initial treatment dose of L-thyroxine in congenital hypothyroidism. *Journal of Pediatrics, 141*(6):786-792, 2002.

Slijper, F.M., Drop, S.L., Molenaar, J.C., de Muinck Keizer-Schrama, S.M.: Long-term psychological evaluation of intersex children. *Archives of Sexual Behavior, 27*(2):125-145, 1998.

Therrell, B.L.: Newborn screening for congenital adrenal hyperplasia. *Endocrinology and Metabolism Clinics of North America, 30*(1):15-29, 2001.

Therrell, B.L., Berenbaum, S.A., Manter-Kapanke, V., et al.: Results of screening 1.9 million Texas newborns for 21-hydroxylase deficient congenital adrenal hyperplasia. *Pediatrics, 101*(4 Pt 1):583-590, 1998.

van Wassenaer, A.G., Briet, J.M., van Baar, A., et al.: Free thyroxine levels during the first weeks of life and neurodevelopmental outcome until the age of 5 years in very preterm infants. *Pediatrics, 109*(3):534-539, 2002.

van Wassenaer, A.G., Kok, J.H., Briet, J.M., et al.: Thyroid function in very preterm newborns: Possible implications. *Thyroid, 9*(1):85-91, 1999.

Warne, G.L. and Kanumakala, S.: Molecular endocrinology of sex differentiation. *Seminars in Reproductive Medicine, 20*(3):169-179, 2002.

CHAPTER

30 Hematologic Disorders

WILLIAM DIEHL-JONES AND DEBBIE FRASER ASKIN

OBJECTIVES

1. Understand the processes of hematopoiesis and erythropoiesis.
2. Recall erythrocyte and leukocyte development from pluripotent stem cells.
3. Relate the consequences of anemia to the management of the infant.
4. Evaluate the clinical presentation of disseminated intravascular coagulation in relation to the coagulation consumption and fibrinolysis.
5. Describe the etiologic factors of hemorrhagic disease of the newborn.
6. Describe key indicators for nursing assessment of the thrombocytopenic infant.
7. Evaluate the neonatal consequences of maternal immune thrombocytopenic purpura.
8. Discuss the role of partial exchange transfusion in the treatment of neonatal polycythemia.
9. Describe current recommendations for use of blood components.
10. Analyze the components of the complete blood cell count and describe the usefulness of each in the determination of neonatal sepsis.

To meet the objectives, the chapter presents an overview of blood cell development and coagulation factors, and includes normal birth values and common diagnostic tests. Blood products and transfusion therapies are discussed with current recommendations for use. Common hematologic problems and therapies affecting the newborn infant are outlined. An evaluation of the components of a complete blood cell count, useful for identification of sepsis, is included.

DEVELOPMENT OF BLOOD CELLS

A. **Hematopoiesis:** formation, production, and maintenance of blood cells (Beardsley and Nathan, 1998; Christensen, 1998; Doyle et al., 1999; Israels and Israels, 2002).
   1. Pluripotent stem cells, from which all blood cells derive, are present in the yolk sac at 16 days' gestation.
   2. Circulation begins by day 22, with primitive cells arising intravascularly from vessel walls.
   3. Extravascular liver hematopoiesis begins with migration of pluripotent stem cells from the yolk sac, well established by 9 weeks' gestation.
   4. Liver hematopoiesis peaks at 4 to 5 months' gestation and then slowly regresses as medullary (bone marrow) hematopoiesis predominates from 22 weeks' gestation.
   5. Sites of extramedullary hematopoiesis (spleen, lymph nodes, thymus, kidneys) aid production of cells during fetal life when long bones are small.

6. Pluripotent cells develop into either colony-forming unit–granulocyte, erythrocyte, monocyte, megakaryocyte (CFU-GEMM), or lymphoid stem cells, which evolve into specific cell lines (Fig. 30-1).
7. Hypoxia, bacterial infection, and other forms of physiologic stress can influence the rate of differentiation of pluripotent cells.
8. Hematopoietic factors include interleukins (e.g., IL-1, IL-3, and IL-5), growth and differentiation factors such as granulocyte colony–stimulating factor (G-CSF), monocyte-colony stimulating factor (M-CSF), granulocyte-monocyte colony-stimulating factor (GM-CSF), thrombopoietin (TPO), and erythropoietin (EPO).

B. **Erythropoiesis:** production of erythrocytes (red blood cells [RBCs]).
1. The erythrocyte precursor or burst-forming unit–erythroid (BFU-E) develops from a myeloid stem cell (CFU-GEMM), which also differentiates to produce a megakaryocyte precursor (CFU-Meg).
2. Erythropoiesis and synthesis of hemoglobin are regulated by a hormone, erythropoietin, which is in turn regulated by hypoxia.
3. Erythropoietin is produced postnatally in the kidneys, but during fetal life extrarenal sites (liver, submandibular glands) predominate.
4. Erythropoietin levels are increased in response to anemia, and low oxygen availability to tissues and are decreased in response to hypertransfusion.
5. Erythropoietin levels are also elevated in infants with Down syndrome, intrauterine growth restriction, and those born to women with diabetes or pregnancy-induced hypertension (PIH).

C. **Hemoglobin:** major iron-containing component of the RBCs.
1. Hemoglobin carries oxygen from the lungs to the tissue cells through the circulation.
2. Hemoglobin synthesis begins around 14 days of embryonic life.
3. Transition from predominant production of fetal hemoglobin (HbF) to production of adult hemoglobin (HbA) begins at the end of fetal life. RBCs contain 70% to 90% HbF at birth.

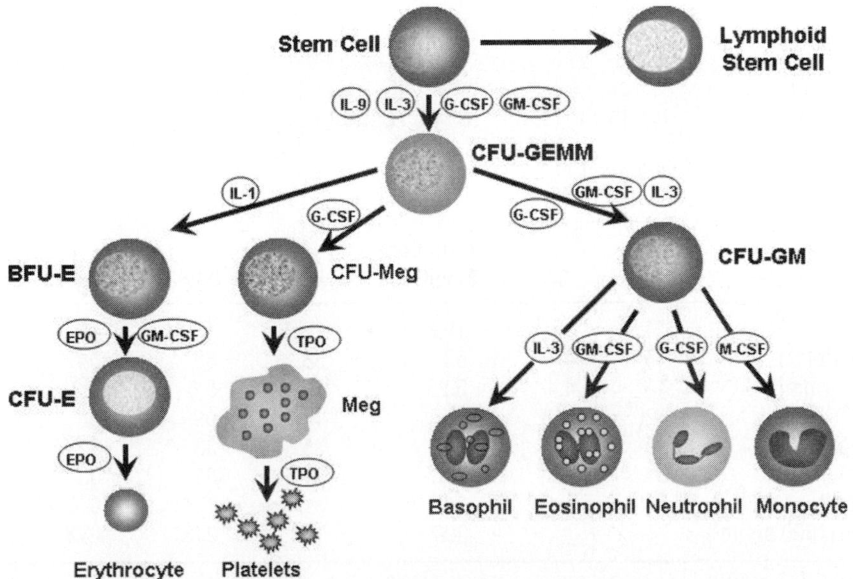

FIGURE 30-1 ■ Hematopoiesis and selected growth factors. (Adapted from Israels, L.G. and Israels, S.J.: *Mechanisms in hematology* [3rd ed.]. Toronto, 2002, Core Health Sciences, Inc., p. 402.)

4. Hemoglobin binds with 2,3-diphosphoglycerate (2,3-DPG), releasing an oxygen molecule.
   a. HbF has far less affinity for 2,3-DPG than does HbA, resulting in a greater affinity for oxygen.
   b. Levels of 2,3-DPG are directly proportional to gestational age.
5. Normal birth values (Table 30-1).
   a. Values depend on gestational age, volume of placental transfusion (timing of cord clamping, infant position), and blood sampling site; Hb in capillary samples may be significantly higher than in venous samples.
   b. Peripheral vasoconstriction and stasis yield higher values from capillary samples.
   c. Hb levels are higher in newborns, and decrease by the end of the first week of life to values similar to cord blood.

D. **Hematocrit:** percentage of RBCs in a unit volume of blood.
1. Values rise immediately after birth and then decline to cord levels in the first week.
2. Normal birth values (see Table 30-1).
   a. Values depend on gestational age and volume of placental transfusion (timing of cord clamping, infant position).
   b. Peripheral vasoconstriction and stasis yield higher values from capillary samples.

E. **RBCs.**
1. The erythrocyte BFU-E differentiates, under hormonal control, to form a CFU-E (colony-forming unit–erythrocyte), which loses its nucleus as it forms erythrocytes (see Fig. 30-1).
2. The CFU-E (or reticulocyte), in the absence of physiologic stress, mature 1 to 2 days in the bone marrow and then another day in the circulation before maturing to erythrocytes.
   a. Reticulocyte count is inversely proportional to gestational age at birth (see Table 30-1) but falls rapidly to less than 2% by 7 days.
   b. Persistent reticulocytosis may indicate chronic blood loss or hemolysis.

TABLE 30-1
Normal Blood Values in Premature and Term Infants

	Gestational Age (wk)						
Value	**28**	**34**	**Term Cord Blood**	**Day 1**	**Day 3**	**Day 7**	**Day 14**
Hb (g/dl)	14.5	15	16.8	18.4	17.8	17	16.8
Hematocrit (%)	45	47	53	58	55	54	52
Red cells (mm^3)	4	4.4	5.25	5.8	5.6	5.2	5.1
MCV (μ^3)	120	118	107	108	99	98	96
MCH (pg)	40	38	34	35	33	32.5	31.5
MCHC (%)	31	32	31.7	32.5	33	33	33
Reticulocytes (%)	5-10	3-10	3-7	3-7	1-3	0-1	0-1
Platelets (1000 s/mm^3)			290	192	213	248	252

Hb, Hemoglobin; *MCH,* mean corpuscular hemoglobin; *MCHC,* mean corpuscular hemoglobin concentration; *MCV,* mean corpuscular volume.
From Klaus, M.H. and Fanaroff, A.A.: *Care of the high-risk neonate* (4th ed.). Philadelphia, 1993, W.B. Saunders.

3. RBC function.
   a. Oxygen transport via oxyhemoglobin.
   b. Carbon dioxide transport via carboxyhemoglobin
   c. Carbon dioxide reacts with water to form carbonic acid; reaction catalyzed by carbonic anhydrase in cytoplasm of RBCs.
   d. Carbonic acid dissociation to form bicarbonate ions.
   e. Buffering protons via binding with hemoglobin to form acid hemoglobin and by reaction with bicarbonate ions.
4. RBC count.
   a. Number of circulating mature RBCs per cubic millimeter (see Table 30-1).
   b. Count equals production versus destruction or loss.
   c. RBC life span proportional to gestational age.
      (1) Adult: 100 to 120 days.
      (2) Term infant: 60 to 70 days.
      (3) Premature infant: 35 to 50 days.
   d. Nucleated RBCs are circulating immature (prereticulocyte) red cells.
      (1) Number is inversely proportional to gestational age and declines rapidly in the first week.
      (2) Increase may indicate hemolysis, acute blood loss, hypoxemia, congenital heart disease, or infection.
5. RBC indices: measure of RBC size and hemoglobin content used for designation of anemias (see Table 30-1).
   a. Mean corpuscular volume (MCV): average size and volume of a single RBC.
      (1) MCV decreases as gestation progresses and continues to decrease after birth to adult size by 4 to 5 years.
      (2) Increased MCV: RBCs referred to as macrocytes.
      (3) Decreased MCV: RBCs referred to as microcytes.
   b. Mean corpuscular hemoglobin (MCH): average amount (by weight) of hemoglobin in each RBC.
      (1) A decrease in MCH parallels a decrease in MCV.
      (2) Increased MCH: RBCs appear hyperchromic.
      (3) Decreased MCH: RBCs appear hypochromic.
   c. Mean corpuscular hemoglobin concentration (MCHC): average concentration of hemoglobin per single RBC, calculated from the amount of hemoglobin per deciliter of cells.
      (1) Adult values for MCHC reached by 6 months.
      (2) Increased MCHC: RBCs appear hyperchromic.
      (3) Decreased MCHC: RBCs appear hypochromic.
   d. Erythrocyte mass: total mass of erythrocytes
      (1) Best measure of anemia.
      (2) Direct correlation between erythrocyte mass and hemoglobin concentration.
      (3) Gold standard is use of chromium-labeled erythrocytes

F. White blood cells (WBCs).

1. Leukocyte precursors mature in the bone marrow and lymphatic tissues, in the absence of physiologic stress, through the CFU-GEMM and granulocyte-macrophage (CFU-GM) stages (see Fig. 30-1).
2. WBCs can leave the circulation to the extravascular tissues, where they function as an important part of the immunologic system in reaction to foreign protein.

3. Granulocytes, lymphocytes, and monocytes are types of WBCs.
   a. Granulocytes: include basophils, eosinophils, and neutrophils.
      (1) Basophils.
         (a) Important in allergic and inflammatory responses.
         (b) Least numerous of the granulocytes: 0.5% to 1% of total WBC count.
      (2) Eosinophils.
         (a) Perform similar functions as neutrophils but are less effective in response.
         (b) Unlike neutrophils, can survive for prolonged periods in extravascular space.
         (c) Important in allergic and anaphylactic responses and most effective granulocyte for parasitic destruction.
         (d) Benign eosinophilia of prematurity, inversely proportional to gestational age, may reflect immaturity of barrier mechanisms in the gastrointestinal and/or respiratory tract (Doyle et al., 1999).
         (e) Normally comprise 1% to 3% of total WBC count.
      (3) Neutrophils.
         (a) Neutrophils function as phagocytes to ingest and destroy small particles such as bacteria, protozoa, cells and cellular debris, and colloids.
         (b) Physiologic stress can increase production and bone marrow release of immature forms.
         (c) Neutrophils are increased at birth but decrease during the first week to reach percentages approximately equal to those of lymphocytes.
   b. Lymphocytes.
      (1) Thymus-derived (T) lymphocytes: important in graft-versus-host disease and delayed hypersensitivity reactions.
      (2) Bone marrow–derived (B) lymphocytes: important in the production and secretion of immunoglobulins and antibodies.
   c. Monocytes.
      (1) Circulating immature macrophages.
      (2) Transformed into macrophages in tissues (i.e., lung, alveolar macrophage; liver, Kupffer cell macrophages).
      (3) Responsible for clearance of old blood cells, cellular debris, opsonized bacteria, antigen-antibody complexes, and activated clotting factors from the circulation.
4. WBC count.
   a. WBC count is the number of circulating WBCs per cubic millimeter (Table 30-2).
   b. WBC count is proportional to gestational age, with the total counts of premature infants approximately 30% to 50% lower than those of term infants.

G. Platelets.

1. Small, nonnucleated, disk-shaped cells aid in hemostasis, coagulation, and thrombus formation.
   a. Platelets are derived from megakaryocytes in the bone marrow.
   b. Disrupted endothelium stimulates platelet plug formation and initiates hemostasis.
2. After release into the bloodstream, platelets will circulate 7 to 10 days before removal by the spleen. In the absence of injury, they circulate freely, without wall adhesion or aggregation with other platelets.

TABLE 30-2
Normal Leukocyte Values in Premature and Term Infants

Age (h)	Total White Cell Count	Neutrophils	Bands/Metas	Lymphocytes	Monocytes	Eosinophils
TERM INFANTS						
0	10.0-26.0	5.0-13.0	0.4-1.8	3.5-8.5	0.7-1.5	0.2-2.0
12	13.5-31.0	9.0-18.0	0.4-2.0	3.0-7.0	1.0-2.0	0.2-2.0
72	5.0-14.5	2.0-7.0	0.2-0.4	2.0-5.0	0.5-1.0	0.2-1.0
144	6.0-14.5	2.0-6.0	0.2-0.5	3.0-6.0	0.7-1.2	0.2-0.8
PREMATURE INFANTS						
0	5.0-19.0	2.0-9.0	0.2-2.4	2.5-6.0	0.3-1.0	0.1-0.7
12	5.0-21.0	3.0-11.0	0.2-2.4	1.5-5.0	0.3-1.3	0.1-1.1
72	5.0-14.0	3.0-7.0	0.2-0.6	1.5-4.0	0.3-1.2	0.2-1.1
144	5.5-17.5	2.0-7.0	0.2-0.5	2.5-7.5	0.5-1.5	0.3-1.2

Data modified from Xanthou (1970) by Glader (1977).
From Oski, F.A. and Naiman, J.L.: *Hematologic problems in the newborn* (3rd ed.). Philadelphia, 1982, W.B. Saunders.

3. Normal range is 150,000 to 400,000/mm^3 in the term and the premature infant. Counts are 20% to 25% lower in infants who are small for gestational age.
4. Neonatal platelets are hypoactive in the first few days after birth; this property protects against thrombosis but may increase risk of bleeding and coagulopathy.

H. Blood volume.

1. Volume of blood is measured in milliliters per kilogram of body weight.
2. Factors affecting blood volume are:
   - **a.** Gestational age.
     - (1) Term infant: approximately 80 to 100 ml/kg.
     - (2) Preterm infant: approximately 90 to 105 ml/kg.
   - **b.** Placental transfusion.
     - (1) Timing of cord clamping.
     - (2) Position of infant relative to placenta (above or below) before cord clamping.
     - (3) Timing and strength of uterine contractions.
     - (4) Onset of respiration and decrease in pulmonary vascular resistance.
     - (5) Cord compression.
   - **c.** Maternal-fetal or fetal-maternal transfusion.
   - **d.** Twin-twin transfusion.
   - **e.** Placenta previa or abruptio placentae.
   - **f.** Nuchal cord.
   - **g.** Iatrogenic loss.

COAGULATION

Hemostasis is accomplished by biochemical and physiologic events initiated to stop the flow of blood when vessel injury occurs (Israels and Israels, 2002).

A. Deficiencies in newborn clotting mechanisms.

1. Transient diminished platelet function.

2. Transient deficiency of clotting factors II, VII, IX, X, XI, and XII.
   a. Immaturity of hepatic enzymes responsible for production.
   b. Transient deficiency of vitamin K, needed for synthesis of factors II, VII, IX, and X.
   c. Factor concentrations: proportional to gestational age.

B. Hemostatic mechanisms.

1. Vascular: damaged vessel contracts, minimizing blood loss.
2. Intravascular: platelet plug formation. Platelet function is stimulated by exposure to damaged endothelial lining. Platelets:
   a. Swell and develop thornlike projections.
   b. Adhere to subendothelial fibers.
   c. Secrete adenosine diphosphate to trigger swelling and adhesiveness in nearby platelets.
   d. Aggregate and form platelet plug.
3. Extravascular.
   a. Compression by surrounding tissue.
   b. Release of tissue thromboplastin by injured tissue.

C. Coagulation process.

1. Cascade of events, requiring both cellular and plasma components (Fig. 30-2).
2. Culminates in the formation of fibrin-based clots, and requires serial activation of precursor zymogens.
3. Calcium, iron, and phospholipids are key components of the coagulation cascade.
   a. Extrinsic system triggered by tissue injury and exposure of cell membrane tissue factor (TF).
   b. Intrinsic system triggered by vascular endothelial injury; amplifies factor X activation, which is a cofactor common to intrinsic and extrinsic pathways.
   c. Factor X activation begins the process of prothrombin-to-thrombin conversion. Conversion hydrolyzes fibrinogen (soluble protein in plasma) to fibrin (insoluble, threadlike polymer) and activates factor XIII, stabilizing fibrin threads into a meshwork to trap platelets and other cells to form the clot.
4. Intravascular clotting is balanced by concurrent fibrinolysis.
   a. Inactive plasminogen synthesized by the liver is converted to plasmin, an active enzyme, when a fibrin clot is present.
   b. Plasmin begins fibrin clot dissolution, releasing fibrin degradation products (FDPs), also called fibrin split products (FSPs), into the circulation.
   c. FDPs exert an anticoagulant effect by interfering with clot formation and the function of platelets, thrombin, and fibrinogen.

D. Coagulation tests (Table 30-3).

1. Platelet count is used to assess platelet number.
2. Prothrombin time (PT) is used to assess extrinsic and common portions of the coagulation cascade.
3. Partial thromboplastin time (PTT) is used to assess intrinsic and common portions of the coagulation cascade.
4. Fibrinogen is used to assess the circulating level of this protein substrate, required for clot formation.
5. FDP/FSP is used to assess fibrinolytic activity.
6. Individual clotting factors may be assayed, depending on results of the tests cited above.

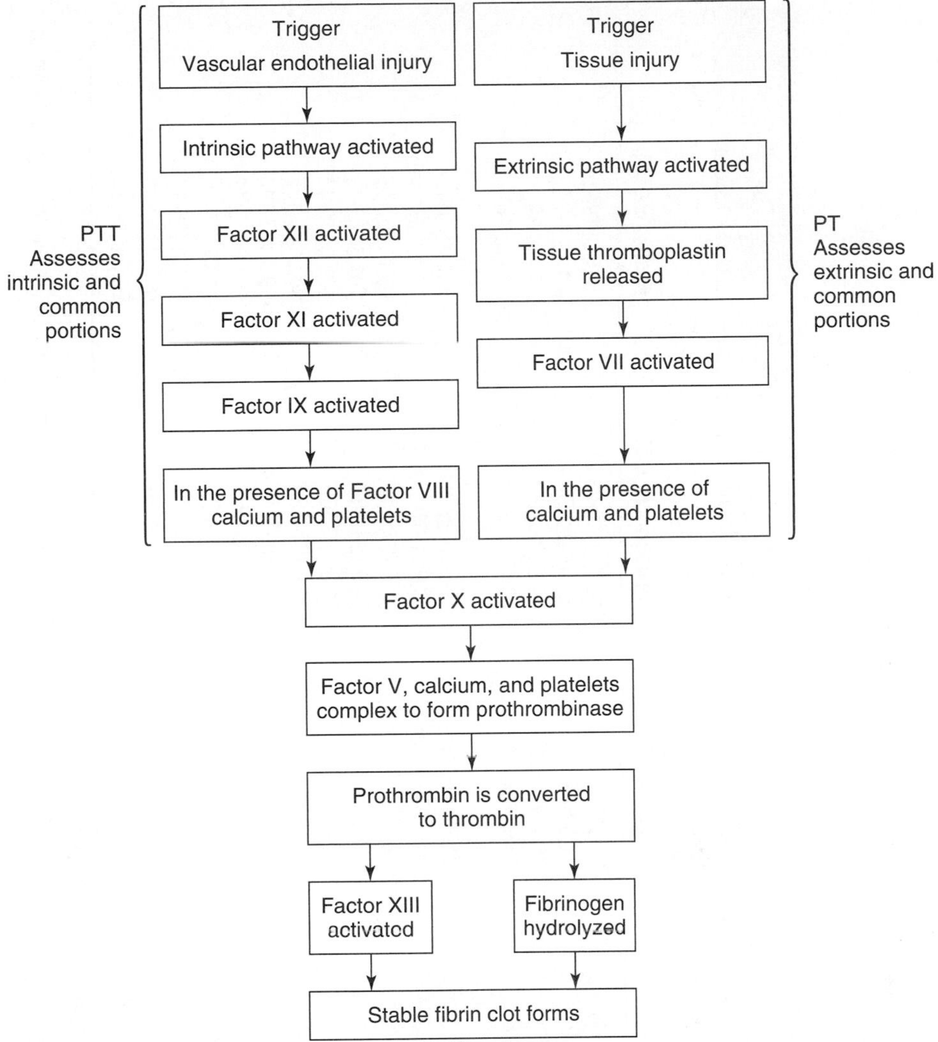

FIGURE 30-2 ■ Fibrin clot formation through activation of intrinsic or extrinsic pathways of coagulation process.

ANEMIA

Low hemoglobin concentration and/or decreased number of RBCs diminishes the oxygen-carrying capacity of the blood and the level of oxygen available to the tissues (Oski et al., 1998). Anemia at birth can be classified into three major causes: (1) the result of blood loss (hemorrhage); (2) hemolysis; or (3) underproduction of erythrocytes (Doyle et al., 1999).

A. Etiologic factors.

1. Hemorrhage.
   - **a.** Fetal-maternal.
     - (1) Spontaneous.
     - (2) Traumatic amniocentesis.
     - (3) External cephalic version.
   - **b.** Twin-to-twin.
     - (1) Monozygotic, monochorionic (single) placenta.
     - (2) Hemoglobin difference between twins greater than 5 g/dl.

TABLE 30-3
Normal Values for Tests of Hemostasis

Parameter	Fetuses (Weeks' Gestation)			Newborns (n = 60)	Adults (n = 40)
	19-23 (n = 20)	24-29 (n = 22)	30-38 (n = 22)		
PT (s)	32.5 (19-45)	32.2 (19-44)†	22.6 (16-30)†	16.7 (12.0-23.5)*	13.5 (11.4-14)
PT (INR)	6.4 (1.7-11.1)	6.2 (2.1-10.6)†	3 (1.5-5)*	1.7 (0.9-2.7)*	1.1 (0.8-1.2)
APTT (s)	168.8 (83-250)	154 (87-210)†	104.8 (76-128)†	44.3 (35-52)*	33 (25-39)
TCT (s)	34.2 (24-44)*	26.2 (24-28)*	21.4 (17-23.3)	20.4 (15.2-25)†	14 (12-16)
Factor					
I (g/L Von Clauss)	0.85 (0.57-1.50)	1.12 (0.65-1.65)	1.35 (1.25-1.65)	1.68 (0.95-2.45)†	3 (1.78-4.50)
I Ag (g/L)	1.08 (0.75-1.50)	1.93 (1.56-2.40)	1.94 (1.30-2.40)	2.65 (1.68-3.60)†	3.5 (2.50-5.20)
IIc (%)	16.9 (10-24)	19.9 (11-30)*	27.9 (15-50)†	43.5 (27-64)†	98.7 (70-125)
VIIc (%)	27.4 (17-37)	33.8 (18-48)*	45.9 (31-62)	52.5 (28-78)†	101.3 (68-130)
IXc (%)	10.1 (6-14)	9.9 (5-15)	12.3 (5-24)†	31.8 (15-50)†	104.8 (70-142)
Xc (%)m	20.5 (14-29)	24.9 (16-35)	28 (16-36)†	39.6 (21-65)†	99.2 (75-125)
Vc (%)	32.1 (21-44)	36.8 (25-50)	48.9 (23-70)†	89.9 (50-140)	99.8 (65-140)
VIIIc (%)	34.5 (18-50)	35.5 (20-52)	50.1 (27-78)†	94.3 (38-150)	101.8 (55-170)
XIc (%)	13.2 (8-19)	12.1 (6-22)	14.8 (6-26)†	37.2 (13-62)†	100.2 (70-135)
XIIc (%)	14.9 (6-25)	22.7 (6-40)	25.8 (11-50)†	69.8 (25-105)†	101.4 (65-144)
PK (%)	12.8 (8-19)	15.4 (8-26)	18.1 (8-28)†	35.4 (21-53)†	99.8 (65-135)
HMWK (%)	15.4 (10-22)	19.3 (10-26)	23.6 (12-34)†	38.9 (28-53)†	98.8 (68-135)

Values are the mean, followed in parentheses by the lower and upper boundaries including 95% of the population.

INR, International Normalized Ratio; *TCT,* thrombin clotting time; *Ag,* antigenic value; *APTT,* activated partial thromboplastin time; *c,* coagulant activity; *HMWK,* high-molecular-weight kininogen; *PK,* protein kinase.

* $p = .05$.

† $p = .01$.

From Nathan, D. G. and Orkin, S.H. (Eds.): *Nathan and Oski's hematology of infancy and childhood* (5th ed.). Philadelphia, 1998, W.B. Saunders.

c. Placental/cord.
(1) Umbilical cord rupture.
(2) Cord or placental hematoma.
(3) Anomalous cord insertion.
(4) Rupture of anomalous vessels of cord or placenta.
(5) Accidental incision of cord or placenta.
(6) Placenta previa or abruptio placentae.

d. Internal.
(1) Intracranial (subdural, subarachnoid, intraventricular), subgaleal.
(2) Organ rupture (liver, spleen, adrenal, kidney).
(3) Pulmonary.

e. External.
(1) Phlebotomy.
(2) Iatrogenic (e.g., catheter losses).

2. Hemolysis.

a. Blood group incompatibilities.
(1) Rh incompatibility: erythroblastosis fetalis (Reid and Toy, 1998).
(a) Sequence of events. Fetal blood cells containing Rh antigen (Rh positive) enter the maternal circulation; maternal red cells have no antigen (Rh negative); maternal immune system produces antibodies against the foreign fetal antigens; in subsequent pregnancies maternal antibodies enter fetal circulation and destroy fetal red cells.
(b) Predisposing factors.
(i) Previous pregnancy or abortion.
(ii) Fetal-maternal hemorrhage during pregnancy.
(iii) Delivery (vaginal, breech, cesarean).
(iv) Amniocentesis, chorionic villus sampling.
(v) External version.
(vi) Manual removal of placenta.
(c) Infant presentation.
(i) Anemia (caused by hemolysis, resulting in increased production of very immature red cells).
(ii) Tissue hypoxia, acidosis (decreased RBC count and decreased oxygen-carrying capacity of immature cells).
(iii) Congestive heart failure and hydrops fetalis (fetus attempts to expand blood volume and cardiac output, resulting in generalized edema).
(iv) Ascites, pleural effusion (fluid collecting in large cavities).
(v) Hepatosplenomegaly (increased extramedullary hematopoiesis).
(vi) Petechiae (thrombocytopenia accompanying severe anemia).
(vii) Hypoglycemia (increased red cell destruction stimulates insulin secretion, resulting in hyperplasia of pancreatic islets and hyperinsulinemia).
(viii) Positive direct Coombs test result.
(d) Prophylactic therapy: anti-D immune globulin (RhoGAM).
(i) Anti-D antibodies injected into maternal circulation (one dose accommodates approximately 15 ml of fetal whole blood or approximately 30 ml of RBCs).
(ii) Destruction of fetal red cells in maternal circulation, blocking maternal antibody production.

(iii) 90% effective in prevention of sensitization.
(iv) Recommended administration at 28 weeks' gestation, within 72 hours after delivery, and after amniocentesis, chorionic villus sampling, percutaneous umbilical blood sampling, or evidence or possibility of fetal-maternal hemorrhage.

(2) ABO incompatibility (Doyle et al, 1999).
(a) More frequently occurring but less severe hemolytic disease than with Rh incompatibility.
(b) Most often seen in mothers with O blood type (absence of antigen) carrying fetus with A or B blood type (see Table 30-4 for other potential incompatibilities).
(c) Maternal exposure to naturally occurring A and B antigens in food, bacteria, and pollen initiates maternal production of anti-A, anti-B antibodies and accounts for severity of disease with first pregnancy.
(d) ABO incompatibility protects against fetal Rh disease because of rapid destruction of fetal A/B cells, preventing Rh antigen exposure and maternal antibody production.
(e) Infant presentation includes:
(i) Mild hemolysis, anemia, reticulocytosis.
(ii) Hyperbilirubinemia (occasionally requiring exchange).

b. Enzymatic defect: glucose-6-phosphate dehydrogenase (G6PD) deficiency (see also Chapter 29).
(1) Most common inherited disorder of red cells (sex-linked disease affecting mainly male offspring, occasionally female carriers).
(2) Interaction of intracellular abnormality (deficiency of red cell enzyme) and extracellular factor (exposure to oxidant stress: drugs, infection), causing hemolysis and shortened erythrocyte life.
(3) Most common occurrence in American black infants (10%-15%) and in infants of Mediterranean, African, and Asian descent.

c. Infection. Intrauterine (viral, protozoan, spirochetal) and postnatal (bacterial) infection may cause neonatal hemolysis, anemia, thrombocytopenia, and disseminated intravascular coagulation.

3. Anemia of prematurity.
a. Hemoglobin concentration at birth varies only slightly in relation to gestational age.
b. During the first 2 to 3 months, hemoglobin concentration falls to the lowest value that occurs at any developmental period.
c. Anemia of prematurity is considered physiologic because it is characteristic of healthy infants.

TABLE 30-4
Potential Maternal-Fetal ABO Incompatibilities

Maternal Blood Group	Incompatible Fetal Blood Group
O	A or B
B	A or AB
A	B or AB

d. Associated factors.
   (1) Rates of decline and nadir are inversely proportional to gestational age.
   (2) Iron concentration is low because of decreased blood volume and decreased concentration of circulating hemoglobin iron.
   (3) Improved extrauterine oxygen delivery causes a temporarily inactive stage of erythropoiesis.
   (4) Erythropoietin production in response to anemia is diminished.
   (5) Shortened red cell life span decreases red cell mass.
   (6) Growth causes dilutional anemia as a result of decreased hemoglobin concentration with expanding blood volume.
   (7) Despite rapid hemoglobin fall, tissue oxygenation is maintained by events responsible for right shift of the hemoglobin-oxygen dissociation curve.
e. Some infants do manifest symptoms of hypoxemia (poor feeding and weight gain, dyspnea, tachypnea, tachycardia, diminished activity, pallor) in the absence of other problems and require transfusion.
f. No direct correlation has been established between low hemoglobin levels and the occurrence of apnea (Westkamp et al., 2002).

4. Iatrogenic postnatal phlebotomy. Critically ill infants who require frequent monitoring may have excessive amounts of blood removed for diagnostic studies, thereby inducing anemia. Removal of greater than 20% of the blood volume over 24 to 48 hours can produce anemia; in a 1500 g infant this represents approximately 25 ml (Doyle et al., 1999).

B. **Clinical presentation:** varies with the volume of hemorrhage and the time period over which the blood is lost.

1. Acute blood loss.
   a. Pallor initially, and then cyanosis and desaturation.
   b. Shallow, rapid, irregular respirations.
   c. Tachycardia.
   d. Weak or absent peripheral pulses.
   e. Low or absent blood pressure, low venous pressure.
   f. Hemoglobin concentration may be normal initially, with rapid decline over 4 to 12 hours with hemodilution.
2. Chronic blood loss.
   a. Pallor without signs of acute distress.
   b. Possible signs of congestive heart failure with hepatomegaly.
   c. Normal blood pressure, normal or elevated venous pressure.
   d. Low hemoglobin concentration.

C. **Clinical assessment.**

1. Family history.
   a. Bleeding, anemia, splenectomy.
   b. Consanguinity.
   c. Ethnic and geographic origins.
   d. Blood group incompatibilities.
2. Maternal history.
   a. Blood type.
   b. Late third-trimester bleeding.

D. **Physical examination.**

1. Signs of acute or chronic blood loss, as above.
2. Jaundice.
3. Cephalohematoma.

4. Abdominal distention or mass: liver, spleen, adrenal, kidney rupture.
5. Petechiae, purpura.
6. Cardiovascular abnormalities: tachycardia, murmur, gallop rhythm.
7. Hydropic changes.

E. **Diagnostic studies.**
1. Hemoglobin concentration. Venous hemoglobin values less than 13 g/dl in infants born at 34 to 35 weeks' gestation or more and in the first week of life are considered abnormal (Oski et al., 1998). Values vary according to birth weight and postnatal age (Table 30-5).
2. Reticulocyte count. This reflects new erythroid activity and is persistently elevated with ongoing red cell destruction.
3. Peripheral blood smear.
   a. Test evaluates alterations in size, shape, and structure of RBCs that might enhance destruction because of decreased deformability.
   b. Fragmentation of RBCs can be identified.
4. Blood type to identify common blood group antigens: A, B, O, and Rh.
5. Coombs test.
   a. Positive result on direct Coombs test indicates presence of maternal IgG antibodies on surface of infant's red cells.
   b. Positive result on indirect Coombs test means that antibodies against the infant's RBCs are present in the maternal serum.
6. Kleihauer-Betke test.
   a. Test identifies fetal hemoglobin in maternal blood.
   b. Calculations indicate volume of fetal-maternal hemorrhage and dose of immune globulin (RhoGAM) required to prevent sensitization.

F. **Differential diagnosis:** diseases that diminish oxygen delivery to the tissues (e.g., pulmonary, cardiac).

G. **Complications.**
1. Inadequate tissue oxygenation, poor growth.
2. Transfusion.
   a. Transfusion reaction.
   b. Overhydration with pulmonary congestion.

H. **Patient care management (see Transfusion Therapies on pp. 750-754).**
1. Emergency treatment for acute blood loss resulting in hypovolemia.
   a. Whole blood or combination of packed RBCs (PRBCs) with crystalloid or colloid.
      (1) Type: group O, Rh negative.
      (2) Amount: 10 to 20 ml/kg.

TABLE 30-5
Serial Hemoglobin Values in Low Birth Weight Infants

	Hemoglobin Concentration (g/dl) by Age (in weeks)				
Birth Weight (g)	**2 wk**	**4 wk**	**6 wk**	**8 wk**	**10 wk**
800-1000	16 ± 0.6	10.2 ± 3.2	8.7 ± 1.5	8 ± 0.9	8 ± 1.1
1001-1200	16.4 ± 2.3	12.8 ± 2.5	10.5 ± 1.8	9.1 ± 1.3	8.5 ± 1.5
1201-1400	16.2 ± 1.3	13.4 ± 2.8	10.9 ± 1.2	9.9 ± 1.9	—
1401-1500	15.6 ± 2.2	11.7 ± 1	10.5 ± 0.7	9.8 ± 1.4	—

Hemoglobin values are presented as grams per deciliter.

From Oski, F.A.: Hematologic problems. In G.B. Avery (Ed.): *Neonatology: Pathophysiology and management of the newborn* (4th ed.). Philadelphia, 1994, J.B. Lippincott.

b. Fresh frozen plasma (FFP), albumin, or saline solution if blood is unavailable.
2. Nonemergency replacement transfusion: clinical decision based on adequacy of tissue oxygenation in the individual infant.
   a. Advantages of transfusion must be weighed against risks, including infection, hypothermia, graft-versus-host disease, and other complications.
   b. Consider gestational and postnatal age, intravascular volume, and coexisting cardiac, pulmonary, or vascular conditions.
3. Exchange transfusion.
   a. Treatment of jaundice caused by blood group incompatibility.
   b. Partial exchange if necessary to treat severe anemia of hydrops without increasing intravascular volume.

I. **Outcome.**
1. Improved tissue oxygenation and resolution of symptoms with replacement transfusion.
2. Long-term outcome varies with degree of anemia and underlying cause.

HEMORRHAGIC DISEASE OF THE NEWBORN

Hemorrhagic disease of the newborn (HDN) is a hemorrhagic tendency caused by vitamin K deficiency and decreased activity of factors II, VII, IX, and X. A new term, vitamin K–dependent bleeding, is thought to describe more accurately the link between vitamin K deficiency and spontaneous hemorrhage and to exclude newborn infants with bleeding from other causes (Andrew and Montgomery, 1998; Bowman, 1997).

A. **Etiologic factors:** primary vitamin K deficiency.
1. Required for activation of clotting factors II, VII, IX, and X and of proteins C and S after liver synthesis.
   a. Vitamin K is important in the formation of calcium-binding sites, which are necessary for functional activation of clotting factors.
   b. In the absence of vitamin K, circulating proteins are decarboxylated; levels of protein induced by vitamin K absence (PIVKA) can be used as an indirect measure of bleeding risk.
2. Suppression of bacterial synthesis.
   a. Intestinal flora is required for vitamin K synthesis.
   b. Newborn intestinal tract is virtually free of bacteria until feedings begin.
   c. Antibiotic therapy can alter normal intestinal bacterial colonization.

B. **Clinical presentation:** bleeding.
1. Begins at 24 to 72 hours of age.
2. May be localized or diffuse.
3. Rarely life threatening.
4. Late-onset bleeding possible at approximately 2 to 3 weeks of age.

C. **Clinical assessment:** oozing.
1. Localized: frequently gastrointestinal (hematemesis, melena).
2. Diffuse: umbilical cord, circumcision, puncture sites.

D. **Physical examination.**
1. Diffuse ecchymosis, petechiae.
2. Oozing puncture sites.
3. Abdominal distention.
4. Jaundice.

E. **Diagnostic studies.**
1. Response to vitamin K administration establishes the diagnosis.

2. PT and PTT are prolonged.
3. Levels of vitamin K–dependent clotting factors are low.
4. PIVKA levels are elevated.

F. **Differential diagnosis.**
1. Decreased absorption of vitamin K.
   a. Biliary atresia.
   b. Cystic fibrosis.
2. Pharmacologic antagonism of vitamin K (Clapp et al., 2001).
   a. Anticonvulsants (hydantoin, phenobarbital) and anticoagulants (coumarin, warfarin).
      (1) Induce hepatic enzymes and increase vitamin K degradation.
      (2) Inhibit vitamin K transport across the placenta.
      (3) Depress vitamin K–dependent coagulation factors.
   b. Coumarol derivatives: replace with heparin during pregnancy.
   c. Maternal supplementation with oral vitamin K_1 from 36 weeks' gestation to delivery might prevent neonatal hemorrhage associated with anticonvulsant therapy; extra vitamin K given to the mother to increase vitamin K available to the fetus.

G. **Complications.**
1. Anemia.
2. Intraventricular/intracranial hemorrhage.

H. **Patient care management.**
1. Prophylactic vitamin K at the time of delivery.
   a. Phytonadione (naturally occurring vitamin K), 0.5 to 1 mg, intramuscular (IM) administration: premature infants may be given the lower dose.
   b. The Canadian Paediatric Society (CPS, 1997) and the American Academy of Pediatrics (AAP, 1993) recommend the use of only IM vitamin K at birth, because of the history of prevention of life-threatening HDN with the parenteral preparation, the unproven risks of cancer, and the need for further research on the efficacy, safety, and bioavailability of oral preparations.
   c. Adequate serum concentrations of vitamin K to prevent classic HDN have been observed after oral administration of 2 mg phylloquinone (vitamin K_1); however, late HDN occurs primarily in breast-fed infants who have not received adequate vitamin K prophylaxis.
      (1) If the oral form is not available, the IV form has been given orally without noted adverse side effects.
      (2) Parental concern with IM administration of vitamin K might stem from:
         (a) Need for injection.
         (b) Readministration of oral dose (2 mg) required at 1 to 2 weeks and again at 4 weeks in breast-fed infants.
            (i) Commercial formulas contain vitamin K supplement.
            (ii) Intestinal flora of breast-fed infant may produce less vitamin K than that of formula-fed infant.
            (iii) Risk of developing HDN after oral dosing is 13:1, compared with IM dosing.
2. Significant bleeding (hemoglobin concentration <12 g/dl). PRBC infusion may be indicated.
3. Persistent bleeding in premature infant.
   a. FFP infusion may be indicated to replace clotting factors.
   b. Repeated doses of vitamin K are needed.

I. **Outcome.** Prophylactic treatment has virtually eliminated the disease.

DISSEMINATED INTRAVASCULAR COAGULATION (DIC)

DIC is an acquired hemorrhagic disorder associated with an underlying disease manifested as uncontrolled activation of coagulation and fibrinolysis. Consumption of clotting factors is thought to be initiated by release of thromboplastic material from damaged or diseased tissue into the circulation. In DIC, fibrinogen converts to fibrin to form microthrombi (Andrew, 1997; Beardsley and Nathan, 1998; Kuehl, 1997; Pugh, 1997).

A. **Common precipitating factors.**
   1. Maternal.
      a. Preeclampsia, eclampsia, placental abruption.
      b. Placental abnormalities.
   2. Intrapartal.
      a. Fetal distress with hypoxia and acidosis.
      b. Dead twin fetus.
      c. Traumatic delivery.
   3. Neonatal.
      a. Infection (bacterial, viral, fungal).
      b. Conditions causing hypoxia, acidosis, and shock.
      c. Severe Rh incompatibility.
      d. Thrombocytopenia.
      e. Tissue injury (birth trauma, breech crush injury).

B. **Clinical presentation (Fig. 30-3).**
   1. Hemorrhage: predominant symptom.
      a. Clotting factors and platelets are depleted.
      b. Fibrinolysis is stimulated.
      c. Endogenous thrombin and plasmin are formed.
   2. Organ and tissue ischemia. Microvascular thrombosis (occlusion) by fibrin thrombi causes potential ischemia and necrosis of any organ, particularly the kidneys.
   3. Anemia.
      a. Blood loss.
      b. Red cell fragmentation by fibrin strands.

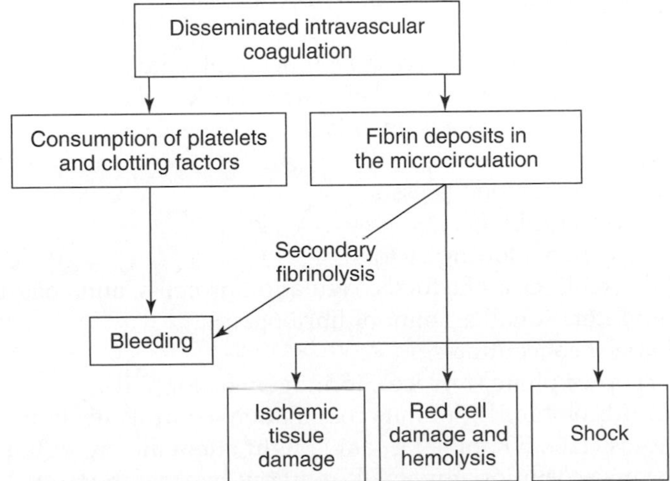

FIGURE 30-3 ■ Sequence of events in pathologic changes of disseminated intravascular coagulation (DIC).

C. **Clinical assessment.**
   1. Review the history for precipitating factors.
   2. Concurrent evidence of coagulation and fibrinolysis.

D. **Physical examination.**
   1. Variable signs, depending on underlying disease process.
   2. Prolonged oozing from puncture sites or umbilicus.
   3. Petechiae, purpura, ecchymosis.
   4. Hemorrhage (pulmonary, gastrointestinal, cerebral).
   5. Localized necrosis and gangrene resulting from microvascular thrombosis of peripheral vessels.

E. **Diagnostic studies.**
   1. Variable diagnostic studies are performed for delineation of the underlying disease process.
   2. Platelet count is low.
   3. PT and PTT are both significantly prolonged.
   4. Peripheral blood smear identifies microangiopathic hemolytic anemia, abnormalities of red cell shape, cell fragmentation, and decreased number of platelets.
   5. Fibrinogen level is low.
   6. Fibrinogen-degradation products are significantly increased.
   7. D-dimer, is a sensitive marker for endogenous thrombin/plasmin production and can detect much milder forms of DIC.
   8. Additional factors and levels might be evaluated: factors VIII and II are decreased, as well as protein C, protein S, and antithrombin III.

F. **Differential diagnosis.**
   1. Parenchymal liver disease.
   2. Vitamin K deficiency.
   3. Microangiopathic disease.
   4. Primary fibrinogenolysis.

G. **Complications.**
   1. Microvascular thrombosis.
   2. Organ failure resulting from ischemia and necrosis, especially renal.
   3. Intraventricular and parenchymal hemorrhage.

H. **Patient care management.**
   1. Aggressive treatment of the underlying disease.
   2. Supportive care.
      a. Replacement transfusion with significant bleeding.
         (1) Whole blood for hypovolemia and shock.
         (2) PRBCs for isovolemic anemia.
         (3) Platelets for consumption.
      b. Maintenance of blood pressure.
   3. Measures to control DIC.
      a. Replacement of clotting factors.
         (1) FFP (replaces all factors, coagulation proteins, and coagulation inhibitors; small amount of fibrinogen).
         (2) Platelet concentrates.
         (3) Cryoprecipitate (replaces fibrinogen, factor VIII).
         (4) Antithrombin III (inhibits coagulation, controls fibrinolysis). High doses (120-250 units/kg/day) might attenuate organ failure and reverse coagulopathy in DIC without heparin therapy.
      b. Heparin therapy remains controversial; use if treatment of underlying disease and replacement of clotting factors fail to reverse the process or with evidence of significant large-vessel thrombosis.

(1) Goals are to interrupt fibrin deposition and to achieve normal fibrinogen levels and platelet counts.
(2) Continuous infusion is more physiologic and is safer because intermittent doses may aggravate existing hemorrhage.
(3) Dosage is adjusted to maintain PTT within 60 to 70 seconds (once achieved, lower-dose heparin therapy may control ongoing consumption).

c. Exchange transfusion.
(1) Rarely tolerated and associated with additional complications (intraventricular hemorrhage, sepsis, thrombocytopenia).
(2) Replaces clotting factors and removes FDP from circulation.
(3) Use fresh heparinized blood or blood stored for less than 72 hours and that has been preserved with citrate-phosphate-dextrose.

I. **Outcome:** related to the prognosis of the underlying disease and the severity of the DIC.

THROMBOCYTOPENIA

Thrombocytopenia is an acquired disease in which there is a significant decrease in the platelet count (<100,000/mm^3) of the term or premature infant (Beardsley and Nathan, 1998; Blanchette and Rand, 1997; Doyle et al., 1999).

A. **Etiologic factors.**
1. Platelet destruction.
a. Maternal autoantibodies (autoimmune): idiopathic thrombocytopenic purpura, systemic lupus erythematosus.
(1) Maternal autoantibodies bind to platelet surface antigens, making them susceptible to premature destruction.
(2) IgG antibodies cross the placenta and destroy fetal platelets.
(a) Approximately 10% to 15% have cord platelet counts of less than 100,000/mm^3 (half of these have counts <50,000/mm^3).
(b) Nadir usually occurs on the second day.
(c) Counts can be depressed for 2 to 4 months (as long as maternal IgG antibodies remain in circulation).
(d) Recent studies show no evidence of severe intracranial hemorrhage.
(3) Maternal platelet count is low.

b. Neonatal conditions.
(1) Neonatal alloimmune thrombocytopenia.
(a) Analogous to Rh incompatibility.
(i) Fetal platelets contain an antigen lacking in the mother.
(ii) Fetal platelets enter the maternal circulation, resulting in maternal production of antibodies against foreign platelets.
(iii) Maternal antibodies cross into the fetal circulation and coat fetal platelets, which are then destroyed.
(b) Fetal thrombocytopenia can occur as early as 20 weeks' gestation.
(c) Nadir occurs in the first few days; counts normalize by the end of the first month.
(d) About 15% to 25% have intracranial hemorrhage (approximately 10% occur in utero).
(e) Maternal platelet count remains normal.
(2) Infection: bacterial or TORCH (*t*oxoplasmosis, *o*ther [congenital syphilis, viruses], *r*ubella, *c*ytomegalovirus, *h*erpes simplex virus).
(a) Megakaryocyte degeneration in bone marrow.
(b) Can cause DIC (platelet consumption).

(c) Activates reticuloendothelial system (increased platelet sequestration).
(d) Platelets may form antigen/antibody complexes with infectious agent.

(3) Thrombotic disorders.
(a) Large-vessel disease (renal vein thrombosis).
(b) Microvascular disease (necrotizing entercolitis, respiratory distress syndrome, persistent pulmonary hypertension of the newborn).
(c) DIC (platelet consumption).

(4) Birth asphyxia. Fetal megakaryocytes may have increased sensitivity to hypoxic injury.

(5) Giant hemangiomas.
(a) Kasabach-Merritt syndrome. Vascular malformation results in platelet and fibrinogen consumption.
(b) Mechanical destruction and sequestration.

(6) Exchange transfusion: shortened survival of transfused platelets.

2. Impaired platelet production (rare, <5%) associated with congenital malformations.
   a. Trisomy syndromes (13, 18). Bone marrow hypoplasia affects megakaryocyte production.
   b. Thrombocytopenia with absent radii (TAR) syndrome.
      (1) Defective megakaryocyte progenitor cell.
      (2) Presentation at birth, improvement thereafter.
      (3) Anomalies of the radius but not the thumb.
   c. Fanconi anemia.
      (1) Thumb, skeletal, renal, and CNS anomalies; café-au-lait spots.
      (2) Thrombocytopenia: presentation rare in neonatal period; worsens with time.
   d. Other, rare syndromes associated with unusually small or giant platelets.
3. Platelet interference: maternal drug ingestion.
   a. Interference with platelet aggregation.
   b. Meperidine (Demerol), promethazine (Phenergan), acetylsalicylic acid, sulfonamides, quinidine, quinine, thiazides.

B. Clinical presentation (platelet-type bleeding).

1. Petechiae, purpura, epistaxis.
2. Ecchymosis over presenting part.
3. Cephalohematoma.
4. Bleeding (mucous membranes, gastrointestinal tract, genitourinary system, umbilical cord, puncture sites, superficial cuts, or abrasions).

C. Clinical assessment.

1. Family history: bleeding complications in previous children, other family members.
2. Maternal history.
   a. History of bruising or bleeding, infections, collagen-vascular disease, splenectomy.
   b. Platelet count (low or normal).
   c. Peripheral blood smear (may show low platelet count, increased immature forms).
   d. Medication history.
3. Birth history.
   a. Hypoxia.
   b. Infection risk.

D. Physical examination.
 1. Signs of clinical presentation.
 2. Jaundice.
 3. Intrauterine growth restriction, microcephaly, hepatosplenomegaly with infectious cause (absent with immune etiology).
 4. Congenital anomalies consistent with syndromes.

E. Diagnostic studies.
 1. Platelet count is low.
 2. Peripheral blood smear shows low platelet count and increased immature forms; may show abnormal size.
 3. PT and PTT are normal.
 4. Bleeding time is prolonged.
 5. Maternal blood can be tested for human platelet antigen (HPA) type and for the presence of platelet-specific antibody (up to 2 weeks postpartum).
 6. In severe cases, platelet typing of mother, father, and infant might be indicated.

F. Differential diagnosis: DIC, vitamin K deficiency.

G. Complications.
 1. Cranial hemorrhage with neurologic sequelae in alloimmune disease.
  a. Associated with approximately 12% mortality rate.
  b. Increased incidence in infants weighing less than 1500 g.
 2. Entrapped hemorrhage.
 3. Anemia.
 4. Hyperbilirubinemia.

H. Infant management (see Table 30-5).
 1. Supportive care and treatment of underlying disease. Majority of neonatal thrombocytopenias are secondary to other disease processes.
 2. Cesarean delivery.
  a. Autoimmune.
   (1) Rarely of benefit for infant.
   (2) Consider if:
    (a) Maternal disease is severe with high antibody levels.
    (b) Prior infant was severely affected.
  b. Alloimmune: maternal HPA typing not routinely done; infants identified postnatally.
 3. Platelet transfusion.
  a. Recommended goal: keep platelet count greater than 30,000 in the first 48 hours, and greater than 50,000 if surgery is necessary or infant is premature and at risk for intraventricular hemorrhage.
  b. Autoimmune.
   (1) Rarely needed; platelet counts greater than 20,000/mm^3 usually benign course.
   (2) Consider cranial ultrasonography if platelet counts less than 50,000/mm^3.
   (3) Consider transfusion if platelet counts less than 20,000/mm^3.
  c. Alloimmune.
   (1) Serial transfusions may be necessary.
   (2) Obtain HPA type for infant before transfusion.
   (3) Transfusion of random donor platelets rarely results in sustained increase because of antibody destruction.
   (4) Transfuse maternal platelets (in absence of HPA) that have been washed and resuspended in AB-negative plasma.
  d. Production defects: repeated transfusions usually necessary.

4. Intravenous immune globulin (IVIG).
    a. 80% effective in increasing platelet count.
    b. Effect delayed 12 to 24 hours.
    c. IgG pooled blood product from multiple donors.
5. Exchange transfusion.
    a. Consider only in infants with life-threatening hemorrhage.
    b. Limited success because IgG has a long half-life and distribution in extravascular tissues.
    c. May be required for hyperbilirubinemia.
6. Steroids.
    a. May be used in infants with platelet counts less than 25,000/mm^3 and clinical bleeding.
    b. May be used for initial treatment of thrombocytopenia resulting from hemangioma.

I. **Outcome**.
1. Varies with underlying disease, presence of congenital malformations.
2. Autoimmune etiology: usually causes only mild, transient problems, with full recovery of platelet count in 8 to 12 weeks.
3. Isoimmune etiology: causes mild to moderate problems with full recovery of platelet count in 6 to 8 weeks.

POLYCYTHEMIA

Polycythemia is a condition in which infants demonstrate an excess in circulating RBC mass. The venous hemoglobin concentration is greater than 22 g/dl or the venous hematocrit is greater than 65% in the first week of life. Blood viscosity increases with hematocrits greater than 60% and leads to a reduction of blood flow to the organs.

A. **Etiologic factors.**
1. Intrauterine hypoxia, placental insufficiency. Hypoxia stimulates erythropoiesis, increasing the fetal red cell mass.
    a. Maternal preeclampsia/eclampsia, placenta previa.
    b. Postmaturity syndrome, intrauterine growth restriction.
2. Maternal-fetal and twin-to-twin transfusion.
3. Placental hypertransfusion.
4. Maternal diabetes: possibly resulting from abnormal fetal erythrocyte deformability.

B. **Clinical presentation.**
1. Many infants are asymptomatic.
2. Plethora.
3. Cyanosis.
4. CNS abnormalities (lethargy, jitteriness, seizures).
5. Respiratory distress (tachypnea, pulmonary edema, pulmonary hemorrhage).
6. Tachycardia, congestive heart failure.
7. Hypoglycemia.
8. Poor feeding behaviors (poor nippling, regurgitation).

C. **Clinical assessment:** history and physical examination usually identify cause.

D. **Physical examination.**
1. Findings may be normal except for plethora and occasionally cyanosis.
2. Symptoms of clinical presentation cannot be attributed to other disease.

E. **Diagnostic studies.** Venous hemoglobin concentration and hematocrit are elevated.

F. **Complications.**
  1. Hyperbilirubinemia.
  2. Hyperviscosity syndrome: elevated whole blood viscosity associated with reduced blood flow, vascular thrombosis (renal, cerebral, mesenteric), neurologic sequelae, fine motor abnormalities, speech delays up to 2 years of age (Drew et al., 1997).

G. **Patient care management.**
  1. Partial exchange transfusion.
    a. Controversial in asymptomatic infants.
    b. Desired reduction of hematocrit to less than 60% (blood viscosity is thought to be relatively normal at this level).
    c. Gastrointestinal symptoms: possibility of bleeding, poor feeding tolerance, necrotizing enterocolitis after partial exchange transfusion (Capasso et al., 2003).
  2. Supportive treatment of persistent symptoms.

H. **Outcome (Capasso et al., 2003).**
  1. Gross motor delays, neurologic sequelae, fine motor abnormalities, speech delays seen at 2 years (Black et al., 1985).
  2. Lower scores on spelling and arithmetic achievement tests and on gross motor skill tests at 7 years (Delaney-Black et al., 1989).

INHERITED BLEEDING DISORDERS

Although inherited bleeding disorders were recognized as early as 600 AD, the specific clotting abnormalities have been delineated only in this century, with the last (deficiency of factor XIII) documented in 1963. These gene disorders are rare, phenotypic expression is extremely variable, and only the most severely affected will be identified in the newborn period (Edwards, 1998; Kisker, 1998).

A. **Etiologic factors.**
  1. Hemophilia.
    a. Ninety percent of infants with hemophilia will have either classic hemophilia (hemophilia A, factor VIII deficiency) or Christmas disease (hemophilia B, factor IX deficiency).
    b. X-linked recessive inheritance.
      (1) Gene is located on the X chromosome.
      (2) Females are carriers; disease is present in male infants because they have only one X chromosome, which carries the abnormal gene (no normal X chromosome as counterbalance).
      (3) Each pregnancy carries a 25% chance of occurrence (50% of the male offspring will be affected).
      (4) 75% percent have a family history of a male with a bleeding disorder.
  2. von Willebrand disease.
    a. Autosomal dominant inheritance.
      (1) Males and females are equally affected.
      (2) Each pregnancy carries a 50% chance of occurrence.
      (3) Transmission is vertical (disease is seen in successive generations).
    b. Gene expression markedly variable (family history may be absent despite dominant inheritance).
  3. Factor XIII deficiency: autosomal recessive inheritance.
    a. Both parents are phenotypically normal carriers.
    b. Males and females are equally affected.

c. In each pregnancy, 25% of the offspring will be affected, 50% will be carriers, 25% will be normal.
d. Expression is horizontal (deficiency is seen in siblings; skips a generation).

B. **Clinical presentation.**
1. Rare newborn presentation except for factor XIII deficiency.
2. Usually well infant with delayed bleeding.
3. Clotting screening results usually normal.

C. **Clinical assessment.**
1. Late bleeding.
   a. Delayed umbilical cord bleeding (>80% with factor XIII).
   b. Circumcision oozing (significant hemorrhage is rare).
   c. Rare intracranial hemorrhage.
2. Family history.

D. **Diagnostic studies.**
1. PT, PTT, platelet count, fibrinogen level (usually normal).
2. Specific factor assays (identification by factor levels and DNA analysis).
   a. Factor VIII levels should be comparable to normal adult levels in the newborn period.
   b. Factor IX levels are normally low in the neonatal period; however, infants with bleeding presentation will be severely affected, with less than 2% activity (clearly abnormal level).

E. **Patient care management.**
1. Initial correction is with FFP (contains adequate amounts of all clotting factors except factor VIII).
2. Cryoprecipitate can be used if bleeding persists after use of FFP (enriched with approximately 20 units of factor VIII per milliliter).
3. Diagnosis allows replacement of specific factor.
   a. Recombinant factor VIII is available for classic hemophilia.
   b. Purified (monoclonal antibody) factor IX is available for Christmas disease.
   c. Prothrombin concentrates are not recommended for neonatal use because of thrombogenicity.

F. **Outcome:** episodic bleeding requiring lifelong replacement.

TRANSFUSION THERAPIES

A. **Recommendations for use of blood components** (CPS, 2002; Doyle et al., 1999; Maier et al, 2000; Manno, 1996; Nugent, 1998; Quirolo, 2002; Reid and Toy, 1998).
1. Develop and document criteria indicating need.
2. Use only the blood components required for therapy.
3. Use crystalloid or nonblood colloid whenever possible.
4. Use universal precautions when handling blood products.

B. **Written, informed consent has been recommended since 1986 to ensure that families understand risks and explore alternatives.**
1. Ethical or religious basis: autonomy—the right of choice.
2. Legal basis: failure to inform adequately and to obtain consent constitutes negligence.
3. Time consuming: start a few days in advance of need (i.e., include in discussion on the first day of life of sick preterm infants).

C. Informed consent includes discussion of the following:

1. Risks.
   a. Infection.
      (1) Blood is screened for human immunodeficiency virus (HIV), hepatitis B virus (HBV), hepatitis C virus (HCV), human T-cell leukemia/lymphoma virus (HTLV), and *Treponema pallidum* (syphilis).
      (2) Cytomegalovirus transmission can be prevented by using leukocyte-depleted, irradiated products.
      (3) Major risks for transmission via transfusion.
         (a) HIV infection incidence is 1:420,000. Nucleic acid testing (NAT) based on polymerase chain reaction (PCR) is routine; a cheaper alternative (but not yet routine) is an enzyme-linked immunosorbent assay (ELISA)–based test for p24 antigen (Schupbach, 2002).
         (b) HBV (hepatitis B surface antigen [HBsAg]) infection incidence is 1:200,000; hepatitis B core antigen (HBcAg) is a marker for non-A, non-B hepatitis.
         (c) HCV infection incidence is 1:80,000.
      (4) Predonation questions foster self-elimination of prospective donors with high-risk behaviors.
      (5) Confidential unit exclusion allows donors to designate the elimination of their donation if they recognize risk but want to avoid the embarrassment of refusing to donate.
   b. Transfusion reactions.
      (1) Febrile reactions (most common).
         (a) Probably caused by transfused (passenger) WBCs and/or their cytokine products (RBC and platelet transfusions).
         (b) Leukocyte reduction might prevent reaction.
            (i) Expensive and time consuming.
            (ii) One unit of PRBCs can contain 1 billion WBCs.
            (iii) WBCs can be removed by centrifugation, or by filtering at donation (prestorage leukocyte depletion), or at transfusion (bedside filtration).
      (2) Allergic reactions.
         (a) Urticaria, angioedema, asthma.
         (b) Higher incidence with multiple transfusions.
         (c) Premedication (antihistamine, antipyretic, steroid) might diminish effect.
      (3) Hemolytic reactions.
         (a) Usually ABO incompatibilities.
         (b) Possible acute or delayed hemolysis.
         (c) Most reactions can be eliminated by typing, screening, and crossmatching.
   c. Graft-versus-host disease.
      (1) Disease may occur in fetus or premature neonate after transfusion.
      (2) Immature immune system may not reject foreign lymphocytes (present in erythrocyte and platelet products); donor lymphocytes proliferate and damage the host (infection and neutropenia).
      (3) Clinical symptoms (within 100 days of transfusion) include rash, diarrhea, hepatic dysfunction, and bone marrow suppression with generalized reduction in all cell lines (pancytopenia).

(4) Gamma irradiation of blood products will prevent lymphocyte proliferation.
  (a) Mature erythrocytes and platelets are resistant to radiation damage.
  (b) Enhances efflux of potassium ion from red cells (store <28 days, wash to remove excess potassium before transfusion).

2. Expected benefits.
- **a.** Whole blood (hematocrit approximately 35%).
  (1) Replacement of blood volume.
  (2) Treatment (massive hemorrhage, exchange transfusion).
- **b.** PRBC (hematocrit approximately 60%-90%).
  (1) Improved oxygen-carrying capacity and tissue oxygenation.
  (2) Relief of symptoms of anemia (tachypnea, apnea, periodic breathing, tachycardia, poor weight gain).
  (3) Treatment (active bleeding, hemolytic disease, extracorporeal membrane oxygenation).
  (4) Minimal fluid administration (approximate red cell mass of a whole unit of blood in one half fluid volume).
- **c.** Platelets.
  (1) Improved coagulation.
  (2) Treatment (hemorrhage caused by thrombocytopenia or platelet dysfunction).
- **d.** FFP: replacement of clotting factor deficiency.
- **e.** Albumin.
  (1) Volume expansion, improved oncotic pressure.
  (2) Treatment (for hypovolemia, third-space losses).
- **f.** Granulocytes.
  (1) Replacement in life-threatening granulocytopenias.
  (2) Improved survival rates in limited studies using granulocyte transfusions in newborn infants who become neutropenic as a result of consumption during infection.

3. Alternatives.
- **a.** Directed donation.
  (1) Family and friends with compatible blood type can donate for infant.
  (2) Blood must be irradiated to prevent graft-versus-host disease.
  (3) There is no evidence of overall increased safety in comparison with anonymous volunteer donations.
    (a) Donors might be more truthful (i.e., regarding acceptability for donation) because they know the recipient.
    (b) Donors might be less truthful because they feel pressure to donate.
  (4) Parental donation.
    (a) Maternal plasma is unacceptable for transfusion to neonates because of the possible presence of antibodies directed against inherited paternal antigens on infant's cells.
    (b) Maternal platelets and RBCs can be used if washed before transfusion.
    (c) Paternal donation might be problematic if infant has circulating maternal antibodies produced by stimulation of inherited paternal antigens.
  (5) All blood products from directed donors should be irradiated. Potential antigen similarities between close family members may impede recognition and destruction of foreign lymphocytes.
- **b.** Erythropoietin (EPO) (Doyle, 1997; Ohls, 2002; Ohls et al., 1997; Ohls et al., 2001; Strauss, 1997).

(1) Recombinant human EPO (r-HuEPO) might be used to treat symptomatic anemia caused by physiologic decline in hematocrit or by blood loss from phlebotomy, or it might be used as a prophylactic therapy to minimize blood product exposure in preterm or sick neonates.
(2) Plasma EPO levels are lower in anemic preterm infants, suggesting responsibility for hematocrit decline.
(a) The liver, the initial site of EPO production at early gestation, is less responsive than the kidney to tissue hypoxia caused by anemia.
(b) EPO pharmacokinetics differ in preterm infants: faster rate of clearance, larger volume of distribution, shorter elimination and mean residence times.
(c) Clearance increases with duration of r-HuEPO therapy, suggesting the need for progressively higher doses.
(3) Variable results and small sample sizes hamper clinical trials testing different doses and treatment schedules.
(a) Therapy with r-HuEPO and iron stimulates erythropoiesis and increases reticulocyte counts.
(b) Increase in reticulocyte count is dose dependent.
(c) Oral iron supplement, adequate to support enhanced erythropoiesis, may not be tolerated. Intravenous iron therapy has not yet been adequately studied to ensure absence of oxidant injury and toxic metabolites; however, preterm infants appear to need a supplement of 4 to 4.5 mg/kg of dietary iron to prevent late anemia (CPS, 2002).
(d) The combination of r-HuEPO and iron stimulates erythropoiesis in infants of less than or equal to 1250 g birth weight; however, the lack of impact on transfusion requirements does not support routine use of r-HuEPO (Ohls et al., 2001).

c. Thrombopoietin. Recombinant human thrombopoietin is currently under development and testing for use as a megakaryocyte enhancer.

d. G-CSF: currently under investigation; stimulates growth of neutrophil colonies and induces maturation of promyelocytes to mature neutrophils.

D. Transfusion volumes.

1. Transfusions with PRBCs. For prevention of overhydration, replacement is usually given in increments of 10 to 15 ml/kg.

2. Partial exchange transfusions.

a. With normal saline solution: treatment of polycythemia (to reduce hematocrit without reducing blood volume).

b. With PRBCs: treatment of hydrops fetalis (to correct anemia without increasing blood volume).

c. Calculations for total exchange volume:

(1) Volume of normal saline solution to exchange =

$$\frac{\text{Blood volume} \times (\text{Measured hematocrit} - \text{Desired hematocrit})}{\text{Measured hematocrit}}$$

(2) PRBC volume to exchange =

$$\frac{\text{Blood volume} \times (\text{Desired hematocrit} - \text{Measured hematocrit})}{\text{PRBC hematocrit} - \text{Measured hematocrit}}$$

3. Exchange transfusions.

a. Single unit of blood (approximately 500 ml) will usually exchange twice the blood volume and remove 70% to 85% of the infant's blood.

   b. For treatment of hyperbilirubinemia, DIC, and autoimmune thrombocytopenia.
   c. Because preservatives provide a significant glucose load, rebound hypoglycemia may occur.
   d. Preservatives contain citrate, which binds calcium and magnesium; hypocalcemia and hypomagnesemia may occur.
   e. Potassium level rises as blood ages; blood should be less than 5 days old.
4. Platelets.
   a. One unit (approximately 40 ml) provides approximately 5×10^{10} platelets; transfusion of 0.2 platelet unit per kilogram should increase the platelet count by 75,000 to 100,000/mm^3 (Kisker, 1998).
   b. Routine volume reduction (platelet concentration) before transfusion is not indicated in infants.
   c. Platelets are separated from single units of whole blood within 6 hours of collection and suspended in small amounts of plasma, or they are obtained by apheresis (single-donor platelets).
5. FFP.
   a. FFP is usually transfused in increments of 10 ml/kg to minimize overhydration.
   b. Transfusion of 15 to 20 ml/kg replaces all coagulation proteins present in adult concentrations (Kisker, 1998).
   c. Plasma is obtained from a unit of whole blood and frozen within 6 hours of collection.
6. Cryoprecipitate.
   a. Transfusion volume is usually 1 unit/kg (approximate volume, 15 ml).
   b. One unit contains approximately 100 to 250 mg of factor I (fibrinogen), approximately 80 to 100 units of factor VIII (von Willebrand), and 50 to 75 units of factor XIII.
7. Albumin.
   a. For volume expansion, 5% albumin is usually administered in increments of 10 ml/kg; for improvement of oncotic pressure, 25% albumin might be used in increments of 1 g/kg (4 ml/kg).
   b. Albumin is a major contributor to oncotic pressure because of molecular size and weight.
8. Granulocytes.
   a. Collected by leukapheresis and selectively harvested from whole blood.
   b. Granulocyte transfusions are now rarely used due to the difficulty in isolation and the efficacy of G-CSF in elevating neutrophil counts (Doyle et al., 1999)

RECOMBINANT HEMATOPOIETIC GROWTH FACTORS

The identification, characterization, and molecular cloning of blood cell growth factors have facilitated production of therapeutic quantities of recombinant hematopoietic growth factors. These include G-CSF, M-CSF, EPO and thrombopoietin (all of which act on committed cell lineages), as well as GM-CSF, IL-3 and IL-11, which act on earlier progenitor cells. The efficacy and safety of these growth factors are currently being evaluated (Clapp et al., 2001).

EVALUATION BY COMPLETE BLOOD CELL COUNT

An evaluation of certain components of the complete blood cell (CBC) count might be helpful as an adjunct in the diagnosis of sepsis, although an organism must be isolated from blood or from other normally sterile body fluid (Baley and Goldfarb, 2001).

A. **Corroboration of clinical impression by supplemental/screening information.**

B. **Serial determinations provide more complete information on trends.**

C. **Automated Coulter counter evaluation.** Factors that can alter results:
   1. Interreader differences in interpretation of the peripheral smear.
      a. Segmented and band neutrophils exist on a continuum of cellular maturation.
      b. Discrete boundaries are artificial and subject to interobserver bias.
   2. Crying for more than 4 minutes: increased WBC count (leukocytosis).
   3. Stress: increased WBC count, left shift.
   4. Birth asphyxia, maternal hypertension and use of tocolytics: neutropenia (first 72 hours).
   5. Hemolytic disease, maternal steroids: neutrophilia (first 72 hours).
   6. Central counts lower than peripheral.

D. **Response to infection.**
   1. Evaluation of the total WBC count is insensitive as a predictor of the infection response.
   2. Neutrophil count: most sensitive indicator of infant sepsis.
      a. Neutrophil release from the bone marrow is increased.
      b. Number of immature neutrophil forms released into the circulating pool is increased.
      c. Neutropenia, rather than neutrophilia, is more common because of depletion of neutrophil storage pool.
         (1) Neutrophil storage pool consists of neutrophils stored outside the circulation in the bone marrow or layered along vessel walls (margination or marginating pool).
         (2) Infant's neutrophil storage pool is diminished in size compared with that of adults.
         (3) Regulation of marrow neutrophil release is disturbed in the neonate.
   3. Absolute neutrophil count (ANC).
      a. Multiply the percentage of total neutrophils by the WBC count.
      b. Normal ranges are:
         (1) Term infants: 1750 to 5400/mm^3.
         (2) Preterm infants: 1200 to 5400/mm^3.
      c. ANC is slightly more sensitive than the total WBC count but, as a single indicator of sepsis, is only approximately 15% predictive.
   4. Absolute band form count (ABC).
      a. Multiply the percentage of band forms by the WBC count.
      b. Normally peaks at 1400/mm^3 by 12 hours of age.
      c. May be elevated early in response to infection but is rarely elevated in fatal infection because of rapid exhaustion of marrow reserves and is therefore insensitive as a single indicator of sepsis.
   5. Immature/total neutrophil (I/T) ratio.
      a. Total number of immature neutrophil forms (bands, myelocytes, metamyelocytes, promyelocytes) divided by the total number of neutrophils (immature forms plus mature segmented or polymorphonuclear leukocytes; Fig. 30-4).
      b. More sensitive indicator of sepsis because it considers the number of metamyelocytes, which indicates accelerated release from the neutrophil storage pool.
      c. I/T ratio greater than 0.2: probable sepsis.

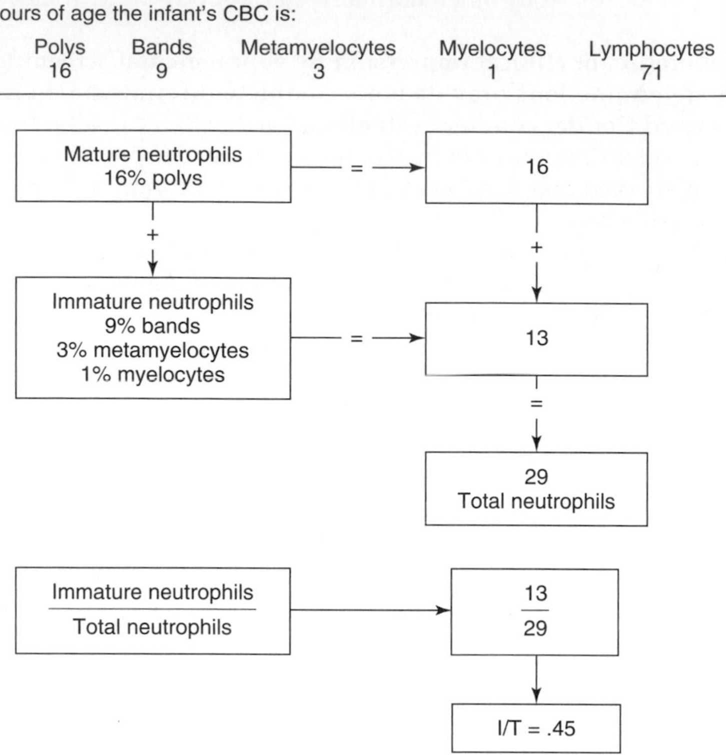

FIGURE 30-4 ■ Calculation of I/T neutrophil ratio. *CBC,* Complete blood cell count.

- **d.** Neutrophil storage pool depletion: I/T ratio greater than 0.8. Immature forms are all released in response to overwhelming infection.
- **e.** Factors associated with increased I/T ratio in the absence of sepsis.
  - (1) Maternal fever.
  - (2) Maternal oxytocin administration.
  - (3) Stressful labor.
  - (4) Asphyxia.
  - (5) Pneumothorax.
  - (6) Intraventricular hemorrhage.
  - (7) Seizures.
  - (8) Prolonged crying (≥4 minutes).
  - (9) Hypoglycemia (blood glucose level <30 mg/dl).
  - (10) Surgical intervention.

E. Evaluation of RBC indices.

1. Identification of diseases affecting synthesis of hemoglobin.
2. RBC morphology.
   - **a.** Anisocytosis: abnormal variation in size of erythrocytes (severe anemia).
   - **b.** Macrocytosis: diameter greater than 9 μm (increased cell volume: vitamin B_{12} and folic acid deficiencies).
   - **c.** Microcytosis: diameter less than 9 μm (decreased cell volume: iron deficiency, spherocytic and hemolytic anemias).
   - **d.** Poikilocytosis: variation in shape (severe anemia).
   - **e.** Spherocytosis: increased thickness and rounding (decreased deformability and greater susceptibility to destruction; seen in congenital spherocytosis, hemolytic anemias, after transfusion of stored blood).

f. Target cells: thin, with large diameter, dark center and periphery, with clear ring between periphery and center (hemoglobinopathies, sickle cell/thalassemia, liver disease).
g. Burr cells: crenations; long spinous processes (hemolytic anemias, DIC, liver disease).
h. Howell-Jolly bodies: spherical blue bodies in or on erythrocytes; nuclear debris (in asplenia, pernicious anemia).
i. Nucleated red blood cells: immature red cells with nuclei still present (in chronic blood loss, significant hemolysis, chronic hypoxia, infection).

REFERENCES

American Academy of Pediatrics Vitamin K Ad Hoc Task Force: Controversies concerning vitamin K and the newborn. *Pediatrics, 91*(5):1001-1003, 1993.

Andrew, M.: The relevance of developmental hemostasis to hemorrhagic disorders of newborns. *Seminars in Perinatology, 21*(1):70-85, 1997.

Andrew, M., Montgomery, R.R.: Acquired disorders of hemostasis. In D.G. Nathan and S.H. Orkin (Eds.): *Nathan and Oski's hematology of infancy and childhood* (5th ed.). Philadelphia, 1998, Saunders, pp. 1677-1718.

Baley, J.E. and Goldfarb, J.: Neonatal infection. In M.H. Klaus and A.A. Fanaroff (Eds.): *Care of the high-risk neonate* (5th ed.). Philadelphia, 2001, Saunders, pp. 363-392.

Beardsley, D.S., and Nathan, D.G.: Platelet abnormalities in infancy and childhood. In D.G. Nathan and S.H. Orkin (Eds.): *Nathan and Oski's hematology of infancy and childhood* (5th ed.). Philadelphia, 1998, Saunders, pp. 1585-1630.

Black, V.D., Lubchenco, L.O., Koops, B.L., et al. Neonatal hyperviscosity: Randomized study of effect of partial plasma exchange transfusion on long-term outcome. *Pediatrics, 75*(6):1048-1053, 1985.

Blanchette, V.S. and Rand, M.L.: Platelet disorders in newborn infants: Diagnosis and management. *Seminars in Perinatology, 21*(1):53-62, 1997.

Bowman, J.: The management of hemolytic disease in the fetus and newborn. *Seminars in Perinatology, 21*(1):39-44, 1997.

Canadian Paediatric Society (Fetus and Newborn Committee): Routine administration of vitamin K to newborns. *Pediatrics & Child Health,* 2(6):429-431, 1997.

Canadian Paediatric Society (Fetus and Newborn Committee): Red blood cell transfusions in newborn infants: Revised guidelines. *Pediatrics & Child Health, 7*(8):553-558, 2002.

Capasso, L., Raimondi, F., Capasso, A. et al.: Early cord clamping protects at-risk neonates from polycythemia. *Biology of the Neonate, 83*(3):197-200, 2003.

Christensen, R.D.: Developmental hematopoiesis. In R.A. Polin and W.W. Fox (Eds.): *Fetal and neonatal physiology* (2nd ed.). Philadelphia, 1998, Saunders, pp. 1737-1802.

Clapp, D.W., Shannon, K.M., and Phibbs, R.H.: Hematologic problems. In M.H. Klaus and A.A. Fanaroff (Eds.): *Care of the high-risk neonate* (5th ed.). Philadelphia, 2001, Saunders, pp. 447-480.

Delaney-Black, V., Camp, B.W., Lubchenco, L.O., et al.: Neonatal hyperviscosity in association with lower achievement and IQ scores at school age. *Pediatrics, 83*(5):662-667, 1989.

Doyle, J.J.: The role of erythropoietin in the anemia of prematurity. *Seminars in Perinatology, 21*(1):20-27, 1997.

Doyle, J.J., Schmidt, B., Blanchette, V., et al.: Hematology. In G.B. Avery, M.A. Fletcher, and M.G. MacDonald (Eds.): *Neonatology: Pathophysiology & management of the newborn.* Philadelphia, 1999, Lippincott Williams & Wilkins, pp. 1045-1091.

Drew, J.H., Guaran, R.L., Cichello, M., and Hobbs, J.B.: Neonatal whole blood hyperviscosity: The important factor influencing later neurologic function is the viscosity and not the polycythemia.

Clinical Hemorheology and Microcirculation, 17(1):67-72, 1997.

Edwards, T.J.: Hemophilia in the newborn: A case presentation. *Neonatal Network, 17*(2):67-71, 1998.

Israels, L.G. and Israels, S.J.: *Mechanisms in hematology* (3rd ed.). Toronto, 2002, Core Health Sciences, Inc., p. 402.

Kisker, C.T.: Pathophysiology of bleeding disorders in the newborn. In R.A. Polin and W.W. Fox (Eds.): *Fetal and neonatal physiology* (2nd ed.). Philadelphia, 1998, Saunders, pp. 1848-1861.

Kuehl, J.: Neonatal disseminated intravascular coagulation. *Journal of Perinatal and Neonatal Nursing, 11*(3):69-77, 1997.

Maier, R.F., Sontag, J., Walka, M.M., et al.: Changing practices of red blood cell transfusions in infants with birth weights less than 1000 g. *Journal of Pediatrics, 136*(2):220-224, 2000.

Manno, C.S.: What's new in transfusion medicine? *Pediatric Clinics of North America, 43*(3):793-808, 1996.

Nugent, D.J.: Platelet transfusion. In D.G. Nathan and S.H. Orkin (Eds.): *Nathan and Oski's hematology of infancy and childhood* (5th ed.). Philadelphia, 1998, Saunders, pp. 1802-1817.

Ohls, R.K.: Erythropoietin treatment in extremely low birth weight infants: Blood in versus blood out. *Journal of Pediatrics, 141*(1):3-6, 2002.

Ohls, R.K., Ehrenkranz, R.A., Wright, L.L., et al.: Effects of early erythropoietin therapy on the transfusion requirements of preterm infants below 1250 grams birth weight: A multicenter, randomized, controlled trial. *Pediatrics, 108*(4):1-18, 2001.

Ohls, R.K., Harcum, J., Schibler, K.R., and Christensen, R.D.: The effect of erythropoietin on the transfusion requirements of preterm infants weighing 750 grams or less: A randomized double-blind, placebo-controlled study. *Journal of Pediatrics, 131*(5):661-665, 1997.

Oski, F.A., Brugnara, C., and Nathan, D.G.: A diagnostic approach to the anemic patient. In D.G. Nathan and S.H. Orkin (Eds.): *Nathan and Oski's hematology of infancy and childhood* (5th ed.). Philadelphia, 1998, Saunders, pp. 375-384.

Pugh, M.: Lab values and diagnostics of DIC screening in the newborn. *Neonatal Network, 16*(7):57-64, 1997.

Quirolo, K.C.: Transfusion medicine for the pediatrician. *Pediatric Clinics of North America, 49*(6):1-23, 2002.

Reid, M.E. and Toy, P.: Erythrocyte blood groups in transfusion. In D.G. Nathan and S.H. Orkin (Eds.): *Nathan and Oski's hematology of infancy and childhood* (5th ed.). Philadelphia, 1998, Saunders, pp. 1760-1783.

Schupbach, J.: Measurement of HIV-1 p24 antigen by signal-amplification-boosted ELISA of heat-denatured plasma is a simple and inexpensive alternative to tests for viral RNA. *AIDS Reviews, 4*(2):83-92, 2002.

Strauss, R.G.: Recombinant erythropoietin for the anemia of prematurity: Still a promise, not a panacea. *Journal of Pediatrics, 131*(5):653-655, 1997.

Westkamp, E., Soditt, V., Adrian, S., et al.: Blood transfusions in anemic infants with apnea of prematurity. *Biology of the Neonate, 82(4):*228-232, 2002.

CHAPTER 31

Immunology and Infectious Disease

KIMBERLY M. HORNS

OBJECTIVES

1. Describe the unique immunodeficiencies in the premature and term infant.
2. Differentiate between humoral and cellular immunologic response in the neonate.
3. Differentiate the three categories of acquisition of infection.
4. Describe clinical signs and symptoms of early- and late-onset bacterial infection.
5. Calculate the absolute neutrophil count and immature/total cell ratio from a complete blood cell count and differential cell count.
6. Identify the common gram-positive and gram-negative organisms responsible for bacterial infections in the neonatal period.
7. Name common broad-spectrum antimicrobial agents used to treat neonatal sepsis and discuss indications for and risks of their use.
8. Differentiate between mucocutaneous, systemic, and cutaneous candidiasis.
9. List several clinical manifestations associated with congenital viral infection.
10. Describe the transmission of human immunodeficiency virus and its effect on the immune system.

Neonatal sepsis is a major cause of death during the first month of life. Neonatal sepsis is a general term used to define actual or potential infection. In the term infant early-onset bacterial infection occurs in 1 to 8 infants per 1000 live births. In several large multicenter studies from the National Institute of Child Health and Human Development Neonatal Research Network, 24% of very low birth weight (VLBW) infants were reported to have significant early-onset infections (Fanaroff et al., 1995; Fanaroff et al., 1998; Hack et al., 1995, Stoll et al., 1996a). The diagnosis of early-onset sepsis, in the first 72 hours of life, remains one of the most difficult diagnostic tasks for neonatal nurses, advanced practice nurses, and physicians. Blood cultures may remain negative in the presence of pneumonia, meningitis, and even in clear indications of clinical signs suggesting fulminant blood-born sepsis. In addition, secondary to the increasing use of intrapartum maternal antibiotics, it is difficult to rely solely on the presence of a positive neonatal blood culture to confirm early-onset sepsis. In contrast to early-onset sepsis, late-onset sepsis or those neonatal infections acquired later by horizontal transmission (nosocomial) may occur in as many as 250 infants per 1000 live births. In late-onset sepsis there is an increased risk of developing meningitis (4-10 per 10,000 live births). Whereas this infection is rare in the neonate, the risk in the first month of life is at the highest risk and 40% of the survivors of meningitis will have some neurologic sequelae.

Failure to identify early-onset sepsis contributes to morbidity, mortality and increased health care costs. The mortality rate is high (4.2%-26%), with the higher rates observed in premature infants and in those with early fulminant clinical signs (Stoll et al., 1996a). A review of the immune system and neonatal infection will aid in the understanding of the unique host-defense limitations of the term and premature infant. Accurate interpretation of hematologic and other studies, and identification of risk factors and clinical signs of sepsis may facilitate early detection of neonatal infection.

Group B streptococci and *Escherichia coli* are currently responsible for the majority of early-onset sepsis. Coagulase-negative staphylococci and *Candida albicans* are presently the most common nosocomial infections in hospitalized low birth weight infants. Antibiotic therapy for bacterial infections must be based on the susceptibility of the organism and the achievement of adequate bactericidal concentrations. Congenital viral infections may be asymptomatic at birth or may involve multiple systems depending on time of acquisition. Human immunodeficiency virus has become a leading cause of immunodeficiency in the neonate, with maternal-infant transmission accountable for the majority of neonatal acquisitions.

This chapter provides the nurse with a comprehensive review of the neonatal immune system and common neonatal infections.

IMMUNE SYSTEM

A. Host defense mechanisms of the immune system.

1. Overall functions of the immune system.
   a. Defense—resistance to infection by microorganisms.
   b. Homeostasis—removal of worn-out cells.
   c. Surveillance—perception and destruction of mutant cells.
2. Components of the immune system.
   a. The nonspecific mechanisms, which include phagocytosis, the inflammatory response, and several amplification systems including complement, coagulation, and kinin systems.
   b. The specific-immune responses, which consist of cell-mediated (T cell) and humoral (B cell) systems.
      (1) Both are interdependent and interrelated, for example, the activation of the complement system by immunoglobulins (IgM and IgG), or the production of chemotactic factors and other lymphokines, plays a significant role in the whole inflammatory response.
      (2) Nonspecific immune mechanisms—function without prior exposure, identified early in gestation, functional development at 32 to 33 weeks.
   c. Embryologic development (Table 31-1).
      (1) The maturation of specific immune responses begins in utero during the 7th to the 12th weeks of gestation.
      (2) Progenitor cells (stem cells) are initially located in the yolk sac, fetal liver, and bone marrow of the developing embryo.
   d. Depending on the type of microchemical environment surrounding the tissue the stem cells will differentiate along at least two pathways:
      (1) The hematopoietic.
      (2) The lymphopoietic.
         (a) The lymphopoietic system develops along two independent pathways leading to morphologically and functionally distinct populations of immune systems:
            (i) The thymus derived or T-system of cell-mediated immunity whose principal effector cells are the T lymphocytes.

■ TABLE 31-1
■ ■ **Development of Immune System in Fetus**

Gestation (Weeks)	Findings
4	First blood centers appear in yolk sac
5.5	Synthesis of complement is detected
7	Lymphocytes appear in peripheral blood, about 1000/mm^3
7-9	Lymphocytes appear in thymus
11	T-cell receptors (E rosette) develop in thymus lymphocytes. B-cell maturation occurs in liver and spleen, with IgG, IgA, IgM, and IgD surface markers. Serum IgG levels can be detected
12	Antigen recognition is demonstrable
13	Graft-versus-host reactivity is present
14	PHA response by thymus lymphocytes occurs
17	Serum IgM levels can be detected
20	Secondary lymphoid complex is present
20-25	Lymphocytes in blood number about 10,000/mm^3
22	Complement levels detectable in serum
30	IgA level detectable in serum

IgG, Immunoglobulin G; *PHA,* pituitary adrenal hypothalmus.
Adapted from Cauchi, M.N.: *Obstetrics and perinatal immunology.* London, 1981, Edward Arnold Publishers.

(ii) The bursal-dependent or B-system of humoral or antibody mediated immunity, which is displayed by the B lymphocytes.

(3) The thymus gland is derived from epithelium of the third and fourth pharyngeal pouches at about 6 weeks.
(4) Concomitantly, the parathyroids also begin their development at about this time from the same location.
(5) Caudal migration occurs, and beginning at about 8 weeks bloodborne stem cells invade the gland and are induced into lymphoid differentiation.
(6) With further development, the thymus is infiltrated by lymphocytes and differentiates into a dense cortex and a less dense loose central medulla with relatively more epithelial tissue.
(7) Within the thymus gland, an intense rate of mitosis occurs, greater than in any other lymphatic organ.

B. Humoral immunity (Blackburn, 2003).

1. Immunoglobulin (McCance and Huether, 2002; Polin et al., 2001).

a. Humoral immunity is a specific antibody-mediated response that functions most effectively if there has been previous exposure.

b. Antibodies are derived from B cells, which have been activated by T cells and antigens (Fig. 31-1).

(1) B cells mature and are stored in lymph tissue and bone marrow.
(2) B cells also produce memory cells that recognize antigens on subsequent exposures and initiate an antibody response.
(3) Antibody functions include:
(a) Recognition of bacterial antigens.
(b) Neutralization or opsonization of foreign substances, rendering them susceptible to phagocytosis.

2. Types of immunoglobulin.

a. Immunoglobulin G (IgG).

(1) Major immunoglobulin of serum and interstitial fluid.
(2) Provides immunity against bacterial and viral pathogens.
(3) Placental transfer to fetus either an active or a passive process.
(4) Increases gradually until 40 weeks' gestation (majority is passed in the third trimester).
(5) Decreased levels in preterm infants, proportional to their gestational age.
(6) Decreased levels in postmature and small for gestational age infants, suggesting inhibition of transfer with placental damage.

b. Immunoglobulin M (IgM).
(1) IgM does not cross the placenta.
(2) Synthesis begins early in fetal life, with detectable levels at approximately 30 weeks' gestation.
(3) Levels may increase (>20 mg/ml) with intrauterine infection.
(4) Serum levels rapidly increase after birth.

c. Immunoglobulin A (IgA).
(1) IgA is the most common immunoglobulin in the gastrointestinal tract, respiratory tract, and is secreted in human colostrum and human milk.
(2) IgA does not cross the placental barrier.
(3) Intrauterine synthesis is minimal in an uninfected fetus.
(4) IgA does not become detectable in the infant until 2 to 3 weeks of postnatal life.
(5) Levels may increase with certain congenital viral infections.

d. Immunoglobulin E (IgE).
(1) Present in very small amounts in serum and secretions.
(2) Major role in allergic reactions.

C. Cellular immunity.

1. Specific cellular immunity is mediated by T lymphocytes, which enhance the efficiency of the phagocytic responses.

a. T lymphocytes migrate to the thymus, where they begin differentiation (see Fig. 31-1).

b. They are activated by antigens to which they have become sensitized and subsequently become memory or activated T cells. However, they must be "processed" and presented on the surface of antigen-presenting cells (i.e., macrophages and monocytes).
(1) Memory cells respond at a later time to the same antigen.
(2) There are three types of activated T cells.

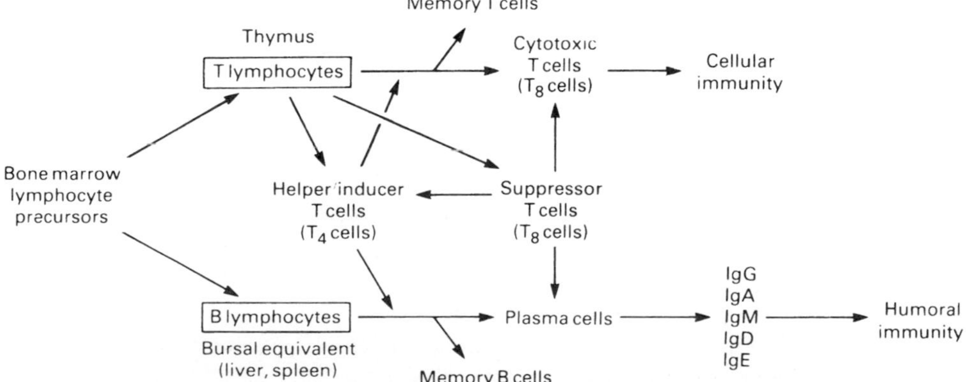

FIGURE 31-1 ■ Development of cellular and humoral immunity. (From Ganong, W.F.: *Review of physiology* [14th ed.]. East Norwalk, CT, 1989, Appleton & Lange.)

(a) Cytotoxic: kill foreign or virus-infected cells.
(b) Helper: enable B or T cells to respond to antigens and activate macrophages.
(c) Suppressor: repress responses of specific T and B lymphocytes to antigens.

(3) T lymphocytes modify the behavior of phagocytic cells, produce a variety of cytokines, and increase their antimicrobial activity.
(4) Depressed T-cell function may occur as a consequence of neonatal viral infection, hyperbilirubinemia, corticosteroid therapy, or maternal medications taken late in pregnancy.

2. Nonspecific cellular immunity is an inflammatory response involving phagocytosis and includes neutrophils, monocytes, and complement. Neutrophilic cell invasion and platelet aggregation are aided by the activation of the three important plasma protein systems (the complement, clotting, and kinin systems) and immunoglobulins. Additionally, some host cells produce soluble factors that contribute to defenses by affecting other neighboring cells. These factors are known as cytokines and include interleukins, interferons, and other proteins. Cytokines are multifunctional proteins, often referred to as "hormones of the immune system."
   a. Neutrophils are phagocytes and must detect them and move toward them (chemotaxis), adhere to them (adhesion), ingest them (phagocytosis), and kill them by intracellular generation of toxic oxygen metabolites such as superoxide ions (respiratory burst).
      (1) Neutrophils mature from the bone marrow from the committed phagocyte stem cells.
      (2) They are the first line of defense against bacterial infection.
      (3) A neutrophil storage pool (reserve) is present and exceeds the circulating pool; however, in a septic neonate, the neutrophil reserve pool quickly becomes depleted because of the following:
         (a) Decrease in proliferation or reproduction.
         (b) Decrease in the immature neutrophil storage pool.
         (c) Decrease in the number of neutrophils that reach the site of infection.
   b. Monocytes are important in the defense against fungal and bacterial infections and are found primarily in the connective tissue.
   c. Complement is a series of proteins that interact or mediate a cascade of synthesis of other proteins responsible for chemotaxis, opsonization, and cell lysis.
      (1) Activation by an antibody-dependent mechanism (classic pathway) or antibody-independent mechanism (alternative pathway).
      (2) Purpose.
         (a) Increase neutrophil mobilization from the bone marrow.
         (b) Draw neutrophils to the site of infection.
         (c) Opsonize bacteria for improved phagocytosis.
         (d) Interleukins (ILs) are biochemical messengers produced by the macrophages or lymphocytes in response to stimulation by an antigen or by products of inflammation (Fig. 31-2). The analysis of immunologic mediators may greatly enhance timely diagnosis of sepsis. Concentrations of the cytokines interleukin-1 receptor antagonist (IL-1ra), interleukin-6 (IL-6), and the circulating adhesion molecule-1 (cICAM-1) are elevated in sepsis. IL-6 plays a critical role in the induction of C-reactive protein (CRP) in the liver.

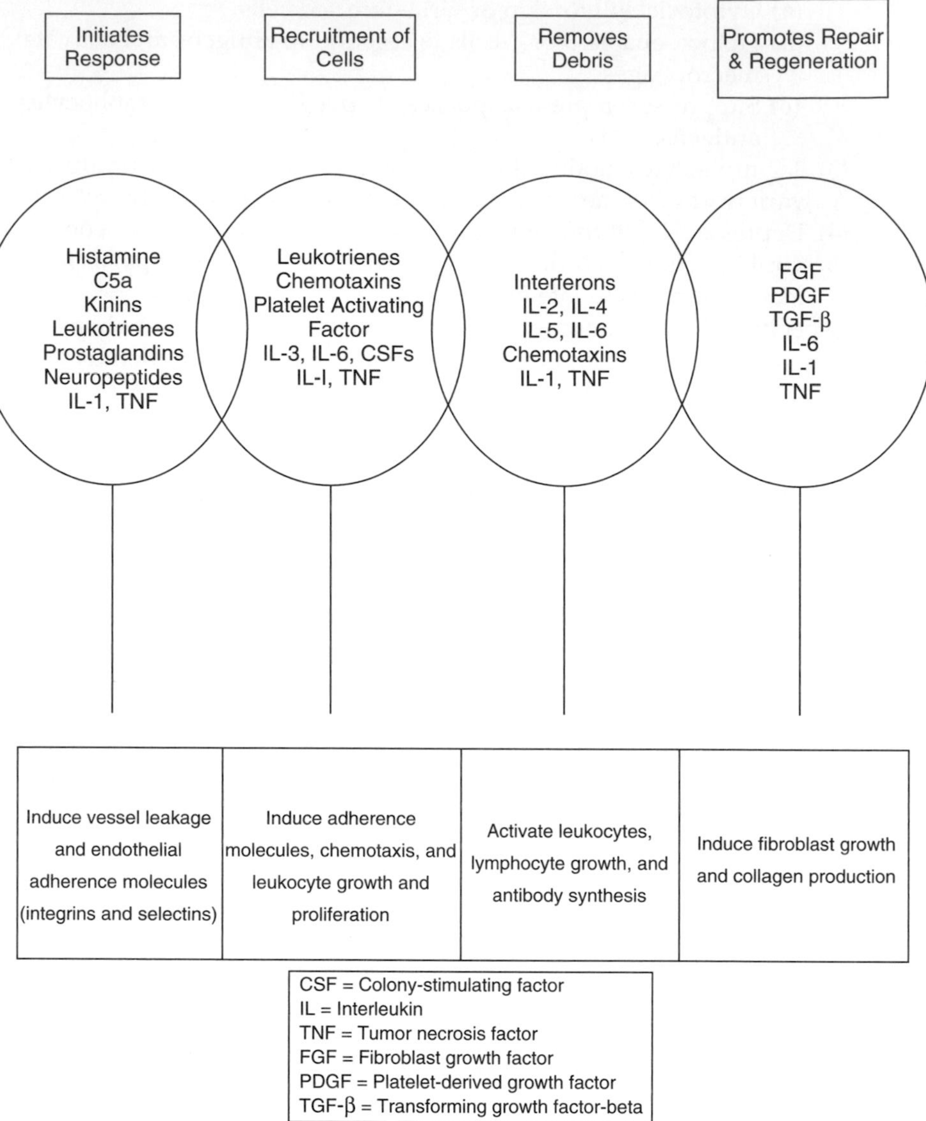

FIGURE 31-2 ■ Mediators associated with stages of inflammation. (Adapted from Rote, N.S.: Inflammation. In K.L. McCance and S.E. Huether [Eds.]: *Pathophysiology: The biologic basis for disease in adults and children* [4th ed.]. St Louis, 2002, Mosby, p. 214.)

Interleukin-6 is an important mediator of the early inflammatory host response to infection; it reaches peak concentrations rapidly after the onset of bacteremia, several hours before the upregulation of CRP by IL-6 begins. IL-6 is a multifunctional polypeptide and is synthesized by an array of cells.

D. Summary of neonatal immunodeficiencies.

1. Humoral immunity.

a. Decreased antibody levels.

(1) Poor response to antigenic stimuli.

(2) No production of type-specific antibodies.

(3) Fewer B cells recognize foreign antibodies.

(4) Delay in the development of cytotoxic T lymphocytes, increasing the risk for viral infections.

b. Decreased opsonic activity.
   (1) Impaired circulating antibody.
   (2) Maternal complement is not transferred.
   (3) Depressed complement (classical and alternate) pathways and decreased levels of components of the complement cascade (50%-80%) of adult values and less in the premature infant.
2. Neutrophil response.
   a. Diminished size of neutrophil storage and proliferative pools.
   b. Reduced numbers of immature neutrophils in the storage pool.
   c. Failure to increase stem cell proliferation during infection.
   d. Abnormal neutrophil function (adhesion, chemotaxis, phagocytosis, and bacterial killing).

TRANSMISSION OF INFECTIOUS ORGANISMS IN THE NEONATE

A. **Vertical transmission:** mother to infant.
   1. Transplacental acquisition.
      a. Transplacental hematogenous transmission (crosses from the placenta to the fetus).
         (1) *Treponema pallidum* and *Listeria monocytogenes*.
   2. Ascending acquisition: into the uterus near time of delivery, when the cervical mucous plug, chorion, and amnion are less than optimal barriers.
   3. Intrapartum acquisition: natal transmission at delivery, during passage of the fetus through a birth canal that is host to a variety of bacteria, as well as chlamydiae, fungi, yeast, and viruses. This mechanism implies colonization of the skin, mucous membranes, gastrointestinal tract, and respiratory tract during parturition.

B. **Horizontal transmission:** from nursery personnel and the hospital equipment to the infant; also known as a nosocomial infection.

DIAGNOSIS AND THERAPY

Clinical Assessment

Identification of Predisposing Risk Factors Found in the Maternal History

A. **Maternal.**
   1. Antepartum.
      a. Inadequate prenatal care.
      b. Inadequate nutrition.
      c. Low socioeconomic status.
      d. Recurrent abortion.
      e. Substance abuse.
      f. History of maternal sexually transmitted diseases.
   2. Intrapartum.
      a. Prolonged rupture of membranes (>12-18 hr).
      b. Vaginal group B streptococcal colonization.
      c. Low levels of maternal group B streptococcus (GBS) antibodies.
      d. Chorioamnionitis: sustained fetal tachycardia, uterine tenderness, purulent amniotic fluid, foul-smelling amniotic fluid, or unexplained maternal temperature higher than 38° C.
      e. Prolonged or difficult labor.
      f. Premature labor.

g. Urinary tract infection.
h. Invasive intrapartum procedures.
i. Maternal fever.
j. Elevated maternal heart rate (>100 beats per minute [bpm]).
k. Elevated fetal heart rate (>160 bpm).

B. Neonatal.

1. Prematurity (infants born <32 weeks' gestation have a 4-25 times increased risk).
2. Low birth weight (<2500 g).
3. Difficult delivery.
4. Birth asphyxia.
5. Meconium staining.
6. Resuscitation.
7. Congenital anomalies (i.e., abdominal wall and spinal defects).
8. Black infants.
9. Male infants.
10. Multiple births.

C. Environmental.

1. Hospital admission.
2. Length of stay.
3. Invasive procedures (i.e., peripheral IV punctures, endotracheal tubes, umbilical catheters, thoracostomy tubes, and other surgical interventions).
4. Common use of broad-spectrum antibiotics.
5. Use of humidification systems in ventilatory or incubator care.

Clinical Manifestations

A. Variable nonspecific presentation of sepsis: appearance of infant "just not right" to nurse or mother, accompanied by subtle changes in feeding and activity. Culture-proven sepsis is relatively rare in the newborn infant; many more infants have signs suggestive of infection at presentation.

B. Thermoregulatory instability.

1. Temperature instability.
2. Fever.
3. Hypothermia.

C. Neurologic clinical signs.

1. Lethargy.
2. Jitteriness.
3. Irritability.
4. Seizures.
5. Hypotonia or hypertonia.
6. Bulging fontanelles.
7. High-pitched cry.

D. Respiratory clinical signs: most common clinical sign occurring in 90% of infants with sepsis (Polin et al., 2001).

1. Grunting.
2. Retractions.
3. Cyanosis.
4. Apnea.
5. Tachypnea.

E. Cardiovascular clinical signs.

1. Tachycardia.
2. Arrhythmias.
3. Hypotension or hypertension.

4. Cold, clammy skin.
5. Decreased peripheral perfusion/vasoconstriction.

F. **Gastrointestinal clinical signs.**
1. Poor feeding.
2. Vomiting, diarrhea.
3. Abdominal distention.
4. Increasing feeding residuals.

G. **Skin.**
1. Rash.
2. Pustules.
3. Jaundice.
4. Pallor.
5. Vasomotor instability.
6. Petechiae.

H. **Internal organ manifestations.**
1. Hepatomegaly.
2. Splenomegaly.

I. **Metabolic disturbances.**
1. Glucose instability.
2. Metabolic acidosis.

Hematologic Evaluation

A. **Complete blood cell count (CBC).**
1. White blood cell (WBC) count: interpretation is often difficult due to the wide range of normal values in the neonate (5000 to 30,000/mm^3) (Oski and Naiman, 1966; Thureen et al., 1999).
   a. Leukocytosis: an elevated WBC count (>25, 000/mm^3); may be a normal finding in the newborn infant.
   b. Leukopenia: a depressed WBC count (<1750/mm^3); generally is an abnormal finding in the newborn infant and may be due to sepsis or pregnancy induced hypertension.
2. Differential cell count (Fig. 31-3).
   a. Neutrophil count.

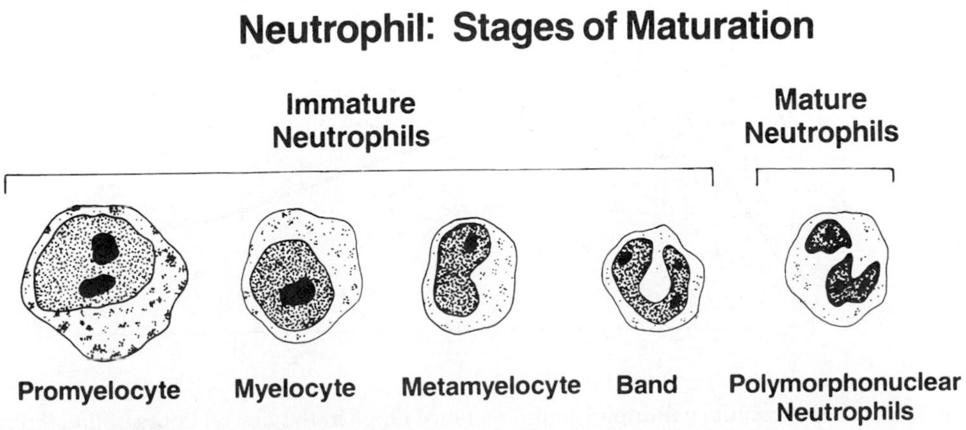

Neutrophil: Stages of Maturation

Immature Neutrophils

Mature Neutrophils

Promyelocyte

Myelocyte

Metamyelocyte

Band

Polymorphonuclear Neutrophils

FIGURE 31-3 ■ Neutrophils represent a percentage of the total white blood cell count and are reported as the differential on a complete blood cell count.

(1) Absolute neutrophil count (ANC) is calculated as:
   (a) ANC = WBC × (% Immature neutrophils + % Mature neutrophils) × 0.01
   (b) Manroe and colleagues (1979) developed a reference range for the absolute neutrophil count in term infants (Fig. 31-4).

(2) Neutropenia: less than 1500/mm^3.
   (a) Most accurate predictor of infection.
   (b) May be associated with maternal hypertension, confirmed periventricular hemorrhage, severe asphyxia, and reticulocytosis (after 14 postnatal days of life).

(3) Neutrophilia.
   (a) Although less predictive, may also suggest presence of infection.
   (b) May be elevated at birth (as high as 26,000/mm^3) because of birth stress, increased neutrophil production, and rates of release and demargination from the circulating neutrophil pool.
   (c) Other clinical conditions associated with neutrophilia include hemolytic disease, asymptomatic hypoglycemia, trisomy 21, use of oxytocin during labor, maternal fever, stress during labor and birth, exogenous steroid administration, pneumothorax, and meconium aspiration.

b. Immature/total neutrophil (I/T) ratio.
   (1) Sensitivity is greater than 90%; however, less specific (having negative results when in fact there is no infection).
   (2) Increase in the I/T ratio also known as a left shift; reflects an increase in immature neutrophils.
   (3) I/T ratio greater than 0.20 is suggestive of infection (Fig. 31-5).

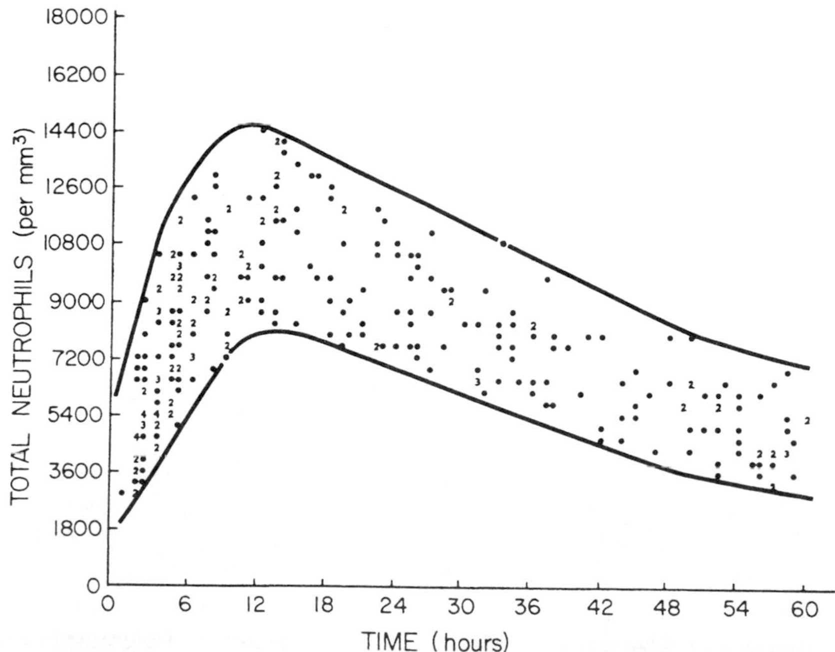

FIGURE 31-4 ■ Absolute neutrophil count reference range in the first 60 hours of life. (From Manroe, B.L., Weinberg, A.G., Rosenfeld, C.R., and Browne, R. et al.: The neonatal blood count in health and disease. *Journal of Pediatrics, 95*[1]:89-98, 1979.)

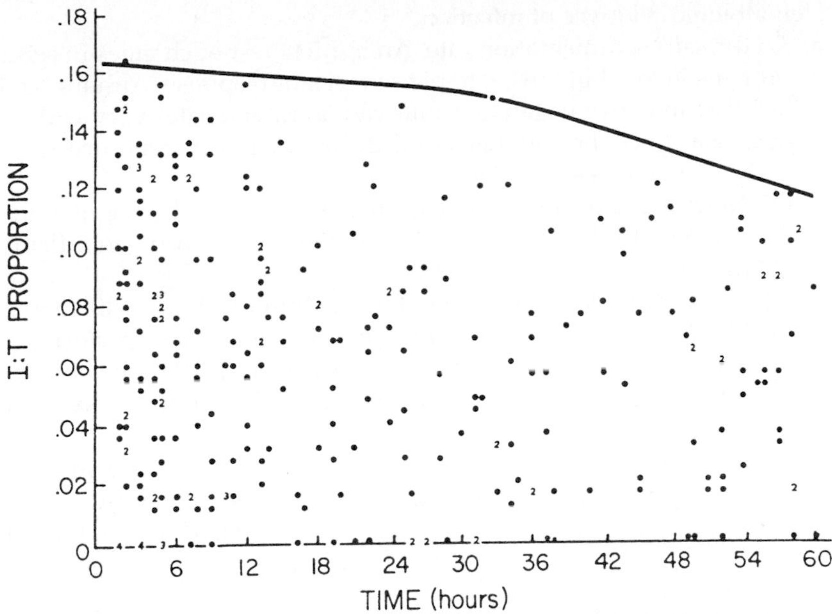

FIGURE 31-5 ■ I/T ratio. Reference range for the proportion of immature to total neutrophils in the first 60 hours of life. (From Manroe, B.L., Weinberg, A.G., Rosenfeld, C.R. and Browne, R et al.: The neonatal blood count in health and disease. *Journal of Pediatrics*, *95*[1]:89-98, 1979.)

(4) Calculation of I/T ratio:

$$\frac{\%\text{ Bands} + \%\text{ Immature forms}}{\%\text{ Mature} + \%\text{ Bands} + \%\text{ Immature forms}}$$

c. Platelet count.
   (1) Normal count: 150,000 to 400,000/mm^3.
   (2) Thrombocytopenia (<100,000/mm^3): possible association with bacterial sepsis or viral infection.
   (3) Severe thrombocytopenia: possible association with disseminated intravascular coagulation (DIC).

B. Additional diagnostic screening tests.

1. Detection of bacterial and viral deoxyribonucleic acid (DNA)–polymerase chain reaction (PCR).
   a. Provides a rapid and sensitive method of diagnosis of a specific bacterial or viral gene (DNA) segment.
   b. Identifies specific bacteria and viruses such as, *Escherichia coli*, methicillin-resistant *Staphylococcus aureus* (MRSA), *Ureaplasma urealyticum*, herpes simplex virus, and hepatitis B virus.
      (1) May be performed on blood, catheter tips, cerebrospinal fluid, joint fluids, and other sterile body sites.
      (2) MRSA remains an important cause of nosocomial infections. Nationally, 5% to 10% of all hospitalized patients will become colonized or infected with MRSA. In addition, coagulase-negative staphylococci are important causes of nosocomial bacteremia, and catheter or other iatrogenic device–associated infections. This PCR test amplifies a segment of the *mec*A gene. This PCR assay should be performed directly on all positive *S. aureus* blood cultures.

2. Hematologic evidence of infection.
   a. Erythrocyte sedimentation rate. An indirect test of changes in serum proteins involed in the acute-phase reactant response. Although false-positive and false-negative results can occur and rates vary widely, levels may rise above the 95th percentile during an infectious process.
   b. CRP (Pourcyrous et al., 1993).
      (1) Nonspecific acute-phase reactant is synthesized by the liver in response to IL-6, which appears in the blood during an inflammatory process.
      (2) Because of a latency period of 6 to 8 hours and a stabilization time of 1 to 2 days after the start of therapy, this test is best performed serially every 12 hours when infection is suspected. CRP is elevated in 50% to 90% of infected infants; however, it has a low positive predictive value (Malik et al., 2003).
      (3) CRP is most useful in determining effectiveness of treatment, resolution of disease, and duration of antibiotic therapy.
   c. IgM levels: may rise in the presence of bacterial and/or viral infections.

Diagnostic Evaluation

A. **Culture:** isolation of a pathogen in a blood culture obtained by using aseptic technique is the gold standard for diagnosing infection (Polin et al., 2001).
   1. Blood.
      a. Culture specimen obtained from peripheral vein or umbilical vessel.
      b. Procedure.
         (1) Carefully clean infant's skin with an antiseptic such as povidone-iodine solution 10%.
         (2) For maximal bactericidal effect, allow skin to dry for 2 minutes before inserting needle and obtaining culture specimen.
         (3) A minimum of 1 ml of blood should be obtained to improve chances for detection of bacteremia. As many as 60% of culture results will be falsely negative if less than 1 ml is drawn (Schelonka et al., 1996).
      c. May be falsely negative if mother received antibiotics in labor.
      d. Blood culture results need to be followed at specified intervals, usually 24, 48, and 72 hours, and a final report at 5 to 14 days.
      e. 92% of positive blood culture will be positive by 24 hours (Byington et al., 2003).
   2. Cerebrospinal fluid (CSF).
      a. Lumbar puncture. Routine use of lumbar puncture is controversial in early sepsis evaluation. It is frequently unsuccessful or bloody (Schwersenski et al., 1991) and may also compromise an unstable infant. Meningitis in the absence of bacteremia is uncommon, especially in the neonate with respiratory disease (Weiss et al., 1991). Lumbar puncture may be reserved for infants with central nervous system signs or proven bacteremia.
      b. Normal CSF findings.
         (1) A normal mean CSF leukocyte count of 9/mm^3 (range = 0-22/mm^3) in premature infants, and 8.2/mm^3 (range = 0-25/mm^3) in term infants.
         (2) A normal mean protein count of 57.2 mg/dl (range = 65-150 mg/dl) in premature infants, and a mean of 61.3 mg/dl (range = 20-170 mg/dl) in term infants.

(3) CSF glucose concentration 55% to 105% in premature infants, 44% to 128% in term infants. Obtain serum level before spinal tap to allow for equilibrium to occur between CSF and blood.
(4) Absence of microorganisms on Gram stain.

c. Positive CSF culture.
(1) Repeat the CSF tap every 24 to 36 hours until culture is sterile.
(2) Duration of antibiotic therapy is based on when the first negative culture is documented.
(3) There is a direct correlation between adverse neonatal outcome and persistence of bacteria in the CSF.

3. Urine.
a. Incidence of contamination with urine obtained by an external collection bag is high. If urine is to be collected, the sample should be obtained by sterile catheterization or suprapubic needle aspiration to avoid contamination and false-positive results.
b. If urine is obtained by urethral catheterization, a count greater than 50,000 to 100,000 organisms per milliliter suggests infection.
c. When culture result is positive, a percutaneous suprapubic bladder tap should be performed because the urine is presumed to be sterile.

4. Superficial cultures: not recommended because:
a. Culture result may indicate colonization, but does not show bacteremia or sepsis.
b. Infant may have sepsis in the absence of a positive surface culture result.

B. Follow-up.

1. If a positive culture result has been obtained from blood, CSF, or urine specimen, a follow-up culture specimen should be obtained to document sterilization.
2. Persistent bacteremia may be caused by:
a. Resistance to antibiotics.
b. Incorrect administration of antibiotics.
c. An occult site of infection that may require surgical intervention (e.g., abscess).
d. Central venous or peripherally inserted central catheters left in place during treatment for bacteremia.

Therapy

A. Antibiotic therapy.

1. Appropriate antibiotic choice depends on the likely organisms, pharmacokinetics, efficacy, and potential toxicity of the antimicrobial agents used.
2. Ampicillin is commonly used in combination with an aminoglycoside for initial broad-spectrum treatment of suspected or confirmed bacterial infection.
3. If meningitis is suspected, ampicillin and cefotaxime are the antibiotics of choice until a specific organism has been identified.
4. Third-generation cephalosporins, including cefotaxime and ceftazidime, have increased antimicrobial activity against gram-negative bacilli and enhanced penetration across the blood-brain barrier over gentamicin.
5. Dosage and frequency of administration of antimicrobial agents vary with gestational age, birth weight, and postconceptual age. A primary drug

reference for pediatric dosing is recommended, such as the *Pediatric Dosage Handbook* (Taketomo et al., 2002).

6. Duration of antibiotic therapy is 10 to 14 days for proven sepsis and 21 days for meningitis.
7. If culture results are negative, antimicrobial agents may be discontinued after 48 to 72 hours.
8. If the mother was treated before delivery, the antimicrobial course may be extended in the face of negative culture results (Polin et al., 2001).

B. Immunotherapy. The neonate is considered immunocompromised, and defense mechanisms to overcome infections are not yet mature. The administration of blood and tissue factors to enhance the neonatal immune system is under investigation.

1. Intravenous immune globulin (IVIG).
   - **a.** Administration of IVIG may be effective in reducing mortality from nosocomial infections, although there is insufficient evidence to support the routine administration of IVIG preparations investigated to date to prevent mortality in infants with suspected or subsequently proved neonatal infection (Ohlsson and Lacy, 2001).
   - **b.** To be useful, IVIG transfusions must contain antibodies specific to the type of infection-causing organism.
   - **c.** IVIG preparations contain protein and varying amounts of IgG, IgA, and IgM (Taketomo et al., 2002).
   - **d.** IVIG acts to neutralize viruses, promote phagocytosis, increase opsonization, and enhance polymorphonucleocyte migration. It prevents neutrophil storage pool depletion by enhancing the neonate's IgG levels for protection against invading bacteria until the immune system is more mature.
   - **e.** Studies continue to determine efficacy of treatment in neonatal infections.
2. Granulocyte transfusion.
   - **a.** Results in an increased number of polymorphonuclear neutrophils, which are responsible for phagocytic action in infection.
   - **b.** May improve survival in infants with sepsis and a decreased neutrophil storage pool (Christensen et al., 1982).
   - **c.** Process is both time consuming and expensive.
   - **d.** Presumed risks include fluid overload, graft-versus-host disease, infections, and blood group sensitization.
   - **e.** Studies continue to determine the potential for reducing morbidity and mortality rates for infection.
3. Exchange transfusion with fresh whole blood.
   - **a.** Used in severe sepsis to remove bacterial endotoxins and decrease the bacterial burden, improve peripheral and pulmonary perfusion, and enhance the immune system.
   - **b.** Used widely before 1980; however, limited prospective studies have been done to support effectiveness (Vain et al., 1980).
   - **c.** Adverse reactions include hypoglycemia, acid-base imbalance, thrombocytopenia, and infection.
4. Granulocyte colony-stimulating factor (G-CSF).
   - **a.** Acts to stimulate proliferation of neutrophils; primes neutrophils, thus enhancing their bactericidal and phagocytic activity.
   - **b.** Early trials have demonstrated neutrophil enhancement in neonates without adverse hematologic, immunologic, or developmental defects.
   - **c.** A recent Cochrane Review concluded (Carr et al., 2003), "There is insufficient evidence to support the introduction of either G-CSF or

granulocyte-macrophage colony-stimulating factor (GM-CSF) into current practice, either as a treatment of established systemic infection or as prophylaxis to prevent systemic infection.

HISTORY, SITES, AND TYPES OF NEONATAL INFECTION

A. Epidemiologic history.

1. In 1930s and 1940s: high incidence of group A streptococcus.
2. In 1940s and 1950s: *E. coli* responsible for majority of infections.
3. In 1950s and 1960s: emergence of *S. aureus*.
4. From 1970s to 1980s: GBS, *E. coli*, *L. monocytogenes*, and *Haemophilus influenzae* responsible for majority of sepsis during first week of life.
5. 1990s: *Staphylococcus epidermidis* and MRSA have emerged as nosocomial pathogens in the nursery.

B. Common sites of neonatal infection: blood, CSF, lungs, and urinary tract.

C. Types of neonatal infections.

1. Sepsis.
   - a. Incidence of neonatal sepsis varies between 1 to 8 in 1000 live term births and 1 in 250 live preterm births.
   - b. Incidence of meningitis is 1:2500 live births.
   - c. Most common organisms responsible for early-onset sepsis:
     - (1) Early onset: *E. coli*, group B streptococcus (GBS), *L. monocytogenes*, and *H. influenzae*, *Enterobacter* spp., *Klebsiella pneumoniae*, *Pseudomonas aeruginosa*, and *S. aureus* (Polin et al., 2001; Stoll et al., 2002).
     - (2) Nosocomial: Coagulase-negative staphylococci, *S. aureus*, *Candida albicans*, *K. pneumoniae*, *P. aeruginosa* and *Serratia marcescens* (Polin et al., 2001; Stoll et al., 1996b).
   - d. Presentation is often nonspecific, with subtle signs of temperature instability, lethargy, poor feeding, and glucose instability.
2. Meningitis.
   - a. More frequent occurrence during neonatal period than at any other time.
   - b. GBS and *E. coli:* are major pathogens identified in neonatal meningitis.
   - c. Acquisition: direct invasion, contamination between CSF space and integumental surfaces, and bacterial dissemination from infected structures.
   - d. Clinical manifestations.
     - (1) General signs and symptoms of infection at presentation.
     - (2) Specific CNS symptoms: increased irritability, alteration in consciousness, poor tone, tremors, seizures, and bulging fontanelle.
   - e. CSF culture.
     - (1) CSF culture result may be positive even though blood culture result is negative.
     - (2) If the CSF culture result is positive, culture must be repeated 24 to 36 hours after initiation of treatment to ensure adequate therapy.
   - f. Antibiotic therapy.
     - (1) Prompt initiation is crucial for optimal outcome, and antibiotic may be administered before CSF specimen is obtained.
     - (2) Choose antimicrobial agents with good CSF penetration.
     - (3) Duration of therapy is dependent on recovered pathogens and clinical response, generally 14 to 21 days.

g. Significant sequelae in 20% to 50% of infants who survive: motor and mental disabilities, convulsions, hydrocephalus, and hearing loss.

3. Pneumonia.
   a. Transmission.
      (1) Vertical.
         (a) Onset usually from birth to 7 days.
         (b) Most common bacterial pathogen responsible for pneumonia: GBS; however, incidence of GBS is changing, any organism present in maternal genital tract can cause pneumonia in neonate.
      (2) Horizontal.
         (a) Onset beyond 1 week of life.
         (b) Through human contact or contaminated equipment.
   b. Clinical manifestations: possibly general but usually specific symptoms of respiratory distress.
   c. Diagnosis.
      (1) May be difficult.
      (2) Chest x-ray examination.
         (a) Possible asymmetric densities and pleural effusion.
         (b) Pulmonary granularity present in GBS-related pneumonia; possibly indistinguishable from respiratory distress syndrome in premature infant.
4. Urinary tract infections.
   a. *E. coli:* most common organism responsible for urinary tract infections; *Klebsiella* and *P. aeruginosa:* less common; gram-positive bacteria: rare.
   b. Clinical manifestations.
      (1) General signs are often nonspecific and may include temperature instability, poor weight gain, poor feeding, cyanosis, abdominal distention, hyperglycemia, hematuria, and proteinuria.
      (2) Localized signs consist of a weak urinary stream and/or bladder distention.
   c. Antimicrobial agents: administer parenterally.
      (1) Oral absorption is erratic.
      (2) There is a 30% association between urinary tract infection and septicemia.
   d. Follow-up.
      (1) Repeat urine culture should be sterile within 36 to 48 hours after initiation of antimicrobial therapy.
      (2) If a urinary tract infection has been documented in an infant, voiding cystourethrogram should be performed to evaluate the possibility of any congenital abnormalities of the urinary tract.
5. Neonatal conjunctivitis.
   a. May be caused by a variety of organisms, including *S. aureus, P. aeruginosa, Neisseria gonorrhoeae*, and *Chlamydia trachomatis*.
   b. Manifestations usually include discharge from the eye and conjunctivitis.
   c. Diagnosis is made by a culture and Gram stain, which reveals leukocytes and the causative organism.
   d. Chemical conjunctivitis is usually due to instillation of prophylactic silver nitrate but may occur with topical antibiotics.
   e. Of the ophthalmic antibiotics, methicillin is the antibiotic of choice for *S. aureus*, and a combination of carbenicillin and gentamicin are used when *P. aeruginosa* has been identified (also refer to *N. gonorrhoeae*, and *C. trachomatis*).

6. Gastrointestinal disease.
   a. Breast-feeding with the transmission of secretory IgA is important in the prevention of illness (Welsh and May, 1979).
   b. Specific gastrointestinal pathogens.
      (1) Rotavirus.
         (a) Virus is acquired by nosocomial transmission in the neonatal intensive care unit (NICU).
         (b) Infection may be asymptomatic; infant may exhibit signs and symptoms of severe gastrointestinal distress.
         (c) Symptoms include fever, vomiting, and watery yellow or green diarrhea.
         (d) Detection of the virus is by radioimmunoassay, immunofluorescence, and/or latex agglutination, enzyme-linked immunosorbent assay (ELISA).
         (e) Management includes:
            (i) Replacement of fluids and electrolytes.
            (ii) Elemental diet: may be needed for improved absorption if mucosal damage has occurred.
            (iii) Parenteral nutrition until feedings are well established.
            (iv) Handwashing after contact with infant is essential. Virus is shed in stool 2 to 3 days before illness is recognized.
            (v) Isolation: may decrease spread of virus.
         (f) Prevention. A rotavirus vaccine (Rv) is now available for the prevention of rotavirus. Rv is administered at 2, 4, and 6 months of age (American Academy of Pediatrics [AAP], 2003).
      (2) *Clostridium difficile.*
         (a) Gram-positive anaerobic bacillus.
         (b) Causative agent for necrotizing enterocolitis and pseudomembranous colitis.
         (c) Manifested by watery diarrhea, abdominal pain and tenderness, nausea and vomiting, fever, and blood in stool.
         (d) Complications: toxic megacolon, dehydration, and electrolyte disturbances.
         (e) Protective effect: possibly from human milk; neutralizing antibody against *C. difficile* in colostrum.
         (f) Associated with long-term administration of antibiotic therapy.
         (g) May be associated with necrotizing enterocolitis.
         (h) Intestinal colonization as high as 50% in neonates who generally remain well.
         (i) Treatment: fluid and electrolyte management, appropriate broad-spectrum antibiotics.

INFECTION WITH SPECIFIC PATHOGENS

Bacterial Infections

A. Gram-positive organisms.
1. Group B streptococci (Centers for Disease Control and Prevention [CDC], 2002; Schrag et al., 2002).
   a. Gram-positive spherical bacteria that form pairs or chains during growth.
   b. 20 identified strains. Groups A, B, and D and *Streptococcus pneumoniae* are responsible for most neonatal infections.
   c. Organism in maternal cervix, vagina, anus, and urethra.

d. Colonization with GBS in 15% to 35% of women, there has been an overall 70% decline in GBS sepsis since the adoption of the 1996 CDC recommendations (Fig. 31-6) (AAP, 2003; Schrag, et al., 2002).

e. Recommendations for intrapartum penicillin therapy: although many of the recommendations in the 2002 guidelines are the same as those in 1996, they include some key changes (www.cdc.gov/mmwr/preview/mmwrhtml/rr5111a1.htm).

(1) Recommendation of universal prenatal screening for vaginal and rectal GBS colonization of all pregnant women at 35 to 37 weeks' gestation, based on recent documentation in a large retrospective cohort study of a strong protective effect of this culture-based screening strategy relative to the risk-based strategy.

(2) Updated prophylaxis regimens for women with penicillin allergy.

(3) Detailed instruction on prenatal specimen collection and expanded methods of GBS culture processing, including instructions on antimicrobial susceptibility testing.

(4) Recommendation against routine intrapartum antibiotic prophylaxis for GBS-colonized women undergoing planned cesarean deliveries that have not begun labor or had rupture of membranes.

(5) A suggested algorithm for management of patients with threatened preterm delivery.

f. Previous and current recommendations for intrapartum penicillin therapy:

(1) History of previous infant with invasive GBS disease.

(2) Maternal GBS bacteremia with current pregnancy.

(3) Intrapartum fever.

(4) Birth at less than 37 weeks' gestation.

(5) Rupture of membranes more than 18 hours before delivery.

g. Colonization/disease ratio: approximately 100 to 200:1.

h. Most common organism responsible for early-onset bacterial infection in the neonate.

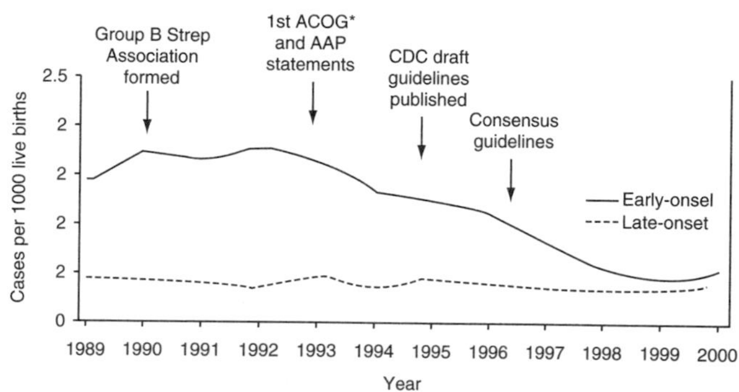

ACOG, American College of Obstetricians and Gynecologists; *AAP*, American Academy of Pediatrics

FIGURE 31-6 ■ Incidence of early- and late-onset invasive group B streptoccocal disease—selected active bacterial core surveillance areas, 1989-2000, and activities for prevention of group B streptococcal disease.(Adapted from Centers for Disease Control and Prevention: Early-onset group B streptococcal disease, United States, 1998-1999. *MMWR Morbidity and Mortality Weekly Report, 49*:793-396, 2000; Schrag, S.J., Zywicki, S., Farley, M.M., et al.: Group B streptococcal disease in the era of intrapartum antibiotic prophylaxis. *New England Journal of Medicine, 342*[1]:15-20, 2000.)

i. Manifestation of infection: asymptomatic bacteremia, septicemia, pneumonia, or meningitis.
j. Early-onset infection with GBS.
  (1) Fulminant presentation, typically within first 24 hours of life.
  (2) Most common presentation is with pneumonia and/or meningitis.
  (3) Acquired by vertical transmission.
  (4) Clinical manifestations: respiratory distress, hypotonia, lethargy, poor feeding, abdominal distention, pallor, tachycardia, temperature instability, shock, and seizures.
k. Late-onset infection with GBS.
  (1) Insidious presentation, usually after 7 to 10 days.
  (2) Common complication: meningitis.
    (a) Mortality rate has declined significantly to 10% in 1997 (Harvey et al., 1999).
    (b) In 12% to 29% of survivors there may be serious neurologic damage such as mental retardation, spastic quadriplegia, cortical blindness, deafness, uncontrolled seizures, hydrocephalus, and diabetes insipidus, and in another 15% to 38% there may be mild neurologic impairment such as neuromotor loss without functional loss, isolated hydrocephalus, epilepsy, and a cognitive IQ score of 70 to 80 (Stevens et al., 2003).
  (3) Acquired by horizontal transmission.
  (4) Symptoms: fever, lethargy, and bulging fontanelle.
l. Treatment.
  (1) Antibiotic therapy.
  (2) Fluid management.
  (3) Volume expansion.
  (4) Seizure control.
  (5) Monitoring of electrolytes, fluid balance status, weight, and intake and output.

2. *Staphylococcus*. These bacteria are gram-positive spherical cells that appear as irregular clusters on a Gram stain. Some species are considered normal flora, and others are pathogenic. Staphylococcal infection can cause mild disease such as local infection from a scalp electrode, or may have widespread manifestations, including osteomyelitis, mastitis, and overwhelming sepsis.
  a. *S. aureus*. A coagulase-positive organism. The major source of infection is through horizontal transmission from hospital personnel, is also associated with umbilical catheters, endotracheal tubes, and central lines. Colonization occurs in 40% to 90% of neonates by the fifth day of life. May have widespread manifestations, including osteomyelitis, mastitis, and overwhelming sepsis. Treatment is with nafcillin or vancomycin. If methicillin resistant, vancomycin is antibiotic of choice. In 2002, two cases of vancomycin-resistant *S. aureus* (VRSA) were documented in two different states. The guidelines for detecting these organisms and preventing the spread of VRSA are available at www.cdc.gov/nicdod/hip/10_20.pdf (AAP, 2003).
  b. *S. epidermidis*. A coagulase-negative staphylococcus (CoNS) organism that is part of the normal skin flora. Nearly all infants are colonized with CoNS by 2 to 4 days of life. In recent years CoNS has emerged as a serious pathogen in the premature low birth weight infant due to invasive procedures such as endotracheal tubes, umbilical catheters, chest tubes, and central lines that contain a slime-producing agent that can erode the

surface of polyethylene catheters and cause colony growth. Many strains are methicillin resistant. Vancomycin is the antibiotic of choice (AAP, 2003).

3. *Listeria monocytogenes.*
   a. Aerobic gram-positive bacillus.
   b. Acquired transplacentally or from the vaginal canal, approximately 65% of women experience clinical symptoms of a prodromal illness prior to a diagnosis of listeriosis (AAP, 2003).
   c. Should be suspected in preterm infant who has passage of meconium or if the maternal history includes prior stillbirth, repeated spontaneous abortions, brown amniotic fluid or amnionitis (infection before 28 weeks' gestation frequently results in fetal death).
   d. May result in fulminant, disseminated early-onset sepsis with multiorgan involvement.
   e. Symptoms: hypothermia, lethargy, and poor feeding. The infant may have a characteristic salmon-colored rash.
   f. Sensitive to ampicillin, an aminoglycoside is recommended for synergy (AAP, 2003).

B. Gram-negative organisms.

1. *E. coli.*
   a. Most common gram-negative organism causing sepsis and meningitis in neonatal period.
   b. Found in female genital tract, with high incidence of colonization in the neonate. Nosocomial acquisition from person to person; nursery environmental sites (i.e., sinks, multiple use solutions, etc.) are also implicated.
   c. Colonization of human gastrointestinal tract soon after birth; predominant fecal flora throughout life.
   d. Many serotypes of *E. coli*. One form of *E. coli* antigen, K1, is associated with neonatal meningitis.
   e. Possible cause of severe, fulminant infection, leading to respiratory distress, cardiovascular collapse, meningitis, and multiorgan failure and death.
   f. In addition to septicemia, possible cause of localized infection, including cellulitis, pneumonia, septic arthritis, urinary tract infection, and otitis media.
   g. Sensitivity to aminoglycosides such as gentamicin and third-generation cephalosporins (such as cefotaxime). Initial treatment should include ampicillin and an aminoglycoside (AAP, 2003).
2. *P. aeruginosa.*
   a. Gram-negative, motile, aerobic rod.
   b. Known as "water bug"; inhabitant of respirators and moist oxygen circuits and humidified environments.
   c. Particular susceptibility to colonization and subsequent development of pneumonia in infant requiring ventilator and receiving antibiotics.
   d. Pathogenic organism in immunocompromised host or where normal defense mechanisms of the skin and mucous membranes are insufficient.
   e. Generally a cause of late-onset disease with respiratory distress.
   f. Treatment: combination of aminoglycoside and an anti-*Pseudomonas* penicillin such as carbenicillin, imipenem, piperacillin, or ticarcillin or by ceftazidime.
   g. Also a cause of conjunctivitis in newborn infant. Generally between 5 and 18 days after birth, mild conjunctivitis begins with edema and erythema

of the lid, with purulent discharge. May progress quickly, causing corneal perforation, and may also result in virulent necrotizing endophthalmitis and blindness. Parenteral therapy is necessary—typically a parenteral aminoglycoside plus antipseudomonal penicillin or cephalosporin—plus topical aminoglycoside therapy for 7 to 10 days (Thureen et al., 1999).

3. *H. influenzae.*
   a. Gram-negative coccobacillus.
   b. Low rate of maternal genital colonization, although passage to fetus is via the ascending transcervical route.
   c. Chorioamnionitis occurs in all placentas but appears more severe among survivors. May also be spread nosocomially through respiratory droplet transmission.
   d. 50% chance of symptomatic infection in colonized infant.
   e. Early-onset fulminant presentation, with pneumonia, respiratory distress, hypotension, and leukopenia.
   f. Mortality rate may be as high as 50%, especially in the very low birth weight (VLBW) infant. Before introduction of the *H. influenzae* vaccine (HiB), *H. influenzae* was the most common cause of bacterial meningitis in children in the United States.
   g. Initial treatment includes a third-generation cephalosporin (cefotaxime or ceftriaxone). Some strains are resistant to ampicillin (AAP, 2003).
   h. The primary series of Hib vaccinations are recommended at 2, 4, and 6 months of age (AAP, 2003).
4. *N. gonorrhoeae.*
   a. Gram-negative diplococcal bacteria.
   b. Most frequently reported sexually transmitted disease in the United States: approximately 1 million cases annually. Concurrent infections with *C. trachomatis* or *T. pallidum* are common.
   c. Ophthalmia neonatorum presents in the first week of life with bilateral copious, mucopurulent eye drainage. Lid and conjunctival edema and erythema are common.
   d. Diagnosis made by Gram stain and confirmed with positive identification on chocolate agar culture. Evaluation for sepsis and meningitis is also necessary.
   e. Sequelae: rare, but permanent visual impairment and/or systemic infection possible.
   f. Treatment: third-generation cephalosporin, such as ceftriaxone, until susceptibility testing can be completed (AAP, 2003). Penicillin G is a secondary choice if the organism is not penicillin resistant. Many *N. gonorrhoeae* pathogens are penicillin and tetracycline resistant. Eye irrigation with saline solution until eye discharge clears is also recommended (Thureen et al., 1999).
   g. Recommended prophylaxis: silver nitrate (1%) aqueous solution or erythromycin (0.5%) ophthalmic ointment in the eyes of all vaginally delivered infants. (NOTE: eye prophylaxis only minimizes the risk of infection; it does not guarantee prevention.)

C. **Bacterial parasite:** *C. trachomatis.*
   1. Parasite is commonly found in the adult female genital tract. *C. trachomatis* has an incidence rate between 6% and 12% in most populations and may be as high as 37% in adolescents; it is the most common sexually transmitted disease in the United States (AAP, 2003).

2. Delivery through an infected vaginal canal may result in neonatal infection.
3. Conjunctivitis usually is manifested at 5 to 4 days of age but may be delayed with eye prophylaxis. Symptoms may be minimal. Findings include copious mucopurulent exudate with frequent pseudomembrane formation. Pneumonia, otitis media, and gastroenteritis may also develop.
   a. Diagnosis is by tissue culture isolation from conjunctival, oropharyngeal, genital, or rectal swabs of cells.
   b. Treatment for conjunctivitis includes ophthalmic and systemic erythromycin (50 mg/kg/day in four divided doses) for 14 days (AAP, 2003). Topical therapy is insufficient to eradicate nasopharyngeal colonization (Thureen et al., 1999).
4. Chlamydial pneumonia is manifested between 4 and 11 weeks postnatally.
   a. Symptoms include a persistent cough, rales, and wheezing.
   b. Chest radiograph may reveal hyperinflation.
   c. Chronic disease may persist even after the acute phase of disease is over.
   d. Treatment is with erythromycin for 14 days.

Fungal Infection: Candidiasis

Candidiasis is caused by *Candida*, a significant neonatal pathogen. The most common species is *C. albicans*.

A. **Mucotaneous candidiasis.**
   1. Most common form of candidiasis in the newborn infant.
   2. Acquired during passage through the birth canal or from mother during breast-feeding.
   3. Appears as pearly white material on the buccal mucosa, dorsum and lateral areas of the tongue, gingivae, and pharynx.
   4. Treatment is with oral nystatin oral suspension (100,000 units/ml) to each side of mouth every 6 hours for 3 days after symptoms have subsided (Taketomo et al., 2002).
   5. May need to treat mother if origin of infection is mother's breast.

B. **Cutaneous candidiasis.**
   1. Presence of oral *Candida* is strongly associated with development of cutaneous candidiasis in the perineal region.
   2. May appear initially as erythematous and vesiculopapular lesions, and then develop into fine white, scaly collarettes.
   3. Therapy.
      a. Use of topical agents such as nystatin four times a day and continued 2 to 3 days after the rash has cleared.
      b. Simultaneous treatment with oral nystatin to minimize the risk of recurrence.
      c. Maintenance of area free from moisture and stool.

C. **Acute disseminated (systemic) candidiasis.**
   1. A serious nosocomial infection occurring in VLBW infants less than 1500 g, with an incidence of 3% to 5% (Faix et al., 1989).
   2. Most frequent sites of infection include the lungs, kidneys, liver, spleen, and brain; several sites may be involved simultaneously.
   3. Risk factors include prematurity (immunocompromised state), use of total parenteral nutrition and intravenous fat emulsions, and prolonged use of broad-spectrum antibiotics.
   4. Presentation includes respiratory deterioration, abdominal distention, apnea, acidosis, carbohydrate intolerance, hypotension, skin abscesses, temperature instability, and/or erythematous rash.

5. Formation of fungus in urine may lead to urinary tract infection.
6. Diagnosis is made by blood cultures, CSF cultures, microscopic examination of urine and the buffy coat of blood, determination of serum *Candida* antigen, ophthalmologic examination, and renal ultrasound.
7. Treatment.
   a. Amphotericin B: initial dose of 0.1 mg/kg IV over 20 to 60 minutes, followed by maintenance doses of 0.25 to 1 mg/kg/day every 24 hours as a daily infusion over 2 to 6 hours. Duration of therapy will vary with the clinical response. Requires close monitoring of hematologic and renal function (Taketomo et al., 2002).
   b. Flucytosine: 50 to 100 mg/kg/day in two divided doses for 3 to 4 weeks; may be used in combination with amphotericin B, if oral administration will be tolerated, especially if there is severe infection or CNS involvement.

Viral Infections

A. Mode of transmission.

1. Congenital: acquired in utero during maternal viral infection with exposure to the fetus. Infant presents with disease at birth or shortly thereafter.
2. Intrapartum: acquired at birth from organisms present in the maternal genital tract; onset of neonatal symptoms occurs within 5 to 7 days or later, depending on incubation period.
3. Postnatal: acquired during neonatal period from breast-feeding (human immunodeficiency virus [HIV], hepatitis B virus, cytomegalovirus), through blood transmission (cytomegalovirus, hepatitis B virus), or from hospital personnel or family members (enterovirus, respiratory syncytial virus).

B. Viral organisms.

1. Rubella virus.
   a. Generally causes a mild and often asymptomatic infection in children and adults. If acquired during pregnancy, can result in any of a wide range of fetal and neonatal outcomes: spontaneous abortion, congenital malformation, stillbirth, and neonatal disease (e.g., hepatitis, hepatosplenomegaly, jaundice, thrombocytopenia, "blueberry muffin" purpura), asymptomatic fetal infection, or no transmission of virus to the fetus (Cooper et al., 1995).
   b. Severity of neonatal disease is increased if infection occurs during the first trimester.
   c. There may be no initial symptoms, although most infected infants will have long-term sequelae such as endocrinopathies, deafness, eye damage, vascular disease, panencephalitis, and developmental delays (Overall, 1992; Sever et al., 1985).
   d. Early manifestations include intrauterine growth restriction, thrombocytopenia, hepatomegaly, jaundice, congenital heart disease (patent ductus arteriosus, peripheral pulmonary artery stenosis, atrial or ventricular septal defect), interstitial pneumonia, cataracts, bone lesions, microphthalmia, lethargy, irritability, bulging fontanelle, and late-onset seizures.
   e. Diagnosis is made by detection of specific rubella IgM; by demonstration of stable or rising rubella IgG titers in serial sera obtained for several months; and/or by cultivation of virus from nasal secretions, throat swab, urine, blood, or CSF. Special cell cultures are required for cultivation of rubella virus.

f. Prevention measures are as follows:
   (1) Pregnant women should be screened for immunity whether or not they have received prior rubella immunization. Susceptible pregnant women should avoid exposure to infected persons. Pregnant women are not given the vaccine because of the small risk of transmission of virus to the fetus (1.2%-1.8%) (CDC, 1987).
   (2) Seronegative women should be vaccinated postpartum, before discharge from the hospital. Vaccine virus is excreted in breast milk, but breast-feeding is not a contraindication to vaccination.
   (3) Routine rubella vaccination should be administered to all infants (AAP, 1998).

g. Isolation procedures are carried out because respiratory and urinary secretion of virus may occur for several months or more after birth. Transmission-Based Precautions, in addition to Standard Precautions, should be used with all infants with suspected congenital rubella during hospitalization.

h. There is no specific antiviral therapy for congenital rubella or for amelioration of progressive disease after birth.

2. Cytomegalovirus (CMV).
   a. CMV causes the most common congenital viral infection that is spread horizontally by salivary or urinary contamination or by sexual transmission. Infection is more common in crowded conditions, in lower socioeconomic groups, and in breast-fed infants (Stagno, 1995). Up to 90% of the adult population and 70% of children in daycare are seropositive. Approximately 2% of women will have a primary CMV infection during pregnancy (Stagno and Whitley, 1985).
   b. Infection may be acquired from cervical secretions at the time of delivery. After birth, the virus may be transmitted in infected maternal secretions or breast milk or through blood transfusions. Overall, with primary maternal infection, 40% of infants are infected, with symptoms manifested at birth in 10% and with late sequelae occurring in another 5% to 10% (Stagno and Whitley, 1985).
   c. Clinical manifestations.
      (1) Congenital infection.
         (a) Symptomatic at birth: growth restriction, hepatosplenomegaly, microcephaly, jaundice, petechiae and purpura, pneumonia, chorioretinitis, and periventricular intracranial calcification. Prognosis is poor, with one third dying in infancy and up to 90% of survivors having severe neurologic sequelae.
         (b) Asymptomatic at birth: 5% to 15% may have long-term sequelae, the majority having hearing loss and decreased IQ, microcephaly, visual difficulties, and school problems (Stagno, 1995).
      (2) Perinatal or postpartum infection. The majority of infections remain asymptomatic and do not appear to result in any long-term sequelae (Stagno, 1995). Severe disease has occurred in premature infants infected with CMV by means of blood transfusion.
   d. Diagnosis is made by viral isolation from the infant's urine or saliva or by a high anti-CMV IgM titer in the first 2 to 3 weeks of life or persistent or rising IgG titers in the first 6 months of life. Infants with both congenital and perinatal/postnatal CMV infection excrete virus in their urine for years (Stagno et al., 1983).
   e. There is no proven treatment.

f. For prevention, pregnant women should be advised to use good handwashing technique. Blood products given to neonates should be treated to reduce the potential for CMV transmission or should be obtained from CMV seronegative donors.
g. Neither infants with symptomatic CMV infection nor those with diagnosed but asymptomatic CMV infection require isolation, but Standard Precautions, particularly for pregnant caretakers, should be enforced.

3. Respiratory syncytial virus (RSV).
   a. Most common respiratory pathogen in infants. It is the major cause of bronchiolitis and pneumonia in infants during the first 3 years of life.
   b. Prevalence. Infection is most prevalent during winter and through early spring (November through April) and is highly contagious. It is transmitted through contact with infected secretions (droplet contamination) resulting from coughing and sneezing. Infection proceeds from the nasal mucosa and spreads from the upper to the lower respiratory tract.
   c. Susceptibility. Initial infection and most serious illness generally occur during the first year of life, especially in infants who were premature or have either chronic lung disease or congenital heart disease.
   d. Presentation.
      (1) Nonspecific: poor feeding, lethargy, apnea, irritability.
      (2) Respiratory symptoms: cough, wheezing, rales, rhonchi, dyspnea, pneumonia, cyanosis, pulmonary infiltrates.
      (3) Increasing respiratory distress, which may result in respiratory failure.
   e. Diagnosis.
      (1) Clinical and epidemiologic findings.
      (2) Rapid viral antigen detection isolated from nasopharyngeal aspirate.
   f. Treatment. Supportive care includes oxygen, hydration, and isolation. High-risk infants may progress to assisted ventilation because of hypoxemia and hypercapnia.
   g. RSV immune globulin (RSVIG). Intravenously administered RSVIG has been approved by the U.S. Food and Drug Administration for use in infants for the prevention of RSV-induced lower respiratory tract disease. RSVIG is ineffective in treating established RSV infection. The AAP (2003) recommends its use in infants and children younger than 24 months of age with a history of bronchopulmonary dysplasia and in infants born at less than 32 weeks' gestation without this disease. Administration begins before onset of the RSV season.
      (1) RSVIG is an IV preparation administered monthly over 4 hours during the RSV season.
      (2) Palivizumab (Synagis), is a monoclonal antibody that should be administered intramuscularly once monthly. A recently completed clinical trial has demonstrated its effectiveness in infants with hemodynamically significant congenital heart disease, although it has not been approved by the FDA for this indication. (see www.aap.org) (Meissner et al., 2002).
   h. Isolation procedures. Transmission-Based Precautions are used, in addition to Standard Precautions. May designate cohort of infected infants to prevent widespread infection.

4. Herpes simplex virus (HSV).
   a. Cause of serious disease in fetus and neonate, with incidence estimated at 1 in 3000 to 1 in 20,000 births (AAP, 2003).

b. Types of HSV infection.
   (1) HSV-1: nongenital type, although it can infect the genital area (accounts for 25% of neonatal disease).
   (2) HSV-2: genital type; more often associated with neonatal disease (accounts for 75% of neonatal disease).

c. Transmission: 85% to 90% of infections are acquired at the time of delivery. More than 75% of infants who acquire neonatal HSV infection have been born to women who had no history or clinical findings suggestive of active HSV infection during pregnancy (AAP, 2003). Infections can also occur in utero or postnatally (Whitley and Arvin, 1995). Postnatal infections can be acquired from breast lesions during breast-feeding, from oral lesions through direct contact, and from other infants with HSV infection. The greatest risk to the neonate is in mothers with a primary infection at birth. Transmission occurs in 40% to 50% of these infants. With reactivation of the disease, transmission occurs in 4% to 5% of deliveries or fewer (Overall, 1992).

d. Presentation.
   (1) Intrapartum or postnatal transmission: vesicular lesions, thermal instability, lethargy, respiratory distress, vomiting, poor feeding, cyanosis, and, if there is CNS involvement, irritability, bulging fontanelle, seizures, opisthotonos, and coma.
   (2) Congenital transmission: early vesicular rash, small for gestational age, low birth weight, chorioretinitis, diffuse brain damage, microcephaly, and intracranial calcification.

e. Diagnosis. Positive culture result with specimen obtained from vesicular fluid, blood, or CSF results in a diagnosis. The diagnostic yield of CSF culture for neonates with CNS disease is less than 50%. The polymerase chain reaction (PCR) test has a much higher yield in CSF and should be performed if available. Other rapid identification tests include direct fluorescent antibody staining of vesicle scrapings and enzyme immunoassay antigen detection in vesicles or body fluids.

f. Treatment.
   (1) Systemic infection: acyclovir, for premature infants, 10 mg/kg/dose every 12 hours for 14 to 21 days. In term infants 10 mg/kg/dose every 8 hours is recommended (Taketomo et al., 2002). Side effects are rare. Phlebitis may occur at the IV site because of alkaline pH of 10.
   (2) Ocular involvement: topical ophthalmic drug such as 3% vidarabine in addition to parenteral antiviral therapy. An ophthalmology consultation should be obtained.

g. Prognosis. Approximately half of all infants with untreated infection die, with high morbidity rates in survivors. Morbidity and mortality rates are highest in infants with CNS or disseminated disease. Antiviral therapy improves prognosis, especially in infants with localized disease.

h. Prevention.
   (1) Maternal history of HSV infection.
      (a) Weekly virologic and clinical screening beginning at 32 weeks.
      (b) Cesarean delivery if lesions are present or a culture result is positive at the time of delivery.
      (c) For known exposure to active recurrent infection at vaginal delivery or cesarean delivery, culture specimens should be obtained from the neonate 24 to 48 hours after birth. Treatment should be considered especially if the infant has symptoms, was

born prematurely, acquired open wounds during delivery, or has other high-risk factors.
(d) Delivery can be vaginal if no clinical or virologic evidence is present. Neonatal surface cultures can be considered but are not routinely recommended.
(2) Primary infection. For infants born vaginally to women with suspected or documented active primary HSV infection at the time of delivery, give prophylactic acyclovir pending neonatal culture results. If delivery is cesarean, acyclovir administration should be considered, especially if rupture of membranes occurred more than 6 hours before delivery or if the neonate has symptoms.
(3) Follow-up of at-risk infants. Infants who are at risk of HSV infection, even if culture result was negative after birth, should be followed up closely for a minimum of 6 weeks.

i. Isolation procedures.
(1) Mothers with HSV infections need to use strict handwashing techniques before touching their infant.
(2) Infants born to mothers with active lesions should be physically separated from other infants and managed with Transmission Precautions in addition to Standard Precautions.
(3) Infants born to mothers with a history of infection but without lesions at delivery do not require isolation. Good handwashing technique should be stressed.
(4) Infants with HSV infection should be isolated and managed with Contact Precautions.

5. Hepatitis B.

a. DNA double-shelled virus.

b. Transmission: vertical. The virus is also found in any bodily secretion, including human milk. There is no added risk to the infant of acquiring HBV infection when the mother is hepatitis B surface antigen (HBsAg) positive; therefore, breast-feeding is not contraindicated if immunoprophylaxis recommendations are followed (Thureen et al., 1999).

c. Presentation. Infants infected in utero are free of symptoms at birth. Infants infected at delivery or after birth do not have HBsAg present for at least 2 to 5 months. Infants who become chronically infected are at risk of having chronic hepatitis, cirrhosis, and/or other hepatocellular carcinoma.

d. Prevention. Routine screening is used for all pregnant women and universal screening for all infants and children. Routine neonatal immunization is with hepatitis B vaccine: Engerix-B, 10 μg, or Recombivax HB, 5 μg (AAP, 2003).
(1) Term infant is immunized at discharge and again at 2 months and 6 months of age (AAP, 2003).
(2) Preterm infant is immunized at discharge if weight is greater than 2 kg or at 2 months of age.

e. Treatment. In the infant born to a HBsAg-positive mother, treatment is 85% to 95% effective in preventing the development of the hepatitis B carrier state and should include the following:
(1) Careful bathing of the neonate to remove blood and secretions that may be contaminated.
(2) Administration of hepatitis B immunoglobulin (HBIG), 0.5 ml intramuscularly, as soon as possible within 12 hours of birth, in

addition to a hepatitis B vaccine: Engerix-B, 10 μg, or Recombivax HB, 5 μg (AAP, 2003).

f. Isolation procedures. Infants born to mothers with HBsAg should be cared for with Standard Precautions. No isolation is required. Immediately after birth the infant should be handled with gloves until all maternal blood is removed.

6. HIV.
   a. Cytopathic human ribonucleic acid (RNA) retrovirus.
   b. Use of reverse transcriptase enzyme. HIV uses the enzyme to produce viral DNA and integrates this into the DNA of the T-helper cells.
   c. Suppression of T-helper lymphocytes. This results in B-cell and suppressor T-cell dysfunction, with subsequent defects in cell-mediated immunity and development of opportunistic infections.
   d. Infection of monocytes and macrophages—also possible.
   e. Symptom-free infection. An infant can have an HIV infection with an absence of symptoms, suggesting that other factors (e.g., genetic predisposition, nutritional status) may contribute to the development of infection.
   f. Transmission.
      (1) Transmission is through blood or blood products.
      (2) Vertical transmission is thought to be the most common method of transfer, although time of transmission is uncertain.
         (a) Transplacental transmission has been demonstrated.
         (b) Intrapartum transmission during drug exposure to infected maternal blood or genital tract secretions is presumed.
         (c) HIV may be transmitted through human milk.
         (d) Risk of infection to an infant born to an HIV-infected mother who did not receive antiretroviral therapy during pregnancy is estimated to be between 13% and 39% (Hutto et al., 1991).
   g. Presentation. Signs and symptoms are rare in the neonatal period but may be seen in infancy.
      (1) Failure to thrive.
      (2) Generalized lymphadenopathy, hepatomegaly, and splenomegaly.
      (3) Recurrent mucosal infections.
      (4) Systemic bacterial infections.
      (5) Recurrent candidiasis.
      (6) Lymphoid interstitial pneumonitis.
      (7) Parotitis, hepatitis, nephropathy, cardiomyopathy.
      (8) Recurrent diarrhea.
      (9) Opportunistic infections.
      (10) Neurodevelopmental delay.
      (11) Malignancies.
   h. Diagnosis. Preferred diagnostic test for neonatal HIV is by PCR (AAP, 2003).
      (1) Antibody-based tests.
         (a) ELISA.
         (b) Western blot.
         (c) Indirect immunofluorescence assay.
      (2) Viral antigen detection: used to detect HIV antigen, usually the p24 antigen.
      (3) Viral nucleic acid detection: PCR and branched-chain DNA assays are used to diagnose and monitor disease progression and therapy efficacy.

(4) Viral culture.
(5) Combination of tests (usually PCR and/or viral isolation). A diagnosis can be made in more than 90% of infants by 2 months of age, and in nearly 100% by 4 months of age (AAP, 2003).

i. Management.

(1) Prompt intervention during bacterial and treatable opportunistic infections.
(2) Adequate nutrition.
(3) Combination antiretroviral therapy (current treatment recommendations for HIV-infected children can be found at www.aidsinfo.nih.gov). The Working Group on Pediatric HIV Infection for the Aids Education and Training Centers (AETC) has current updates of the medication recommendations for infants less than 12 months of age. Treatment recommendations for initial therapy have been revised, based on current clinical trial and pharmacokinetic data.
Several complete regimens are strongly recommended for initial therapy (Table 31-2).
Several protease inhibitor (PI) and nonnucleoside reverse transcriptase inhibitor (NNRTI)–based regimens are listed as "alternative recommendations," as is one triple nucleoside reverse transcriptase inhibitor (NRTI) regimen. The guidelines also include discussion of regimens and individual drugs that are "not recommended" or that have "insufficient data to recommend" (included in the latter category are the newer antiretrovirals tenofovir, emtricitabine, atazanavir, and enfuvirtide) (www.aidsetc.org).
(4) Perinatal prophylaxis (CDC, 2002).
  (a) Zidovudine (ZDU), 200 mg by mouth three times per day, or 300 mg two times per day, initiated at 14 to 34 weeks' gestation and continued throughout the pregnancy.
  (b) Intrapartum loading dose of ZDU is 2 mg/kg IV over 1 hour, followed by continuous infusion of 1 mg/kg/hour until delivery.
  (c) Neonatal administration is 2 mg/kg/dose by mouth every 6 hours for 6 weeks, beginning at 8 to 12 hours of age (Taketomo et al., 2002).

■ TABLE 31-2
■ ■ **Highly Active Antiretroviral Combination Regimens**

Mechanism of Action	Recommended Medication Combinations
Protease inhibitor based	Lopinavir/ritonavir + 2 NRTIs* Nelfinavir + 2 NRTIs* Ritonavir + 2 NRTIs*
Nonnucleoside reverse transcriptase inhibitor (NRTI) based	Children >3 years: efavirenz + 2 NRTIs* Children ≤3 years or unable to take capsules: Nevirapine + 2 NRTIs*

*The nucleoside analog (NRTI) pairs of zidovudine + lamivudine, zidovudine + didanosine, and stavudine + lamivudine are strongly recommended for use in combination therapy regimens.
Data from Working Group on Antiretroviral Therapy and Medical Management of HIV-Infected Children convened by the National Pediatric and Family HIV Resource Center (NPHRC), The Health Resources and Services Administration (HRSA), and The National Institutes of Health. *Guidelines for the Use of Antiretroviral Agents in Pediatric HIV Infection.* Washington, DC, 2003, Authors.
Available from: www.aidsetc.org or http://aidsinfo.nih.gov.

(5) Prevention.
 (a) Cesarean delivery has not been shown to prevent transmission of HIV to the infant.
 (b) Breast-feeding concerns (AAP, 2003).
  (i) Transmission of HIV infection to infants from breast-feeding occurs at rates of 27% to 40% in women with primary infection postpartum (Palasanthiran et al., 1993).
  (ii) Women who are known to be HIV infected should be advised not to breast-feed (AAP, 2003).
(6) Isolation procedures. Standard Precautions should be strictly followed.

Other Infections

A. Toxoplasmosis.

1. Caused by intracellular protozoan parasite, *Toxoplasma gondii*, which is an important human pathogen.
2. Maternally acquired from consumption of poorly cooked meat or by exposure to infected cat feces. Only women who become acutely infected during pregnancy can give birth to a newborn infant with congenital toxoplasmosis. Estimated incidence of acute maternal infection in pregnancy is 1.1 in 1000 (Sever et al., 1988).
3. Congenitally acquired disease in the newborn infant by vertical transmission. Approximate neonatal incidence is 0.1 to 1 in 1000 live births.
4. Manifestations may include maculopapular rash, hepatomegaly, splenomegaly, jaundice, and thrombocytopenia
5. CNS involvement includes microcephaly or hydrocephalus accompanied by convulsions; cerebral calcifications may be seen on radiographs.
6. Sequelae include mental retardation, learning disabilities, impaired vision, and blindness.
7. Toxoplasmosis may be asymptomatic at birth but may be manifested as intellectual impairment in late infancy or childhood.
8. Diagnosis may be made by a number of methods: isolation or histologic demonstration of the organism, detection of *Toxoplasma* antigens in tissues and body fluids, detection of *Toxoplasma* nucleic acid by PCR, and serologic tests.
9. Treatment consists of pyrimethamine, trisulfapyrimidines, and a folic acid supplement to prevent bone marrow suppression.
10. Isolation procedures consist of Standard Precautions.

B. Syphilis.

1. Cause: *T. pallidum*, a thin, motile spirochete.
2. Transmission: through sexual contact or by maternal-fetal transmission.
3. Presentation.
   a. Sometimes asymptomatic.
   b. Petechiae.
   c. Skin lesions: copper-colored maculopapular rash that is most severe on the hands and feet and appears at 1 to 3 weeks of age, with subsequent desquamation. Lesions present at birth may be bullous.
   d. Hepatosplenomegaly.
   e. Respiratory distress.
   f. CNS involvement.
   g. Rhinitis.
   h. Periostitis of long bones, with guarding of extremities.

4. Diagnosis.
   a. U.S. Public Health Service recommendation: all pregnant women screened with Venereal Disease Research Laboratory (VDRL) or rapid plasma reagin (RPR) test early in pregnancy and at the time of delivery.
   b. Diagnosis of active disease in the neonate.
      (1) High VDRL titer (four times higher than maternal titer).
      (2) Reactive RPR.
      (3) Serum IgM level greater than 20 mg/dl.
      (4) Confirmation with a positive result on fluorescent treponemal antigen-antibody absorption (FTA-ABS) test.
   c. Prevention. Uninfected infants possess maternally acquired antibodies at concentrations similar to those of infected infants. It may be difficult to interpret neonatal laboratory data; therefore, it is important to determine adequacy of maternal treatment, possibility of reexposure, and family compliance with follow-up.
5. Treatment.
   a. Penicillin.
      (1) Benzathine penicillin G, 50,000 units/kg given intramuscularly once if infection is asymptomatic and CSF is normal (Bhatt et al., 1997).
      (2) Procaine penicillin G, 50,000 international units/kg/dose given intramuscularly once daily for 10 to 14 days if infection is symptomatic and CSF is abnormal (Young and Mangum, 2003); alternatively, aqueous crystalline penicillin G, 50,000 international units/kg/day divided every 8 to 12 hours (interval based on gestational age and postnatal age) and administered IV for 10 to 14 days (Young and Mangum, 2003).
      (3) Procaine and benzathine penicillins are administered intramuscularly only, providing tissue depots from which drug is absorbed for hours or days.
   b. Neonatal therapy: should be instituted if maternal treatment is uncertain or if treatment was given within the last 4 weeks of pregnancy.
6. Isolation procedures: Standard Precautions.

INFECTION CONTROL

A. In 1996 the Hospital Infection Control Practices Advisory Committee of the CDC issued new guidelines for isolation practices for hospitalized patients. Comprehensive guidelines for preventing and controlling health care–associated infections, including isolation precautions, personnel health recommendations, and guidelines for the prevention of postoperative and device-related infections can be found on the CDC website (www.cdc.gov/ncidod/hip/guide/guide.htm).
B. Two major categories of infection control practices were designated (AAP, 2003; Garner, 1996):
   1. Standard Precautions: expanded set of previously designated Universal Precautions. Developed to protect patients and health care workers from blood-borne and other body fluid–borne infections; designed to prevent cutaneous and mucous membrane exposure to blood and body fluids. Guidelines include:
      a. Immediate handwashing or washing of other body surfaces if contaminated with blood and body fluids. This applies even if gloves are used, and hands should be washed immediately after glove removal.

Hands should be thoroughly washed after all patient contact regardless of whether or not there was obvious contact with body fluids.

b. Barrier precautions to prevent cutaneous and mucous membrane exposure to blood, body fluids, secretions, excretions, and contact with any items that might be contaminated with these fluids. Barriers include:
   (1) Gloves: should be worn when contacting blood and body fluids, mucous membranes, open skin, or items soiled by blood and body fluids. Hands should be washed immediately after glove removal. New gloves should be used with new patient contact and before touching noncontaminated items or surfaces.
   (2) Masks, face shields, and protective eyewear: should be used when patient contact or procedures can potentially generate splashes, sprays, or droplets of blood, body fluids, secretions, or excretions that might come in contact with the mucous membranes of the eyes, nose, or mouth.
   (3) Nonsterile gowns or aprons should be worn when patient contact or procedures likely to generate splashes, sprays, or droplets of blood, body fluids, or secretions, which may contaminate the caregiver's skin or clothing.

c. Cleaning of patient care equipment that might be contaminated, to prevent skin and mucous membrane exposure and clothing contamination.

d. Correct handling, transport, and cleaning of soiled linen to prevent skin and mucous membrane exposure and clothing contamination.

e. "Sharps program" in place to prevent exposure by needlestick and other sharp object injuries during cleaning, using, or disposing of these items.

f. Avoidance of mouth-to-mouth resuscitation; replacement by readily available resuscitation and ventilation equipment.

2. Transmission-Based Precautions: guidelines for the care of patients infected with specific pathogens or with syndromes in which the pathogenic organism may be spread by airborne, droplet, or contact routes. Measures additional to standard precautions are needed to prevent spread of infection. They are based on preventing transmission by one of three types of infection:
   a. Airborne transmission. Prevention requires special air handling and ventilation.
      (1) Private room with negative air pressure ventilation.
      (2) Masks.
      (3) Not required: gowns or gloves.
   b. Droplet transmission. Droplets do not remain suspended, so special air handling and ventilation measures are not required.
      (1) Private room preferred but not required; cohorting of infants with same infection is acceptable.
      (2) Masks.
      (3) Not required: gowns and gloves.
   c. Contact transmission. Contact is the most common type of transmission of hospital-acquired infections.
      (1) Direct contact: person-to-person transmission. This frequently involves transmission that occurs during patient care.
      (2) Indirect contact: contact with a contaminated object such as gloves, dirty dressings, dirty linen, or instruments, or transmission by personnel from one patient to another because of failure to wash hands thoroughly between patients.

(3) Preferred but not required: private room. Cohorting of infants with same infection is acceptable.
(4) Not required: masks.
(5) Required: gowns and gloves.

d. Nursery infection control measures (AAP and American College of Obstetricians and Gynecologists [ACOG], 2002).
(1) Routine, thorough handwashing: initially on entering the nursery, between patient contacts, and after touching contaminated objects.
(2) Clothing worn by nursery personnel: short-sleeved hospital attire laundered in hospital. A long-sleeved gown should be worn over clothing when infant is held by nursing staff, other personnel, or parents.
(3) Cover gowns: to be worn when caring for infants with known or suspected infection. Gowns should be discarded before another patient is handled.
(4) Sterile long-sleeved gowns, caps, and mask for surgical procedures.
(5) Hand jewelry should not be worn in nursery while caring for patients.
(6) Disposable, nonsterile gloves: use, if desired, for care of patients in isolation or to protect caregiver from contamination during procedures.
(7) Dirty diapers: handle with gloved hands.

e. Screening of visitors for contagious infections before admission to the nursery.

3. Linen and trash disposal (AAP and ACOG, 2002).
a. Linen provided does not need to be sterile but should be clean.
b. Cloth or disposable diapers are acceptable.
c. Soiled linen should be placed in plastic bags in hampers.
d. Linen and all diapers should be removed from the nursery at least once every 8 hours.
e. Nursery linens and cloth diapers should be laundered separately from other hospital linen.

4. Intravascular flush solutions (AAP and ACOG, 1997—update reference).
a. Sterile, unpreserved flush solution should be provided by the pharmacy.
b. Flush solution containers should be timed and dated and kept no longer than 8 hours at room temperature before being discarded.

REFERENCES

American Academy of Pediatrics, Committee on Infectious Diseases: Age for routine administration of the second dose of measles-mumps-rubella vaccine. *Pediatrics, 101*(1 Pt 1):129-133, 1998.

American Academy of Pediatrics, Committee on Infectious Diseases. *2003 Red Book: Report of the Committee on Infectious Diseases* (24th ed.). Elk Grove Village, IL, 2003, AAP.

American Academy of Pediatrics: Respiratory syncytial virus immune globulin intravenous: Indications for use. *Pediatrics, 99*(4):645-651, 1997.

American Academy of Pediatrics and American College of Obstetricians and Gynecologists: Guidelines for Perinatal Care, 5th edition. Elk Grove Village, IL, and Washington, DC, 2002, Authors.

Bhatt, D.R., Reber, D.J., Wirtschafter, D.D., et al.: *Neonatal drug formulary* (4th ed.). Los Angeles, 1997, N.D.F. Los Angeles Publishers.

Blackburn, S.T.: *Maternal, fetal, and neonatal physiology: A clinical perspective* (2nd ed.). St Louis, 2003, Saunders.

Byington, C.L., Rittichier, K.K., Bassett, K.E., et al.: Serious bacterial infections in febrile infants younger than 90 days of age: The importance of ampicillin-resistant pathogens. *Pediatrics, 111*(5 Pt 1):964-968, 2003.

Carr, R., Modi, N., and Doré, C.: G-CSF and GM-CSF for treating or preventing neonatal infections. *Cochrane Database of Systematic Reviews*, (3):CD003066, 2003.

Centers for Disease Control and Prevention: Rubella vaccination during pregnancy—United States, 1971-1986. *MMWR Morbidity and Mortality Weekly Report, 36*:457-461, 1987.

Centers for Disease Control and Prevention: Prevention of perinatal group B streptococcal disease in newborns. *MMWR Morbidity and Mortality Weekly Report, 51* (No. RR-11):1-12, 2002.

Christensen, R.D., Rothstein, G., Anstall, H.B., and Bybee, B.: Granulocyte transfusions in neonates with bacterial infection, neutropenia and depletion of mature marrow neutrophils. *Pediatrics, 70*(1):1-6, 1982.

Cooper, L.Z., Preblud, S.R., and Alford, C.A., Jr.: Rubella. In J.S. Remington and J.O. Klein (Eds.): *Infectious diseases of the fetus and newborn infant* (4th ed.). Philadelphia, 1995, Saunders, pp. 268-311.

Faix, R.G., Kovarik, S.M., Shaw, T.R., and Johnson, R.V.: Mucotaneous and systemic candidiasis among very low birth weight (<1500 grams) infants in intensive care nurseries: A prospective study. *Pediatrics, 83*(1):101-107, 1989.

Fanaroff, A.A., Korones, S.B., Wright, L.L., et al.: Incidence, presenting features, risk factors and significance of late onset septicemia in very low birth weight infants. The National Institute of Child Health and Human Development Neonatal Research Network. *Pediatric Infectious Disease Journal, 17*(7):593-598, 1998.

Fanaroff, A.A., Wright, L.L., Stevenson, D.K., et al.: Very-low-birth-weight outcomes of the National Institute of Child Health and Human Development Neonatal Research Network, May 1991 through December 1992. *American Journal of Obstetrics and Gynecology, 173*(5):1423-1431, 1995.

Garner, J.S.: Hospital Infection Control Practices Advisory Committee: Guidelines for isolation precautions in hospitals. *Infection Control and Hospital Epidemiology, 17*(1):53-80, 1996.

Hack, M., Wright, L.L., Shankaran, S., et al.: Very-low-birth-weight outcomes of the National Institute of Child Health and Human Development Neonatal Network, November 1989 to October 1990. *American Journal of Obstetrics and Gynecology, 172*(2 Pt 1):457-464, 1995.

Harvey, D., Holt, D. E., and Bedford, H.: Bacterial meningitis in the newborn: A prospective study of mortality and morbidity. *Seminars in Perinatology, 23*(3):218-225, 1999.

Hutto, C., Parks, W.P., Laik, S., et al.: A hospital-based prospective study of perinatal infection with HI modifier virus type 1. *Journal of Pediatrics, 118*(3):347-353, 1991.

Malik, A., Hui, C.P., Pennie, R.A., and Kirpalmi, H.: Beyond the complete cell count and C-reactive protein. *Archives of Pediatrics and Adolescent Medicine, 157*(6):511-516, 2003.

Manroe, B.L., Weinberg, A.G., Rosenfeld, C.R., et al.: The neonatal blood count in health and disease. *Pediatrics, 95*:89-98, 1979.

McCance, K.L. and Huether, S.E. (Eds.). *Pathophysiology: The biologic basis for disease in adults and children* (4th ed.). St Louis, 2002, Mosby.

Meissner, H.C., Sarah, S.L., and the Committee on Infectious Diseases and the Committee on Fetus and Newborn: Revised Indications for the Use of Palivizumab and Respiratory Syncytial Virus Immune Globulin Intravenous for the Prevention of Respiratory Synctial Virus Infections. American Academy of Pediatrics Technical Report, 2002, pp. 1-12.

Ohlsson, A. and Lacy, J.B.: Intravenous immunoglobulin for suspected or subsequently proven infection in neonates. *Cochrane Database of Systematic Reviews*, (2):CD001239, 2001.

Oski, F. and Naiman, J.: *Hematologic problems in the newborn*. Philadelphia, 1966, Saunders.

Overall, J.C., Jr.: Viral infections of the fetus and neonate. In R.D. Feigin and J.E. Cherry (Eds.): *Textbook of pediatric infectious diseases* (3rd ed.). Philadelphia, 1992, Saunders, pp. 924-959.

Palasanthiran, P., Ziegler, J.B.V., Stewart, G.J., et al.: Breastfeeding during primary maternal human immunodeficiency virus infection and risk of transmission from mother to infant.

Journal of Infectious Disease, 167(2):441-444, 1993.

Polin, R.A., Yoder, M.C., and Burg, F.D.: *Workbook in practical neonatology* (3rd ed.). Philadelphia, 2001, Saunders.

Pourcyrous, M., Bada, H.S., Korones, S.B., et al.: Significance of serial C-reactive protein responses in neonatal infections and other disorders. *Pediatrics, 92*(2):431-435, 1993.

Schelonka, R.L., Chai, M.K., Yoder, B.A., et al.: Volume of blood required to detect common pathogens. *Journal of Pediatrics, 129(2)*:275-278, 1996.

Schrag, S.J., Zell, E.R., Lynfield, R., et al.: A population based comparison of strategies to prevent early-onset group B streptococcal disease in neonates. *New England Journal of Medicine, 347*(4):233-239, 2002.

Schwersenski, S., McIntyre, L., and Bauer, C.R.: Lumbar puncture frequency and cerebrospinal fluid analysis in the neonate. *American Journal of Diseases in Children, 145*(1):54-58, 1991.

Sever, J.L., Ellenberg, J.H., Ley A.C., et al.: Toxoplasmosis: Maternal and pediatric findings in 23,000 pregnancies. *Pediatrics, 82*(2):181-192, 1988.

Sever, J.L., South, M.A., and Shaver, K.A.: Delayed manifestations of congenital rubella. *Reviews of Infectious Diseases,* 7(Suppl 1):S164-S169, 1985.

Stagno, S.: Cytomegalovirus. In J.S. Remington and J.O. Klein (Eds.): *Infectious diseases of the fetus and newborn infant* (4th ed.). Philadelphia, 1995, Saunders, pp. 312-353.

Stagno, S., Pass, R.F., Dworsky, M.E., et al.: Congenital and perinatal cytomegaloviral infections. *Seminars in Perinatology,* 7(1):31-42, 1983.

Stagno, S. and Whitley, R.J.: Herpesvirus infections of pregnancy. Part I. Cytomegalovirus and Epstein-Barr virus infections. *New England Journal of Medicine, 313*(20):1270-1274, 1985.

Stevens, J.P., Eames, M., Kent, A., et al.: Long term outcome of neonatal meningitis. *Archives of Disease in Childhood, Fetal and Neonatal Edition, 88*(3):F179-F184, 2003.

Stoll, B.J., Gordon, T., Korones, S.B., et al.: Early-onset sepsis in very low birth weight infants: A report from the National Institute of Child Health and Human Development Neonatal Research Network. *Journal of Pediatrics, 129*(1):72-80, 1996a.

Stoll, B.J., Gordon, T., Korones, S.B., et al.: Late-onset sepsis in very low birth weight neonates: A report from the National Institute of Child Health and Human Development Neonatal Research Network. *Journal of Pediatrics, 129*(1):63-71, 1996b.

Stoll, B.J., Hansen, N., Fanaroff, A.A., and Wright, L.L.: Changes in pathogens causing early-onset sepsis in very-low-birth-weight-infants. *New England Journal of Medicine, 347*(4):240-247, 2002.

Taketomo, C.K., Hodding, J.H., and Kraus, D.M.: *Pediatric dosage handbook* (9th ed.). Hudson, OH, 2002, Lexi-Comp.

Thureen, P.J., Deacon, J.M., O'Neill, P.A., and Hernandez, J.: *Assessment and care of the well newborn*. Philadelphia, 1999, Saunders.

Vain, N.E., Mazlumian, J.R., Swarner, O.W., and Cha, C.C.: Role of exchange transfusion in neonatal septicemia. *Pediatrics, 66*(5):693-697, 1980.

Weiss, M.G., Ionides, S.P., and Anderson, C.L.: Meningitis in premature infants with respiratory distress: Role of admission lumbar puncture. *Journal of Pediatrics, 119*(6):973-975, 1991.

Welsh, J.K. and May, J.T.: Anti-infective properties of breast milk. *Journal of Pediatrics, 94*(1):1-9, 1979.

Whitley, R.J. and Arvin, A.M.: Herpes simplex virus infections. In J.S. Remington and J.O. Klein (Eds.): *Infectious diseases of the fetus and newborn infant* (4th ed.). Philadelphia, 1995, Saunders, pp. 354-376.

Young, T.E., and Mangum, O.B. (Eds).: Neofax, 16th edition. Raleigh, NC, Acorn Pubishers.

CHAPTER

32 Renal and Genitourinary Disorders

CAROL BOTWINSKI

OBJECTIVES

1. Relate congenital renal/genitourinary disorders to embryologic development.
2. Apply knowledge of normal renal anatomy and physiology to renal pathophysiology that presents in the neonatal period.
3. Explain the etiology of selected neonatal renal/genitourinary disorders.
4. Describe clinical manifestations and complications that may be associated with selected neonatal renal/genitourinary disorders.
5. Determine the appropriate management of each disorder discussed.
6. Formulate an appropriate plan of care for each disorder discussed.

Homeostasis of the newborn is dependent upon a functioning renal system. In utero the placenta is the organ responsible for fluid and electrolyte homeostasis. Postnatally the kidney must assume its role as the regulator. However, the immature renal system of the newborn responds slowly and erratically to physiologic changes and demands that are placed on it. Knowledge of renal physiology and embryological development is essential in caring for these newborns. This chapter presents information on the anatomy and physiology of the kidney as a base from which to discuss selected renal/genitourinary disorders.

EMBRYOLOGY

A. Introduction.

1. Embryologic development of the urinary system begins within the first weeks after conception and progresses through three stages.
2. Both the urinary and the genital systems develop from the same germ layer of the embryo.

B. Kidney.

1. The kidneys develop in three sequential stages.
   a. Pronephros.
      (1) Plays a primary role in normal organogenesis.
      (2) Appears during 3 to 4 weeks' gestation.
      (3) Degenerates by the fifth week.

b. Mesonephros.
   (1) Originates during 4 to 5 weeks' gestation, just before degeneration of the pronephros, and is fully developed by 37 days.
   (2) Consists of 30 to 40 glomerulotubular units.
   (3) Capsule and glomerulus form the mesonephros (renal) corpuscle.
   (4) Develops into genital glands.
   (5) Regresses at the end of the second month.

c. Metanephros.
   (1) Develops early in the fifth week and functions within a few weeks.
   (2) Permanent kidney develops from the metanephric diverticulum (ureteric bud) and the metanephric mesoderm (metanephrogenic blastema).
   (3) Normal differentiation of the ureteric bud is essential for initiation of branching, which leads to formation of the urinary collecting system (ureter, pelvis, calyces, and collecting ducts) and to the start of nephron formation within the metanephric blastema.
   (4) Nephroblastic cells differentiate into the glomerulus, proximal convoluted tubule, loop of Henle, and distal convoluted tubule.
   (5) Nephrons form from the proximal end of the renal/metanephric tubules, beginning at about 8 weeks and continuing until approximately 34 to 36 weeks. Approximately one million nephrons result.
   (6) Minor calyces and their communicating papillary ducts are well delineated and resemble those of a mature kidney by 13 to 14 weeks' gestation.
   (7) By 4 months the kidney contains 14 to 16 lobes, equivalent to the mature kidney.
   (8) The kidney begins urine production and glomerular filtration at 9 to 10 weeks' gestation.

C. **Urinary tract.**
   1. Differentiation of the urinary tract occurs synchronously with the early stages of metanephric development.
   2. Urinary bladder develops at approximately 6 weeks' gestation.
   3. Formation of the urethra is completed by the end of the first trimester.
   4. Fetal ureter does not open functionally into the bladder until the ninth week.

D. **Development of vascular supply.**
   1. The vascular pattern of the fetal kidney resembles that of the mature kidney by 14 to 15 weeks' gestation.
   2. Renal blood flow in the fetus is low due to high renal vascular resistance and low systemic blood pressure.

RENAL ANATOMY

A. **Gross anatomy.**
   1. **Cortex:** outermost portion of the kidney, which contains the glomeruli, proximal, and distal convoluted tubules, and collecting ducts of the nephron.
   2. **Medulla:** middle section of the kidney, which contains renal pyramids, straight portions of tubules, loops of Henle, vasa recta, and terminal collecting ducts.
   3. **Renal sinus and pelvis:** innermost portion of the kidney. The renal sinus contains the uppermost part of the renal pelvis and calyces, surrounded by some fat in which branches of the renal vessels and nerves are embedded.
   4. **Ureter:** excretory duct of the kidney, which transports urine from kidney to bladder.

B. Microscopic renal anatomy: the nephron.
1. Structural and functional unit of the kidney.
2. Composed of glomerulus, Bowman capsule, and the tubules.
3. All nephrons are present by 32 to 34 weeks' gestation; functional maturation and hypertrophy continue into infancy (Huether, 2002; Vogt and Avner, 2002).
4. Functional component of the nephron is the renal corpuscle, which consists of the glomerulus and the glomerular (Bowman) capsule.
   a. Glomerulus is formed by a capillary network.
   b. Glomerular/Bowman capsule is a membrane surrounding the glomerulus, which serves as a filter mechanism through which nonprotein components of blood plasma can enter the renal tubules.
5. Tubular system consists of proximal convoluted tubule, loop of Henle, distal convoluted tubule, and collecting duct.

RENAL HEMODYNAMICS

A. Renal blood flow (Huether, 2002; Porth, 2002).
1. Renal blood flow comprises 4% to 6% of the cardiac output during the first 12 hours of life and 8% to 10% of the cardiac output during the first week of life.
2. The rate of renal blood flow is determined by the cardiac output and the ratio of renal to systemic vascular resistance. Developmental changes in these parameters contribute to the postnatal increase in renal blood flow.
3. The primary factor responsible for maturational increase in renal blood flow and redistribution of intrarenal blood flow from the inner cortex to the outer cortex is decreased renal vascular resistance.
4. Renal plasma flow.
   a. Flow is 150 ml/minute/1.73 m^2 at term and increases to 200 ml/minute/1.73 m^2 in the first weeks of life.
   b. The low renal plasma flow in the neonate is due mainly to high renal vascular resistance but also to low perfusion pressure.

B. Regulation of renal blood flow (Huether, 2002; Porth, 2002).
1. Autoregulation of renal blood flow.
   a. Autoregulation refers to the ability of the kidney to maintain a relatively constant glomerular filtration rate (GFR) over a range of systemic blood pressure.
   b. Mechanisms.
      (1) Myogenic mechanism is the dilation or constriction of the afferent arteriole in response to changes in vascular wall tension for the purpose of maintaining normal blood flow.
      (2) Tubuloglomerular feedback mechanism consists of afferent and efferent feedback mechanisms.
         (a) Afferent arteriolar vasodilator feedback mechanism is activated by decreased glomerular filtrate in the tubules, which results in dilation of the afferent arteriole and increased GFR. When renal blood flow increases, the afferent arterioles constrict and return GFR to normal.
         (b) Efferent arteriolar vasodilator feedback mechanism is activated by decreased volume. This stimulates renin release and causes constriction of the efferent arteriole to a greater degree than constriction of the afferent arteriole and thus maintains the GFR.

2. Hormonal regulation of renal blood flow.
   a. Renin-angiotensin-aldosterone system.
      (1) Major renal hormonal system.
      (2) Well developed in the newborn infant; renin is present from 3 months' gestation onward.
      (3) Responsible for regulation of systemic blood pressure, sodium, potassium, and regional blood flow.
   b. Prostaglandins.
      (1) Synthesized in both cortex and medulla, and by glomerulus and tubules.
      (2) Renal medulla seems to be the major site of prostaglandin synthesis in the kidney.
      (3) Most important prostaglandins in the kidney are prostaglandins E_2 and $F_{2-\alpha}$, prostacyclin (prostaglandin I_2, epoprostenol), and thromboxane A_2.
      (4) Role in regulation of renal function and control of systemic blood pressure.
         (a) Vasodilation.
         (b) Natriuresis.
         (c) Inhibition of the distal tubule's response to antidiuretic hormone.

RENAL PHYSIOLOGY

A. Postnatal changes (Kim and Emma, 1998; Swinford et al., 2002; Vogt and Avner, 2002).
   1. GFR doubles in the first 2 weeks of life in term and preterm neonates to 30 to 40 ml/minute/1.73 m^2 and increases to adult values of 100 to 120 ml/minute/1.73 m^2 between 1 and 2 years of life. Factors responsible for this increase are:
      a. Increasing mean arterial blood pressure.
      b. Increasing renal blood flow.
      c. Increasing glomerular permeability and filtration surface area.
   2. Fractional excretion of sodium decreases due to increasing tubular reabsorption.
   3. Infant has an increasing ability to concentrate urine.
   4. Renal vasoactive hormones are initially increased.
   5. Renal vascular resistance decreases.
   6. Renal blood flow increases.

B. Glomerular filtration (Kim and Emma, 1998; Swinford et al., 2002; Vogt and Avner, 2002).
   1. As blood passes through the capillaries, plasma is filtered through the glomerular capillary walls. Filtrate is collected in Bowman space and enters the tubules, where composition is modified until it is excreted as urine.
   2. Glomerular filtration rate (GFR).
      a. Factors that may contribute to decreased GFR at birth are:
         (1) Small glomerular capillary area available for filtration.
         (2) Structural immaturity of glomerular capillary, which is associated with decreased water permeability.
         (3) Decreased blood pressure.
         (4) Increased hematocrit.
         (5) Renal vasoconstriction, which results in decreased glomerular plasma flow.

b. Neonates born at less than 34 weeks' gestation have low GFR (0.5 ml/min) until nephrogenesis is completed.

3. Three primary factors determine GFR.
   a. Glomerular capillary hydrostatic pressure.
   b. Hydrostatic pressure in Bowman capsule.
   c. Capillary colloid osmotic pressure.
4. Glomerular capillary hydrostatic pressure is the major controller of GFR.
5. Additional factors that affect GFR are:
   a. Capillary surface area.
   b. Permeability of capillary basement membrane.
   c. Rate of renal plasma flow.
   d. Changes in renal blood flow.
   e. Changes in blood pressure.
   f. Vasoactive changes in afferent or efferent arterioles.
   g. Ureteral obstruction.
   h. Edema of kidney.
   i. Changes in the concentration of plasma proteins.
      (1) Dehydration.
      (2) Hypoproteinemia.
   j. Increased permeability of the glomerular filter.
   k. Decrease in total area of glomerular capillary bed.

C. Tubular function (Kim and Emma, 1998; Swinford et al., 2002; Vogt and Avner, 2002).

1. Components of tubular system include proximal tubule, loop of Henle, distal tubule, and collecting ducts.
2. Tubules modify glomerular ultrafiltrate, leading to production of urine, which is accomplished by the process of tubular reabsorption and secretion.
   a. Tubular reabsorption is the movement of substances into the peritubular capillary plasma from the tubular epithelium, which occurs by diffusion and active transport. The proximal tubule is the major site of reabsorption.
   b. Tubular secretion is the movement of substances into the tubular epithelium from the peritubular capillary plasma. Tubular secretion is necessary for regulation of fluid and electrolyte balance, along with other renal processes.
3. Regulation of fluids and electrolytes is an important tubular function.
4. Tubular function is altered in the neonate due to decreased renal blood flow and GFR.
5. Tubular portions of the neonatal nephron are smaller and less functionally mature, resulting in an altered ability to transport sodium, urea, chloride, and glucose, with decreased renal thresholds for many substances.
6. Rapid maturation of proximal tubular cells occurs between 32 and 35 weeks' gestation.

D. Concentration and dilution mechanism (Kim and Emma, 1998; Swinford et al., 2002; Vogt and Avner, 2002).

1. Maintenance of osmolality. The term and preterm infant's ability to dilute urine is fully developed, but concentrating ability is limited. A major function of the kidney is to maintain osmolality of extracellular fluid within the narrow range compatible with optimal cellular function.
2. Sites of urinary concentration and dilution.
   a. Loop of Henle.
   b. Collecting duct.

3. Factors responsible for the limited ability of the neonatal kidney to concentrate urine:
   a. Anatomic immaturity of the renal medulla.
   b. Decreased medullary concentration of sodium chloride and urea.
   c. Diminished responsiveness of the collecting ducts to arginine vasopressin.
4. Normal range of neonatal specific gravity: 1.002 to 1.010.
5. Maximum concentrating ability.
   a. Term infants: 700 mOsm of water per kilogram of body weight.
   b. Preterm infants: 600 to 700 mOsm of water per kilogram of body weight.
6. Capacity for urine dilution.
   a. 30 to 50 mOsm/kg of water.
   b. Ability of neonate to excrete a hypotonic load is limited, presumably due to the low GFR.

E. **Acid-base balance.**
1. Regulation of acid-base balance by the kidneys occurs in conjunction with the lungs and blood buffers. The role of the kidneys in regulating acid-base balance involves regulating the plasma bicarbonate by reabsorbing filtered bicarbonate and affecting hydrogen ion secretion through the formation of titratable acids and ammonium (Askin, 1997; Kim and Emma, 1998; Porth, 2002).
2. Renal response to acidosis.
   a. Reabsorption of bicarbonate in the proximal tubule.
   b. Increased secretion of hydrogen ions in the distal convoluted tubule.
   c. Production of ammonia.
3. Renal response to alkalosis.
   a. Excretion of bicarbonate.
   b. Decreased production of ammonia.
   c. Decreased hydrogen ion secretion in the distal tubule.
4. Neonatal limitations in maintaining acid-base homeostasis.
   a. Decreased ability to handle an acid load and compensate for acid-base abnormalities.
   b. Decreased renal threshold for bicarbonate, and decreased capacity to reabsorb bicarbonate results in slightly lower serum bicarbonate and pH.
   c. Decreased GFR.
   d. Decreased production of ammonia.
   e. Decreased ability to secrete organic acids.

ACUTE RENAL FAILURE (ARF)

A. **Definition.** ARF is the loss of the kidneys' ability to maintain water and electrolyte homeostasis. It is associated with an abrupt and severe decrease in GFR, a decrease in urine output, and a progressive increase in BUN and creatinine (Vogt and Avner, 2002).

B. **Incidence.** The incidence of acute renal failure in the neonatal intensive care unit (NICU) has been reported to range from 6% to 8%, with some estimates as high as 23% (Vogt and Avner, 2002).

C. **Etiology.** The causes of ARF in the newborn are multiple and can be divided into prerenal, intrinsic, and postrenal categories.
1. Prerenal: results from a state of relative hypoperfusion in an otherwise normal kidney. It is the most common cause of acute renal failure in the neonate (Kim and Emma, 1998; Vogt and Avner, 2002).
   a. Hemorrhage.
   b. Sepsis.

c. Congestive heart failure.
d. Dehydration.
e. Necrotizing enterocolitis.
f. Respiratory distress syndrome.
g. Hypoxia.
h. Drugs: angiotensin-converting enzyme (ACE) inhibitors, indomethicin, amphotericin B.

2. Intrinsic: renal cellular damage involving functional compromise to the glomerular, tubular, and collecting system due to prolonged prerenal insult, use of nephrotoxic agents or congenital anomaly (Kim and Emma, 1998; Vogt and Avner, 2002). Perinatal asphyxia is the most common cause of acute tubular necrosis in the term neonate (65%); sepsis is the most common in the preterm neonate (35%). Conditions resulting in intrinsic failure can be categorized into four broad groups.
   a. Congenital anomalies.
      (1) Agenesis.
      (2) Renal dysplasia.
      (3) Polycystic kidney disease.
   b. Thromboembolic disease.
      (1) Renal vein thrombosis.
      (2) Renal artery thrombosis.
      (3) Disseminated intravascular coagulation (DIC).
   c. Infection/inflammatory disease.
      (1) Acute pyelonephritis.
      (2) Congenital syphilis and toxoplasmosis.
   d. Acute tubular necrosis.
      (1) Perinatal asphyxia.
      (2) Cardiac surgery.
      (3) Prolonged prerenal state.
      (4) Nephrotoxic drug administration.
      (5) Uric acid nephropathy.
3. Postrenal: obstruction to urinary flow distal to the kidney (Kim and Emma, 1998; Vogt and Avner, 2002).
   a. Posterior urethral valves.
   b. Bilateral ureteropelvic junction (UPJ) obstruction.
   c. Neurogenic bladder.
   d. Obstructive nephrolithiasis.

D. Clinical presentation (Kim and Emma, 1998; Vogt and Avner, 2002).

1. Oliguric ARF is characterized by urinary excretion of less than 1 ml/kg/hour, whereas in nonoliguric ARF, the urinary flow rate is maintained above this level.
2. Azotemia with a blood urea nitrogen (BUN) greater than 20 mg/dl or rising more than 10 mg/dl/day.
3. Elevated serum creatinine greater than 1.5 mg/dl or rising more than 0.2 mg/dl/day.

E. Clinical assessment.

1. Careful review of perinatal history.
   a. History of renal disease in family.
   b. Perinatal asphyxia.
   c. Renal abnormalities on antenatal sonogram.
   d. History of oligohydramnios.

2. Careful physical examination of infant can be revealing.
   a. Abdominal palpation is important because renal masses are the most common abdominal masses in the newborn.
   b. Bilateral renal enlargement may reflect cystic disease, hydronephrosis, or renal vein thrombosis.
   c. Edema, ascites, or hydrops at birth, which may be associated with congenital renal disease.
   d. Isolated ear anomalies can be associated with obstructive uropathy.
3. Urine output less than 0.5 to 1 ml/kg/hour after first 24 hours of life.
4. Increase in daily weight greater than that predicted on basis of infant's condition and caloric intake.
5. Blood pressure.
   a. Hypotension: may contribute to acute renal failure.
   b. Hypertension: may be observed in cases of acute renal failure.

F. Diagnostic studies can be useful to differentiate between prerenal, intrinsic, and postrenal failure.

1. Urine studies.
   a. Urinalysis.
      (1) Presence of casts, tubular cells, and proteinuria suggests intrinsic renal failure.
   b. Culture and Gram stain to rule out urinary tract infection/sepsis.
   c. Urine sodium and creatinine.
      (1) Used in determining the fractionated excretion of sodium (FeNa) (urine Na/plasma Na × plasma creatinine/urine creatinine × 100).
      (2) Values greater than 3% generally indicate intrinsic ARF, whereas those with a value of less than 2.5% indicate prerenal failure.
         (a) These values will have limited significance in neonates born at less than 32 weeks' gestation because of these infants' limited ability to conserve sodium.
         (b) Urinary indices lose their diagnostic usefulness after therapy for oliguria has begun, particularly with diuretics.
2. Blood.
   a. BUN and creatinine.
      (1) BUN/creatinine ratio. A disproportionate rise in the BUN/creatinine ratio suggests a prerenal etiology, whereas a proportionate rise indicates an intrinsic etiology.
      (2) BUN greater than 20 mg/dl or rise greater than 1 mg/dl/day.
      (3) Creatinine concentration greater than 1.5 mg/dl or increase greater than 0.2 mg/dl/day. A rising serum creatinine level is never normal.
   b. Serum electrolytes to evaluate for metabolic abnormalities associated with ARF.
      (1) Hyperkalemia.
      (2) Hyponatremia.
      (3) Hypocalcemia.
      (4) Hyperphosphatemia.
3. Renal ultrasound is helpful in identification of congenital renal disease and urinary tract obstruction.
4. Voiding cystourethrography to rule out obstructive disease and reflux.
5. Radionuclide renal scans may be used to evaluate renal perfusion and function.
   a. Fluid challenge should be administered to exclude prerenal ARF.
   b. 10 to 20 ml/kg of normal saline is administered over 1 hour.

c. Rapid and sustained diuresis within 1 to 2 hours indicates a prerenal cause.
d. Urine output of less than 2 ml/kg/hour after furosemide administration suggests an intrinsic or postrenal cause.

G. Management.

1. Most important principle in treating ARF is to identify the cause and provide appropriate care for the primary condition (Kim and Emma, 1998; Vogt and Avner, 2002).
   a. Prerenal → treat specific causes of renal hypoperfusion.
   b. Intrinsic → supportive care until kidney function returns.
   c. Postrenal → surgery/nephrology.
2. Strict management of intake and output.
   a. With intrinsic failure fluids are restricted to insensible water loss plus urine output.
   b. Full-term infants → 30 ml/kg/day + urinary losses.
   c. Premature infants → up to 70 ml/kg/day + urinary losses.
3. Monitor body weight once or twice daily.
   a. Newborns with ARF should either maintain steady weight or lose 20 to 30 g per day.
4. Monitor serum glucose and electrolytes.
   a. Sodium and potassium intake may need to be restricted.
   b. Newborns with anuria require no electrolyte intake.
   c. Treat acidosis.
5. Provide adequate nutrition.
   a. Provide 100 cal/kg with fat and carbohydrates.
   b. Provide 1 to 2 g/kg/day of protein.
6. Monitor blood pressure and treat hypertension.
   a. Hypertension occurs secondary to renal damage or fluid overload.
   b. Can be treated with restriction of sodium and fluid, or with antihypertensive agents (Kenner et al., 1998).
7. Observe for signs and symptoms of congestive heart failure.
8. Assess for bleeding diathesis.
9. Avoid nephrotoxic medications and those with a high sodium content.
10. Dialysis treatment is indicated for protracted course of ARF or if conservative treatment fails to prevent complications.
    a. Symptomatic hyponatremia.
    b. Hyperkalemia.
    c. Congestive heart failure.
    d. Hypertension.
    e. Hypervolemia.

H. Outcome (Vogt and Avner, 2002).

1. Prognosis for neonates with ARF is variable with mortality rates ranging from 14% to 73%.
2. Reversal of underlying condition is the most important factor in determining prognosis.
   a. Best prognosis is for patients who receive prompt treatment for renal hypoperfusion.
   b. Long-term sequelae.
      (1) Chronic renal failure.
      (2) Decreased GFR.
      (3) Impaired tubular function.
      (4) Chronic hypertension.

(5) Renal tubular acidosis.
(6) Nephrocalcinosis.
(7) Impaired renal growth.

HYPERTENSION

Blood pressures vary by gestational age, body weight, cuff size, and state of alertness. Hypertension is diagnosed when blood pressure is consistently greater than the 95th percentile (Ettinger and Flynn, 2002; Flynn, 2000).

A. Etiology.
1. The most common causes of neonatal hypertension include renovascular anomalies and intrinsic renal disease (Ettinger and Flynn, 2002; Flynn, 2000).
2. Additional causes include endocrine disorders, medications, and various other disease states.

B. Incidence (Ettinger and Flynn, 2002).
1. Incidence of neonatal hypertension is approximately 0.08%.
2. Incidence of neonatal hypertension has been reported to be 2% of NICU admissions.

C. Disease states (Ettinger and Flynn, 2002).
1. Renal vascular.
   a. Thromboembolism.
   b. Renal artery stenosis.
   c. Renal vein thrombosis.
2. Cardiac.
   a. Coarctation of the aorta.
3. Pulmonary.
   a. Bronchopulmonary dysplasia.
4. Renal disease.
   a. Congenital.
      (1) Polycystic kidney disease.
      (2) Multicystic-dysplastic kidney disease.
      (3) Ureteropelvic junction obstruction.
   b. Acquired.
      (1) Acute tubular necrosis.
      (2) Hemolytic-uremic syndrome.
      (3) Obstruction by tumor.
5. Endocrine.
   a. Congenital adrenal hyperplasia.
   b. Pseudohypoaldosteronism type II.
   c. Thyrotoxicosis.
6. Medications/intoxications.
   a. Maternal.
      (1) Cocaine.
      (2) Heroin.
   b. Infant.
      (1) Dexamethasone.
      (2) Theophylline.
      (3) Caffeine.
      (4) Pancuronium.
      (5) Phenylephrine.
7. Neoplasms.
   a. Wilms tumor.

    b. Mesoblastic nephroma.
    c. Neuroblastoma.
  8. Neurologic.
    a. Pain.
    b. Intracranial hypertension.
    c. Seizures.
  9. Miscellaneous.
    a. Closure of abdominal wall defect.
    b. Fluid overload.
    c. Hypercalcemia.
    d. Adrenal hemorrhage.
    e. Birth asphyxia.
    f. Extracorporeal membrane oxygenation.

D. Clinical presentation (Ettinger and Flynn, 2002; Vogt and Avner, 2002).

1. Presenting symptoms may be nonspecific including feeding difficulties, unexplained tachypnea, lethargy, mottling of skin; mild to moderate hypertension may be asymptomatic.
2. Life-threatening presentations of hypertension include congestive heart failure and cardiogenic shock.

E. Clinical assessment.

1. Arterial blood pressure: persistent elevation of blood pressure (BP) to greater than 90/60 mm Hg in term infant and 80/50 mm Hg in preterm infant.
2. Careful review of perinatal history to identify history of umbilical artery catheter, renal disease, or congenital heart disease; maternal history of medications or illicit drug use during pregnancy; family history of renal or endocrine disease.
3. Physical examination should focus on cardiac and abdominal evaluations.
4. Obtain set of four extremity BPs and careful palpation of femoral pulses to rule out coarctation of aorta.
5. Dysmorphic features may indicate the diagnosis of congenital adrenal hyperplasia or Turner syndrome.
6. Presence of flank mass may indicate UPJ obstruction or renal cystic disease.

F. Diagnostic studies (Ettinger and Flynn, 2002).

1. Initial laboratory tests include urinalysis, complete blood count (CBC), electrolytes, BUN, creatinine, calcium, urine culture if infection is suspected, plasma renin level.
2. Renal ultrasonography with Doppler flow study to rule out renovascular hypertension.
3. Renal scan to detect renal thrombosis and surgically amenable lesions (e.g., UPJ obstruction).
4. Magnetic resonance imaging or CT scan to detect tumors or masses.

G. Management.

1. Measure resting blood pressure, using a cuff of the appropriate size.
2. Correctable causes of hypertension should be addressed initially before considering medications (Ettinger and Flynn, 2002).
    a. Treat pain.
    b. Correct volume overload.
    c. Wean inotropic agents if present.
3. Antihypertensive medications (Young and Mangum, 2003).
    a. Hydralazine: 0.10 to 0.5 mg/kg/dose every 6 to 8 hours, IV bolus; or 0.25 to 1.5 mg/kg/dose twice to four times a day, by mouth (maximum dose 7.5 mg/kg/day).

b. Propranolol: 0.025 to 1 mg/kg/dose twice a day, IV; or 1 to 4 mg/kg/dose twice to four times a day, by mouth.
c. Captopril: 0.01 to 0.5 mg/kg/dose every 8 to 12 hours, by mouth.
d. Enalapril: 0.1 to 0.3 mg/kg/dose every 12 to 24 hours; maximum dose, 0.15 mg/kg/dose every 6 hours.
e. Sodium nitroprusside: 0.5 to 10 μg/kg/minute by continuous infusion.

H. Complications.

1. Congestive heart failure.
2. Left ventricular hypertrophy.
3. Hypertensive retinopathy.
4. Intracranial hemorrhage.
5. Cerebrovascular accident.
6. Encephalopathy.

I. Outcome.

1. Prognosis depends primarily on the etiology; however, time of diagnosis, presence of neurologic complications, and response to therapy are also factors (Vogt and Avner, 2002).
2. Poor renal growth may ensue on the side with renal artery pathologic changes, and renal scans may show abnormalities (Swinford et al., 2002).

POTTER SYNDROME (OLIGOHYDRAMNIOS SYNDROME)

A. Bilateral renal agenesis with Potter facies (Fig. 32-1).

B. Etiology: failure of ureteric bud to divide and develop (Kenner, 1998).

C. Incidence.

1. Approximately 1:4800 to 1:10,000 births (Housley and Harrison, 1998; Vogt and Avner, 2002).
2. Male predominance.
3. Approximately 40% of affected infants are stillborn (Huether, 2002).

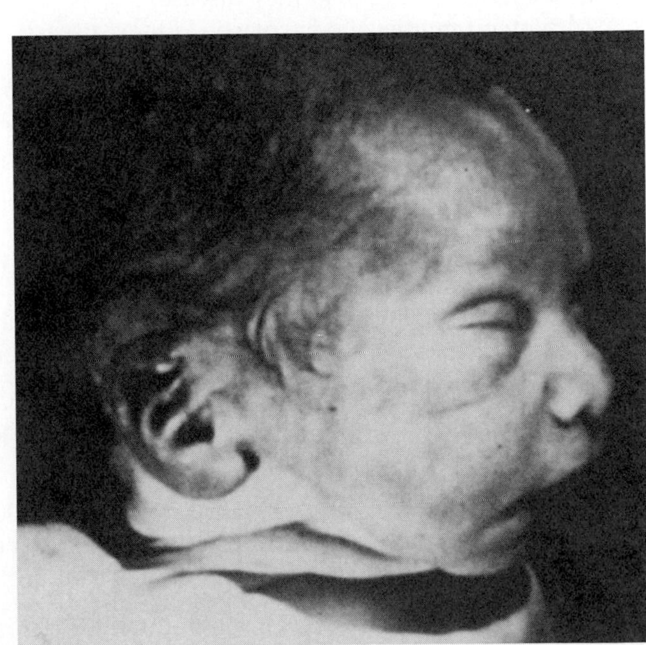

FIGURE 32-1 ■ Potter facies. Note epicanthal folds, hypertelorism, low-set ears, crease below lower lip, and receding chin. (From Fanaroff, A.A. and Martin, R.J.: *Neonatal-perinatal medicine: Diseases of the fetus and infant* [7th ed.]. St Louis, 2002, Mosby.)

D. **Clinical presentation.**
   1. Anuria.
   2. Potter facies.
      a. Blunted nose.
      b. Receded chin.
      c. Prominent depression between lower lip and chin.
      d. Low-set ears.
      e. Widely spaced eyes.
      f. Depressed nasal bridge.
      g. Prominent skinfold arising from epicanthus, progressing interiorly, and extending laterally beneath the eyes.
   3. Small for gestational age.
   4. Pulmonary hypoplasia.
   5. Excessively dry skin.
   6. Relatively large and clawlike hands.
   7. Bell-shaped chest.
   8. History of oligohydramnios.
   9. Bowed legs and clubbed feet possible.

E. **Clinical assessment.**
   1. Urinary output: anuria after the first 24 hours without bladder distention.
   2. Potter facies.
   3. Signs and symptoms of respiratory distress.
   4. Perinatal history of oligohydramnios.
   5. Presence of other associated anomalies.
      a. Abnormal genitalia.
      b. Gastrointestinal malformations.

F. **Physical examination:** palpation of abdomen for presence of kidneys.

G. **Diagnostic studies.**
   1. Renal ultrasonography: to rule out renal agenesis.
   2. Renal scan: if ultrasonography is inconclusive.

H. **Differential diagnosis.**
   1. Bilateral polycystic kidney disease.
   2. Bilateral multicystic dysplastic kidney disease.

I. **Complications.**
   1. Respiratory distress.
   2. Pneumothorax.
   3. Complications associated with acute renal failure.

J. **Patient care management.**
   1. Palliative care measures for neonate.
   2. Support for the grieving family.

K. **Outcome (Huether, 2002; Swinford et al., 2002).**
   1. Death usually occurs within hours to several days.
   2. Most die of respiratory distress caused by associated pulmonary hypoplasia.

AUTOSOMAL RECESSIVE POLYCYSTIC KIDNEY DISEASE

A. **Etiology:** autosomal recessive.

B. **Incidence:** 1:10,000 to 1:40,000 (Vogt and Avner, 2002).

C. **Clinical presentation (Swinford et al., 2002; Vogt and Avner, 2002).**
   1. History of oligohydramnios.
   2. Bilateral flank masses.
   3. Oliguria.

4. Abdominal distention from the massively enlarged kidneys.
5. Respiratory distress and spontaneous pneumothorax.
6. Hypertension.
7. Renal insufficiency.
8. Some degree of congenital hepatic fibrosis with biliary dysgenesis.

D. **Diagnostic studies.** Renal ultrasonography shows symmetrically enlarged hyperechoic kidneys with loss of corticomedullary junction (Levine et al., 1997).

E. **Differential diagnosis.**
1. Multicystic dysplasia.
2. Hydronephrosis.
3. Renal vein thrombosis.
4. Renal tumor.
5. Autosomal dominant polycystic kidney disease.
6. Tuberous sclerosis.

F. **Complications.**
1. Renal failure.
2. Hepatic failure.
3. Hypertension.
4. Portal hypertension with palpable liver and esophageal varices.
5. Congestive heart failure.

G. **Patient care management.**
1. Genetic counseling for parents.
2. Supportive care.
   a. Treat hypertension.
   b. Treat congestive heart failure.
   c. Give adequate nutrition to support normal growth and development.
3. Infants surviving neonatal period: close monitoring for inevitable decrease in renal function.
4. Consideration of renal transplant once renal failure develops.

H. **Outcome (Levine et al., 1997; Vogt and Avner, 2002).**
1. Those who survive the perinatal period have varying degrees of renal insufficiency and hypertension.
2. Long-term consequences of hepatic fibrosis may include portal hypertension and liver failure.
3. Death usually results from a combination of renal and respiratory failure.
4. Survival time varies: 86% of affected children survive to 3 months; 79% to 1 year; 51% to 10 years; and 46% to 15 years.

MULTICYSTIC DYSPLASTIC KIDNEY DISEASE

A. **Definition:** a nonfunctional, dysplastic kidney with multiple large cysts and ureteral atresia. It is the most severe form of renal dysplasia (Vogt and Avner, 2002).

B. **Etiology.**
1. Developmental anomaly.
2. Nongenetic.

C. **Incidence.**
1. Reported as 1:4300 (Vogt and Avner, 2002).
2. Males and females equally affected.
3. Most common form of renal cystic disease in neonates: unilateral multicystic dysplasia (Swinford et al., 2002).

D. **Clinical presentation.**
   1. Abdominal mass.
   2. History of oligohydramnios.
   3. Frequently associated with contralateral renal and extrarenal abnormalities, including cardiac, gastrointestinal, and central nervous system (CNS) abnormalities, and several malformation syndromes (Levine et al., 1997; Vogt and Avner, 2002).

E. **Physical examination:** abdominal palpation.
   1. Irregular mass.
   2. Usually unilateral.
      a. More often on left side.
      b. Possible hypertrophy of contralateral kidney; also risk of other abnormality, most commonly vesicoureteral reflux or ureteropelvic junction obstruction (Swinford et al., 2002).

F. **Diagnostic studies (Vogt and Avner, 2002).**
   1. Renal ultrasonography shows noncommunicating cysts of varying size; lack of normal renal parenchyma.
   2. Renal scan: absence of renal function.
   3. Voiding cystourethrogram to rule out reflux.

G. **Differential diagnosis.**
   1. Polycystic kidney disease.
   2. Hydronephrosis.
   3. Renal vein thrombosis.
   4. Renal tumor.

H. **Complications.**
   1. Hypertension.
   2. Hematuria.
   3. Infection.

I. **Patient care management.**
   1. Nonoperative approach
      a. Serial ultrasonography.
      b. Monitoring of blood pressure.
      c. Monitoring for infection.
      d. Monitoring for hematuria.
      e. Assessment for signs and symptoms of renal failure.
   2. Surgical removal of kidney may be indicated if its size causes severe abdominal distention preventing provision of adequate nutrition (Swinford et al., 2002).

J. **Outcome (Vogt and Avner, 2002).**
   1. Bilateral involvement is incompatible with life.
   2. Most unilateral disease undergoes spontaneous involution.
   3. Contralateral kidney (if unaffected) develops a compensatory hyperplasia.
   4. There is small but increased risk of the development of Wilms tumor.

HYDRONEPHROSIS

A. **Definition:** dilation of the pelvis and calyces of one or both kidneys, resulting from obstruction of urine flow (Swinford et al., 2002).

B. **Etiology.** The etiology of most types of hydronephrosis is unclear. However, a urinary tract obstruction causes a retrograde increase in hydrostatic pressure and dilation above the lesion, resulting in impaired renal structure and function (Swinford et al., 2002).

C. **Incidence.**
   1. Most common congenital condition detected by prenatal ultrasound, occurring in 1 of 500 to 700 deliveries (Vogt and Avner, 2002).
   2. The abnormality occurs predominantly in males and most often on the left side (Housley and Harrison, 1998; Reddy and Mandell, 1998).

D. **Clinical presentation.**
   1. Palpable abdominal mass.
   2. Decreased urinary output.
   3. Poor urinary stream.
   4. Urinary tract infection: common.

E. **Clinical assessment.**
   1. Urinalysis.
      a. Findings possibly within normal limits.
      b. Proteinuria.
      c. Hematuria.
      d. Leukocyturia.
   2. Serum creatinine: may be elevated.
   3. BUN: may be elevated.
   4. Antenatal ultrasonography: evidence of hydronephrosis.

F. **Physical examination.**
   1. Abdominal palpation reveals enlarged kidney.
   2. Observe for other genitourinary or associated anomalies that may occur outside the urinary tract.
      a. Imperforate anus.
      b. Congenital vertebral anomalies.
      c. Facial and skeletal anomalies.
      d. Malformed ears.
      e. Myelodysplasia.
      f. Absent or decreased abdominal musculature.
      g. Unexplained pneumonia.
      h. Absence or dysplasia of the radius.
      i. Hypoplasia of the pelvis.
      j. Unexplained septicemia.

G. **Diagnostic studies (Kenner, 1998; Reddy and Mandell, 1998; Vogt and Avner, 2002).**
   1. Renal ultrasonography.
   2. Voiding cystourethrogram.
   3. Renal scan.

H. **Differential diagnosis.**
   1. Obstructive.
      a. Ureteropelvic junction obstruction: most common cause of hydronephrosis in neonates (Vogt and Avner, 2002; Ward et al., 1998).
      b. Ureterovesical junction obstruction.
      c. Multicystic dysplastic kidney disease.
      d. Ureterocele/ectopic ureter.
      e. Duplicated collecting system.
      f. Posterior urethral valves: most common cause of severe obstructive uropathy in children (Vogt and Avner, 2002).
      g. Urethral atresia.
   2. Nonobstructive.
      a. Physiologic dilation (Vogt and Avner, 2002).
         (1) Unassociated with anatomic abnormality of urinary tract.

(2) May be caused by delay in maturation of the ureter leading to transient urinary flow obstruction.

b. Vesicoureteral reflux.

c. Prune-belly syndrome (also known as Eagle-Barrett syndrome).

I. Complications.

1. Urinary tract infection.
2. Hypertension.
3. Damage to renal parenchyma.

J. Specific patient care management.

1. Ureteropelvic junction obstruction (Shalaby-Rana et al., 1997).
   - a. Management depends on age and affected kidney's function.
   - b. Evidence of obstruction on diuretic renogram and preserved renal function may not require immediate pyeloplasty. Treat with antibiotics and follow up with a diuretic renogram in 3 months to determine any change in drainage pattern or deterioration in function of affected kidney.
   - c. Pyeloplasty (excision of stenotic segment; normal ureter and renal pelvis are reattached) is indicated for obstruction with compromised renal function.
2. Posterior urethral valves.
   - a. Catheterize initially to provide drainage of urinary tract.
   - b. Correct fluid and electrolyte or other metabolic imbalances.
   - c. Neonates whose diagnosis was made after 24 weeks' gestation or postnatally are treated in the neonatal period with endoscopic fulguration of the posterior urethral valves or decompression by various methods (i.e., percutaneous nephrostomy drainage, vesicostomy, or ureterostomies with later valve ablation) (Housley and Harrison, 1998).
3. Vesicoureteral reflux (Belman, 1997).
   - a. Catheterize initially.
   - b. Nonsurgical treatment.
     - (1) Antibiotic prophylaxis: amoxicillin for first 2 months, followed by trimethoprim-sulfamethoxazole or nitrofurantoin daily.
     - (2) Cystography should be repeated every 12 to 18 months to determine resolution of reflux.
     - (3) Circumcision is recommended for male neonates to decrease the risk of urinary tract infection (Elder, 1997).
   - c. Surgical repair is indicated for higher reflux grade and breakthrough infection, lack of compliance, and unlikely resolution (Greenfield et al., 1997).
4. For obstruction at ureterovesical junction, management is similar to that for obstruction of the ureteropelvic junction (Shalaby-Rana et al., 1997).

K. Outcome.

1. Success rates for pyeloplasty: reported as 91% to 98% (Elder, 1997).
2. Posterior urethral valves.
   - a. Neonates identified after 24 weeks' gestation or postnatally have a 5% mortality rate.
   - b. Long-term outcome depends on degree of associated renal dysplasia.
   - c. 30% of boys with posterior urethral valves (PUV) who present in infancy are at risk for progressive renal insufficiency in childhood (Vogt and Avner, 2002).
3. Vesicoureteral reflux.
   - a. Most reflux resolves; 60% to 80% of grades 1 through 3 cases resolve spontaneously (Belman, 1997).
   - b. The generally accepted rate for complication-free correction of reflux, including all grades, is more than 95% when carried out by an experienced urologist (Belman, 1997).

RENAL VEIN THROMBOSIS

A. Predisposing conditions (Vogt and Avner, 2002).
1. Hyperviscosity.
2. Polycythemia.
3. Hypovolemia.
4. Hypercoagulable states.
5. Dehydration.
6. Presence of indwelling umbilical arterial catheters.
7. Perinatal asphyxia.
8. Any condition resulting in decreased blood flow to the kidneys.

B. Clinical triad of symptoms (Kim and Emma, 1998; Vogt and Avner, 2002).
1. Hematuria.
2. Flank mass.
3. Thrombocytopenia.
4. Additional signs include:
   a. Hypertension.
   b. Oliguria.
   c. Gross hematuria.

C. Diagnostic studies.
1. Renal ultrasound shows enlarged kidney with diffuse homogeneous hyperechogenicity.
2. Doppler flow study may show renal venous or vena caval thrombosis.
3. Renal scan may show absent or decreased uptake indicating nonfunctioning kidney.

D. Patient care management.
1. Treat underlying illness.
2. Supportive treatment.
   a. Correct electrolyte imbalances.
   b. Correct fluid imbalances.
   c. Treat for renal insufficiency.
   d. Treat coagulation disorders.
3. Thrombolytic therapy with streptokinase, urokinase, and recombinant tissue plasminogen activator remain controversial (Kim and Emma, 1998; Vogt and Avner, 2002).

E. Outcome.
1. Kidney may recover or show signs of damage; depends in part on severity of underlying medical condition.
2. Long-term consequences can include renal insufficiency, renal tubular dysfunction, and systemic hypertension (Vogt and Avner, 2002).

URINARY TRACT INFECTIONS (UTIs)

A. Etiology.
1. Abnormality of the urinary tract.
2. Sepsis, although there is debate as to whether the UTI is the cause or effect of bacteremia (Edwards, 2002).
3. *Escherichia coli* accounts for approximately 75% of the UTIs. Pathogens causing hospital-acquired infections also include other gram-negative bacilli (*Klebsiella, Enterobacter,* and *Proteus*), gram-positive cocci (enterococci, *Staphylococcus epidermidis, S. aureus*), and fungal organisms (Ahmed and Swedlund, 1998; Edwards, 2002; Kim and Emma, 1998).

B. Incidence (Edwards, 2002; Guerina, 1998).
  1. Reported to range from 0.1% to 1% in all newborn infants and to be as high as 3% in low birth weight infants.
  2. Occurs more frequently in males than females.

C. Clinical presentation (Edwards, 2002; Kenner et al., 1998; Rushton, 1997).
  1. May be asymptomatic.
  2. Symptomatic manifestations are usually nonspecific.
    a. Abnormal weight loss during the first days of life.
    b. Poor feeding.
    c. Irritability.
    d. Lethargy.
    e. Jaundice.

D. Diagnostic studies (Edwards, 2002; Kim and Emma, 1998; Ross and Kay, 1999)
  1. Urine culture: urine specimen should be obtained for culture via suprapubic aspiration or bladder catheterization (Edwards, 2002).
    a. Bacterial counts of 10^3 higher colony-forming units (CFUs) per milliliter of catheterized urine are considered significant.
    b. Isolation of any bacteria from a suprapubic tap is considered significant.
  2. Urinalysis may show pyuria (>10-15 white blood cells/high-power field [WBC/hpf] and hematuria.
  3. Blood culture.
  4. Complete blood cell count with differential cell count.
  5. Renal ultrasonography to rule out urologic abnormalities.
  6. Voiding cystourethrogram (VCUG) to rule out reflux.
    a. Vesicoureteral reflux (VUR) occurs in 40% of neonates with UTIs.
    b. VUR is associated with renal scarring.
  7. If renal abnormalities are detected by VCUG, a renal scan to detect renal inflammation and scarring may be warranted.

E. Management (Edwards, 2002; Kim and Emma, 1998, Ross and Kay, 1999).
  1. Administer antibiotic therapy for 10 days.
    a. Empiric treatment for neonatal UTI includes broad-spectrum antibiotics (e.g., ampicillin and aminoglycoside) in dosages used for sepsis.
    b. Consider vancomycin and an aminoglycoside for empiric treatment of nosocomial UTIs.
    c. Final choice of antibiotic is based on sensitivity of the cultured organism.
    d. Prophylaxis antibiotic coverage may be instituted in infants with an abnormal urinary tract after an initial urinary tract infection until VCUG is done.
  2. Sterilization of urine should be documented posttreatment.
  3. VCUG should be done as soon as infection has resolved to assess for VUR.
    a. Neonates who demonstrate reflux should be maintained on prophylaxis antibiotic therapy.
    b. VCUG should be repeated in 6 months if reflux was initially present.

F. **Outcome:** excellent with prompt and adequate treatment.

PATENT URACHUS

A. **Definition:** a communication between the bladder and the umbilicus, causing a leakage of urine from the umbilicus.

B. **Etiology:** failure of normal closure of epithelialized urachal tube, resulting in patent urachus.

C. **Incidence:** more common in males than in females.

D. **Clinical presentation.**
   1. Discharge of urine from umbilicus at birth or later.
   2. Wet umbilicus.
   3. Enlarged/edematous umbilicus.
   4. Delayed sloughing of cord.

E. **Physical examination:** observation of umbilicus.

F. **Diagnostic studies (Atala and Retik, 1997).**
   1. Analysis of fluid for urea and creatinine.
   2. Bladder ultrasonography.
   3. Voiding cystourethrography.
   4. Transurethral injection of methylene blue.

G. **Differential diagnosis.**
   1. Patency of vitelline/omphalomesenteric duct.
   2. Omphalitis.
   3. Simple granulation of a healing umbilical stump.
   4. Infected umbilical vessel.
   5. External urachal sinus.

H. **Complications.**
   1. Urinary tract infection.
   2. Excoriation.
   3. Infection.

I. **Patient care management.**
   1. Nonintervention: spontaneous closure may occur if defect is small and drainage is intermittent.
   2. Operative intervention.
      a. Treatment of distal obstructive uropathy, if present, before surgical closure of urachal duct.
      b. Extraperitoneal surgical excision of urachal tract with bladder cuff (Atala and Retik, 1997).

J. **Outcome:** good with surgical procedure.

HYPOSPADIAS

A. **Definition:** urethral meatus is located on ventral surface or undersurface of penis (Fig. 32-2). The condition varies in severity from a slightly malpositioned meatus still within the glans and without chordee to extreme genital ambiguity with hypoplastic phallus, bifid scrotum, and scrotal or perineal meatus.

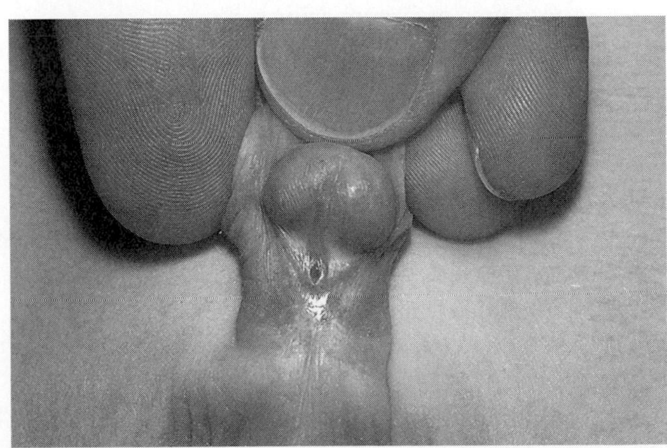

FIGURE 32-2 ■ Hypospadias. (Courtesy H. Gil Rushton, M.D., Children's National Medical Center, Washington, DC. In M.J. Hockenberry (Ed.): *Wong's nursing care of infants and children* [7th ed.]. St Louis, 2003, Mosby.)

B. **Etiology.**
  1. Deficient anterior urethral development.
  2. Delay or arrest in normal sequence of development, causing the urethra to open proximally and the prepuce to be incomplete ventrally.
  3. Probably multifactorial mode of inheritance.

C. **Incidence:** reported as approximately 1:300 newborn boys (Huether, 2002).

D. **Clinical presentation.**
  1. Urinary meatus located on undersurface of penis.
  2. Deviation of urinary stream.

E. **Clinical assessment.**
  1. Direction of urinary stream.
  2. Voiding pattern.

F. **Physical examination.**
  1. Observation of external genitalia.
    a. Meatal location.
    b. Quantity of ventral shaft skin and dorsal foreskin; usually incomplete formation of ventral prepuce.
    c. Chordee: downward curving of penis.
      (1) Association with chordee variable.
      (2) Severity of chordee generally proportional to degree of hypospadias.
    d. Assess for presence of associated anomalies (e.g., inguinal hernia, cryptorchidism, hydrocele, and meatal stenosis) (Danish and Dahms, 2002). Undescended testes and inguinal hernias are the most commonly associated anomalies (Zaontz and Packer, 1997).
  2. Palpation.
    a. Descent of testes.
    b. Presence of inguinal hernia.

G. **Complications.**
  1. Without repair.
    a. Difficulty in voiding while standing.
    b. The presence of chordee may cause painful erection.
  2. With postsurgical repair.
    a. Urethrocutaneous fistula.
    b. Balanitis xerotica obliterans.
    c. Meatal stenosis.
    d. Urethral stricture.
    e. Urethral diverticulum.

H. **Patient care management.**
  1. Avoidance of circumcision.
  2. Genotypic evaluation if only one gonad is palpated; congenital adrenal disease must be ruled out when no gonads are palpable (Belman, 1997; Danish and Dahms, 2002).
  3. Surgical repair.
    a. Move meatus distally.
    b. Improve cosmetic appearance of genitalia.
    c. Straighten curved penis.
    d. Most cases can be corrected with single-stage repair (Atala and Retik, 1997; Huether, 2002).
    e. Repair between 6 and 12 months of age is generally recommended (Belman, 1997).

I. **Outcome:** good for surgical correction of simple hypospadias.

EXSTROPHY OF THE BLADDER

A. **Definition:** the bladder is exposed and protruding onto the abdominal wall due to failure of the anterior abdominal walls to close at the point of the bladder (Fig. 32-3). The umbilicus is displaced downward, and the pubic rami (bony projections of the pubic bone) are widely separated in the midline, and the rectus muscles are separated (Huether, 2002).
   1. Virtually all affected male infants have associated epispadias (opening of the urinary meatus onto the dorsal aspect of the penis).
   2. The remainder of the urinary tract is usually normal.

B. **Etiology.**
   1. Part of the spectrum of conditions resulting from abnormal development of the cloacal membrane.
   2. Failure of the mesoderm to invade cephalad extension of the cloacal membrane.
   3. Variant of exstrophy-epispadias complex determined by the position and timing of rupture of the cloacal membrane.

C. **Incidence.**
   1. Approximately 1:24,000 to 1:40,000 (Huether, 2002; Kenner, 1998).
   2. More common in males by a ratio of 3:1 (Huether, 2002).

D. **Clinical presentation:** external presentation of bladder.

E. **Physical assessment.**
   1. Observation of external presentation of bladder.
   2. Assessment of associated anomalies.
      a. Epispadias.
      b. Bifid clitoris.
      c. Anteriorly located vagina.
      d. Anteriorly located anus.
   3. Palpation.
      a. Testes: to assess descent.
      b. Groin: to assess for presence of inguinal hernias.
      c. Symphysis pubis: to assess widening.

F. **Differential diagnosis:** complete exstrophy-epispadias complex.

G. **Complications.**
   1. Infections.
   2. Postoperative hydronephrosis.

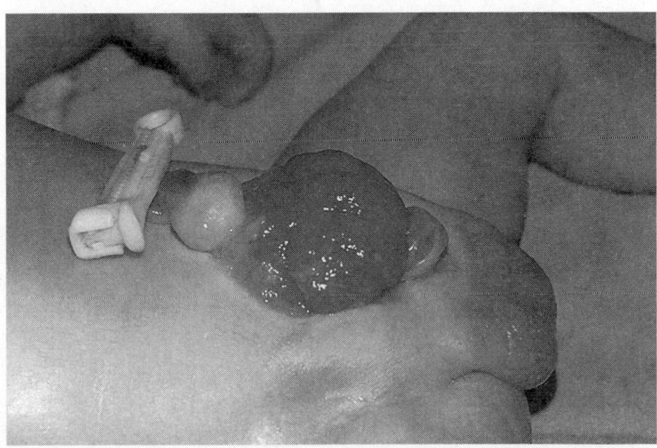

FIGURE 32-3 ■ Exstrophy of bladder. (Courtesy H. Gil Rushton, M.D., Children's National Medical Center, Washington, DC. In M.J. Hockenberry (Ed.): *Wong's nursing care of infants and children* [7th ed.]. St Louis, 2003, Mosby.)

3. Vesicoureteral reflux after bladder closure.
4. Swelling and edema in the bladder wall after surgery, which obstructs ureteral drainage and can lead to anuria, hypertension, or hydroureteronephrosis.
5. Urinary incontinence.
6. Anal incontinence.
7. Malignancy occurring 10 or more years later.

H. Patient care management.

1. Prevent cord clamp from damaging bladder by using cord tie.
2. Cover exposed bladder with clear plastic wrap.
3. Irrigate bladder surface with sterile saline solution and replace the plastic wrap at each diaper change.
4. Surgical closure is needed within 48 hours.
5. Administer antibiotic therapy (Kenner, 1998).
   a. Therapy continued for at least 7 days postoperatively.
   b. 42% of wound dehiscence is due to infections.
6. Renal ultrasonography or radionuclide scan is performed to determine presence or absence of upper tract abnormalities.
7. Assess for possible hydronephrosis and infections postoperatively.
8. Modified Bryant traction for immobilization is used for 4 weeks in patients who have undergone closure without osteotomy or with only a posterior osteotomy; light Buck traction, with legs supported on a pillow, is used if the approach was anterior.
9. Bladder is drained with a 10F suprapubic Malecot catheter for 4 weeks and with 3.5F ureteral stents for 2 weeks to prevent ureteral obstruction hypertension.
10. Antispasmodics, analgesics, and sedatives are administered to prevent bladder spasm and excessive crying, which may disrupt closure.
11. Ultrasonography is performed to assess the upper tracts, and catheterization is performed to obtain residual urine and urine culture specimens before discharge.
12. The condition of the upper tracts is followed up with ultrasonography every 6 months.
13. Subsequent repair of epispadias is performed at about 2 to 3 years of age as are bladder neck reconstruction, ureteral implantation, and bladder augmentation (Huether, 2002).

I. Outcome.

1. Results of functional closure of bladder exstrophy can be expected to be as high as a 75% to 85% continence rate with preservation of renal function.
2. May have lifelong problem with incontinence.
3. Precise prognosis is directly related to the presence of other deformities (Kenner, 1998).

UNDESCENDED TESTICLES (CRYPTORCHIDISM)

A. Etiology.

1. Endocrine dysfunction of the hypothalamic-pituitary-gonadal axis.
2. Abnormal epididymal development, with failure to induce testicular descent.
3. Anatomic abnormality preventing descent.

B. Incidence (Danish and Dahms, 2002).

1. Reported as 3.7% of term male infants.

2. Increased incidence of 21% in preterm infants, approaching 100% in the very preterm.
3. At 1 year of age: 0.8%.

C. Disease states.

1. Specific types of cryptorchidism.
   a. Abdominal: testes located inside the internal inguinal ring.
   b. Canalicular: testes located between the internal and external inguinal rings.
   c. Ectopic: testes located away from the normal pathway of descent, between the abdominal cavity and the base of the scrotum.
2. Genetic syndromes.
   a. Klinefelter syndrome.
   b. Noonan syndrome.
   c. Prader-Willi syndrome.
3. Vasal and/or epididymal abnormalities.
4. Prune-belly syndrome.

D. Clinical presentation: absence of the testes in the scrotum.

E. Clinical assessment. Associated abnormalities may be present. There is an increased incidence of CNS abnormalities and hypospadias.

F. Physical examination.

1. Palpation of scrotum for presence of testes or associated hernia.
2. Palpation of inguinal area for presence of hernia.

G. Diagnostic studies.

1. Ultrasonography: identification of intraabdominal testes.
2. Magnetic resonance imaging: identification of intraabdominal testes.
3. Laparoscopy: identification of intraabdominal testes.
4. Complete endocrine and electrolyte evaluation and chromosome analysis to rule out hypothalamic-pituitary insufficiency, female adrenogenital syndrome, and anorchism in phenotypic male infants with bilateral impalpable gonads (Gill and Kogan, 1997).

H. Differential diagnosis.

1. Specific type of cryptorchidism.
   a. Abdominal.
   b. Canalicular.
   c. Ectopic or maldescended.
2. Anorchia: absence of testes.

I. Complications (Danish and Dahms, 2002; Gill and Kogan, 1997).

1. Testicular torsion.
2. Hernia.
3. Infertility.
4. Postoperative complications.
   a. Obstruction of the testicular vascular supply by direct injury.
   b. Compression from twisting of the vascular supply resulting from direct injury.
   c. Tight closure of the abdominal musculature.
   d. Narrowing of vessels by placing them under significant tension as the testis is brought into the scrotum.
   e. Transient testicular swelling from partial obstruction of lymphatic and venous drainage.
5. Increased risk of testicular cancer.

J. Patient care management.

1. Orchiopexy.

a. Surgical procedure that alters the course of the spermatic artery and creates a direct line from the renal pedicle to the scrotum.
b. Surgical repair is to be performed at 1 to 2 years of age

2. Hormonal treatment (Danish and Dahms, 2002).
   a. Consists of administration of human chorionic gonadotropin (hCG), and/or gonadotropin-releasing hormone (GnRH), also referred to as luteinizing hormone-releasing hormone (LH-RH).
   b. May be attempted in an effort to avoid orchiopexy.
   c. May make technical aspects of orchiopexy easier.
3. Reevaluation of testicular location, size, and viability after 1 year.

K. **Outcome (Danish and Dahms, 2002; Gill and Kogan, 1997).**
   1. Success rates for orchiopexy by anatomic testicular position have been reported as 74% for abdominal, 87% for canalicular, and 92% for those located beyond the external ring.
   2. Fertility may be impaired.

CIRCUMCISION

A. **Indications.** There are no absolute medical indications for routine circumcision in the newborn period, although the advantages, disadvantages, and risks of the procedure have been reviewed in the literature (American Academy of Pediatrics [AAP] Task Force on Circumcision, 1999; Bartman et al., 2001; Canadian Paediatric Society [CPS] Fetus and Newborn Committee, 1996; Schoen et al., 2000).

B. **Incidence.** Percentage of male infants circumcised varies by geographic location, by religious affiliation, and to some extent by socioeconomic classification. The National Center for Health Statistics estimated that 64.1% of male infants were circumcised in the United States in 1995 (AAP Task Force on Circumcision, 1999).

C. **Physical examination.**
   1. Observation. Assess for the presence of abnormalities of the glans, foreskin, or urethral meatus.
   2. Gestational age assessment. Circumcision should not be performed on premature infants until they meet discharge criteria.

D. **Complications.**
   1. Bleeding.
   2. Infection.
   3. Injury to the glans.
   4. Meatal stenosis.
   5. Urethrocutaneous fistula.
   6. Formation of skin bridge.
   7. Adhesions.
   8. Phimosis.
   9. Concealed penis.
   10. Inflammation of the meatus or meatal ulcer.
   11. Chordee.
   12. Inclusion cysts.
   13. Lymphedema.
   14. Necrosis.

E. **Patient care management.**
   1. Circumcision should not be performed on infants with bleeding disorders or on those with abnormalities of the glans, foreskin, or urethral meatus.

2. Vitamin K should be administered within 1 hour after birth.
3. Eutectic Mixture of Local Anesthetic (EMLA) cream, dorsal penile nerve block, and a subcutaneous ring block have been shown to alleviate the discomfort associated with the procedure. The subcutaneous ring block may provide the most effective analgesia (AAP Task Force on Circumcision, 1999; CPS Fetus and Newborn Committee, 1996; Mohan et al., 1998; Taddio et al., 1997).
4. Risks and benefits should be discussed with parents and informed consent obtained.
5. Postoperative care.
   a. Check the site for bleeding, redness, or pus.
   b. Check for voiding.
   c. Avoid prone position.
   d. Change diapers frequently.
   e. Apply petroleum gauze to the site for 24 hours.
   f. Apply petroleum to site until healed.
6. Teach parent how to care for circumcision before discharge.

F. **Outcome.** The precise incidence of complications after circumcision is unknown; however, data indicate that the rate is low and that the most common complications are local infection and bleeding (AAP Task Force on Circumcision, 1999; CPS Fetus and Newborn Committee, 1996).

REFERENCES

Ahmed, S.M. and Swedlund, S.K.: Evaluation and treatment of urinary tract infections in children. *American Family Physician, 57*(1):1573–1580, 1998.

American Academy of Pediatrics Committee Task Force on Circumcision. Circumcision policy statement. *Pediatrics, 103*(3): 686-693, 1999.

Askin, D.F.: Interpretation of neonatal blood gases. I. Physiology and acid-base homeostasis. *Neonatal Network, 16*(5):17-21, 1997.

Atala, A. and Retik, A.B.: Congenital urologic anomalies. In R.W. Schrier and C.W. Gottschalk (Eds.): *Diseases of the kidney* (vol. 3.). Boston, 1997, Little, Brown.

Bartman, T., Frank, R., Goldenring, J., et al.: Newborn circumcision and urinary tract infections. *Pediatrics, 107*(7):210b-214, 2001.

Belman, A.B.: Hypospadias update. *Urology, 49*(2):166-172, 1997.

Canadian Paediatric Society Fetus and Newborn Committee: Neonatal circumcision revisited. *Canadian Medical Association Journal, 154*:769-780, 1996.

Danish, R.K. and Dahms, W.T.: Abnormalities of sexual differentiation. In A.A. Fanaroff and R.J. Martin (Eds.): *Neonatal-perinatal medicine: Diseases of the fetus and infant* (7th ed., vol. 2.). St Louis, 2002, Mosby, pp. 1416-1467.

Edwards, M.S.: Postnatal bacterial infections. In A.A. Fanaroff and R.J. Martin (Eds.): *Neonatal-perinatal medicine: Diseases of the fetus and infant* (7th ed., vol. 2.). St Louis, 2002, Mosby, pp. 706-745.

Elder, J.S.: Antenatal hydronephrosis: Fetal and neonatal management. *Pediatric Clinics of North America, 44*(5):1299-1321, 1997.

Ettinger, L. and Flynn, J.: Hypertension in the neonate. *NeoReviews, 3*(8):e151-154, 2002.

Flynn, J.T.: Neonatal hypertension: Diagnosis and management. *Pediatric Nephrology, 14*(4):332-341, 2000.

Gill, B. and Kogan, S.: Cryptorchidism. *Pediatric Clinics of North America, 44*(5):1211-1227, 1997.

Greenfield, S.P., Manyan, N.G., and Wan, J.: Experience with vesicoureteral reflux in children: Clinical characteristics. *Journal of Urology, 158*(2):574-577, 1997.

Guerina, N.: Bacterial and fungal infections. In J. Cloherty and A. Stark (Eds.): *Manual of neonatal care* (4th ed.). Philadelphia, 1998, Lippincott-Raven.

Housley, H.T. and Harrison, M.R.: Fetal urinary tract abnormalities: Natural history, pathophysiology and treatment. *Urologic Clinics of North America, 25*(1):63-73, 1998.

Huether, S.E.: Alterations of renal and urinary tract function in children. In K.L. McCance and S.E. Huether (Eds): *Pathophysiology: The biologic basis for disease in adults and children* (4th ed.). St Louis, 2002, Mosby, pp. 1217-1230.

Kenner, C.: Assessment and management of genitourinary dysfunction. In C. Kenner, J.W. Lott, and A.A. Flandermeyer (Eds.): *Comprehensive neonatal nursing: A physiologic perspective* (2nd ed.). Philadelphia, 1998, Saunders, pp. 620-647.

Kenner, C., Amlung, S.R., and Flandermeyer, A.A.: *Protocols in neonatal nursing,* Philadelphia, 1998, Saunders.

Kim, M. and Emma, F.: Renal conditions. In J. Cloherty and A. Stark (Eds.): *Manual of neonatal care* (4th ed.). Philadelphia, 1998, Lippincott-Raven.

Levine, E., Hartman, D.S., Meilstrup, J.W., et al.: Current concepts and controversies in imaging of renal cystic diseases. *Urologic Clinics of North America, 24*(3):523-543, 1997.

Mohan, C., Risucci, D.A., Casimir, M., and Gulrajani-LaCorte, M.: Comparison of analgesics in ameliorating the pain of circumcision. *Journal of Perinatology, 18*(1):13-19, 1998.

Porth, C.: *Pathophysiology: Concepts of altered health states* (6th ed.). Philadelphia, 2002, Lippincott Williams & Wilkins.

Reddy, P.P. and Mandell, J.: Prenatal diagnosis: Therapeutic implications. *Urologic Clinics of North America, 25*(2):171-180, 1998.

Ross, J.: Pediatric urinary tract infections and reflux. *American Family Physician, 56*(6): 1-8, 1996.

Ross, J.H. and Kay, R.: Pediatric urinary tract infections and reflux. *American Family Physician,* 59(6):1472-1478, 1485-1486, 1999.

Rushton, H.: Urinary tract infections in children: Epidemiology, evaluation, and management. *Pediatric Clinics of North America, 44*(5):1133-1169, 1997.

Schoen, E., Colby, C., and Ray, G.: Newborn circumcision decreases incidence and costs of urinary tract infections during the first year of life. *Pediatrics, 105*(4): 789-793, 2000.

Shalaby-Rana, E., Lowe, L.H., Blask, A.N., and Majd, M.: Imaging in pediatric urology. *Pediatric Clinics of North America, 44*(5):1065-1089, 1997.

Swinford, R.D., Bonilla-Felix, M., Cerda, R.D., and Portman, R.J.: Neonatal nephrology. In G.B. Merenstein and S.L. Gardner (Eds.): *Handbook of neonatal intensive care* (5th ed.). St Louis, 2002, Mosby, pp. 609-643.

Taddio, A., Stevens, B., Craig, K., et al.: Efficacy and safety of lidocaine-prilocaine cream for circumcision. *New England Journal of Medicine, 336*(17): 1197-1201, 1997.

Vogt, B.A. and Avner, E.D.: The kidney and urinary tract. In A.A. Fanaroff and R.J. Martin (Eds.): *Neonatal-perinatal medicine: Diseases of the fetus and infant* (7th ed., vol. 2.). St Louis, 2002, Mosby, pp. 1517-1536.

Ward, A.M., Kay, R., and Ross, J.H.: Ureteropelvic junction obstruction in children: Unique considerations for open operative intervention. *Urologic Clinics of North America, 25*(2):211-217, 1998.

Young, T. and Mangum, B.: *Neofax 2002* (16th ed.). Raleigh, NC, 2003, Acorn Publishing, Inc.

Zaontz, M.R. and Packer, M.G.: Abnormalities of the external genitalia. *Pediatric Clinics of North America, 44*(5):1267-1297, 1997.

CHAPTER

33 Neurologic Disorders

LYNN LYNAM AND M. TERESE VERKLAN

OBJECTIVES

1. Identify the six primary stages of neurodevelopment and the congenital anomalies that result from defective development at each stage.
2. Define autoregulation.
3. Review a complete neurologic examination.
4. Examine birth injuries and patient care management.
5. Differentiate between the different types of intracranial hemorrhages and their origins, clinical presentation, and outcomes.
6. Recognize neonatal seizures, their distinguishing characteristics, and issues in patient care management.
7. Describe hypoxic-ischemic encephalopathy.
8. Describe the clinical implications of periventricular leukomalacia.
9. Distinguish pathophysiologic factors, clinical presentation, and patient care management of early- and late-onset meningitis.

The human brain is an intricate, fragile organ requiring precise development from the moment of conception. Several crucial developmental landmarks pinpoint major events in the development of the human brain. If the process is interrupted, difficulties ranging from simple, easily treatable conditions to major neurologic malformations may occur. Neurologic problems account for a significant number of admissions into the neonatal intensive care unit each year. This chapter provides a comprehensive review of neurodevelopment, neurophysiology, and neuromalformations.

ANATOMY OF THE NEUROLOGIC SYSTEM (Moore and Persaud, 2003; Volpe, 2001).

A. Embryologic development (Table 33-1).

1. Primary neurulation (dorsal induction).
   a. Occurs within the first month of life, ending between 24 and 28 days' gestation.
   b. Neural tube is formed by the invagination and curling of the distal neural plate.
   c. Closure of the neural tube gives rise to the central nervous system, including the cranial nerves.
   d. This evolution results in the formation of the skull and vertebrae.
   e. Inaccuracies of primary neurulation result in anencephaly, occipital encephalocele, myelomeningocele, and Arnold-Chiari malformation.

TABLE 33-1
Major Events in Human Brain Development and Peak Times of Occurrence

Major Developmental Event	Peak Time of Occurrence
Primary neurulation	3 to 4 weeks of gestation
Prosencephalic development	2 to 3 months of gestation
Neuronal proliferation	3 to 4 months of gestation
Neuronal migration	3 to 5 months of gestation
Organization	5 months of gestation to years postnatal
Myelination	Birth to years postnatal

From Volpe, J.J.: *Neurology of the newborn* (4th ed.). Philadelphia, 2001, W.B. Saunders.

2. Prosencephalic development.
   - a. Peak development is in the second and third months of gestation.
   - b. This influences the formation of the face, forebrain, corpus callosum and septum pallucidum, optic nerves/chiasm, the hypothalamic structures (thalamus and hypothalamus [diencephalon]), and the cerebral hemispheres (telencephalon).
   - c. Absence of olfactory bulbs and tracts is not uncommon.
   - d. Disturbance in prosencephalic development causes facial and forebrain alterations.
     - (1) Holoprosencephaly (abnormal formation of telencephalon and diencephalon).
     - (2) Midline and midfacial defects.
       - (a) Hypotelorism (less common: hypertelorism).
       - (b) Cyclopia.
       - (c) Cleft lip with or without cleft palate.
     - (3) Agenesis of corpus collusum, corpus pellucidum.
   - e. Most common karyotype is normal (chromosomal disorder is possible).
3. Neuronal proliferation.
   - a. Occurs between 3 and 4 months' gestation.
   - b. Toxins and inherited diseases can significantly alter the number of neurons.
   - c. Chemical and environmental substances can reduce the number of neurons, causing microcephaly vera.
   - d. Excess neurons can produce macrencephaly.
   - e. Disorders of proliferation of small veins cause Sturge-Weber syndrome (6% unilateral, 24% bilateral facial lesions).
4. Neuronal migration.
   - a. Can occur as early as 2 months; peaks between 3 and 5 months.
   - b. By 6 months' gestation, the neurons have migrated to their final, permanent place in the cortex.
   - c. Neurons follow glial paths outward.
   - d. Cells migrate and differentiate into six cortical layers.
   - e. Migration is critical for development of the cerebral cortex and the deeper nuclear structures.
     - (1) Basal ganglia.
     - (2) Hypothalamus.

(3) Thalamus.
(4) Brainstem.
(5) Cerebellum.
(6) Spinal cord.

f. Dysfunction at this stage results in cortical malformation with abnormalities of neurologic function.
g. Seizures may be the first clinical manifestation in the early postnatal period.
h. Defects associated with abnormal migration range in severity and may be associated with other neurologic development.
i. Abnormal development of gyrus denotes a neuronal migration disorder.
j. Disorders include lissencephaly ("smooth brain"), agenesis of the corpus callosum, and schizencephaly (clefts found in the cerebral wall).

5. Neuronal organization.
a. Peaks at 5 months' gestation to several years after birth.
b. Provides the basis for brain function and its complex circuitry.
c. Includes cell differentiation, cell death, synaptic development, neurotransmitters, and myelination.
d. Achieves stabilization of cell connections.
e. Disorders due to organizational deficits and detrimental retardation (as with Down syndrome, fragile-X syndrome, and mild Duchenne muscular dystrophy).

6. Myelination.
a. Begins in the second trimester and continues into adult life.
b. Involves myelin deposition around axons.
c. Myelin, a fatty covering, insulates the circuitry; prevents leakage of current and enables rapid, efficient transmission of nerve impulses.
d. Enhances intercellular communication.
e. Deficiencies occur in some acquired and inherited diseases.

B. Brain anatomy (Fig. 33-1) (Moore and Persaud, 2003; Volpe, 2001).

1. Cerebellum.
a. Promotes integrative muscle function.
b. Maintains balance.
c. Enables smooth, purposeful movements.

2. Cerebrum: main components of cerebral hemisphere.
a. Contains four lobes: frontal, parietal, occipital, and temporal.
(1) Frontal lobes make up command center; concerned with decision making and other "executive" tasks.
(2) Parietal lobes are responsible for hearing, understanding speech, and forming an integrated sense of self.
(3) Occipital lobes process vision.
(4) Temporal lobes: center for smell, with association areas for memory and learning.

b. Corpus callosum: fiber bundles connecting the cerebral hemispheres.
c. Cerebral cortex.
(1) Encompasses the mind, the intellect.
(2) Gray matter.

d. Lateral ventricles.
e. Third ventricle: fluid-filled space.
f. Thalamus: integrates sensory input.
g. Hypothalamus: regulates body temperature.

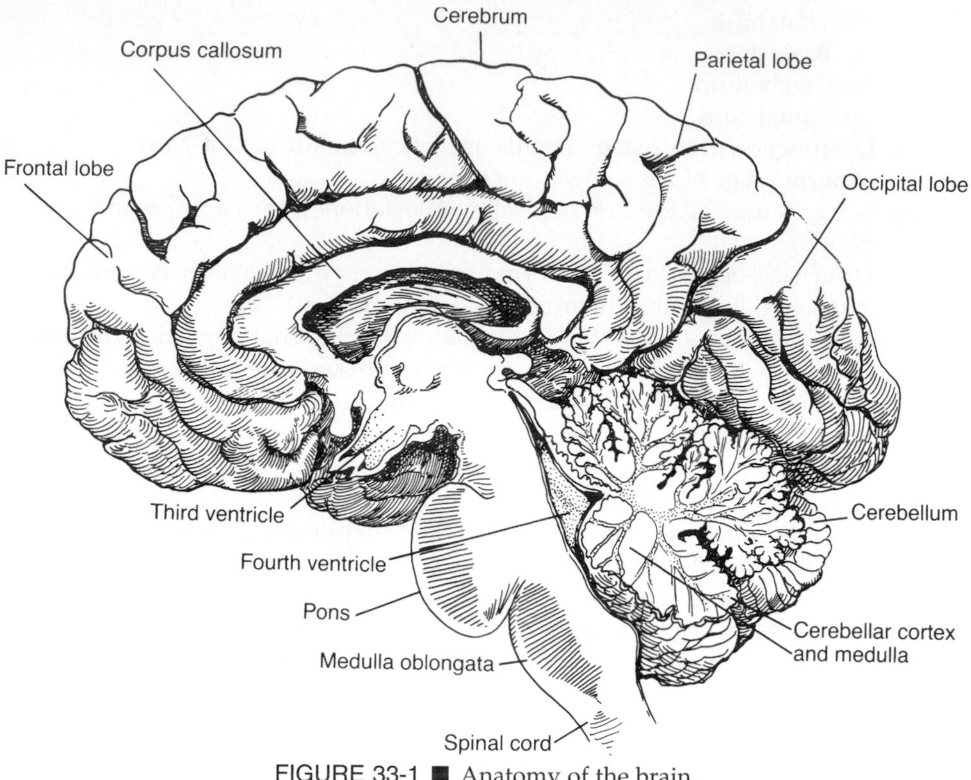

FIGURE 33-1 ■ Anatomy of the brain.

3. Brainstem.
   a. Relays input and output signals between higher brain centers and the spinal cord.
   b. Three main components.
      (1) Medulla oblongata.
         (a) Implicated within cranial nerves VIII, IX, X, XI, and XII.
         (b) Controls areas of the abdomen, thorax, throat, and mouth.
      (2) Pons: carries information between the brainstem and the cerebellum.
      (3) Midbrain: involved in eye movements.

PHYSIOLOGY OF THE NEUROLOGIC SYSTEM

A. Glucose metabolism.

1. Cerebral metabolism is influenced by the availability of glucose and oxygen.
2. Glucose is transported from blood to brain by a glucose transporter found in capillaries (Volpe, 2001).
3. Serum glucose provides the brain with a glucose pool.
4. The neonatal brain is glucose dependent. The central nervous system (CNS) is quickly and significantly affected by hypoglycemia (Volpe, 2001).
5. Glycogen stores are minimal or nonexistent in the premature baby.
6. The brain depends on adequate circulation to supply both oxygen and glucose to create enough energy for normal growth and metabolism.
7. Anaerobic metabolism causes lactic acid buildup.
8. Anaerobic metabolism produces significantly smaller amounts of energy.

9. Newborn blood glucose levels less than 30 mg/dl are associated with significant increases in cerebral blood flow.
10. Defining the lower limit of the neonatal blood glucose level is difficult because the infant's ability to present overt symptoms of hypoglycemia is not developed.

B. Cerebral blood flow.

1. Cerebral blood flow is affected by pH (controlled by hydrogen ions and carbon dioxide levels), potassium, hypoxemia, osmolarity, and calcium ion concentrations.
   a. The brain increases cerebral blood flow to spare itself inadequacies.
   b. As pH decreases, cerebral blood flow increases.
   c. As potassium levels increase, cerebral blood flow increases.
   d. Hypoxemia causes an increase in cerebral blood flow to provide adequate oxygenated blood to the brain.
   e. Increased osmolarity causes increased cerebral blood flow.
   f. An increase in calcium ions causes a decrease in cerebral blood flow.
   g. Cerebral blood flow increases when blood glucose levels fall to less than 30 mg/dl; the hypoglycemic brain recruits previously unperfused capillaries to maintain glucose levels (Volpe, 2001).
   h. Degree and duration of hypoglycemia are significant (Volpe, 2001).
   i. Studies have shown that neonatal neurologic signs can be minimal or absent with subsequent abnormal cognitive development.
2. Autoregulation (Volpe, 2001).
   a. Maintains steady-state cerebral blood flow over a broad range of perfusion pressures.
   b. Important vasoactive factors in the brain: hydrogen ions, potassium ions, adenosine, prostaglandins, osmolarity, calcium.
   c. Cerebral blood flow increases with advancing gestational age and concomitant cerebral metabolic demands.
   d. Normal arterial blood pressure in the preterm neonate is thought to be near or at the lower autoregulatory limit. This suggests an increased vulnerability to ischemic brain injury with modest hypotension, especially with decreasing gestational age.
   e. Cerebral vasculature vasodilates maximally in response to hypoxemia, hypercapnia, and acidosis.
      (1) Hypotension leads to ischemia.
         (a) Ischemia damages blood vessels and surrounding elements supporting the blood vessels.
         (b) Blood flow to cerebral white matter restored only after reperfusion of other brain regions (Szymonowicz et al., 1990).
         (c) Once adequate blood supply resumes, hemorrhage can occur into ischemic areas.
      (2) Hypertension leads to hemorrhage.

NEUROLOGIC ASSESSMENT (Rennie, 1999; Volpe, 2001)

A. History.

B. Observation.

1. Determine state (Table 33-2).
2. Note posture.
   a. Gestational age determines posture.
      (1) Premature infants: open, extended position reflecting diminished tone.
      (2) Term infants: flexed position reflecting adequate tone.

TABLE 33-2
Summary of Neurologic States

Neurologic State	Physical Findings
Deep sleep	No observable movement
REM sleep	Eye movement, body movement, and irregular respiratory activity
Drowsy	
Quiet-alert	
Active	
Crying	

REM, Rapid eye movement.

b. Sequelae of intrauterine position may be evident.
c. Abnormal findings are:
   (1) Hyperextension.
   (2) Asymmetry.
   (3) Flaccidity.
3. Note movements.
   a. Symmetric or asymmetric body movements.
   b. Note movement quality (jitteriness, seizures, tremors, and clonus).
   c. Quantity (absent or pronounced).
4. Note respiratory activity.
   a. Signs of distress.
   b. Hypoventilation (apnea).
   c. Quality of cry.
      (1) High pitched (consider meningitis, drug withdrawal, neurologic abnormalities).
      (2) Stridor (consider vocal cord damage or paralysis).
5. Observe skin.
   a. Lesions (note number, size, shape, color, and texture).
      (1) Café-au-lait spots (six or more lesions of ≥ 1.5 cm; may indicate neurofibromatosis).
      (2) Port-wine facial hemangioma (consider Sturge-Weber syndrome).
      (3) Areas of depigmentation.
   b. Abrasions, lacerations, bruises, and forceps marks (consider intracranial bleeding, injury).

C. **Physical examination** (Volpe, 2001).
1. Check the skull size, shape, symmetry, hair whorls, fontanelles, and sutures.
2. Measure occipital frontal circumference (OFC).
   a. Document less than 10th percentile (symmetric vs. asymmetric compared with total body growth; may indicate microcephaly).
   b. Document greater than 90th percentile (symmetric vs. asymmetric compared with total body growth; may indicate macrocephaly).
3. Examine the face for abnormalities in structure.
   a. Placement of ears.
   b. Neck skinfolds.
4. Spine (intact, openings, masses).
5. Cranial nerve function.
   a. Refer to Table 33-3.
   b. Blink reflex requires intact cranial nerves III and VII.

■ TABLE 33-3
■ ■ **Cranial Nerves**

Cranial Nerve	Bedside Testing Mechanisms
I. Olfactory (smell)	Place ammonia under nose; response is startle, grimace
II. Optic	Check PERL
III. Oculomotor (muscles of the eye)	PERL, EOM full and conjugate
IV. Trochlear (superior oblique muscle of the eye)	
V. Trigeminal (sensory to face, motor to jaw)	Touch cheek; should turn cheek toward stimulus
VI. Abducens (lateral gaze, abducts eyeball)	Rotate infant; eyes look in the direction of travel
VII. Facial	Asymmetric facial movements
VIII. Auditory	Infant quiets to voice; blinks to clap of hand
IX. Glossopharyngeal (taste)	Strong gag response
X. Vagus (pharynx, larynx, esophagus)	Cry is not hoarse
XI. Accessory (sternocleidomastoid muscles)	Turn supine infant's head to one side; infant attempts to bring head to midline
XII. Hypoglossal (muscles of tongue)	Insert finger in mouth while sucking; note force of tongue; note vesiculations or quivering tongue (uncommon)

EOM, Extraocular movements; *PERL,* pupils equal and reactive to light.
Adapted from Scanlon, J.W., Nelson, T., Grylack, L.J., and Smith, Y.F.: *A system of newborn physical examination.* Baltimore, 1979, University Park Press; Whaley, L.F. and Wong, D.L.: *Nursing care of infants and children.* St Louis, 1979, Mosby.

c. Corneal reflex requires intact cranial nerves V and VII.
   (1) Generally elicited only if one suspects brain or eye damage (Whaley and Wong, 1999).
   (2) Cranial nerves IX, X, and XII regulate the tongue, swallow, gag, and cry.
6. Muscle tone.
   a. Evaluate head lag, ventral suspension, clonus, and recoil from extension.
   b. Check symmetry; briskness versus flaccidity.
7. Reflexes.
   a. Check grasp (bilaterally), Babinski, Moro, gag, suck, root, and tonic neck.
   b. Evaluate symmetry and strength of response.
   c. Abnormal Moro reflex: consider clavicular or humeral fractures or brachial plexus injury.
   d. Grasp varies with gestational age; if grasp is absent, consider nerve damage (refer to Birth Injuries, on pp. 836-841).

NEUROLOGIC DISORDERS

A. Anencephaly (Volpe, 2001).
1. Risk factors: thought to be due to a combination of genetic and environmental influences.
   a. Risk appears to increase with low socioeconomic status, history of affected siblings.
   b. More common in whites.
   c. Females affected more often than males.
2. Pathophysiology.
   a. Failure of anterior neural tube closure.
   b. Malfunction of the first stage of neurologic development, primary neurulation.

c. Most commonly involves the forebrain and variable amounts of upper brainstem.
d. Partial absence of skull bones, with absent cerebrum and with or without missing cerebellum, brainstem, and spinal cord.
3. Incidence: Approximately 0.2 per 1000 live births.
4. Clinical presentation.
a. Exposed neural tissue with little definable structure.
b. The anomalous skull has a froglike appearance from en face view.
c. Amniotic fluid reveals high levels of alpha-fetoprotein late in the first trimester.
5. Diagnostic evaluation.
a. Identified by prenatal cranial ultrasonography in the second trimester.
b. Apparent upon visual inspection after birth.
6. Patient care management.
a. Provide comfort measures for the infant.
b. Obtain genetic consultation; encourage parents to seek genetic counseling.
c. Support the grieving process.
d. Encourage the family to see their baby because the family's imaginary impressions may be worse than reality.
e. Clinicians must maintain a delicate balance between benefit and harm.
7. Outcome.
a. Stillbirth occurs in 75%
b. Survival is unlikely beyond the neonatal period.

B. **Microcephaly** (DeMyer, 1999).
1. Definition.
a. Occipital-frontal circumference ≥ 2 standard deviations below the mean for age and gender.
b. Small brain implies neurologic impairment.
2. Risk factors.
a. Maternal:
(1) Viral infections *Toxoplasmosis*; Other [Syphillis], Rubella, Cytomegalovirus, Herpes [TORCH].
(2) Exposure to radiation.
(3) Metabolic conditions such as diabetes, phenylketonuria.
(4) Prescription and street drugs, especially in first trimester.
(5) Genetic: autosomal recessive; autosomal dominant; X-linked.
(6) Malnutrition: most common worldwide cause.
b. Fetal:
(1) Prenatal/perinatal insult: inflammation; hypoxia; birth trauma.
c. Neonatal:
(1) Very low birth weight infant.
(2) Hypoxic ischemic encephalopathy.
(3) Nutrition: most common worldwide cause.
3. Pathophysiology.
a. Neuronal proliferation defect.
b. Occurs between 3 and 4 months' gestational age (Volpe, 2001).
c. Destructive microcephaly occurs when the normal brain suffers prenatal/perinatal insult.
4. Clinical presentation.
a. Small head, backward sloping of the forehead, small cranial volume.
b. Neurologic deficits rarely evident at birth.

5. Diagnostic evaluation.
   a. Perform a complete physical examination including neurologic assessment.
   b. Elicit a thorough maternal history.
   c. Use tests to confirm or rule out etiologic factors aligned with maternal history.
   d. Computed tomography (CT) or magnetic resonance imaging (MRI) is performed.
6. Patient care management.
   a. Record accurate measurement of OFC, length, and weight weekly.
   b. Note percentiles and alert physician to abnormalities.
   c. Document clearly any deviations from normal.
   d. Obtain tests as ordered; note dates to follow up results.
   e. Ensure that the family is informed.
   f. Obtain consultations as needed: genetics, infectious diseases.
7. Outcome.
   a. Dependent on severity.
   b. May be associated with developmental delays.

C. **Hydrocephalus (Ashwal, 1999).**
1. Definition: excess cerebrospinal fluid (CSF) in the ventricles of the brain due to a decrease in reabsorption or overproduction.
   a. CSF is in balance between formation and absorption.
   b. CSF is produced at a rate of 0.35 cc/minute from brain parenchyma, cerebral ventricles, areas along the spinal cord, and the choroid plexus (70% is from the choroid plexus).
2. Incidence: estimated that there are approximately 125,000 individuals with shunts, and that 33,000 shunts are placed annually in the United States (Bondurant and Jimenez, 1995).
3. Pathophysiology.
   a. Excessive CSF production (rare).
   b. Inadequate CSF absorption secondary to abnormal circulation.
   c. Excess ventricular CSF secondary to aqueductal outflow obstruction causes obstructive, noncommunicating hydrocephalus (refer to Fig. 33-2 for a simplified diagram of the brain).
      (1) The condition is most common in newborn infants.
      (2) Obstructive hydrocephalus may progress rapidly.

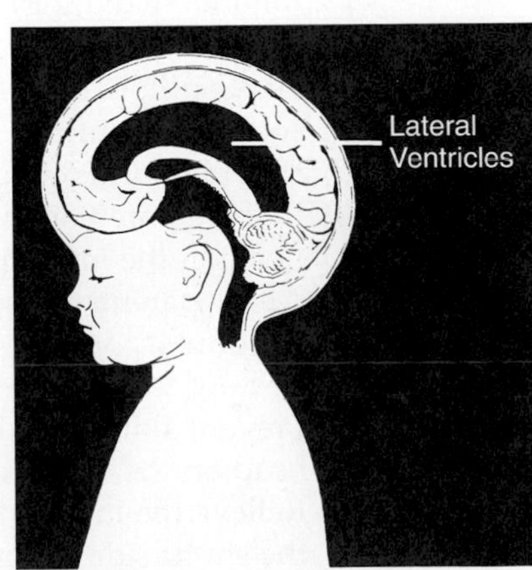

FIGURE 33-2 ■ Hydrocephalus. (From Ross Laboratories: *New perspectives on intraventricular hemorrhage*, Columbus, OH, 1988, Ross Laboratories.)

d. Excess ventricular CSF with flow between the lateral ventricles and the subarachnoid space results in communicating, nonobstructive hydrocephalus.

4. Congenital hydrocephalus.
   a. Risk factors.
      (1) Aqueductal stenosis.
      (2) Dandy-Walker cyst (cystic transformation of fourth ventricle).
      (3) Myelomeningocele with Arnold-Chiari malformation (herniation of the hindbrain, usually causing obstructive hydrocephalus).
      (4) Congenital masses and tumors.
      (5) Congenital infection (toxoplasmosis, cytomegalovirus [CMV] infection).
   b. Associated etiologies and/or congenital defects.
      (1) Spina bifida.
      (2) Encephalocele.
      (3) Holoprosencephaly.
   c. Clinical presentation.
      (1) Large head.
      (2) Widened sutures.
      (3) Full (bulging) and tense fontanelles.
      (4) Increasing OFC.
      (5) Setting-sun eyes (may signify brain tissue damage).
      (6) Vomiting, lethargy, irritability.
      (7) Visible scalp veins.
   d. Diagnostic evaluation.
      (1) Serial intracranial ultrasonography.
      (2) Neuroimaging techniques: CT, MRI, and cranial ultrasonography.
   e. Patient care management.
      (1) Intrauterine diagnosis affords the family more options and allows time for preparation and anticipation.
      (2) Perform a thorough physical examination, assessing for further anomalies.
      (3) Obtain neurosurgery and genetics consultation.
      (4) Confirm diagnosis and cause.
      (5) Consider the possible need for reservoir placement versus ventriculoperitoneal (VP) shunt placement.
      (6) Support the infant by decreasing noxious stimuli (dim lights, minimal handling).
      (7) Position the head carefully.
      (8) Water-pillow beds diminish skin breakdown and may provide a source of comfort.
      (9) Provide normal infant care as much as possible.
      (10) Involve parents in infant's care as soon as family is ready.
      (11) Position the infant prone for oral feedings.
      (12) Allow parents to view an infant with a VP shunt or review pictured handouts.
      (13) Review VP shunt with parents preoperatively and postoperatively.
      (14) Prevent skin breakdown by not allowing the infant to put his or her head on the shunt side postoperatively.
      (15) Relieve the infant's probable stiff neck by holding the child's neck on the shunt side during feedings.

(16) Review signs of infection or blocked shunt with the family.
  (a) Irritability.
  (b) Vomiting.
  (c) Increasing head size.
  (d) Lethargy.
  (e) Changes in feeding patterns.
  (f) Bulging fontanelle.
(17) If incision site reddens, position infant on opposite side to relieve pressure from this area.

f. Outcome.

5. Posthemorrhagic hydrocephalus (PHH) (Ashwal, 1999).

a. Etiology.
(1) Progressive dilation of the ventricles after intraventricular hemorrhage (IVH) caused by injury to the periventricular white matter.
(2) Two types: acute and chronic.
  (a) Acute.
    (i) Rapidly appears—within days of the initial hemorrhage.
    (ii) Probably occurs secondary to malabsorption of CSF secondary to a blood clot.
  (b) Subacute, chronic.
    (i) Inhibition of CSF flow.
    (ii) Blood from IVH.

b. Incidence.
(1) Approximately 45% of infants with IVH have no evidence of hydrocephalus (Volpe, 2001).
(2) Acute ventricular dilation develops in approximately 50% of surviving infants with hemorrhage; in the majority, it resolves spontaneously or remains static (Papile, 1997).

c. Clinical presentation.
(1) Insidious following mild ventricular dilatation.
(2) May be profound following severe ventricular dilatation.
  (a) Rapid increase in head size (begins days to weeks after ventricular dilatation present).
  (b) Episodic apnea and bradycardia.
  (c) Lethargy.
  (d) Increased intracranial pressure.
  (e) Tense, bulging anterior fontanelle.
  (f) Cranial sutures separating.
  (g) Ocular movement abnormalities.

d. Diagnostic evaluation.
(1) Graph of weekly OFC measurements.
(2) CT scan.
(3) Cranial ultrasonography.
(4) MRI.

e. Patient care management (Madsen and Frim, 1999).
(1) Obtain daily OFC measurements.
(2) Serial cranial ultrasonography.
(3) Neurosurgical consultation.
(4) Interventions to maintain lumbar or ventricular pressure at approximately 5 cm H_2O while evaluating for shunt placement.
  (a) Serial lumbar punctures or direct ventricular access may be helpful.

(b) Administer medications that diminish CSF production rates:
(i) Furosemide (Lasix): 1 mg/kg/day.
(ii) Acetazolamide (Diamox): up to 100 mg/kg/day.
(5) Consideration given to placing a reservoir or ventriculoperitoneal (VP) shunt.
(6) Observe the infant for signs of increasing intracranial hemorrhage and hydrocephalus.
(7) Support the family: neonate is very susceptible to shunt infections and shunt malfunction.

f. Outcome.
(1) Poor outcomes are likely when cerebral decompression does not occur after VP shunt placement.
(2) Initial IVH severity is the major determining factor in PHH development.
(3) In slightly more than 50% of the cases, severe hemorrhage results in progressive ventricular dilatation (Volpe, 2001).
(4) Without therapy, a considerable number of infants exhibit halted progression, with or without resolution (Volpe, 2001).
(5) Deficits are motor and/or cognitive.

D. Myelomeningocele (Volpe, 2001).

1. Definition.

a. Neural tube defect.
(1) Spina bifida occulta involves vertebral bone.
(2) Defect is invisible (may be found if problems develop in later infancy or in childhood).
(3) Meningocele is the protrusion of the meninges lying directly under the skin.
(4) Myelocele is the exposure of the internal surface of the spinal cord or the nerve roots.

b. In myelomeningocele, the spinal cord and meninges are exposed through the skin and onto the surface of the back.

c. In myeloschisis, large areas of the spinal cord are without dermal or vertebral covering.

2. Risk factors and/or associated disease states.

a. Hydrocephalus.
(1) With OFC at greater than the 90th percentile, 95% of infants will have hydrocephalus.
(2) All newborn infants with myelomeningocele should be evaluated for hydrocephalus with CT scan and cranial ultrasonography shortly after birth.

b. Arnold-Chiari malformation.
(1) Hindbrain malformation with or without aqueductal atresia.
(2) Almost always present with myelomeningocele (Goddard-Finegold, 1998).
(3) Hydrocephalus present in 70 percent.
(4) Common features.
(a) Reflux and aspiration.
(b) Laryngeal stridor.
(c) Central hypoventilation, apnea.

3. Pathophysiology.

a. Results from failure of posterior neural tube to close.

b. 80% of cases occur in the lumbar region (the last region of the neural tube to close).

c. Environmental factors, maternal nutrition, genetics, and teratogens, including maternal hyperthermia, are implicated.

4. Incidence: Approximately .2 to .4/1000 live births.
5. Clinical presentation.
   a. The majority of cases occur in the thoracolumbar, lumbar, and lumbosacral regions.
   b. A herniated sac, sealed or leaking, protrudes from the back.
   c. Defects include vascular networks surrounding abnormal neural tissue.
   d. Most lesions have incomplete skin coverage.
6. Diagnostic evaluation.
   a. Radiographic evaluation.
   b. Spinal ultrasound.
   c. MRI.
7. Patient care management.
   a. Prenatal diagnosis helpful.
   b. Examine lesion and measure size.
   c. Culture specimen from lesion if sac is open.
   d. Wrap lesion with sterile gauze moistened with warm sterile saline solution; place a sterile feeding tube within the gauze mesh for intermittent infusion of warm saline solution.
   e. Maintain the infant in a prone kneeling position, and protect the knees from skin breakdown.
   f. Place a drape over the buttocks below the lesion; utilize the drape's adhesive backing to secure the drape to the body.
   g. Obtain immediate consultation.
      (1) Neurosurgery.
      (2) Urology.
   h. Perform a thorough physical examination to assess the level of the injury, sensory involvement, and anal wink; include an OFC measurement.
   i. Encourage an open discussion among the family, the consultants, and the primary care team, providing the following:
      (1) Underlying physiology.
      (2) Physical examination findings.
      (3) Consultant reports.
      (4) Prognosis.
      (5) Complications.
      (6) Long-term care.
      (7) Options.
   j. Begin preparing the family for discharge.
      (1) Suggest that the parents contact a support group.
      (2) Involve the parents in their infant's care.
   k. Postoperatively, follow positioning instructions from the neurosurgeon.
   l. Spend time making eye contact with the infant.
   m. Observe for signs of hydrocephalus (refer to section C, Hydrocephalus, on p. 829).
   n. Observe for development of Arnold-Chiari malformation that may present with feeding problems (reflux, aspiration), laryngeal stridor (due to vocal cord paralysis), or central hypoventilation or apnea.
   o. Maintain meticulous hygiene by clearing stool and urine quickly.
   p. Provide adequate nutrition.
   q. Orthopedic consultation is appropriate for maximal function of lower extremities.
   r. Physical therapy encourages maximal range of motion.

8. Outcome.
   a. Survival in 90%, with 80% or more having normal intelligence and 85% being ambulatory with or without special aids.
   b. Optimistic outlook with meningocele because of normal spinal cord.
   c. Varying degrees of paralysis: commonly in the lower extremities (Volpe, 2001).
      (1) Lesions below the first sacral vertebra: infants can learn to walk unaided.
      (2) Lesions between the fourth and fifth lumbar vertebrae: infants may be able to walk with crutches or braces.
      (3) Lesions above the second lumbar vertebra: infants usually become wheelchair dependent.
   d. If surgery for defect closure is not performed, 80% die by 8 weeks and 100% are dead by 10 months.

E. **Encephalocele** (Volpe, 2001).
1. Definition.
   a. Neural herniation.
   b. May or may not contain meninges or brain parenchyma.
2. Risk factors.
   a. Environmental and genetic factors.
   b. May be multifactorial.
3. Pathophysiology.
   a. Precise pathogenesis is unknown, but is thought of as a restricted disorder of neurulation that involves the closure of the anterior neural tube.
   b. About 70% to 80% of encephaloceles occur in the occipital region.
   c. About 10% to 20% of lesions in the occipital region contain no neural elements.
4. Clinical presentation.
   a. Protruding midline skin-covered sac from the head or base of neck.
   b. Majority of sacs occur in the occipital region.
5. Diagnostic evaluation.
   a. Second-trimester intrauterine ultrasonography.
   b. Cranial ultrasonography.
   c. CT scan.
   d. MRI.
6. Patient care management.
   a. Examine the infant closely.
   b. Obtain neurosurgery consultation.
   c. Educate and support the family.
   d. Treat seizure activity.
7. Outcome.
   a. Early surgery recommended.
   b. Prognosis more favorable if encephocele is anterior.
   c. Possible motor deficits.
   d. Possible impaired intellectual function.
   e. 50% complicated by hydrocephalus.

F. **Craniosynostosis (Ashwal, 1999; Sun and Persing, 1999).**
1. Definition.
   a. Premature closure of cranial sutures.
   b. Occurs along one or more suture lines (see Fig. 33-3 for names and placement of cranial sutures).
2. Risk factors. Usually sporadic and without associated anomalies.

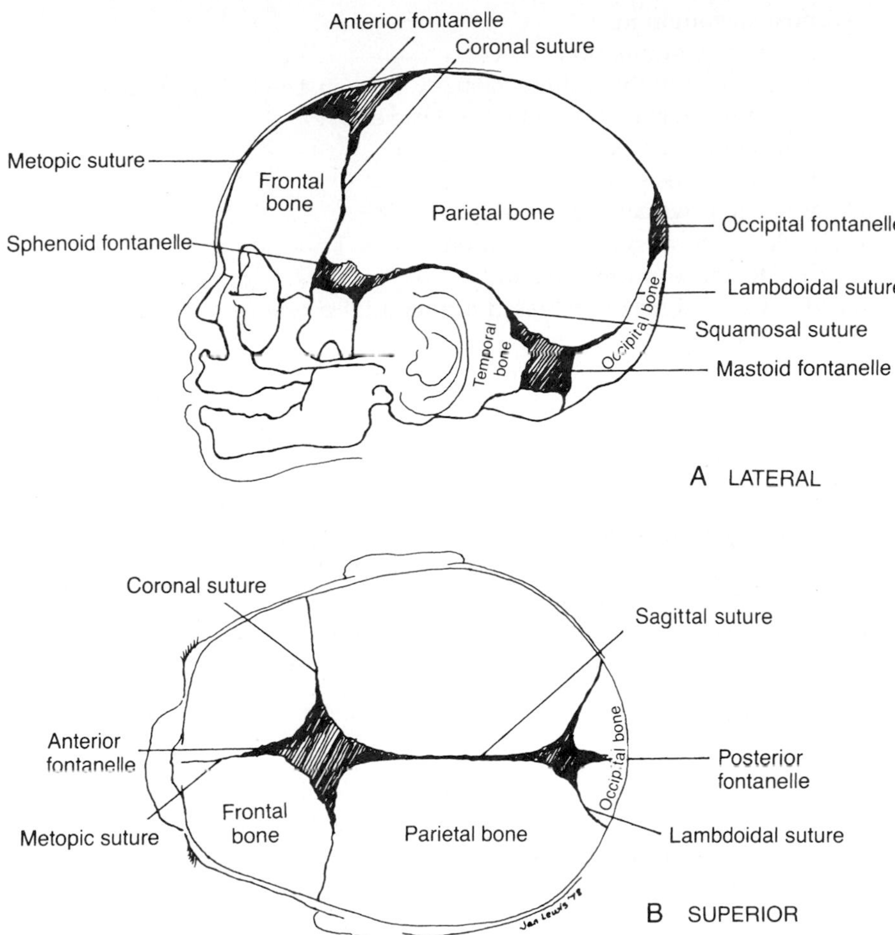

FIGURE 33-3 ■ *A* and *B*, Two views of neonatal skull, showing clinically important fontanelles and sutures. (From Scanlon, J.W., Nelson, T., Grylack, L., and Smith, Y.F.: *A system of newborn physical examinations*. Baltimore, 1979, University Park Press, p. 47.)

3. Pathophysiology.
   a. Cause unclear. May be a defect in the mesenchymal layer of the ossification center within the skull.
   b. Etiology includes developmental, mechanical, metabolic, and genetic factors that influence skull growth.
4. Incidence.
   a. Reported as 1 in 2000 to 2500 births.
   b. Sagittal craniosynostosis most common.
5. Clinical presentation.
   a. Asymptomatic.
   b. Cranial suture line reveals bony prominence; even and smooth bilaterally.
   c. Inability to move the suture.
   d. Abnormal cranial shape.
   e. Later signs:
      (1) Increased intracranial pressure.
      (2) Increased irritability.
      (3) Possible separation of other sutures.

6. Diagnostic evaluation.
   a. Skull x-ray examination.
   b. High resolution three-dimensional CT reconstruction scanning to determine the extent of premature bone fusion.
   c. Weekly graph of OFCs.
7. Patient care management.
   a. Thorough physical examination.
   b. Obtain neurosurgery consultation.
   c. Educate and support the family.
   d. Observe for signs of increased intracranial pressure.
      (1) Irritability.
      (2) Lethargy.
      (3) Vomiting.
      (4) Bulging fontanelle.
   e. Early surgical treatment is recommended.
8. Outcome.
   a. Surgically correctable.
   b. Good outcome; possible absence of sequelae.
   c. Cosmetically pleasing outcome.
   d. Multiple craniosynostoses associated with numerous syndromes.

G. **Birth injuries.**
1. Definition.
   a. Any injury that occurs during the entire phase of the birth process, comprising labor and delivery.
   b. Classification of the injury is anatomic or etiologic.
2. Risk factors.
   a. Abnormal labor time (long or short).
   b. Large size for gestational age.
   c. Cephalopelvic disproportion.
   d. Prematurity.
   e. Birth dystocia.
   f. Abnormal presentation (transverse, breech, face, and brow).
   g. Instrument-assisted extraction (vacuum or forceps).
3. Pathophysiology (see specific injury).
4. Incidence.
   a. Ranges from less than 2% of live births to about 6:1000 to 8:1000.
   b. Ranked eleventh in major causes of neonatal death (3.7 deaths per 100,000 live births) (Mangurten, 2002).
   c. Varies with specific injury.
5. Specific injuries.
   a. Cephalohematoma.
      (1) Pathophysiology.
         (a) Subperiosteal hemorrhage.
         (b) Does not extend across the cranial suture lines.
         (c) Usually unilateral.
      (2) Incidence approximates 0.4% to 2.5% of deliveries (Mangurten, 2002).
      (3) Clinical presentation.
         (a) Enlarges during the first few days after birth.
         (b) Feels firm.
         (c) Does not transilluminate.
      (4) Diagnostic evaluation.

(5) Patient care management.
  (a) Provide supportive care to the family and their baby.
  (b) Watch for hyperbilirubinemia.
  (c) If sudden enlargement occurs, question infection.
  (d) Educate the family.
  (e) Assess neurologic status.
(6) Outcome (Volpe, 2001).
  (a) Bony calcified ring may develop; usually disappears within 6 months.
  (b) Usually takes 2 weeks to 3 months for resolution.
  (c) Essentially all cases resolve.

b. Caput succedaneum.
(1) Pathophysiology.
  (a) Hemorrhagic edema crossing cranial suture lines.
  (b) Commonly seen after vaginal delivery.
(2) Clinical presentation.
  (a) Evident at birth.
  (b) Hemorrhagic scalp edema, causing discoloration at the site.
  (c) Does not grow in size after birth.
(3) Diagnostic evaluation.
(4) Patient care management.
  (a) No treatment is given.
  (b) Educate and counsel the family.
(5) Outcome: resolution occurs during first few days of life.

c. Subgaleal hemorrhage (Levene, 1999).
(1) Pathophysiology.
  (a) Hemorrhage beneath the scalp into the loose connective tissue below the aponeurotic membrane.
  (b) Possible entry of blood into the subcutaneous tissue of the neck.
  (c) Hematoma may cross suture lines in sufficient quantities to lead to exsanguination of the infant.
(2) Incidence.
  (a) 1:1250 deliveries and 1:150 vacuum-assisted deliveries.
  (b) Occurs much less often than caput succedaneum.
  (c) Usually associated with a difficult delivery requiring midforceps or vacuum extraction (Mangurten, 2002).
(3) Clinical presentation.
  (a) History of fetal distress noted in 50% of cases.
  (b) Often a fluctuant mass of the scalp.
  (c) May increase in size postnatally.
  (d) Hypotonia, pallor, lethargy, seizures.
  (e) Falling hematocrit levels.
(4) Diagnostic evaluation.
  (a) Palpate: hemorrhage crosses suture lines, is firm but fluctuant to palpation.
  (b) Vital signs: monitor for symptoms of shock.
  (c) Serial hematocrit levels.
  (d) Monitor bilirubin levels during recovery.
(5) Patient care management.
  (a) Rapid diagnosis and blood replacement is key to management.
    (i) Observe for signs/symptoms of shock/hypovolemia.

(ii) Monitor blood pressure, heart rate, and serial CBCs.
(iii) Management for supporting organs, such as kidney, if shock occurs.
(b) Infant may need blood transfusion on an emergent basis.
(c) Ensure that infant receives vitamin K promptly.
(d) Observe for hyperbilirubinemia.
(6) Outcome: once the infant has survived the acute phase, recovery occurs in 2 to 3 weeks (Volpe, 2001).

d. Skull fractures.
(1) Pathophysiology.
(a) Linear fracture can occur.
(b) Depressed fractures occur secondary to excessive force used with forceps and extreme molding.
(2) Incidence.
(a) Unknown.
(b) Linear fracture fairly common finding.
(c) Depressed fracture much less common than linear.
(3) Clinical presentation.
(a) Linear fracture: asymptomatic.
(b) Depressed fracture.
(i) Presents with depressed surface of skull; indented, without craniotabes.
(ii) Does not cross the suture lines.
(iii) Possible marked separation of adjacent sutures.
(iv) Most often occurs in right parietal bone.
(4) Diagnostic evaluation.
(a) X-ray examination.
(b) CT scan.
(5) Patient care management.
(a) Obtain neurosurgery consultation.
(b) Assess closely for neurologic deficits.
(c) If lesion is less than 2 cm and patient is without neurologic deficits, follow clinically; spontaneous resolution expected within a few weeks.
(6) Outcome.
(a) Linear fractures usually heal completely within 3 months.
(b) Depressed fracture outcome is dependent on degree of cerebral injury and success of therapy.

e. Brachial nerve plexus injuries (Hensinger and Jones, 1999).
(1) Pathophysiology.
(a) Excessive stretching of brachial plexus during delivery.
(b) Erb palsy, involving cervical nerves 5 and 6. Denervation of the deltoid, supraspinatus, biceps, and brachioradialis leads to upper arm paralysis.
(c) Klumpke paralysis, involving cervical nerve VI to thoracic nerve I. Denervation of the intrinsics of the hand, flexors of the wrist, fingers, and sympathetics (Horner syndrome) leads to lower arm paralysis.
(d) Combination of Erb-Duchenne-Klumpke paralysis, involving the entire arm from cervical nerve V to thoracic nerve I (entire arm paralyzed). Paralysis of the diaphragm will occur if injury involves cervical nerve IV.

(2) Incidence: .38 per 1000 live births.
(3) Risk factors.
  (a) Multiparous mother.
  (b) Prolonged labor.
  (c) Large size for gestational age.
  (d) Shoulder dystocia.
(4) Clinical presentation.
  (a) Erb palsy.
    (i) Affected arm is abducted and internally rotated.
    (ii) The elbow is extended, with arm pronation and wrist flexion (waiter's tip position).
    (iii) Asymmetric Moro reflex (absent in the affected arm), with a normal grasp.
  (b) Klumpke paralysis.
    (i) Swelling in shoulder and supraclavicular fossa; clavicle may be fractured.
    (ii) Involves intrinsic muscles of the hand, with a claw-hand deformity.
    (iii) No grasp in the affected hand.
  (c) Erb-Duchenne-Klumpke paralysis.
    (i) A combination of the above.
    (ii) Occurs more often than isolated Klumpke paralysis.
    (iii) Entire affected arm is flaccid.
    (iv) Moro and grasp reflexes are absent.
(5) Diagnostic evaluation.
  (a) Obtain x-ray examination of affected arm and shoulder.
  (b) Obtain serial electromyographic studies.
  (c) Rule out fracture of the clavicle or humerus.
  (d) Rule out shoulder dislocation.
  (e) Rule out cerebral injury.
(6) Patient care management.
  (a) Obtain neurology consultation.
  (b) Obtain serial electromyographic examinations to note improvements.
  (c) Primary goal: avoid contractures of involved joints:
    (i) Begin passive range of motion exercise, beginning after the swelling and inflammation subside.
    (ii) Exercise the arm with every diaper change.
    (iii) Request a physical therapy consultation (infant may be able to benefit from splints at some point).
    (iv) Educate the family about the importance of maintaining normal joint function.
      a. Reinnervated musculature needs supple joints.
      b. Will have wider choice of reconstructive procedures in the absence of contractures in the event there is no recovery.
(7) Outcome.
  (a) Generally spontaneous recovery occurs.
  (b) About 88% fully recover by 4 months, and 92% fully recover by 12 months (Volpe, 2001).
  (c) If no appreciable recovery is noted by 3 months, surgical exploration may be warranted (Volpe, 2001).

f. Phrenic nerve paralysis (Volpe, 2001).
  (1) Pathophysiology.
    (a) Diaphragmatic paralysis involving overstretching of cervical nerves III, IV, and V.
    (b) Results from torn nerve sheaths with edema and hemorrhage.
    (c) 80% to 90% occur in association with brachial plexus injury, but it may also occur in isolation.
  (2) Clinical presentation.
    (a) History of traumatic delivery, especially difficult breech delivery.
    (b) First hours after birth.
      (i) Respiratory distress with cyanosis, tachypnea, hypoxemia, hypercapnia, and acidosis.
      (ii) Diagnosis may be missed as the elevated hemidiaphragm may not be present early in the course, especially with use of positive pressure ventilation.
    (c) Next several days.
      (i) Improvement with oxygen and ventilatory support.
  (3) Diagnostic evaluation.
    (a) Chest x-ray examination may not be useful, especially if positive pressure ventilation is in use.
    (b) Ultrasonographic or fluoroscopic examination will show elevated hemidiaphragm and the paradoxical movement of the affected side with breathing.
    (c) Serial ultrasonography to evaluate diaphragmatic function.
  (4) Patient care management.
    (a) Administer oxygen and ventilatory support as needed.
    (b) Place the infant affected side down (splint the affected side).
    (c) Follow physical examination closely to note improvements.
    (d) Family education and support because prolonged ventilatory support may be required.
  (5) Outcome.
    (a) Mortality rate 10% to 15%.
    (b) Majority recover within the first 6 to 12 months.
    (c) Prolonged ventilatory support associated with 50% mortality rate.

g. Traumatic facial nerve palsy (Volpe, 2001).
  (1) Pathophysiology.
    (a) Trauma causes hemorrhage and edema into the nerve sheath, rather than a true disruption of the nerve fiber (Volpe, 2001).
    (b) Site of the lesion typically at or near the exit of the nerve from the stylomastoid foramen.
    (c) Weakness of the facial muscles results.
  (2) Incidence: Approximately 0.75% of term infants.
  (3) Clinical presentation.
    (a) Varies with the degree of nerve involvement.
    (b) Usually presents the first 2 days after birth.
    (c) Persistently open eye on the affected side.
    (d) Suck with drooling.
    (e) Mouth drawn to normal side during crying.
    (f) Corner of mouth does not pull down on affected side.
    (g) Eyeball may roll up behind open eyelid.
    (h) Usually does not increase in severity.

(4) Patient care management.
  (a) Artificial tears for the open eye.
  (b) Possible need to tape or patch affected eye to protect cornea.
  (c) Support of parents.
  (d) Necessary to watch for signs of improvement.
(5) Outcome.
  (a) High rate of spontaneous recovery by 7 to 10 days, especially between 1 and 3 weeks of age.
  (b) Detectable deficits rarely evident after several months.
  (c) For persistence beyond a few weeks, pediatric neurology referral (Goddard-Finegold et al., 1998).

INTRACRANIAL HEMORRHAGES

A. Subdural hemorrhage.

1. Definition (Hill and Volpe, 1999).
   - **a.** Due to laceration of the major veins and sinuses, usually associated with a tear of the dura overlying the cerebral hemispheres or cerebellum.
   - **b.** Occurs in both preterm and term neonates.
   - **c.** Occurrence with or without laceration of the dura.
2. Risk factors (Volpe, 2001).
   - **a.** Large fetal head in comparison with size of birth canal and with rigid pelvic structures.
   - **b.** Vaginal breech delivery.
   - **c.** Malpresentation (breech, face, brow, foot).
   - **d.** Skull is unusually compliant and/or pelvic structures unusually rigid.
   - **e.** Labora is either very short (not enough time for dilation) or too long (head subjected to prolonged compression/molding)
   - **f.** Forceps, vacuum extraction, or rotational maneuvers required to effect delivery.
3. Pathophysiology (Volpe, 2001).
   - **a.** Excessive vertical molding and frontal-occipital elongation, or oblique expansion of the head results in stretching of the falx and tentorium.
   - **b.** Venous sinuses are stretched, with possible rupture of the vein of Galen or cerebellar bridging veins.
   - **c.** Tear of the dura, including the falx or tentorium may also occur.
4. Incidence.
   - **a.** Uncommon occurrence, accounts for <10% of intracranial hemorrhages.
5. Clinical presentation.
   - **a.** Decreased level of consciousness.
   - **b.** Seizure activity.
   - **c.** Asymmetry of motor function.
   - **d.** Determined by the extent of associated hypoxic-ischemic encephalopathy injury.
   - **e.** Often minimal to no clinical symptoms for first 24 hours due to slowly enlarging hematoma.
   - **f.** On day 2 or 3: signs of increasing intracranial pressure due to block in CSF flow in posterior fossa.
     (1) Full fontanel, irritability, lethargy.
   - **g.** Signs of brainstem disturbance
     (1) Dilated, poorly reactive pupil on same side as the hemorrhage.
     (2) Respiratory abnormalities, facial paralysis.
     (3) Doll's eye reflex: normal to abnormal.

h. Chronic subdural effusion: present within the first 6 months of life with enlarging OFC.

6. Diagnostic evaluation.
   a. CT scan.
   b. MRI scan more effective if hemorrhage is in the posterior fossa.
   c. Skull radiographs demonstrate skull fractures.
7. Outcome.
   a. Major laceration of tentorium and falx with massive hemorrhage have poor prognosis.
   b. Mortality rate approximately 45%.
   c. Survivors develop hydrocephalus and other sequelae.
   d. Concomitant hypoxic-ischemic injury critical factor in determining outcome.

B. **Subarachnoid hemorrhage (primary)** (Hill and Volpe, 1999; Volpe, 2001).
1. Definition: an intracranial hemorrhage into the CSF-filled space between the arachnoid and pial membranes on the surface of the brain.
2. Pathophysiology.
   a. Bleeding of venous origin in the subarachnoid space due to rupture of small vessels in the leptomeningeal plexus or bridging veins in the subarachnoid space.
   b. Bleeding is not secondary to an extension of subdural hemorrhage, intraventicular hemorrhage, or cerebellar hemorrhage.
   c. Self-limited.
   d. May be precipitated by trauma (term infant) or hypoxia (preterm infant).
3. Incidence: common type of neonatal intracranial hemorrhage.
4. Clinical presentation.
   a. Most commonly no symptoms develop.
   b. Seizure activity may begin on day 2 of life, especially in the term infant.
   c. Infant looks healthy between seizures: "well baby with seizures" (Volpe, 2001).
   d. Recurrent apnea (more common in preterm infants).
5. Diagnostic evaluation.
   a. Diagnosis of exclusion. Other forms of intracranial bleeding are eliminated by CT scan.
   b. Lumbar puncture demonstrates uniformly blood-stained CSF.
6. Outcome.
   a. Sequelae very uncommon.
   b. 90% of term infants who exhibited seizures have normal follow-up.

C. **Intracerebellar hemorrhage.**
1. Definition: hemorrhage(s) within the cerebellum resulting from primary bleeding or extension of intraventricular or subarachnoid hemorrhage into the cerebellum.
2. Risk factors: association exists with respiratory distress, hypoxic events, prematurity, and traumatic delivery.
3. Pathophysiology.
   a. Intravascular, vascular, and extravascular factors (Volpe, 2001).
      (1) Breech presentation and difficult forceps delivery secondary to a compliant skull, with external pressure causing occipital pressure.
      (2) Vitamin K deficiency, thrombocytopenia.
      (3) Vulnerable cerebral capillaries exposed to rapid colloid infusion, causing hypertensive spikes.

(4) Richly vascularized subpial and subependymal locations.
(5) Poor vascular support for subependymal and subpial germinal matrices.
(6) Extension of blood into the cerebellum associated with:
(i) Large volume of blood present with IVH.
(ii) Increased intracranial pressure.
(iii) Incomplete myelination of the cerebellum.

4. Incidence (Volpe, 2001).
a. About 5% to 10% of neonatal deaths studied by autopsy.
b. Higher in preterm infants than in term.
c. Occurrence of 15% to 25% in premature infants born at less than 32 weeks' gestation or weighing less than 1.5 kg at birth.

5. Clinical presentation (Hill and Volpe, 1999).
a. May have a history of hypoxic-ischemic insult.
b. Catastrophic deterioration with apnea, bradycardia, decreasing hematocrit values and blood CSF may occur.
c. Signs appear within the first 3 weeks, most commonly within the first 2 days of life.
d. Term infants may have a history of difficult breech delivery.

6. Diagnostic evaluation.
a. Cranial ultrasonography (lack of symmetric echogenicity may be important).
b. CT scan necessary to define the hemorrhage.
c. MRI only if CT scan is unable to provide definitive diagnostic information.

7. Outcome.
a. More favorable in term infant than in premature infant.
b. Poor outcome in premature infant.
c. Probable neurologic deficits.

D. Periventricular-intraventricular hemorrhage (Volpe, 2001).

1. Definition.
a. Occurs once subependymal germinal matrix hemorrhage extends into lateral ventricles.
b. Most extensive periventricular-intraventricular hemorrhage is a parenchymal intracerebral hemorrhage (Papile, 1997).
(1) Involves bleeding into the periventricular (i.e., intracerebellar) white matter and may also precipitate cerebral infarction.
(2) Only 10% to 15% of infants with hemorrhages.
(3) With time, on follow-up scans, may see formation of porencephalic cyst at original hemorrhage site.
c. See Figure 33-4 for description and grading system.
(1) Small hemorrhage: grade I or II (Papile, 1997).
(2) Moderate hemorrhage: grade III (Papile, 1997).
(3) Severe hemorrhage: grade IV (Papile, 1997).

2. Risk factors.
a. Prematurity: birth at less than 34 weeks' gestation; respiratory failure requiring mechanical ventilation.
b. Associated with increasing arterial blood pressure and perinatal asphyxia.
c. Associated clinical factors (DeVries and Rennie, 1999).
(1) Maternal general anesthesia.
(2) Low 5-minute Apgar score.
(3) Asphyxia.

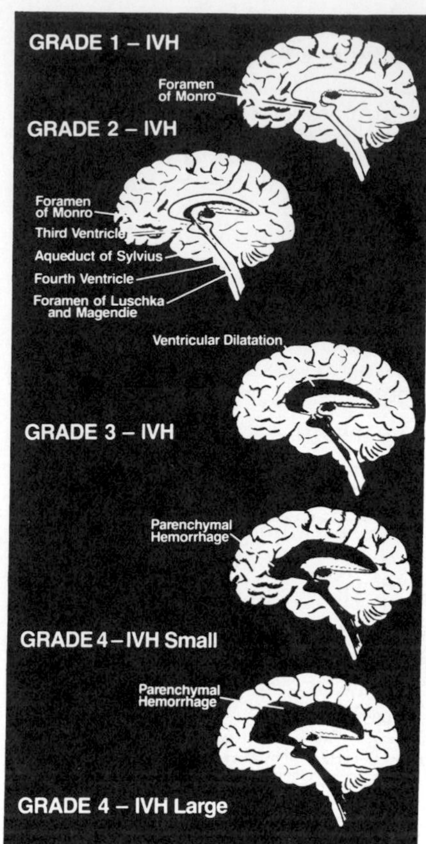

Grade I IVH: Subependymal hemorrhage in the Periventricular Germinal Matrix. Often localized at the Foramen of Monro.

Grade 2 IVH: Partial filling of lateral ventricles without ventricular dilatation.

Grade 3 IVH: Intraventricular hemorrhage with ventricular dilatation.

Grade 4 IVH (small and large): Parenchymal involvement or extension of blood into the cerebral tissue itself. Can be present to a lesser degree.

Correlation between the severity or extent of involvement and subsequent impairment is not absolute. Because outcomes are so varied, assessment of early symptoms and the practice of purposeful interventions are extremely important.

FIGURE 33-4 ■ Quantification of extent of intraventricular hemorrhage (IVH). Four grades of hemorrhagic involvement categorized IVH as differentiated by Papile and Burstein. (From Ross Laboratories: *New perspectives on intraventricular hemorrhage,* Columbus, OH, 1988, Ross Laboratories.)

(4) Low birth weight.
(5) Acidosis.
(6) Hypotension or hypertension.
(7) Low hematocrit.
(8) Respiratory distress requiring mechanical ventilation.
(9) Rapid administration of sodium bicarbonate.
(10) Rapid volume expansion.
(11) Infusion of hyperosmolar solution.
(12) Coagulopathy.
(13) Pneumothorax.
(14) Ligation of patent ductus arteriosus.
(15) Transport.

3. Pathophysiology.
   a. Occurs once subependymal germinal matrix hemorrhage extends into lateral ventricles.
   b. Most extensive periventricular-intraventricular hemorrhage is a parenchymal intracerebral hemorrhage (Papile, 1997).
      (1) Involves bleeding into the periventricular (i.e., intracerebellar white matter and may also precipitate cerebral infarction).

(2) Only 10% to 15% of infants with hemorrhages.
(3) With time, on follow-up scans, may see formation of porencephalic cysts at original hemorrhage site.

4. Incidence.

a. Occurs in 30% to 40% of infants weighing <1500 grams or approximately 30 weeks' gestation (Rutherford, 2002).

b. Infants born at less than 28 weeks' gestation have three times higher risk than infants born at 28 to 31 weeks' gestation (Sheth, 1998).

c. Only 2% to 3% normal term infants have a periventricular-intraventricular hemorrhage.
(1) More than half of these hemorrhages originated at the subependymal germinal matrix.
(2) The remainder originated at the choroid plexus.
(3) Timing of onset (Volpe, 2001).
(a) About 50% occur by 24 hours of age.
(b) About 80% occur by 48 hours of age.
(c) About 90% occur by 72 hours of age.
(d) By 7 days of age, 99.5% have occurred.
(e) 20% to 40% exhibit progression of the hemorrhage over 3 to 5 days.

5. Clinical presentation.

a. Presentation ranges from unnoticeable to dramatic.
(1) Sudden deterioration.
(2) Oxygen desaturation.
(3) Bradycardia.
(4) Metabolic acidosis.
(5) Significant decrease in hematocrit.
(6) Hypotonia.
(7) Shock.
(8) Hyperglycemia.
(9) Tense anterior fontanelle.

b. Symptoms of worsening hemorrhage.
(1) Full, tense fontanelles.
(2) Increased ventilatory support.
(3) Seizure activity.
(4) Apnea.
(5) Decrease in level of consciousness and/or activity.

6. Diagnostic evaluation.

a. Optimal time to screen: 7 days of age because >90% of all hemorrhages have occurred.
(1) If test result is normal, there is no need to recheck.
(2) If test result is positive for periventricular-intraventricular hemorrhage, repeat test in 2 weeks.

b. Serial cranial ultrasonography replaces CT as the principle diagnostic technique.

c. Lumbar puncture (CSF studies show elevated red blood cells, increased protein concentration, xanthochromia, and decreased glucose concentration).

d. Rule out septic shock or meningitis.

7. Patient care management.

a. Prevent preterm birth, perinatal asphyxia, and birth trauma.

b. Promote in utero transport.

c. Promote nonstressful intrapartum course.

d. Provide efficient, expedient intubation.

e. Appropriate handling; minimal stimulation with clustering of care activities as tolerated.
f. Minimize noxious stimuli (dim the lights, quiet the environment).
g. Avoid noxious procedures when possible.
h. Avoid events associated with wide swings in arterial and venous pressures.
   (1) Seizures.
   (2) Excess motor activity.
   (3) Apnea.
   (4) Crying.
   (5) Pneumothorax.
i. Avoid administration of hyperosmolar solutions.
j. Prevent blood pressure swings: give volume replacement slowly.
k. Avoid overventilation leading to pneumothorax.
l. Use two people for endotracheal suctioning.
m. Use noninvasive monitoring of oxygen and carbon dioxide levels (maintain within normal limits).
n. Monitor and maintain normal pH.
o. Correct abnormal clotting.
p. Be alert to signs of a hemorrhage.
q. Educate and support the parents.

8. Outcome.
   a. Mortality rate is 50% with severe hemorrhage, 15% with moderate hemorrhage, and 5% with small hemorrhage.
   b. These hemorrhages are an important cause of morbidity and death in low birth weight infants.
   c. Hemorrhage alone does not account for all neurologic deficits.
   d. Approximately 50% of premature infants are free of neurologic symptoms.
   e. Approximately 25% to 30% of very low birth weight infants discharged from a level III neonatal intensive care unit (NICU) have a periventricular-intraventricular hemorrhage without major neurodevelopmental sequelae.
   f. Outcome depends on degree of severity of hemorrhage (Hill and Volpe, 1999; Volpe, 2001.)
      (1) Small hemorrhage.
         (a) Neurodevelopmental disability similar to that in premature infants without hemorrhage.
         (b) Major neurodevelopmental disability in 10%.
      (2) Moderate hemorrhage.
         (a) Major neurodevelopmental disability in 40% during infancy.
         (b) Mortality rate 10%, with progressive hydrocephalus in less than 20%.
      (3) Severe hemorrhage.
         (a) Major neurodevelopmental disability in 80%.
         (b) Mortality rate 50% to 60%, with hydrocephalus common in survivors.

SEIZURES (Hill and Volpe, 1999; Rennie, 1999A)

A. **Definition:** symptom of neurologic dysfunction (not a disease).

B. **Risk factors.**
   1. Metabolic encephalopathies.
      a. Decreased production of adenosine triphosphate.

(1) Ischemia.
(2) Hypoxemia.
(3) Hypoglycemia.

b. Hyponatremia or hypernatremia.
c. Hypocalcemia, hypomagnesemia.
d. Inborn errors of metabolism.
e. Pyridoxine dependency.
f. Hyperammonemia.

2. Structural.
a. IVH.
b. Intrapartum trauma.
c. Cerebral cortical dysgenesis: result of abnormal neuronal migration.
d. Hypoxic-ischemic encephalopathy, the most common diagnosis of neonatal seizures.

3. Intracerebral meningitis.
a. Bacterial infection.
(1) Group B beta-streptococci and *Escherichia coli:* 65% of cases.
(2) *Listeria monocytogenes.*
b. Nonbacterial infection: TORCH.

4. Withdrawal from maternal drugs.
a. Uncommon cause of seizures (may cause jitteriness).
b. Onset during first 3 days of life.
c. Drugs.
(1) Narcotic-analgesics.
(2) Sedative-hypnotics.
(3) Alcohol.

5. Familial (genetic).
a. Onset in second and third days of life.
b. Infant appears well between seizures.
c. Self-limiting: within 1 to 6 months, seizures stop.
d. Autosomal dominant inheritance.

C. Pathophysiology: seizures result from excessive simultaneous electrical discharge or depolarization of neurons.

D. Incidence (Rennie, 1999a).
1. 6% to 13% of very low birth weight infants.
2. 1 to 2 per 1000 term infants.

E. Clinical presentation.
1. Subtle.
a. Most frequent of neonatal seizures.
b. Present at some degree in most term and premature newborn infants having seizures.
c. Often unrecognized.
d. Presentation varies.
(1) Horizontal deviation of the eyes.
(2) Pedaling movements.
(3) Rowing, stepping movements.
(4) Eye blinking or fluttering.
(5) Nonnutritive sucking.
(6) Smacking of lips.
(7) Drooling.
(8) Apnea (convulsive apnea usually does not occur by itself).

2. Tonic.
   a. Characteristic in premature infants weighing ≤500 g.
   b. Often seen with severe IVH.
   c. Generalized tonic extension of all extremities or flexion of upper limbs with extension of lower extremities.
   d. Often mimics decorticate posturing.
3. Multifocal clonic.
   a. Characteristic in term infants with hypoxic-ischemic encephalopathy.
   b. Clonic movements migrating from one limb to another without a specific pattern.
4. Focal clonic.
   a. Uncommon.
   b. Presents as localized clonic jerking.
5. Myoclonic.
   a. Very rare in neonatal period.
   b. Multiple jerks of upper or lower limb flexion.

F. Diagnostic evaluation.
1. Perform physical examination.
   a. Rule out jitteriness.
      (1) Characterized by trembling of hands and feet.
      (2) No involvement of eye movements.
      (3) Stopped by gentle, passive flexion of affected extremity.
   b. Note infant's history, which may provide a predisposed underlying etiology.
2. Laboratory work.
   a. Serum glucose level.
   b. Electrolyte levels (sodium, potassium, chloride, calcium, magnesium).
   c. Arterial blood gas analysis.
   d. Urea, ammonia.
3. Diagnostic study for sepsis.
   a. Lumbar puncture.
   b. Culture of blood, urine, and CSF specimens; bacterial and viral.
   c. Complete blood cell count and platelet count.
4. Electroencephalography, CT scan, cranial ultrasonography, MRI.
5. Skull films if etiology is trauma.
6. 12-lead electrocardiography.
7. Consideration of following laboratory tests:
   a. Blood pyruvate.
   b. Lactate.
   c. TORCH.
   d. Urinary drug screen.
8. Neurology consultation.

G. Patient care management.
1. Determine underlying etiology.
2. Resuscitate as necessary.
3. Obtain diagnostic studies as ordered.
4. Provide pharmaceutical therapy (Young and Mangum, 2003).
   a. Phenobarbital.
      (1) Load: 20 mg/kg slow IV for 10 to 15 minutes.
      (2) Close monitoring of respiratory status.

(3) Maintenance dosage: 3 mg/kg/day, beginning 12 to 24 hours after the loading dose.
(4) Therapeutic range: 15 to 30 μg/ml.
(5) Excretion.
(a) Metabolized by liver: 50% to 70%.
(b) Unchanged in urine: 20% to 30%.
(6) Consider as the drug of choice (Young and Mangum, 2003).

b. Phenytoin. Many facilities are replacing phenytoin with fosphenytoin. Check with your physician or pharmacist.
(1) Load: 15 to 20 mg/kg IV (for 30 min or longer).
(2) Maintenance dosage: 4 to 8 mg/kg/day.
(3) Recommended administration routes, by slow IV push or by mouth.
(4) Therapeutic range: 6 to 15 μg/cc in the first weeks, then 10 to 20 μg/cc due to changes in protein binding. First trough should be obtained 48 hours after the IV loading dose.
(5) Excretion.
(a) Protein bound (approximately 90%).
(b) Displaced by bilirubin, increasing free drug levels.

c. Fosphenytoin (Young and Mangum, 2003).
(1) Load: 15 to 20 mg PE/kg IV over at least 10 minutes [PE = phenytoin equivalents; Fosphenytoin 1 mg PE = phenytoin 1 mg]. Continuous electrocardiographic, blood pressure, and respiratory monitoring with loading doses.
(2) Maintenance.
(a) Dosage: 4 to 8 mg PE/kg/day.
(b) Rate of administration: up to 1.5 mg PE/kg/minute.
(c) Flush the IV with saline before and after administration.
(d) Term infants > 1 week of age may need up to 8 mg PE/kg per dose every 8 to 12 hours.
(e) Therapeutic range and excretion. See section (b) Phenytoin, above.
(i) Peak plasma concentrations: about the time that the IV infusion is complete; half-life is 4 to 10 minutes.
(ii) Rapidly converted by the body to generate therapeutic levels of phenytoin.

d. Lorazepam.
(1) Administer: 0.05 to 0.1 mg/kg slow push IV (for status epilepticus).
(2) Repeat dose based on clinical response.
(3) Note routes of excretion.
(a) By kidneys.
(b) Lipid soluble.
(4) Lorazepam produces anticonvulsant effect in minutes after administration.
(5) Monitor oxygenation and vital signs.
(6) Document precisely.
(7) Educate and inform the family.
(8) Provide support as needed.

H. Outcome.

1. Related to underlying etiology.

2. Refer to Table 33-4.

TABLE 33-4
Prognosis for Infant with Neonatal Seizures: Relation to Neurologic Disease

Neurologic Disease*	Normal Development†
Hypoxic-ischemic encephalopathy	50
Intraventricular hemorrhage‡	10
Primary subarachnoid hemorrhage	90
Hypocalcemia	
Early onset	50§
Later onset	100
Hypoglycemia	50
Bacterial meningitis	50
Developmental defect	0

*Prognosis is for those cases with the stated neurologic disease when seizures are a manifestation (thus value usually will differ from *overall* prognosis for the disease).
†Values are rounded off to nearest 5%.
‡Usually severe intraventricular hemorrhage associated with major periventricular hemorrhagic infarction.
§Represents primarily the prognosis of complicating illness; prognosis approaches that of later-onset hypocalcemia if no or only minor neurologic illness is present.
From Volpe, J.J.: *Neurology of the newborn* (3rd ed.). Philadelphia, 1995, W.B. Saunders.

HYPOXIC-ISCHEMIC ENCEPHALOPATHY

A. Definition of hypoxic-ischemic encephalopathy (HIE).
1. Hypoxemia and anoxia (diminished oxygen in blood supply; partial or complete). Moderate to severe hypoxia leads to metabolic acidosis.
2. Ischemia (diminished blood supply perfusing the brain).
   a. Systemic hypotension.
   b. Occlusive vascular disease.
3. Hypoxia and ischemia, which lead to neurologic dysfunction.
4. Asphyxia.
   a. Impairment of gas exchange of respiratory gases—oxygen and carbon dioxide.
   b. Mixed respiratory and metabolic acidosis.
   c. Failure of systemic multiorgan systems, including heart, lungs, liver, and kidneys.

B. Incidence of HIE (Volpe, 2001).
1. About 2% to 4% of term infants.
2. Approximately 60% of very low birth weight infants.
3. Timing of occurrence.
   a. Antepartum occurrence: 20%.
   b. Intrapartum occurrence: 30%.
   c. Antepartum-intrapartum occurrence: 35%.
   d. Postpartum occurrence: 10%.

C. Clinical presentation and staging (Hill and Volpe, 1999; Volpe, 2001).
1. Stage I (mild encephalopathy): characteristic features.
   a. Hyperalert state.
   b. Normal muscle tone, active suck, strong Moro reflex, normal/strong grasp, and normal doll's-eye reflex.
   c. Increased tendon reflexes.
   d. Myoclonus present.

e. Hyperresponsiveness to stimulation.
f. Tachycardia possible.
g. Dilation of pupils, reactive.
h. Sparse secretions.
i. No convulsions (unless due to hypoglycemia or preexisting conditions that predisposed the infant to the perinatal distress).
j. Electroencephalographic findings: within normal limits.

2. Stage II (moderate encephalopathy).
a. Characteristic features.
(1) Lethargy.
(2) Hypotonia.
(3) Increased tendon reflexes.
(4) Myoclonus.
(5) Seizure activity frequent.
(6) Weak suck.
(7) Incomplete Moro reflex.
(8) Strong grasp.
(9) Overactive doll's-eye reflex.
(10) Pupils constrictive and reactive.
(11) Respirations variable in rate and depth; respirations may be periodic.
b. Critical period: infant's condition either improves or deteriorates.
c. Indications of deterioration.
(1) No signs of improvement.
(2) Development of:
(i) Seizures.
(ii) Cerebral edema.
(iii) Lethargy.
(iv) Abnormalities on electroencephalogram.
d. Recovery.
(1) No further seizure activity.
(2) Electroencephalographic findings return to normal.
(3) Transient jitteriness.
(4) Improvement in level of consciousness.

3. Stage III (severe encephalopathy).
a. Clinical course.
(1) Level of consciousness deteriorates from obtunded to stuporous to comatose.
(2) Mechanical ventilation is required to sustain life.
b. Clinical features.
(1) Apnea/bradycardia.
(2) Seizures appearing within the first 12 postnatal hours. Seizures occur in 50% to 60% of patients who do ultimately seize within the first 6 to 12 hours. Premature infants present with generalized seizures. Term infants demonstrate multifocal clonic seizures. All these infants display subtle seizures (Volpe, 2001).
(3) Severe hypotonia and flaccidity; suck, Moro, and grasp reflexes absent.
(4) Stuporous to comatose.
(5) Absent or depressed reflexes.
(6) Doll's-eye reflex weak or absent.
(7) Pupils often unequal; variable reactivity and poor light reflex.

c. Deterioration (Volpe, 2001).
   (1) Deterioration occurs within 24 to 72 hours.
   (2) Severely affected infants often worsen, sinking into deep stupor or coma.
   (3) Death may ensue.
d. Survivors.
   (1) Infants who survive to this point often improve in the next several days to months.
   (2) Feeding difficulties often develop secondary to abnormalities of suck and swallow. These are due to the poor muscle tone connected to involvement of cranial nerves for these functions.
   (3) Generalized hypotonia is common; hypertonia is uncommon.
   (4) Severe neurologic disabilities may ensue.

D. Diagnostic studies (Hill and Volpe, 1999; Volpe, 2001).

1. Valuable in assessing the nature of the brain insult and the extent of the brain injury.
2. Used to track the evolution of HIE.
   a. Precise history.
   b. Complete neurologic examination.
   c. Electroencephalography.
      (1) Confirm or deny clinical diagnosis of seizures.
      (2) Provide prognostic information regarding severity of permanent brain damage.
   d. Evoked potentials.
   e. Creatinine kinase and other biochemical/enzyme markers.
   f. Lumbar puncture, CSF analysis.
   g. CT scan.
   h. Cranial ultrasonography.
   i. Technetium scan.
   j. MRI.
   k. Intracranial pressure monitoring.

E. Patient care management.

1. Prevent perinatal hypoxia, ischemia, and asphyxia (anticipation of risk factors, appropriate intervention).
2. Perform prompt, efficient resuscitation by trained staff.
3. Maintain physiologic oxygenation and acid-base balance.
4. Correct fluid, electrolyte, and caloric abnormalities.
5. Monitor blood volume; avoid blood pressure swings and hypotension.
6. Maintain optimal perfusion.
7. Treat seizures.
8. Consider cerebral hypothermia (Gunn and Bennett, 2002).
9. Perform a thorough neurologic examination.
10. Monitor and manage disturbances of other body organs.
    a. Pulmonary.
    b. Cardiac.
    c. Hepatic.
    d. Renal.
11. Educate and support the family.
12. Obtain neurology consultation.

F. Outcome (Volpe, 2001).

1. Based on severity of brain insult; selective neuronal necrosis.
2. Death within newborn period in 20% to 50% of asphyxiated infants who exhibit HIE.

3. Overall neurologic sequelae with HIE at 3½ years of age: approximately 17%.
4. Factors associated with poor outcome.
   a. Apgar score.
      (1) If score is 0 to 3 for 20 minutes or more, approximately 60% die.
      (2) If score is less than 3 at 1 minute and less than 5 at 5 minutes, with abnormal neurologic signs (feeding difficulties, apnea, hypotonia, seizures):
         (a) About 20% die.
         (b) About 40% are normal.
         (c) About 40% have neurologic sequelae.
   b. Encephalopathy.
      (1) Mild: no subsequent deficits.
      (2) Severe: 75% die, 25% have sequelae.
      (3) Term infants: 60% normal, 30% abnormal, and 10% die.
      (4) Premature infants: 50% normal, 20% abnormal, and 30% die.
      (5) Duration of abnormal neurologic signs: good indicator of severity of HIE injury.
      (6) Disappearance of abnormal neurologic signs by 1 to 2 weeks: good chance of being normal (possibility of learning disabilities not ruled out).
5. Seizures early (first 12 hours of life) and/or difficult to control: associated with poorer prognosis.
6. Hyperactivity and attention difficulties: in infants with less severe encephalopathy.
7. Rapid initial improvement indicative of better outcomes.
8. Long-term sequelae based on:
   a. Site.
   b. Extent of cerebral injury.
   c. Duration of abnormal clinical presentation.

PERIVENTRICULAR LEUKOMALACIA (DeVries and Rennie, 1999; Hill and Volpe, 1999; Volpe, 2001)

A. Definition of periventricular leukomalacia (PVL).
1. Ischemic, necrotic periventricular white matter.
2. Principally ischemic lesion of arterial origin.
3. Multicystic encephalomalacia with or without secondary hemorrhage into ischemic area.

B. Pathophysiology.
1. Predisposition.
   a. Systemic hypotension severe enough to impair cerebral blood flow.
   b. Occurrence of focal cerebral infarction and cerebral ischemia.
   c. Major systemic hypotension.
   d. Episodes of apnea and bradycardia.
2. Occurrence secondary to inadequate cerebral perfusion.
3. Manifestation of hypoxic-ischemic encephalopathy in premature infants.

C. Incidence.
1. Unknown.
2. Approximately 3% to 10% of those with bilateral cystic leukomalacia.
3. Increases to approximately 26% if non-cystic PVL is included.

D. Clinical presentation.
1. Acute phase: hypotension and lethargy
2. 6 to 10 weeks later characteristic picture:
   a. Irritable, hypertonic, increased flexion of arms and extension of legs.
   b. Frequent tremors and startles.
   c. Moro reflex may be abnormal.

E. Diagnostic evaluation.
1. Cranial ultrasonography.
2. CT scan.
3. MRI.

F. Outcome.
1. Spastic dysplegia (major motor deficit common in premature infants with PVL).
2. Motor deficits in premature infants; possible spontaneous resolution in first several years of life.
3. Significant upper arm involvement associated with intellectual deficits.
4. Visual impairment.
5. Lower limb weakness.
6. Outcome based on:
   a. Location.
   b. Extent of injury.

MENINGITIS

A. Definition.
1. Infection of central nervous system (CNS).
2. Early-onset infection from pathogens in vaginal flora (e.g., group B beta-streptococci and *Escherichia coli*).
3. Late-onset infection from environmental microbes found in nursery environment (e.g., *Pseudomonas aeruginosa* and *Staphylococcus aureus*).

B. Risk factors.
1. Maternal infection.
2. Prolonged ruptured membranes.
3. Prematurity.

C. Pathophysiology.
1. Organisms reach the fetus or newborn.
   a. Transplacental organisms lead to congenital infection.
   b. Ascending organisms from the vagina or cervix lead to early-onset infection.
   c. Late-onset infection develops in infants infected by passage through birth canal.
   d. Organism introduction after birth from surrounding environment leads to iatrogenic infection.
2. Organisms.
   a. Bacteria.
      (1) Aerobic.
         (a) Group B beta-streptococci (most common).
         (b) *E. coli* (second most common).
         (c) *Listeria monocytogenes* (third most common).
      (2) Anaerobic.
   b. Viruses.
      (1) TORCH infection.
      (2) Enterovirus.
   c. Fungi.

D. Clinical presentation.
1. Congenital viral infection.
   a. Preterm delivery.
   b. Possible low birth weight.
   c. Blueberry muffin rash.
   d. Inflammation of other affected organs.
   e. Microcephaly.
2. Early-onset bacterial meningitis.
   a. Presentation with shock in first 24 hours.
   b. Possible rapid progression to shock.
   c. Respiratory distress.
   d. Hypotension.
   e. Apnea.
   f. Seizures.
   g. Temperature instability.
   h. Diarrhea.
   i. Hepatomegaly.
   j. Jaundice.
3. Late-onset meningitis.
   a. Nonspecific symptoms.
   b. Lethargy.
   c. Feeding intolerance.
   d. Irritability.
   e. Posturing.
   f. Temperature instability.
   g. Apnea.
   h. Bradycardia.
   i. Bulging fontanelles.
   j. Nuchal rigidity.

E. Diagnostic evaluation.
1. CSF.
   a. Organism found on Gram stain.
   b. Low glucose level.
   c. Elevated protein concentration and white blood cell count.
   d. Culture for specific identification of organism.
   e. Counterimmune electrophoresis.
2. Complete diagnostic study for sepsis.

F. Patient care management.
1. Promote prevention.
2. Detect early and treat.
3. Perform thorough physical examination.
4. Observe for seizure activity.
5. Obtain infectious disease consultation.
6. Provide pharmaceutical agents (Nelson, 1996).
   a. Initial therapy.
      (1) Ampicillin or penicillin G (IV).
      (2) *In addition*, aminoglycoside (IV or IM).
      (3) Ampicillin and cefotaxime recommended for aminoglycoside-resistant organism.
      (4) Treatment 7 to 10 days for sepsis without a focus; minimum of 21 days for gram-negative meningitis.

b. Group B beta-streptococci.
(1) Ampicillin or penicillin G (IV or IM).
(2) *In addition:* gentamicin (IV or IM) (discontinue if sensitivities warrant).

c. Coliform bacteria (e.g., *E. coli*).
(1) Cefotaxime (IM or IV).
(2) *In addition,* aminoglycoside as a suitable alternative.

d. *L. monocytogenes* and enterococci.
(1) Ampicillin (IV or IM).
(2) *In addition,* aminoglycoside (IV or IM).

e. *Staphylococcus epidermidis.*
(1) Vancomycin (IV or IM).
(2) Methicillin resistance in many strains.

f. *S. aureus.*
(1) Methicillin (IV or IM).
(2) Vancomycin if methicillin-resistant strain.
(3) Rarely cause of meningitis in the newborn infant (vancomycin for meningitis).

g. *P. aeruginosa.*
(1) Mezlocillin or ticarcillin (IV or IM).
(2) *In addition,* aminoglycoside (IV or IM).

h. Bacteroides fragilis (anaerobic).
(1) Metronidazole, clindamycin, mezlocillin, or ticarcillin (IV or IM).
(2) For CNS infection, metronidazole recommended.

7. Sample CSF at specific intervals until sterile.
8. Treat at least 2 weeks after sterilization of CSF.
9. Obtain and test CSF sample 48 hours after antibiotic therapy has been discontinued.
10. Educate and support the family.

G. Outcome.

1. Dependent on rapidity of detection and initiation of adequate drug therapy.
2. Survivors of bacterial meningitis: 50% have significant neurologic sequelae.
a. Hydrocephalus.
b. Seizures.
c. Sensorineural hearing loss.
d. Visual losses.
e. Mental and motor disabilities.

REFERENCES

Ashwal, S.: Congenital structural defects. In Swaiman, KF and Ashwal, S. (Eds). *Pediatric neurology: Principles and practice,* (3rd ed.). St Louis, 1999, Mosby, pp. 234-300.

Bondurant, C.P. and Jimenez, D.F. Epidemiology of cerebrospinal fluid shunting. *Pediatric Neurosurgery, 23*(5): 254-258, 1995.

DeMyer, W. Microcephaly, micrencephaly, megalocephaly and megalencephaly. In K.F. Swaiman and S. Ashwal (Eds). *Pediatric neurology: Principles and practice* (3rd ed.) St Louis, 1999, Mosby, pp. 301-311.

DeVries S.L. and Rennie, J.M.: In J.M. Rennie and N.R.C. Roberton (Eds.). *Textbook of neonatology* (3rd ed.). Edinburgh, 1999, Churchill Livingstone, pp. 1252-1271.

Goddard-Finegold, J.: The intrauterine nervous system. In W.H. Taeusch and R.A. Ballard (Eds). *Avery's diseases of the newborn,* (7th ed.). Philadelphia, 1998, W.B. Saunders, pp. 802-832.

Goddard-Finegold, J., Mizrahi, E.M., and Lee, R.T.: The newborn nervous system. In W.H. Taeusch and R.A. Ballard (Eds.). *Avery's diseases of the newborn,* (7th ed.). Philadelphia, 1998, W.B. Saunders, pp. 839-891.

Gunn, A.J. and Bennett, L.: Cerebral hypothermia in the management of hypoxic-ischemic encephalopathy. *NeoReviews, 3*(6):e116-122, 2002.

Hensinger, R.N. and Jones, E.T.: Orthopaedic Problems in the Newborn. In J.M. Rennie and N.R.C. Roberton (Eds.). *Textbook of neonatology* (3rd ed.). Edinburgh, 1999, Churchill Livingstone, pp. 1063-1088.

Hill, A. and Volpe, J.J.: Neurological and neuromuscular disorders. In G.A. Avery., M.A. Fletcher, and M.G. MacDonald. (Eds.). *Neonatalogy: Pathophysiology and management of the newborn* (5th ed.). Philadelphia, 1999, J.B. Lippincott, pp. 1231-1252.

Levene M.I.: Intracranial haemorrhage at term. In J.M. Rennie and N.R.C. Roberton (Eds). *Textbook of Neonatology* (3rd ed). Edinburgh, 1999, Churchill Livingstone, pp. 1223-1231.

Madsen J.R. and Frim, A.M.: Neurosurgery of the newborn. In G.A. Avery, M.A. Fletcher and M.G. MacDonald (Eds.). *Neonatalogy: Pathophysiology and management of the newborn* (5th ed.). Philadelphia, 1999, J.B. Lippincott, pp. 1213-1268.

Mangurten H.H. Birth injuries. In A.A. Fanaroff and R.J. Martin (Eds.). *Neonatal-perinatal medicine: Diseases of the fetus and infant* (7th ed.). St. Louis, 2002, Mosby, pp. 425-454.

Moore, K.L. and Persaud, T.V.N.: The neurological system. In K.L. Moore and T.V.N. Persaud (Eds.). *The developing human: clinically oriented embryology* (7th ed.). Philadelphia, 2003, W.B. Saunders, pp. 427-463.

Nelson, J.D. Pocketbook of Pediatric Antimicrobial Therapy (12th ed.), Baltimore, 1996, Williams & Wilkins.

Papile L. Intracranial hemorrhage. In A.A. Fanaroff and R.J. Martin (Eds). *Neonatal-Perinatal medicine: Diseases of the fetus and infant.* (6th ed.). St Louis, 1997, Mosby, pp. 891-899.

Rennie, J.M.: Assessment of the neonatal nervous system. In J.M Rennie and N.R.C. Roberton (Eds.). *Textbook of neonatology* (3rd ed). Edinburgh, 1999, Churchill Livingstone, pp. 1203-1213.

Rennie, J.M. Seizures in the newborn. In J.M. Rennie and N.R.C. Roberton (Eds.). *Textbook of neonatology* (3rd ed). Edinburgh, 1999a, Churchill Livingstone, pp. 1213-1223.

Rutherford M.A. Hemorrhagic lesions of the newborn brain. In M. Rutherford (Ed.). *MRI of the neonatal brain.* London, 2002, W.B. Saunders, pp. 171-200.

Sheth R.D.. Frequency of neurologic disorders in the neonatal intensive care unit. *Journal of Child Neurology,* 13(9):424-428, 1998.

Sun P.P. and Persing, J.A.. Craniosynostosis. In A.L. Albright, I.F. Pollach, and P.D. Adelson (Eds.). *Principles and practice of pediatric neurosurgery.* New York, 1999, Theime Medical Publishers Inc., pp. 219-242.

Szymonowicz, W., Walker, A.M., Yu, V.Y., et al.: Regional cerebral blood flow after hemorrhagic hypertension in the preterm, near-term, and newborn neonatal lamb. *Pediatric Research, 28*(4):361-366, 1990.

Wong D.L. *Whaley & Wong's nursing care of infants and children,* (6th ed.). St. Louis, 1999, Mosby.

Volpe, J.J. *Neurology of the newborn* (4th ed.). Philadelphia, 2001, W.B. Saunders.

Young, T.E. and Mangum, B. *Neofax* (16th ed.). Raleigh, 2003, Acorn Publishing, Inc.

CHAPTER

34 Congenital Anomalies

LEANN STERK

OBJECTIVES

1. Describe assessment strategies for diagnosis of infants experiencing a congenital defect.
2. Identify methods of initial management and care for individual congenital anomalies.
3. List possible causative factors that result in common congenital abnormalities.
4. Verbalize the importance of parental involvement on the development of infants affected with congenital anomalies.

Throughout gestation the fetus negotiates through genetic, metabolic, mechanical, chemical, and environmental forces. The interaction of one or more of these forces can result in the development of a congenital anomaly.

This chapter presents information concerning incidence, etiology, clinical presentation, and treatment modalities for common congenital abnormalities.

A congenital abnormality is defined as an alteration of normal anatomic structure that is present at birth (McClean, 1999) (Box 34-1).

A. Incidence of occurrence.

1. Congenital anomalies account for greater than 20% of infant deaths in North America (Moore et al., 2000). These defects can present as single or multiple defects, all with varying clinical significance.
2. Incidence of major malformations present at birth is estimated at 2% to 3% (McLean, 1999). This suggests that occult anomalies eventually detected by midchildhood raise the cumulative incidence to 5% to 6%.
3. Moore and colleagues (2000) relate that single minor abnormalities occur in approximately 14% of all newborns.
4. 90% of infants that have three or more minor anomalies will also have one or more major defects (Moore et al., 2000).

B. Factors influencing the development of congenital anomalies.

1. The fundamental cause of nearly half of all birth defects is unknown (McLean, 1999).
2. Anomalies for which a cause has been identified fall into three main categories
   a. Chromosomal abnormalities
      (1) Account for 6% to 7% of all anomalies (Moore et al., 2000).
      (2) Abnormal karyotypes are identified in 1 of 170 live-born infants (McLean, 1999).
      (3) Chromosomal aberrations result in defective zygotes, blastocysts, and early embryos, which are usually spontaneously aborted in the first weeks of pregnancy.
      (4) Chromosomal abnormalities occur secondary to numerical or structural changes in chromosomes.

(5) Both sex chromosomes and/or autosomes may be affected.
(6) Numerical defects result in characteristic phenotypic expression (Moore et al., 2000), e.g., Down syndrome.

b. Environmental factors.
(1) Dosage and the timing of exposure within the pregnancy determine effects of known teratogens on the fetus.
(a) During blastocyst formation exposure to a teratogen will likely end in spontaneous abortion and fetal death. (Cole, 2001).
(b) The fetus is most vulnerable to the effects of teratogens during organogenesis. Structural defects are the most common result.
(c) Later exposure may have little or no effect.
(2) Majority of teratogens act by interfering with cellular metabolic activity. The end result is cell death, failure in replication, migration, or fusion of cells (Cole, 2001).
(3) Known teratogenic agents including medications, alcohol, radiation, and infections, as well as disease states such as diabetes mellitus.

c. Multifactorial disorders.
(1) Anomalies result as a combination of genetic and environmental factors. In order for an abnormality to be expressed a threshold of traits must be exceeded.
(a) Disorders are familial, but lack inheritance traits of single-gene defects.
(b) Recurrence risk for first-degree relatives is higher than for second- or third-degree relatives.
(c) Recurrence risk is higher if the malformation is severe.

d. The etiology of a defect or syndrome may never be discovered despite in-depth evaluation.
(1) Determination of the type of defect may provide the first step in investigation of an anomaly.

BOX 34-1
TERMINOLOGY

Syndrome	A recognized pattern of abnormalities that occur together, e.g., Down syndrome
Sequence	Pattern of anomalies that result from a single or primary defect, e.g., Potter sequence
Malformation	Defect occurs as a result of intrinsic developmental problems, e.g., neural tube defects
Deformation	Defect in shape, form, or function of body parts secondary to mechanical forces, e.g., clubfeet
Disruption	Extrinsic factors acting on developing structures resulting in abnormalities in normal tissue, e.g., amniotic banding sequence
Mosaicism	Two different cell lines in the same individual resulting from nondisjunction of an anaphase lag during mitosis
Translocation	Transfer of all or a portion of a chromosome to another location after chromosome breakage
Nondisjunction	Failure of paired chromosomes to separate equally during cell division, resulting in abnormal chromosome numbers in gametes or somatic cells

C. **Diagnosis.** Investigation of a congenital anomaly must take into account the prenatal, perinatal, and postnatal cause.

1. Family history, including the last three generations, provides the basis for study. Reproductive history, possible consanguinity, and previous patterns of inheritable disease must be included.
   a. Prenatal history.
      (1) Length of gestation.
      (2) Maternal exposure to teratogens, infections, fever, illness, medications, drugs.
      (3) Obstetric factors: uterine malformations, complications of labor.
      (4) Neonatal factors: birth weight, length, and head circumference.
   b. Physical examination of the infant providing detailed study of physical characteristics.
      (1) Assess defects in a detailed systematic fashion including clinical photographs.
      (2) Measure features that are abnormal in size, shape, or symmetry (McLean, 1999).
      (3) Head: size of fontanelles, prominence of frontal bone, occiput flattened or prominent; microcephaly.
      (4) Face: configuration, elfin, coarse, flat, triangular, round, birdlike, expressionless characteristics, smooth philtrum, micrognathia.
      (5) Nose: one nare, beaked, pinched, upturned, flattened bridge, centered on face.
      (6) Eyes: iris color, colobomas, hypotelorism or hypertelorism, ptosis, degree/direction of slanting.
      (7) Mouth: size of tongue, intact palate, teeth, shape of mouth.
      (8) Hair: hairline, whorls, texture, pigmented areas, eyelash length, eyebrow length.
      (9) Skin: open areas, tracts, skin tags.
      (10) Ears: location, rotation, unilateral/bilateral defect, protruding/prominent shape.
      (11) Neck: short, webbed/redundant skinfolds.
      (12) Chest: shape and size, number of accessory nipples.
      (13) Examine parents for similar variation.
      (14) If one to three minor abnormalities are present suspect further abnormalities or possibility of a syndrome.
   c. A detailed study of all body systems in an infant diagnosed with a congenital anomaly is essential.
      (1) During the clinical examination associated renal, cardiac, or other organ system defects may be discovered, e.g., infants with Turner syndrome and known coarctation of the aorta require renal ultrasounds secondary to higher incidence of renal abnormalities.
2. Chromosomal analysis should be undertaken for those infants with multiple anomalies or a recognized syndrome.
   a. Chromosomal testing for infants exhibiting intrauterine growth restriction (IUGR), abnormal neurologic examination, occurrence of multiple minor malformations accompanied by a major malformation may prove valuable in diagnosis (McLean, 1999).
3. Metabolic studies to determine the presence of inborn errors of metabolism may be of value because some metabolic disorders result in distinctive phenotypes, e.g., Zellweger syndrome or Smith-Lemli-Opitz syndrome.

FAMILY ISSUES

A. The birth of an infant with congenital anomalies presents a crisis to the family; understanding of their response to this event can assist caregivers in their support of the family.
  1. Parents may feel responsible and have undeserved guilt. Reassurance over their lack of control over events causing the anomaly may allow parents to work beyond unreasonable guilt.
  2. Grief in all stages: shock, denial, bargaining, and acceptance is normal and to be expected as they grieve the loss of the perfect infant.
  3. Encourage parents to verbalize feelings, provide unconditional support.
  4. Identify normal features of their baby that coexist with the anomalies.
  5. Offer opportunities for parents to provide care and to be part of choices in care and interventions.
  6. Enable parents by providing them with routes to obtain further information concerning the anomaly their child experiences.
  7. Facilitate support systems on local and national levels.
  8. Encourage genetic counseling when appropriate.

SPECIFIC DISORDERS

Chromosomal Abnormalities

Trisomy 21

A. **Incidence and etiology.**
  1. Overall incidence of 1 per 700 live births (Rudolph, 1997).
    a. Incidence related to maternal age is as follows:
      (1) Ages 20 to 24: 1:1400.
      (2) Ages 25 to 29: 1:1100.
      (3) Ages 30 to 34: 1:700.
      (4) Age 35: 1:350.
      (5) Age 39: 1:140.
      (6) Age 43: 1:50.
      (7) Age 45+: 1:25.
  2. Affected individuals have 47 chromosomes (3 of chromosome 21) (Moore et al. 2000) (Fig. 34-1).
    a. Complete trisomies account for 95% of affected infants with 2% mosaics and 3% translocation (Alman and Goldberg, 2001).
      (1) For women less than 30 years of age, the incidence of translocation is higher — 6.9%.
      (2) Chromosome studies should be done on every Down syndrome infant to determine if a translocation is present. If translocation is confirmed, parental studies should be done to determine who is the carrier (Herring, 2002).
      (3) Down chromosome region is located on q22.2.
      (4) Greater than 50% of trisomy 21 fetuses abort in early pregnancy.
      (5) Expression of affect may be variable.
      (6) If balanced translocation exists, no abnormality is seen.

B. **Clinical presentation.**
  1. Characteristic phenotype.
    a. Head: skull small rounded with flat occiput. Flat facies due to lack of orbital ridges, flat nose, and micrognathia.

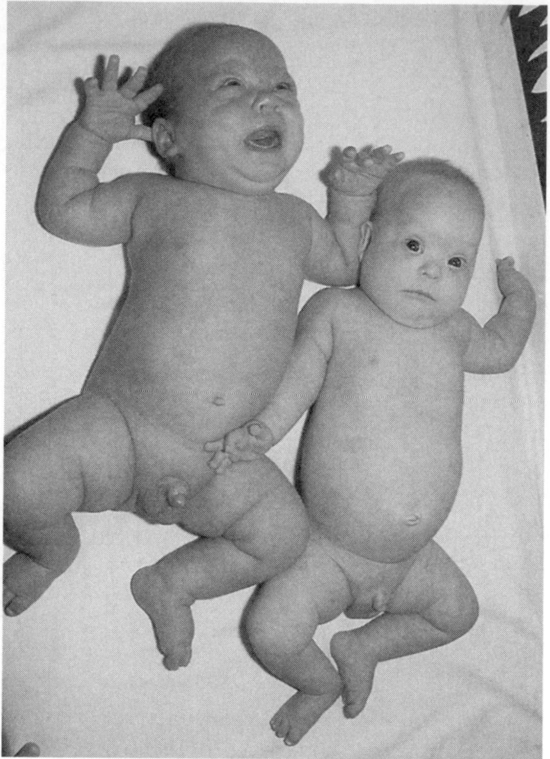

FIGURE 34-1 ■ Anterior view of dizygotic (fraternal) male twins discordant for Down syndrome (trisomy 21). The twin at right is smaller and hypotonic compared with the unaffected twin. The twin at right developed from a zygote that contained an extra 21 chromosome. (Courtesy Dr. A.E. Chudley, Department of Pediatrics and Child Health, University of Manitoba, Children's Hospital, Winnipeg, Manitoba, Canada.)

(1) Eyes: upward slanting of palpebral fissures. Iris may be specked with gold to gray Brushfield spots. Colobomatous cataracts and glaucoma are common. Prominent epicanthal folds.
(2) Ears: low-set; boxy appearance.
(3) Mouth: narrow short palate with protruding tongue.

b. Skin: excess at nape of neck.

c. Musculoskeletal.

(1) General hypotonia with poor Moro reflex present in 80% of infants.
(2) Hyperflexibility of joints.
(3) Square hands with short fingers. Bilateral or single simian creases.
(4) Fifth fingers are short, curving inward due to absent or hypoplastic middle phalanx.
(5) Thumbs are low-set with greater than usual separation from the second finger.
(6) Dysplasia of pelvis: narrow acetabular angle.
(7) Foot: wide space between great toe and second toe with deep crease that curves toward medial edge of foot.
(8) Short stature.

2. Associated findings.

a. Prematurity: occurs in 20% (Schiefelbein, 1999).

b. Mental retardation: IQ range 25 to 70.

c. Cardiac abnormalities.

(1) Endocardial cushion defects (atrioventricular canal), ventricular septal defect, patent ductus arteriosus.
(2) Gastrointestinal.
 (a) Duodenal atresia/stenosis, imperforate anus.

(3) Hematologic: leukemoid reaction, polycythemia, congenital leukemia.
(4) Endocrine: hypothyroidism.

C. Complications and outcomes.

1. In order to optimize potential functioning of these infants, ongoing assessment and integration of family, social and physical resources is vital.

2. Affected infants are mildly to severely retarded: IQ range from 25 to 70 (Schiefelbein, 1999).

3. Parent education and support are essential for continuing treatment of common continuing health issues.

a. Frequent upper respiratory and ear infections.
b. Cardiac/sequelae, including congestive heart failure.
c. Developmental delays.

Trisomy 18

A. Incidence and etiology.

1. Overall occurrence: 1 of 5000 newborns (McLean, 1999).

a. Advanced maternal age is a causative factor.
b. Most affected fetuses and neonates are female—4:1 ratio (McLean, 1999).

2. Affected individuals have 47 chromosomes (3 of chromosome 18) (Fig. 34-2).

a. Nondisjunction during meiosis accounts for 90% of trisomy 18 infants.
b. Various translocations, mosaicism, and isochromosomal anomalies account for the remainder.

B. Clinical presentation.

1. Characteristic phenotype.

a. Growth deficiency.
b. Head: microcephaly with prominent occiput.

(1) Eyes: microphthalmia with narrow palpebral fissures. Colobomas and corneal opacities and hypoplasia of orbital ridges. Ptosis of one or both eyes.
(2) Ears: low-set, poorly developed, often cupped in shape with large pinna. Atresia of auditory canals also seen.
(3) Mouth: micrognathia and microstomia. High arched palate.
(4) Skin: excessive skin at nape of neck, widely spaced nipples, decreased dermal creases secondary to decreased fetal movement.

c. Musculoskeletal.

(1) Hands have a typical appearance in 50% of affected infants. Hand is clenched with index finger overlapping the third finger and fifth finger overlapping the fourth.
(2) Rocker-bottom appearance of feet (Moore et al., 2000). Prominent heels, hammertoes, syndactyly between toes two and three (McLean, 1999). Hypoplastic nails.

d. Short sternum with slender ribs.
e. Narrow pelvis with hip dislocation.

2. Associated findings.

a. Cardiac abnormalities: varied. Ventricular septal defect and patent ductus arteriosus.
b. Renal anomalies: horseshoe kidneys, ectopic kidneys, double ureters, cystic kidneys.
c. Genital abnormalities: cryptorchidism in males. Hypoplasia of labia and prominent clitoris in females.
d. Umbilical hernias.
e. Severe psychomotor retardation.

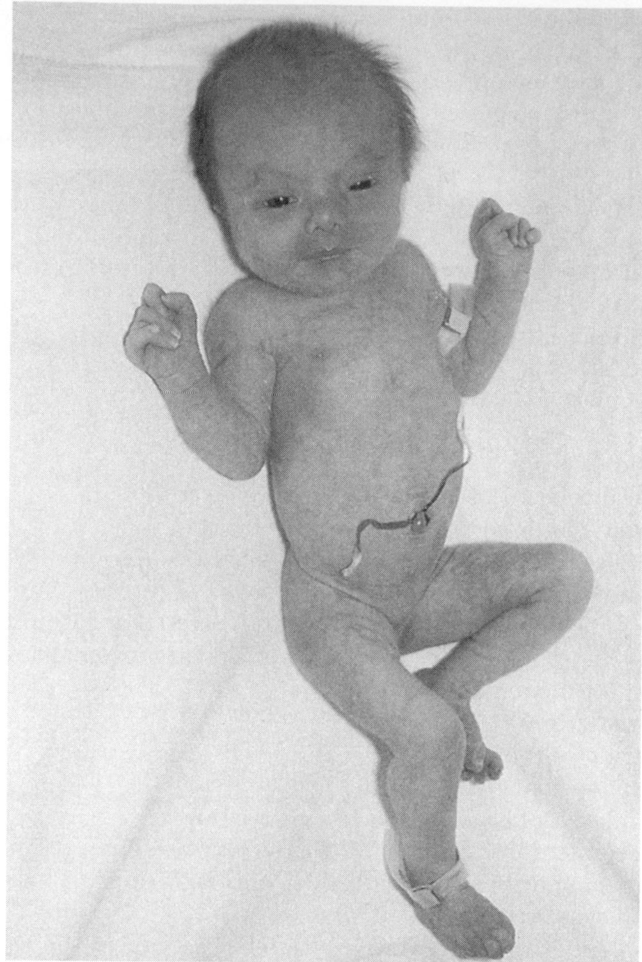

A

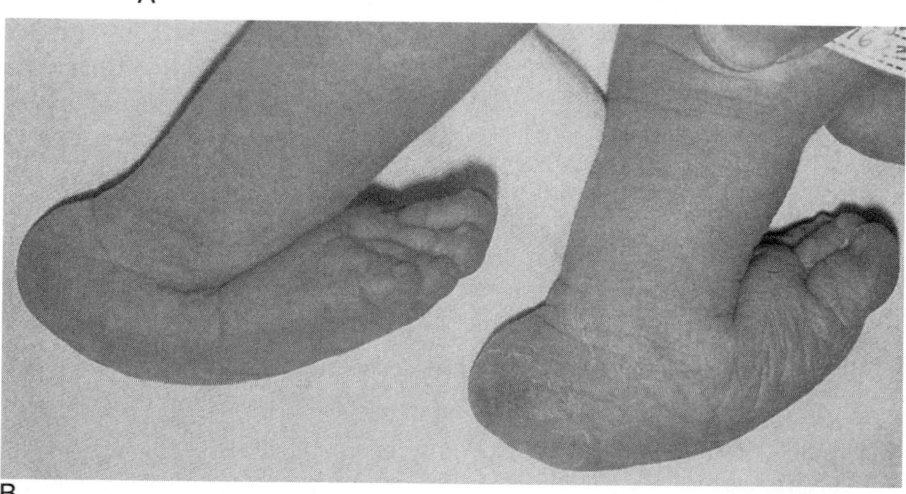

B

FIGURE 34-2 ■ **A,** Female neonate with trisomy 18. Note growth retardation, clenched fists with characteristic positioning of fingers (second and fifth digits overlap third and fourth digits. **B,** Feet of another trisomy 18 infant showing characteristic rocker-bottom appearance as a result of vertical position of tali (ankle bones). Also observe prominent calcanei (heel bones). (Courtesy Dr. A.E. Chudley, Department of Pediatrics and Child Health, University of Manitoba, Children's Hospital, Winnipeg, Manitoba, Canada.)

C. Complications and outcomes.

1. Life expectancy decreased: 90% mortality in the first year (McLean, 1999). Anomalies are severe, multiple.
2. No treatment beyond supportive care.
3. Parental involvement is essential, focusing on education concerning known defects, and assistance in providing supportive care.

Trisomy 13

A. Incidence and etiology.

1. Affects 1 of 12,000 newborns (McLean, 1999).
   a. Maternal age thought to be a causative agent.
2. Infants have 47 chromosomes (3 of chromosome 13).
   a. Majority of defects result from nondisjunction during the first division of maternal meiosis (Moore et al., 2000).
   b. 20% of defects are caused by translocations, some familial.
   c. 5% occur as a result of mosaicism.

B. Clinical presentation.

1. Characteristic phenotype.
   a. Growth deficiency.
   b. Head: microcephaly with sloping forehead. Midline scalp defects.
      (1) Eyes: ocular hypotelorism, colobomas, microphthalmia, glaucoma.
      (2) Ears: low-set, malformed ears, atresia of external auditory canals.
      (3) Nose: prominent nasal bridge.
      (4) Mouth: bilateral cleft lip and/or palate.
      (5) Neck: short neck with excessive skin.
   c. Musculoskeletal.
      (1) Polydactyly (Fig. 34-3).
      (2) Overlapping of fingers with single palmar creases. Flexion deformities of hands and wrists.
      (3) Prominent heel resulting in rocker-bottom feet.
      (4) Genitals: female—bicornate or septate uterus. Male—cryptorchidism, small scrotum.
2. Associated anomalies.
   a. Cardiac: ventricular septal defects, dextroposition, patent ductus arteriosus.
   b. Renal abnormalities: cystic kidneys.
   c. Cutaneous hemangiomas.
   d. Holoprosencephaly.
   e. Seizure activity.
   f. Severe deficits in cognitive and motor development.

C. Complications and outcomes.

1. Life expectancy is 130 days, though 14% survive to 1 year of age (McLean, 1999).
2. Care is supportive.
3. Parental education and support are essential.

Osteogenesis Imperfecta

Clinically and genetically heterogeneous hereditary disease involving connective tissue and bone (Zaleske, 2001).

A. Incidence and etiology.

1. Generalized disturbance of the skeletal system with varied expression. Four clinical types are identified:
   a. Type I: autosomal dominant, frequency 1:25,000. Characterized by bone fragility, blue sclera, possible hearing loss, and onset of fractures at birth.

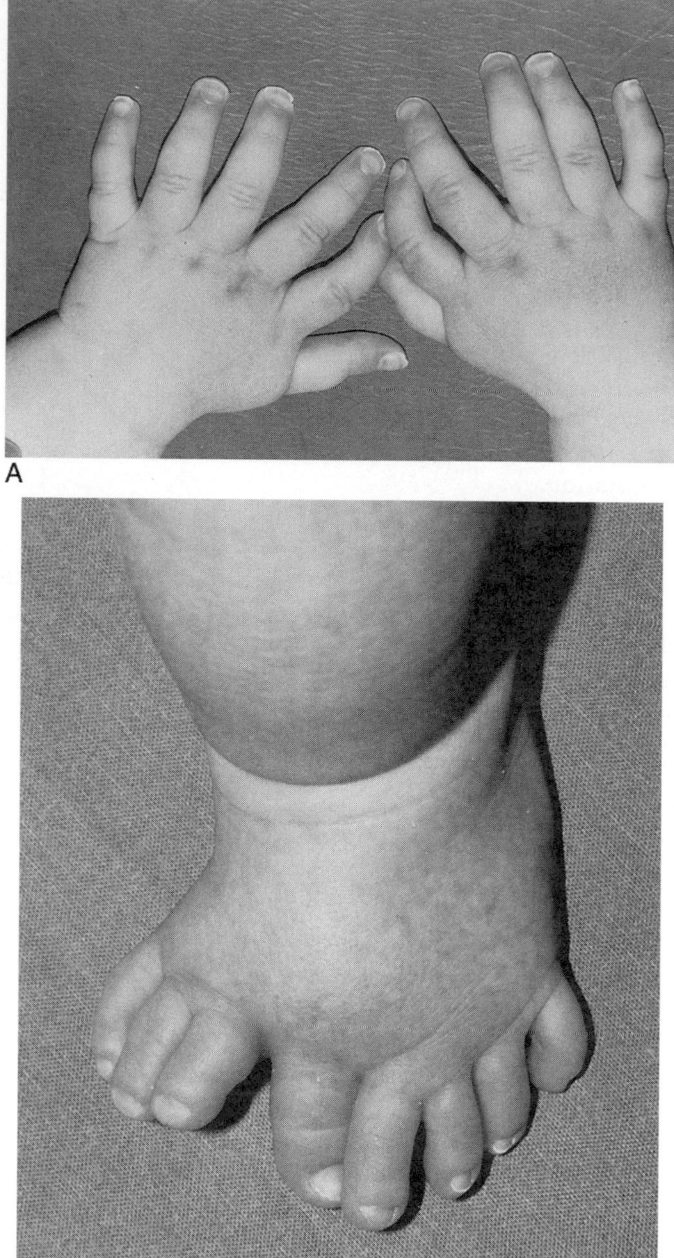

FIGURE 34-3 ■ Polydactyly of hands (**A**) and feet (**B**). This condition results from formation of one or more extra digital rays during the embryonic period. (Courtesy Dr. A.E. Chudley, Department of Pediatrics and Child Health, University of Manitoba, Children's Hospital, Winnipeg, Manitoba, Canada.)

b. Type II: autosomal dominant, frequency 1.6:100,000. Lethal in perinatal period; characterized by dark blue sclerae, concertina femurs, beaded ribs, and extreme bone fragility (Wiedemann and Kunze, 1997).

c. Type III: autosomal recessive. Fractures present at birth and deformities are progressive. Normal sclerae and hearing.

d. Type IV: autosomal dominant inheritance with fragile bones. Normal sclerae and hearing.
2. Most types of osteogenesis have been linked to mutations in type I collagen (Zaleske, 2001).

B. Clinical presentation. Physical findings vary with type and severity of defect.
1. Characteristic phenotype.
   a. Stature affected by incidence of fractures, shorted extremities, bowed extremities.
      (1) Head: small triangular facies, large head with wide intertemporal measurements, soft misshapen skull secondary to wormian bone development.
      (2) Eyes: bluish sclera secondary to lack of collagen.
      (3) Nose: low nasal bridge, small nose.
      (4) Skin: thin, translucent and easily distensible.
      (5) Teeth: delayed and defective dentition with soft, brownish, translucent teeth.
      (6) Musculoskeletal
         (a) Chest: normal length trunk often with multiple fractures.
         (b) Bones are mineral deficient. Vertebrae fracture easily. Long bones have narrow diaphyses with bowing and frequent fractures (Zaleske, 2001).
         (c) Laxity of the ligaments results in hypermobile joints that are easily dislocated (Wiedemann and Kunze, 1997).

C. Associated anomalies.
1. Eye abnormalities: corneal clouding, farsightedness.
2. Otosclerotic hearing disorders (Wiedemann and Kunze, 1997).
3. Hydrocephalus and intracranial hemorrhage.
4. Short stature secondary to multiple fractures and hyperplastic callus formation.
5. Platelet function is decreased secondary to defects in adhesion and clot retraction.
6. Resting tachycardia and tachypnea, hyperthermia, and diaphoresis.
7. Inguinal, umbilical, and diaphragmatic hernias are common (Zaleske, 2001).

D. Complications and outcomes.
1. Treatment is dependent on the type of osteogenesis imperfecta. Type I patients may require little or no treatment. Type II patients die early before treatment can be done. Types III and IV are the most complex, requiring intensive involvement and support.
   a. Treatment is aimed toward prevention and treatment of fractures as well as supporting function and ambulation.
   b. Treatment of fractures is difficult due to ligamentous laxity and structural abnormalities of the bone. New bone forms readily but new bone is the same in structure as preceding bone—plastic and easily deformed by muscle or weight bearing forces (Zaleske, 2001).
      (1) Lightweight splints or braces provide first-line treatment followed by corrective surgeries to provide support. Treatment of recurrent fractures minimizes deformities and promotes function.
      (2) Scoliosis is difficult to treat as the curves advance quickly and bracing is ineffective. Early fusing appears to offer the best relief.
2. The variability of expression of this disease poses a challenge for all concerned. Detailed assessment, examination, and education are essential first steps.

3. Involvement of parents from diagnosis to discharge is needed to provide the basis of continuing care of not only orthopedic issues but other anomalies as well. The value of parental involvement cannot be understated.

Beckwith-Wiedemann

A. Incidence and etiology.

1. Autosomal dominant inheritance pattern with variable expression.
2. Gene localized on the short arm of chromosome 11p15 (Wiedemann and Kunze, 1997).
3. Some cases occur as sporadic mutation and carry a low risk for recurrence. With familial occurrence, risk for recurrence is 50%.
4. Incidence 1:12 to 15,000 newborns (Wiedemann and Kunze, 1997).
5. 60% of affected infants are female.

B. Clinical presentation.

1. Characteristic phenotype: triad of organomegaly omphalocele and large tongue (Alman and Goldberg, 2001).
   - **a.** Head: prominent occiput, relatively small head, hypoplasia of midface, large fontanelle.
   - **b.** Eyes: mild exophthalmos, relative infraorbital hypoplasia tissue folds under eyes.
   - **c.** Ears: transverse ear creases located on earlobes.
   - **d.** Mouth: macroglossia, prognathism and malocclusion.
   - **e.** Skin: telangiectasia nevi in upper half of face in infancy.
   - **f.** Musculoskeletal: scoliosis common, asymmetric growth, postnatal gigantism.

C. Associated findings.

1. Polycythemia.
2. Hypoglycemia: severe prolonged resistance to treatment secondary to pancreatic cell hyperplasia.
3. Omphalocele or other umbilical anomaly.
4. Mild to moderate mental deficiency: normal intelligence possible.
5. Cardiomegaly.
6. Hyperplasia of pancreas and pituitary.
7. Increased kidney size with renal medullary dysplasia.

D. Complications and outcome.

1. Symptomatic treatment of hypoglycemia and polycythemia.
2. At birth the tongue is gigantic, presenting airway and feeding challenges.
3. Over time the tongue may recess, but hemiglossectomy is sometimes needed (Alman and Goldberg, 2001).
4. Affected infants are at greater risk for development of tumors, most frequently Wilms' tumor.
5. Treatment of hypoglycemia is essential to avoid seizures and subsequent central nervous system damage and a cerebral palsylike picture (Alman and Goldberg, 2001).
6. Parental education and support are vital as close follow-up for progression of orthopedic conditions.

Cornelia de Lang Syndrome

A. Etiology and incidence.

1. Cause of the syndrome is unknown. Majority of cases are sporadic (Wiedemann and Kunze, 1997).
2. Syndrome is felt to be related to duplication or deletion of chromosome band 3q25-29, the mother being the transmitting parent (Alman and Goldberg, 2001).
3. Incidence: 1:10,000 to 1:30,000.

B. Clinical presentation.

1. Overall: shortness of stature with growth failure.
   a. Head: narrow forehead, microcephaly, distinctive facies.
   b. Eyes: downward slanting of palpebral fissures.
   c. Ears: low-set, malformed.
   d. Nose: short nose with anteverted nostrils, flat nasal bridge.
   e. Mouth: micrognathia, thin lips with small midline beak of upper lip, long philtrum, small mandible, growling cry, down-turned corners of mouth.
   f. Skin: hirsutism, single bushy eyebrows, curly eyelashes, cutis marmorata.
   g. Musculoskeletal: micromelia, small hands with proximal thumb due to first metacarpal shortening, single palmar crease, clinodactyly of fifth finger, flexion contractures.
   h. Genital: undescended testicles, hypospadias, hypoplastic genitalia.

C. Associated findings.

1. Mental retardation: usually severe. Features of autism common (Herring, 2002).
2. Syndactyly of second and third toes.
3. IUGR with subsequent failure to thrive: children remain small with delayed skeletal age (Alman and Goldberg, 2001).
4. Gastrointestinal reflux (Alman and Goldberg, 2001).
5. Cardiac defect: present in 30% of infants.
6. Sensorineural hearing loss is common.

D. Complications and outcome.

1. Infants are a higher mortality risk due to poor feeding and defective swallowing mechanisms, gastroesophageal reflux, aspiration, and respiratory infections (Alman and Goldberg, 2001).
2. Mental retardation, failure of speech development, and lack of communication lead to further disability.
3. Treatment of orthopedic abnormalities is supportive: most infants will walk but milestones are frequently delayed.
4. This complex syndrome requires continued support and multiple resources. Parents must be aware of the need for continued follow-up of numerous abnormalities.

Crouzon Syndrome

A. Incidence and etiology.

1. Autosomal dominant pattern of inheritance. De novo mutations in up to 50%.
2. Possible association with increased paternal age.
3. Gene locus on chromosome 10q25-q26 (Wiedemann and Kunze, 1997). Gene responsible for fibroblast growth factor receptor-2 gene.
4. Frequency 1:25,000 births.

B. Clinical presentation.

1. Head: bulging of anterior fontanelle region, flat occiput.
2. Eyes: exophthalmos, antimongolian slant of palpebral fissures.
3. Nose: parrot-beak nose.
4. Mouth: short upper lip, high narrow palate, narrowly spaced teeth.
5. Upper cervical fusions (Loder, 2001).

C. Associated findings.

1. Craniosynostosis.
2. Optic atrophy with decreased visual activity.
3. Impaired hearing, primarily middle ear deafness (Zaleske, 2001).
4. Mild to moderate mental retardation.

D. Complications and outcome.

1. Prognosis is dependent on the presence and degree of mental retardation.
2. Initial treatment is symptomatic. Craniotomy within the first months of life may be necessary, depending on the infant's condition.
3. Cosmetic surgery may be done at later date to mitigate facial deformity (Wiedemann and Kunze, 1997).
4. Optic nerve damage with subsequent decreased visual acuity requires initial assessment and ongoing treatment.
5. Cervical fusions are progressive with age. There are no standard recommendations for treatment. Safety and stability of cervical spine must be ensured; lateral flexion and extension radiographs should be obtained for those children in question (Loder, 2001).

Abnormalities of the Sex Chromosomes

Turner Syndrome

A. Incidence and etiology.

1. Affects 1:2500 newborn girls (McLean, 1999).
2. Caused by complete or partial absence of one X chromosome.
   - a. Two thirds of affected infants have XO karyotype. Parental origin is maternal in 70% of cases (Alman and Goldberg, 2001).
   - b. Remainder of infants have other X chromosome abnormalities: simple, deletions, ring chromosomes, mosaics.
   - c. Affect of the single X chromosome varies depending on which parent is responsible for transmission. Rate of intrauterine lethality is 95%. XO is the most common genotype identified in spontaneously aborted fetuses (Alman and Goldberg, 2001).
   - d. Individuals with partial loss of the X chromosome suggest a critical region at X p11.2-p22 (Alman and Goldberg, 2001).

B. Clinical presentation.

1. Characteristic phenotype.
   - a. Short stature common in older girls. Mean birth length is 47 cm, and thus, may be small for gestational age.
   - b. Head.
     - (1) Low posterior hairline with appearance of short neck, micrognathia.
     - (2) Eyes: ptosis of eyelids, epicanthal folds.
     - (3) Ears: low-set, often malformed.
     - (4) Nose: broad nasal bridge.
     - (5) Neck: webbing of neck due to redundant skin.
   - c. Chest.
     - (1) Shape: broad, shieldlike with widely spaced hypoplastic or inverted nipples.
   - d. Musculoskeletal.
     - (1) Marked lymphedema of extremities.
     - (2) Skeletal abnormalities.
   - e. Genital.
     - (1) Gonadal dysplasia.
     - (2) Lack of secondary sexual characteristics.
   - f. Skin: pigmented nevi, nails are narrow hyperconvex, deep-set.
2. Associated findings.
   - a. Cardiac: coarctation of aorta, aortic valvular stenosis.
   - b. Renal: horseshoe kidneys, unilateral renal agenesis.
   - c. Learning disabilities: normal intelligence.

C. **Complications and outcome.**
   1. Initial care supportive: dependent on clinical findings.
   2. Only one third of the cases of Turner syndrome are diagnosed as newborns. Remainder are diagnosed in early adolescence: common cause of primary amenorrhea.
   3. Early education and need for continued follow-up support essential.
   4. Outcome good despite failure of sexual development.

Klinefelter Syndrome XXY

A. **Incidence and etiology.**
   1. Affects 1:500 to 1000 male newborns born with some variation of the syndrome (Wiedemann and Kunze, 1997).
   2. Extra X chromosome results from abnormal chromosome separation during oogenesis or spermatogenesis.
   3. Increased maternal age may be causative; in two thirds of affected infants both X chromosomes are of maternal origin.

B. **Clinical presentation.**
   1. Characteristic phenotype.
      a. Growth: affected individuals frequently tall in stature with mildly eunuchoid body proportions (Cole, 2001).
      b. Genital: male hypogonadism, cryptorchidism, hypospadias.
   2. Associated findings.
      a. Below average intelligence: IQ may be 10 to 15 points below siblings.
      b. Behavioral disorders including anxiety, impulsive behavior, and poor social adjustment.

C. **Complications and outcome.**
   1. Most patients are diagnosed after 14th year of life; late onset of puberty.
   2. Infertility is common.
   3. Life expectancy is normal.

Single Gene Disorders

Single gene disorders are produced when a defect alters one or both copies of a gene.

Achondroplasia

A. **Incidence and etiology.**
   1. Incidence 1:10,000 live births.
   2. Transmission of defect as an autosomal dominant trait, though 80% of cases result from spontaneous mutation (Sponseller, 2001).
   3. Defect localized to chromosome 4p16.3 (McLean, 1999). Affects fibroblast growth factor receptors resulting in limited endochondral bone formation.

B. **Clinical presentation.**
   1. Characteristic phenotype.
      a. Growth: small at birth with increasingly apparent postnatal growth deficiency secondary to failure of endochondral ossification.
      b. Head.
         (1) Large square head with frontal bossing, foramen magnum hypoplasia.
         (2) Midface hypoplasia with a depressed nasal bridge and relative prognathism.
         (3) Nose: short, flat with broad tip, anteverted nares, and long philtrum.
         (4) Eyes: epicostal folds, hypertelorism.
      c. Musculoskeletal.
         (1) Trunk: normal height arm span; decreased standing height; vertebral abnormalities with thoracolumbar kyphosis, spinal stenosis secondary to abnormal growth of pedicles in spine.

(2) Limbs: rhizomelic shortening of bones. Upper limbs: shortened flexion contractures evident at elbows. Hands are short and broad with fingers of equal length referred to as starfish hands (Herring, 2002) and trident hand.
(3) Muscular development sometimes increased with skin and soft tissues overabundant in relation to length of limbs.
(4) Joints may be hyperextensible.
(5) Lumbar lordosis common.
(6) Muscle tone in trunk and extremities low in infancy.

2. Associated findings.
   a. Hearing defects are present in two thirds of patients (Wiedemann and Kunze, 1997).
   b. Speech problems related to maxillary hypoplasia.
   c. Recurrent otitis media.
   d. Gait abnormalities.
   e. Intelligence is normal but motor development may be delayed.
   f. Two thirds of achondroplastic infants will exhibit ventriculomegaly but only a small fraction will have clinically significant hydrocephalus.

C. **Complications and outcome.**
1. Infants with known achondroplasia must be closely monitored for developmental delay, hypotonia, and spasticity. Sleep apnea may be a symptom of foramen magnum stenosis.
2. Obesity is often an ongoing problem and should be monitored closely.
3. Upper respiratory problems as a result of midfacial hypoplasia are common.
   a. Dental crowding.
   b. Recurrent otitis media and resultant hearing loss.
   c. Obstructive sleep apnea.
   d. Decreased pulmonary function and respiratory drive (Sponseller, 2001).
4. Kyphosis is frequently present but improves after walking begins. For those children that retain kyphosis, bracing, support sitting, and surgical correction offer relief.

Limb Abnormalities

Polydactyly. Development of supernumerary digits.

A. **Incidence and etiology.**
1. Inherited as an autosomal dominant trait.
2. Incidence is common: anomaly results from a duplication error in which a stimulus induces excessive limb bud formation.

B. **Clinical presentation** (see Fig. 34-3).
1. Characteristic presentation.
   a. Frequently involves the ulnar aspect of the hand.
   b. Affected digits are often incomplete and lacking in muscular development.
   c. Bilateral defects are common.
   d. Abnormalities are divided into three classifications: soft tissue mass connected by a tissue pedicle; partial duplication involving the phalanges; and complete duplication of the digit with bony formation (Mosca, 2001). Defects are further classified according to the anatomic placement.
      (1) Preaxial, or duplicate, thumbs occur most commonly as an isolated lesion. Defect has been associated with Holt-Oram, Fanconi, and Ellis-van Crevald syndromes.

(2) Triphalangeal thumb also referred to as a thumbless, five-fingered hand. Demonstrated equally between sexes and is bilateral in 80% of affected children (Mosca, 2001). Trisomies 13 and 15, Blackfan-Diamond, and Fanconi syndromes are associated with this lesion.

C. **Complications and outcome.**
1. Treatment: dependent on specific defect.
2. Therapy is aimed toward preservation of function and motion, as well as provision of cosmetic remedy.
3. Radiography is useful in identifying bony defects and guiding treatment.
4. Parental involvement and support of continuing care are essential.

Syndactyly. Webbing or fusion of any portion of two or more digits.

A. **Incidence and etiology.**
1. Occurs in about 1:2200 births (Moore et al., 2000).
2. Males are affected twice as often as females.
3. 50% of defects are manifested bilaterally.
4. Feet are more commonly affected than hands.
5. Familial incidence may be as high as 20% to 40%.
6. Etiology: believed to be sporadic in 80% of cases (Moore et al., 2000).

B. **Clinical presentation.**
1. Defect occurs as a result of a failure of mesenchyme between developing digits to complete apoptosis, resulting in fusion of one or more fingers or toes.
2. Defect involves both physical and functional development.
3. Anomaly is considered complete if webbing exists along entire length of the digit or incomplete if webbing occurs only distally (Mosca, 2001).
4. The defect is further classified as single if the skin alone is affected, or complex if bones of adjacent fingers are fused.
5. Syndactyly most often affects the third web space of the hand.

C. **Associated abnormalities.**
1. Commonly seen in infants with Apert, Turner, Smith-Lemli-Opitz, and trisomy 18 (Rudolph, 1997).

D. **Complications and outcome.**
1. Treatment is dependent on physical findings. Radiographs assist in classification of the abnormality as simple or complex.
2. Timing of surgical relief is related to extent of involvement and size discrepancy and growth rates of affected digits. Surgery is generally performed in infancy between 6 and 12 months of age. Delays in surgery may result in bowing of the longer digit.
3. Surgical remedy is not without risk due to the potential for damage to the neurovascular bundle, underlying joints, tendons, and underlying bony abnormalities. Complete separation of digits in the neonatal period has a higher rate of complications (Griffin and Robertson, 1999).
4. Parents must be aware of the seriousness of surgical remedy as well as the need for staged repairs depending on the extent of syndactyly.
5. Genetic counseling is offered in light of described patterns of inheritance, frequency of associated anomalies, and risk of reoccurrence.

Talipes Equinovarus. Developmental deformity of the hind foot.

A. **Incidence and etiology.**
1. Occurs in 1:1000 births (Moore et al., 2000).
2. Clubfoot is bilateral in 50% of cases, males being affected twice as often as females.

3. Multifactorial pattern of inheritance. Increased incidence of idiopathic clubfoot in siblings of affected infant.
   a. Extrinsic: related to changes within the uterine environment, uterine abnormalities, oligohydramnios as well as the effects of uterine pressure during critical periods of development.
   b. Mendelian: usually part of a syndrome. Autosomal dominant and recessive, as well as X-linked recessive patterns found. Associated with Smith-Lemli-Opitz, Larsen, and Freeman-Sheldon syndromes.
   c. Neural origin: neuromuscular pathologic condition resulting in muscle imbalance. Changes in innervations lead to muscle fibrosis, shortening of muscles, and development of joint contractures affecting embryonic development of the talus (Mosca, 2001).

B. Clinical presentation.
1. Abnormal position of foot prevents normal weight bearing.
2. Sole of the foot is turned medially and inverted, varus deformity of hindfoot, equinus of ankle. Radiography may be helpful for identification of bony defect (Fig. 34-4).

C. Associated abnormalities.
1. Poland, Freeman-Sheldon, Larsen, and Smith-Lemli-Opitz syndromes.
2. Congenital hip dysplasia, myelomeningocele.
3. Neural tab defects.
4. Neuromuscular conditions: myotonic dystrophy.

D. Complications and outcome.
1. Highly individualized according to severity of defect.

Talipes Calcaneovalgus. Positional deformity characterized by marked dorsiflexion of the entire foot at the ankle joint (Mosca, 2001). Deformity is relatively common, benign, and flexible resulting from intrauterine positioning.

A. Incidence and etiology.
1. Incidence reported at 30% to 50%: felt to be the most common deformity of the foot present at birth (Mosca, 2001).
   a. More common in girls, first-born children, and children of young mothers.
2. Etiology uncertain but felt to be secondary to positioning of the sole of the foot against the uterine wall and the dorsal skin of the foot resting against the anterior surface of the tibia.
3. Physical examination reveals free mobility of the foot to passive manipulation.
   a. Soft tissues of the dorsal and lateral aspects of the foot are contracted, limiting plantar flexion and inversion (Mosca, 2001).
4. Condition must be differentiated from more serious deformities such as congenital vertical talus.
5. Radiographs are not needed for diagnosis as interosseous relationships are normal and the diagnosis is generally easily differentiated from a structural defect.
6. Treatment consists primarily of passive stretching exercises for infants with difficulty in manipulating the foot to a neutral position. Majority of cases resolve spontaneously.

B. Clinical presentation.
1. Presents as hyperdorsiflexion of the foot against the anterior surface of the tibia (Herring, 2002).
2. Plantar flexion limited due to contracture of the ankle and foot structures.
3. Heel of the foot is often in a valgus position with the forefoot appearing abductus.

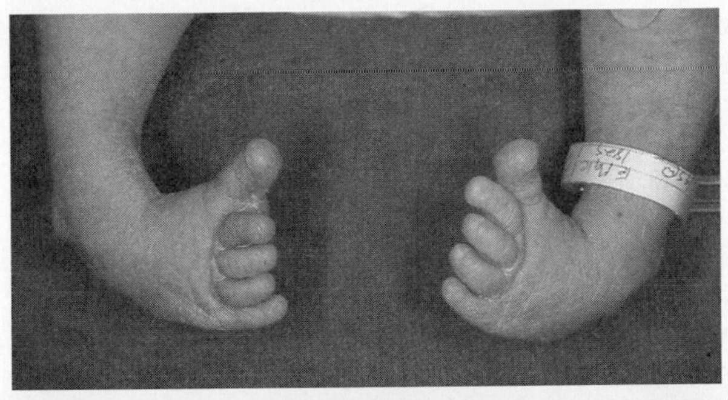

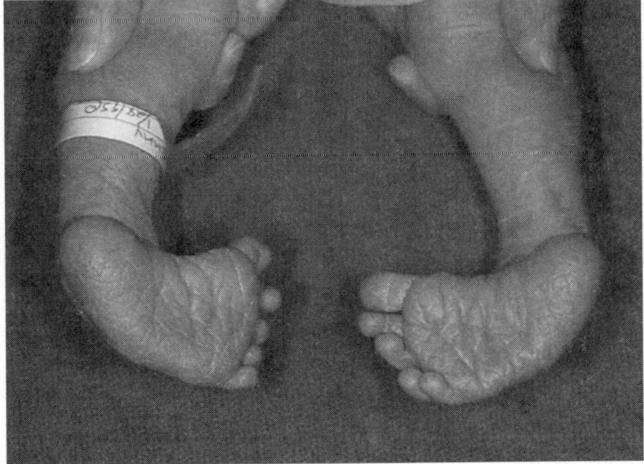

FIGURE 34-4 ■ Bilateral talipes equinovarus. Note structural deformity of hind part of foot. (Courtesy Jane Deacon, RNC, MS, NNP, The Children's Hospital, Denver, CO.)

4. Calcaneus is palpable in the heel pad, maintained in dorsiflexion (Herring, 2002).

C. **Associated findings.**
   1. Hip dysplasia is sometimes associated, presenting with no hip instability initially.
   2. External rotation of the lower extremities is felt to be the most commonly associated finding (Herring, 2002).
      a. Felt to exist secondary to persistent eversion of the calcaneovalgus or from external rotation contracture of the hip.

D. **Complications and outcome.**
   1. Cases commonly resolve with gentle stretching exercises within 3 to 6 months.
   2. Only in severe cases with marked restriction of plantar flexion and supination is further intervention needed.
      a. Casting and splinting in association with stretching exercises provide relief in most cases.
      b. Occasionally ankle-foot orthosis splint may be needed to ensure appropriate resolution.
   3. Parental support and education is important for improvement.
      a. Clarification of this as a mechanical defect.
      b. Need for ongoing support with exercises and follow-up evaluations.

Developmental Dysplasia of the Hip (DDH). Wide spectrum of abnormalities that affect the femoral head and acetabulum. Involves embryonic, fetal, and infantile periods.

A. **Incidence and etiology.**
   1. Incidence: 1:1000 to 2:1000 live births.
   2. DDH is more common in females than in males.
   3. Genetic and ethnic factors play an important role. Weinstein (2001) relates DDH as high as 25 to 50 cases per 1000 in Native American and Lapp populations, whereas southern Chinese, Korean, and people of African descent have very low rates.
   4. Etiology is believed to be multifactorial.
      a. Prenatal breech positioning, especially frank breech with hip flexed and knees extended, increases the risk.
      b. Ligamentous laxity resulting from circulating maternal hormone (relaxin) exerts an effect, resulting in hip dislocation. Familial ligamentous laxity has also been described.
      c. Postnatal positioning fostering hip extension may also be a factor in development of DDH.
      d. Genetic factors possible as recurrence rate for siblings of an affected neonate are increased.

B. **Clinical presentation.**
   1. Differences in adduction, apparent shortening of the affected femur, and extra skinfolds can indicate dislocation.
   2. Detection may be difficult in the neonatal period as asymmetry of gluteal and other skinfolds may not be clearly evident.
   3. Manipulation of hip utilizing Ortolani or Barlow maneuver is meant to elicit dislocation and reduction of the hip.
   4. Anatomic changes are minimal in the neonate. As the hip becomes permanently dislocated, pathologic changes of the acetabulum, femoral head, hip capsule joints, and ligaments become progressive. End result is degenerative changes in femoral head and acetabulum.

C. **Associated abnormalities.**
   1. Congenital hip dysplasia is associated with other congenital postural adductus deformities such as torticollis, talipes equinovarus, and metatarsus (Herring, 2002).
   2. Strong association with congenital cutis laxa syndrome and Larsen syndrome.
   3. In cases of unilateral dislocations, secondary problems with limb-length inequality, ipsilateral knee deformity scoliosis, and disturbances in gait commonly develop (Weinstein, 2001).

D. **Complications and outcome.**
   1. Physical examination including detailed family history is essential.
   2. Radiographs may provide diagnostic clues but may be difficult to obtain. Ultrasonography may be useful in detection of DDH as well as monitoring response to treatment.
   3. Most unstable hips in newborns will stabilize soon after birth (Weinstein, 2001). Others may progress to subluxation or dislocation. Outcome of the hip instability cannot be predicted. All newborns with clinical hip instability should be treated.
      a. Initial goal of treatment of DDH is reduction of the displaced femoral head and support of acetabular and femoral head growth.
         (1) Early diagnosis results in improved outcome.
         (2) Triple diapers and abduction diapers are generally ineffective.

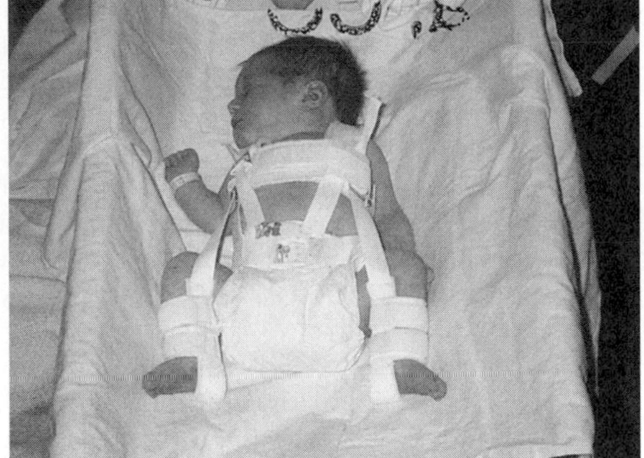

FIGURE 34-5 ■ Infant with dislocated hips in a Pavlik harness. (Courtesy Jane Deacon, RNC, MS, NNP, The Children's Hospital, Denver, CO.)

4. The Pavlik harness is the most commonly used device to prevent adduction while allowing flexion and abduction. Treatment is provided for 6 weeks on a full-time basis (Fig. 34-5).
   a. Proper prescribing, fit, and adjustment of the harness are essential to monitor treatment success or failure.
   b. Improper use may result in pathologic changes to the femoral head acetabulum and bone growth.
   c. Frequent clinical assessment is necessary to assess hip stability and to adjust the harness to allow for growth.
   d. Care must be taken to avoid skin breakdown.
5. Parental involvement in treatment is essential because they will play an integral role in early treatment success.
6. Closed reduction with traction and open reduction are reserved for those infants/children for whom early harness intervention has been unsuccessful.

Neural Tube Defects

A. **Incidence and etiology.** Congenital defects of the spine or skull resulting from defective closure of the neural tube.
   1. Neural tube defects are among the most commonly occurring human congenital malformations of the central nervous system (Paige and Carney, 2002).
   2. Incidence of neural tube defects in the United States estimated at 1:1000 live births (Paige and Carney, 2002).
      a. Fetuses with neural tube defects often spontaneously abort before the end of the embryonic period (Paige and Carney, 2002).
   3. Etiology of neural tube defects varied.
      a. Polygenic: several genes exerting a singular effect.
      b. Multifactorial: interaction of genetic and environmental factors to produce a defect.
      c. Single gene disorders: identified gene responsible for defect, e.g., Meckel syndrome.
      d. Chromosome abnormalities: improper distribution of chromosomes.
      e. Teratogenic exposure: substance triggers malformation, e.g., valproic acid results in neural tube defects.

   f. Maternal diseases states: conditions that are associated with formation of defects, e.g., diabetes (Wynbrandt and Ludman, 2000).
4. The form and severity of the neural tube defect depend on the location and extent of the defect. Lumbar and sacral lesions are most commonly occurring.
   a. The spinal column and brain develop from a process called neurulation.
      (1) Primary neurulation begins with folding of the neural plate to form the neural tube. The neural folds meet and fuse with the rostral (anterior) and caudal (posterior) ends (neuropore) between 18 and 28 embryonic days (Volpe, 2001).
      (2) Secondary neurulation is a process of cavitation and differentiation of lower sacral and coccygeal segments. This process begins at about 26 days and continues through 8 weeks postovulatory (Volpe, 2001).
      (3) Disturbances in the events of neurulation result in various errors in neural tube closure (Volpe, 2001).

Anencephaly

Lethal malformation secondary to defective closure of the rostral end of the neural tube resulting in complete or incomplete formation of the cranium and brain.

A. Incidence and etiology.
1. Defect relatively common with marked variation in frequency within:
   a. Geographic location.
   b. Sex.
   c. Age.
   d. Race: white infants experience increased frequency.
   e. Ethnic group: infants of Irish descent have increased incidence.
   f. Maternal age.
   g. History of other previously affected siblings (Volpe, 2001). Incidence in the United States is estimated at 1:1000 live births (Wynbrandt and Ludman, 2000).
2. Onset of anencephaly is estimated to be no greater than 24 days of gestation.
   a. 75% of infants are stillborn; the remainder die within the neonatal period.
3. Anencephaly is felt to be a multifactorial condition though some autosomal recessive and X-linked patterns have been reported (Wynbrandt and Ludman, 2000).

B. Clinical presentation.
1. Absence of most of the brain and in extreme cases, the spinal cord.
   a. Cranial vault absent, exposing brain tissue.
   b. Cerebral hemispheres usually missing; lower brainstem is present.
   c. Bones in the skull are often deformed, resulting in typical froglike appearance: protruding eyes with prominent nose; cleft lip with or without cleft palate.
2. Associated anomalies include malformations of limbs, thoracic cage, abdominal wall, gastrointestinal tract, and genitourinary system (Wynbrandt and Ludman, 2000).
3. Polyhydramnios is a common finding (Volpe, 2001).
4. Prenatal screening for elevated maternal serum, alpha-fetoprotein levels, amniocentesis, and ultrasound enable diagnosis in 90% of cases (Wynbrandt and Ludman, 2000).

C. Complications and outcome.
1. Most anencephalic infants are either stillborn or die within a few days of delivery.

2. With life support, some anencephalic infants have provided organs for transplantation, usually liver, heart, heart valves and corneas.
3. Ethical and legal concerns surrounding the diagnosis of brain death and persistent clinical signs of brainstem function have limited the donation of organs of anencephalic infants (Volpe, 2001).
4. Parents of infants with one affected infant have a 3% to 5% risk of recurrence of a neural tube defect (Wynbrandt and Ludman, 2000). Appropriate counseling must be undertaken for all families experiencing this anomaly.
5. Prevention therapies such as folic acid 600 mg orally daily have reduced the occurrence of neural tube defects when taken before conception and in early pregnancy.
6. Though rates of neural tube defects have decreased, total prevention is not possible because these defects occur from environmental as well as genetic factors (Paige and Carney, 2002).
7. Postnatal treatment is primarily symptomatic, comfort measures.
8. Encouraging parents to see their infant may be vital to the grieving process.

Encephalocele

Defect caused by limited failure of the rostral portion of the neural tube to close, resulting in extension of brain tissue through the defect in the skull.

A. Incidence and etiology.
1. 1:2000 to 1:5000 live births (Wynbrandt and Ludman, 2000).
2. Precise pathogenesis unknown.
   a. Autosomal recessive patterns of inheritance have been reported (Volpe, 2001).
3. Onset of serious defects no later than 26 days' gestation, at the time of anterior neural tube closure. Less serious lesions may have a later onset (Volpe, 2001).
4. Encephaloceles account for approximately 10% of all neural tube defects (Paige and Carney, 2002).
   a. Infants affected have a higher risk for associated anomalies then other forms of neural tube defects (Wynbrandt and Ludman, 2000).
   b. Incidence of encephalocele is increased when associated with maternal teratogens, specifically maternal rubella, diabetes, and warfarin embryopathy (Wynbrandt and Ludman, 2000).

B. Clinical presentation.
1. Defect presents as a protrusion of brain tissue through congenital defect in the skull. Anomaly affects brain, membranes surrounding the brain, as well as the bone.
2. Occipital encephaloceles are the most common occurring in 70% to 80% of affected infants; frontal, temporal, and parietal encephaloceles comprise the remainder (Volpe, 2001).
   a. Occipital encephaloceles are associated with microcephaly, posterior defects with hydrocephaly.
3. Size and severity of lesion dictate immediate treatment course.
4. Prenatal diagnosis aided by elevated alpha-fetoprotein levels and ultrasound assay.

C. Associated findings.
1. Hydrocephalus occurs in 50% of cases (Volpe, 2001).
2. Partial or complete absence of the corpus callosum in two thirds of patients (Volpe, 2001).
3. Occur as a component of other syndromes, e.g., Meckel syndrome or amniotic band syndrome (Paige and Carney, 2002).

D. Complications and outcome.

1. Neurosurgical intervention is indicated for most cases.
   a. Mortality ranges from 60% when hydrocephaly is present to 100% when a large occipital defect with microcephaly is present (Wynbrandt and Ludman, 2000).
   b. Surgical relief is undertaken within the first 48 hours for lesions leaking cerebral spinal fluid.
      (1) Of those infants surviving, 50% will experience disabilities including paralysis, blindness, seizures, and defects in muscular coordination.
      (2) Mental retardation of varying degrees exists in 40% of affected infants (Wynbrandt and Ludman, 2000).
      (3) Outcomes are more favorable for infants with anterior encephaloceles.
2. Genetic counseling is essential.
   a. Recurrence range from 3% to 5%.
   b. Recognition of encephalocele as part of a large syndrome is important when considering recurrence risk (Wynbrandt and Ludman, 2000).
      (1) Care provided to families includes education about the individual patient, problem, and counseling for immediate and long-term support.

Spina Bifida

Congenital condition resulting from failure of the neural plate to join together to form the neural tube. Bone and muscle are unable to grow over the open section of the spinal column.

A. Incidence and etiology.

1. Precise etiology unknown, believed to be a multifactorial trait (Wynbrandt and Ludman, 2000).
   a. Evidence suggests a strong genetic component as parents with one child with spina bifida have an increased risk of giving birth to another affected child (Wynbrandt and Ludman, 2000).
   b. A greater number of females than males are affected (Volpe, 2001).
   c. Variation exists between ethnic and racial groups; Egyptians, Irish, and English having higher occurrence rates.
2. Incidence of spina bifida has decreased over the past two decades; occurrence is estimated at 0.2 to 0.4 per 1000 live births in the United States (Volpe, 2001).
3. Onset of the disorder is felt to be no greater than 26 days postovulatory age (Volpe, 2001).
4. Leading disabler of newborns in America.
   a. Nerves responsible for relaying sensation and movement in legs, bladder, and bowel are damaged or incompletely developed (Wynbrandt and Ludman, 2000).
   b. Degree of damage or underdevelopments of individual nerves determine severity of symptoms.
5. Prenatal diagnosis aided by ultrasound, elevated alpha-fetoprotein levels, and amniocentesis.

B. Clinical presentation.

1. Two categories of disorder.
   a. Spina bifida occulta: mildest form of the defect with skin covering the opening of spinal column.

(1) Defect may be limited to a dermal sinus between adjacent vertebrae indicating the point at which fusion is not complete.
(a) Hairy patch or birthmark may be above the defect.
(2) Defect may present as a bulge under the skin as spinal cord ends terminate in fatty tissue.
(a) If several vertebrae are involved and a fatty area, hairy patch or dimpled skin is evident, bowel, bladder, or motor problems may develop (Wynbrandt and Ludman, 2000).

b. Spina bifida manifesta: defect is clearly evident as a secular protrusion on the infant's back.

2. Defects are divided into two categories:

a. Meningocele: spinal column develops normally but bulges through incompletely developed vertebrae.
(1) Minor muscle paralysis or incontinence can result if nerves protrude into the sac.
(2) Occurs in approximately 1 out of 20,000 live births, equally distributed between males and females (Wynbrandt and Ludman, 2000).

b. Myelomeningocele: undeveloped spinal cord protrudes through spinal column defect resulting in a saccular protrusion containing neural tissue.
(1) Accounts for 90% of spina bifida (Wynbrandt and Ludman, 2000).
(2) Position of the defect dictates degree of defect. The higher up in the spinal column, the greater the possibility for neural damage including paralysis, sensory loss, and bowel-bladder incontinence.
(3) 80% lesions occur in the lumbar area (Volpe, 2001).

C. Associated findings.

1. Hydrocephalus occurs frequently: between 70% and 90% either at birth or shortly following.
2. Chronic bladder infections and subsequent kidney deterioration.
3. Kyphosis at birth, scoliosis later in childhood.
4. Clubfeet: occurs secondary to neurologic and orthopedic abnormalities.
5. Dislocated hips.
6. Mental retardation: 30% of infants with myelomeningocele (Volpe, 2001).
7. Arnold-Chiari malformation secondary to inferior placement of the medulla and fourth ventricle in the cervical canal.

D. Outcome and complication.

1. Assessment of the functional level of the lesion allows for estimates of potential capabilities.
a. Detailed examination of motor sensory and sphincter function are vital to immediate as well as long-term care.

2. Surgical repair is dependent on lesion.
a. Surgical repair of myelomeningocele within the first year of life carries a favorable prognosis.
b. Repair of myelomeningocele is complicated if the lesion is open, exposed to amniotic fluid and labor stressors.
c. Subsequent surgeries may be needed to improve function.

3. Recurrence risk is estimated to be between 1% and 5%, increasing to 4% to 9% after having two affected infants (Wynbrandt and Ludman, 2000).

4. Supplemental folic acid appears to exert some preventive role when taken before conception and early pregnancy.

5. Educational support for families is essential because these defects can produce long-term health issues.
a. Access to community support resources can provide vital support.

STRUCTURAL ABNORMALITIES

Defects result from breakage of chromosomes or faulty repair mechanisms. Environmental factors appear to induce the defect. The type of abnormality is dependent on the fate of broken chromosome pieces.

Cri du Chat Syndrome

A. **Incidence and etiology** (McLean, 1999; Wiedemann and Kunze, 1997).
   1. Affects 1:37,000 to 1:50,000 live births
   2. Etiology secondary to deletion of chromatin from the short arm of chromosome 5. Clinical features correlate with specific regions on the 5p chromosome.
   3. De novo deletion present in 85%; 10% to 15% familial with greater than 90% due to translocations.

B. **Clinical presentation.**
   1. Characteristic phenotype dependent on the size of the chromosomal deletion.
      a. Infants with full deletions are usually low birth weight with marked hypotonia.
      b. Head.
         (1) Craniofacial disproportion with rounded faces, microcephaly.
      c. Eyes: hypertelorism, epicanthic focus, strabismus, and antimongoloid slant of palpebral fissures.
      d. Nose: low broad nasal bridge.
      e. Ears: low-set, dysplastic.
      f. Mouth: micrognathia, high-pitched mewing cry secondary to narrow larynx.
   2. Associated abnormalities.
      a. Severe psychomotor dysfunction.
      b. Congenital scoliosis.
      c. Partial syndactyly.
      d. Hypotonia.

C. **Complications and outcome.**
   1. Accurate cytogenic analysis is essential to ongoing development and treatment (McLean, 1999; Wiedemann and Kunze, 1997).
      a. Critical regions on chromosome 5 have been mapped for characteristic findings: cat-like cry, speech delay, severe intellectual impairment.
      b. Individuals have been shown to have 5p deletions, which result in a more favorable intellectual outcome but other common clinical findings (McLean, 1999; Wiedemann and Kunze, 1997).
   2. Feeding difficulties and associated failure to thrive are common. Enteral feeding support may be needed.
   3. Affected children are prone to respiratory infections, otitis media, and dental problems (McLean, 1999; Weidemann and Kunze, 1997).
   4. Cardiovascular complications include atrial and ventral septal defects.
   5. Developmental language and speech disorders are varied dependent on specific area of chromosome deletion.
      a. Typical IQ scores fall into the moderate to severe learning disability range (McLean, 1999; Weidemann and Kunze, 1997). Verbal IQ develops with age and peaks at about 10 years of age.
      b. Receptive language appears to be better than expressive language.

c. Early intervention to enhance communication skills may lead to improvement in behavior problems.
6. Family support is essential to deal with behavioral problems of affected children and their siblings.
   a. Sleep disorders and detection and treatment are essential.
   b. Provision of behavioral routines that support optimal development has been found to be effective (McLean, 1999; Wiedemann and Kunze, 1997).

DiGeorge Sequence

A. **Incidence and etiology.**
   1. Sequence results secondary to deletion of band q11 on chromosome 22. Effects of deletion affect several adjacent genes.
   2. Primary defect of the fourth brachial arch and the third and fourth pharyngeal pouches.
   3. Defects occur as a result of partial monosomy of chromosome 22 due to a microdeletion.

B. **Clinical presentation.**
   1. Head: microcephaly, abnormal facies (Rudolph, 1997).
   2. Eyes: hypertelorism, small fissures.
   3. Nose: anteverted nares, short philtrum.
   4. Neck: hypoplasia to aplasia of the thymus, parathyroids.

C. **Associated findings.**
   1. Cardiac: aortic arch abnormalities, interrupted aorta, ventricular septal defect (VSD), tetralogy, patent ductus arteriosus (PDA), peripheral pulmonary stenosis (Flanagan et al., 1999).
   2. Hypocalcemia secondary to lack of parathyroid.
   3. Imperforate anus.
   4. Defect in cellular immunity owing to thymic hypoplasia.
   5. Mental retardation: mild to moderate.

D. **Complications and outcome.**
   1. Significant mortality and morbidity are related to cardiac defects, immunodeficiency, and hypocalcemia (Leane-Cox, 1996)
   2. Treatment is aimed at specific problems after accurate diagnosis of cardiac anomalies.

Multifactorial Defects

Abnormalities occur secondary to multiple genes coupled with environmental factors. These defects are responsible for 25% of major congenital anomalies (Fix and Dudek, 1995).

Cleft Lip and Cleft Palate

A. **Etiology and incidence.**
   1. Cleft lip results from failure of mesenchymal masses in the medial nasal and maxillary prominences to come together (Moore et al., 2000).
   2. Cleft palate results secondary to failure of mesenchymal masses in the palatal shelves to meet and fuse (Moore et al., 2000).
   3. Multifactorial inheritance is felt to be causative. Factors interfere with migration of cells to the maxillary prominences, resulting in a decrease in the number of cells and hence the defects.

4. Overall incidence of clefts of the lip are 1:1000.
5. 60% to 80% of affected infants are males (Moore et al., 2000).
6. Defect more common in white and Asian populations.

B. Clinical presentation.
1. Defect may occur as a single defect or part of a syndrome of anomalies.
2. Defect varies in degree with associated nasal distortion and alterations in dentition.
   a. Unilateral cleft lip occurs most commonly on the left side.
   b. Bilateral cleft lip is usually accompanied by a cleft palate.

C. Associated findings.
1. Impaired speech.
2. Impaired hearing secondary to upper respiratory track infections with recurrent otitis media.
3. Orthodontic issues.

D. Complications and outcome.
1. Nutritional support challenging dependent on degree of defect.
   a. Nipple selection for most appropriate fit is key.
   b. Creation of dental appliance to provide palatal surface.
   c. Increased risk of aspiration.
2. Need for parent education concerning defect and associated anomalies provides the basis for continuing care.
   a. In order to maximize the infant's potential for growth and development, parents must be involved and recognize the importance of their role.
3. Good outcome with surgical correction.

MULTIFACTORIAL DISORDERS

Amniotic Band Syndrome

A syndrome of multiple malformations resulting from bands of fibrous tissue that encircles body parts (Wiedemann and Kunze, 1997).

A. Etiology and incidence.
1. Approximately 1:5000 to 10,000 newborns (MacKenzie and Gabos, 2001).
2. Primary event is thought to be a vascular disruption of the amnion (Moore et al., 2000).
3. Considered to be a disruption sequence due to external mechanical forces with little risk of recurrence.

B. Clinical presentation. Anomalies are variable: may occur alone or in varied combinations depending on timing of amniotic rupture (Fig. 34-6). Constriction bands most commonly found in distal portion of limbs with upper extremities affected twice as often as lower extremities.
1. Defects are classified into four types:
   a. Simple ring constriction.
   b. Constriction ring with distal deformity.
   c. Constriction plus fusion of distal parts.
   d. Complete amputation.
2. Pieces of amnion or other material may be found with tissue. Multiple bands may occur on a single extremity.
3. Neurologic defects distal to the defect may occur.
4. Defect may involve veins, arteries, nerves compromising circulation, and growth of affected extremities (MacKenzie and Gabos, 2001).
5. Head, neck, or trunk constriction bands are very common.

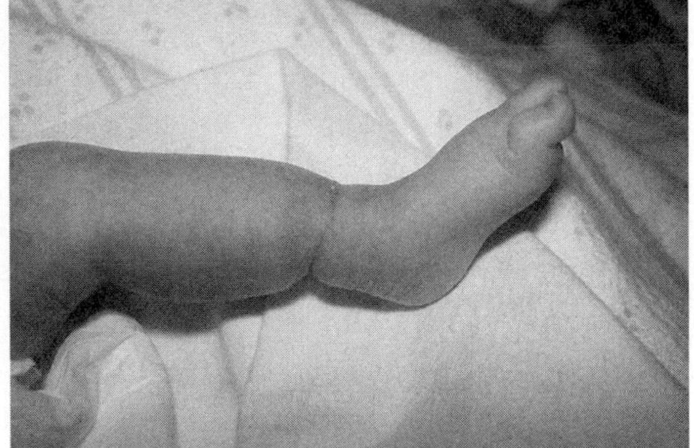

FIGURE 34-6 ■ Amniotic band constriction of lower leg. (Courtesy Jane Deacon, RNC, MS, NNP, The Children's Hospital, Denver, CO.)

C. **Associated anomalies.**
   1. Clubfeet: occurring in 12% to 56% of affected infants. Treatment may be more difficult secondary to rigid position and paralysis secondary to nerve damage.
   2. Angular deformity, bone dysplasia, pseudarthrosis, and anterolateral bowing of the tibia can occur deep to constriction bands in upper and lower extremities (MacKenzie and Gabos, 2001).
   3. Leg length discrepancy exceeding 2.5 cm occurs in 25% of children with constriction bands (Mosca, 2001).
   4. Syndactyly, brachydactyly.
   5. Cranial vault defects.

D. **Complications and outcome.**
   1. Life expectancy is normal unless brain malformations or deep facial clefts are present.
   2. Treatment is symptomatic.
      a. Physical examination must include a careful evaluation of vascular supply to the affected extremities.
      b. Assessment of joint function: if lymphedema is present. Joints may be stiff and immobile.
      c. Radiographs assist with classification of the type of defect.
      d. Surgical remedy is aimed at releasing constrictions and improving contour of affected parts. Those defects with greater constrictive forces are aimed at improving venous and lymphatic drainage.
      e. Timing of repair is dependent on severity of lesion. Acute constriction may require emergent care while less involved deformities can be corrected at 1 to 2 years of age.
   3. Parents must be aware of the need for staged surgical repair as surgery is seldom completed in one stage.

Inborn Errors of Metabolism

Inborn errors of metabolism are genetic biochemical disorders, which if left untreated can cause brain damage and death.

A. **Etiology.**
   1. Individual inborn errors are relatively uncommon, but collectively they are not rare. More than 100 inborn errors have neonatal onset.
   2. Inborn errors of metabolism are genetically transmitted, usually autosomal recessive or X-linked recessive (Burton, 1999).

3. Gene mutations responsible for inborn errors of metabolism produce deficiencies in enzymes, cofactors, transport proteins, and cell function (Stokowski, 1999).
4. The pathophysiology of metabolic disorders has been divided into three categories:
   a. Disruption of the synthesis or catabolism of complex molecules. Symptoms are progressive, leading to permanent damage.
   b. Interference with intermediary metabolism, resulting in accumulation of toxic compounds. Symptoms are related to food intake and nutritional status.
   c. Deficiency of energy production or use. Symptoms result from accumulation of toxin compounds and deficient energy production (Stokowski, 1999).

B. Clinical presentation.

1. Fetus is normally unaffected because placenta removes toxins. Newborns with inborn errors appear normal at birth, but may quickly present with life-threatening symptoms as the underlying metabolic defect manifests itself.
2. Timing of the onset and progression of symptoms may assist with diagnosis of inborn errors of metabolism.
   a. Symptoms occur acutely with rapid progression.
   b. Symptoms occur after a period of normal health.
   c. Symptoms correspond with the introduction of feeds.
3. Symptoms of inborn errors commonly include:
   a. Metabolic encephalopathy: lethargy, changes in muscle tone, seizures, irritability, weak suck, and apnea.
   b. Respiratory distress secondary to metabolic encephalopathy and underlying metabolic acidosis: most commonly tachypnea and apnea.
   c. Gastrointestinal symptoms: vomiting secondary to protein intolerance, failure to gain weight despite formula changes.
   d. Cardiac symptoms: cardiomyopathy, arrhythmias.
   e. Hepatic symptoms: appear during the first 2 weeks of life. Jaundice: usually direct reacting associated with vomiting, diarrhea, poor weight gain, hepatomegaly, cataract formation, and hypoglycemia. Most commonly associated disease is galactosemia (Burton, 1999).
   f. Unusual body or urinary odor. Phenylketonuria (PKU) infant's urine has a musty odor, whereas maple syrup urine disease infant's urine has a sweet odor secondary to isovaleric academia.
   g. Eye findings include cataracts: usually associated with galactosemia, glaucoma, corneal clouding, and dislocated lenses.

C. Complications and outcome.

1. Diagnostic tests.
   a. Blood gases, plasma ammonia, lactic acid, blood glucose, urinary ketones, and reducing substances (Stokowski, 1999).
   b. Urine screening for mucopolysaccharides, and oligosaccharides.
   c. Enzyme analysis, molecular and deoxyribonucleic acid (DNA) testing of urine, skin, blood.
2. General care.
   a. Supportive care of acute symptoms.
   b. Elimination of metabolites, toxic substances.
   c. Provision of nutrition either through high-calorie infusion of glucose or defect-specific formula.

d. Administration of vitamins to serve as cofactors to increase residual enzyme activity.

3. Mandatory screening of newborns.
   a. Screening of newborns must be undertaken early, before 7 days of life.
      (1) Sample should be drawn before transfusions or dialysis.
      (2) Battery of tests obtained varies from state to state, but all states test for PKU and hypothyroidism.

DISORDERS OF METABOLISM

Disorders of Amino Acid Metabolism

Phenylketonuria

A. Incidence and etiology.

1. Occurs in 1:10,000 to 15,000 live births (Stokowski, 1999). Autosomal recessive.
2. Results from a deficiency of the liver enzyme required for the conversion of phenylalanine to tyrosine.
   a. Phenylalanine results from breakdown of tissue protein and digestion of dietary protein.

B. Clinical presentation.

1. Symptoms occur following birth to 3 months of age.
   a. Early symptoms include vomiting, poor feedings, overactivity, and irritability.
   b. Later symptoms include: infantile eczema and musty-smelling urine.

C. Complications and outcome.

1. Diet must be altered to restrict phenylalanine.
2. Families must be aware of the need for continued dietary restrictions: the defect can only be managed.
3. Mental retardation results if treatment is not undertaken. Following a diet low in phenylalanine and high in other amino acids can prevent serious health and learning problems.

Maple Syrup Urine Disease (MSUD)

A. Incidence and etiology.

1. Defect results from a deficiency of enzymes necessary for breakdown of leucine, isoleucine, and valine. These amino acids accumulate in the blood as toxic ketoacids.
2. Incidence 1:150,000 in general U.S. population (Stokowski, 1999). Risk in the Mennonite population is 1:760. Familial risk: autosomal recessive.
3. Males and females equally affected.

B. Clinical presentation.

1. Metabolic acidosis with increased anion gap, greater than 16.
2. Elevated plasma and urine ketones, abnormal amino acids, and positive ferric chloride test (Burton, 1999).
3. Infant appears normal for first 48 to 72 hours then presents with vomiting, shrill cry, shallow respirations, hypertonicity, seizures, and coma (Stokowski, 1999). This is the classic MSUD category.
4. Urine may have sweet maple syrup odor.

C. Complications and outcome.

1. This disease is quickly fatal if untreated: immediate treatment must be initiated.

2. Treatment goals include removal of circulating ketoacids via peritoneal dialysis, exchange transfusion or, if possible, hemodialysis. Treatment must be instituted before waiting for lab confirmation.
3. Dietary manipulation to decrease protein.
4. Aggressive treatment may be life-saving and reduce the neurologic consequences of this disorder.

Disorders of Organic Acid Metabolism

A. **Incidence and etiology.**
   1. Enzyme defect prevents metabolism of intermediate metabolites of amino acids. The resulting organic acids accumulate and cause central nervous system (CNS) damage and kidney damage (Stokowski, 1999).

B. **Clinical presentations.**
   1. Metabolic acidosis, elevated plasma and urine ketones, elevated ammonia lactate, abnormal urine organic acids (Burton, 1999).
   2. Presents commonly with metabolic acidosis, hypoglycemia, feeding problems, vomiting, CNS depression, and seizures.
   3. Hematologic findings include leukopenia and thrombocytopenia.
   4. Example: multiple carboxylase deficiency.

C. **Complications and outcome.**
   1. Vitamin B_{12} should be given in case the defect is a responsive form of methylmalonic acidemia.
   2. If acidosis exists, sodium bicarbonate is utilized. Continuing management of acid-base status is essential.
   3. Prevention of catabolism is essential: appropriate support with glucose, lipids, amino acids must be provided based on individual infant needs.

Urea Cycle/Hyperammonemia

A. **Incidence and etiology.**
   1. The urea cycle provides the major pathway for detoxification of ammonia. The cycle is complex, having five stages. Any defect affecting any part of the process can result in accumulation of ammonia.
   2. Rare, but represents a substantial cause of brain damage/death in neonates.
   3. Exact incidence unknown, but estimated at 1:10,000 births (Summar and Tuchman, 2001).

B. **Clinical presentation.**
   1. Infants with urea cycle defects become symptomatic after 24 hours.
   2. Poor feeding, vomiting, and dehydration are initial findings. Majority is thought to be presenting with signs of sepsis.
   3. Further symptoms include seizures, coma, cardiovascular disease, and collapse (Stokowski, 1999).
   4. Variable respiratory alkalosis, elevated plasma ammonia greater than 1000 μg/dl, and elevated plasma amino acids are present.
   5. Associated findings include liver dysfunction, sepsis, perinatal asphyxia, and herpes simplex.

C. **Complications and outcome.**
   1. Protein intake is stopped immediately and dialysis begun to decrease ammonia (NH_3) levels.
   2. Neurologic sequela is dependent on the timing of initiation of therapy.

3. Carnitine therapy may be undertaken to provide cofactor support by providing a mechanism for excretion of accumulated metabolites (Burton, 1999).
4. Patients with urea cycle defects require supplemental oral arginine.
5. Patients with these defects are at risk for intercurrent episodes of hyperammonemia. Death or serious neurologic sequelae can occur.

Disorders of Carbohydrate Metabolism

Galactosemia

A. **Incidence and etiology.**
   1. Galactosemia is the most common disorder in this category
   2. Lactose is a disaccharide composed of galactose and glucose (Burton, 1999). If the enzyme that converts galactose to glucose is absent, infants cannot metabolize lactose.
   3. Incidence 1:40,000 to 1:60,000 (Burton, 1999).
B. **Clinical presentation.**
   1. Laboratory studies: urine-reducing substances, red blood cell galactose-1-phosphate uridylic transferase (classic).
   2. Jaundice and liver dysfunction are commonly found, usually at the end of the first or second week of life. Indirect hyperbilirubinemia may be present (Burton, 1999).
   3. Vomiting, diarrhea, poor weight gain, and hypoglycemia are common findings.
   4. Cataracts develop early in life.
   5. Gram-negative sepsis is common secondary to damage of intestinal mucosa by galactose-1-phosphate.
C. **Complications and outcome.**
   1. Galactose-containing feeds must be discontinued and replaced by soy formula or other lactose-free formula.
   2. If untreated, infants have persistent liver disease, cataracts, and severe mental retardation.
   3. With appropriate treatment, intellectual development may be normal or near normal, but even in treated infants, the rate of mental retardation remains higher.
   4. Long-term problems encountered by affected infants include premature ovarian failure.

Disorders of Fatty Acid Oxidation

A. **Incidence and etiology.**
   1. Considered to be the most common of the inborn errors of metabolism. Incidence 1:15,000 (Burton, 1999).
      a. 18 distinctive disorders have been identified: medium-chain-acyl-CoA deficiency (MCAD) is the most common defect (Stokowski, 1999).
   2. Fatty acid oxidation provides energy during periods of neonatal caloric deprivation. When normal metabolism of lipids is disrupted, hypoglycemia results.
      a. Triglycerides accumulate, leading to organ damage and failure.
      b. Infants have impaired capacity to use stored fat for fuel, and depleted glycogen stores quickly.

B. Clinical presentation.
   1. Hypoglycemia occurring within 48 hours of life.
      a. Characterized as nonketotic.
      b. Can occur as an isolated finding.
   2. Additional symptoms include vomiting, lethargy, hyperammonemia, liver function abnormalities, and metabolic acidosis.
      a. Similar to Reye-like symptoms.
   3. May present as a life-threatening event
   4. Fat accumulation in liver or muscle of an infant who dies unexpectedly suggests a disorder of fatty acid oxidation.
   5. Secondary carnitine deficiency develops as a result of excretion of excess acylcarnitine in the urine (Burton, 1999).

C. Complications and outcome.
   1. Treat hypoglycemia aggressively.
   2. Avoid times of fasting: provided glucose during times of illness or infection.
   3. A strong family association exists within these defects. Not uncommonly, infants who have a fatty acid oxidation defect have a sibling who has died of sudden infant death syndrome (SIDS) (Burton, 1999).

Congenital Adrenal Hyperplasia (CAH)

This defect results from a failure of an enzyme used by the adrenal cortex to produce cortisol and aldosterone (Ruble and Flores, 2000).

A. Incidence and etiology.
   1. In the United States incidence is 1:5000 (Ruble and Flores, 2000).
   2. 90% of the CAH is caused by 21-hydroxylase deficiencies (21-OHD).
   3. Inherited as an autosomal recessive genetic trait, believed to be located on the short arm of chromosome 6.
   4. Cortisol production is blocked in patients with CAH. This blockage of normal adrenal production of glucocorticoids results in high adrenocorticotropic hormone (ACTH) levels, which stimulate adrenal glands inappropriately. The end result of this process leads to adrenal hypertrophy, buildup of cortisol precursors, and overproduction of adrenal androgens (Ruble and Flores, 2000).
      a. Block of aldosterone synthesis increases activity levels of plasma renin.

B. Clinical presentation.
   1. Two forms of classic 21-hydroxylase deficiencies are present.
      a. Salt losing: both cortisol and aldosterone production are blocked, resulting in excess sodium loss through the kidneys. Accounts for 75% of cases (Stokowski, 1999).
         (1) Electrolyte imbalances are common: elevated serum potassium and decreased sodium levels may not be evident for 1 week. As aldosterone is used up, effects become evident.
      b. Non–salt-losing: only cortisol production is blocked. Aldosterone production is usually sufficient.
         (1) Mild deficit of aldosterone production presents as an elevated plasma renin activity or mild hyponatremia during periods of stress (Ruble and Flores, 2000)
   2. Nearly all female infants with CAH will display virilization, which is apparent on physical examination at birth.
   3. Infants of both types of CAH have significant elevations in 17-OHP (cortisol precursor) levels by 24 to 36 hours of age.

4. If diagnosis and treatment are not provided at birth, symptoms of acute adrenal insufficiency and salt-losing crisis occur (Ruble and Flores, 2000).
   a. Symptoms include weakness, vomiting, and dehydration.
   b. Hyponatremia.
   c. Hyperkalemia: secondary to failure of potassium excretion.
   d. Hypoglycemia secondary to impaired carbohydrate metabolism.
5. Mortality for these conditions may be high because symptoms are nonspecific. Additional symptoms include apnea, seizures, shock, and eventual cardiovascular collapse.
   a. Males are at highest risk for nondiagnosis and death.
6. Children with non–salt-losing CAH are frequently undiagnosed for years.
   a. These children are frequently unable to withstand stress, resulting in prolonged course of illness for minor illness or acute adrenal insufficiency with severe stressors.

C. **Complications and outcome.**
1. All infants with ambiguous genitalia should be screened for CAH.
2. Clinical consequences of these defects can be controlled by provision of the blocked end products of cortisol and aldosterone (Ruble and Flores, 2000).
   a. Goals of therapy include:
      (1) Prevent acute adrenal crises.
      (2) Prevent further virilization.
      (3) Maintain fluid and electrolyte homeostasis.
      (4) Achieve normal growth and normal fertility.
   b. Hydrocortisone is given in both types of CAH as a replacement for cortisol; doses are increased during times of stress.
   c. Mineralocorticoids are given in salt-losing CAH as a replacement for aldosterone.
   d. Sodium supplements for these times when salt loss exceeds intake.
3. Parents of infant girls affected with CAH must deal with issues of ambiguous genitalia.
   a. Incorrect or delayed gender assignment.
   b. Need for corrective surgery, often beginning before 2 years of age.
4. Support of family as they cope with acceptance of this diagnosis and their need for lifelong support for an infant with a complex disorder.
5. Parents can be screened for carrier state. Additionally all newborn siblings should be evaluated because multiple siblings' involvement is common (Stokowski, 1999).

REFERENCES

Alman, B., and Goldberg, M.: Syndromes of orthopaedic importance. In R. Morrissy and S. Weinstein (Eds.): *Lovell and Winter's pediatric orthopaedics*. Philadelphia, 2001, Lippincott Williams & Wilkins, pp. 288-338.

Burton, B.: Inherited metabolic disorders. In G. Avery, M.A. Fletcher, and M. MacDonald (Eds.): *Neonatology: Pathophysiology and management of the newborn* (5th ed.). Philadelphia, 1999, Lippincott Williams & Wilkins, pp. 821-839.

Cole, W.: Genetic aspects of orthopaedic conditions. In R. Morrissy and S. Weinstein (Eds.): *Lovell and Winter's pediatric orthopaedics*. Philadelphia, 2001, Lippincott Williams & Wilkins, pp. 158-176.

Fix, J.D. and Dudek, R.W.: *Human birth defects in embryology*. Baltimore, 1995, Williams & Wilkins, pp. 221-229.

Flanagan, M., Yeager, S., and Weindling, S.: Cardiac disease. In G. Avery, M.A. Fletcher, and M. MacDonald (Eds.):

Neonatology: Pathophysiology and management of the newborn (5th ed.). Philadelphia, 1999, Lippincott Williams & Wilkins, p. 580.

Griffin, P. and Robertson, W.: Orthopedics. In G. Avery, M.A. Fletcher, and M. MacDonald, (Eds.): *Neonatology: Pathophysiology and management of the newborn*, (5th ed), Philadelphia, 1999, Lippincott Williams & Wilkins, pp. 1269-1284.

Herring, J.: Orthopaedic related syndromes. In J.A. Herring and M.O. Tachdjian, (Eds.). *Tachdjian's pediatric orthopaedics* (3rd ed.). Philadelphia, 2002, Saunders, pp. 1585-1683.

Leana-Cox, J., Pangkanon S., Eanet K.R. et al. Familial DiGeorge/velocardiofacial syndrome with deletions of chromosomes area 22q11.2: Report of five families with a review of the literature. *American Journal of Medical Genetics, 65*(4):309-316, 1996.

Loder, R.: The cervical spine. In R. Morrissy and S. Weinstein (Eds.): *Lovell and Winter's pediatric orthopaedics*. Philadelphia, 2001, Lippincott Williams & Wilkins, pp. 821-822.

MacKenzie, W. and Gabos, P.: Localized disorders of bone and soft tissue. In R. Morrissy and S. Weinstein (Eds.): *Lovell and Winter's pediatric orthopaedics*. Philadelphia, 2001, Lippincott Williams & Wilkins, pp. 337-377.

McLean, S.: Congenital anomalies. In G. Avery, M.A. Fletcher, and M. MacDonald (Eds.): *Neonatology: Pathophysiology and management of the newborn* (5th ed.). Philadelphia, 1999, Lippincott Williams & Wilkins, pp. 839-858.

Moore, K.L., Persaud, T.V.N., and Shiota, K.: Congenital anomalies or birth defects. In K.L. Moore, T.V.N. Persaud, and K. Shiota: *Color atlas of clinical embryology* (2nd ed.). Philadelphia, 2000, Saunders, pp. 69-99, 100-119, 218-231.

Mosca, V.: The foot. In R. Morrissy and S. Weinstein (Eds.): *Lovell and Winter's pediatric orthopaedics*. Philadelphia, 2001, Lippincott Williams & Wilkins, pp. 1151-1215.

Paige, P. and Carney, P.: Neurologic disorders. In G.B. Merenstein and S.L. Gardner (Eds.): *Handbook of neonatal intensive care* (5th ed.). St Louis, 2002, Mosby, pp. 644-655.

Ruble, J. and Flores, B.: Congenital adrenal hyperplasia. In P.L. Jackson and J.A. Vessey (Eds.): *Primary care of the child with a chronic condition* (3rd ed.). St Louis, 2000, Mosby, pp. 352-373.

Rudolph, A.J.: *Atlas of the newborn: Musculoskeletal disorders and congenital deformities* (vol. 2). Hamilton, BC, 1997, Decker.

Schiefelbein, J. Genetics and fetal anomalies. In J. Deacon and P. O'Neill (Eds.): *Core curriculum for neonatal intensive care nursing* (2nd ed.). Philadelphia, 1999, Saunders, pp. 540-559.

Sponseller, P.: Skeletal dysplasias. In R. Morrissy and S. Weinstein (Eds.): *Lovell and Winter's pediatric orthopaedics*. Philadelphia, 2001, Lippincott Williams & Wilkins, pp. 243-285.

Stokowski, L.: Metabolic disorders. In J. Deacon and P. O'Neill (Eds.): *Core curriculum for neonatal intensive care nursing* (2nd ed.). Philadelphia, 1999, Saunders, pp. 349-355.

Summar, M. and Tuchman, M.: Proceedings of a consensus conference for the management of patients with urea cycle disorders. *Journal of Pediatrics, 183*(1): S6-S10, 2001.

Volpe, J.: Neural tube formation on prosencephalic development. In J. Volpe: *Neurology of the newborn* (4th ed.) Philadelphia, 2001, Saunders, pp. 3-44.

Weinstein, S.: Developmental hip dysplasia and hip dislocation. In R. Morrissy and S. Weinstein (Eds.): *Lovell and Winter's pediatric orthopaedics*. Philadelphia, 2001, Lippincott Williams & Wilkins, pp. 905-956.

Wiedemann, H.R. and Kunze, J.: *Clinical syndromes* (3rd ed.) London, England, 1997, Mosby-Wolfe.

Wynbrandt, J. and Ludman, M.: *The encyclopedia of genetic disorders and birth defects* (2nd ed.). New York, 2000, Facts On File, Inc., pp. 237-239, 293-295.

Zaleske, D.: Metabolic and endocrine abnormalities. In R. Morrissy and S. Weinstein (Eds.): *Lovell and Winter's pediatric orthopaedics*. Philadelphia, 2001, Lippincott Williams & Wilkins, pp. 177-241.

CHAPTER

35 Neonatal Dermatology

CATHERINE L. WITT

OBJECTIVES

1. Name three functions of the skin.
2. Describe two ways in which the skin of a newborn or preterm infant differs from that of an adult.
3. Identify three factors that affect the appearance of the neonate's skin.
4. Identify two nursing interventions that provide protection for the preterm infant's skin.
5. Recognize three common skin lesions that are normal variations in the newborn infant. Describe their appearance and treatment, if any.
6. Describe three common vascular lesions in the neonate, their appearance, and appropriate treatment.
7. Identify two syndromes associated with vascular lesions.
8. Evaluate two pigmented lesions occurring in the newborn infant and list implications associated with each.
9. Name two types of infectious skin lesions and select the appropriate treatment.

Careful assessment of the skin is an important element of the neonatal physical examination. The appearance of the skin gives the nurse important clues regarding gestational age, nutritional status, function of organs such as the heart and liver, and the presence of cutaneous or systemic disease. It is important for the clinician to be familiar with normal variances in the skin of the newborn infant, as well as those variances that signify disease.

Proper care of the neonate's skin can directly affect mortality and morbidity, especially in the preterm infant. The skin is the first line of defense against infection. Proper skin care can protect the integrity of the skin and prevent breakdown.

ANATOMY AND PHYSIOLOGY OF THE SKIN

A. Anatomy of the skin—three main layers (Fig. 35-1).

1. Epidermis: outermost layer, which functions as a barrier from outside penetration. The epidermis is subdivided into:
   a. Stratum corneum: outermost layer, consisting of closely packed dead cells that are consistently brushed off and replaced by lower levels of the epidermis. These cells are flatter and have thicker walls than other cells. The cells are held together by intracellular lipids, which aid in forming the protective barrier of the skin.
   b. Lower layers of epidermis: contain keratin-forming cells that create the outer layer of skin; as well as melanocytes, which produce melanin, or pigment. Despite racial differences in pigmentation, the number of melanocytes in a given surface area of skin is the same (Weston et al., 2002).

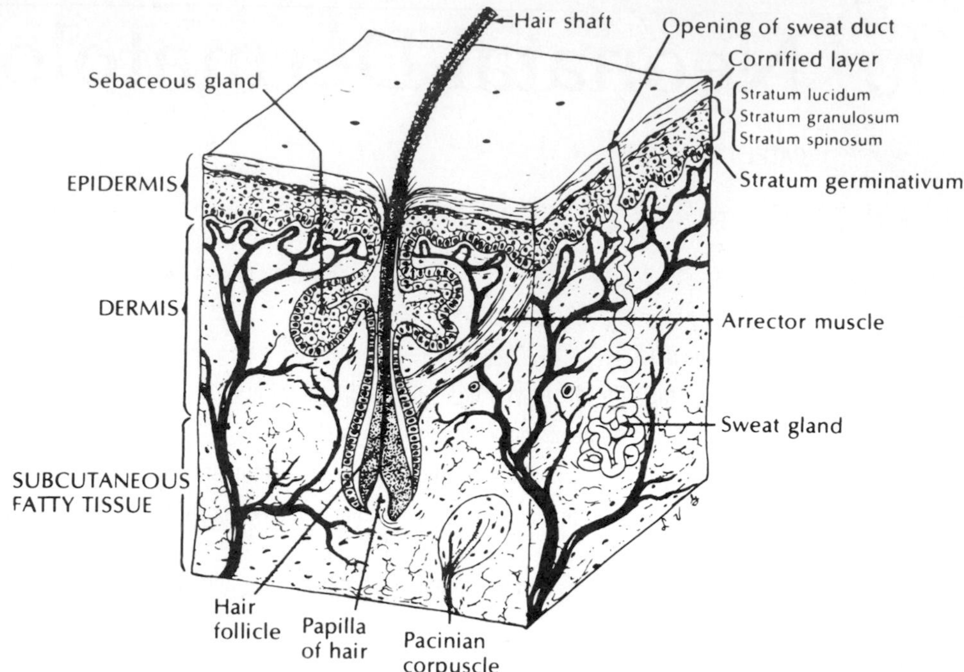

FIGURE 35-1 ■ Several layers and structures of human skin. (From Francis, C.C. and Martin, A.H.: *Introduction to human anatomy* [7th ed.]. St Louis, 1975, Mosby.)

2. Dermis: directly under epidermis; 2 to 4 mm thick at birth. The dermis is composed of:
   a. Collagen and elastic fibers that connect the epidermis and dermis, and provide the skin with the ability to stretch and then to return to normal shape.
   b. Blood vessels and nerves that carry sensations of heat, touch, pain, and pressure from the skin to the brain and provides protection against injury, infections, or other invasions.
   c. Sweat glands, sebaceous glands, and hair shafts.
3. Subcutaneous layer: fatty tissue functions as insulation, protection of internal organs, and calorie storage.

B. Functions of the skin.

1. Physical protection.
   a. Mechanical.
      (1) Tightly packed, thick-walled cells, held together by intercellular lipids, provide a protective barrier against transepidermal water loss and external invasions.
      (2) Process of constant sloughing and replacement of stratum corneum prevents colonization of the skin surface by bacteria and other organisms.
   b. Chemical/bacterial.
      (1) Acidic surface of skin (pH 5-6) provides defense against bacteria and other microorganisms (Giusti et al., 2001).
      (2) Production of melanin protects against damage from ultraviolet-light radiation.

2. Heat regulation.
   a. Production and evaporation of sweat.
   b. Dilation and constriction of blood vessels.
   c. Insulation of body by subcutaneous fat.
3. Sense perception: heat, touch, pain, and pressure.

C. **Differences in newborn/preterm skin.**
1. Basic structure is same as that of the adult; the less mature the infant, the less mature is the functioning of the skin.
2. The earlier the gestational age, the more thin and gelatinous is the skin, with fewer layers in the stratum corneum and a thinner dermis with fewer elastic fibers. The skin gradually matures after birth; however, even at 4 weeks of age, a 25-week infant has twice the transepidermal water loss as a term infant (Hoeger and Enzmann, 2002; Siegfried, 1998). Maturation of skin is accelerated after preterm delivery, but may take as long as 8 weeks in an infant of 24 to 25 weeks (Kalia et al., 1998; Williams, 2001).
3. Subcutaneous fat is accumulated predominantly during the third trimester.
   a. Preterm babies have little fat, resulting in an inability to maintain body temperature and blood glucose level.
   b. Brown fat, which is important for temperature regulation in the newborn infant, begins to differentiate during the seventh month of gestation (Williams, 2001).
4. Immature skin is thinner and therefore more permeable.
   a. An infant, especially a preterm infant, quickly absorbs topically applied medications and chemicals (Siegfried, 1998; Williams, 2001).
   b. Greater permeability allows for greater insensible water loss in the preterm infant.
   c. Higher surface area/body weight ratio allows for greater absorption of chemicals and greater transepidermal water loss.
5. Fewer fibrils connect the dermis and epidermis, and they are more fragile in term and preterm skin than in the skin of an adult. The stratum corneum is thinner in the term and preterm infant. Risk of injury from tape, monitors, and handling is increased, especially in the preterm infant; this type of injury includes removal of the outermost layer of the dermis with removal of tape or electrodes (Lund et al., 1997).
6. Sweat glands are present at birth, but full adult functioning is not present until the second or third year of life. Though present in the preterm infant, sweat glands are immature and function poorly before 36 weeks' gestation (Mancini, 2001).
   a. The newborn infant has limited ability to tolerate excessive heat.
   b. Vasodilatation to increase heat loss can result in hypotension and dehydration caused by increased insensible water loss.

CARE OF THE NEWBORN INFANT'S SKIN

A. **Term newborn infant.**
1. Initial bath with water and a mild soap.
   a. Avoid strong alkaline soaps to minimize alteration of surface pH.
   b. Soaps containing hexachlorophene should not be used. The hexachlorophene has been shown to be absorbed through the skin (Kopelman, 1973).
   c. Safety of other bacteriostatic soaps has not been determined. These should be used with caution and rinsed off completely (Siegfried, 1998).

d. As soon as the body temperature is stable (>36.5° C) it is advisable to bathe the healthy term infant to decrease the caregiver's risk of exposure to blood-borne pathogens. Standard precautions, including the use of gloves, should be adhered to when handling the infant who has not been bathed after delivery and during any invasive procedure in which the caregiver may be exposed to body fluids (Darmstadt and Dinulos, 2000; Varda and Behnke, 2000).

2. Parents may prefer to give the first bath themselves.
3. Vernix caseosa contains large amounts of fats, which protect the skin from the amniotic fluid and bacteria in utero. Vernix insulates the stratum corneum and should not be scrubbed off during the initial bath (Bautista et al., 2000; Pickens et al., 2000).
4. When possible, avoid puncturing the skin of babies with suspected maternal infections.
5. Routine use of emollients is not recommended in the term infant. Creams and emollients that contain perfumes are drying and may irritate the infant's skin. Products that change the pH of the skin decrease the bacteriostatic properties (National Association of Neonatal Nurses [NANN], 1997). If cracking or fissures develop in the skin, a nonperfumed product should be used.

B. Preterm infant.

1. Keep skin clean with water. Mild, nonalkaline soap may be used. Preterm infants should be bathed infrequently during the first 2 months of life to avoid excessive drying of the skin and to avoid overstimulation, stress, and fatigue (Lund and Kuller, 2003; NANN, 1997).
2. Handle infant gently and minimally to avoid trauma.
3. Minimize use of tape as much as possible. Use care when removing tape to avoid stripping the epidermis (Lund et al., 1997).
   a. Safety of adhesive solvents is uncertain. Cotton balls soaked with warm water can be used effectively for removing tape and other adhesives.
   b. Gelled adhesives and pectin-based barriers have been found to be helpful in avoiding trauma to the skin during their removal (Lund et al., 1997).
   c. Pectin or hydrocolloid layers applied before adhesives may protect the skin from damage when endotracheal tubes or catheters are secured.
   d. Benzoin and other adhesive bonding agents form a strong bond between the adhesive and the epidermis, increasing the risk of stripping the epidermis when the adhesive is removed. Use of these agents with preterm infants should be avoided.
   e. Increased permeability of the skin allows absorption of some medications and products such as alcohol and povidone-iodine (Betadine) (Linder et al., 1997). When these substances are used for an invasive procedure, it is recommended that they be removed completely with water as soon as possible to prevent absorption or chemical burns.
4. Emollient creams that are free of preservatives and perfumes may be of benefit to the preterm infant by decreasing transepidermal water loss and skin breakdown when cracking, excessive dryness, or fissures are present (Lund and Kuller, 2003; Lund et al., 2001).
5. A tent with warm mist may protect the skin and decrease insensible water loss in the very low birth weight infant.
6. Transparent adhesive dressings can be used over wounds and abrasions and to secure intravenous (IV) catheters and central lines (Lund and Kuller, 2003).

C. **Umbilical cord care.**
1. Sterile cutting of cord at delivery, rapid drying of umbilical cord, and keeping cord clean is the most effective way to prevent umbilical infections. If cord is not treated, diligent follow-up and attention to the signs and symptoms of omphalitis is required (Janssen et al., 2003).
2. Isopropyl alcohol and triple dye (a solution containing crystal violet, brilliant cresyl green, and proflavine hemisulfate) are the agents most commonly used for cord care. Alcohol may result in cord separating sooner, and appears to be just as effective in keeping cord clean and promoting drying.
3. Tub bath should be delayed until cord has fallen off, generally 10 to 14 days.

ASSESSMENT OF THE NEWBORN INFANT'S SKIN

A. **Factors affecting the appearance of the skin.**
1. Gestational age.
2. Postnatal age.
3. Nutritional status and hydration.
4. Racial origin.
5. Type and amount of available light.
6. Hemoglobin and bilirubin levels.
7. Environmental temperatures.
8. Oxygenation status.

B. **Definitions used to describe skin lesions (Kim and Honig, 2001).**
1. Macule: a pigmented, flat spot that is visible but not palpable. Macules greater than 1 cm in diameter may be referred to as a patch.
2. Papule: a solid, elevated, palpable lesion, with distinct borders less than 1 cm in diameter.
3. Plaque: a solid, elevated, palpable lesion, with distinct borders, greater than 1 cm in size.
4. Nodule: a solid lesion, elevated with depth, up to 2 cm in size
5. Tumor: a solid lesion, elevated with depth, greater than 2 cm in size.
6. Vesicle: an elevated lesion or blister filled with serous fluid and less than 1 cm in diameter.
7. Bulla: a fluid-filled lesion larger than 1 cm.
8. Pustule: a vesicle filled with cloudy or purulent fluid.
9. Petechiae: subepidermal hemorrhages, pinpoint in size. They do not blanch with pressure.
10. Ecchymosis: a large area of subepidermal hemorrhage.
11. Wheal: area of edema in the upper dermis, creating a palpable, slightly raised lesion.
12. Ulcer: erosion of skin with damage of the epidermis into the dermis. Will leave a scar after healing.

COMMON SKIN LESIONS

A. **Normal variations in newborn skin.**
1. Cutis marmorata (Fig. 35-2).
   a. Bluish mottling or marbling effect of the skin.
   b. Physiologic response to chilling caused by dilation of capillaries and venules.
   c. Disappears when infant is rewarmed.
   d. May be sign of stress or overstimulation in newborn infant.

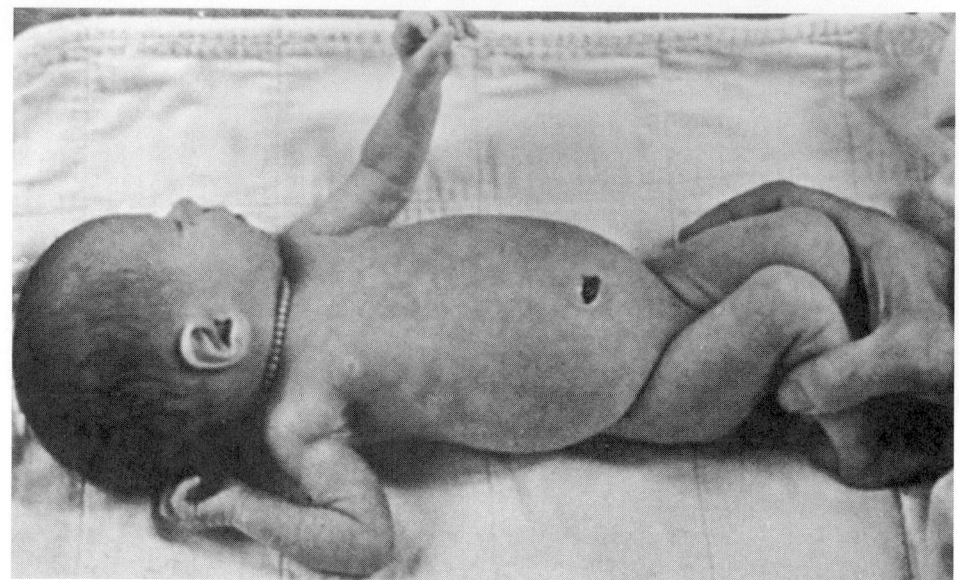

FIGURE 35-2 ■ Cutis marmorata. (Courtesy Jacinto Hernandez, M.D., The Children's Hospital, Denver, CO.)

e. Common in infants with trisomies 18 and 21.
f. If condition persists in infants 6 months of age or older, it may be a symptom of hypothyroidism or a vascular abnormality such as cutis marmorata telangiectasia (Mazereeuw-Hautier et al., 2002).

2. Harlequin color change (Fig. 35-3).

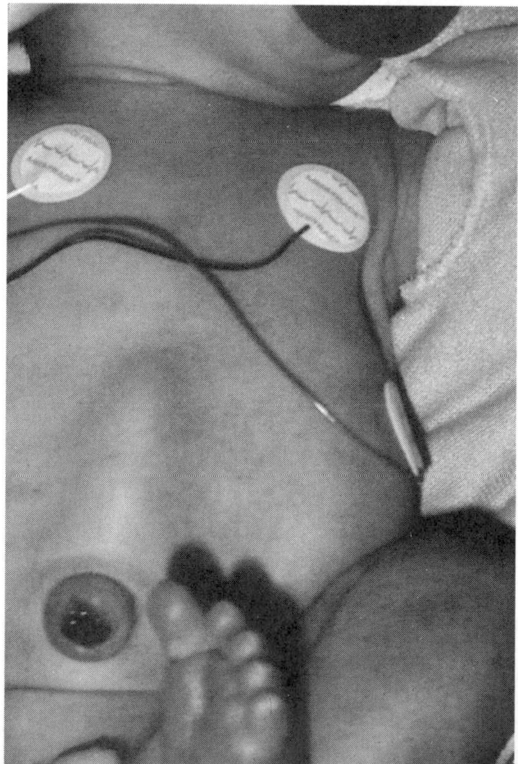

FIGURE 35-3 ■ Harlequin color change. (Courtesy Jane Deacon, RNC, MS, NNP, The Children's Hospital, Denver, CO.)

a. A sharply demarcated red color seen in the dependent half of the body when the infant is lying on its side. When the infant's position is reversed, the color changes to the other side. This condition may also be seen when the infant is lying flat.
b. Caused by immaturity or temporary disturbance of the autonomic regulation of the cutaneous vessels.

3. Erythema toxicum (newborn rash) (Fig. 35-4).
   a. Small white or yellow pustules surrounded by an erythematous base (erythematous base caused by a histamine release) (Marchini et al., 2001).
   b. Benign, found in up to 70% of newborn infants (Margileth, 1999).
   c. Seen in neonates and infants up to 3 months of age.
   d. Lesions come and go on various sites of face, trunk, and limbs, although they are never seen on the palms of the hands or soles of the feet.
   e. Cause unknown, but condition may be exacerbated by handling or by chafing from linen.
   f. Differential diagnosis: may resemble a staphylococcal infection. Diagnosis can be confirmed by smear of aspirated pustule showing numerous eosinophils.
   g. No treatment is necessary. Lotions or creams may exacerbate condition.
4. Milia (Fig. 35-5).
   a. Multiple yellow or pearly white papules about 1 mm in size; epidermal inclusion cysts composed of laminated, keratinous material. They occur on the brow, cheeks, and nose.
   b. Milia are observed in about 40% of term infants (Margileth, 1999).
   c. No treatment is necessary. They resolve spontaneously during the first few weeks after birth.
5. Epstein pearls (Fig. 35-6).
   a. Oral counterpart of facial milia. They can be seen on the midline of the palate or on the alveolar ridges.
   b. Epstein pearls occur in approximately 60% of neonates (Weston et al., 2002).
6. Sebaceous gland hyperplasia.
   a. Tiny (<0.5 mm) white or yellow papules found on the nose, cheeks, and upper lips of newborn infants.

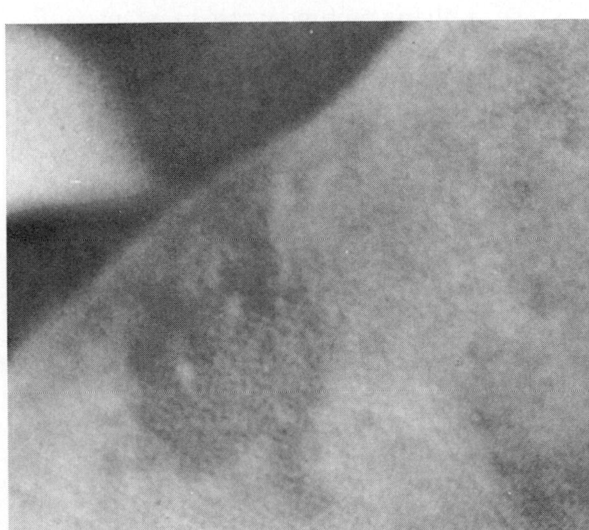

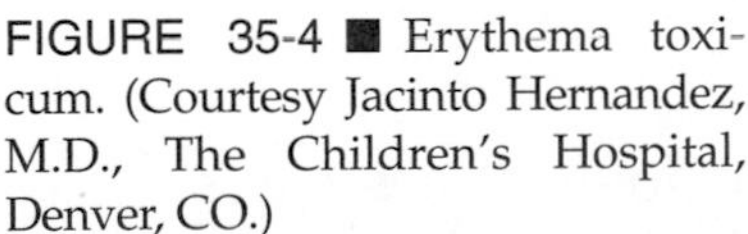
FIGURE 35-4 ■ Erythema toxicum. (Courtesy Jacinto Hernandez, M.D., The Children's Hospital, Denver, CO.)

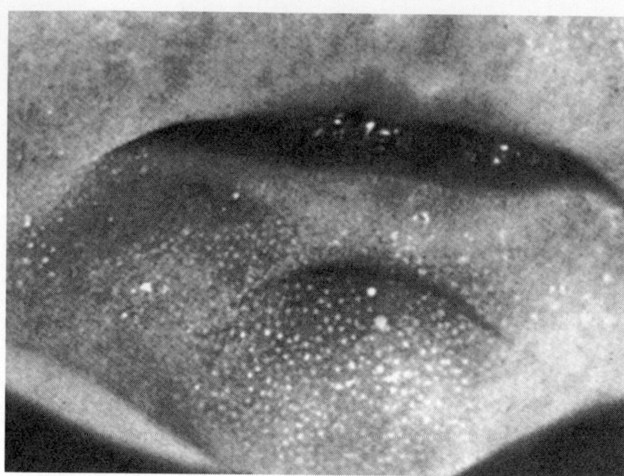

FIGURE 35-5 ■ Milia. (Courtesy Jacinto Hernandez, M.D., The Children's Hospital, Denver, CO.)

   b. Common in term infants but rarely seen in preterm infants.
   c. Represent overactivity of the sebaceous follicles and are a manifestation of maternal androgen stimulation.
   d. They resolve without treatment within a few weeks.
7. Miliaria. Caused by occlusion of sweat ducts by keratin, resulting in retention of sweat. There are four types of miliaria.
   a. Miliaria crystallina: clear, thin vesicles, 1 to 2 mm in diameter that develop in the epidermal portion of the sweat glands. They are seen over the head, neck, and upper aspect of the trunk in newborn infants. Can be present at birth (Haas et al., 2002).
   b. Miliaria rubra: commonly referred to as prickly heat; results from prolonged occlusion of pores, leading to release of sweat into the lower epidermis. Condition appears as pink or white papules and vesicles 2 to 4 mm in diameter, with an erythematous base. The lesions are generally found in the flexure areas, such as the neck, groin, and axillae, as well as on the face and the upper aspect of the chest.
   c. Miliaria pustulosa: resulting from continued exposure to heat, which leads to infiltration of the vesicles with leukocytes. This is rare in most climates and resolves with change to a dry, cool environment.
   d. Miliaria profunda: rare in infants; infection of lower portion of sweat glands in the dermis. Treatment consists of avoidance of further sweating and keeping the skin cool and dry.

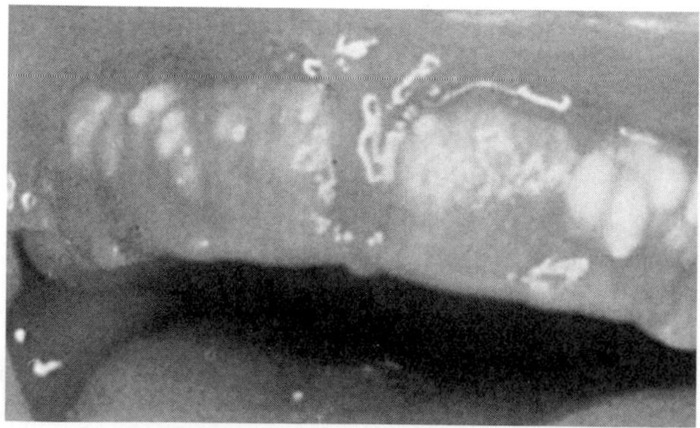

FIGURE 35-6 ■ Epstein pearls. (Courtesy Jacinto Hernandez, M.D., The Children's Hospital, Denver, CO.)

8. Diaper dermatitis.
   a. May be caused by chafing from diapers, by prolonged contact with urine or feces, or by sensitivity to chemicals in disposable diapers or in detergent used in laundering cloth diapers.
   b. The best treatment is prevention by frequent diaper changes and by protection of the skin with a barrier product containing zinc oxide. The skin should be cleansed with warm water after voiding or stooling. Avoid diaper wipes that contain alcohol.
   c. Cornstarch and baby powder should not be used. They provide a medium for growth of bacteria and yeast, and inhaled particles are irritating to the respiratory tract (NANN, 1997).
   d. *Candida* diaper dermatitis: see item 2 under section E, Infectious Lesions, page 907.

B. Lesions resulting from trauma.

1. Forceps marks.
   a. Forceps marks are red or bruised areas seen over the cheek, scalp, or face of infants after forceps delivery.
   b. The infant should be examined for underlying tissue damage or other signs of birth trauma such as scalp abrasions, fractured clavicles, or facial palsy.
2. Subcutaneous fat necrosis.
   a. A hard, circumscribed, red or purple nodule under the dermis in the subcutaneous tissue. Nodules appear on the trunk, extremities, or face, usually during the first 2 weeks of life. They may grow larger initially and then resolve spontaneously within several weeks.
   b. Subcutaneous fat necrosis has been attributed to trauma, cold stress, shock, and asphyxia and is caused by crystallization of the subcutaneous fat cells.
   c. Hypercalcemia may be associated with subcutaneous fat necrosis in infants with multiple nodules. Serum calcium levels should be monitored (Cunningham and Paes, 1991).
3. Scalp lacerations.
   a. Scalp lacerations may be caused by trauma during delivery, placement of scalp electrodes, or fetal blood pH sampling.
   b. Treatment consists of keeping the area clean and dry, and assessing for infection.
4. Intravenous extravasations.
   a. Vascular access sites in the infant should be assessed hourly to evaluate line patency and detect extravasation. The IV catheter should be removed immediately if patency is not certain or if signs of extravasation are apparent.
   b. If extravasation occurs, the extremity should be elevated. Heat or moist dressings are not recommended.
   c. Topical antimicrobial ointment may aid in healing (Lund and Kuller, 2003).

C. Pigmented skin lesions.

1. Hyperpigmented macules (mongolian spots) (Fig. 35-7).
   a. Large macules or patches, gray or blue-green, seen most commonly over the buttocks, flanks, or shoulders.
   b. Most common pigmented lesion seen at birth, occurring in 90% of black, Asian, and Hispanic infants and in 1% to 5% of white infants (Margileth, 1999).
   c. Hyperpigmented macules are caused by the increased presence of melanocytes dispersed in the dermis.

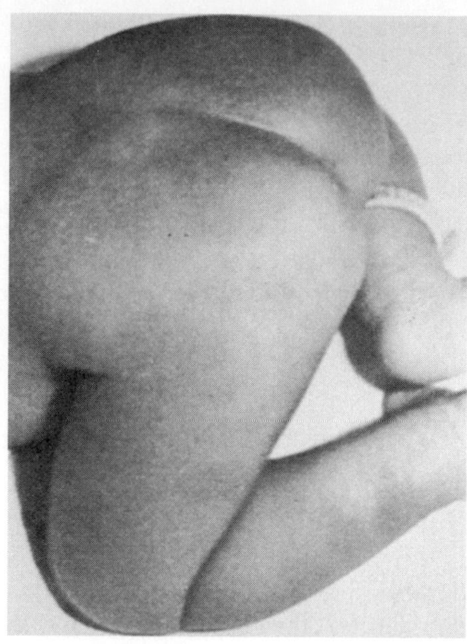

FIGURE 35-7 ■ Hyperpigmented macules (mongolian spots). (Courtesy Jacinto Hernandez, M.D., The Children's Hospital, Denver, CO.)

d. The spots fade somewhat during the first few years after birth, particularly as surrounding skin darkens, but may persist into adulthood.
e. It is important to document size and location to avoid question of nonaccidental trauma.

2. Congenital melanocytic nevi (pigmented nevi) (Fig. 35-8).
    a. Dark brown or black macules that may or may not be hairy. Nevi may occur anywhere on the body, with the "bathing trunk" area being the most common site.
    b. Caused by collection of melanocytes under the skin.
    c. Most are small, less than 2 cm, with smooth surfaces. Large nevi (>10 cm) are rare (Weston et al., 2002).
    d. Pigmented nevi are generally benign, but malignant changes occur in approximately 8% to 10% of larger lesions (Dohil et al., 2000; Margileth, 1999).
    e. Close observation for changes in size or shape is indicated, with possible surgical excision. Large, unusually shaped nevi may be difficult to assess for changes and should be followed closely (Weston et al., 2002). Surgical

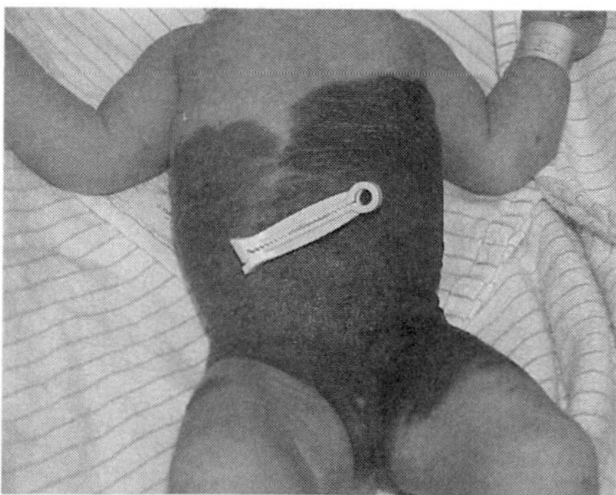

FIGURE 35-8 ■ Giant pigmented nevus. (Courtesy Catherine L. Witt, Aurora, CO.)

excision of at least part of the lesion may be necessary, although it can be difficult in large lesions. (De Raeve and Roseeuw, 2002).

f. Pigment specific lasers such as the Q switched ruby laser have been used with some success, although complete clearance is rare. May be useful to clear edges of lesion prior to surgical excision (Morelli, 1998).

g. A hairy nevus present over the spine may be associated with spina bifida or meningocele (Drolet, 1998).

h. Pigmented nevi may also be associated with neurofibromatosis or tuberous sclerosis.

3. Transient neonatal pustular melanosis (Fig. 35-9).
   a. Superficial vesiculopustular lesions that rupture during the first 12 to 48 hours after birth, leaving small, brown, hyperpigmented macules. The macules may be surrounded by very fine white scales. They often rupture before delivery, presenting as macules.
   b. Benign; found in up to 5% of black infants and in about 0.2% of white neonates (Ramamurthy et al., 1976).
   c. No treatment is necessary. The macules generally fade during the first few weeks or months after birth.
   d. Aspirating the contents of the vesicles will reveal a variable number of neutrophils and few or no eosinophils.
4. Café-au-lait spots (Fig. 35-10).
   a. Tan or light brown patches with well-defined borders.
   b. When less than 3 cm in length and fewer than six in number, they are of no pathologic significance.
   c. Six or more spots may be an indication of neurofibromatosis (Eichenfield and Gibbs, 2001).
      (1) Neurofibromatosis is a condition in which tumors form on cutaneous nerves and along the thoracic, brachial, and lumbar nerve trunks. Cranial nerves may also be affected.
      (2) It is an autosomal dominant disorder.
      (3) Café-au-lait spots may be the only finding of this disease in the neonatal period.
5. Ash leaf macules.
   a. White macules in the shape of an ash leaf or thumbprint; seen primarily over the trunk or buttocks.

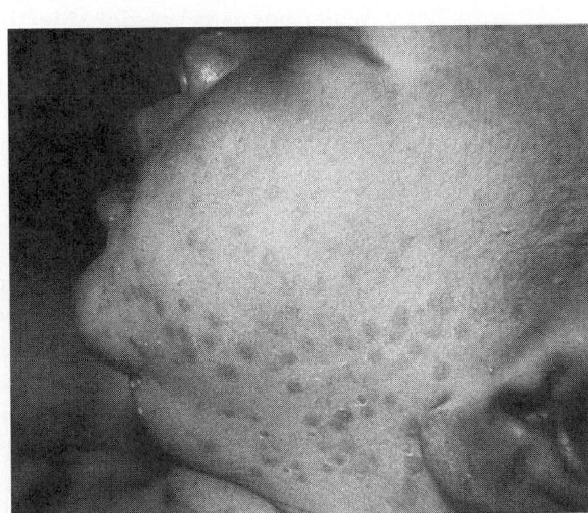

FIGURE 35-9 ■ Neonatal pustular melanosis. (Courtesy Jane Deacon, RNC, MS, NNP, The Children's Hospital, Denver, CO.)

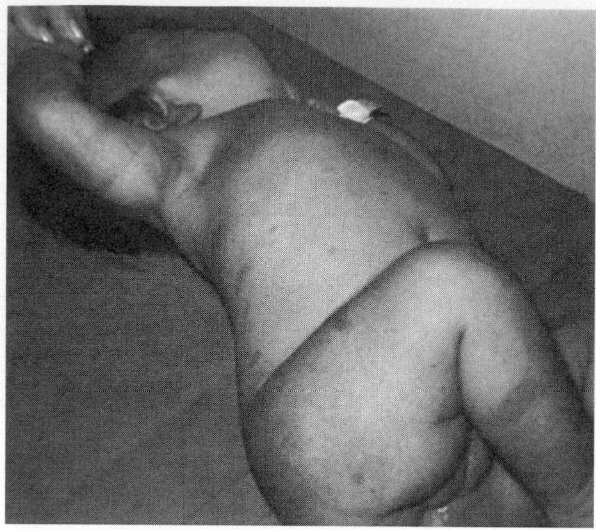

FIGURE 35-10 ■ Café-au-lait spots. (Courtesy Jacinto Hernandez, M.D., The Children's Hospital, Denver, CO.)

b. Found in 90% of infants with tuberous sclerosis (Margileth, 1999).
c. May be difficult to see in fair-skinned infants. Use of a Wood (ultraviolet) lamp will aid in examination.
d. Infants with unexplained seizures should be examined for these macules.
e. May also be a normal finding or may be associated with neurofibromatosis.

D. Vascular lesions.

1. Nevus simplex.
   a. Nevus simplex (stork bite) refers to macular pink areas of distended capillaries found on the nape of the neck, the upper eyelids, the nose, or the upper lip. They have diffuse borders, blanch with pressure, and become pinker with crying.
   b. These are the most common of vascular birthmarks, seen in 30% to 50% of newborn infants (Weston et al., 2002).
   c. The lesions tend to fade by the first or second year, with the exception of those on the nape of the neck, which may persist.
2. Port-wine stain.
   a. A flat vascular nevus is present at birth. It is usually pink in infancy, but may be red or purple. The nevus may be small or may cover almost half of the body. It is flat, sharply delineated, and blanches minimally. Facial lesions are the most common.
   b. Port-wine stains consist of mature capillaries that are dilated and congested directly below the epidermis. The cause is unknown.
   c. The nevus does not grow in area or size. It will not resolve and should be considered permanent. The lesion may become darker and thicker with age.
   d. The pulsed-dye laser has been successful in lightening most port-wine stains by up to 50%. The laser works by causing intravascular coagulation (Morelli, 1998). Light-colored facial lesions have the best results; red or purple lesions that are thick and nodular respond less well. Most infants require five or more treatments. Other methods of surgical excision have been largely unsatisfactory.
   e. Sturge-Weber syndrome (Fig. 35-11).
      (1) Port-wine stains are confined to a pattern similar to that of the branches of the trigeminal nerve.

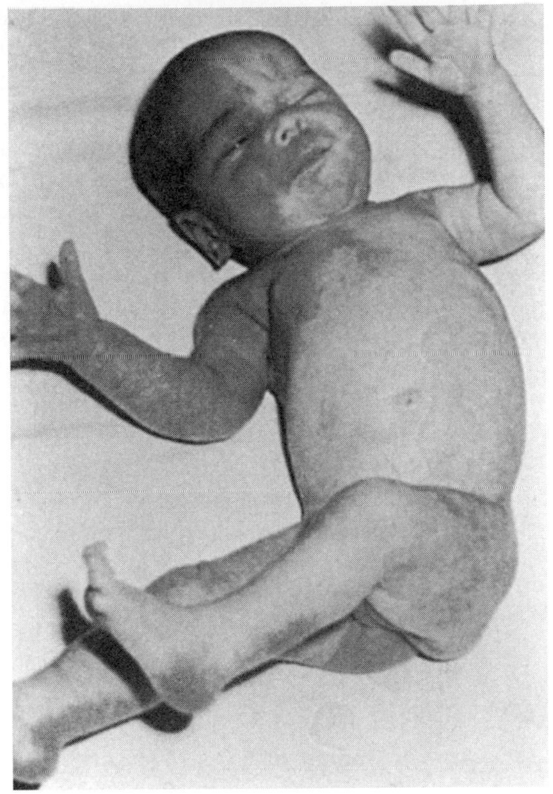

FIGURE 35-11 ■ Sturge-Weber syndrome. (Courtesy Jacinto Hernandez, M.D., The Children's Hospital, Denver, CO.)

(2) Central feature is disordered proliferation of endothelial cells, particularly in the small veins. It is associated with atrophic changes in the cerebral cortex and calcium deposits in the walls of small vessels and areas of affected cortex (Margileth, 1999).

(3) Manifested by glaucoma, focal seizures, hemiparesis, and mental retardation (Morelli, 1998).

3. Strawberry hemangioma (Fig. 35-12).

a. Raised, lobulated, soft, bright red tumor located on the head, neck, trunk, or extremities. These lesions may also occur in the throat, where they can cause airway obstruction, requiring a tracheostomy in extreme cases.

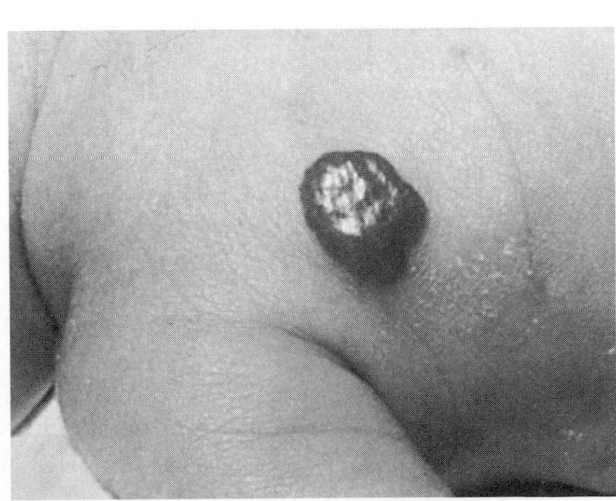

FIGURE 35-12 ■ Strawberry hemangioma. (Courtesy Jacinto Hernandez, M.D., The Children's Hospital, Denver, CO.)

b. Caused by dilated capillaries occupying the dermal and subdermal layers, in association with endothelial proliferation.
c. About 20% to 30% are present at birth, and 90% are evident by 2 months of age (Drolet et al., 1999; Margileth, 1999). The lesions occur in approximately 1% to 2% of newborn infants and are more common in preterm infants with females predominating (Blei et al., 1998; Chiller et al., 2002; Freiden et al., 1997). The lesions may also be familial (Blei et al., 1998).
d. Strawberry hemangiomas will generally increase in size during the first 6 months, and then become stable in size before undergoing gradual spontaneous regression, with most leaving no trace. This may take several years. Infants will often have more than one lesion.
e. Treatment of choice is to allow the lesion to regress spontaneously. If the lesion is interfering with vision, is bleeding or ulcerating, or is impinging on other vital functions, treatment should be considered.
   (1) Systemic corticosteroid therapy is the treatment of choice for most hemangiomas (Freiden et al., 1997).
   (2) Flash-lamp pumped pulsed-dye laser may be effective on some lesions (Morelli, 1998).
   (3) Cryosurgery may be helpful, but concerns about scarring have prevented this option from becoming widespread (Freiden et al., 1997).
   (4) Interferon-α-2b may be effective in treating steroid-resistant lesions (Tamayo et al., 1997).
f. The infant should be monitored for signs of impingement on vital organs or functioning, such as stridor, poor feeding, and difficulty in swallowing, which would make treatment necessary.
g. The cosmetic concerns of parents require a caring, supportive approach. Pictures illustrating spontaneous regression may be helpful.

4. Cavernous hemangioma.
   a. This lesion is composed of large venous channels and vascular elements lined by endothelial cells.
   b. It involves the dermis and subcutaneous tissue and appears as a bluish red discoloration under the overlying skin.
   c. The cavernous hemangioma has poorly defined borders and may feel cystic, like a "bag of worms," when palpated (Margileth, 1999). Like the strawberry hemangioma, the cavernous hemangioma will increase in size during the first 6 to 12 months and then involute spontaneously.
   d. Treatment is not indicated unless the lesion is interfering with vital functions, including airway obstruction, in which case systemic corticosteroid treatment or interferon-α may be helpful (Enjolras and Garzon, 2001).
   e. Kasabach-Merritt syndrome.
      (1) Giant cavernous hemangiomas may be associated with sequestration of platelets and thrombocytopenia.
      (2) Treatment consists of systemic corticosteroid therapy. Transfusions of platelets and blood are frequently necessary (Enroljas and Garzon, 2001; Weston et al., 2002). The lesions may resolve spontaneously.
      (3) Surgical excision has been successful in isolated cases (George et al., 2002).
      (4) It has been suggested that infants with Kasabach-Merritt syndrome do not have true cavernous hemangiomas but rather a different type of vascular malformation (Enjolras et al., 1997).

f. Klippel-Trenaunay-Weber syndrome.
   (1) Syndrome consists of hypertrophy of a limb with associated vascular nevi and hypertrophy of underlying bone and soft tissue.
   (2) Rare congenital abnormality, seen mostly in males (Margileth, 1999).
   (3) No specific treatment for the disease. Severe limb hypertrophy may require orthopedic consultation, with possible amputation of affected limb.

E. Infectious lesions.

1. Thrush.
   a. A fungal infection of the mouth or throat, caused by *Candida albicans*.
   b. Very common in infants.
   c. Manifested as patches of adherent white material scattered over the tongue and mucous membranes.
   d. Treated with an oral antifungal preparation such as nystatin (Mycostatin).
2. *Candida* diaper dermatitis.
   a. Fungal infection of skin in the diaper area; may include buttocks, groin, thighs, and abdomen.
   b. Caused by organism *C. albicans*.
   c. Manifested as a moist, erythematous eruption, often with white or yellow satellite pustules.
   d. Treatment consists of an antifungal cream or ointment preparation such as nystatin (Mycostatin), applied to the rash several times per day. Oral antifungal treatment may be recommended in cases of persistent *Candida* dermatitis.
3. Systemic *Candida* infection.
   a. Very low birth weight infants are at risk of having systemic, invasive fungal infections, with invasion of the fungus beyond the stratum corneum.
   b. Improving the barrier function of the skin by minimizing trauma and maintaining a sterile environment may help prevent onset of this infection.
4. Herpes.
   a. Neonatal herpes simplex infection is one of the most serious viral infections in the neonate.
   b. Rash appears as vesicular or pustular rash (Fig. 35-13).
   c. 70% of infants with herpes will have subsequent rash, but not necessarily before other signs and symptoms of illness develop. Therefore the absence of vesicles does not eliminate the possibility of disease.

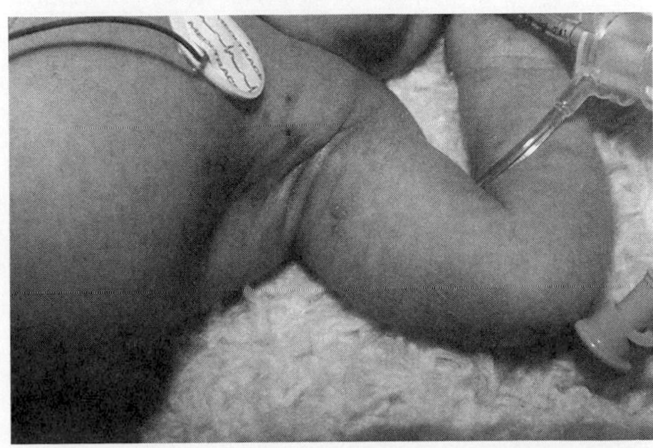

FIGURE 35-13 ■ Herpes simplex vesicles. (Courtesy Jane Deacon, RNC, MS, NNP, The Children's Hospital, Denver, CO.)

d. Treatment with an antiviral agent such as acyclovir should begin immediately. The earlier treatment is begun, the better the outcome (Weston et al., 2002).

5. "Scalded skin" syndrome (also known as bullous impetigo, toxic epidermal necrolysis, Ritter disease, and nonstreptococcal scarlatina).
   a. An inflammatory skin disorder generally caused by the phage strain of group II staphylococcus. May follow an upper respiratory tract infection or otitis media.
   b. Manifested as a widespread, tender erythema, followed by blisters ranging from small vesicles to large bullae. Caused by the release of an endotoxin that acts on the stratum granulosa of the epidermis. The blisters, which frequently begin in the diaper area and spread to the rest of the body, rupture, leaving large, raw, scaldlike areas.
   c. Treatment includes isolation and aseptic handling to prevent further infection in the infected infant and the spread of bacteria to others. The infant is treated systemically with methicillin because of the number of penicillin-resistant strains in the phage strain of group II staphylococcus. A topical antibiotic ointment such as bacitracin may be applied locally.
6. Congenital viral infection.
   a. Petechiae and purpuric macules erupt on the head, trunk, and extremities of affected infants. The lesions are often described as "blueberry muffin" spots and are caused by dermal erythropoiesis (Fig. 35-14).
   b. The lesions generally disappear in 2 to 3 weeks. Treatment is based on the underlying disorder.
   c. Although the lesions are most often associated with rubella, they are also seen in association with other congenital infections such as cytomegalovirus, toxoplasmosis, syphilis, and herpes.
   d. Affected infants may also have growth restriction, jaundice, hepatosplenomegaly, and thrombocytopenia.

F. **Hereditary and miscellaneous lesions.**
   1. Epidermolysis bullosa.
      a. Disease characterized by the formation of vesicles and bullae over various parts of the body. Skin is extremely fragile. The underlying genetic defect

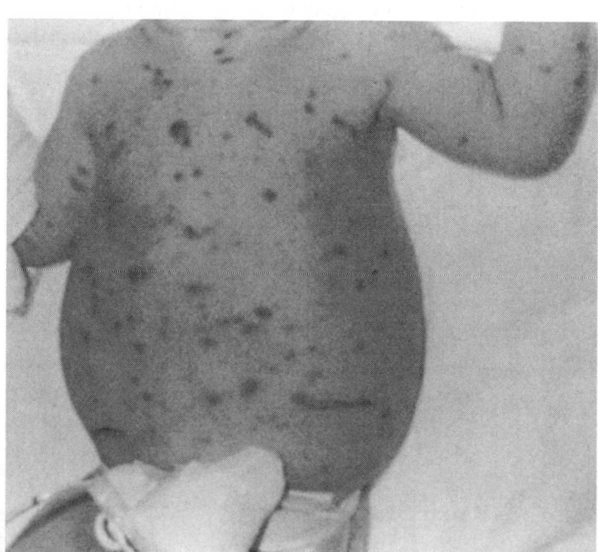

FIGURE 35-14 ■ Blueberry muffin rash. (Courtesy Jacinto Hernandez, M.D., The Children's Hospital, Denver, CO.)

may be autosomal dominant or recessive (Campbell and Banta-Wright, 2000).

b. Vesicles may appear spontaneously or in response to minor trauma such as routine handling.

c. Lesions may appear at birth or a few weeks later.

d. Three types of vesicles may appear at birth.

(1) Simple, nonscarring: bullae form in small numbers throughout childhood and heal without scarring. Often disappear at puberty. Prevention of trauma and infection is important.

(2) Dystrophic, scarring: more severe form of the disease, with lesions forming scars, loss of nails, and contractures. Death may result from secondary infections.

(3) Epidermolysis bullosa lethalis: most severe form, with large, numerous lesions, usually present at birth. Large areas of epidermis are lost, leaving red, weeping erosions. Esophageal lesions may also occur. The life span of these patients is generally short. Treatment is supportive care, minimizing trauma and infection (Weston et al., 2002).

2. Collodion baby.

a. Term describes an appearance rather than a disease. These babies are born covered with a tight, shiny, transparent membrane that cracks and peels off after a few days. A few infants will have no underlying disorder, but many will have some form of ichthyosis (Weston et al., 2002) (Fig. 35-15).

b. Treatment consists of liberal application of sterile olive or mineral oil several times a day to hydrate and lubricate the skin, careful handling, and prevention of infection.

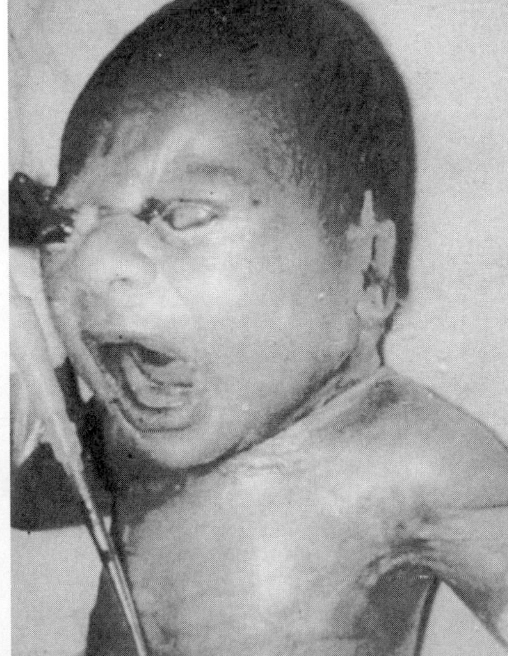

FIGURE 35-15 ■ Collodion infant. (From Solomon, L.M. and Esterly, N.B.: *Neonatal dermatology.* Philadelphia, 2001, Saunders, p. 115.)

3. Ichthyosis.
   a. Ichthyosis is a disease involving excessive scaling of the skin, caused by excessive production of stratum corneum cells or faulty shedding of the stratum corneum (Weston et al., 2002). There are four types of ichthyosis.
      (1) Ichthyosis vulgaris: an autosomal dominant disease, usually appearing after 3 months of age. This is the most common and most benign of the ichthyosis disorders, occurring in approximately 1 in 250 infants (Margileth, 1999). It consists of fine white scales and excessively dry skin (Campbell and Banta-Wright, 2000).
      (2) X-linked ichthyosis: appears at birth or during the first year of life. It occasionally occurs in a collodion baby. The disorder consists of large, thick, dark brown scales over the entire body, with the exception of the palms and soles. It occurs in males only.
      (3) Lamellar ichthyosis: an autosomal recessive trait that is manifested at birth as bright red erythema and universal desquamation. Some infants resemble collodion babies. Scales are large, flat, and coarse and may be less prominent in infancy than later in childhood. Eversion of the lips and eyelids may occur, and the palms and soles may be thickened. Hyperkeratosis may be seen on skin biopsy, although this is not diagnostic of the disorder (Weston et al., 2002).
      (4) Bullous ichthyosis: autosomal dominant disorder characterized by recurrent formation of bullous lesions, erythroderma, and excessive dryness and peeling. As the child grows the involvement generally becomes limited to small, thick, hard scales, most often found in the flexure regions. Hyperkeratosis may be seen on the palms and soles (Campbell and Banta-Wright, 2000). Infection in the neonatal period with *Staphylococcus aureus* is of primary concern because of the widespread skin breakdown.
   b. Treatment of ichthyosis is limited to use of topical preparations to hydrate and lubricate the skin. Daily baths with a water-dispersible bath oil, with use of alpha hydroxy acid ointments, may be helpful (Weston et al., 2002).
   c. Drying soaps and detergents should be avoided.
   d. Care must be taken to prevent infection of dry or cracked skin.

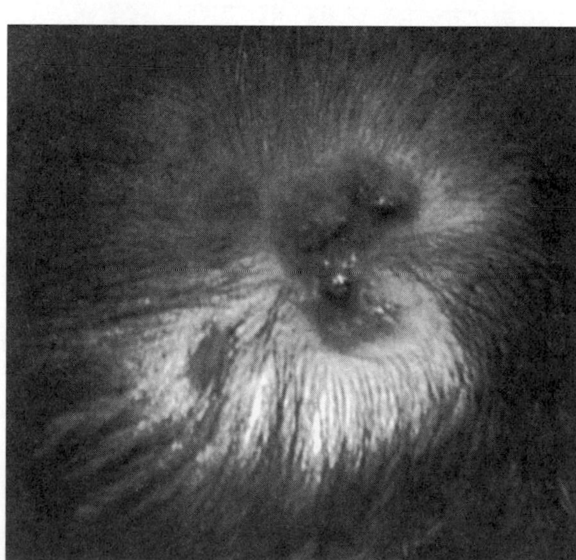

FIGURE 35-16 ■ Cutis aplasia. (Courtesy Jacinto Hernandez, M.D., The Children's Hospital, Denver, CO.)

4. Harlequin fetus.
   a. The harlequin fetus previously was considered to have a severe form of ichthyosis but may in fact have a separate rare autosomal recessive disease (Weston et al., 2002). The harlequin fetus has hard, thick, gray or yellow scales that cause severe deformities of skeletal and soft tissues.
   b. The condition is untreatable, and most infants die within a few hours or days of life.
5. Cutis aplasia.
   a. Term refers to congenital absence of skin, either as a midline defect, a posterior scalp defect, or several small or large defects involving the upper and lower extremities (Fig. 35-16).
   b. Lesions heal slowly over several months, leaving a hypertrophic or atrophic scar.
   c. May be associated with other defects such as cleft lip and palate, heart disease, tracheoesophageal fistula, and other midline defects. It is commonly seen in infants with trisomy 13.

REFERENCES

Bautista, M.I.B., Wickett, R.R., Visscher, M.O., et al.: Characterization of vernix caseosa as a natural biofilm: Comparison to standard oil-based ointments. *Pediatric Dermatology, 17*(4):253-260, 2000.

Blei, F., Walter, J., Orlow S.J., and Marchuk, D.A.: Familial segregation of hemangiomas and vascular malformations as an autosomal dominant trait. *Archives of Dermatology, 134*(6):718-742, 1998.

Campbell, J.M. and Banta-Wright, S.A.: Neonatal skin disorders: A review of selected dermatologic abnormalities. *Journal of Perinatal and Neonatal Nursing, 14*(1):63-83, 2000.

Chiller, K.G., Passaro, D., Freiden, I.J.: Hemangiomas of infancy: Clinical characteristics, morphologic subtypes, and their relationship to race, ethnicity, and sex. *Archives of Dermatology, 138*(12): 1567-1576, 2002.

Cunningham, K. and Paes, B.A.: Subcutaneous fat necrosis of the newborn with hypercalcemia: A review. *Neonatal Network, 10*(3):7-14, 1991.

Darmstadt, G.L. and Dinulos, J.G.: Neonatal skin care. *Pediatric Clinics of North America, 47*(4):757-782, 2000.

De Raeve, L.E. and Roseeuw, D.I.: Curettage of giant congenital melanocytic nevi in neonates. A decade later. *Archives of Dermatology, 138*(7):943-947, 2002.

Dohil, M.A., Baugh, W.P., and Eichenfield, L.F.: Vascular and pigmented birthmarks. *Pediatric Clinics of North America, 47*(4):783-812, 2000.

Drolet, B.A.: Birthmarks to worry about. *Dermatologic Clinics, 16*(3):447-453, 1998.

Drolet, B.A., Esterly, N.B., and Freiden, I.J.: Hemangiomas in children. *New England Journal of Medicine, 341*(3):173-181, 1999.

Eichenfield, L.F. and Gibbs, N.F.: Hyperpigmentation disorders. In L.F. Eichenfield, I.J. Freiden, and N.B. Esterly (Eds.): *Textbook of neonatal dermatology*. Philadelphia, 2001, Saunders, pp. 370-394.

Enroljas, O. and Garzon M.C.: Vascular stains, malformations, and tumors. In L.F. Eichenfield, I.J. Freiden, and N.B. Esterly (Eds.): *Textbook of neonatal dermatology*. Philadelphia, 2001, Saunders, pp. 324-352.

Enjolras, O., Wassef, M., Mazoyer, E., et al.: Infants with Kasabach-Merritt syndrome do not have "true" hemangiomas. *Journal of Pediatrics, 130*(4): 631-640, 1997.

Freiden, I.J., Eichenfield, L.F., Esterly, N.B., et al.: Guidelines for care of hemangiomas of infancy. *Journal of the American Academy of Dermatology, 37*(4):631-637, 1997.

George, M., Singhal, V., Sharma, V., and Nopper, A.J.: Successful surgical excision of a complex vascular lesion in an infant with Kasabach-Merritt Syndrome. *Pediatric Dermatology, 19*(4):340-344, 2002,

Giusti, F., Martella A., Bertoni L., and Seidenari S.: Skin barrier, hydration, and pH of the skin of infants under 2 years of age. *Pediatric Dermatology, 18*(2):93-96, 2001.

Haas, N., Henz, B.M., and Weigel, H.: Congenital miliaria crystallina. *Journal of the American Academy of Dermatology, 47*(5 Suppl):S270-S272, 2002.

Hoeger, P.H. and Enzmann, C.C.: Skin physiology of the neonate and young infant: A prospective study of functional skin parameters during early infancy. *Pediatric Dermatology, 19*(3):256-262, 2002.

Janssen, P.A., Selwood, B.L., Dobson, S.R., et al.: To dye or not to dye: A randomized, clinical trial of a triple dye/alcohol regime versus dry cord care. *Pediatrics, 111*(1):15-20, 2003.

Kalia, Y.N., Nonato, L.B., Lund, C.H., et al: Development of skin barrier function in preterm infants. *Journal of Investigative Dermatology, 111*(2):320-326, 1998.

Kim, H.J. and Honig, P.J.: Lesional morphology and assessment. In L.F. Eichenfield, I.J. Freiden, and N.B. Esterly (Eds.): *Textbook of neonatal dermatology*. Philadelphia, 2001, Saunders, pp. 33-45.

Kopelman, A.E.: Cutaneous absorption of hexachlorophene in low birth weight infants. *Journal of Pediatrics, 82*(6):972-975, 1973.

Linder, N., Davidovitch, N., Reichman, B., et al.: Topical iodine-containing antiseptics and subclinical hypothyroidism in preterm infants. *Journal of Pediatrics, 131*(3):434-439, 1997.

Lund, C.H. and Kuller, J.M.: Assessment and management of the integumentary system. In C. Kenner and J.W. Lott (Eds.): *Comprehensive neonatal nursing: A physiologic perspective* (3rd ed.). Philadelphia, 2003, Saunders, pp. 700-724.

Lund, C.H., Kuller, J.M., and Lott, J.W.: Neonatal skin care: Clinical outcomes of the AWHONN/NANN evidenced-based clinical practice guideline. *Journal of Obstetric, Gynecologic, and Neonatal Nursing, 30*(1):41-51, 2001.

Lund, C.H., Nonato, L.B., Kuller, J.M., et al.: Disruption of barrier function in neonatal skin associated with adhesive removal. *Journal of Pediatrics, 131*(3):367-372, 1997.

Mancini, A.J.: Structure and function of newborn skin. In L.F. Eichenfield, I.J. Freiden and N.B. Esterly (Eds.): *Textbook of neonatal dermatology*. Philadelphia, 2001, Saunders, pp. 18-32.

Marchini, G., Ulfgren, A.K., Lore, K., et al.: Erythema toxicum neonatorum: An immunohistochemical analysis. *Pediatric Dermatology, 18*(3):177-187, 2001.

Margileth, A.: Dermatologic conditions. In C.B. Avery (Ed.): *Neonatology: Pathophysiology and management of the newborn* (5th ed.). Philadelphia, 1999, Lippincott Williams & Wilkins, pp. 1323-1360.

Mazereeuw-Hautier, J., Carel-Caneppele, S., and Bonafe, J.L.: Cutis marmorata telangiectatica congenital: Report of two persistent cases. *Pediatric Dermatology, 19*(6):506-509, 2002.

Morelli, J.G.: Use of lasers in pediatric dermatology. *Dermatologic Clinics, 16*(3):489-495, 1998.

National Association of Neonatal Nurses. *Guidelines for practice: Neonatal skin care*. Petaluma, CA, 1997, Author.

Pickens, W.L., Warner, R.R., Boissy, Y.L., et al.: Characterization of vernix caseosa: Water content, morphology, and elemental analysis. *Journal of Investigative Dermatology, 115*(5):875-881, 2000.

Ramamurthy, R.S., Reveri, M., Esterly, N.B., et al.: Transient neonatal pustular melanosis. *Journal of Pediatrics, 88*(5): 831-835, 1976.

Siegfried, E.C.: Neonatal skin and skin care. *Dermatologic Clinics, 16*(5):437-446, 1998.

Tamayo, L., Ortiz, D.M., Orozco-Covarrubias L, et al.: Therapeutic efficacy of interferon alfa-2b in infants with life-threatening giant hemangiomas. *Archives of Dermatology, 133*(12):1567-1571, 1997.

Varda, K. and Behnke, R.: The effect of timing of initial bath on newborn's temperature. *Journal of Obstetric, Gynecologic, and Neonatal Nursing, 29*(1):27-32, 2000.

Weston, W.L., Lane, A.T., and Morelli, J.T.: *Color textbook of pediatric dermatology* (3rd ed.). St Louis, 2002, Mosby.

Williams, M.L.: Skin of the premature infant. In L.F. Eichenfield, I.J. Freiden, and N.B. Esterly (Eds.): *Textbook of neonatal dermatology*. Philadelphia, 2001, Saunders, pp. 46-61.

CHAPTER 36

Ophthalmologic and Auditory Disorders

DEBBIE FRASER ASKIN AND WILLIAM DIEHL-JONES

OBJECTIVES

1. Describe the normal anatomy of the eye.
2. Identify the normal anatomy of the ear.
3. Identify the major function(s) of each structure.
4. Describe the components of a nursing assessment of the eyes and ears in the neonate.
5. Describe the nurse's role in assisting the physician with neonatal eye examinations.
6. Discuss the factors to consider in universal hearing screening of newborns.
7. For each of six types of eye disorders in the neonatal period—traumatic injuries to the eye, conjunctivitis, nasolacrimal duct obstruction, cataracts, infections (TORCH diseases), and retinopathy of prematurity—(1) provide an overview of the pathogenesis and (2) describe commonly used treatment modalities, outlining the specific nursing care measures designed to meet the needs of neonates with these disorders.
8. Outline the most common causes of hearing loss in the newborn.

An examination of the neonate's eyes and ears is an important, though often neglected, portion of a physical assessment. There is a great deal of clinically significant information that the astute nurse can glean from a thorough evaluation of these systems. Evidence of intrauterine infection, birth trauma, congenital malformations, disease, and a variety of genetic abnormalities can be detected during the course of the nurse's assessment of the neonate's eyes and ears.

This chapter provides the neonatal nurse with a review of normal anatomy of the eye and ear, together with the major function(s) of each structure; the essential components of an assessment of the newborn's eyes and ears; an overview of the most common eye disorders in the neonate; and common treatment modalities and nursing measures used in the treatment of various ocular disorders in the newborn infant. The essential elements of a universal hearing screening program for newborns is addressed as are the most common causes of hearing loss in neonates.

ANATOMY OF THE EYE (Fig. 36-1)

Protective Structures

A. **Eyelids:** shade the eyes during sleep; protect from excessive light or foreign objects; spread lubricating secretions over the eyeball.
B. **Conjunctiva:** mucous membrane lining the inner aspect of the eyelids (palpebral) and onto the eyeball to the periphery of the cornea (bulbar).

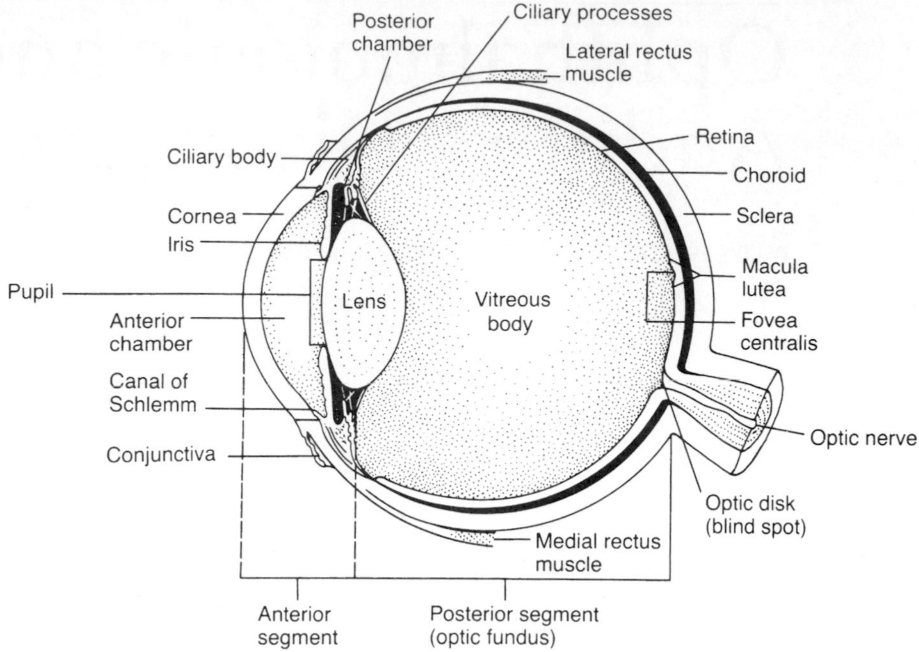

FIGURE 36-1 ■ Cross section of eyeball. (From Boyd-Monk H: The structure and function of the eye and its adnexa. *Journal of Ophthalmic Nursing and Technology,* 6[5]:176-183, 1987.)

C. **Lacrimal system:** manufactures and drains away tears; cleans, lubricates, and moistens the eyeball.
D. **Bony orbit or socket:** surrounds and protects the eyeball. Most important opening within the orbit is the optic foramen, through which the optic nerve, ophthalmic artery, and ophthalmic vein from each eye pass en route to the brain.

The Eyeball

A. **Outer layer (fibrous tunic).**
   1. Cornea: transparent; reflects light rays.
   2. Sclera: the "white" of the eye; normal bluish appearance in newborn infants; gives shape to the eyeball and protects the inner parts.
B. **Middle layer (vascular tunic): the uveal tract.**
   1. Iris and pupil: a circular pigmented diaphragm with a central hole; controls the amount of light entering the eye.
   2. Ciliary body: the anterior portion of the choroid.
   3. Choroid: a vascular, pigmented membrane that lines most of the internal surface of the sclera, absorbs light rays, and nourishes the retina.
C. **Inner layer: the retina.**
   1. Extends from the ora serrata to the optic nerve.
   2. Functions in image formation.
      a. Photoreceptors: rods and cones.
      b. Bipolar cells.
      c. Ganglion cells.

3. Optic disc: retinal blood vessels enter the eye, and optic nerve exits the eye. Blind spot in field of vision because optic disc has no photoreceptors.
4. Optic nerve: second cranial nerve.
5. Macula: exact center of the retina and location of sharpest vision.

D. **Anterior cavity (filled with aqueous humor).**
  1. Anterior chamber: behind the cornea, in front of the iris.
  2. Posterior chamber: behind the iris, in front of the suspensory ligament and lens.

E. **The lens:** a biconvex, transparent capsule that refracts light; the most important focusing mechanism of the eye.

F. **Posterior cavity (filled with vitreous humor):** lies between the lens and the retina. Contributes to intraocular pressure, gives shape to the eyeball, and holds the retina in place.

Extraocular Muscles

A. **Musculature.** Six muscles move each globe. The muscles of each eye work in conjunction with each other.

B. **Innervation.** The extraocular muscles are innervated by the oculomotor (third cranial) nerve, the abducens (sixth cranial) nerve, and the trochlear (fourth cranial) nerve.

PATIENT ASSESSMENT

History

A. **Pregnancy:** first-trimester infections (e.g., rubella), unknown rashes, fever, venereal disease, vaginal discharge, medications.

B. **Birth history:** gestational age, duration of labor, use of forceps.

C. **Family history:** incidence of ocular disorders, especially retinoblastoma; systemic diseases.

Examination

The examination is performed with the baby in a quiet, alert state. To facilitate the spontaneous eye-opening, use an auditory stimulus, change the infant's position from supine to upright, or dim the lights (Johnson, 2003). Eye prophylaxis may make the examination more difficult.

A. **External assessment.**
  1. General facial configuration: should be symmetric. Note distance between the eyes; an abnormal width between the eyes is referred to as hypertelorism.
  2. Spontaneous eye movements: note range of motion and conjugation (the ability of the eyes to move together). Infants can track and follow objects with both eyes. Erratic or purposeless movements may be observed during the first few weeks of life. Median focal distance for the term neonate is about 8 inches (20 cm).

B. **Reaction to light or visual stimuli:** strong blink reflex to bright light or stimulation of the lids, lashes, or cornea. A somewhat unsteady gaze can be observed shortly after birth, with ability to fixate on a stimulus for 4 to 10 seconds and refixate every 1 to 1.5 seconds. Ability to maintain fixation and to follow does not occur until 5 to 6 weeks of age.

C. **Pupils:** shape should be round and reaction to light should be equal; constriction to both direct and contralateral stimulation should occur. The red reflex should be elicited bilaterally; normally appears as a homogeneous bright red-orange. Opacities or interruptions may indicate cataracts or retinoblastoma.

D. **Eyelids:** note symmetry, epicanthal folds, bruising or edema, lacerations, ptosis, presence of lacrimal puncta.
E. **Conjunctiva:** should be pink and moist; redness or exudate is abnormal.
F. **Cornea:** may be somewhat less than transparent or slightly hazy in the first few days of life in both premature and term infants. Sclerae may be bluish in premature or small babies as a result of thinness.
G. **Irises:** should be similar in appearance; note pigmentation. A coloboma, or keyhole pupil, may be associated with congenital anomalies. Brushfield spots are silvery gray spots scattered around the circumference of the iris. Strongly associated with Down syndrome.
H. **Lens:** should be clear and black with direct illumination. Examination of the anterior vascular capsule of the lens is a useful adjunct to determination of gestational age in preterm infants between 27 and 34 weeks.
I. **Doll's-eye reflex:** as head is turned *toward* each shoulder, eyes move in opposite direction.

PATHOLOGIC CONDITIONS AND MANAGEMENT

Birth Trauma

Pathophysiology

A. Direct result of duration and difficulty of delivery.
B. Improperly applied forceps.
C. Compression of cranial nerves.

Clinical Presentation

A. Petechiae; ecchymoses; edema; and/or lacerations of pinna, lids, conjunctiva, or globe.
B. Bright red patches on conjunctiva (subconjunctival hemorrhage). Occurs in up to 13% of births (Isenberg, 1999).
C. Droopy eyelids.

Complications

These injuries are generally mild and transient, often resolving spontaneously.

Conjunctivitis

Conjunctivitis is an inflammatory reaction resulting from invasion of conjunctiva by pathologic organisms.

Etiology

A wide variety of infectious agents are capable of producing conjunctivitis in the newborn infant. The most common causes in North America include the following:

A. *Neisseria gonorrhoeae:* peripartum transmission.
B. *Chlamydia trachomatis:* peripartum transmission.
C. *Staphylococcus aureus:* acquired during the neonatal period.
D. **Enteric pathogens.**

NEISSERIA GONORRHOEAE

A. **Incidence.** 30% to 35% of neonates born vaginally to infected women develop ophthalmic gonococcal infection (Gutman, 2001). May be higher in areas with poor perinatal care or irregular antibiotic eye prophylaxis after birth.
B. **Onset of infection:** onset of symptoms usually between days 2 and 5 of life.
C. **Clinical presentation.**

1. Edema of the eyelids.
2. Purulent discharge.
3. Redness/hyperemia of the conjunctiva.

D. **Diagnostic findings.**
1. History.
   a. Maternal history of sexually transmitted disease.
   b. Age at onset of infection.
2. Physical examination.
   a. Clinical signs of inflammation.
   b. Purulent discharge.
3. Laboratory.
   a. Gram stain shows gram-negative diplococci.
   b. Culture positive for gonococci from conjunctival surface or exudate.

E. **Nursing care.**
1. Isolate infant in accordance with infection control guidelines.
2. Irrigate eyes with sterile normal saline solution hourly until discharge is eliminated.
3. Promptly administer appropriate systemic therapy. Topical antimicrobial therapy is *not* required.
   a. Penicillin-sensitive *N. gonorrhoeae:* aqueous crystalline penicillin G, intravenous (IV) or intramuscular (IM), 50,000 to 100,000 units/kg/day in two or three divided doses for 7 days based on postconceptional and postnatal age (consult a drug manual for specific information).
   b. Penicillin-resistant *N. gonorrhoeae:* ceftriaxone, 50 mg/kg (maximum 125 mg) IV or IM in a single daily dose (Zenk, 2003).
4. Parents of infected infant should be referred for evaluation and treatment.

F. **Complications.**
1. Infants with gonococcal conjunctivitis are at risk of having corneal ulceration, perforation, and subsequent visual impairment.
2. Systemic complications involving the blood, joints, or central nervous system (CNS) may occur in a small number of infants.

CHLAMYDIA TRACHOMATIS

A. **Incidence.**
1. The most common cause of conjunctivitis in the neonatal period, especially in areas with poor perinatal care or irregular administration of erythromycin eye prophylaxis after delivery. Chlamydial eye infections occur in up to 1% of births in developed countries (Isenberg, 1999).
2. About 20% to 50% of babies born to mothers who are colonized with *C. trachomatis* will develop the disease (Schachter and Grossman, 2001).
3. Prevention of infection in the newborn infant is dependent on prenatal detection and treatment of the mother or on the use of an effective form of eye prophylaxis at birth (e.g., erythromycin ointment).

B. **Onset.** Symptoms are usually observed between 5 and 14 days of age.

C. **Clinical presentation.** Symptoms vary from mild conjunctivitis to intense edema of the lids with purulent discharge.

D. **Diagnostic findings.**
1. Identification of *Chlamydia* antigen.
2. Stains of conjunctival scrapings.
3. Culture of conjunctival scrapings.

E. **Patient management.**
1. Therapy of choice is ophthalmic and oral erythromycin (estolate preparation), 20 mg/kg/day (Zenk, 2003).

2. Topical therapy alone is *inadequate* to eradicate the organism from the upper respiratory tract.
3. Parents of infected infants should be referred for evaluation and therapy.

F. **Complications.** Infection is spread via the nasolacrimal system to the nasopharynx, leading to *Chlamydia*-related pneumonia.

Nasolacrimal Duct Obstruction

Pathophysiology

A. **Lacrimal apparatus** consists of structures that produce tears (lacrimal glands) and structures responsible for drainage of tears (upper and lower puncta, canaliculi, lacrimal sac, and nasolacrimal duct). System functions to clean, lubricate, and moisten the eyeball.
B. **Term and preterm newborn infants have the capacity to secrete tears** (reflex tearing to irritants) but usually do not secrete emotional tears until 2 to 3 months of age.
C. **Congenital obstruction** is usually caused by an imperforate membrane at the distal end of the nasolacrimal duct.
D. **Congenital nasolacrimal obstruction is the most common abnormality of the neonate's lacrimal apparatus.** Incidence of this condition ranges between 2% and 6% of all newborn infants.

Clinical Presentation

A. **Usually within the first few weeks of life.**
B. **Persistent tearing (epiphora).** Need to rule out congenital glaucoma.
C. **Crusting or matting of the eyelashes:** "sticky eye."
D. **Spilling of tears over the lower lid and cheek;** a "wet look" in the involved eye(s).
E. **Absence of conjunctival infection.**
F. **Mucopurulent material** refluxing from either punctum when gentle pressure is applied over the involved nasolacrimal sac.

Complications

A. **Acute dacryocystitis:** inflamed, swollen lacrimal sac.
B. **Fistula formation.**
C. **Orbital or facial cellulitis.**

Nursing Care

A. **Conservative management,** with daily massage of the nasolacrimal sac in an attempt to rupture the membrane at the lower end of the duct.
B. **Technique.** Technique consists of placing the index finger over the common canaliculus to block the exit of material through the puncta, and stroking downward firmly.
C. **Digital pressure increases hydrostatic pressure in the nasolacrimal sac,** which may cause a rupture of the membranous obstruction.
D. **If a mucopurulent discharge is present,** antibiotic eyedrops (sodium sulfacetamide) or ointment (erythromycin) may be required.
E. **Cleansing of eyes.** Eyes should be cleaned with moist compresses, with secretions mechanically removed.
F. **Duration of conservative management.** Conservative management is advocated for the first year of life.
G. **Resolution.** The majority of nasolacrimal obstructions resolve spontaneously or with massage by 1 year of age.
H. **Surgical treatment.** Unresolved obstructions can be successfully treated surgically: tear duct probing is done, with the infant under general anesthesia, after the first year of life.

Cataracts

Congenital cataracts are the main treatable cause of visual impairment in infancy. The sooner in life the cataracts are removed surgically and proper optics are restored, the better the child's visual prognosis.

Pathophysiology

A. **Lens.** The lens is a biconvex, transparent capsule that refracts light. It is the most important focusing mechanism of the eye.
B. **Cataract.** A cataract is an opacity of any size or degree in the lens of the eye.
C. **Path of light.** Normally the light from an object passes directly through the lens to a focal point on the retina, producing a sharp image. Cataracts result in a degraded image or no image at all.
D. **Visual impairment.** Cataracts lead to varying degrees of visual impairment, from blurred vision to blindness, depending on the location and extent of the opacity. In neonates, cataracts are often transient, disappearing spontaneously within a few weeks.

Etiology or Precipitating Factors

A. **Idiopathic:** developmental variation, not associated with other abnormalities.
B. **Genetically determined:** most common mode of inheritance—autosomal dominant.
C. **Congenital rubella:** cataracts in 50% of newborn infants with congenital rubella syndrome.
D. **Other congenital infections.**
   1. Toxoplasmosis.
   2. Cytomegalovirus infection.
   3. Herpes simplex.
   4. Varicella.
E. **Metabolic disorders** (e.g., galactosemia).
F. **Chromosomal abnormalities** (e.g., Down syndrome).
G. **Clinical syndromes** (e.g., Crouzon disease, Pierre Robin syndrome).
H. **Prematurity.**

Clinical Presentation

A. **White pupil** (leukocoria).
B. **Searching nystagmus** (at 1-2 months of age).

Diagnostic Findings

A. **History.**
   1. Family history of ocular disease or systemic disorders.
   2. Pregnancy, especially first-trimester TORCH infections (see explanation of acronym under Congenital Infections, on p.920).
B. **Physical examination.**
   1. Normally the pupils look black to the bare eye of the examiner when light is directed at them.
   2. Examine to detect a white pupil by shining a light into each eye, with the light source held to one side.
   3. If the opacity is small, it may be identified only when the pupils are dilated, and with the use of an ophthalmoscope.
   4. Consider other diseases of the eye that may produce a white pupil (e.g., retinoblastoma).

Complications

A. **Varying degrees of visual impairment,** leading to developmental delay.
B. **Presence and/or severity of associated ocular defects,** such as microphthalmos and glaucoma.

Nursing Care

A. **Eye examination.** Assist the physician in carrying out a thorough eye examination of the newborn infant. This includes administering drops to dilate the pupils before the examination and supporting the infant's head to facilitate examination.
B. **Parental education.** In collaboration with the physician, assist parents in understanding the nature, possible cause, and treatment of cataracts in the newborn infant, together with the prognosis for future vision. Surgery is indicated whenever the cataract is likely to interfere with vision.
C. **Explore any feelings of guilt the parents may have** in relation to the cause of the cataracts; provide appropriate support.
D. **Encourage parent-infant attachment.** Neonate may not be able to see the parents but can learn to know their voices, smell, and touch.
E. **Care for the patient postoperatively.**
   1. Prevent increased intraocular pressure. Keep the neonate comfortable, well fed, and free of pain to decrease crying.
   2. Administer eyedrops or ointments as ordered postoperatively.
   3. Apply clean eyepatches or protective shields to protect the eye from rubbing or bumping and to prevent irritation from light.
   4. Monitor for complications of cataract surgery. These are relatively infrequent but include infection within the eye, glaucoma, and retinal detachment. Note any increased redness or haziness of the eye, increased tearing, photophobia, or cloudiness of the cornea. Increased crying, irritability, disruption in sleeping patterns, or rubbing of the eye may indicate pain.
   5. Assist the parents in understanding the essential role of optical correction devices, such as glasses or contact lenses, on their infant's vision and development.
   6. Promote appropriate visual stimulation and foster normal infant development by teaching parents about newborn visual preferences (e.g., black-and-white contrast or medium-intensity colors; the human face; geometric shapes; checkerboard designs).

Outcome

Visual prognosis depends not only on the extent of cataracts, age at removal, surgical outcome, and rapid optical correction but also on the nature of other associated anomalies of the eye or syndromes.

Congenital Infections

The developing eyes are highly vulnerable to the damaging effects of prenatal infection (Allen et al., 2002), and ocular abnormalities may in fact be the predominant manifestation of the disease. A number of the congenitally acquired infections are associated with abnormal ocular conditions, including cataracts, chorioretinitis, corneal opacities, and glaucoma.

The most common of these infections is referred to by the acronym TORCH: *t*oxoplasmosis, *o*ther (e.g., congenital syphilis and viral infections), *r*ubella, *c*ytomegalovirus, and *h*erpes. (See also Chapter 31).

Congenital Rubella Syndrome

Pathophysiology

A. **Timing of infection.** Consequences of the transplacental infection are determined primarily by the timing of the viral insult.
B. **Infection in the first trimester of pregnancy presents the greatest hazard to organogenesis, including that of the eyes.**

Incidence

Ocular abnormalities are the cardinal manifestations of congenital rubella, occurring in 50% to 75% of patients with cataracts being the most common ocular abnormality (Cooper and Alford, 2001).

Clinical Presentation

A. **Gestational age.** Findings in the infant exposed to rubella in utero depend on the gestational age at which the infection occurred.
B. **Ocular manifestations.**
   1. Cataracts: in approximately 50% to 75% of patients.
   2. Pigmentary retinopathy.
   3. Microphthalmos.
   4. Glaucoma: in 20% to 50% of patients.
C. **Other common manifestations** include intrauterine growth restriction, hepatomegaly, thrombocytopenia, and cardiac anomalies (see also Chapter 31).

Nursing Care

A. **Virus shedding may continue for months after birth.** Infants with suspected congenital rubella should be isolated from other newborn infants and from pregnant women (both in the hospital and at home after discharge).
B. **Parents need to understand the immediate and long-term effects of this disease.**
C. **See Nursing Care section,** under Cataracts, on p. 920.

Outcome

A. **Prognosis:** depends on severity of symptoms and number of organ systems involved.
B. **Mortality rate:** in first year of life may approach 80% when multisystem involvement occurs.
C. **Multiple disabilities:** common in surviving infants.
D. **Consequences of congenital rubella:** may not be evident at birth but may become apparent in subsequent months.
E. **Follow-up:** ongoing follow-up and evaluation after discharge of infant from hospital. Major problems after the neonatal period include communication disorders, hearing defects, and mental or motor retardation.

Cytomegalovirus

Pathophysiology

A. **Cytomegalovirus (CMV) can cause a perinatal viral infection.**
B. **Congenital illness is most severe if infection occurs early in pregnancy,** the period of greatest susceptibility of the developing fetus.

Etiology

A. **Ubiquitous virus.** CMV can cause infection in all age groups.
B. **Route of transmission.** Infection may be acquired transplacentally, during birth (via the cervix), or through breast milk.
C. **Transfusion.** An important possible cause of morbidity in premature infants is transfusion-acquired CMV. All premature infants should receive seronegative blood products.

Incidence

A. **The *most common* congenital viral infection.**
B. **In the presence of primary acute maternal infection,** 30% to 50% of fetuses are affected (Stagno, 2001).

Clinical Presentation

A. **A diagnosis of congenital CMV infection can rarely be made on the basis of clinical findings alone.** Only 5% to 10% of neonates infected with CMV will have symptoms at birth.
B. **Laboratory diagnostic methods** (e.g., isolation of the virus from the urine) must be employed if this condition is suspected.
C. **Chorioretinitis** is present in 10% to 20% of infants with symptoms and is the *single most common finding* in congenitally infected infants.
D. **Other eye abnormalities** include conjunctivitis, corneal clouding, cataracts, and optic atrophy.
E. **Other manifestations** include intrauterine growth restriction, hepatosplenomegaly, and bleeding disorders (see also Chapter 31).

Complications

A. **Cytomegalic inclusion disease.**
B. **Sensorineural hearing loss,** the most important late sequela and the most common cause of congenital hearing loss (Stagno, 2001).

Nursing Care

A. **No effective treatment exists.** Supportive nursing care measures, aimed at specific symptoms, are employed.
B. **Use of gowns and good handwashing technique are essential** to prevent the spread of infection.
C. **Seronegative pregnant women should not care for infants with known or suspected infection.**
D. **These infants require long-term follow-up.**

Outcomes

A. **Mortality rate.** Overall mortality rate for symptomatic congenital infection is up to 30% (Kuhlmann and Autry, 2001, Whitley and Kimberlin, 1997).
B. **Few survivors are normal.** In 10% to 20% of infants who are free of symptoms at birth, neurologic sequelae, such as mental retardation or sensorineural deafness, may develop in the first years of life.

Toxoplasmosis

Pathophysiology

Fetal damage occurs as a direct result of inflammation caused by the presence of cysts in the tissues, including the eyes.

Etiology

A. **Maternal infection by the protozoan *Toxoplasma gondii*** in the first and second trimesters of pregnancy is often associated with transplacental infection of the fetus.
B. **Infection is acquired through contact with the excrement of infected cats and ingestion of improperly cooked meat.**

Incidence

A. **The incidence of maternal infection ranges from 2 to 12 per 1000** (Isaacs and Moxon, 1999).
B. **Congenital infection rates are approximately 1 to 7 per 1000 live births** (Isaacs and Moxon, 1999).

Clinical Presentation

A. **Chorioretinitis** is the most common manifestation.
B. **Other manifestations** include hepatosplenomegaly, jaundice, and bleeding disorders (see also Chapter 31).

Specific Nursing Care

A. **Nursing care includes pharmaceutical treatment of *Toxoplasma* infection by administering *sulfadiazine* and *pyrimethamine*.** These agents will eradicate the cysts but will not reverse damage already done.
B. **Give supportive care to the family,** with sensitivity to feelings of guilt they might have.
C. **Teach parents to recognize the signs of visual impairment in infancy** (e.g., failure to fix and focus on objects or faces).

Outcome

A. **Prognosis for infants with congenital infection:** poor.
B. **Mortality rate:** roughly 10% to 15% of infected infants.
C. **Psychomotor retardation:** severe in 85% of survivors.
D. **Visual disturbances:** develop in 50% of surviving infants.

Retinopathy of Prematurity

Formally referred to as retrolental fibroplasia, retinopathy of prematurity (ROP) is a vasoproliferative retinopathy that occurs primarily in premature infants less than 28 weeks' gestational age (American Academy of Pediatrics [AAP], 2001).

Pathophysiology

A. **Human retina is avascular until 16 weeks' gestation.** After this time a capillary network begins to grow, starting at the optic nerve and branching outward toward the ora serrata (edge of the retina).
B. **Nasal periphery is vascularized by about 32 weeks' gestation,** but the process is not complete in the more distant temporal periphery until 40 to 44 weeks.
C. **After premature birth,** this process of normal vasculogenesis may be arrested as a result of injury from some noxious agent(s) or stressor(s).
D. **Vasoproliferation.** This arrest of normal vasculogenesis is later followed by a phase of rapid, excessive, irregular vascular growth and shunt formation (vasoproliferation), stimulated by a "vasoactive factor."
E. **Area of new growth generally forms an abrupt ridge between the vascular and avascular retina,** particularly in the temporal periphery.
F. **ROP may resolve if the vasculature in the area recovers and resumes advancing normally,** allowing the retina to become completely vascularized.
G. **If the new vasculature proceeds to develop abnormally,** these capillaries may extend into the vitreous body and/or over the surface of the retina (where they do not belong). Leakage of fluid or hemorrhage from these weak, aberrant blood vessels may occur.
H. **Blood and fluid leakage** into various parts of the eye can result in scar formation and traction on the retina.
I. **Traction may pull the macula out of its normal position, thus affecting visual acuity.** If the macula is slightly out of position, vision will be mildly affected.
J. **Tractional exudative retinal detachment results in blindness.**

Etiology

A. **Complex multifactorial disorder.**
B. **Possible risk factors (Hagedorn et al., 2002).**
   1. Prematurity/low birth weight: *most important clinical factor associated with ROP.*
   2. Hyperoxia.
   3. Hypoxia.
   4. Multiple births.
   5. Blood transfusions.
   6. Intraventricular hemorrhage.
   7. Apnea/bradycardia episodes.

8. Sepsis.
9. Hypercapnia/hypocapnia.
10. Patent ductus arteriosus.
11. Vitamin E deficiency.
12. Lactic acidosis.
13. Prenatal complications: maternal hypertension; diabetes; bleeding; smoking.
14. Duration of mechanical ventilation and oxygen therapy.
15. Exposure to bright light.

Incidence

A. **Incidence of ROP appears to increase significantly as birth weight and gestational age decrease.** Up to 82% of neonates weighing less than 1 kg will develop ROP; 9.3% of these infants will progress to vision threatening disease (Isenberg, 1999).

Stages of Retinopathy

A. **Standardized approach for describing ROP,** developed by the Committee for the Classification of Retinopathy of Prematurity (1984) according to five stages.
   1. Stage 1: demarcation line within the plane of the retina separating the avascular and vascular retinal regions.
   2. Stage 2: ridge or elevation extending out of the plane of the retina.
   3. Stage 3: ridge with extraretinal fibrovascular proliferation, either:
      a. Continuous with the posterior edge of the ridge.
      b. Posterior but disconnected from the ridge.
      c. Into the vitreous.
   4. Stage 4: subtotal retinal detachment.
      a. Extrafoveate.
      b. Involving the foveae.
   5. Stage 5: total retinal detachment.

B. **"Plus" disease:** an indicator of activity. Signs (in increasing severity) include:
   1. Engorgement and tortuosity of the posterior pole retinal vessels.
   2. Iris vessel engorgement.
   3. Pupil rigidity.
   4. Vitreous haze.

C. **Rush disease,** an aggressive type of ROP. Rush disease develops between 3 and 5 weeks after delivery and may progress rapidly to severe ROP.

D. **Zones for classification of ROP (Fig. 36-2).**
   1. Zone 1: extends from the optic disc to twice the disc-foveal distance—a radius of 30 degrees.
   2. Zone 2: extends from the periphery of the nasal retina (ora serrata) in a circle around the anatomic equator.
   3. Zone 3: anterior to zone 2; present temporally, inferiorly, and superiorly but not in the nasal retina.

Physical Examination

A. **Examination of the high-risk neonate.** All newborn infants born at *less than 28 weeks' gestation or with a birth weight of less than 1500 g, and selected infants between 1500 and 2000 g with an unstable clinical course* should have their eyes examined by a trained pediatric ophthalmologist when in stable clinical condition, 4 to 6 weeks after birth (approximately 31-33 weeks' postconceptional age) (AAP, 2001; Canadian Paediatric Society, 1998; Joint Working Party of the Royal College of Ophthalmologists and the British Association of Perinatal Medicine, 1996).

B. **Dilation of pupils.** Infant's pupils should be dilated with a mydriatic agent before examination, to facilitate optimal evaluation. Cycloplegic mydriatic

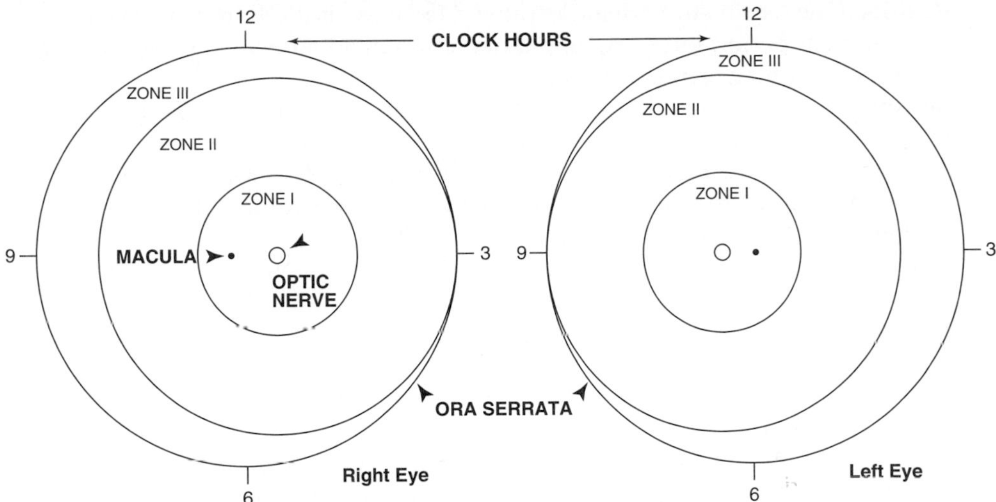

FIGURE 36-2 ■ Zones in retinopathy of prematurity. (From George, D.S.: The latest on retinopathy of prematurity. *MCN American Journal of Maternal Child Nursing, 13*[4]:254-258, 1988.)

agents (e.g., cyclopentolate, tropicamide) have rapid onset of action, with peak ophthalmic effects between 20 and 60 minutes. The excess eyedrops should be wiped away promptly to avoid systemic absorption. Absorption can also be minimized by applying gentle pressure over the nasolacrimal duct for 1 minute following instillation of the eyedrops. It is necessary to protect eyes from bright light after mydriasis. Assess for symptoms of systemic absorption (e.g., tachycardia, restlessness) and notify physician immediately if symptoms are present.

C. **Documentation.** Location and extent of any retinopathy should be precisely documented and classified according to the guidelines developed by the international Committee for the Classification of Retinopathy of Prematurity (1984).

D. **Follow-up.**
   1. Infants who are found to have areas of retinal immaturity on initial examination should have repeated examinations every other week and, subsequently, every 2 to 3 weeks until vascularization has reached the ora serrata.
   2. If ROP is present during the initial examination, the infant should be examined weekly or every other week, depending on the severity of clinical findings.

Prevention

A. **Precautions while using oxygen.** Although the role of oxygen in the pathogenesis of ROP is unclear, cautious and judicious administration and monitoring of oxygen remains one possible preventive measure.
   1. Continuous assessment and monitoring of the infant receiving oxygen to control arterial oxygenation. Cautious administration of oxygen while carrying out nursing procedures such as suctioning.
   2. Ongoing assessment of the oxygen delivery system, including calibration of oxygen analyzers, monitoring fractional inspired oxygen, checking/recording ventilator settings, circuit, and oxygen saturation monitors.
   3. Use of oxygen blenders to deliver precise oxygen concentrations.

B. **Results.** One recent study demonstrated a decrease in ROP from 12.5% to 2.5% over a 5-year period following implementation of an education program and changes in O_2 management strategies (Chow et al., 2003).
C. **Sensory stimulation.** Provide a variety of forms of sensory stimulation to the infant, appropriate to level of development and behavioral cues.
D. **Assessment.** Assess newborn infant's ability to fix and focus.
E. **Assistance.** Assist the physician in carrying out a safe, minimally stressful eye examination of the newborn infant.
F. **Protection against bright light.** Protect the infant's eyes from bright light by shielding the incubator with a blanket and reducing the light in the nursery. The use of eye pads should be evaluated according to the principles of developmental care.
G. **Parent education.** Provide accurate parent education about the possibility of ROP (when parents are ready to receive information about potential non–life-threatening complications). Ensure that parents understand that ROP is essentially a problem of immaturity whose cause is yet unknown.

Treatment

A. **Timing of treatment.** Treatment is indicated when ROP reaches threshold stage, defined as stage 3 disease in zone 1 or 2—involving 5 or more contiguous clock hours or 8 or more total clock hours with "plus" disease (AAP, 2001).
B. **Laser photocoagulation.**
   1. Uses either an argon or diode laser to coagulate the avascular periphery of the retina.
   2. With results similar to cryotherapy results, laser surgery can be performed in the nursery with sedation rather than general anesthesia.
   3. Is more difficult when the retina is not readily visualized (pupils can't be dilated, presence of hemorrhage)
   4. Has fewer systemic and ocular side effects than cryotherapy and carries less risk of damage to adjacent structures (Isenberg, 1999). Is less painful than cryotherapy.
   5. Complications: cataracts (Isenberg, 1999); burns to the cornea, iris, or lens; retinal, periretinal, or vitreous hemorrhage; photocoagulation of the fovea; and late-onset retinal detachment (Christiansen and Bradford, 1995).
C. **Nursing care for the infant undergoing laser photocoagulation.**
   1. Preoperatively, the infant should be given nothing by mouth for 4 to 6 hours; phenylephrine with cyclopentolate (Cyclomydril) and sedation should be given as ordered.
   2. Intraoperatively, monitor the baby and give medications as indicated.
   3. After laser photocoagulation, the infant's respiratory status, oxygen saturation, and vital signs should be monitored.
   4. Assess the eyes for drainage and edema.
   5. Medications such as cyclopentolate and the combination dexamethasone, neomycin, and polymyxin B sulfate (Maxitrol) may be ordered to reduce postoperative complications (Hunsucker et al., 1995).
D. **Cryotherapy.**
   1. Although the use of cryotherapy is decreasing, it continues to be used in some centers. Cryotherapy can be used in special circumstances such as when the retina cannot be visualized (Lee, 1999).

2. Supercooled probe is used to freeze the avascular retina, preventing vessel proliferation.
3. Invasive procedure requires anesthesia.
4. Complications include scarring of the retina; periorbital edema; conjunctival hematoma or laceration; elevation of intraocular pressure; retinal, periretinal, or vitreous hemorrhage; central renal artery occlusion; freezing of the optic nerve; and late-onset retinal detachment (Isenberg, 1999; Vander, 1994).

E. **Nursing care of the infant undergoing cryotherapy.**
1. Monitor the infant closely for possible risks of the procedure.
   a. Risks of undergoing general anesthesia.
   b. Arrhythmias induced from the use of lidocaine (Xylocaine).
   c. Bradycardia caused by vagal stimulation created by pressure on the eyeball.
   d. Edema of the eyelids.
   e. Infection.
   f. Intraocular bleeding.
2. Ensure patient safety and comfort during the treatment.
   a. Place baby in supine position.
   b. Maintain adequate heat source throughout the procedure.
   c. Monitor vital signs and oxygenation status throughout the procedure.
   d. Provide comfort measures and analgesia as needed.
3. Provide postoperative care after the treatment.
   a. Administer eyedrops or ointments as ordered.
   b. Shield infant from unnecessary direct light.
   c. If mydriatic agents were used, observe infant for signs of feeding intolerance, gastric distention, and/or aspirates when feedings are resumed.

F. **Vitreoretinal surgery** results in reattachment of the retina in 30% of cases; however, following macular detachment visual prognosis is poor even if the retina is successfully reattached (Isenberg, 1999).

G. **Provide emotional support and appropriate community referrals** for parents whose infant will have significant visual impairment.

Complications

A. **Mydriatic eyedrops and eye examinations can produce hypertension, reflex bradycardia, and apnea as a result of drug effects and vagal stimulation.**

B. **Varying degrees of visual impairment** (e.g., myopia) may require corrective lenses to improve visual acuity.

C. **Additional complications include:**
1. Strabismus.
2. Glaucoma.
3. Cataracts
4. Amblyopia.
5. Retinal detachment and blindness.

Outcome

A. **90% (or more) cases of acute ROP resolve spontaneously, with little or no visual loss.**

B. **Laser and cryotherapy have been shown to decrease the risk of blinding complications of ROP by 50%.** A significant number of visual impairments may result, especially in the presence of disease in zone 1.

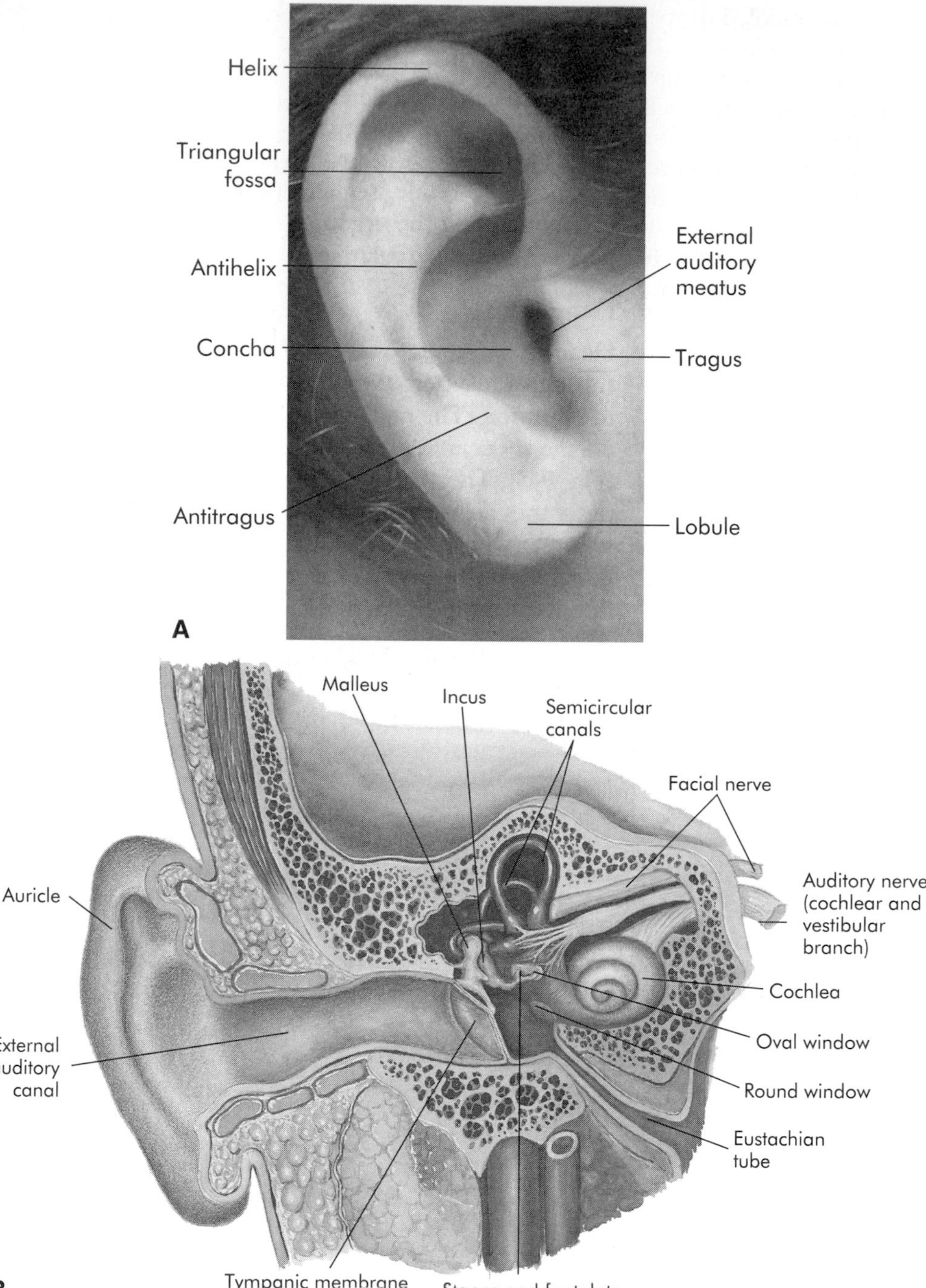

FIGURE 36-3 ■ **A,** Different parts of the auricle of the external ear. **B,** Anatomy of the ear. (From Seidel, H.M., Ball, J.W., Dains, J.E., and Benedict, G.W.: *Mosby's guide to physical examination* [5th ed.]. St Louis, 2003, Mosby.)

ANATOMY OF THE EAR (Fig. 36-3)

External Ear

A. Auricle.

1. Thin plate of elastic cartilage covered by skin.
2. Collects air vibrations.

3. Possesses extrinsic and intrinsic muscle.
4. Supplied by branches of facial nerve.
5. Consists of tragus, helix, concha, and lobule.

B. External auditory meatus.

1. Curved tube leading to tympanic membrane
2. Framework composed of elastic cartilage (outer one third) and bone (inner two thirds).
3. Lined by skin; outer one third has hair, sebaceous, and ceruminous glands.
4. Auriculotemporal nerve and auricular branch of vagus nerve provide sensory output.
5. Lymph drainage is to parotid, mastoid, and cervical lymph nodes.
6. At birth, meatus is shorter and less curved than in the adult.

Middle Ear

A. Slitlike air-containing cavity within petrous (bony) portion of temporal bone

B. Has roof, floor, anterior, posterior, medial, and lateral walls.

C. Lateral wall is the tympanic membrane.

1. Tympanic membrane is thin, fibrous membrane.
2. Sound waves move tympanic membrane medially.
3. Obliquely placed, concave laterally.
   a. Depression in concavity is called the umbo.
   b. Umbo is produced by the tip of the handle of the malleus ("hammer").

D. Contains the auditory ossicles.

1. Ossicles include malleus, incus (anvil), and stapes (stirrup).
2. Malleus and incus can be recognized on otoscopic examination.
   a. Tensor tympani muscle inserts on malleus; dampens vibrations.
3. Stapes inserts on the oval window of the semicircular canal.
   a. Stapedius muscle inserts on stapes; dampens vibrations.
4. Movement of tympanic membrane moves ossicles.
5. Movement of ossicles induces compression waves in fluid (perilymph) in cochlea.

E. Communicates to the nasopharynx via the eustachian (auditory) canal.

1. Eustachian tube equalizes air pressure between the middle ear and the nasopharynx.

Inner Ear

A. Cavity in petrous portion of temporal bone, medial to middle ear.

B. Consists of bony labyrinth and membranous labyrinth; the latter is lodged within the former.

1. Membranous labyrinth filled with endolymph.
2. Bony labyrinth consists of vestibule, semicircular canals, and cochlea.
   a. Vestibule forms base of semicircular canals.
   b. Semicircular canals (superior, posterior, and lateral) arise from vestibule; filled with perilymph.
   c. Movement of perilymph in semicircular canals induced by axial movement.
   d. Transduced by vestibular branch of cochlear nerve.
   e. Cochlea composed of two continuous chambers (scala tympani and scala vestibule) filled with perilymph and a medial chamber (cochlear duct) filed with endolymph.

f. Sensory ("hair") cells stimulated by compression waves that cause relative movement of membranes within cochlea.

INNERVATION

A. **Sensory afferents from cochlea and vestibule transmitted by branches of vestibulocochlear (eighth cranial) nerve.**
   1. Vestibular branch forms vestibular ganglion, which receives nerves from different regions of the vestibule.
   2. Cochlear nerve has motor and sensory branches.
B. **Motor efferents to tensor tympani and stapedius muscles.**
   1. Tensor tympani supplied by mandibular branch of trigeminal nerve.
   2. Stapedius supplied by the facial nerve.
C. **Vestibulocochlear and facial nerves enter inner ear via internal acoustic meatus.**

PATIENT ASSESSMENT

History

A. **Pregnancy:** first trimester infections (e.g., cytomegalovirus), unknown rashes, fevers, flulike illnesses.
B. **Family history**: incidence of hearing loss, ocular disorders.
C. **History of risk factors**: identified on p. 931.

Examination

During all interactions care providers should observe the neonate's response to sound. A more focused assessment is performed with the baby in a quiet, alert state.

A. **General assessment.**
   1. General facial configuration: the ears should be symmetrically positioned with the helix of the ear on or above an imaginary line drawn from the inner to the outer canthus of the eye toward the ear. Ears that fall below that line are termed "low-set" and often associated with genetic syndromes and other congenital malformations.
   2. The development of the pinna correlates with the infant's gestational age. The pinna of a term infant is firm with prompt recoil.
   3. Presence of preauricular pits or skin tags may be familial or associated with other anomalies especially of the renal system. Pits may also communicate with the brain or inner ear and lead to infection
   4. Poorly developed or malformed ears are associated with hearing loss and other anomalies (Johnson, 2003).
   5. Otoscopic examination of the newborn ear is not part of a routine examination. Visually inspect the auditory canal to ensure patency.
   6. As part of a complete assessment, physical features of syndromes associated with sensorineural hearing loss should be identified.

Hearing Loss

Hearing loss in the newborn population is estimated to occur at a rate of between 1 and 6 in 1000 live births (AAP, 1999; Stein, 1999). Hearing loss occurs across a continuum and can be classified as mild, moderate, or severe. Some types of hearing loss such as those caused by congenital infections are progressive or manifest well beyond the newborn period. Ongoing monitoring is needed for those infants with risk factors but who have normal hearing at birth.

Pathophysiology

A. **Conductive:** dysfunction of the outer or middle ear prevents sound transmission.
B. **Sensorineural:** results from damage to the sensory nerve endings in the cochlea or impairment of the auditory nerve.
C. **Mixed:** a combination of conductive and sensorineural hearing loss.

Etiology

RISK FACTORS (Stein, 1999)

A. **Familial.**
B. **Craniofacial anomalies:** especially those involving the pinna and ear canal.
C. **Hyperbilirubinemia**: at levels requiring exchange transfusion.
D. **Bacterial meningitis.**
E. **Low Apgar scores** (less than 5 at 1 minute, less than 6 at 5 minutes).
F. **Ototoxic drugs.**
   1. Gentamicin.
   2. Vancomycin.
G. **Intrauterine infections.**
   1. Cytomegalovirus.
   2. Rubella.
   3. Syphilis.
   4. Herpes.
   5. Toxoplasmosis.
H. **Syndromes associated with hearing loss.**
I. **Idiopathic (up to 50% of cases).**

Hearing Screening

Examination of all newborns. The AAP and the Joint Committee on Infant Hearing recommend universal hearing screening for all newborns (AAP, 1999; Joint Committee on Infant Hearing, 2000). Prompt detection of hearing loss facilitates interventions aimed at preventing speech, language, and cognitive development impairments.

Methodology

A. **Evoked otoacoustic emissions (EOAE).**
   1. Measures sound waves generated in the inner ear in response to clicks or tone bursts generated by small microphones placed in the infant's auditory canals.
   2. Advantages: results are specific to each ear; not dependent of the infant's state; short test time.
   3. Disadvantages: inaccurate in the presence of debris in the ear canal; infant must be relatively inactive during the test; does not test neural transmission of sound.
B. **Auditory brainstem response (ABR).**
   1. Using three scalp electrodes, measures brain waves generated in response to mechanically generated ticks.
   2. Advantages: ear-specific results; unaffected by ear canal debris.
   3. Disadvantages: infant must be in a quiet state.
C. **Follow-up:** hearing screening identifies infants at risk for hearing loss but is not diagnostic. Infants who fail screening tests must be referred for further testing and intervention.

REFERENCES

Allen, M.C., Donohue, P.K., and Porter, M.: Follow-up of the NICU Infant. In G.B. Merenstein and S.L. Gardner (Eds.): *Handbook of neonatal intensive care* (5th ed.). St Louis, 2002, Mosby, pp. 787-800.

American Academy of Pediatrics. Newborn and Infant Hearing Loss: Detection and Intervention. *Pediatrics, 103*(2):527-530, 1999.

American Academy of Pediatrics, American Association for Pediatric Ophthalmology and Strabismus, and American Academy of Ophthalmology: Screening examination of premature infants for retinopathy of prematurity. *Pediatrics, 108*(3):809-811, 2001.

Canadian Paediatric Society: Retinopathy of prematurity: Recommendations for screening. *Pediatric Child Health, 3*(3): 173-180, 1998.

Chow, L.C., Wright, K.W., and Sola, A.: Can changes in clinical practice decrease the incidence of severe retinopathy of prematurity in very low birth weight infants? *Pediatrics, 111*(2):339-346, 2003.

Christiansen, S.P. and Bradford, J.D.: Cataracts in infants treated with argon laser photocoagulation for threshold retinopathy of prematurity. *American Journal of Ophthalmology, 119*(2):175-180, 1995.

Committee for the Classification of Retinopathy of Prematurity. An international classification of retinopathy of prematurity. *AMA Archives of Ophthalmology, 102*:1130-1134, 1984.

Cooper, L.Z. and Alford, C.A.: Rubella. In J.S. Remington and J.O. Klein (Eds.): *Infectious diseases of the fetus and newborn infant.* Philadelphia, 2001, Saunders, pp 347-388.

Gutman, L.T.: Gonococcal infections: Epidemiology and control. In J.S. Remington and J.O. Klein (Eds.): *Infectious diseases of the fetus and newborn infant.* Philadelphia, 2001, Saunders, pp. 1199-1216.

Hagedorn, M.I., Gardner, S.L., and Abman, S.: Respiratory diseases. In G.B. Merenstein and S.L. Gardner (Eds.): *Handbook of neonatal intensive care* (5th ed.). St Louis, 2002, Mosby, pp. 525-531.

Hunsucker, K., King, C., Stamm, S., and Cisneros, N.: Laser surgery for retinopathy of prematurity. *Neonatal Network, 14*(4):21-26, 1995.

Isaacs, D. and Moxon, E.R.: *Handbook of neonatal infections: A practical guide.* London, 1999, Saunders.

Isenberg, S.J.: Eye disorders. In G.B. Avery, M.A. Fletcher, and M.G. MacDonald (Eds.): *Neonatology: Pathophysiology and management of the newborn* (5th ed.). Philadelphia, 1999, Lippincott Williams & Wilkins, pp. 1285-1300.

Johnson, C.B.: Head, eyes, ears, nose, mouth and neck assessment. In E. Tappero and M.E. Honeyfield (Eds.): *Physical assessment of the newborn* (3rd ed.). Santa Rosa, CA, 2003, NICU Ink.

Joint Committee on Infant Hearing. Year 2000 Position Statement: Principles and guidelines for early hearing detection and intervention program. *Pediatrics, 106*(4):798-817, 2000.

Joint Working Party of the Royal College of Ophthalmologists and the British Association of Perinatal Medicine. Retinopathy of prematurity: Guidelines for screening and treatment. *Early Human Development, 46*(3):239-258, 1996.

Kuhlmann, R.S. and Autry, A.M.: An approach to nonbacterial infections in pregnancy. *Clinics in Family Practice, 3*(2):1-17, 2001.

Lee, S.: Retinopathy of prematurity in the 1990s. *Neonatal Network, 18*(2):31-38, 1999.

Schachter, J. and Grossman, M.: Chlamydia. In J.S. Remington and J.O. Klein (Eds.): *Infectious diseases of the fetus and newborn infant.* Philadelphia, 2001, Saunders, pp. 769-778.

Stagno, S.: Cytomegalovirus. J.S. Remmington and J.O. Klein (Eds.): *Infectious diseases of the fetus and newborn infant.* Philadelphia, 2001, Saunders, pp. 389-424.

Stein, L.K.: Hearing loss in children: Factors influencing the efficacy of universal newborn hearing screening. *Pediatric Clinics of North America, 46*(1):95-105, 1999.

Vander, J.: Retinopathy of prematurity: Diagnosis and management. *Journal of Ophthalmic Nursing and Technology, 13*(5):207-212, 1994.

Whitley, R.J. and Kimberlin, D.W.: Treatment of viral infections during pregnancy and the neonatal period. *Clinics in Perinatology, 24*(1):267-283, 1997.

Zenk, K.: *Neonatal medications and nutrition* (3rd ed.). Santa Rosa, CA, 2003, NICU Ink.

SECTION FOUR

Professional Practice

CHAPTER

37 Research

KAREN A. THOMAS

OBJECTIVES

1. Describe the role of research in neonatal nursing.
2. Identify roles of nurses engaged in research based on educational preparation.
3. Describe the research process and key components of research studies.
4. Identify nurses as research consumers who implement research utilization strategies in clinical practice.
5. List questions to ask when critiquing research literature.
6. Be informed about the rights of research subjects and the ethical conduct of research.

RESEARCH AND GENERATION OF NURSING KNOWLEDGE

Research refers to systematic inquiry or investigation governed by scientific principles and conducted to expand knowledge and increase understanding. The research process describes a logical and orderly progression from a question through conduct of a study and resultant findings and conclusions. The questions asked and the methodology that guide inquiry reflect underlying values and beliefs, worldview, or philosophy (Young et al., 2001). Scientific method describes prescribed rules of logic and imposed controls ensuring that the knowledge generated is truthful. Research generates empirical (i.e., experienced) knowledge. Although nursing, as a science-based profession, strongly subscribes to empirical research, the body of nursing knowledge is enriched by diversity in ways of knowing (Gillis and Jackson, 2002; LoBiondo-Wood and Haber, 2002; Young et al., 2001). Nonresearch bases for nursing knowledge—tradition, authority, trial and error, personal experience, intuition, and commonsense reasoning—have a powerful influence and are part of nursing tradition; however, nonresearch knowledge does not permit scientific predictability, nor does it provide for scientific rationale and justification for nursing actions (Gillis and Jackson, 2002). Within the nursing profession, research promotes health and well-being of client populations through a variety of applications. Research improves practice by providing answers to clinical questions, evaluating the effectiveness of nursing interventions, and expanding the body of nursing knowledge (Lanuza, 1999). Increasing emphasis on evidence-based practice, research-based practice, best practices, practice guidelines, and outcomes focus mandate that research occupy a central role in nursing (Lindsey, 1999).

"There is a research role for every nurse practicing in the twenty-first century" (LoBiondo-Wood and Haber, 2002, p. 9). Every nurse is a consumer of research, an extremely important function. Research roles vary from using research findings in practice to independently planning and conducting research. There is an unfortunate myth that anyone can do research (Beyea and Nicoll, 1998). Assuming that any nurse can do research is like assuming any nurse can insert a peripherally inserted central catheter (PICC) line. Both require specific education and skill development. The conduct of research requires expertise in research design and methods as well as statistical analysis. Research is differentially emphasized in the curriculum of nursing academic programs. Table 37-1 illustrates general research roles based on educational preparation. The American Association of Colleges of Nursing (AACN) specifies emphasis on critical thinking, application of research-based knowledge, and data-driven evaluation of nursing care outcomes as essentials in baccalaureate education (AACN, 1998). The AACN also specifies a central core of research for the utilization of new knowledge to provide high-quality health care, initiate change, and improve nursing practice in master's education (AACN, 1996).

Various nursing organizations have published standards emphasizing the importance of research in nursing practice. Box 37-1 illustrates the research standards of the Canadian Orthopaedic Nurses Association. Nurse practitioner professional role competencies, written by the National Organization of Nurse Practitioner Faculties (2002) and AACN, speak of using research to implement the nurse practitioner role.

RESEARCH PROCESS AND COMPONENTS OF A RESEARCH STUDY

The nursing process and research process both represent an organized approach to critical thinking and share several similarities (Table 37-2). Regardless of the topic investigated, a research study contains several key elements (Brink and Woods, 2001; Gillis and Jackson, 2002; LoBiondo-Wood and Haber, 2002):

A. **Question.** All research begins with a problem or general question, which is refined to form specific research questions or hypotheses.
   1. The research questions or hypotheses are the focal point of a research study, driving all other aspects of the investigation including choice of design and analysis.
   2. Each element of a research project fits the stated questions or hypotheses.

B. **Background.** Framework is derived from a review of the literature that establishes what is currently known regarding the study topic and identifies the gaps in knowledge that the study will address.
   1. When a study is derived from an existing theory the theoretical framework portrays the variables and their relationships as prescribed by the theory.
   2. A conceptual framework is a description of concepts, defined for the purposes of the research and their relationships.

TABLE 37-1
Research Roles of Nurses and Educational Preparation

Associate degree in nursing	Appreciates the importance of research in nursing and assists in problem identification and data collection
Baccalaureate in nursing	Critically applies research findings to practice, participates in development and conduct of research projects, and uses research approaches to improve nursing practices
Master's degree in nursing	Facilitates the conduct of research in clinical settings, collaborates with other investigators, develops research problems based on practice expertise, evaluates quality of care and best practices, promotes research utilization in nursing practice
Doctoral degree	Capable of independently planning and conducting theory-based research, provides leadership in research activities, and expands scientific basis for nursing

Adapted from American Nurses Association, Commission on Nursing Research: *Guidelines for the Investigative Function of Nurses.* Kansas City, MO, 1989, American Nurses Association.

■ BOX 37-1
■ **STANDARDS FOR RESEARCH IN NURSING**

Understand and appreciate the research process
Identify researchable questions in nursing practice
Use professional literature to examine nursing problems
Work collegially in solving identified problems
Participate in research activities, based on educational preparation
Support nursing research activities
Share research outcomes through presentation and publication
Comply with ethical standards in the conduct of research
Advocate for protection from harm for research participants
Use research findings to implement change in nursing practice

Adapted from Canadian Orthopaedic Nurses Association: *Orthopaedic Nursing Standards,* 2002.

C. **Method.** In some readings the term method is used to define what was done to collect the data (e.g., observation, questionnaire, interview, physiologic measure); however, here method is defined as the entire description of how the study is conducted.
   1. Design. The plan for data collection, much like a recipe or pattern. There are two general types of research design:
      a. Descriptive (sometimes divided into descriptive and exploratory).
         (1) Designs involve depicting the study sample "as is."
      b. Experimental.
         (1) The investigator manipulates independent variables and measures the response in dependent variables.
      c. The design determines the number of subject groups, the timing of data collection, and control of extraneous variables.
      d. These design choices reduce bias in the study and are related to how subjects are selected, the degree of the investigator's control over the independent variables, and whether the outcome of interest was present at the time of enrollment (Jacob and Carr, 2000).
      e. Designs are described according to internal and external validity. Designs offer differing strengths and weaknesses relative to internal and external validity (Table 37-3).

■ TABLE 37-2
■ ■ **Similarities of the Research Process and the Nursing Process**

Nursing Process	Research Process
Client assessment	Identification of problem
Nursing diagnosis	Questions or hypotheses
Plan of care	Method
Evaluation	Findings
Revision of plan	Implications and dissemination

Adapted from Gillis, A. and Jackson, W.: *Research for nurses: Methods and interpretation.* Philadelphia, 2002, F.A. Davis.

TABLE 37-3
Levels of Bias Control in Research Design

Level	Designs	Independent Variable Control*	Control Group	Outcomes Present at Enrollment
A	Randomized concurrent controlled trial Quasi-randomized concurrent trial Randomized pre-post design	Yes	Yes (concurrent)	No
B	Cohort concurrent study Pre-post study	No	Yes (may or may not be concurrent)	No
C	Ex-post facto study Case control study	No	Yes (may or may not be concurrent)	Yes
D	Descriptive	No	No	Yes or no

* Independent variable or intervention controlled by investigator.
Adapted from Jacob, R.F. and Carr, A.B.: Hierarchy of research design used to categorize the "strength of evidence" in answering clinical dental questions. *Journal of Prosthetic Dentistry, 83*(2):137-152, 2000.

(1) Internal validity refers to lack of bias and random variation that support obtaining accurate results obtained in the population studied.
(2) External validity refers to the generalizability of results to a wider population.

2. Sample. Represents who or what is studied.
   a. Made up of units of analysis, such as individuals, nursing units, or hospitals.
   b. Typically selected from a larger population.
   c. Specific strategies for sampling determine if results from a sample can reasonably be generalized to the larger population.
      (1) Probability sampling: each individual in the population has an equal chance of being included in the sample. Probability sampling is not always feasible, particularly in nursing research dealing with small client populations. In this situation, nonprobability sampling is employed.
   d. Sample size is a factor in the selection of analysis strategies.
3. Variables. The attribute or property measured in a research study.
   a. Variables are defined both conceptually and operationally.
      (1) Operational definition defines the variable in measurable terms. For example, hypertension will be defined as a systolic blood pressure greater than 100 mm Hg in the term neonate.
      (2) Conceptual definition: variable is described in the abstract, e.g., hypertension.
   b. Instruments and tools are terms used interchangeably to indicate operational measures.
   c. The quality of measurement is critical to research. Validity and reliability describe instrument measurement characteristics.
      (1) Validity is the degree to which an instrument measures what it is purported to measure.
      (2) Reliability refers to ability of the instrument to obtain consistent results (i.e., reproducibility).

4. Setting. Portrays where the study is conducted and the conditions surrounding the study.
5. Procedure. Describes in step-wise fashion how the study was carried out.
6. Analysis. Uses statistical techniques on the data collected to answer the research questions or compare findings with stated hypotheses.
   a. Quantitative research: numerical data are analyzed using a statistical approach specified as part of the planning for the research project.
      (1) Descriptive statistics include measures of central tendency (mean, median, mode) and dispersion (standard deviation, variance, range).
      (2) Inferential statistics are based on probability and allow judgments to be made about the population and to test hypotheses. In general inferential statistics test either how things differ or how things are related.
      (3) Statistical significance means that the particular finding is not likely due to chance alone. The investigator sets an alpha or probability level that will be acceptable in interpreting results (often alpha is set at $p < 0.05$). The p value is the probability associated with the test statistic calculated from the study data. If the p value is less than alpha, the test is statistically significant.
      (4) Statistical significance, however, is not always consistent with clinical significance, meaning that the magnitude of the effect is not relevant or important in clinical practice.
      (b) Qualitative research (see next section).
7. Results. Include a description of the study sample as well as findings from the analysis.
8. Conclusion. Includes discussion of study findings, implications, limitations, and recommendations for future research.

QUALITATIVE RESEARCH

A. Maintains the same rigor as quantitative research.
B. Focus is in-depth understanding of a phenomenon with particular emphasis on the subject's reports of personal experience.
C. Participant observation, focus groups, and interviews are methods frequently employed in qualitative research.
D. The specific research approach stems from an underlying philosophical perspective. Three perspectives commonly used in nursing qualitative research include phenomenology, grounded theory, and ethnography (Gillis and Jackson, 2002).
   1. Phenomenology: seeks to understand the lived experience of individuals.
   2. Grounded theory: symbolic interaction forms the basis for understanding social processes and behavior.
   3. Ethnographic: describes a cultural group.
E. The analysis is inductive and interpretive.
F. The process of conducting qualitative research and components of the research project are parallel with those of quantitative research.

NURSES AS CONSUMERS OF RESEARCH

A. Every nurse is a consumer of research whether or not direct participation in research activities occurs (Box 37-2).

BOX 37-2
RESEARCH APPLICATIONS IN PRACTICE

Clinical practice committee	Critical pathways
Quality improvement committee	Protocols
Process improvement protocol	Guidelines
Policies	Journal club
Procedures	Product review committee
Standards	

Adapted from Granger, B.B. and Chulay, M.: *Research strategies for clinicians.* Stamford, CT, 1999, Appleton & Lange.

B. Consumption of research may occur informally or formally and varies in scope (Kirchhoff, 1999).
   1. Reading current research articles and attending conference research presentations expand nurses' knowledge base, supporting practice.
   2. Conducting a focused literature review provides information addressing a clinically defined problem area. In an integrated literature review the findings from several research publications are summarized and synthesized establishing the current knowledge base for a specific topic.
   3. Skill in searching the literature and critical appraisal are essential to nurses (Jennings and Loan, 2001). Research critique is a systematic approach to reading and assessing research articles to assess applicability of knowledge in practice and use in further research. Key questions to ask when reviewing a research article are provided in Box 37-3.

C. There are several formal, structured ways of using research findings in nursing.
   1. The concept of evidence-based practice is derived from evidence-based medicine. The principles guiding evidence-based medicine entail assessment of intervention effectiveness through systematic review of data-based literature, grading studies according to level of evidence with highest priority given to randomized controlled trials (Box 37-4), and aggregation of findings, typically using metaanalysis.
   2. Evidence-based medicine is exemplified by the Cochrane Collaboration, an organization that has established robust criteria for the systematic evaluation of research studies resulting in production of practice.
   3. Evidence-based practice in general refers to established criteria for sources of knowledge and acceptable research methods (Jennings and Loan, 2001). Unfortunately there is confusion and misconception within the nursing community regarding evidence-based medicine, evidence-based practice, research utilization, best practices, and research-based practice (Jennings and Loan, 2001). Jennings and Loan (2001) suggest that research use and research-based practice are subsets of the wider term evidence-based practice. Evidence-based practice has been criticized for negating the full range of knowledge used in practice and the multiple sources of knowledge that constitute nursing.

D. Research utilization refers to specific application of research findings, irrespective of research method, in practice and includes critique of studies, synthesis of findings, assessing applicability to practice, development and implementation of research-based guidelines, and evaluation of practice change (Titler et al., 2001).

BOX 37-3
RESEARCH CRITIQUE

Is there a clear statement of the problem and purpose?
Are the research questions or hypotheses unambiguous and stated in measurable terms?
Does the background establish a theoretical or conceptual framework and show gaps in knowledge?
Does the background define key concepts and their measures and describe relationships among study concepts?
Is the literature review comprehensive and current?
Do the purpose, questions/hypotheses, design, method, analysis fit together logically?
Is the design clearly described?
Are possible extraneous variables identified and controlled?
Are the sample characteristics described and sampling exclusion and inclusion criteria reported?
To whom can study results be generalized?
Is the sample size adequate to address the research questions or hypotheses?
Is loss of subjects explained?
Is the measurement of study variables described?
Are study measures valid and reliable?
Are study procedures described?
How were extraneous variables controlled?
Is the analysis described and are the statistics appropriate for addressing the questions/hypotheses?
Do the reported results address the research questions/hypotheses?
Are the findings interpreted and compared with current knowledge?
Are conclusions justifiable based on the stated findings?
Are statistically significant findings also clinically significant?
Are limitations of the study presented?
Is application of findings discussed?
Are future research directions outlined?

BOX 37-4
LEVELS OF RESEARCH EVIDENCE

Metaanalysis of randomized controlled trials
Single randomized controlled trial
Single well-designed controlled study without randomization
Single well-designed quasi-experimental study
Well-designed nonexperimental study
Expert opinions, committee reports, consensus panels

Adapted from Agency for Health Care Policy and Research: *Clinical practice guideline, Number 9, Management of cancer pain* (AHCPR Publication No. 94-0592). Rockville, MD, 1994, Department of Health and Human Services; Jennings, B.M. and Loan, L.A.: Misconceptions among nurses about evidence-based practice. *Journal of Nursing Scholarship, 33*(2):121-127, 2001.

1. Several models of research utilization have been implemented in nursing (Gillis and Jackson, 2002).
   a. The Iowa Model (Fig. 37-1) is an example of research-based practice that includes generation of practice-related questions and systematic assessment of research findings used to change caregiving.

(1) The Iowa Model emphasizes a variety of research sources of data, and is not limited to randomized controlled trials.
(2) AWHONN has been instrumental in establishing research-based practice programs, addressing such issues as transition of the preterm to an open crib and neonatal skin care (AWHONN, 2002).

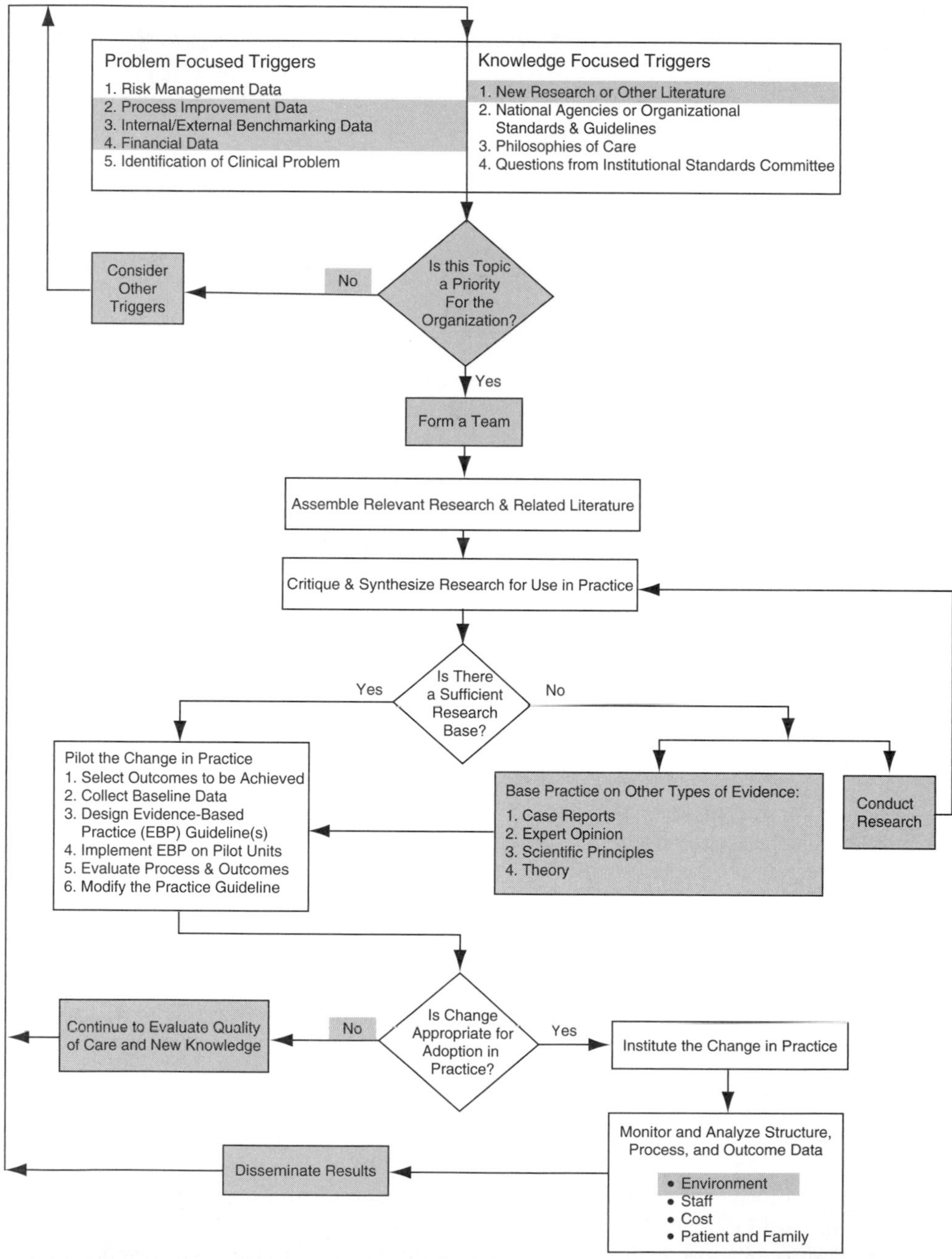

FIGURE 37-1 ■ Iowa Model of research-based practice to promote quality care. (From Titler, M.G., Steelman, V.J., Budreau, G., et al.: The Iowa Model of evidence-based practice to promote quality of care. *Critical Care Nursing Clinics of North America*, 13[4]: 497-509, 2001.)

ETHICS IN RESEARCH AND NURSES AS ADVOCATES

A. Whether nurses are investigators conducting research or caring for clients who are research participants, careful consideration of ethics in research is essential.

B. It is important that nurses maintain a clear distinction between research and practice and of role of researcher and care provider (American Association of Critical-Care Nurses [AACN], 2001). Practice is aimed at caregiving to aid the well-being of an individual, whereas research involves gathering of data to generate knowledge (AACN, 2001).

C. The ethical principles guiding human research include autonomy, beneficence, and justice (AACN, 2001).

1. Autonomy: the ability to make an informed choice, free of coercion, regarding participation in research. The components of informed consent are provided in Box 37-5. Consent for research participation must be obtained by a member of the research team who is qualified to explain the study and answer questions. In neonatal research, parents provide consent for infant participation.
2. Beneficence: the research benefits must outweigh the risks. Children are considered to be a vulnerable group and federal mandates require that risks to a child must be minimal when there is no direct benefit to the child. When a research project involves more than minimal risk, the direct benefit to the child must outweigh the risk.
3. Justice: relates to who is represented in the research sample. Groups that bear the burden for research participation should also be groups that will ultimately benefit from the results.

D. Subject selection should be free of discrimination and represent a broad population.

E. Several documents provide guidelines for the protection of human subjects in the United States.

BOX 37-5
ELEMENTS OF INFORMED CONSENT

Complete explanation of study purpose and procedures
Duration of involvement and time commitment clearly stated
Full disclosure of study risks
Potential adverse effects described and how they will be treated
Identification of any costs that are subject's responsibility
Accurate description of potential benefit to self and/or society
Description of deviations from standard care
Indication of alternatives if an intervention is to be tested
Permission for use of medical records
Protection of confidentiality
Specify possible limits to confidentiality (e.g., mandatory reporting)
Duration of identifiable data retention
Permission to withdraw at any time
Permission to refuse to answer any questions
No coercion including assurance that refusal will not change care or other entitlements
Opportunity to ask questions
Consent language and literacy at level of signatory's understanding
Receive copy of consent

1. The Belmont Report (National Commission for the Protection of Human Subjects of Biomedical and Behavioral Research, 1979) was developed within the Department of Health and Human Services (DHHS).
2. All research sponsored by any of 17 federal agencies, including the National Institute for Nursing Research (an institute under the National Institutes of Health and part of the DHHS), must comply with standards for human participation in research listed under Title 45, Code of Federal Regulations, Part 46, "Protection of Human Subjects" (Code of Federal Regulations, 1991).
3. The Office for Human Research Protections (OHRP) is specifically charged with ensuring the safety and welfare of people participating in DHHS research (OHRP, 2003).
4. To ensure the protection of human subjects all research should be approved by a peer review group. All research supported by federal funds requires review by an internal review board (IRB), a specific type of peer review group established according to federal regulations.
5. Nurses conducting research should become familiar with regulations protecting human subjects. For nurses in practice, understanding of rights in research, particularly informed consent, provides a basis for advocacy and ensuring the protection of clients who are also research participants (AACN, 2001). Concerns about research ethics should be raised with the local peer review group or IRB.

REFERENCES

American Association of Colleges of Nursing: *The essentials of master's education for advanced practice nursing.* Washington, DC, 1996, AACN.

American Association of Colleges of Nursing: *The essentials of baccalaureate education for professional nursing practice.* Washington, DC, 1998, AACN.

American Association of Critical-Care Nurses: *Research: Ethics in critical care nursing research,* 2001. Retrieved March 16, 2003, from wysiwyg://64/ https:www.aacn.org.

AWHONN: *Research-based practice programs,* 2002. Retrieved March 16, 2003, from www.awhonn.org/awhonn/?pg=0-874-2190.

Beyea, S.C. and Nicoll, L.H.: Debunking research myths—Anyone can do research. *AORN Online,* 1998. Retrieved March 16, 2003, from www.aoarn.org/journal/research/rc1098.htm.

Brink, P.J. and Woods, M.J.: *Basic steps in planning nursing research: From question to proposal* (5th ed.). Boston, 2001, Jones and Bartlett.

Code of Federal Regulations: *Title 45 Public Welfare, Part 46 Protection of Human Subjects,* Washington, DC, 1991, DHHS. Retrieved March 16, 2003, from http://ohrp.osophs.dhhs.gov/humansubjects/guidance/45cfr46.htm.

Gillis, A. and Jackson, W.: *Research for nurses: methods and interpretation.* Philadelphia, 2002, F.A. Davis.

Jacob, R.F. and Carr, A.B.: Hierarchy of research design used to categorize the "strength of evidence" in answering clinical dental questions. *Journal of Prosthetic Dentistry, 83*(2):137-152, 2000. Retrieved March 16, 2003, from www.us.elsevierhealth.com.

Jennings, B.M. and Loan, L.A.: Misconceptions among nurses about evidence-based practice. *Journal of Nursing Scholarship, 33*(2):121-127, 2001.

Kirchhoff, K.T.: Strategies in research utilization, one form of evidence-based practice. In M.A. Mateo and K.T. Kirchhoff (Eds.): *Using and conducting nursing research in the clinical setting* (2nd ed.). Philadelphia, 1999, Saunders, pp. 56-63.

Lanuza, D.M.: Research and practice. In M.A. Mateo and K.T. Kirchhoff (Eds.): *Using and conducting nursing research in the clinical setting* (2nd ed.). Philadelphia, 1999, Saunders, pp. 2-12.

Lindsey, A.M.: Integrating research and practice. In M.A. Mateo and K.T. Kirchhoff (Eds.): *Using and conducting nursing research in the clinical setting* (2nd ed.). Philadelphia, 1999, Saunders, pp. 42-55.

LoBiondo-Wood, G. and Haber, J.: *Nursing research: methods, critical appraisal, and utilization* (5th ed.). St Louis, 2002, Mosby.

National Commission for the Protection of Human Subjects of Biomedical and Behavioral Research: *The Belmont Report: Ethical principles and guidelines for the protection of human subjects of research*, Washington, DC, 1979, DHHS. Retrieved March 16, 2003, from http://ohrp.osophs.dhhs.gov/humansubjects/guidance/belmont.htm.

National Organization of Nurse Practitioner Faculties: *Nurse practitioner primary care competencies in specialty areas: adult, family, gerontological, pediatric, and women's health*, 2002, pp. 1-84. The U.S. Department of Health and Human Services, Health Resource and Services Administration, Bureau of Health Professions, Division of Nursing, Washington, DC.

Office for Human Research Protections (2003). Date retrieved: February 11, 2004.http://ohrp.osophs.dhhs.gov/.

Titler, M.G., Steelman, V.J., Budreau, G., et al.: The Iowa Model of evidence-based practice to promote quality of care. *Critical Care Nursing Clinics of North America*, 13(4):497-509, 2001.

Young, A., Taylor, S.G., and McLaughlin-Renpenning, K.: *Connections: Nursing research, theory, and practice*. St Louis, 2001, Mosby.

CHAPTER

38 Ethical Issues

TANYA SUDIA-ROBINSON

OBJECTIVES

1. Explore how the principles of biomedical ethics can be applied in the neonatal intensive care unit (NICU).
2. Identify alternate theoretical and case analysis approaches to examining ethical issues in the NICU.
3. Examine the nurse's role when ethical issues arise in the NICU.
4. Recognize the role of hospital ethics committees in exploring and resolving ethical issues in the NICU.

Ethical issues are ever present in the NICU. Each technologic advance brings ethical questions to the forefront of care. How far can and should the limits of viability be extended? How can we minimize the social, emotional, and financial costs associated with NICU care? Are we providing adequate palliative care in the NICU? These are just a few of the poignant questions that warrant ongoing ethical analysis.

EXAMINING ETHICAL ISSUES

Nurses, physicians, and other members of the NICU health care team need to have a framework for understanding and resolving the ethical issues that arise in the NICU. Although there are many different philosophical perspectives one can use to examine ethical issues, health care professionals need to be able to directly translate those theories to bedside care. Thus this chapter's discussion of ethical approaches focuses on models from the field of applied ethics.

PRINCIPLES OF BIOMEDICAL ETHICS

The most well-known framework for examining biomedical ethical issues was developed by Beauchamp and Childress in 1979. Commonly referred to as the Principle Approach or the Principles of Biomedical Ethics, this model provides the health care team with four key principles to examine: beneficence, nonmaleficence, autonomy, and justice. All four principles must be taken into account when examining an ethics case.

Beneficence

The principle of beneficence focuses on the act of doing good or performing actions with the intent of benefiting another person (Beauchamp and Childress, 2001). Under this principle the health care team must examine their actions and overall plan of care to determine the intended direct benefit for the neonate. An important point to remember is that as the neonate's condition changes, an ongoing consideration of beneficence should occur.

To illustrate the principle of beneficence in the NICU, consider the case of a neonate who is born extremely premature and with an extremely low birth weight. The parents are in agreement with a plan of aggressive treatment. However, at approximately 4 days of age, the neonate has a grade IV intraventricular hemorrhage, severely distended abdomen, poor perfusion, and signs of failing organs. The plan of care that was benefiting this neonate several days ago no longer has the same effect. The care measures are not having a direct beneficial effect and must be reexamined with the parents.

Nonmalcficence

The principle of nonmaleficence obligates health care providers to avoid directly causing harm to a patient. Specifically, the plan of care must avoid causing *intentional* harm. Using the above example, the NICU team would need to evaluate the continuing use of aggressive therapies when the neonate is in the dying process. The plan of care should not involve measures directly intended to cause the neonate's death, nor should the care plan cause harm without any direct benefit.

The key aspect of this principle resides in the intent of the action. The health care provider cannot perform an action that is intrinsically wrong to yield a positive outcome. This is known as the principle of double effect or the rule of double effect (RDE) (Beauchamp and Childress, 2001). According to Beauchamp and Childress (2001), for an act to be considered morally justifiable under the RDE, the following four conditions must be met: (1) the actual act must be good or morally neutral; (2) the intent must be limited to the good effect; (3) the bad effect cannot serve as the means to the good effect; and (4) the good effect must outweigh the bad effect.

The RDE is best illustrated by the administration of increasing amounts of morphine in a dying patient. A nurse administers morphine with the intent of relieving the patient's pain and in the process the patient's respirations slow considerably to the point of cessation. The nurse's intent was not to cause the patient to stop breathing and die. Rather, the nurse's intent was to ease the patient's pain. Thus this nurse did not act in a maleficent manner toward the patient.

Autonomy

The principle of autonomy emphasizes the right of an individual to make decisions for himself/herself. In health care, this principle is reflected in both the right to make decisions about a treatment plan as well as the right to refuse treatment.

In the NICU, parents serve as the legal surrogate decision makers for their neonate. NICU staff can assist parents in their decision-making role by keeping them well informed of the neonate's condition and by objectively presenting treatment options. Parents' preferences for care must be reassessed as the neonate's condition warrants.

Justice

The principle of justice focuses on the fair distribution of the benefits, risks, and costs among members of society in relation to health care needs. In the NICU, questions of justice frequently arise. For example, two mothers are about to give birth to neonates who will require care in the NICU. The births will occur within an hour of each other. One neonate is extremely premature and will have a less than 20% chance of survival. The other neonate will have a 75% chance of survival. If the neonate with only a 20% chance of survival is born first, should he/she occupy the last available NICU bed or should that bed be reserved for the more viable neonate?

Questions of justice are difficult to resolve at the bedside. Yet pursuing these questions is an important step in achieving balance in health care. Further, moving toward examining justice from a societal perspective provides an opportunity to develop and refine health policy that will shape hospital policy and translate back to the bedside.

Utilization of Principle Approach in the NICU

When ethical issues arise in the NICU, the principle approach can assist the health care team to organize its assessment and analysis of the situation. Examining the proposed plan of care with full consideration of benefits and burdens to the neonate can provide insight into competing goals. Fully engaging the parents in the decision-making process as early as possible will assist them in exercising their rights as surrogate decision makers for their neonate. Raising justice-related questions will help clarify how this neonate's case affects the institution and how related cases affect public policy.

OTHER APPROACHES TO ETHICAL ISSUES

In addition to the principle approach to ethical issues, there are many ethical theories and case analysis models. It is beyond the scope of this chapter to adequately address all of these perspectives. However, NICU nurses should be encouraged to further explore these in any clinical ethics textbook.

Ethical Theories

Three of the theories commonly referenced in bioethics are kantianism, utilitarianism, and liberal individualism. Whereas these theories can assist nurses in examining ethical issues broadly, they do not provide direct guidance for resolving issues at the bedside.

Kantianism

Kantianism, or deontology, is an obligation-based theory from the 1700s. This theory requires that individuals act with a sense of obligation, yet does not address how to act when there are conflicting obligations (Beauchamp and Childress, 2001). For example, a father may have a child who needs a kidney donation as well as his own parent who needs a kidney. The father may wish to donate, and may have an obligation to donate. Yet to whom does he owe the greatest obligation? This theory does not directly help resolve such dilemmas.

Utilitarianism

The focus of utilitarianism is on utility, or the maximization of the goodness of an act (Beauchamp and Childress, 2001). According to this theory, the decision maker has to identify greatest good while balancing the interests of all affected individuals. For example, the health care team may desire to provide aggressive treatment to a neonate who will require a succession of expensive surgical repairs. The family may be unable to pay for any of the treatment. Under utilitarianism, it may be determined that providing care for this infant would not maximize utility of resource allocation for the community and thus this infant would not receive the extensive care recommended. Although this theory provides a means of examining issues, it was developed in the late 1700s and is not easily adapted to daily NICU decision making.

Liberal Individualism

Liberal individualism addresses the rights, both positive and negative, that individuals in our society possess. A *positive right* requires someone to do something for another individual; such as a health care provider's duty to treat those in need of immediate care. A *negative right* keeps individuals from being directly harmed by others. For example, an individual requests that no experimental treatments be performed on him. Without his explicit consent, his right cannot be overridden.

CASE ANALYSIS MODEL

Apart from ethical theories and principles, a model for analyzing ethical cases was developed and refined for bedside use by Jonsen, et al (2002). Their model provides four components that health care providers should examine for each case: the medical indications, patient preferences, quality of life, and contextual features.

Medical Indications

Health care providers can begin by summarizing the neonate's diagnosis and prognosis. The treatment plan, along with the benefits and burdens, would also be discussed.

Patient Preferences

In the NICU, the health care providers would obtain the parents' preferences for their neonate's treatment plan. It would be important to ask the parents what their goals are for the infant. In light of the current and/or proposed treatment plan, the NICU team should also ask parents how they view the benefits and burdens for their infant.

Quality of Life

This component of the model provides an opportunity to examine the quality of life from the perspective of the health care team and to relate those to the stated parental preferences. This may require additional conversation with the parents to ensure correct interpretation of their values by the NICU team.

Contextual Features

The contextual features incorporate a variety of factors, including religious beliefs and practices, financial concerns, family issues, potential conflicts of interest among the care providers or the institution, and the legal implications of treatment options (Jonsen, Siegler, et al., 2002).

The case analysis model can be useful as an initial step in examining or identifying ethical issues in the NICU. It does not provide a directive for decision making, but it illuminates the issues so that further steps can be taken toward resolution.

THE NURSE'S ROLE IN ETHICAL ISSUES

The NICU nurse plays a critical role in both direct care of the neonate and support for the parents. The nurse can help prevent some ethical issues from arising by engaging the parents from the time of admission throughout the neonate's hospitalization. Parents will need help understanding and coping with their infant's NICU admission.

Adequate Communication with Parents

In the NICU, nurses along with other members of the health care team have an obligation to keep the parents thoroughly informed of the options for care and the associated risks and benefits (Sudia-Robinson and Freeman, 2000). To adequately involve parents in the decision-making process, health care providers need to move beyond merely imparting information. Parents must have the information but also know how to interpret the information they receive. This has been described in various health care situations as the *transparency model* (King, 1992).

Nurses can assist in this process by incorporating the transparency model into their daily interactions with parents. Telling parents what the neonate's ventilator settings or latest blood gas results were represent simply giving information, which parents may or may not know how to interpret. However, when a nurse explains what the ventilator settings mean for this particular neonate in relation to the course of the neonate's disease process, then parents can begin to better understand and think about the information. Nurses need to remember that knowledge is different than comprehension or understanding. Therefore when parents are helped to understand their neonate's condition, they will be better prepared to make decisions for their neonate.

Not all parents will want to be fully engaged in the decision-making process for their neonate. Sometimes parental preferences for involvement will change during the course of the neonate's hospitalization. For example, some parents may be so intimidated by the NICU initially that they may not ask many questions and agree with whatever is presented to them. As time passes they may begin to ask more questions and become more involved in daily care. It is important to recognize differences in parental preferences while reassessing parental desire for involvement as the neonate's condition changes.

Supporting the NICU Team

At times the NICU nurse may feel torn between support for the parents and support for the health care team. This can occur when the health care team advocates one plan of care and the parents disagree with the team's recommendation. For example, the NICU team may recognize that the neonate is in multiorgan system failure and that death is imminent; yet the parents continue to request that aggressive medical intervention continue. The nurse has an obligation to support the team and the parents while ensuring that the infant's best interests are being met. This is where ethical dilemmas arise, and the nurse may find it helpful to seek ethical consultation.

CONSULTING THE HOSPITAL ETHICS COMMITTEE

When significant differences in the desired plan of care arise between the parents and NICU team, it can be beneficial to initiate an ethics consultation. In most institutions, a nurse, physician, social worker, other staff, or a parent can request an ethics consultation. The focus of the consultation should be the actual process rather than the outcome. Ethics committee members can sometimes aid in clarifying the issues and various perspectives presented. The process must be respectful of all perspectives and give full consideration of all possible options. The product of an ethics consultation will be a set of recommendations, not a mandate for a particular trajectory of care.

The ethics committee can be of assistance to the NICU in situations other than actual case consultation. Hospital ethics committees can serve as important resources about both ethically and legally permissible courses of action that can guide policy development in the NICU. Some ethics committees also prepare educational materials for families to make them aware of the process and how to access committee members (Mitchell and Truog, 2000).

REFERENCES

Beauchamp, R.L. and Childress, J.F.: *Principles of biomedical ethics* (5th ed.). New York, 2001, Oxford University Press.

Jonsen, A.R., Siegler, M., and Winslade, W.J.: *Clinical ethics* (5th ed.). New York, 2002, McGraw-Hill.

King, N.M.: Transparency in neonatal intensive care. *Hastings Center Report*, *22*(3):18-25, 1992.

Mitchell, C. and Truog, R.D.: From the files of a pediatric ethics committee. *Journal of Clinical Ethics*, *11*(2):112-120, 2000.

Sudia-Robinson, T. and Freeman, S.B.: Communication patterns and decision-making among parents and health care providers in the neonatal intensive care unit: A case study. *Heart & Lung*, *29*(2):143-148, 2000.

CHAPTER

39 Legal Issues

M. TERESE VERKLAN

OBJECTIVES

1. Identify how an attorney may use the nursing process for litigation.
2. Define standards of care and guidelines for establishing the standard of care.
3. Define malpractice and the conditions that constitute malpractice.
4. Define concepts of liability and negligence.
5. Discuss the importance of documentation in the patient's record and guidelines for charting.
6. Discuss the nurse's role in informed consent.
7. Identify scope of practice issues in providing patient care functions.
8. Identify the risks and benefits of possessing professional liability insurance.

In the past, the specialty of obstetrics was considered the "high risk" area for malpractice suits and loss of licensure. Today litigation is not uncommon in our own area of specialization. Neonates are seen as a "special" population that are afforded extra protection (Verklan, 2001). Thus neonatal nurses must be cognizant of the minimum standards of professional conduct that they, as health care providers, must adhere to. The purpose of this chapter is to familiarize the nurse with the concepts and ramifications of legal concerns as they pertain to the realm of neonatal intensive care nursing. Topics that will be discussed include standards of care, liability, documentation, informed consent, scope of practice, and professional liability insurance.

NURSING PROCESS

A. **The nursing process forms the foundation for nursing education, practice, and documentation, regardless of whether the nurse graduated from a diploma, associate degree, or baccalaureate program.** Although the phrase "nursing process" is often omitted from practice standards and teaching strategies, nursing documentation should continue to be reflective of the nursing process. Failure to follow the following five steps of the nursing process is the number one cause of all patient injuries:
   1. **Assessment:** gathers data related to the neonate's physiologic and psychosocial status.
      a. Vital sign records, flowsheets, and nursing progress records.
      b. Body and organ-system findings (e.g., cardiopulmonary findings).
      c. Laboratory and diagnostic reports.
      d. Medical progress notes.
      e. Intake and output.

   f. Progress notes from other disciplines (e.g., respiratory, social work, pharmacy).
   g. Information from the family.
2. **Diagnosis:** correctly identifies the neonate's condition using the data obtained from the assessment step, documents on the nursing care plan and in the progress notes.
3. **Planning:** develops a plan of care that incorporates all aspects of the neonate's condition.
   a. Uses multidisciplinary approach.
   b. Documents interventions and anticipated outcomes for the targeted diagnosis on the nursing care plan.
   c. Incorporates research-based findings into practice.
4. **Implementation:** carries out the plan of care.
   a. Follows neonatologist and/or advanced practice nurse orders, provides direct care, supervises the care given by another, teaches and/or counsels the family, provides referrals for care by other disciplines.
   b. Documents all pertinent information on the neonate's medical record.
5. **Evaluation:** evaluates the neonate's response to the plan of care as outlined by the multidisciplinary team, noting any revisions or changes to the plan.
   a. Implementation process is not complete without evaluating the effectiveness of the intervention.
   b. Communicates patient response to treatment to members of the multidisciplinary team.
   c. Documents pertinent findings in the patient's medical record.
   d. Revises plan of care based on the patient's response and anticipated outcomes.

B. The attorney, as well as all interested parties involved in the legal process, will use the steps of the nursing process to:
1. Interpret the medical record.
2. Identify possible deviations from the standard of care.
3. Speak the same language as the nurse.
4. Generate questions that will be used to depose a nurse defendant.
5. Use the reports of expert witnesses who will outline how the nurse did or did not follow the nursing process.

STANDARD OF CARE

The standard of care outlines the minimum criteria by which proficiency is defined in the clinical area. When the standard is not specifically referred to in the state nurse practice act, it becomes a guideline for practice rather than law. In the legal system, the standard of care is established by defining what a reasonable and prudent nurse would have done in the same or similar circumstances (Brent, 2001). The issue of excellence in practice or quality of care given does not pertain to the argument—what is being sought is reasonableness and prudence. A reasonable and prudent nurse is a nurse with like education, background, and experience who would behave in a corresponding manner, given a parallel set of events. The plaintiff attorney has the burden to prove that the standard(s) does exist and that the defendant nurse failed to meet the standard(s).

In addition, it is expected that the standard of care given to neonates everywhere is the same. "A neonatal nurse is a professional nurse who provides skilled nursing care for low-risk, high-risk and critically ill neonates, high-risk neonates, and their families. The neonatal nurse has specialized knowledge and develops and maintains clinical competence through standardized practice and continuing education" (Association of Women's Health, Obstetric and Neonatal Nurses [AWHONN] and National Association of Neonatal Nurses [NANN], 1997, p. 8). "In addition to providing basic neonatal care, neonatal nurses may focus on one or more areas of expertise, such as intensive or critical neonatal care, transport, lactation, grief, extracorporeal membrane oxygenation or developmental care" (AWHONN and NANN, 1997, pp. 8-9).

Ewing v. Aubert (1988) set out that a maternal-child nurse is held to the standard of care of a nurse practicing in the maternal-child specialty. Neonatal nurses, a subspecialty within maternal-child nursing, must be cognizant of what the professional practice standards are for that subspecialty:

> "A nurse who practices her profession in a particular specialty owes to her patients the duty of possessing the degree of knowledge or skill ordinarily possessed by members of her profession actively practicing in such a specialty under similar circumstances. It is the nurse's duty to exercise the degree of skill ordinarily employed, under similar circumstances, by members of the nursing profession in good standing who practice their profession in the same specialty and to use reasonable care and diligence, along with his/her best judgment, in the application of his/her skill to the case" (*King v. Department of Health & Hospitals*, 1999).

The quality of the nursing care provided is judged according to national standards, making obsolete the "locality rule." The locality rule permitted nurses to be judged according to the standard of care evidenced by nurses working in the same geographic area, reflecting the community's accepted practices. Recognition of national standards by professional neonatal nursing organizations and accreditation agencies is reflected in clinical policy and procedure manuals. In addition, accredited schools of nursing across the nation have similar curricula and textbooks, and nurses attend similar continuing education conferences. Thus it is expected that the professional nurse will be and remain competent and continually updated on the standards of care and practice (American Nurses Association, [ANA], 1991).

Five basic types of evidence are used to establish the legal standard of care: (1) state and federal regulations, (2) institutional policies, procedures, and protocols, (3) testimony from expert witnesses, (4) standards of professional organizations, and (5) current professional literature.

State and Federal Regulations

These agencies establish the standards of care and scope of practice. The national standards tend to be written in broad language to permit flexibility without compromising standards to accommodate differences within each state. The standard of practice is also defined by the state nurse practice act as mandated by each state's legislature. Here the scope of practice is delineated for each level of nursing (e.g., licensed vocational nurse, registered nurse, advanced practice nurse). For example, a registered nurse may not delegate the act of assessment and the formulation of a nursing diagnosis to any assistive personnel who are unqualified to perform this task (American Nurses Association [ANA], 1994). In addition, standards of nursing practice are also regulated by the state board of nursing, the department of health, the Joint Commission on Accreditation of Healthcare Organizations (JCAHO), and the Health Care Financing Administration, in addition to other regulatory agencies (Iyer, 2001a).

Institutional Policies, Procedures, and Protocols

The hospital's policies, procedures, and protocols also outline the standard of care. The policy establishes the purposes for performing a procedure, whereas the procedure is the guideline for how that procedure should be carried out. These guidelines must reflect the national and state standards of care, should be reviewed at least annually, and should be revised to reflect current acceptable nursing practice (JCAHO, 2000). In addition, these guidelines must also be (1) prepared by a qualified committee of professionals who practice in the specialty, (2) consistent with current research and practice literature, (3) archived for the length of liability, and (4) accessible to staff (Park and Speid, 2001). The policy and procedure manual should be approved by both the unit and the hospital's nursing and medical administrations.

Being unaware of the policy and procedures for the standard clinical practice at your institution is not an acceptable excuse for not being held accountable for your practice. The policy and procedures manual is often one of the first documents requested by both the plaintiff and defense attorneys because it is the best source for specific standards by which to evaluate a specific nurse's care. Because the statutes of limitations endure for 18 to 21 years and standard care practices change dramatically across the years, keeping the policy and procedures manual will also help to determine what the standard of care was at the time the neonate was hospitalized.

Testimony from Expert Witnesses

A nurse expert is typically required to articulate what the standard of care is or was in the situation in which the nurse has deviated from the usual and customary standard of care. A nursing expert opinion requires that the person expressing that opinion possess special skill, knowledge, and experience in the neonatal area, and knowledge of the standards applicable at the time of the occurrence (Iyer and Banes-Gerritzen, 2001). The judge and jury have little knowledge related to neonatal physiology, pathophysiology, and the relevant neonatal nursing care. They therefore need assistance in understanding just what a reasonable and prudent nurse would have done in the given circumstances. (For example, did the nurse meet the accepted standard of care?)

Both liability and damages have to be proved in nursing malpractice cases. Thus two types of experts are usually necessary: a nurse to address the nursing standard of care, and a physician to determine causation, that is, to link the breach of standard to the injuries suffered by the neonate. Professional nursing philosophies dictate that nurses be the only witnesses permitted to testify as experts outlining what the nursing standard of care is in a nursing malpractice suit. However, it is the quality of the expert's experience and education that determines the competency and credibility of the testimony (Guido, 2001).

Standards of Professional Organizations

Professional associations represent the interests of nurses. The ANA has developed standards with measurable criteria that define professional nursing practice. Specialty organizations such as the NANN, AWHONN, American Association of Critical Care Nurses (AACN), and National Association of Pediatric Nurse Associates and Practitioners (NAPNAP) have adapted these standards to define the standards of care and professional practice guidelines applicable to the care of neonates. For example, AWHONN publishes *Standards and Guidelines for Professional Nursing Practice in the Care of Women and Newborns* (1998).

Current Professional Literature

Current texts and journal articles, although technically hearsay, aid in establishing the legal standard of care. A number of journals specific to the care of neonates focus on clinical, management, and research articles. Clinical articles are useful in helping to determine the applicable standard of care at the time of the malpractice suit, whereas nursing textbooks provide information related to the standard of care associated with nursing techniques and care (Iyer, 2001a). Research articles are beginning to assume more importance in the legal arena because of the desire to document evidence-based practice. Evidence-based practice is defined as the incorporation of the current best evidence in clinical decision making. Increased use of websites for research/clinical information such as MEDLINE and CINHAL have led to an increase in the critique of published literature by nurses. Hospitals holding "magnet" status, must demonstrate that nurses participate in research utilization or they will lose their designation. Despite this, the integration of research findings into clinical practice is slow, taking as long as 10 years (Pinkerton, 1999). However, keeping theory and clinical practice on par with the literature and remaining current with regard to continuing education will assist the nurse in ensuring that his or her professional standards are synonymous with those of his or her peers.

Further Issues: Practice Guidelines and Ethical Standards

Standards of care are often confused with practice guidelines. Standards of care are the basis for proving that the nurse had a duty to the patient and that there was a breach of that duty. Clinical practice guidelines, with reference to the standards of care, are meant to assist the health care provider in the delivery of care in specific clinical circumstances. For example, *Guidelines for Perinatal Care* outlines recommendations regarding nurse providers, nursing ratios, staffing guidelines, and outreach education for inpatient perinatal care facilities providing basic, specialty, and subspecialty care (American Academy of Pediatrics and American College of Obstetricians and Gynecologists [AAP/ACOG], 2002). Critical pathways are another example of a practice guideline that is modified to reflect the neonate's clinical progress. Therefore the difference between a standard of care and a practice guideline is that the standard always must be adhered to, whereas the guideline suggests a voluntary approach to achieve a desirable patient outcome (Iyer, 2001a).

The ethical standards of nursing practice may also be the issue in a malpractice suit:

> The Mississippi Board of Nursing charged Terry Lynn Hanson, a registered nurse, with abuse of neonatal patients. It was noted that her clinical practices included holding a baby around its neck with only one hand, carrying babies by holding them under their axillae, carrying naked babies around the NICU and washing them in the unit's sinks, and that she endangered the babies by rapidly flipping the levers on the incubators when attempting to stimulate them. The Board, finding her guilty on all charges, revoked her license. Nurse Hanson appealed to the Supreme Court of Mississippi, who held that her behavior constituted a reckless disregard of the health and safety of the neonates. The Court also ruled that she was negligent by holding babies under the axillae, permitting their bodies to dangle, removing them naked from incubators to bathe and weigh them in different areas of the NICU compromised thermoregulation and exposed them to risks of infection, and that overstimulation increased the risk of intraventricular hemorrhage (Tammelleo, 1998, page 1).

MALPRACTICE

The term "malpractice" means negligence on the part of the nurse, in that she or he has violated the standards of ordinary nursing practiced by nurses of similar background in the same specialty of nursing. Malpractice is professional misconduct that may be intentional or unintentional (Monarch, 2002). If the individual is acting in a personal capacity, then the individual would be subject to negligence, as malpractice is limited to the omission, lack or misuse of a professional skill.

> By undertaking professional services to the patient, a nurse represents that she/he possesses, and it is her/his duty to possess only that degree of learning of skill ordinarily possessed by nurses of good standing practicing in the same community under similar circumstances. It is her/his further duty to use the care ordinarily exercised in like cases by reputable members of her/his profession practicing in the same or a similar locality and under similar circumstances. She/he is to use reasonable diligence and her/his best judgment in the exercise of her/his skill and application of her/his learning in an effort to accomplish the purpose for which she/he is employed. A defendant nurse must violate one of these duties before she/he is guilty of malpractice (Davis et al., 2001, p. 802).

It must be emphasized that the nurse need possess only the knowledge and skill possessed by the *average* reasonable, prudent nurse and to exercise reasonable care, skill, and judgment in carrying out her/his professional work:

> Difficulties and uncertainties in nursing make guaranteed results impossible. Absent negligence, a nurse is not responsible for unexpected occurrences or unsuccessful results during the course of treatment or care she/he provides (Davis et al., 2001, p. 802).

Occasionally an unexpected situation arises so quickly that one's actions on hindsight may not be considered to have been the perfect course of action. These behaviors do not automatically constitute malpractice:

> A nurse, suddenly and unexpectedly confronted with an actual or apparent dangerous emergency for her/his patient, is not expected or required to use the same judgment and prudence required in a calmer and more deliberate moment. Her/his duty is to exercise only the care that an ordinarily prudent nurse would exercise under the same circumstances. If, at that moment she/he does what an ordinarily prudent nurses would have done under the circumstances, she/he does all that the law requires (Davis et al., 2001, p. 802).

A mistake in judgment is not considered malpractice:

> A mistake in judgment on the part of the nurse is not evidence of negligence. If a nurse possesses reasonable and ordinary skill and uses care ordinarily used in like or similar situations by nurses of reasonable and average skill, practicing in the community at the time in question, she/he is not guilty of negligence even though her/his judgment may be subsequently proven incorrect (Davis et al., 2001, p. 803).

LIABILITY

Today nurses are recognized as professionals who are responsible and accountable for the care they give to their patients. If the nurse is liable to the patient because of negligent conduct, that nurse can be held legally responsible for the harm caused to that patient (Brent, 2001). Harm must result from the act, because without damage, no legal wrong has been committed.

> A newborn male was discharged from the defendant XYZ hospital two days after birth with a diagnosis of physiologic jaundice. Four days later, he was admitted to ABC hospital with a diagnosis of *Escherichia coli* sepsis and meningitis. The boy was later diagnosed with galactosemia that had not been diagnosed when he was treated for meningitis. The plaintiffs alleged that the neonate's jaundice was the first sign of infection and should have led the XYZ hospital to conduct further tests. It was also claimed that the XYZ hospital failed to communicate results of a newborn screening that was done while the child was hospitalized for meningitis at the second hospital. The plaintiffs further alleged that ABC hospital failed to

recognize symptoms and the results of diagnostic testing which should have led to a diagnosis of galactosemia. Furthermore, this delay resulted in brain damage, mild retardation and right-sided weakness. According to the *Ohio Trial Reporter*, a $1,200,000 settlement was reached (*Anonymous Minor, et al., v. Anonymous Pediatricians, ABC Hospital and XYZ Hospital*, Cuyahoga County [OH] Court of Common Pleas, Case No. 280713 [Laska, 1997a]).

The plaintiff, the party bringing the suit, must prove the following four elements in a malpractice case:

1. The nurse had a duty to her or his patient.
2. There was a breach of that duty.
3. Harm or damages did occur to the patient.
4. Breach of that duty resulted in harm (proximal cause).

An infant, born in a depressed state, had Apgars of 3 and 8 at 1 and 5 minutes, respectively. Although his condition was improving, he continued to have raspy breathing that required suctioning. It was alleged that the defendants failed to provide adequate special care and observation, causing the baby to suffocate on its own secretions. The neonate was discovered in a cyanotic state two hours after birth. Resuscitative techniques restored the heartbeat in eighteen minutes. He was transferred to another hospital, declared to be brain-dead, and was removed from life support four days later. The plaintiff claimed that resuscitation was both delayed and improperly performed. The defendants argued that the baby appeared normal, that the cause of the respiratory arrest was unknown, and that inborn errors of metabolism caused the death. They also countered that failure to respond to resuscitation does not imply negligence (Du Page County [IL] Circuit Court, Case No. 94L-318 [Laska, 1997b]).

In this case the plaintiff proved that the defendant owed a duty to the neonate, in that the baby and his parents should expect the care received to be at least equal to the standard of care. However, the plaintiff was not able to prove that the defendant breached the duty (failure to respond to resuscitation does not imply negligence) or that there was proximal cause (inborn errors of metabolism may have contributed to or caused the injury). Thus, despite the neonate's death (damages), a malpractice suit cannot be won if all four elements are not present.

A. **The costs of liability when a neonate is involved are high for three reasons:**
   1. The costs of health care for a damaged infant with a normal life expectancy are high.
   2. The longer statute of limitations for minors may permit charges to be made years later, applicable to other medical malpractice actions.
   3. There is sympathy toward the family, who may not be able to afford the needed care for the child, as opposed to the deep pockets of a corporation, who may be seen as uncaring and will not miss the money anyway.

B. **Although an individual nurse is accountable only for his or her own practice, there are three additional theories of liability that may be pursued against a facility or its management (Guido, 2001; Park and Speid, 2001):**
   1. *Respondeat superior*, which, in essence, says that the employer is given the responsibility and accountability for the actions or intentions of the employee. This doctrine:
      a. Holds an employer liable for the negligent acts of employees that arise in the course of the employment (i.e., employers are held responsible for the acts of those whom they have a right to supervise or control).
      b. Holds the institution responsible for ensuring that the policies and procedures meet the standard of care, and that employees follow these policies.
      c. Will not impose liability in most circumstances on a nursing supervisor for negligent acts of the nursing personnel he or she is supervising. This

responsibility rests with the person who makes changes in the policies and procedures.

d. Obligates the nursing supervisor to ensure that the licensed and unlicensed nursing personnel under his or her supervision is able to provide patient care safely. If the supervisor does not document the personnel's deficiencies and use the chain of command, she or he can be held liable for any damages that befall a patient.

e. Holds that negligent employees are always liable for their own conduct.

2. *Corporate negligence* holds the institution's management and board of trustees liable for any breach of its duties:

a. The institution must provide a safe physical setting and monitor the quality of care provided, along with the equipment necessary for patient care.

b. An equipment standard must be implemented.

(1) The institution must have a management plan documenting competency validation for the proper use of medical equipment by the institution's employees (JCAHO, 2000).

(2) The institution may also name the equipment manufacturer as a third-party defendant in an attempt to shift the blame (Verklan, 2001).

In a case in which a neonate was burned while being warmed under an infrared lamp, it was the plaintiff's contention that the neonatal intensive care unit negligently monitored the preterm infant. The neonate sustained second- and third-degree burns to her legs, resulting in the amputation of her leg. It was further contended that the neonate will need surgery to her breast area, and further surgeries, including prosthetic devices for her leg, as she continues to grow. The hospital named the company that assembled and distributed the lamp as a third-party defendant, contending that the company did not provide sufficient education with respect to the procedures to follow when using the lamp. The hospital also contended that the intensity of the heat was poorly controlled because of a defective switch. The third party contended that the design was proper and that if the nurse had provided appropriate observation and monitoring of the neonate, the incident would not have occurred. The third-party defendant argued that the information contained in the accompanying literature was adequate, because this hospital had previous experience with similar equipment. The case was settled before summations for $4,500,000, with the third-party defendant responsible for $500,000 (Zarin, 1995).

c. The facility may be found liable for advertising a service for which it lacks the proper equipment or personnel or for failure to keep these services at the acceptable standard of care.

d. The institution must verify the credentials of those who apply for clinical privileges (e.g., advanced practice nurses) and must also query the National Practitioner Data Bank at the time clinical privileges are requested, and subsequently every 2 years, regarding those who hold practice privileges. The data bank maintains records of disciplinary action taken on licenses, hospital privileges, and payment in conjunction with malpractice suits. In addition to health care organizations, professional societies and attorneys have access to the data bank. Each advanced practice nurse should be familiar with the data bank and should periodically verify that the information it contains regarding herself/himself is accurate.

e. Clinical competencies must also be evaluated and documented every 2 years (JCAHO, 2000).

3. *Apparent/ostensible authority* holds an institution liable for the acts and omissions of an independent contractor (Guido, 2001; Park and Speid, 2001).

a. The hospital should maintain a file for each agency nurse that contains her/his nursing license, required certifications, and a current competency skills checklist.
b. Advanced practice nurses working within the hospital must be aware that patients view them as hospital employees even if they are in private practice, and as such the hospital may be held liable for their acts.

C. **An area of considerable controversy in the liability arena relates to risk management and quality assurance activities (Brent, 2001).**
1. Quality assurance, more commonly called quality management today, focuses on evaluation of the quality of patient care, continuous quality improvement, and total quality management. The department and its activities may or may not be integrated with risk management.
2. Risk management is an internal systematic process aimed at preventing injuries and accidents, and reducing financial liability for the institution. Occurrence, variance, or incident reports are reviewed to evaluate and anticipate risk associated with the provision of services.
   a. By documenting occurrences and maintaining related records, such as the organization's claims history, quality assurance and utilization review activities, and risk management and analysis, this area may have information valuable for a plaintiff's malpractice case.
   b. Many jurisdictions have provided a protective shield for quality assurance and risk management activities, which renders the materials generated and the thought processes engaged in during those activities "privileged" or otherwise nondiscoverable (defendant cannot be asked to produce the materials) (Ament, 1997; Scott, 2000).
3. Risk management works closely with quality assurance as information from risk management activities may be helpful in improving the quality of patient care. JCAHO links these areas in that such information must be accessible to all components of the quality assessment departments (JCAHO, 2000).

D. **Scope of practice.** Each state has its own nurse practice act, composed of statutes passed by its legislature and defining the boundaries of nursing practice. These laws vary from state to state in their demarcation of nursing practice. In contrast to state medical practice acts, the nurse practice statutes delineate nursing responsibilities in broad, universal nomenclature that generally must be examined with reference to the pertinent local law. The crucial issue regarding the scope of practice is whether the procedure performed by the nurse is legally within or beyond the scope of a nursing license to practice (Verklan, 2001).

There are numerous areas of medical and nursing practice that overlap one another, especially in the NICU. Depending on the unit and its written protocols, the same procedure may be considered within the realm of medicine when performed by a physician and within the realm of nursing when performed by a nurse. These gray areas have evolved partly in response to the nurse's increased level of educational preparation and advanced practice role and partly in response to the high-tech environment found in the NICU. Neonatal nursing is considered a specialty area of practice, and the high-risk neonatal nursing in the NICU is considered a subspecialty area of practice. Certification for both the low-risk and the high-risk neonatal nurse is available through several specialty organizations (ANA, AACN, National Certification Corporation [NCC], NAPNAP).

Increasing the scope of practice, autonomy, and authority is likely to result in greater exposure to liability situations. Critical legal-liability and scope-of-practice problems arise whenever the nurse assumes patient care functions of an independent nature that:

1. Have long been held to be solely within the province of physicians.
2. Are not the subject of standing orders.
3. Lack definition in the nurse practice act.
4. Are not generally recognized as legitimate nursing functions by accredited professional organizations.

The standard of care and liability for negligence may be determined by (Brent, 2001):

1. Nurse's level of training and experience.
2. Manuals and textbooks written for the specialty.
3. Actions and inactions of the nurse.
4. Protocols and instructions referred to by the nurse.
5. The accepted professional nursing practice.

The following case highlights many of these principles.

Dr. Seal remained with Baby T, born at 0130 after a difficult labor and traumatic forceps delivery, for approximately one hour before the baby was taken to the nursery. He left the hospital at approximately 0300, with instructions to the nurse that the medical student was in charge, but that he was to be called if needed. Nurse Bowles was concerned about Baby T from the outset, taking vital signs every 15 minutes. She called the medical student at 0345 and 0400, both times at which she was reassured that the baby looked "fine." Nurse Bowles did not call Dr. Seal. The nurse's aide assigned to Baby T did not take vital signs as ordered, and fell asleep twice during the shift. Baby T's condition required transport to another hospital, where he was diagnosed with hypovolemic shock related to a subgaleal hematoma, likely the result of the forceps delivery. The plaintiffs brought a negligence suit against the hospital after the baby's death alleging that the hospital personnel failed to take proper action when Baby T displayed signs of distress. The jury returned a verdict against the hospital of $800,000, which was reduced to $650,000 because Dr. Seal agreed to a pre-trial settlement of $150,000 (Tammelleo, 1995).

The reasonable, prudent nurse besides being responsible to the patient, is also accountable to herself or himself and to the profession (Verklan, 2001). Both the nurse and the employer have the responsibility to determine the level of competence of the nurse who is asked to provide care outside her or his specialty area. The right of a nurse's refusal to "float" has been upheld by the Wisconsin Supreme Court (*Winkelman v. Beloit Memorial Hospital*, 1992):

A nursery nurse, Nurse Winkelman, was asked to float to a unit that provided postoperative and geriatric care. She discussed the situation with the supervisor, indicating that she had never floated, that she was exclusively a nursery nurse, and that she was not qualified to provide the type of care being requested. It was her opinion that the floating would put the patients and her license at risk, and thus, the hospital in jeopardy. The supervisor gave her three options, (a) float; (b) find another nurse to float; or (c) take an unexcused absence day. Nurse Winkelman left the hospital, and later received a letter informing her that the hospital took her actions to be a voluntary resignation. Although she denied that she had ever resigned, the hospital refused to reinstate her. Nurse Winkelman filed a complaint of wrongful discharge against the hospital. The case was decided in her favor, and the hospital appealed. The Supreme Court affirmed that she had identified the fundamental policy that provides for only qualified nurses to render care, and that nurses who provide care for which they are not qualified are subject to sanctions under the law (Tammelleo, 1992).

ADVANCED PRACTICE

Coincident with evolving health care delivery systems, neonatal advanced practice nurses can be found in hospitals, ambulatory care centers, and private practice. The advanced practice nurse (APN) is often the only health care provider in many rural areas. According to the American Nurses Association (ANA) APNs are those who have further knowledge and practice experiences that have prepared them for specialization, expansion, and advancement in the practice role (ANA, 1993).

1. Specialization: focusing on one aspect of the field of nursing.
2. Expansion: acquisition of new practice skills.
3. Advancement: encompassing both specialization and expansion and involving:
   a. New integration of theories and skills.
   b. Graduate education.

The licensing statute in each state controls advanced practice and thereby protects the use of the title of APN. All states have defined the scope of the APN by the board of nursing, with several states having the state board of nursing and the state medical board jointly oversee licensing and scope of practice for APNs. The ANA defined APNs as:

> nurses in advanced clinical practice with a graduate degree in nursing. They conduct comprehensive health assessments, and demonstrate a high level of autonomy and expert skill in the diagnosis and treatment of complex responses of individuals, families, and communities to actual or potential health problems. They formulate clinical decisions to manage acute and chronic illness and promote wellness. Nurses in advanced practice integrate education, research, management, leadership, and consultation into their clinical role and function in collegial relationships with nursing peers, physicians, and others who influence the health environment (ANA, 1993, p. 1).

In the neonatal area, the two recognized APNs are the neonatal nurse practitioner (NNP) and the clinical nurse specialist (CNS). As APN roles continue to expand, there will be further debate on what constitutes nursing functions.

A. **Neonatal nurse practitioner.**
   1. One of the most common APNs found in the tertiary care setting.
   2. Is responsible for managing a caseload of neonatal patients with general supervision, collaboration, and consultation from a physician.
   3. Exercises independent judgment in the assessment, diagnosis, and initiation of delegated medical processes and procedures by using extensive knowledge of pathophysiology, pharmacology, and physiology (NANN, 1992).
   4. Is involved in education, consultation, and research.
   5. Has successfully graduated from a master's program (after year 2000) with certification through the NCC.

B. **Clinical nurse specialist.**
   1. Focuses on patient care, staff education, research, and consultation.
   2. Responsibilities are (AWHONN and NANN, 1997):
      a. Acting as a resource for neonatal nurses, NNPs, and other care providers.
      b. Establishing and evaluating patient care standards.
      c. Assessing and identifying educational needs of the family, nursery, and community.
      d. Designing and implementing appropriate educational programs based on identified needs.
      e. Providing consultation to health care providers.
      f. Initiating research projects, participating in data collection, and instituting changes based on research findings (evidence-based practice).

By virtue of the necessary education and training required to become an APN, they are held to a higher standard than a registered nurse. Thus the standard of care expected of the APN is the degree of care expected of any reasonable and prudent APN who practices in the same specialty.

A major legal issue relates to the permissible scope of practice and how independent of physician oversight the APN may be. The nurse practice act, in reference to the APN, has been broadened to include diagnosis and treatment, areas that were exclusive to those holding medical credentials. All states have passed legislation that defines the scope of practice. Although the majority still require physician supervision or mandated collaboration, many are moving toward removing these statutory requirements to permit full independent practice (Flanagan, 1998).

Most common areas in which APNs have incurred liability (Guido, 2001):

1. Conduct exceeding their scope of expertise resulting in damages.
2. Conduct exceeding physician-delegated authority resulting in damages.
3. Practicing independently in a state that stipulates that APNs must have a sponsoring physician.
4. Failure to refer the patient to a physician when the APN's skills are exceeded.
   a. Is the most common cause of action.
   b. APNs must also refer the patient in a timely manner when they recognize the patient's condition requires increased medical attention.
5. Negligence in their delivery of health care.
6. Failure to adequately diagnose the patient's condition.

DOCUMENTATION

A. **It is a professional responsibility of the nurse to document on the medical record. This will:**
   1. Facilitate care.
   2. Enhance continuity and coordination of care.
   3. Assist in the evaluation of the patient's response to treatment.
   4. Provide a legal and official record of the care provided.

B. **Thus the medical record is used by the attorney as a tool to provide evidence in legal proceedings because it also verifies that the nurse (Iyer, 2001b):**
   1. Provided the standard of care.
   2. Did so within the scope of his or her nursing practice act.
   3. Provided "routine care." Negligence could be proved if this information is absent or inappropriate. Flowsheets that list these routines, along with times, dates, patient and caregiver identification, and nursing care outcomes are valuable in providing a means of documenting repetitious nursing activities.

C. **Although nursing notes need to be as complete as possible, the comment "If it's not documented, then it wasn't done" doesn't always hold true.** Patient care is always the number one priority. Once the emergency is past, the nurse should strive to document the events, using as much detail as possible. However, if the needs of other patients were placed on hold during a crisis, those needs must be met immediately once the crisis is past. When the medical record is incomplete, the nurse may testify as to what constitutes her or his usual practice.

D. **The most common charting systems in the NICU are (Iyer, 2001b):**
   1. Flowsheets.
      a. Decrease the need to document repetitive, *routine* nursing functions in the narrative notes.
      b. Have column-and-row format organized according to time and/or shift.
      c. Use abbreviations, symbols, and checkmarks to enter information.
   2. Narrative charting.
      a. Patient care is documented by using chronologic format.

b. Entries describe the neonate's status, interventions, evaluation of care, medical treatments, and equipment (e.g., ventilator, bed, phototherapy lights) used, and the neonate's response to care.

3. Problem-oriented charting.
   a. Problem list outlines the patient's priority problems.
   b. Updates should be entered on a regular basis as problems resolve and new ones emerge.
   c. Documentation may be directly on the care plan or in the narrative notes.
   d. Specific format is followed:
      (1) S = subjective information that the patient tells the nurse.
      (2) O = objective information the nurse observes (including laboratory results).
      (3) A = assessment of the above-mentioned data, leading to a nursing diagnosis.
      (4) P = plan that the nurse will implement to address the care issue.
4. *P*roblem, *i*ntervention, and *e*valuation of problems (PIE) charting: uses flowsheets, progress notes, and nursing diagnoses.
5. Charting by exception.
   a. Narrative notes are completed only when the neonate's progress and/or condition deviates from the expected or when an untoward occurrence arises.
   b. Charting system contains nursing care plans, nursing database, flowsheets, and progress notes.
   c. Standards of practice, determined by the institution, are incorporated into the charting system to record routine, repetitive nursing interventions (e.g., observation of intravenous site, checking ventilator settings).

E. Table 39-1 outlines the advantages and disadvantages of each charting strategy.

F. Guidelines for documentation (Iyer, 2001b; Scott, 2000).

1. Sign at the end of every entry by using full name and credentials or only initials (full name and credentials noted in the appropriate space). Ensure that no vacant lines are left. An empty space may later prompt someone to fill in a "missing" piece of information.
2. Cosigning means that you have observed and/or approved the care given and that you are accepting joint responsibility (and liability) for that care. Nurses who are required by hospital policy routinely to countersign documents or information in the patient's chart should protect themselves in one of two ways:
   a. By personally verifying the information being recorded.
   b. By noting in the record that the signature is included in accordance with hospital policy and is not based on personal knowledge of the information in question.
3. Illegible, sloppy handwriting with spelling and grammatical errors will convey a negative impression of the nurse.
4. Late charting is always suspect because it is typically key information that is added. Chart the information as soon as possible, beginning with the words "late entry for [date and time]."
5. To correct a mistaken entry:
   a. Draw one line through the entry.
   b. Write "mistaken entry" above the line. (The term "error" is no longer advised because juries tend to associate it with a clinical error.)
   c. Initial or sign document and add date next to "mistaken entry."
   d. What if a nurse is instructed *not to chart* an error by the attending physician? Nurses who accede to the demands of a physician to cover up

■ TABLE 39-1
■ ■ **Advantages and Disadvantages of Charting Systems**

Charting Systems	Advantages	Disadvantages
Flowsheets	Easy to use Decrease time spent	No note on narrative sheet Duplication of documentation on narrative sheet
Narrative charting	Easy to document events as they occur in time	Information may be disorganized and may not contain all elements of nursing process Key patient issues may vary from shift to shift and from nurse to nurse, thus it may be difficult, years later, for hospital, nurse, and/or attorney to tease out relevant information related to specific patient complaint
Problem-oriented charting	Documentation is organized	Continuing same format on all patient problems becomes redundant, with same information appearing over and over
	All disciplines use same progress notes, permitting increased collaboration and continuity of care	Time consuming because of repetitious nature of note
PIE charting	Documentation is organized	Novice nurses may have difficulty where there is no traditional care plan but instead an ongoing plan of care that is documented daily
	Evaluation of each problem requires only the information that is specific to that particular problem, intervention, and evaluation	
Charting by exception	Complete, detailed patient information is easily accessible to the health care provider Standard of practice for documentation outlines expected normal findings	Exceptions to the standards of practice may not be documented because nurses become accustomed to "checking off" the flowsheets

PIE, Problem, intervention, and evaluation.
Data from Iyer, P. (Ed.): *Nursing malpractice.* Tucson, 2001, Lawyers & Judges Publishing, pp. 85-143.

the true facts of an unusual clinical episode by deliberately not mentioning it in the patient's chart not only may be subject to possible loss of licensure but also, in flagrant circumstances, even subject themselves to criminal action, leading to a fine or jail sentence.

6. Avoid inappropriate comments concerning:
   a. The patient's or family's personality traits or idiosyncrasies (unless such remarks are relevant to the infant's treatment).
   b. Subjective views to the effect that the patient or family is a potential litigant.
   c. Admissions of legal liability with respect to untoward medical or nursing events. Examples are:
      (1) "The IV infiltrated because the night staff forgot to check it" (Solberg, 1986, p. 13).
      (2) "Patient going into shock. Could not get Dr. Jones to come. We never can!!!" (Fox and Imbiorski, 1979).

7. Document occurrences accurately and concisely. For example, the neonate's parents (plaintiffs) may have a different view of what actually took place. In a malpractice action the burden of proof rests with the plaintiff. In the case of *Coleman v. Touro Infirmary of New Orleans* (506 So. 2d 571-LA, 1993), the plaintiff alleged that the defendants had been negligent by failing to treat an abruptio placentae before the premature delivery of the infant and that the defendants' actions or inaction had caused the child's death. There were several discrepancies between the patient's recollection of events and the medical record. The court consulted the chart and the physician, determined that the nurses' notes stated another set of events, and concluded that the plaintiff failed to prove any act or omission by the obstetrician or hospital that resulted in the wrongful death of the Coleman infant.
8. Document objectively.
   a. Avoid using "appears to be" and "seems to be." These phrases are not consistent with the judgments/diagnosis made by the critical thinking nurse of today.
   b. Quantify in measurable aliquots when possible. For example, "approximately 30 cc emesis" gives more information than "large emesis."
   c. The patient record is not an appropriate place to refer to an incident report's having been made. What should be documented is a factual account of what transpired and what was done. Incident reports enable the hospital or agency to make necessary investigations of the situation while the patient is still hospitalized, to identify situations of increased risk, and to trend these events to determine whether they are preventable (Iyer, 2001b; Scott, 2000).
9. Document promptly:
   a. Any significant changes in the patient's status.
   b. Nursing actions undertaken to intercede in the situation, including notifying the physician of the concern. Note the time of the phone call notifying the physician, the information relayed, any orders received, and what you did next.

The case of *Mark and Debbie Easter, etc. v. Baylor University Medical Center* (Laska, 1993) illustrates the way in which nurses can place themselves in a liability situation by ignoring the above-noted standard of conduct.

The defendant was a 29-week gestational age neonate delivered by cesarean section at the defendant hospital. His serum potassium was not measured during the first 6 days of his life, and the blood glucose level was measured once on the day of his birth. As a result, hyperkalemia and hypoglycemia were undetected until he had a severe episode of bradycardia and/or cardiac arrest, stopped breathing, and required cardiopulmonary resuscitation. He suffered permanent brain damage. A subsequent laboratory report revealed severe hyperkalemia and hypoglycemia; however, the report was not forwarded to the neonatologists for approximately 7 hours. The plaintiff brought a complaint of gross negligence for failure to properly diagnose and timely treat the hyperkalemia and hypoglycemia. The jury returned a $4,500,000 verdict.

Medical records are crucial in a court case because they provide the sequence of events, the time frame in which they occurred, and the participants in the care of the patient.

Dylan Keene was born at 0107 May 15, 1986. He was discharged from the NICU to the regular nursery at 0630 with a one-page discharge note that noted "watch for sepsis, hold antibiotics pending complete blood count [CBC] results and cultures." The medical records for the next 24 hours went missing. Dylan was diagnosed with septic shock and seizures at 0230 May 16, 1986. Testing determined he had sepsis and meningitis that resulted in profound brain damage. He was discharged from the hospital June 18, 1986. His parents brought a malpractice suit against the hospital on May 12, 1995, alleging that there was a failure to properly diagnose and treat for sepsis and meningitis. The plaintiffs requested names of health care providers involved in the treatment and care of Dylan on May 14, 15 and 16, 1986, included those involved in the decision to not give antibiotics on those dates. The hospital records for these dates could not be located. The judge applied a default sanction against the hospital as the loss of the records for which the hospital was responsible had deprived the plaintiffs of their day in court. The plaintiffs were awarded $4,108,311.66. *Keene v. Brigham and Women's Hospital*, 755 N.E.2d 725-MA (2002) (Tammelleo, 2002).

If a nurse is named in a suit or is called to testify with regard to what took place, sometimes many years later, the chart serves as a memory aid. Statements contained in the medical record are not, in themselves, admitted into evidence; rather, the testimony of the witness concerning the particular event, as reinforced by the medical record, becomes the direct evidence given under oath. Most cases in which the hospital records cannot be located appear to be those in which the amount of damages in question is significant and the hospital appears to be liable; seldom do "missing" records ever favor the defendant hospital (Tammelleo, 2002).

INFORMED CONSENT

Legally, for a person to be able to give informed consent, that person must have the capability of "capacity." This usually entails that the person (1) has reached the age of majority and (2) can understand the information that is being given by the health care provider. Neonates therefore do not meet the criteria to give informed consent legally. Thus the parents typically are the surrogate decision makers for the neonate, as long as they appear to be acting in the best interests of their infant. If the parents are married (to each other), either may consent on behalf of the neonate. However, in situations involving divorce, custody battles, and teenaged and foster parenting, issues related to informed consent and patient privacy can become convoluted (Guido, 2001). A *guardian ad litum* may be appointed by the court to act in the neonate's best interests, instead of or in addition to the parent(s). To meet the legal standard of informed consent, the surrogate decision maker must receive sufficient information regarding the proposed plan of treatment, including the risks and benefits of treatment, alternative treatment strategies, and the repercussions of not consenting (Brent, 2001). The only exception to treating before obtaining informed consent is when delay of treatment could place the neonate at risk of further harm, such as in an emergency situation.

It is outside the boundaries of nursing practice to provide the patient and/or family with information regarding medical-surgical risks and benefits of treatment or to suggest alternative medical-surgical therapies. It is appropriate for the nurse to inform the physician that the family members need further clarification to enable them to come to a decision comfortably. Obtaining the informed consent is the responsibility of the physician providing the treatment. Ideally, this physician should also be responsible for obtaining the signatures on the appropriate form once the parent(s) has consented, because she or he is truly the only one who can ensure that the parent(s) has no further questions and fully comprehends all treatment issues (Scott, 2000).

A. If nurses are required to obtain patient and/or family signatures on consent forms, they should limit their clarification of patient and/or family understanding to two questions:

1. Has your physician discussed your baby's surgery (i.e., treatment approach) with you?
2. Are you ready to sign this consent form? This means that you consent to the procedure.

B. It is recommended that the name of the person able to give informed consent on behalf of the neonate be recorded in the medical record or nursing care plan once identified (Scott, 2000).

C. What if the parents or guardian will not give consent?

1. If physicians heed the parents' wishes and do not treat the infant, they may be guilty of child abuse or neglect, because laws stipulate that parents must provide needed medical care. Denial of this care can constitute a form of child neglect or abuse.
2. If physicians proceed to treat the infant, ignoring parental objections, they could be liable for battery because their touching of the infant was intentional and there was a lack of consent.
3. Physicians may petition the court for an authorization to provide the infant with the necessary treatment (i.e., obtain a court order). The most common example of physicians' seeking court orders to intervene in treatment is that of refused consent for blood transfusions based on religious beliefs. This request is almost always granted—certainly in emergency situations.

D. When parents refuse treatment for other reasons, the court will base its decision on several factors (Brent, 2001; Guido, 2001; Scott, 2000).

1. The infant's overall health and development.
2. The immediacy of danger to the infant if treatment is withheld.
3. The risks and benefits of the proposed treatment.

PROFESSIONAL LIABILITY INSURANCE

There is a growing trend to hold nurses personally liable for their acts of negligence, especially when they have assumed additional responsibility as APNs. Some believe that nurses should not carry insurance because this only provides them with "deep pockets," making them more attractive to the plaintiff. Others insist that being well insured will serve as good protection. How much insurance is enough? Is the insurance coverage provided by the employer enough, or should nurses also invest in a personal policy for additional protection? These questions need to be answered by the individual nurse after examination of her or his practice.

A. Principal benefits afforded by an individual malpractice policy (Guido, 2001).

1. Insurer's agreement to defend *all* malpractice claims filed against the nurse. Also generally included are claims alleging assault, battery, invasion of privacy, and defamation of character and claims that the nurse/APN practiced outside the scope of his or her license.
2. Insurer's agreement to pay the amount that the nurse is legally liable to pay the plaintiff, up to the limits of the policy.
3. Coverage of all costs associated with an appeal of an adverse verdict.
4. Coverage for instructional and supervisory activities, as well as off-duty and non–hospital-related nursing activities, such as volunteer work.

B. Reasons to obtain malpractice insurance (Guido, 2001).

1. The hospital may have liability insurance policies that limit coverage and cover employees only when they work as hospital employees. No institutional policy covers a nurse for any acts or omissions that occur outside the normal work environment.
2. Hospital's policy is designed to meet its needs, and may not be able to protect the nurse's best interests.

3. If the hospital decides that what you did was not covered under its policy, it will not defend you. In fact, the hospital may actually assume an adversarial position to demonstrate that you are the legally responsible party. The institution may bring an *indemnity* claim against the nurse for monetary contributions if the nurse's actions or failure to act resulted in the patient's original injury. You will now have to defend yourself on your own.
4. Hospital policies do not have supplementary payments for the nurse's additional expenses related to investigating the claim or loss of work while defending the claim. The nurse will have to pay for his or her own out-of-pocket expenses.
5. You will be protected if the hospital is not insured.

The case of *Wake County Hospital System v. National Casualty Co.* (1992) involved alleged nursing malpractice of a neonatal nurse. The hospital had a self-insured retention, or a deductible, of up to $750,000 per person/event before its commercial insurance coverage became effective. The defendant nurse's policy was deemed to be excess coverage over other valid and collectible insurance. The U.S. District Court ruled that self-insurance by a hospital is not really insurance in the legal sense. It also ruled that the nurse's insurer had to pay the full amount awarded in the case. This case is a good illustration of a nurse's needing her or his own malpractice coverage.

6. When an insurance carrier makes payment to a plaintiff on the basis of malpractice, the insurer is legally entitled to sue the nurse to obtain reimbursement for the amount paid.
7. Cost of a policy for staff nurses is low; however, the insurance for the APN may cost several hundred dollars a year.

C. **Most health care providers do carry their own professional liability insurance.** There are two types of insurance policies (Guido, 2001).
   1. Claims-made policy: covers damages only when the damages occurred during the policy period (when the policy was in effect) and only if the claim is reported to the insurance company during the policy period or the extending reporting endorsement (tail). This is typical of policies held by institutions.
   2. Occurrence-basis policy: covers damages occurring during the period covered by the policy, even if the claim is made after the policy period has ended. This is typical of policies held by *individuals*.
      a. Preferable for neonatal nurses because the lawsuit may not be filed until an extended period after the infant is discharged from the hospital.

D. **There are differences in coverage between an institutional and an individual liability policy (Guido, 2001).**
   1. Institutional liability policy.
      a. Employer purchased and provided as typical "claims-made" coverage.
      b. Institution is the primary insured party, holding fullest rights and responsibilities.
      c. Policy covers specific professional activities in the work environment.
      d. Institution may be able to sue the nurse for all or part of the money paid in settlement, judgment, and legal fees.
      e. Insurance company employs the attorney; the individual nurse may not have a right to select counsel.
      f. Individual nurse has no right to refuse or authorize settlement.
   2. Individual liability policy.
      a. Commercially purchased insurance that typically has an "occurrence" coverage.
      b. Individual nurse is the primary insured party.
      c. Policy covers specific professional activities of the insured at any time and place.

E. All nurses can practice preventive legal maintenance by avoiding eighteen legal pitfalls (Guido, 2001; Monarch, 2002; Rostant and Cady, 1999; Scott, 2000):

1. Neglecting to make safety a high priority.
2. Failing to spot and report possible violence. For example, the number of kidnapping occurrences has increased in recent years. Nurses play a role in the security plan by wearing photographic identification badges, enforcing visiting policies, and, along with risk management, developing a preventive program to anticipate neonatal kidnapping.
3. Not following institutional policies and standards of care.
4. Responding unwisely in a short-staffing or floating situation. Courts have generally upheld the validity of the hospital's floating policy, thus a nurse's refusal to accept the assignment may place the nurse in jeopardy. It is suggested that the prudent course is to accept the assignment after clearly informing the nurse manager or charge nurse concerning your limitations and concerns.
5. Neglecting to use due care in physical procedures, such as the dispensing of medications.
6. Not checking equipment.
7. Assuming that others are responsible for your duties.
8. Assuming responsibility for informed consent.
9. Wrongfully disclosing confidential information.
10. Making reckless accusations.
11. Failing to act like a professional.
12. Confusing licensure issues with malpractice.
13. Failing to communicate.
14. Failing to monitor and assess.
15. Failing to listen to information provided by family and friends, and to patient's or parent's requests for assistance.
16. Neglecting to follow principles of risk management.
17. Not following documentation principles.
18. Confusing legal and ethical questions.

REFERENCES

Ament, L.A.: Risk management and continuous quality improvement. In S.L. Gardner and M.I.E. Hagedorn (Eds.): *Legal aspects of maternal-child nursing practice: Concepts and strategies in risk management*. Menlo Park, CA, 1997, Addison-Wesley, pp. 51-66.

American Academy of Pediatrics and the American College of Obstetricians and Gynecologists: *Guidelines for perinatal care* (5th ed.). Elk Grove Village, IL, 2002, American Academy of Pediatrics.

American Nurses Association: *Standards of clinical nursing practice*. Washington, DC, 1991, Author.

American Nurses Association: *Nurses in advanced practice*. Washington, DC, 1993, Author.

American Nurses Association: *Registered nurses and unlicensed assistive personnel*. Washington, DC, 1994, Author.

Association of Women's Health, Obstetric, and Neonatal Nurses and National Association of Neonatal Nurses: *Neonatal nursing: Orientation and development for registered and advanced practice nurses in basic and intermediate care settings*. Washington, DC, 1997, Author.

Association of Women's Health, Obstetric and Neonatal Nurses. *Standards and guidelines for professional nursing practice in the care of women and newborns* (5th ed.). Washington, DC, 1998, Author.

Brent, J. N.: *Nurses and the law: A guide to principles and applications* (2nd ed.). Philadelphia, 2001, Saunders.

Coleman v. Touro Infirmary of New Orleans, 506 So.2d 571-LA, 1993.

Davis, S.L., Weisgal, H.G., and Neggers, W.F.: Trial techniques. In P. Iyer (Ed.): *Nursing malpractice.* Tucson, 2001, Lawyers & Judges Publishing, pp. 773-806.

Ewing v. Aubert, 532 S.2d 876 (Lo. App. 1988).

Flanagan, L.: Nurse practitioners: Growing competition for family physicians? *Family Practice Management, 5*(9):34-36, 41-43, 1998.

Fox, L. and Imbiorski, W.: *The record that defends its friends.* Chicago, 1979, Care Communications.

Guido, G.W.: *Legal and ethical issues in nursing* (3rd ed.). Upper Saddle River, NJ, 2001, Prentice Hall, pp. 44-46.

Iyer, P.: Foundations of nursing practice. In P. Iyer (Ed.): *Nursing malpractice.* Tucson, 2001a, Lawyers & Judges Publishing, pp. 3-23.

Iyer, P.: Nursing documentation. In P. Iyer (Ed.): *Nursing malpractice.* Tucson, 2001b, Lawyers & Judges Publishing, pp. 75-114.

Iyer, P. and Banes-Gerritzen, C.: Working with nursing expert witnesses. In P. Iyer (Ed.): *Nursing malpractice.* Tucson, 2001, Lawyers & Judges Publishing, pp. 627-650.

Joint Commission on Accreditation of Healthcare Organizations: *2000 Hospital accreditation standards.* Oakbrook Terrace, IL, 2000, Author.

Keene v. Brigham and Women's Hospital, 755 N.E.2d 725-MA, 2002.

King v. Department of Health & Hospitals (1999). 728 So. 2d 1027, 1030 (La. Ct. App.), *writ denied,* 741 So. 2d 656 (La. 1999).

Laska, L. (Ed.): Failure to timely diagnose and treat hyperkalemia and hypoglycemia in premature infant: Brain damage—$4.5 million Texas verdict. *Medical Malpractice Verdicts, Settlements & Experts* 9:1, 1993.

Laska, L. (Ed.): Ohio boy's retardation blamed on failure to recognize signs of galactosemia. *Medical Malpractice Verdicts, Settlements & Experts,* 13:8, 1997a.

Laska, L. (Ed.): Newborn suffers cyanosis soon after birth due to lack of suctioning: Brain damage leads to death—Defense verdict. *Medical Malpractice Verdicts, Settlements & Experts,* 1:25-26, 1997b.

Monarch, K.: The nurse as a civil litigation defendant. In K. Monarch (Ed.): *Nursing and the law: Trends and issues.* Washington, DC, 2002, American Nurses Association, pp. 53-94.

National Association of Neonatal Nurses: *Role definitions for advanced practice.* Petaluma, CA, 1992, Author.

Park, D.B. and Speid, M.H.: An inside look at today's health care environment. In P. Iyer (Ed.): *Nursing malpractice.* Tucson, 2001, Lawyers & Judges Publishing, pp. 47-73.

Pinkerton, S.: Best nursing practices and best hospitals. *Journal of Professional Nursing, 15*(4):207, 1999.

Rostant, D.M. and Cady, R.F.: *Liability issues in perinatal nursing.* Philadelphia, 1999, Lippincott.

Scott, R.W.: *Legal aspects of documenting patient care* (2nd ed.). Gaithersburg, MD, 2000, Aspen Publishers.

Solberg, P.: *Legal implications of patient charting.* Fayetteville, NC, 1986, Nursing Business News.

Tammelleo, A.D.: Court upholds nurse's refusal to float. *Regan Report on Nursing Law, 33*(2):2, 1992.

Tammelleo, A.D.: Nurses fail to "go over doctor's head": Death results. *Regan Report on Nursing Law, 36*(4):4, 1995.

Tammelleo, A.D.: Neonatal nurse's reprehensible conduct results in revocation. *Regan Report on Nursing Law, 38*(9):4, 1998.

Tammelleo, A.D.: "Lost" hospital records lead to default and 4 million-dollar award. *Nursing Law's Regan Report, 43*(5):2, 2002.

Verklan, M.T.: Neonatal and pediatric malpractice issues. In P. Iyer (Ed.): *Nursing malpractice.* Tucson, 2001, Lawyers & Judges Publishing, pp. 159-189.

Wake County Hospital System v. National Casualty Co., 804 F. Supp. 768 (N.C. 1992).

Zarin, I. (Ed.): $4,500,000 recovery. *New Jersey Jury Verdict Review and Analysis, 16*(2):27, 1995.

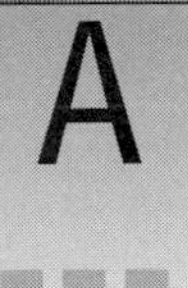

APPENDIX A Newborn Metric Conversion Tables

TABLE A-1
Temperature

FAHRENHEIT (F) TO CENTIGRADE (C)

°F	°C	°F	°C	°F	°C	°F	°C
95.0	35.0	98.0	36.7	101.0	38.3	104.0	40.0
95.2	35.1	98.2	36.8	101.2	38.4	104.2	40.1
95.4	35.2	98.4	36.9	101.4	38.6	104.4	40.2
95.6	35.3	**98.6**	**37.0**	101.6	38.7	104.6	40.3
95.8	35.4	98.8	37.1	101.8	38.8	104.8	40.4
96.0	35.6	99.0	37.2	102.0	38.9	105.0	40.6
96.2	35.7	99.2	37.3	102.2	39.0	105.2	40.7
96.4	35.8	99.4	37.4	102.4	39.1	105.4	40.8
96.6	35.9	99.6	37.6	102.6	39.2	105.6	40.9
96.8	36.0	99.8	37.7	102.8	39.3	105.8	41.0
97.0	36.1	100.0	37.8	103.0	39.4	106.0	41.1
97.2	36.2	100.2	37.9	103.2	39.6	106.2	41.2
97.4	36.3	100.4	38.0	103.4	39.7	106.4	41.3
97.6	36.4	100.6	38.1	103.6	39.8	106.6	41.4
97.8	36.6	100.8	38.2	103.8	39.9	106.8	41.6

Note: °C = (°F – 32) × 5/9. Centigrade temperature equivalents are rounded to one decimal place by adding 0.1 when second decimal place is 5 or greater.
The metric system replaces the term "centigrade" with "Celsius" (the inventor of the scale).

TABLE A-2
Length

INCHES TO CENTIMETERS

1-inch increments. Example: to obtain centimeters equivalent to 22 inches, read "20" on top scale, "2" on side scale; equivalent is 55.9 cm.

Inches	0	10	20	30	40
0	0	25.4	50.8	76.2	101.6
1	2.5	27.9	53.3	78.7	104.1
2	5.1	30.5	55.9	81.3	106.7
3	7.6	33.0	58.4	83.8	109.2
4	10.2	35.6	61.0	86.4	111.8
5	12.7	38.1	63.5	88.9	114.3
6	15.2	40.6	66.0	91.4	116.8
7	17.8	43.2	68.6	94.0	119.4
8	20.3	45.7	71.1	96.5	121.9
9	22.9	48.3	73.7	99.1	124.5

One-quarter (¼) Inch increments. Example: to obtain centimeters equivalent to 14¾ inches, read "14" on top scale, "¾" on side scale; equivalent is 37.5 cm.

10 TO 15 INCHES

	10	11	12	13	14	15
0	25.4	27.9	30.5	33.0	35.6	38.1
¼	26.0	28.6	31.1	33.7	36.2	38.7
½	26.7	29.2	31.8	34.3	36.8	39.4
¾	27.3	29.8	32.4	34.9	37.5	40.0

16 TO 21 INCHES

	16	17	18	19	20	21
0	40.6	43.2	45.7	48.3	50.8	53.3
¼	41.3	43.8	46.4	48.9	51.4	54.0
½	41.9	44.5	47.0	49.5	52.1	54.6
¾	42.5	45.1	47.6	50.2	52.7	55.2

Note: 1 inch = 2.540 cm. Centimeter equivalents are rounded one decimal place by adding 0.1 when the second decimal place is 5 or greater; for example, 33.48 becomes 33.5.

■ TABLE A-3

■ ■ Weight (Mass)

Pounds and Ounces to Grams

Example: to obtain grams equivalent to 6 pounds, 8 ounces, read "6" on top scale, "8" on side scale; equivalent is 2948 g.

	Pounds														
Ounces	**0**	**1**	**2**	**3**	**4**	**5**	**6**	**7**	**8**	**9**	**10**	**11**	**12**	**13**	**14**
0	0	454	907	1361	1814	2268	2722	3175	3629	4082	4536	4990	5443	5897	6350
1	28	482	936	1389	1843	2296	2750	3203	3657	4111	4564	5018	5471	5925	6379
2	57	510	964	1417	1871	2325	2778	3232	3685	4139	4593	5046	5500	5953	6407
3	85	539	992	1446	1899	2353	2807	3260	3714	4167	4621	5075	5528	5982	6435
4	113	567	1021	1474	1928	2381	2835	3289	3742	4196	4649	5103	5557	6010	6464
5	142	595	1049	1503	1956	2410	2863	3317	3770	4224	4678	5131	5585	6038	6492
6	170	624	1077	1531	1984	2438	2892	3345	3799	4252	4706	5160	5613	6067	6520
7	198	652	1106	1559	2013	2466	2920	3374	3827	4281	4734	5188	5642	6095	6549
8	227	680	1134	1588	2041	2495	2948	3402	3856	4309	4763	5216	5670	6123	6577
9	255	709	1162	1616	2070	2523	2977	3430	3884	4337	4791	5245	5698	6152	6605
10	283	737	1191	1644	2098	2551	3005	3459	3912	4366	4819	5273	5727	6180	6634
11	312	765	1219	1673	2126	2580	3033	3487	3941	4394	4848	5301	5755	6209	6662
12	340	794	1247	1701	2155	2608	3062	3515	3969	4423	4876	5330	5783	6237	6690
13	369	822	1276	1729	2183	2637	3090	3544	3997	4451	4904	5358	5812	6265	6719
14	397	850	1304	1758	2211	2665	3118	3572	4026	4479	4933	5386	5840	6294	6747
15	425	879	1332	1786	2240	2693	3147	3600	4054	4508	4961	5415	5868	6322	6776

Note: 1 pound = 453.59237 g; 1 ounce = 28.349523 g; 1000 g = 1 kg. Gram equivalents have been rounded to whole numbers by adding 1 when the first decimal place is 5 or greater.

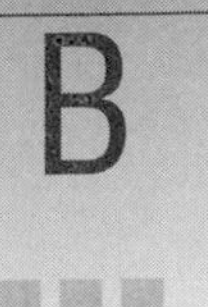

Recommended Childhood Immunization Schedule, United States, 2004

Range of recommended ages | Catch-up vaccination | Preadolescent assessment

Vaccine	Birth	1 mo	2 mos	4 mos	6 mos	12 mos	15 mos	18 mos	24 mos	4-6 yrs	11-12 yrs	13-18 yrs
Hepatitis B[1]	HepB #1	only if mother HBsAg(-)								HepB series		
			HepB #2			HepB #3						
Diphtheria, Tetanus, Pertussis[2]			DTaP	DTaP	DTaP		DTaP			DTaP	Td	Td
Haemophilus influenzae Type b[3]			Hib	Hib	Hib	Hib						
Inactivated Poliovirus			IPV	IPV		IPV				IPV		
Measles, Mumps, Rubella[4]						MMR #1				MMR #2	MMR #2	
Varicella[5]							Varicella				Varicella	
Pneumococcal[6]			PCV	PCV	PCV	PCV			PCV	PPV		
Vaccines below this line are for selected populations												
Hepatitis A[7]										HepA series		
Influenza[8]									Influenza (yearly)			

FIGURE B-1 ■ Recommended childhood immunization schedule—United States, 2004.

This schedule indicates the recommended ages for routine administration of currently licensed childhood vaccines, as of December 1, 2003, for children through age 18 years. Any dose not given at the recommended age should be given at any subsequent visit when indicated and feasible. ▨ Indicates age groups that warrant special effort to administer those vaccines not previously given. Additional vaccines may be licensed and recommended during the year. Licensed combination vaccines may be used whenever any components of the combination are indicated and the vaccine's other components are not contraindicated. Providers should consult the manufacturers' package inserts for detailed recommendations. Clinically significant adverse events that follow immunization should be reported to the Vaccine Adverse Event Reporting System (VAERS). Guidance about how to obtain and complete a VAERS form can be found on the Internet: http://www.vaers.org or by calling 1-800-822-7967.

1. **Hepatitis B (HepB) vaccine.** All infants should receive the first dose of hepatitis B vaccine soon after birth and before hospital discharge; the first dose may also be given by age 2 months if the infant's mother is hepatitis B surface antigen (HBsAg) negative. Only monovalent HepB can be used for the birth dose. Monovalent or combination vaccine containing HepB may be used to complete the series. Four doses of vaccine may be administered when a birth dose is given. The second dose should be given at least 4 weeks after the first dose, except for combination vaccines, which cannot be administered before age 6 weeks. The third dose should be given at least 16 weeks after the first dose and at least 8 weeks after the second dose. The last dose in the vaccination series (third or fourth dose) should not be administered before age 24 weeks. <u>Infants born to HBsAg-positive mothers</u>

should receive HepB and 0.5 ml of Hepatitis B Immune Globulin (HBIG) within 12 hours of birth at separate sites. The second dose is recommended at age 1 to 2 months. The last dose in the immunization series should not be administered before age 24 weeks. These infants should be tested for HBsAg and antibody to HBsAg (anti-HBs) at age 9 to 15 months. Infants born to mothers whose HBsAg status is unknown should receive the first dose of the HepB series within 12 hours of birth. Maternal blood should be drawn as soon as possible to determine the mother's HBsAg status; if the HBsAg test is positive, the infant should receive HBIG as soon as possible (no later than age 1 week). The second dose is recommended at age 1 to 2 months. The last dose in the immunization series should not be administered before age 24 weeks.

2. **Diphtheria and tetanus toxoids and acellular pertussis (DTaP) vaccine.** The fourth dose of DTaP may be administered as early as age 12 months, provided 6 months have elapsed since the third dose and the child is unlikely to return at age 15 to 18 months. The final dose in the series should be given at age ≥4 years. **Tetanus and diphtheria toxoids (Td)** is recommended at age 11 to 12 years if at least 5 years have elapsed since the last dose of tetanus and diptheria toxoid-containing vaccine. Subsequent routine Td boosters are recommended every 10 years.
3. ***Haemophilus influenzae* type b (Hib) conjugate vaccine.** Three Hib conjugate vaccines are licensed for infant use. If PRP-OMP (PedvaxHIB or ComVax [Merck]) is administered at ages 2 and 4 months, a dose at age 6 months is not required. DTaP/Hib combination products should not be used for primary immunization in infants at ages 2, 4, or 6 months but can be used as boosters following any Hib vaccine. The final dose in the series should be given at age ≥12 months.
4. **Measles, mumps, and rubella vaccine (MMR).** The second dose of MMR is recommended routinely at age 4 to 6 years but may be administered during any visit, provided at least 4 weeks have elapsed since the first dose and both doses are administered beginning at or after age 12 months. Those who have not previously received the second dose should complete the schedule by the 11- to 12 year-old-visit.
5. **Varicella vaccine.** Varicella vaccine is recommended at any visit at or after age 12 months for susceptible children (i.e., those who lack a reliable history of chickenpox). Susceptible persons aged >13 years should receive 2 doses, given at least 4 weeks apart.
6. **Pneumococcal vaccine.** The heptavalent **pneumococcal conjugate vaccine (PCV)** is recommended for all children age 2 to 23 months. It is also recommended for certain children age 24–59 months. The final dose in the series should be given at age ≥12 months. **Pneumococcal polysaccharide vaccine (PPV)** is recommended in addition to PCV for certain high-risk groups. See *MMWR* 2000;49(RR-9):1–38.
7. **Hepatitis A vaccine.** Hepatitis A vaccine is recommended for children and adolescents in selected states and regions, and for certain high-risk groups; consult your local public health authority. Children and adolescents in these states, regions, and high-risk groups who have not been immunized against hepatitis A can begin the hepatitis A immunization series during any visit. The 2 doses in the series should be administered at least 6 months apart. See *MMWR* 1999;48(RR-12):1-37.
8. **Influenza vaccine.** Influenza vaccine is recommended annually for children age >6 months with certain risk factors (including but not limited to children with asthma, cardiac disease, sickle cell disease, human immunodeficiency virus infection, and diabetes, and household members of persons in high-risk groups (see *MMWR* 2003;52[RR-8]:1–36), and can be administered to all others wishing to obtain immunity. In addition, healthy children age 6 to 23 months are encouraged to receive influenza vaccine if feasible, because children in this age group are at substantially increased risk of influenza-related hospitalizations. For healthy persons age 5 to 49 years, the intranasally administered live-attenuated influenza vaccine (LAIV) is an acceptable alternative to the intramuscular trivalent inactivated influenza vaccine (TIV). See *MMWR* 2003;52(RR-13): 1-8. Children receiving TIV should be administered a dosage appropriate for their age (0.25 ml if age 6 to 35 months or 0.5 ml if age >3 years). Children age <8 years who are receiving influenza vaccine for the first time should receive 2 doses (separated by at least 4 weeks for TIV and at least 6 weeks for LAIV).

For additional information about vaccines, including precautions and contraindications for immunization and vaccine shortages, please visit the National Immunization Program Web site at www.cdc.gov/nip/or call the National Immunization Information Hotline at 800-232-2522 (English) or 800-232-0233 (Spanish). Approved by the **Advisory Committee on Immunization Practices** (www.cdc.gov/nip/acip), the **American Academy of Pediatrics** (www.aap.org), and the **American Academy of Family Physicians** (www.aafp.org).

Index

ote: Page numbers followed by "b" indicate boxes. Page numbers followed by "f" indicate figures. Page numbers followed by "t" dicate tables.

J

K

L

N

U

V